DISCLAIMER

Every effort has been made to ensure the accuracy of this text, and that the best information available has been used. However, palliativedrugs.com Ltd neither represents nor guarantees that the practices described herein will, if followed, ensure safe and effective patient care. The recommendations contained in this book reflect the editors' judgement regarding the state of general knowledge and practice in the field as of the date of publication. Information in a book of this type can never be all-inclusive, and therefore will not cover every eventuality.

Thus, those who use this book must make their own determinations regarding specific safe and appropriate patient-care practices, taking into account the personnel, equipment, and practices available at the hospital or other facility at which they are located. Neither palliativedrugs.com Ltd nor the editors can be held responsible for any liability incurred as a consequence of the use or application of any of the contents of this book. Mention of specific product brands does not imply endorsement.

Particularly when prescribing a drug for the first time, a doctor (or other independent prescriber) should study the contents of the manufacturer's Summary of Product Characteristics (SPC), paying particular attention to indications, contra-indications, cautions, drug interactions, and undesirable effects.

EDITORIAL STAFF

Staffan Lundstrom MD, PhD
>Department of Palliative Medicine, Stockholms Sjukhem Foundation and Karolinska Institute, Stockholm, Sweden

Tim Morgan BSc, FRCP, FRCS
>Macmillan Consultant and Lead Physician in Palliative Medicine, Roxburghe House and Aberdeen Royal Infirmary, NHS Grampian and Honorary Senior Lecturer, Aberdeen University, UK

Simon Noble MD, FRCP, Dip Pall Med
>Clinical Reader in Palliative Medicine, Cardiff University, UK

Victor Pace FRCP, FRCS, DipPallMed
>Consultant in Palliative Medicine, St Christopher's Hospice, London, UK

Rachel Quibell MRCGP, FRCP
>Consultant in Palliative Medicine, Newcastle upon Tyne Hospitals FT and Marie Curie Hospice, Newcastle, UK

Joy Ross PhD, MRCP
>Consultant in Palliative Medicine, Royal Marsden Hospital, London, UK

John Shaw PhD
>Hayward House Study Centre, Nottingham University Hospitals NHS Trust, City Campus, Nottingham, UK

Anna Spathis MA, MSc, MRCP, MRCGP, FHEA
>Consultant in Palliative Medicine, Cambridge University Hospitals NHS Foundation Trust, Cambridge, UK

Mark Taubert MRCGP, MSc, DipPallMed
>Consultant in Palliative Medicine, Holme Tower Marie Curie Centre, Penarth, UK

Jillian Wall MRCP
>Registrar in Palliative medicine, Hayward House Specialist Palliative Care Unit, Nottingham University Hospitals NHS Trust, Nottingham, UK

Rebecca White BSc, MSc, MRPharmS (IPresc), FFRPS
>Consultant Pharmacist: Nutrition & Intestinal Failure, Oxford University Hospitals NHS Trust, Oxford, UK

Zbigniew Zylicz MD, PhD
>Consultant in Palliative Medicine, Hildegard Hospiz, Basel, Switzerland

CONTENTS

PREFACE

Welcome to the latest edition of the *Palliative Care Formulary* (*PCF*), written primarily for the UK. Regional adaptations include German and Japanese editions (see *www.palliativedrugs.com* for details).

The target audience comprises doctors, nurses and pharmacists involved in the care of patients receiving palliative/hospice care. *PCF* is a core textbook for medical registrars in Palliative Medicine in the UK. It is used in some areas to fulfil the NHS National Cancer Standards requirement for specialist palliative care services within a Cancer Centre and Network to have a core palliative care drug formulary and is referred to in many official healthcare documents, e.g. NICE CKS guidelines.

Although written primarily with cancer patients in mind, *PCF* contains specific material relating to a number of other life-limiting diseases, e.g. COPD, congestive heart failure, renal failure, and Parkinson's disease. *PCF* also includes a number of *Quick Clinical Guides* and *Quick Prescribing Guides* (listed inside the back cover and in the Supplementary topic index). To enhance user-friendliness, each *Guide* is limited to no more than two pages, and references are not normally included. We welcome feedback on these. We also encourage the donation of clinical guidance from other sources for posting on our website (e-mail copies to hq@palliativedrugs.com).

The production of a book of this nature depends partly on the help and advice of numerous colleagues, both past and present. We acknowledge with gratitude the support of clinical colleagues, and members of the palliativedrugs.com community who have provided feedback, particularly via surveys or by contributing to the *Syringe Driver Survey Database*.

We acknowledge with thanks the advice provided by various correspondents, including: Victoria Barnett, Claudia Bausewein, James Beattie, Christopher Blick, Ronald Elin, Bethany Foster, Philippa Hawley, Sue Hollingsworth, Aleksandra Kotlinska–Lemieszek, Louise Lynch, Mary Mihalyo, Eva Murphy, Renee Page, Russell Portenoy, Constanze Remi, Jan Rémi, John Shuster, Nigel Sykes, and by Medical Information Departments in the pharmaceutical industry.

We are grateful to Sarah Keeling for co-ordinating production, John Shaw for assistance in copy-editing, and to Karen Isaac for secretarial support.

Robert Twycross
Andrew Wilcock
Paul Howard
Editors-in-chief
July 2014

SUMMARY OF MAIN CHANGES IN PCF5

Since the publication of *PCF4* in 2011, every drug monograph has been reviewed and updated. With the anticipated demise of *Symptom Management in Advanced Cancer*, several items have been transferred into the *Formulary*:

- *Chapter 2 in Haemostatics*: a section about Haematuria, including a Table of bladder instillations and irrigations for haemorrhagic cystitis
- *Chapter 10 in Skeletal muscle relaxants*: a list of drugs which can cause cramps, and a Box detailing the use of anti-epileptics for treating cramp
- *Chapter 11 in Drugs for oral inflammation and ulceration*: a list of drugs which can cause oral ulceration.

New Chapters
25 Variability in response to drugs (replaces Cytochrome P450)
28 Drugs for pruritus

Deleted monographs
Dextropropoxyphene has been withdrawn in the UK, Europe, the USA, and other countries because of its relatively common use in intentional overdose and its potential fatal toxicity in accidental overdose. Accordingly, the monograph in earlier editions of PCF is now redundant, and has been removed.

Other monographs have been subsumed into generic drug class monographs, e.g.:
- Dalteparin and Enoxaparin (→ LMWH)
- Flecainide (→ Systemic local anaesthetics)
- Methylphenidate and Modafinil (→ Psychostimulants)
- Naloxone and Naltrexone (→ Opioid antagonists)

Monographs
Either new or amalgamations:
- Anticoagulants
- Low molecular weight heparin (LMWH)
- Haemostatics
- Gabapentin and pregabalin
- Psychostimulants
- Cannabinoids
- Tapentadol
- Opioid antagonists
- Bisphosphonates

Quick Practice Guides
These have been renamed as either *Quick Clinical Guides* (e.g. Heparin-Induced Thrombocytopenia) or *Quick Prescribing Guides* (e.g. Depression, Opioid-induced constipation). For full list, see inside the back cover.

HOW PCF IS CONSTRUCTED

There is continual review and updating of the contents of *PCF* over a three year cycle. These updates are published regularly on-line, with the whole book published in print every three years.

The *Palliative Care Formulary* (*PCF*) is a unique independent professional publication which provides essential information for prescribers and health professionals involved in palliative and hospice care. *PCF* contains authoritative independent guidance on best practice, and helps to ensure that drugs are used appropriately, safely, and optimally.

Recommended International Non-proprietary Names (rINN) are used for drugs. The order of drug monographs broadly follows that of the *British National Formulary* (*BNF*).

Editorial team

The *PCF* editorial team is co-ordinated by three medically qualified Editors-in-chief who are (or have been) accredited specialists in Palliative Medicine and a specialist palliative care pharmacist. For each print edition, every section of *PCF* is reviewed and updated with the help of an Editorial Board. Suggestions for new monographs are discussed by the *PCF* editorial team, and experts identified to assist in the preparation of new documents.

The Editorial Board

The Editorial Board mainly comprises palliative care physicians appointed on the basis of their clinical knowledge and expertise. Editorial Board members have committed to reviewing one or more drug monographs or chapters, and work in liaison with the editorial team. Responsibilities include scrutinizing literature databases such as PubMed, and accessing and studying relevant new publications.

Correspondents

Correspondents are drawn from a range of medical specialties. They include doctors, pharmacists, nurses, and others who provide advice on the text by:
- checking amendments for scientific accuracy, and to enhance clarity
- providing additional expert opinion in areas of controversy or when reliable evidence is lacking
- advising on areas when the *PCF* diverges from a manufacturer's Summary of Product Characteristics (SPC)
- providing additional validation and clinical evidence about unauthorized (off-label) use.

Sources of *PCF* information

PCF uses various sources for its information, including:

Summary of product characteristics (SPC)

The SPCs are the principal source of product information and are carefully reviewed to ensure that *PCF* monographs are fully up-to-date in this respect.

Literature

Research papers and reviews relating to the drugs featured in *PCF* are carefully processed. When a difference between the advice in the *PCF* and a paper is noted, the new information is evaluated for reliability and relevance to UK clinical practice. If necessary, new text is drafted and thoroughly reviewed by the editorial team with support, as needed, from the Editorial Board and/ or Correspondents.

PCF also has access to many on-line information resources (see p.xviii). For example, www.azcert.org is used to flag drugs which have the potential to prolong QT interval to a clinically relevant degree, and www.psychotropical.com is used to help adjudicate whether a report about serotonin toxicity is reliable.

Systematic reviews
PCF monitors various databases of systematic reviews, including the *Cochrane Library* and several other web-based resources. Reviews published in *Clinical Evidence* are used to validate PCF advice.

Consensus guidelines
The advice in PCF is checked against consensus guidelines produced by expert bodies including the National Institute for Health and Care Excellence (NICE), the Scottish Medicines Consortium (SMC), and the Scottish Intercollegiate Guidelines Network (SIGN).

PCF also takes note of other expert bodies which produce clinical guidelines relevant to palliative care, e.g. Association for Palliative Medicine, British Lymphology Society.

Statutory information
PCF routinely processes relevant information from various Government bodies, including Statutory Instruments and regulations affecting the Prescription only Medicines Order, Controlled Drugs and from the Medicines and Healthcare products Regulatory Agency (MHRA). Safety warnings issued by the Commission on Human Medicines (CHM) and guidelines on drug use issued by the UK health departments are routinely processed.

Relevant professional statements issued by the Royal Pharmaceutical Society (RPS), Nursing and Midwifery Council (NMC) and General Medical Council (GMC) are included in PCF as are guidelines from the medical Royal Colleges.

Pricing information
Drug prices are net prices based on those in the online edition of the *BNF* at the time of the monograph update. For products not included in the *BNF*, prices are checked directly with suppliers. However, particularly in hospitals, heavily discounted contract prices radically alter both the absolute and relative acquisition costs.

Prices worked out for 28 days' supply are generally based on the most convenient strength for the patient and cheapest pack size. Costs for broken bulk, dispensing/sourcing fees and delivery charges are *not* included. Costs under £5 have been rounded up to the next 50p; prices over £5 are rounded up to the next full pound.

Comments from industry
Manufacturers are contacted directly if there are queries about the content of an SPC.

GETTING THE MOST OUT OF PCF

Information in a book of this type can never be all-inclusive, and thus will not cover every eventuality. Readers should satisfy themselves as to the appropriateness of the information before applying it in practice.

Particularly when prescribing a drug for the first time, a doctor (or other independent prescriber) should study the contents of the manufacturer's Summary of Product Characteristics (SPC), paying particular attention to indications, contra-indications, cautions, drug interactions, and undesirable effects (also see p.xvii).

PCF often refers to the use of drugs beyond the scope of their marketing authorization (product licence). The use of drugs in this way clearly has implications for the prescriber (see p.xix).

A cautious approach is always necessary when prescribing for the frail, the elderly, and patients with hepatic impairment, renal impairment or respiratory insufficiency (see Chapter 14, p.639). Further, if caring for a woman who is pregnant or breast-feeding, or someone with porphyria, it is crucial to double-check a drug's suitability in both the *BNF* and its SPC.

The literature on the pharmacology of pain and symptom management in end-stage disease is growing continually, and it is impossible for anyone to be familiar with all of it. This is where a book like *PCF* comes into its own as a major accessible resource for prescribing clinicians involved in palliative care.

PCF is not an easy read, indeed it was never intended that it would be read from cover to cover. It is essentially a reference book – to study the monograph of an individual drug, or class of drugs, with specific questions in mind.

In Part 1, the sections generally follow the systematic order of the *British National Formulary* (*BNF*). Drugs marked with an asterisk (*) should generally be used only by, or after consultation with, a specialist palliative care service.

Part 2 and the appendices deal with themes that transcend the drug monographs, e.g. pre-emptive prescribing in the community, continuous subcutaneous infusions, administering drugs via enteral tubes, the use of nebulized drugs.

Reliable knowledge, levels of evidence and strength of recommendations

Research is the pursuit of reliable knowledge. The gold standard for drug treatment is the randomized controlled trial (RCT) or, better, a systematic review of homogeneous RCTs.

Over the last 20–30 years, numerous systems have been published for categorizing levels of evidence and the strength of the derived recommendations. Box A reproduces the system used by the British Medical Journal. This checklist is based on material published by three main sources, namely the US Agency for Health Care Policy and Research, the NHS Management Executive, and the North of England Guidelines Group.[1–3]

However, it is important to recognize that the RCT is *not* the only source of reliable knowledge. Broadly speaking, sources of knowledge can be conveniently grouped under three headings:
- *instrumental*, includes RCT data and data from other high-quality studies
- *interactive*, refers to anecdotal data (shared clinical experience), including retrospective and prospective surveys
- *critical*, data unique to the individual in question (e.g. personal choice) and societal/cultural factors (e.g. financial and logistic considerations).[5]

Relying on one type of knowledge alone is *not* good practice. All three sources must be exploited in the process of therapeutic decision-making.

Box A	A scheme for categorizing evidence and grading recommendations[4]		
Category	Level of evidence	Grade	Strength of recommendations
Ia	Evidence obtained from a meta-analysis of RCTs	A	Directly based on Category I evidence without extrapolation
Ib	Evidence from at least one RCT		
IIa	Evidence obtained from at least one well-designed controlled study without randomization	B	Directly based on Category II evidence or by extrapolation from Category I evidence
IIb	Evidence obtained from at least one other well-designed quasi-experimental study		
III	Evidence obtained from well-designed non-experimental descriptive studies, such as comparative studies, correlation studies and case studies	C	Directly based on Category III evidence or by extrapolation from Category I or II evidence
IV	Evidence obtained from expert committee reports or opinions and/or clinical experiences of respected authorities	D	Directly based on category IV evidence or by extrapolation from Category I, II, or III evidence
			This grading indicates that directly applicable clinical studies of good quality are absent or not readily available

Pharmaceutical company information

Although the manufacturer's SPC is an important source of information about a drug, it is important to remember that many published studies are sponsored by the drug company in question. This can lead to a conflict of interest between the desire for objective data and the need to make one's own drug as attractive as possible.[6] It is thus best to treat information from company representatives as inevitably biased. The information provided by PCF is commercially independent, and should serve as a counterbalance to manufacturer bias.

Remember: it is often safer to stick with an 'old favourite', and not seek to be among the first to prescribe a newly released product – which may simply be a 'me-too' drug rather than true innovation.[6]

Generic drugs

PCF encourages generic prescribing.[7] Apart from occasional exceptions, e.g. m/r formulations of diltiazem, nifedipine, theophylline and some anti-epileptics, there is little reliable evidence that different preparations of the same drug are significantly different in terms of bio-availability and efficacy.[8] However, particularly for oral morphine preparations, the Department of Health (London) recommends including the brand name of opioid analgesics on the prescription and dispensing label, to avoid unwittingly switching brands and confusing the patient.[9]

Indications

PCF often refers to the use of drugs beyond the scope of their marketing authorization (product licence). The use of drugs in this way clearly has implications for the prescriber (see p.xix). As always, readers should satisfy themselves as to the appropriateness of the information before applying it in practice.

In PCF generally, only those indications which are relevant to palliative care are listed, with unauthorized indications or uses preceded by a † sign. However, a succinct summary is not always

possible because the Marketing Authorization reflects what the manufacturer applied for. Thus, authorized indications can vary between drugs within a therapeutic class or for the same drug by different:
- manufacturers
- routes of administration, e.g. haloperidol tablets and injection
- formulations, e.g. buprenorphine TD patches, desmopressin tablets
- pack sizes, e.g. buprenorphine tablets.

We have endeavoured to indicate such circumstances with the statement: 'Authorized indications vary between products; consult SPC for details'. In any event, before using a product for the first time, the SPC should be studied.

Contra-indications and cautions

Contra-indications and cautions listed in SPCs sometimes vary between different manufacturers of the same drug. Thus, a contra-indication in one SPC may be styled a caution in another, and vice versa.

In *PCF*, we do *not* include universal contra-indications (e.g. history of hypersensitivity to the drug), and have generally *not* included a contra-indication from the SPC if the use of the drug in the stated circumstance is accepted prescribing practice in palliative care.

Advice regarding dosing a drug in renal impairment can vary. When this occurs, *PCF* favours the opinion of the independent *Renal Drug Handbook* over the manufacturer's SPC.

However, as always, a cautious approach is necessary when prescribing for the frail, the elderly, and patients with organ impairment or respiratory insufficiency (see Chapter 14, p.639). If caring for a woman who is pregnant or breast-feeding, or for someone with porphyria, it is crucial to check a drug's suitability in both the *BNF* and SPC.

Pharmacokinetics
Generally, pharmacokinetic data are taken from *Martindale: the complete drug reference*[10] or from a manufacturer's SPC. Other sources are referenced in the text.

Drug interactions
Generally, information on drug interactions is taken from *Stockley's drug interactions*[11] or from a manufacturer's SPC. Other sources are referenced in the text.

It is assumed that clinicians are aware of the risk of commonsense pharmacodynamic interactions, e.g. that the concurrent prescription of two or more drugs with sedative properties is likely to result in more sedation than if each drug was prescribed alone. On the other hand, pharmacokinetic interactions (leading to either increased or reduced effect) are generally covered in individual drug monographs and in Chapter 25, p.767.

Undesirable effects of drugs
As recommended by the European Commission, the term 'undesirable effect' is used rather than 'side effect' or 'adverse drug reaction'. Wherever possible, undesirable effects are categorized as:
- very common ($>10\%$)
- common ($<10\%$, $>1\%$)
- uncommon ($<1\%$, $>0.1\%$)
- rare ($<0.1\%$, $>0.01\%$)
- very rare ($<0.01\%$).

PCF generally includes information on the very common and common undesirable effects. Selected other undesirable effects are also included, e.g. uncommon or rare ones which may have serious consequences. The manufacturer's SPC should be consulted for a full list of undesirable effects.

Supply

The list of products in the Supply section is *not* exhaustive. Generally, generic products and selected proprietary ones are included, e.g. an alternative proprietary formulation not available as a generic.

Literature references

In choosing references, articles in hospice and palliative care journals have frequently been selected preferentially. Such journals are likely to be more readily available to our readers, and often contain detailed discussion.

It is not feasible to reference every statement in *PCF*. However, readers are invited to enter into constructive dialogue with the Editors via the Bulletin Board on *www.palliativedrugs.com*. This is currently accessed by > 25,000 health professionals worldwide.

Online sources of information

Website references are not routinely given for articles available in traditionally published journals. However, various full-text core journals are available free to UK NHS staff with an Athens password through the NHS Evidence Services website at https://www.evidence.nhs.uk.

Information from the *BNF* and *BNFc* is freely available, after registration, from www.bnf.org.uk for users in the UK and the HINARI group of developing countries. References to manufacturer's SPCs and PILs are generally *not* included. However, most can be freely accessed from www.medicines.org.uk or obtained directly from the manufacturer.

Online sources of information are referenced when this is the usual route of publication and access is freely available, e.g. UK Department of Health guidelines, MHRA Drug Safety Updates, NICE guidance, SIGN guidance. The website address quoted is for the homepage or the page from which the guidance can be found and downloaded.

Whenever possible, subscription websites have been avoided. However, to ensure that the most current information is included when revising *PCF*, the following standard reference texts are consulted from subscribed access to Medicines Complete (www.medicinescomplete.com):

- *Amercian Hospital Formulary Service (AHFS)*
- *Handbook of drug administration via enteral feeding tubes*
- *Handbook on injectable drugs*
- *Martindale: the complete drug reference*
- *Stockley's drug interactions.*

These are available in all UK Medicines Information Services.

1 Eccles M, et al. (1996) North of England evidence based guidelines development project: methods of guideline development. *British Medical Journal.* **312**: 762–762.
2 DoH (1996) *Clinical Guidelines: Using Clinical Guidelines to Improve Patient Care Within the NHS.* Department of Health: NHS Executive, Leeds.
3 Agency for Health Care Policy and Research (1992) Acute pain management, operative or medical procedures and trauma 0032–0032. In: *Clinical Practice Guideline Quick Ref Guide for Clinicians.* AHCPR Publications, Rockville, Maryland, USA, pp. 22–22.
4 BMJ Publishing Group (2009) Resources for authors. Checklists and forms: clinical management guidelines. Available from: http://resources.bmj.com/bmj/authors/checklists-forms/clinical-management-guidelines
5 Aoun SM and Kristjanson LJ (2005) Challenging the framework for evidence in palliative care research. *Palliative Medicine.* **19**: 465–465.
6 Angell M (2004) *The Truth About the Drug Companies: how they deceive us and what to do about it.* Random House, New York.
7 National Prescribing Centre (2011) Generic prescribing in primary care. *MeReC Bulletin.* **21**: 6–6.
8 National Prescribing Centre (2000) Modified-release preparations. *MeReC Bulletin.* **11**: 16–16.
9 Smith J (2004) Building a Safer NHS for Patients - Improving Medication Safety. pp. 111–111. Department of Health, London. Available from: www.dh.gov.uk/assetRoot/04/08/49/61/04084961.pdf
10 Sweetman SC. *Martindale: The Complete Drug Reference.* London: Pharmaceutical Press www.medicinescomplete.com
11 Baxter K and Preston CL. *Stockley's Drug Interactions.* London:- Pharmaceutical Press www.medicinescomplete.com

THE USE OF DRUGS BEYOND (OFF-LABEL) AND WITHOUT MARKETING AUTHORIZATION

The use of drugs for off-label purposes is widespread. Surveys suggest that up to one quarter of all prescriptions in palliative care come into this category.[1,2] In *PCF*, the symbol † is used to indicate such use. However, it is impractical to highlight all cases of off-label use, particularly when it is simply a matter of the route or dose being different from those in the manufacturer's Summary of Product Characteristics (SPC).

It is important for prescribers to understand that *marketing authorization* for drugs regulates the *marketing activities* of pharmaceutical companies, and not the prescriber's clinical practice. Even so, off-label use does have implications for prescribers, and these are discussed in this section.

Definitions
Marketing authorization
Marketing authorization (MA) means that a drug has been approved by a regulatory body for use in humans and authorized for specific indications, and can be marketed by the relevant pharmaceutical company.

Off-label use
Off-label describes the use of a drug beyond the specifications of its MA, e.g. for an unauthorized indication, or in doses, preparations, patient population or route not covered by the MA.

Unauthorized drug
There is no simple definition of an unauthorized drug. Essentially it is a drug which does not have MA for medicinal use in humans. Unauthorized drugs include:
- the final product when two or more drugs are mixed together for administration e.g. in a syringe for CSCI (see below and Chapter 20, p.697)
- 'specials' obtained from a commercial company with a 'specials' manufacturing licence, e.g. alfentanil solution for nasal/buccal administration (see Alfentanil, p.385)
- preparations made in a local pharmacy at the request of a prescriber for an individual named patient
- drugs that have had a MA withdrawn but special provision has been made by the MHRA for a continued supply, e.g. co-proxamol or for which MA has been abandoned, suspended or revoked, e.g. cisapride, oxetacaine, thioridazine
- drugs that are authorized in another country but not in the UK and are imported into the UK by a specialist importing company, e.g. hydromorphone injection
- new drugs undergoing clinical trials or awaiting a MA, e.g. if a patient wishes to continue an investigational product after a clinical trial.

The authorization (licensing) process
Before a drug can be marketed in the UK, it requires MA (previously product licence). There are four application procedures in the European Union:
- *centralized*, application evaluated by the European Medicines Agency (EMEA); the European Commission grants a single MA valid for the whole European Union
- *decentralized*, simultaneous application made by several member states, with one taking the lead; if successful, national MA then being granted in each state

- *mutual recognition*, application for authorization in a member state when MA exists in another member state; the new member state relies on the original member state's evaluation as a basis for its decision
- *national*, application for MA in only one member state; in the UK the application is evaluated by the Medicines and Healthcare products Regulatory Agency (MHRA) on behalf of the Licensing Authority, a body consisting of UK health ministers.[3]

Certain drugs, e.g. for HIV/AIDS, cancer, neurodegenerative diseases, must be authorized through the centralized procedure. The UK Parallel Import Licensing Scheme also allows a drug authorized in other European Union states to be imported and marketed in the UK, if it has labels and a Patient Information Leaflet (PIL) in English.

In the UK, the MHRA evaluation comprises an evaluation of the efficacy, safety and quality of the drug from a medical, pharmaceutical and scientific viewpoint to ensure that it satisfies predefined criteria. Advice is sought from the Commission on Human Medicines (CHM), an independent advisory body, which in turn is assisted by specialist expert advisory groups.

At a European level, the Committee for Medicinal Products for Human Use (CHMP) fulfils a similar role to the CHM. New drugs will have relatively limited safety information and the pharmaceutical company is generally required to outline a risk management plan.

Restrictions are imposed if evidence of safety and efficacy is unavailable in particular patient groups, e.g. children. MA is granted for up to 5 years and then renewed following re-evaluation of the risks and benefits.[3]

Thus, the process ensures that in relation to the drug's authorized uses, there has been due consideration of its efficacy, safety and quality, that the benefits outweigh the potential risks, and that there is appropriate accompanying product information and labelling.[4] The MA defines the conditions and patient groups for which a pharmaceutical company can market and supply the drug, with more information about the drug's authorized uses provided by the manufacturer in the Summary of Product Characteristics (SPC).

However, the MA does not limit what the drug could be used for (i.e. off-label use), and clinical experience may reveal other indications. For these to receive a MA, additional evidence would need to be gathered and submitted. The considerable expense of this, perhaps coupled with a small market for a new indication, often means that a revised application is not made.

Prescribing for off-label indications or unauthorized drugs

In the UK, the following may legally prescribe authorized drugs for off-label indications and unauthorized drugs:[5–7]
- doctors, specifically safeguarded in the UK Medicines Act 1968
- nurses, pharmacists, podiatrists, physiotherapists and radiographers who are registered as *supplementary prescribers*, provided it is done within the framework of an agreed Clinical Management Plan for a specific patient in partnership with a doctor or dentist
- nurses or pharmacists who are registered as *independent prescribers* if this is accepted clinical practice and within their clinical competence.

These prescriptions can be dispensed by pharmacists[8] and administered by nurses or midwives.[9]

In addition to clinical trials, such prescriptions may be justified:
- when prescribing generic formulations for which indications are not described
- with established drugs for proven but unauthorized indications
- with drugs for conditions for which there are no other treatments (even in the absence of strong evidence)
- when using drugs in individuals not covered by the MA, e.g. children
- when mixing drugs before administration, e.g. two or more drugs in a syringe for administration by continuous infusion.[10,11]

Any *independent prescriber*, including non-medical prescribers, can mix drugs and direct others to mix, as can *supplementary prescribers* when the preparation is part of the Clinical Management Plan for an individual patient. Legislation on mixing now extends to controlled drugs. Existing good practice recommendations should be followed in relation to mixing all drugs.[10] Preparations resulting from mixing drugs, other than when one product is a vehicle for the administration of the other, cannot be supplied or administered under Patient Group Direction arrangements.

The responsibility for the consequences of prescribing a drug under such circumstances lies with the prescriber, who must be competent, operate within the professional codes and ethics of their statutory bodies and the prescribing practices of their employers.[4–6] The prescriber must be

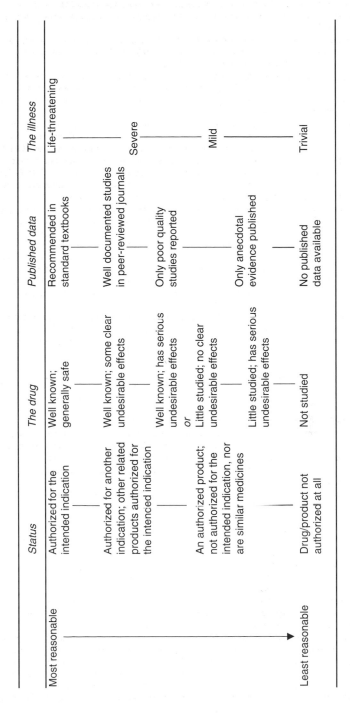

Figure I Factors influencing the reasonableness of prescribing decisions.

fully informed about the actions and uses of the drug, be assured of the quality of the particular product, and in the light of published evidence, balance both the potential good and the potential harm which might ensue.

It is possible to draw a hierarchy of degrees of reasonableness relating to off-label and unauthorized drug use (Figure 1). The more dangerous the medicine and the more flimsy the evidence the more difficult it is to justify its prescription.

The PIL will not contain information about unauthorized indications. Thus, it is important that prescribers (or those authorizing treatment on their behalf) provide sufficient information to patients about the drug's expected benefits and potential risks (undesirable effects, drug interactions, etc.) to enable them to make an informed decision (Box A). The GMC also recommends that when prescribing a drug off-label, doctors should:

- be satisfied that such use would better serve the patient's needs than an authorized alternative (if one exists)
- be satisfied that there is sufficient evidence/experience of using the drug to show its safety and efficacy, seeking the necessary information from appropriate sources
- record in the patient's clinical notes the drug prescribed and, when not following common practice, the reasons for the choice
- take responsibility for prescribing the drug and for overseeing the patient's care, including monitoring the effects of the drug, or arrange for another suitable doctor to do so.[12]

Non-medical prescribers should ensure that they are familiar with their own profession's prescribing standards, e.g. NMC. Although the advice is broadly similar to that of the GMC, there are some differences.[13,14]

Box A Providing information for patients about the use of drugs beyond and without marketing authorization[12]

Patients (or their proxy) should be given sufficient information about any proposed drug treatment to allow them to make an informed decision. Questions must be answered fully and honestly.

Some drugs are routinely used beyond their licence, e.g. when treating children and in palliative care.

In emergencies, or when there is no realistic alternative treatment and such information is likely to cause distress, it may not be practical or necessary to draw attention to the licence.

In other situations, when the prescription of an unauthorized drug is supported by authoritative clinical guidance, it may be sufficient to describe in general terms why the drug is not authorized for the proposed use.

When prescribing a drug which is unauthorized or off-label in a non-routine way, or when suitable authorized alternatives exist, the reason for this should be explained to the patient.

In palliative care, off-label drug use is so widespread that concerns have been expressed that a detailed explanation on every occasion is impractical, would be burdensome for the patient and increase anxiety, and could result in the refusal of beneficial treatment.[15] A UK survey of over 220 palliative medicine doctors showed that, when using a drug for a routine off-label indication, <5% *always* mention this to their patients, and 20% *never* do. However, in situations where there is little evidence and limited clinical experience to support a drug's off-label use, these figures change to 75% and 5% respectively.[16]

This is a grey area and each clinician must decide how explicit to be; an appropriate level of counselling and a sensitive approach is essential. Some NHS Trusts and other institutions have policies in place and have produced information cards or leaflets for patients and caregivers (Box B). A joint position statement has also been produced by the British Pain Society and the Association for Palliative Medicine (Box C),[17] together with a patient information booklet.[18]

Box B Example of a patient information leaflet about the off-label use of a drug

Use of medicines beyond their licence (off-label)

This leaflet contains important information about your medicines, so please read it carefully.

Generally, medicines prescribed by your doctor or bought over-the-counter from a pharmacist are licensed for use by the Medicines and Healthcare products Regulatory Agency (MHRA).

The licence (or marketing authorization) specifies the conditions and patient groups for which the medicine should be used, and how it should be given.

Patient Information Leaflets (PILs) supplied with medicines reflect the licensed uses. When a medicine is used beyond its licence, the information in the PIL may not be relevant to your circumstances.

In palliative care, medicines are commonly used for conditions or in ways that are not specified on the licence.

Your doctor will use medicines beyond the licence only when there is research and experience to back up such use.

Medicines used very successfully beyond the licence include some antidepressants and anti-epileptics (anti-seizure drugs) when given to relieve some types of pain. Also, instead of injecting into a vein or muscle, medicines are often given subcutaneously (under the skin) because this is more comfortable and convenient.

If you would like more information, please ask your doctor or pharmacist.

Alternatively, contact:

Dr/Nurse ....

Hospital..

....

....

Tel ....

1 Atkinson C and Kirkham S (1999) Unlicensed uses for medication in a palliative care unit. *Palliative Medicine.* **13**: 152–152.
2 Todd J and Davies A (1999) Use of unlicensed medication in palliative medicine. *Palliative Medicine.* **13**: 466.
3 Anonymous (2009) The licensing of medicines in the UK. *Drug and Therapeutics Bulletin.* **47**: 48–48.
4 Anonymous (2009) Off-label or unlicensed medicines: prescribers' responsibilities. *MHRA Drug Safety Update.* **2 (9)**: 7–7.
5 Department of Health (2005) Supplementary prescribing by nurses, pharmacists, chiropodists/podiatrists, physiotherapists and radiographers within the NHS in England: a guide for implementation. HMSO, London. Available from: *www.dh.gov.uk/en/PublicationsandstatisticsPublications/PublicationsPolicyAndGuidance/DH_4110032*
6 Department of Health (2006) Improving patients' access to medicines: a guide to implementing nurse and pharmacist independent prescribing within the NHS in England. HMSO, London. Available from: *www.dh.gov.uk/assetRoot/04/13/37/47/04133747.pdf*
7 Department of Health (2010) Changes to medicines legislation to enable Mixing of Medicines prior to administration in clinical practice. Available from: *www.dh.gov.uk/en/Healthcare/Medicinespharmacyandindustry/Prescriptions/TheNon-MedicalPrescribing-Programme/DH_110765*
8 Royal Pharmaceutical Society of Great Britain (2007) Fitness to practise and legal affairs directorate fact sheet: five. The use of unlicensed medicines in pharmacy. Royal Pharmaceutical Society of Great Britain. Available from: *www.rspgb.org/pdfs/factsheet5.pdf*
9 Anonymous (1992) Prescribing unlicensed drugs or using drugs for unlicensed indications. *Drug and Therapeutics Bulletin.* **30**: 99–99.
10 Department of Health (2010) Mixing of medicines prior to administration in clinical practice: medical and non-medical prescribing. HMSO, London. Available from: *www.gov.uk*
11 National Prescribing Centre (2010) Mixing of medicines prior to administration in clinical practice - responding to legislative changes. Liverpool. Available from: *www.npc.nhs.uk*
12 General Medical Council (2013) Good practice in prescribing medicines. Available from: *www.gmc-uk.org*

Box C Recommendations of the Association for Palliative Medicine of Great Britain and Ireland and the British Pain Society[17]

Use of medicines beyond (off-label) and without (unlicensed) Marketing Authorization (MA) in palliative care and pain medicine

1 This statement should be seen as reflecting the views of a responsible body of opinion within the clinical specialties of palliative medicine and pain medicine

2 The use of medicines beyond and without a MA in palliative care and pain medicine practice is both necessary and common and should be seen as a legitimate aspect of clinical practice.

3 Organizations providing palliative care and pain medicine services should support therapeutic practices that are underpinned by evidence and advocated by a responsible body of professional opinion.

4 Health professionals involved in prescribing medicines beyond or without MA should select those medicines that offer the best balance of benefit against harm for any given patient.

5 Choice of treatment requires partnership between patients and health professionals, and informed consent should be obtained, whenever possible, before prescribing any medicine.

6 Patients should be offered accurate, clear and specific information that meets their needs about the use of medicines beyond or without a MA in accordance with professional regulatory body guidance. The information needs of carers and other health professionals involved in the care of the patient should also be considered and met as appropriate. The use of information cards or leaflets may help with this. It is often unnecessary to take additional steps when recommending medicines beyond or without MA.

7 Health professionals should inform, change and monitor their practice with regard to medicines beyond or without MA in the light of evidence from audit and published research.

8 The Department of Health should work with health professionals and the pharmaceutical industry to enable and encourage the extension of product licences where there is evidence of benefit in circumstances of defined clinical need.

---

13 Nursing and Midwifery Council (2006) Standards of proficiency for nurse and midwife prescribers. Available from: *www.nmc-uk.org*

14 Royal Pharmaceutical Society of Great Britain (2010) Professional Standards and Guidance for Pharmacist Prescribers. Available from: *www.rpharms.com/archived-documents/archived-documents.asp#law*

15 Pavis H and Wilcock A (2001) Prescribing of drugs for use outside their licence in palliative care: survey of specialists in the United Kingdom. *British Medical Journal.* **323:** 485–485.

16 Culshaw J et al. (2013) Off-label prescribing in palliative care: a survey of independent prescribers. *Palliative Medicine.* **27:** 319–319.

17 British Pain Society (2012) Use of medicines outside of their UK Marketing Authorization in pain management and palliative care. Available from: *www.britishpainsociety.org*

18 British Pain Society (2012) Use of medicines outside of their UK Marketing Authorisation in pain management and palliative medicine - information for patients. Available from: *www.britishpainsociety.org*

DRUG NAMES

All drugs marketed in Europe are now known by their recommended International Non-proprietary (generic) Name (rINN). In the past, most publications in the UK used the now outdated British Approved Name (BAN). To aid understanding of the older literature, significant differences between BANs and rINNs are listed in Table 1. However, when the difference is simply, e.g. 'f' instead of 'ph', 'e' instead of 'oe', or 't' instead of 'th', these generally have *not* been included.

In the USA, United States Adopted Names (USANs) take precedence over rINNs. USANs are also included in Table 1 where these differ significantly from rINNs.

Note: in the UK, the BANs **adrenaline** and **noradrenaline** are still used in conjunction with the corresponding rINNs, i.e. **adrenaline (epinephrine)** and **noradrenaline (norepinephrine)**.

Care should be taken with proprietary drug names in different countries. Some proprietary names are similar in spelling or pronunciation but contain different drugs. Further, some products with identical proprietary names contain different drugs, e.g. Urex® in the USA contains **methenamine** but, in Australia, **furosemide**.[1]

Table 1 Drug names relevant to palliative care for which the rINN, BAN and/or USAN differ

rINN	BAN	USAN
Alimemazine	Trimeprazine	Trimeprazine
Amobarbital	Amylobarbitone	
Bendroflumethiazide	Bendrofluazide	Bendroflumethiazide
Benzylpenicillin		Penicillin G
Calcitonin (salmon)	Salcatonin	Calcitonin
Carmellose		Carboxymethylcellulose
Chlorphenamine	Chlorpheniramine	Chlorpheniramine
Clomethiazole	Chlormethiazole	
Dexamfetamine	Dexamphetamine	Dextroamphetamine
Dextropropoxyphene		Propoxyphene
Dicycloverine	Dicyclomine	Dicyclomine
Diethylstilbestrol	Stilboestrol	Diethylstilbestrol
Dosulepin	Dothiepin	Dothiepin
Epinephrine	Adrenaline	Epinephrine
Glibenclamide		Glyburide
Glycerol	Glycerine	Glycerin
Glyceryl trinitrate		Nitroglycerin
Hyoscine		Scopolamine
Isoprenaline		Isoproterenol
	Ispaghula	Psyllium
Levomepromazine	Methotrimeprazine	
Levothyroxine	Thyroxine	
Liquid paraffin		Mineral oil
Methenamine hippurate	Hexamine hippurate	
Paracetamol		Acetaminophen
Pethidine		Meperidine

continued

Table I Continued

rINN	BAN	USAN
Phenobarbital	Phenobarbitone	
Phenoxymethylpenicillin		Penicillin V
Phytomenadione		Phytonadione
Retinol	Vitamin A	Vitamin A
Rifampicin		Rifampin
Salbutamol		Albuterol
Simeticone[a]	Simethicone	Simethicone
Sodium cromoglicate	Sodium cromoglycate	Cromolyn sodium
Tetracaine	Amethocaine	
Trihexyphenidyl	Benzhexol	Trihexyphenidyl

a. silica-activated dimeticone; known in some countries as activated dimethylpolysiloxane.

1 FDA (2006) Consumers filling U.S. prescriptions abroad may get the wrong active ingredient because of confusing drug names. *Public Health Advisory.* www.fda.gov/Drugs/DrugSafety/PostmarketDrugSafetyInformationforPatientsandProviders/default.htm

ABBREVIATIONS

Drug administration

In 2005, the Joint Commission on Accreditation of Healthcare Organizations (JCAHO) in the USA published National Patient Safety Goals. These include a series of recommendations about ways in which confusion (and thus errors) can be reduced by avoiding the use of certain abbreviations on prescriptions. The full set of recommendations is available at http://www.jointcommission.org/standards_information/npsgs.aspx.

Although some traditional abbreviations remain acceptable (e.g. Table 1), other commonly used ones are not. Thus, it is now recommended that the following are written in full:
- at bedtime
- once daily
- each morning
- every other day.

These four recommendations have also been adopted in *PCF*.

Although the following conventions have *not* been adopted in PCF, readers should be aware of the following recommendations for handwritten and printed prescriptions, and other printed medical matter, e.g. packaging, patient records:
- include a space between the drug dose and the unit of measure, e.g. 25 mg, not 25mg
- write 'per' instead of an oblique (mistaken for a figure 1), e.g. 200 mg per day, not 200mg/day
- use 'subcut' or 'subcutaneous' instead of SC (mistaken for SL)
- write 'less than' or 'greater than' instead of < and > (mistaken for a letter L or figure 7; or written the wrong way round and thus signifying the opposite of the intended meaning).

Further, although it has been recommended in the UK that 'PR' (prolonged-release) should become the generic term for 'slow-release', 'extended-release' etc., PR is a time-honoured abbreviation for 'per rectum'. It is in this latter sense that PR will be used in *PCF*. As in earlier editions, 'm/r' (modified-release) will be used.

Note: in earlier editions, 'normal-release' was used for non-modified products. However, because of international popular usage, in this edition the term 'immediate-release' is used (without abbreviation).

Table 1 Abbreviations used in *PCF* for the times of drug administration

Times	UK	Latin
Twice per day	b.d.	*bis die*
Three times per day	t.d.s.	*ter die sumendus*
Four times per day	q.d.s.	*quarta die sumendus*
Every 4 hours etc.	q4h	*quaque quarta hora*
Rescue medication (as needed/required)	p.r.n.	*pro re nata*
Give immediately	stat	*stat*

a.c.	ante cibum (before food)
amp	ampoule containing a single dose (cf. vial)
CD	controlled drug; preparation subject to prescription requirements under the Misuse of Drugs act (UK); for regulations see BNF
CIVI	continuous intravenous infusion

CSCI	continuous subcutaneous infusion
e/c	enteric-coated (gastroresistant)
ED	epidural
IM	intramuscular
IT	intrathecal
IV	intravenous
IVI	intravenous infusion
m/r	modified-release; alternatives, controlled-release, extended-release, prolonged-release, slow-release, sustained-release
NHS	not prescribable on NHS prescriptions
OTC	over the counter (i.e. can be obtained without a prescription)
p.c.	post cibum (after food)
PO	per os, by mouth
POM	prescription-only medicine
PR	per rectum
PV	per vaginam
SC	subcutaneous
SL	sublingual
TD	transdermal
TM	transmucosal
vial	sterile container with a rubber bung containing either a single or multiple doses (cf. amp)
WFI	water for injections

General

*	specialist use only
†	unauthorized (unlicensed) use
ACBS	Advisory Committee on Borderline Substances
AHFS	American Hospital Formulary Service
BNF	British National Formulary
BP	British Pharmacopoeia
CHM	Commission on Human Medicines
CSM	Committee on Safety of Medicines (now part of CHM)
DH	Department of Health (UK)
EMEA	European Medicines Agency
EORTC	European Organisation for Research and Treatment of Cancer
FDA	Food and Drug Administration (USA)
IASP	International Association for the Study of Pain
IDIS	International Drug Information Service
MCA	Medicines Control Agency (now MHRA)
MHRA	Medicines and Healthcare products Regulatory Agency (formerly MCA)
NICE	National Institute for Health and Care Excellence
NPF	Nurse Prescribers' Formulary
NPSA	National Patient Safety Association
NYHA	New York Heart Association
PCS/PCU	palliative care service/unit
PEG	percutaneous endoscopic gastrostomy
PIL	Patient Information Leaflet (UK)
rINN	recommended International Non-proprietary Name
RPS	Royal Pharmaceutical Society
SIGN	Scottish Intercollegiate Guidelines Network
SPC	Summary of Product Characteristics (UK)
UK	United Kingdom
UKMI	UK Medicines Information
USA	United States of America
USP	United States Pharmacopoeia
VAS	visual analogue scale, 0–100mm
WHO	World Health Organization

Medical

ACE	angiotensin-converting enzyme
ADH	antidiuretic hormone (vasopressin)
ATP	adenosine triphosphate
AUC	area under the plasma concentration-time curve
β_2	beta 2 adrenergic (receptor)
CHF	congestive heart failure
C_{max}	maximum plasma drug concentration
CNS	central nervous system
COX	cyclo-oxygenase; alternative, prostaglandin synthase
COPD	chronic obstructive pulmonary disease
CKD	chronic kidney disease
CRP	C-reactive protein
CSF	cerebrospinal fluid
CT	computed tomography
δ	delta-opioid (receptor)
D_2	dopamine type 2 (receptor)
DIC	disseminated intravascular coagulation
DVT	deep vein thrombosis
ECG (EKG)	electrocardiogram
EFT	enteral feeding tube
ERCP	endoscopic retrograde cholangiopancreatography
FBC	full blood count
FEV_1	forced expiratory volume in 1 second
FRC	functional residual capacity
FSH	follicle-stimulating hormone
FVC	forced vital capacity of lungs
GABA	gamma-aminobutyric acid
GI	gastro-intestinal
Hb	haemoglobin
HIV	human immunodeficiency virus
H_1, H_2	histamine type 1, type 2 (receptor)
Ig	immunoglobulin
INR	international normalized ratio
κ	kappa-opioid (receptor)
LABA	long-acting β_2-adrenergic receptor agonist
LFTs	liver function tests
LH	luteinizing hormone
LMWH	low molecular weight heparin
MAOI	mono-amine oxidase inhibitor
MARI	mono-amine re-uptake inhibitor
MRI	magnetic resonance imaging
MSU	mid-stream specimen of urine
μ	mu-opioid (receptor)
NaSSA	noradrenergic and specific serotoninergic antidepressant
NDRI	noradrenaline (norepinephrine) and dopamine re-uptake inhibitor
NG	nasogastric
NJ	nasojejunal
NMDA	N-methyl D-aspartate
NNH	number needed to harm, i.e. the number of patients needed to be treated in order to harm one patient sufficiently to cause withdrawal from a drug trial
NNT	number needed to treat, i.e. the number of patients needed to be treated in order to achieve 50% improvement in one patient compared with placebo
NO	nitric oxide
NRI	noradrenaline (norepinephrine) re-uptake inhibitor
NSAID	non-steroidal anti-inflammatory drug
$PaCO_2$	arterial partial pressure of carbon dioxide
PaO_2	arterial partial pressure of oxygen

PCA	patient-controlled analgesia
PE	pulmonary embolus/embolism
PEF	peak expiratory flow
PG	prostaglandin
PPI	proton pump inhibitor
RCT	randomized controlled trial
RIMA	reversible inhibitor of mono-amine oxidase type A
RTI	respiratory tract infection
SaO_2	oxygen saturation
SNRI	serotonin and noradrenaline (norepinephrine) re-uptake inhibitor
SRE	skeletal-related events
SSRI	selective serotonin re-uptake inhibitor
TCA	tricyclic antidepressant
TIBC	total iron-binding capacity; alternative, plasma transferrin concentration
Tl_{CO}	transfer factor of the lung for carbon monoxide
T_{max}	time to reach C_{max}
UTI	urinary tract infection
VEGF	vascular endothelial growth factor
VIP	vaso-active intestinal polypeptide
WBC	white blood cell
w/v	weight of solute (g) per 100mL

Units

cm	centimetre(s)
cps	cycles per sec
dL	decilitre(s)
g	gram(s)
Gy	Gray(s), a measure of radiation
h	hour(s)
Hg	mercury
kcal	kilocalories
kg	kilogram(s)
L	litre(s)
mg	milligram(s)
microL	microlitre(s)
micromol	micromole(s)
mL	millilitre(s)
mm	millimetre(s)
mmol	millimole(s)
min	minute(s)
mosmol	milli-osmole(s)
msec	millisecond
nm	nanometre(s)
nmol	nanomole(s); alternative, nM
sec	second(s)

1: GASTRO-INTESTINAL SYSTEM

ANTACIDS   BNF 1.1.1

Indications: Occasional dyspepsia and/or acid reflux; H₂-receptor antagonists (see p.26) and PPIs (see p.31) are used when continuous gastric acid reduction is indicated.[1]

Pharmacology
Antacids taken by mouth to neutralize gastric acid include:
- magnesium salts
- aluminium hydroxide
- hydrotalcite (aluminium magnesium carbonate hydroxide hydrate)
- calcium carbonate
- sodium bicarbonate.

Magnesium salts are *laxative and can cause diarrhoea; aluminium salts* constipate. Most proprietary antacids contain a mixture of **magnesium salts** and **aluminium salts** so as to have a neutral impact on intestinal transit. With doses of 100–200mL/24h or more, the effect of **magnesium salts** tends to override the constipating effect of **aluminium**.[2]

The sodium content of some antacids and alginate products may be detrimental in patients on salt-restricted diets, e.g. those with hypertension, heart failure or renal impairment. **Magnesium trisilicate mixture BP**, Gaviscon® Liquid, Acidex® liquid, and Peptac® oral suspension all contain 6mmol/10mL; Gaviscon® Advance liquid contains 4.6mmol/10mL. This compares with < 1mmol/10mL in **co-magaldrox**.

Regular use of **sodium bicarbonate**, an ingredient in many OTC products, may cause sodium loading and metabolic alkalosis. **Calcium carbonate** may cause rebound acid secretion about 2h after each dose, and regular use may cause hypercalcaemia, particularly if taken with **sodium bicarbonate**.

Aluminium hydroxide binds dietary phosphate. It is of benefit in patients with hyperphosphataemia in renal failure. Long-term complications of phosphate depletion and osteomalacia are not an issue in advanced cancer. **Hydrotalcite**, an aluminium-magnesium complex, binds bile salts and is of specific benefit in patients with bile salt reflux, e.g. after certain forms of gastroduodenal surgery.

In post-radiation oesophagitis and candidosis which is causing painful swallowing, an **aluminium hydroxide-magnesium hydroxide** suspension containing **oxetacaine**, a local anaesthetic, can be helpful; this is unauthorized in the UK. Give 5–10mL (without fluid) 15min a.c. & at bedtime, and p.r.n. before drinks. This should be regarded as short-term symptomatic treatment while time and specific treatment of the underlying condition permits healing of the damaged mucosa.

Other agents which are added to antacid products include alginates (see p.3) and **simeticone** (silica-activated **dimeticone**; see p.4).

Most antacid tablets feel gritty when sucked; some patients dislike this. Some proprietary products contain peppermint oil which masks the chalky taste of the antacid and helps belching by decreasing the tone of the lower oesophageal sphincter. Some are fruit-flavoured, e.g. Tums® (chewable tablet).

Cautions

Risk of hypermagnesaemia if magnesium-containing antacids are used in patients with renal impairment; **calcium carbonate** is preferable.

The administration of antacids should be separated from the administration of e/c tablets because direct contact between e/c tablets and antacids can result in damage to the enteric coating with consequential exposure of the drug to gastric acid, and of the stomach mucosa to the drug.

Antacids tend to delay gastric emptying and thus may modify drug absorption; if possible avoid administration at the same time as other drugs. Antacids should not be administered by enteral feeding tube as they can coagulate with the feed (see Chapter 22, Table 2, p.733).

Drug interactions

Antacids will temporarily increase the pH of the stomach contents, and this may affect drug absorption. These interactions can generally be avoided by separating administration of the antacid and the affected drug by ⩾2h, e.g.:

- reduced absorption: some antiretrovirals (**atazanavir, delavirdine, tipranavir**), **cefpodoxime, fexofenadine, itraconazole** capsules (but not oral solution)
- increased absorption: **flurbiprofen, ibuprofen**.[3]

With certain drugs, magnesium salts form an insoluble complex in the GI tract, thereby decreasing absorption, e.g.:

- oral bisphosphonates (**alendronic acid, ibandronic acid, risedronate**): take magnesium salts ⩾30min after the bisphosphonate
- quinolone antibacterials (e.g. **ciprofloxacin**): take the quinolone 2h before or ⩾4h after the magnesium salt
- **tetracycline** antibacterials: separate administration by ⩾2h.[3]

Magnesium hydroxide interacts with **sodium polystyrene sulfonate** resin (used to treat hyperkalaemia) and creates an excess of bicarbonate ions, which can lead to metabolic alkalosis; avoid by giving the resin rectally.[3]

If magnesium salts lead to alkalinization of the urine, the excretion of round-the-clock anti-inflammatory doses of **aspirin** is increased. Occasional doses of **aspirin** are not affected.[3]

Supply

The cheapest single-ingredient products are **magnesium trisilicate mixture BP** and **aluminium hydroxide** capsules; if a combination is required, the cheapest liquid product is Mucogel®. Note: Low Na$^+$ is defined as <1mmol/tablet or 10mL dose.

Aluminium hydroxide
Alucap® (Meda)
Capsules 475mg, 28 days @ 1 t.d.s. & at bedtime = £4.50; low Na$^+$.

Magnesium trisilicate mixture BP (generic)
Oral suspension (magnesium trisilicate 250mg, **magnesium carbonate** 250mg and **sodium hydrogen carbonate** 250mg/5mL) 28 days @ 10mL t.d.s. & at bedtime = £5; *peppermint flavour, 6mmol $Na^+/10mL$.*

Co-magaldrox
Maalox® (Sanofi-Aventis)
Oral suspension (sugar-free) co-magaldrox 195/220 (**magnesium hydroxide** 195mg, **aluminium hydroxide** 220mg/5mL), 28 days @ 10mL t.d.s. & at bedtime = £6.50; *low Na^+.*

Mucogel® (Chemidex)
Oral suspension (sugar-free) co-magaldrox 195/220 (**magnesium hydroxide** 195mg, **aluminium hydroxide** 220mg/5mL), 28 days @ 10mL t.d.s. & at bedtime = £4; *low Na^+.*

Calcium carbonate is available either on its own as an OTC product e.g. Tums®, or in combination with an **alginate** (see Compound alginate products, p.4).

Hydrotalcite (aluminium-magnesium complex) is available only in combination with **simeticone** (see p.5).

Sodium bicarbonate is present in many OTC products.

With oxetacaine
Oral suspension oxetacaine 10mg, **aluminium hydroxide** 200mg, **magnesium hydroxide** 100mg/5mL, 28 days @ 10mL t.d.s. a.c. & at bedtime = £117; *low Na^+* (Unauthorized product, available as a special order from Rosemont; see Appendix 1, p.817. *Available as Mucaine suspension (Wyeth) in some countries.*

Also see Compound alginate products, p.4 and **simeticone**, p.5.

---

1 NICE (2004) Dyspepsia. Management of dyspepsia in adults in primary care. *Clinical Guideline.* **CG17**. www.nice.org.uk
2 Morrissey J and Barreras R (1974) Antacid therapy. *New England Journal of Medicine.* **290**: 550–554.
3 Baxter K and Preston CL (2014). *Stockley's Drug Interactions (online edition).* Pharmaceutical Press, London. Available from: www.medicinescomplete.com

Updated (minor change) June 2014

COMPOUND ALGINATE PRODUCTS   BNF 1.1.2

Included for general information. Alginate products are generally *not recommended* as antacids for palliative care patients.

Class: Alginate.

Indications: Acid reflux ('heartburn').

Pharmacology
Antacid products containing alginic acid or sodium alginate prevent oesophageal reflux pain by forming an inert low-density raft on the top of the acidic stomach contents. Both acid and air bubbles are necessary to produce the raft. Compound alginate products may thus be less effective if used with drugs which reduce acid (e.g. an H_2-receptor antagonist or a PPI) or products which reduce air bubbles (i.e. an antifoaming agent/antiflatulent).

   Gaviscon® products, Peptac® and Acidex® oral suspensions are sodium alginate products and weak antacids; most of the antacid content adheres to the alginate raft. This neutralizes acid which seeps into the oesophagus around the raft but does nothing to correct the underlying causes, e.g. lax lower oesophageal sphincter, hyperacidity, delayed gastric emptying, obesity. Indeed, alginate-containing products are no better than **simeticone**-containing antacids in the treatment of acid reflux.[1] Compound alginate products have been largely superseded by acid suppression with PPIs and H_2-receptor antagonists.

Onset of action <5min.
Duration of action 1–2h.

Cautions

Gaviscon® Liquid, Peptac® and Acidex® oral suspensions contain approximately Na^+ 6mmol/10mL. Gaviscon®Advance oral suspension and tablets contain Na^+ 4.6mmol/10mL and 2.3mmol/tablet, respectively. They should not be used in patients on a salt-restricted diet, e.g. those with fluid retention, heart failure or renal impairment.

Do not administer antacid products containing alginates at the same time of day as e/c tablets, or via enteral feeding tubes. Preferably avoid co-administration with other drugs (see Antacids, p.2).

Dose and use
Several products are available but none is recommended.

Supply
Gaviscon® products, Peptac® and Acidex® oral suspensions all contain sodium alginate 250mg, sodium bicarbonate 133.5mg and calcium carbonate 80mg/5mL and are prescribable on the NHS and available OTC (for full details see BNF and SPCs).

Other compound alginate products are also available (see BNF); some have high sugar content.

---

1 Pokorny C et al. (1985) Comparison of an antacid/dimethicone mixture and an alginate/antacid mixture in the treatment of oesophagitis. *Gut.* **26**: A574.

Updated October 2012

SIMETICONE   BNF 1.1.1

Class: Antifoaming agent (antiflatulent).

Indications: Acid dyspepsia (including acid reflux), gassy dyspepsia, †hiccup (if associated with gastric distension).

Pharmacology
Simeticone (silica-activated dimeticone or dimethylpolysiloxane) is a mixture of liquid dimeticones with silicon dioxide. It is an antifoaming agent present in several proprietary combination antacids, e.g. Altacite Plus®, Maalox Plus®. It alters the surface tension of bubbles, causing them to coalesce. This facilitates belching, easing flatulence, distension and postprandial gastric discomfort. Simeticone-containing antacids are as effective as alginate-containing products in the treatment of acid reflux.[1] Altacite Plus® or Maalox Plus® should be used in preference to Gaviscon® products or Acidex® and Peptac® oral suspensions because they contain much less sodium and are cheaper.

Onset of action <5min.
Duration of action 1–2h.

Cautions
Although Maalox Plus®contains both **aluminium** and **magnesium**, at higher doses (e.g. >100–200mL/day) the laxative effect of **magnesium** tends to override the constipating effect of **aluminium**.[2]

Do not administer antacid products containing simeticone at the same time of day as e/c tablets, or via enteral feeding tubes. Preferably avoid co-administration with other drugs (see Antacids p.2).

Dose and use
Altacite Plus® is preferred because it contains a higher dose of simeticone than Maalox Plus®.
• 10mL p.r.n. or 10mL q.d.s

Supply
Altacite plus® Peckforton
Oral suspension (sugar-free) simeticone 125mg, **hydrotalcite** 500mg/5mL, 28 days @ 10mL q.d.s. = £7; *low Na⁺*.

Maalox Plus® (Sanofi Aventis)
Oral suspension (sugar-free) simeticone 25mg, dried **aluminium hydroxide** 220mg, **magnesium hydroxide** 195mg/5mL, 28days @ 10mL q.d.s. = £9; *low Na⁺*.

---

1 Pokorny C et al. (1985) Comparison of an antacid/dimethicone mixture and an alginate/antacid mixture in the treatment of oesophagitis. *Gut.* **26**: A574.
2 Morrissey J and Barreras R (1974) Antacid therapy. *New England Journal of Medicine.* **290**: 550–554.

Updated April 2013

ANTIMUSCARINICS   BNF 1.2, 4.6 & 15.1.3

Indications: Smooth muscle spasm (e.g. bladder, intestine), motion sickness (**hyoscine hydrobromide**), drying secretions (including surgical premedication, †sialorrhoea, †drooling, †death rattle/noisy respiratory secretions, and †inoperable intestinal obstruction), †paraneoplastic pyrexia and sweating.

Pharmacology
Chemically, antimuscarinics are classified as tertiary amines or quaternary ammonium compounds. The naturally-occurring belladonna alkaloids, **atropine**, **hyoscyamine (l-atropine)** and **hyoscine hydrobromide**, are tertiary amines, whereas the numerous semisynthetic and synthetic derivatives fall into both categories. Thus, **dicycloverine**, **oxybutynin** and **tolterodine** are tertiary amines, and **glycopyrronium**, **propantheline** and **hyoscine butylbromide** are quaternary ammonium compounds. **Hyoscyamine (l-atropine**, not UK) is twice as potent as racemic **atropine**.

Numerous other drugs have antimuscarinic effects (Box A). In addition, some drugs generally not considered antimuscarinic have been shown to have detectable antimuscarinic activity by means of a radioreceptor assay, including **codeine**, **digoxin**, **dipyridamole**, **isosorbide**, **nifedipine**, **prednisolone**, **ranitidine**, **theophylline**, **warfarin**.[1] Theoretically, these drugs could exacerbate toxicity, particularly in debilitated elderly patients.

At least five different types of muscarinic receptors have been identified,[2] and newer drugs tend to be more selective in their actions. Thus, **oxybutynin** and **tolterodine** are relatively selective for muscarinic receptors in the urinary tract (see p.551).

At toxic doses, all the tertiary amines, including **hyoscine hydrobromide**, cause CNS stimulation resulting in mild central vagal excitation, respiratory stimulation, agitation and delirium. However, in contrast to **atropine**, **hyoscine hydrobromide** causes CNS depression at typical therapeutic doses.

Synthetic tertiary amines generally cause less central stimulation than the naturally-occurring alkaloids. Quaternary ammonium compounds do not cross the blood-brain barrier in any significant amount, and accordingly do not have any central effects.[3] They are also less well absorbed from the GI tract.

Box A   Drugs with antimuscarinic effects used in palliative care

Analgesics
  pethidine (*not* recommended)
  nefopam (mostly postoperative)
Antidepressants
  TCAs, e.g. amitriptyline, imipramine
  paroxetine (SSRI)
Antihistamines, e.g.
  chlorphenamine
  cyclizine
  dimenhydrinate (not UK)
  promethazine
Antiparkinsonians, e.g.
  orphenadrine
  procyclidine
Antipsychotics (atypical)
  clozapine
  olanzapine

Antipsychotics (typical)
  phenothiazines, e.g.
   chlorpromazine
   levomepromazine
   prochlorperazine
Antisecretory drugs
  belladonna alkaloids
   atropine
   hyoscine
   hyoscyamine (l-atropine, not UK)[a]
  glycopyrronium
Antispasmodics, e.g.
  dicycloverine
  mebeverine
  oxybutynin
  propantheline
  tolterodine

a. because the d-isomer is virtually inactive, hyoscyamine is twice as potent as racemic atropine.

Box B   Peripheral antimuscarinic effects

Visual
Mydriasis
Loss of accommodation   }   blurred vision (and thus may impair driving ability)

Cardiovascular
Tachycardia, palpitations
Extrasystoles   }   also related to noradrenaline (norepinephrine)
Arrhythmias   potentiation and a quinidine-like action

Gastro-intestinal
Dry mouth (inhibition of salivation)
Heartburn (relaxation of lower oesophageal sphincter)
Constipation (decreased intestinal motility)

Urinary tract
Hesitancy of micturition
Retention of urine

Skin
Reduced sweating
Flushing

Peripheral antimuscarinic effects are a class characteristic (Box B), and have been summarized as:

     'Dry as a bone, blind as a bat, red as a beet, hot as a hare, mad as a hatter.'

The muscarinic receptors in salivary glands are very responsive to antimuscarinics and inhibition of salivation occurs at lower doses than required for other antimuscarinic effects.[4] In some patients, a reduction in excess saliva results in improved speech.[5]

In the UK, parenteral antimuscarinics are widely used to reduce death rattle (noisy respiratory secretions) in those close to death (see Quick Prescribing Guide p.11). Although the use of antimuscarinics for this purpose has been questioned,[6,7] such use is often, although not always, beneficial.[8–10] For example, a prospective clinical survey concluded that antimuscarinics reduce death rattle in 1/2–2/3 of patients.[11]

In relation to death rattle, belladonna alkaloids are generally equally effective,[8,9] although **glycopyrronium** may sometimes be effective when belladonna alkaloids have not been.[12] Although one study reported that **hyoscine hydrobromide** acts faster than **glycopyrronium**, there is no detectable difference between the two drugs after 1h.[13]

Antimuscarinics used as antispasmodics and/or antisecretory drugs differ in their pharmacokinetic characteristics (Table 1). In relation to death rattle, availability, fashion, familiarity and cost are probably the main influences in choice of drug.

Table 1 Pharmacokinetic details of antimuscarinic drugs used for death rattle (noisy respiratory secretions)[4]

	Bio-availability	Plasma halflife	Duration of action (antisecretory)
Atropine	50% PO	2–2.5h[a]	no data
Glycopyrronium	<5% PO	1–1.5h[a]	7h
Hyoscine butylbromide	<1% PO[14]	1–5h[14]	<2h[b15]
Hyoscine hydrobromide	60–80% SL	1–4h[a]	1–9h

a. after IM injection into deltoid muscle
b. in volunteers; possibly longer in moribund patients.

Cautions

Myasthenia gravis, conditions predisposing to tachycardia (e.g. thyrotoxicosis, heart failure, β agonists), and bladder outflow obstruction (prostatism). Use in hot weather or pyrexia may lead to heatstroke. Likely to exacerbate acid reflux. Narrow-angle glaucoma may be precipitated in those at risk, particularly the elderly.

The increased GI transit time produced by antimuscarinics may allow increased drug absorption from some formulations, e.g. **digoxin** and **nitrofurantoin** from tablets and **potassium** from m/r tablets, but reduced absorption from others, e.g. **paracetamol** tablets. Dissolution and absorption of SL tablets (e.g. **glyceryl trinitrate**) may be reduced because of decreased saliva production.

Concurrent treatment with two antimuscarinic drugs will increase the likelihood of undesirable effects, and of central toxicity, i.e. restlessness, agitation, delirium. Children, the elderly, and patients with renal or hepatic impairment are more susceptible to the central effects of antimuscarinics.

Both antimuscarinics and opioids cause constipation (by different mechanisms) and, if used together, will result in an increased need for laxatives, and may even result in paralytic ileus. On the other hand, **morphine** and **hyoscine butylbromide** or **glycopyrronium** are sometimes purposely combined in terminally ill patients with inoperable intestinal obstruction in order to prevent colic and to reduce vomiting.

Drug interactions

Because antimuscarinics competitively block the final common (cholinergic) pathway through which prokinetics act,[16] concurrent prescription with **metoclopramide** and **domperidone** should be avoided as far as possible.

Undesirable effects

What is a desired effect becomes an undesirable effect in different circumstances (see Box B). Thus, dry mouth is an almost universal *undesirable* effect of antimuscarinics except when a reduction of oropharyngeal secretions is intended, as in death rattle.

Dose and use

By injection, there is no good evidence to recommend one antimuscarinic in preference to another.[9] However, because **atropine** and **hyoscyamine** (not UK) tend to stimulate the CNS rather than sedate, concurrent prescription of **midazolam** or **haloperidol** is more likely to be necessary. In the UK where alternatives are available, these two antimuscarinics are *not* recommended.

When given IM, **atropine**, **hyoscine** *hydrobromide* and **glycopyrronium** are all absorbed faster from the deltoid muscle than from the gluteal muscles.[4]

Antispasmodic

Antimuscarinics are used to relieve smooth muscle spasm in the bladder (see **oxybutynin**, p.551) and rectum.

Antispasmodic and antisecretory

Antimuscarinics are used to reduce intestinal colic and intestinal secretions, particularly gastric, associated with inoperable organic intestinal obstruction in terminally ill patients (Table 2).

Table 2 Antisecretory and antispasmodic drugs: typical SC doses

Drug	Stat and p.r.n. doses	CSCI dose/24h
Glycopyrronium	200microgram	600–1,200microgram
Hyoscine *butylbromide*	20mg	20–300mg[a]
Hyoscine *hydrobromide*[b]	400microgram	1,200–2,000microgram

a. death rattle 20–60mg, some centres use up to 120mg; intestinal obstruction 60–300mg.
b. atropine doses are generally the same as hyoscine hydrobromide.

Antisecretory

Drooling (and sialorrhoea)
Seen particularly in patients with ALS/MND, advanced Parkinson's disease and with various disorders of the head and neck. A recent survey of UK neurologists[17] with a special interest in MND/ALS showed that their preferred first-line drugs for sialorrhoea are:
* **hyoscine** *hydrobromide*, e.g. 1mg/3 days TD[18]
* **amitriptyline**, e.g. 10–25mg at bedtime
* **atropine**, e.g. 1% ophthalmic solution, 4 drops on the tongue or SL q4h p.r.n.

In relation to the latter, drop size varies with applicator and technique. Thus, the dose varies from 200–500microgram per drop (800microgram–2mg/dose). It is important to titrate the dose upwards until there is an adequate effect; in an RCT, 500microgram q.d.s. was no better than placebo.[19]

Glycopyrronium is the most popular second-line drug, typically PO or SL.[17] It has also been used for drooling in other conditions (see Glycopyrronium, p.12).

In patients in whom antimuscarinics are contra-indicated, ineffective or not tolerated, the parotid ± submandibular glands can be injected with **botulinum toxin**.[17] Injections are generally effective within 2 weeks, and benefit lasts 3–4 months.[20–24] In patients with a relatively long prognosis (years rather than months), radiotherapy and surgery are further options.[17]

Death rattle (noisy respiratory secretions)

In end-stage renal failure, do *not* use **hyoscine** *hydrobromide* for death rattle because of an increased risk of delirium. Instead, use **hyoscine** **butylbromide** (dose unchanged) or **glycopyrronium** (dose halved).

Treatment regimens are all unauthorized and based mainly on local clinical experience. In the UK antimuscarinic drugs for death rattle are generally given SC.[25] See Table 2 and Quick Prescribing Guide, p.11.

In some countries the SL route is preferred, particularly in home care because it circumvents the need for injections, e.g. **glycopyrronium** 100microgram/mL oral solution, 1mL (100microgram) SL q6h p.r.n. (prepared locally from **glycopyrronium** powder, see p.13).

Paraneoplastic pyrexia and sweating

Antimuscarinic drugs are used in the treatment of paraneoplastic pyrexia (Box C).

Box C   Symptomatic drug treatment of paraneoplastic pyrexia and sweating

Prescribe an antipyretic:
- paracetamol 500–1,000mg q.d.s. or p.r.n. (generally less toxic than an NSAID)
- NSAID, e.g. ibuprofen 200–400mg t.d.s. or p.r.n. (or the locally preferred alternative).

If the sweating does not respond to an NSAID, prescribe an antimuscarinic drug:
- amitriptyline 25–50mg at bedtime. (may cause sedation, dry mouth, and other antimuscarinic effects)
- hyoscine *hydrobromide* 1mg/3 days TD[26]
- glycopyrronium up to 2mg PO t.d.s.[27]

If an antimuscarinic fails, other options include:
- propranolol 10–20mg b.d.–t.d.s.
- cimetidine 400–800mg b.d.[28]
- olanzapine 5mg b.d.[29]
- thalidomide 100mg at bedtime.[30,31]

Thalidomide is generally seen as the last resort even though the response rate appears to be high.[31] This is because it can cause an irreversible painful peripheral neuropathy; it may also cause drowsiness (see p.543).

Overdose

In the past, **physostigmine** (not UK), a cholinesterase inhibitor, was sometimes administered to correct antimuscarinic toxicity/poisoning. This is no longer recommended because **physostigmine** itself can cause serious toxic effects, including cardiac arrhythmias and seizures.[32–34] A benzodiazepine can be given to control marked agitation and seizures. Phenothiazines should not be given because they will exacerbate the antimuscarinic effects, and could precipitate an acute dystonia (see Drug-induced movement disorders, p.781). Anti-arrhythmics are not advisable if arrhythmias develop; but hypoxia and acidosis should be corrected.

Supply

See individual monographs: **hyoscine** *butylbromide* (p.15), **hyoscine** *hydrobromide* (p.17), **glycopyrronium** (p.12), **propantheline** (p.19), **oxybutynin** (p.551).

---

1   Tune I et al. (1992) Anticholinergic effects of drugs commonly prescribed for the elderly; potential means of assessing risk of delirium. *American Journal of Psychiatry.* **149**: 1393–1394.
2   Caulfield M and Birdsall N (1998) International Union of Pharmacology. XVII. Classification of muscarinic acetylcholine receptors. *Pharmacological Review* **50**: 279–290.
3   Sweetman SC (ed) (2005) Martindale: The Complete Drug Reference. (34e). Pharmaceutical Press, London, p. 475.
4   Ali-Melkkila T et al. (1993) Pharmacokinetics and related pharmacodynamics of anticholinergic drugs. *Acta Anaesthesiologica Scandinavica.* **37**: 633–642.
5   Rashid H et al. (1997) Management of secretions in esophageal cancer patients with glycopyrrolate. *Annals of Oncology.* **8**: 198–199.
6   Wee B and Hillier R (2012) Interventions for noisy breathing in patients near to death. *Cochrane Database of Systematic Reviews.* **1**: CD005177.
7   Lokker ME et al. (2014) Prevalence, impact, and treatment of death rattle: a systematic review. *Journal of Pain and Symptom Management.* **47**: 105–122.
8   Likar R et al. (2008) Efficacy of glycopyrronium bromide and scopolamine hydrobromide in patients with death rattle: a randomized controlled study. *Wiener Klinische Wochenschrift.* **120**: 679–683.
9   Wildiers H et al. (2009) Atropine, hyoscine butylbromide, or scopolamine are equally effective for the treatment of death rattle in terminal care. *Journal of Pain and Symptom Management.* **38**: 124–133.
10 Hugel H et al. (2006) Respiratory tract secretions in the dying patient: a comparison between glycopyrronium and hyoscine hydrobromide. *Journal of Palliative Medicine.* **9**: 279–284.
11 Hughes A et al. (2000) Audit of three antimuscarinic drugs for managing retained secretions. *Palliative Medicine.* **14**: 221–222.
12 Mirakhur R and Dundee J (1980) A comparison of the effects of atropine and glycopyrollate on various end organs. *Journal of the Royal Society of Medicine.* **73**: 727–730.
13 Back I et al. (2001) A study comparing hyoscine hydrobromide and glycopyrrolate in the treatment of death rattle. *Palliative Medicine.* **15**: 329–336.
14 Boehringer Ingelheim GmbH Data on file.
15 Herxheimer A and Haefeli L (1966) Human pharmacology of hyoscine butylbromide. *Lancet.* **ii**: 418–421.

16 Schuurkes JAJ et al. (1986) Stimulation of gastroduodenal motor activity: dopaminergic and cholinergic modulation. *Drug Development Research.* **8**: 233–241.

17 Hobson EV et al. (2013) Management of sialorrhoea in motor neuron disease: A survey of current UK practice. *Amyotrophic Lateral Sclerosis Frontotemporal Degeneration.* **14**: 521–527.

18 Talmi YP et al. (1990) Reduction of salivary flow with transdermal scopolamine: a four-year experience. *Otolaryngology Head and Neck Surgery.* **103**: 615–618.

19 De Simone GG et al. (2006) Atropine drops for drooling: a randomized controlled trial. *Palliative Medicine.* **20**: 665–671.

20 Ondo WG et al. (2004) A double-blind placebo-controlled trial of botulinum toxin B for sialorrhea in Parkinson's disease. *Neurology.* **62**: 37–40.

21 Jongerius P et al. (2004) Effect of botulinum toxin in the treatment of drooling: a controlled clinical trial. *Pediatrics.* **114**: 620–627.

22 Mancini F et al. (2003) Double-blind, placebo-controlled study to evaluate the efficacy and safety of botulinum toxin type A in the treatment of drooling in parkinsonism. *Movement Disorders.* **18**: 685–688.

23 Lipp A et al. (2003) A randomized trial of botulinum toxin A for treatment of drooling. *Neurology.* **61**: 1279–1281.

24 Ellies M et al. (2004) Reduction of salivary flow with botulinum toxin: extended report on 33 patients with drooling, salivary fistulas, and sialadenitis. *Laryngoscope.* **114**: 1856–1860.

25 Bennett M et al. (2002) Using anti-muscarinic drugs in the management of death rattle: evidence based guidelines for palliative care. *Palliative Medicine.* **16**: 369–374.

26 Mercadante S (1998) Hyoscine in opioid-induced sweating. *Journal of Pain and Symptom Management.* **15**: 214–215.

27 Klaber M and Catterall M (2000) Treating hyperhidrosis. Anticholinergic drugs were not mentioned. *British Medical Journal.* **321**: 703.

28 Pittelkow M and Loprinzi C (2003) Pruritus and sweating in palliative medicine. In: D Doyle et al. (eds) *Oxford Textbook of Palliative Medicine* (3e). Oxford University Press, Oxford, pp. 573–587.

29 Zylicz Z and Krajnik M (2003) Flushing and sweating in an advanced breast cancer patient relieved by olanzapine. *Journal of Pain and Symptom Management.* **25**: 494–495.

30 Deaner P (2000) The use of thalidomide in the management of severe sweating in patients with advanced malignancy: trial report. *Palliative Medicine.* **14**: 429–431.

31 Calder K and Bruera E (2000) Thalidomide for night sweats in patients with advanced cancer. *Palliative Medicine.* **14**: 77–78.

32 Aquilonius SM and Hedstrand U (1978) The use of physostigmine as an antidote in tricyclic anti-depressant intoxication. *Acta Anaesthesiologica Scandinavica.* **22**: 40–45.

33 Caine ED (1979) Anticholinergic toxicity. *New England Journal of Medicine.* **300**: 1278.

34 Newton RW (1975) Physostigmine salicylate in the treatment of tricyclic antidepressant overdosage. *Journal of the American Medical Association.* **231**: 941–943.

Updated April 2014

Quick Prescribing Guide: Management of death rattle (noisy respiratory secretions)

Death rattle is a term used to describe noisy rattling breathing which occurs in about 50% of patients near the end of life. It is caused by fluid pooling in the hypopharynx which arises from one or more sources:

- saliva (most common)
- bronchial mucosa
- respiratory tract infection
- pulmonary oedema
- gastric reflux.

Rattling breathing can also occur in patients with a tracheostomy and infection. Because the patient is generally semiconscious or unconscious, drug treatment for death rattle is mainly for the benefit of relatives, other patients and staff.

Non-drug treatment

- ease the family's distress by explaining that the semiconscious/unconscious patient is not distressed by the rattle
- position the patient semiprone to encourage postural drainage; but upright or semirecumbent if the cause is pulmonary oedema or gastric reflux
- oropharyngeal suction but, because it can be distressing, generally restrict use to unconscious patients.

Drug treatment

Note: because atropine tends to stimulate rather than sedate, concurrent prescription of midazolam or haloperidol is more likely to be necessary. In the UK, atropine is *not* recommended for death rattle.

Saliva

Because they do not affect existing secretions, an antisecretory drug should be given SC as soon as the rattle begins (see Table).

Antimuscarinic antisecretory drugs for death rattle: typical SC doses

Drug	Stat and p.r.n. SC dose	CSCI dose/24h
Glycopyrronium	200microgram	600–1,200microgram
Hyoscine *butylbromide*	20mg	20–120mg
Hyoscine *hydrobromide*	400microgram	1,200–2,000microgram

In end-stage renal failure, do *not* use **hyoscine *hydrobromide*** because of an increased risk of delirium. Use **hyoscine *butylbromide*** (dose unchanged) or **glycopyrronium** (dose halved) instead.

Respiratory tract infection

Occasionally it is appropriate to prescribe an antibiotic in an imminently dying patient if death rattle is caused by profuse purulent sputum associated with an underlying chest infection:

- e.g. ceftriaxone, mix 1g ampoule with 2.1mL lidocaine 1% (total volume 2.6–2.8mL), and give 250–1000mg SC/IM once daily
- some centres use larger volumes of lidocaine 1% (up to 4mL) and administer a divided dose at separate SC/IM sites once daily, or give b.d.

Pulmonary oedema

Consider furosemide 20–40mg SC/IM/IV q2h p.r.n.
Note: beware precipitating urinary retention.

Gastric reflux
Consider metoclopramide 20mg SC/IV q3h p.r.n., but do not use concurrently with an antimuscarinic because the latter blocks the prokinetic effect of the former.

Rattling breathing causing distress to a patient
In a semiconscious patient, if rattling breathing is associated with breathlessness, supplement the above with an opioid (e.g. morphine) ± an anxiolytic sedative (e.g. midazolam).

Updated April 2014

GLYCOPYRRONIUM   BNF 15.1.3

Class: Antimuscarinic (anticholinergic).

Indications: Drying secretions (including surgical premedication, control of upper airway secretions, COPD (Seebri Breezhaler®), †sialorrhoea, †drooling, †death rattle (noisy respiratory secretions), †smooth muscle spasm (e.g. intestine, bladder), †inoperable intestinal obstruction), †paraneoplastic pyrexia and sweating, †hyperhidrosis.[1,2]

Pharmacology
Glycopyrronium is a synthetic ionized quaternary ammonium antimuscarinic which penetrates biological membranes slowly and erratically.[3] In consequence it rarely causes sedation or delirium.[4,5] Absorption PO is poor and the IV to PO potency ratio is about 35:1.[6] Even so, glycopyrronium 200–400microgram PO t.d.s. produces plasma concentrations associated with an antisialogogic effect lasting up to 8h.[7–9] By injection, glycopyrronium is 2–5 times more potent than **hyoscine hydrobromide** as an antisecretory drug,[6] and may be effective in some patients who fail to respond to **hyoscine**. However, the efficacy of **hyoscine hydrobromide**, **hyoscine butylbromide** and glycopyrronium as antisialogogues is generally similar, with death rattle reduced in 1/2–2/3 of patients.[10] Further, provided that time is taken to explain the cause of the rattle to the relatives and there is ongoing support, relatives' distress is relieved in >90% of cases.[11]

The optimal parenteral single dose is 200microgram.[12,13] It has fewer cardiac effects because of a reduced affinity for muscarinic-type 2 receptors.[14–16] Although at standard doses glycopyrronium does not change ocular pressures or pupil size, it can precipitate narrow-angle glaucoma. It is excreted by the kidneys and lower doses are effective in patients with renal impairment.[3,17]

Glycopyrronium PO or SL has been used to reduce drooling in MND/ALS,[18] head and neck cancer,[9,19] and oesophageal cancer.[20] It has also been given by nebulizer.[21] It is also used as a bronchodilator (inhaled or nebulized) in asthma and COPD.[22]
Bio-availability <5% PO.
Onset of action 1min IV; 30–40min SC, PO.
Time to peak plasma concentration immediate IV; no data SC, PO.
Plasma halflife 1–1.5h.
Duration of action 7h.

Cautions
Increases the peripheral antimuscarinic toxicity of antihistamines, phenothiazines and TCAs (see Antimuscarinics, Box B, p.6). Use with caution in conditions predisposing to tachycardia (e.g. thyrotoxicosis, heart failure, concurrent β_2 agonists), and bladder outflow obstruction (prostatism). Likely to exacerbate acid reflux. Narrow-angle glaucoma may be precipitated in those at risk, particularly the elderly. Use in hot weather or pyrexia may lead to heatstroke.

Drug interactions
Competitively blocks the prokinetic effect of **metoclopramide** and **domperidone**.[23]

Undesirable effects
Peripheral antimuscarinic effects (see Antimuscarinics, Box B, p.6). The US Product Information lists the following effects, which are not included in the UK SPC:

Very common (>10%): inflammation at the injection site.
Common (<10%, >1%): dysphagia, photosensitivity.

Dose and use

Glycopyrronium is an alternative to **hyoscine hydrobromide, hyoscine butylbromide** and **atropine.**[19,20,24] For CSCI, dilute with WFI, 0.9% saline or 5% glucose.

CSCI compatibility with other drugs: There are 2-drug compatibility data for glycopyrronium in WFI with **alfentanil, clonazepam, diamorphine, haloperidol, hydromorphone, levomepromazine, metoclopramide, midazolam, morphine sulfate** and **oxycodone.**

Glycopyrronium is *incompatible* with **dexamethasone** and **ketorolac.** For more details and 3-drug compatibility data, see Appendix 3 (p.821).

Compatibility charts for mixing drugs in 0.9% saline can be found in the extended appendix section of the on-line PCF on www.palliativedrugs.com

Drooling

Administer as a locally prepared solution PO:
- start with 200microgram PO stat and q8h
- if necessary, increase dose progressively every 2–3 days to 1mg q8h[25]
- occasionally doses of ≤2mg q8h are needed.

A subsequent reduction in dose may be possible, particularly when initial dose escalation has been rapid. Can be given by enteral feeding tube (also see p.733).[9,20]

Examples of locally prepared formulations for PO use are shown in Box A.[26,27] Unauthorized products (tablets, solutions, suspensions) are available as Specials (see Supply). The tablets will disperse in water, but they are not suitable for administration via an enteral feeding tube.

Box A   Examples of locally prepared glycopyrronium formulations for PO use

From glycopyrronium powder

Glycopyrronium concentrated solution 1mg/mL[28]
Dissolve 100mg of glycopyrronium powder (obtainable from AMCo) in 100mL of sterile or distilled water.

This concentrate is stable for approximately 28 days if stored in a refrigerator.

Dilute the required volume of the concentrate 1 part with 9 parts sterile or distilled water (i.e. for every 1mL of concentrate, add 9mL of water) to give a *glycopyrronium oral solution 100microgram/mL.*

To avoid microbial contamination, store in a refrigerator and discard any unused diluted solution after 1 week.

Glycopyrronium oral suspension 500microgram/mL[26]
Add 5mL of glycerol to 50mg of glycopyrronium powder and mix to form a smooth paste. Add 50mL of Ora-Plus® in portions and mix well. Add sufficient Ora-Sweet® or Ora-Sweet SF® to make a total volume of 100mL.

This suspension is stable for 90 days at room temperature or in a refrigerator.

From glycopyrronium injection[a]

Glycopyrronium oral suspension 100microgram/mL[27]
Combine 25mL of Ora-Plus® and 25mL of Ora-Sweet®; add to 50mL of preservative-free glycopyrronium injection 200microgram/mL to make up to 100mL, and mix well.

Stable for 35 days at room temperature or in a refrigerator (refrigeration minimizes risk of microbial contamination).

In a taste test, this formulation masked the bitter taste of glycopyrronium better than water or syrup-based vehicles, and was preferred by most patients.

---

a. this is an expensive option, particularly for long-term use (see Supply).

Death rattle (noisy respiratory secretions)
- 200microgram SC stat and p.r.n.[29] and/or
- 600–1,200microgram/24h CSCI or
- 100microgram SL q6h p.r.n.

Antispasmodic and inoperable intestinal obstruction
- 200microgram SC stat and p.r.n. and/or
- 600–1,200microgram/24h CSCI.

Paraneoplastic pyrexia and sweating
- start with 200microgram PO t.d.s.
- if necessary, increase progressively to 2mg PO t.d.s.

Localized hyperhidrosis
- apply topically as a 0.5–4% cream (Box B) or aqueous solution once daily–b.d. avoiding the nose, mouth and particularly the eyes; do not wash treated skin for 3–4h[2,30]
- if severe, or if alternative treatments fail, 1–2mg PO b.d.–t.d.s., titrated to response.[1]

Box B   Locally prepared glycopyrronium cream 10mg/mL (1%)

Mix 1g of glycopyrronium powder with propylene glycol to make a paste. Incorporate into a water-washable cream base until smooth, making a total of 100g. Refrigerate after preparation. Stable for 60 days.

Supply
Glycopyrronium bromide (generic)
Oral solution or oral suspension 200microgram/5mL, 1mg/5mL, 2mg/5mL, 2.5mg/5mL and 5mg/5mL, 7 days or 28 days @ 1mg t.d.s. = £146 and £150 respectively (unauthorized, available as a special order, see Appendix 1, p.817). *Note price based on 1mg/5mL oral solution specials tariff in community; prices vary significantly between formulations and quantities ordered.*
Tablets 1mg, 2mg, 28 days @ 1mg t.d.s. = £27 (unauthorized, available to import as a special order via IDIS, see Appendix 1, p.817).
Injection 200microgram/mL, 1mL amp = £0.50, 3mL amp = £1.50. *Note: using the injection to make an oral solution 7 days @ 1mg t.d.s. = £53 worth of glycopyrronium injection.*

Robinul® (AMCo)
Glycopyrronium bromide
Powder for local preparation of oral solutions and topical formulations (see Box A and Box B), 3g = £266.
Note: *using the powder to make the concentrated oral solution = £9 (but need to buy 3g).*

Seebri Breezhaler® (Novartis)
Dry powder inhalation each 50microgram capsule delivers 44microgram glycopyrronium; for use with Seebri Breezhaler device, 28 days @ 1 puff once daily = £28.

---

1 Solish N et al. (2007) A comprehensive approach to the recognition, diagnosis, and severity-based treatment of focal hyperhidrosis: recommendations of the Canadian Hyperhidrosis Advisory Committee. Dermatologic Surgery. 33: 908–923.
2 Kim WO et al. (2008) Topical glycopyrrolate for patients with facial hyperhidrosis. British Journal of Dermatology. 158: 1094–1097.
3 Mirakhur R and Dundee J (1983) Glycopyrrolate pharmacology and clinical use. Anaesthesia. 38: 1195–1204.
4 Gram D et al. (1991) Central anticholinergic syndrome following glycopyrrolate. Anesthesiology. 74: 191–193.
5 Wigard D (1991) Glycopyrrolate and the central anticholinergic syndrome (letter). Anesthesiology. 75: 1125.
6 Mirakhur R and Dundee J (1980) A comparison of the effects of atropine and glycopyrrollate on various end organs. Journal of the Royal Society of Medicine. 73: 727–730.
7 Ali-Melkkila T et al. (1989) Glycopyrrolate; pharmacokinetics and some pharmacodynamics findings. Acta Anaesthesiologica Scandinavica. 33: 513–517.
8 Blasco P (1996) Glycopyrrolate treatment of chronic drooling. Archives of Paediatric and Adolescent Medicine. 150: 932–935.
9 Olsen A and Sjogren P (1999) Oral glycopyrrolate alleviates drooling in a patient with tongue cancer. Journal of Pain and Symptom Management. 18: 300–302.
10 Hughes A et al. (2000) Audit of three antimuscarinic drugs for managing retained secretions. Palliative Medicine. 14: 221–222.
11 Hughes A et al. (1997) Management of 'death rattle'. Palliative Medicine. 11: 80–81.

---

12 Mirakhur R et al. (1978) Evaluation of the anticholinergic actions of glycopyrronium bromide. British Journal of Clinical Pharmacology. 5: 77–84.

13 Back I et al. (2001) A study comparing hyoscine hydrobromide and glycopyrrolate in the treatment of death rattle. Palliative Medicine. 15: 329–336.

14 Scheinin H et al. (1999) Spectral analysis of heart rate variability as a quantitative measure of parasympatholytic effect-integrated pharmacokinetics and pharmacodynamics of three anticholinergic drugs. Therapeutic Drug Monitoring. 21: 141–151.

15 Warren J et al. (1997) Effect of autonomic blockade on power spectrum of heart rate variability during exercise. American Journal of Physiology. 273: 495–502.

16 Mirakhur R et al. (1978) Atropine and glycopyrronium premedication. A comparison of the effects on cardiac rate and rhythm during induction of anaesthesia. Anaesthesia. 33: 906–912.

17 Ali-Melkkila T et al. (1993) Pharmacokinetics and related pharmacodynamics of anticholinergic drugs. Acta Anaesthesiologica Scandinavica. 37: 633–642.

18 Hobson EV et al. (2013) Management of sialorrhoea in motor neuron disease: A survey of current UK practice. Amyotrophic Lateral Sclerosis Frontotemporal Degeneration. 14: 521–527.

19 Lucas V and Amass C (1998) Use of enteral glycopyrrolate in the management of drooling. Palliative Medicine. 12: 207.

20 Rashid H et al. (1997) Management of secretions in esophageal cancer patients with glycopyrrolate. Annals of Oncology. 8: 198–199.

21 Strutt R et al. (2002) Nebulized glycopyrrolate for drooling in a motor neuron patient. Journal of Pain and Symptom Management. 23: 2–3.

22 Hansel TT et al. (2005) Glycopyrrolate causes prolonged bronchoprotection and bronchodilatation in patients with asthma. Chest. 128: 1974–1979.

23 Schuurkes JAJ et al. (1986) Stimulation of gastroduodenal motor activity: dopaminergic and cholinergic modulation. Drug Development Research. 8: 233–241.

24 Davis M and Furste A (1999) Glycopyrrolate: a useful drug in the palliation of mechanical bowel obstruction. Journal of Pain and Symptom Management. 18: 153–154.

25 Arbouw ME et al. (2010) Glycopyrrolate for sialorrhea in Parkinson disease: a randomized, double-blind, crossover trial. Neurology. 74: 1203–1207.

26 Anonymous (2004) Glycopyrrolate 0.5mg/mL oral liquid. International Journal of Pharmaceutical Compounding. 8: 218.

27 Landry C et al. (2005) Stability and subjective taste acceptability of four glycopyrrolate solutions for oral administration. International Journal of Pharmaceutical Compounding. 9: 396–398.

28 Amass C (2007) Personal communication. Pharmacist, East and North Hertfordshire NHS Trust.

29 Bennett M et al. (2002) Using anti-muscarinic drugs in the management of death rattle: evidence based guidelines for palliative care. Palliative Medicine. 16: 369–374.

30 Kavanagh GM et al. (2006) Topical glycopyrrolate should not be overlooked in treatment of focal hyperhidrosis. British Journal of Dermatology. 155: 477–500.

31 Glasnapp A and BJ S (2001) Topical therapy for localized hyperhidrosis. International Journal of Pharmaceutical Compounding. 5: 28–29.

Updated April 2014

HYOSCINE BUTYLBROMIDE   BNF 1.2

Class: Antimuscarinic.

Indications: Smooth muscle spasm (e.g. bladder, GI tract), †drying secretions (including †sialorrhoea, †drooling, †death rattle (noisy respiratory secretions) and †inoperable bowel obstruction), †paraneoplastic pyrexia and sweating.

Contra-indications: Narrow-angle glaucoma (unless moribund), myasthenia gravis (unless moribund).

Pharmacology

Hyoscine *butylbromide* is an antimuscarinic (see p.5) and has both smooth muscle relaxant (antispasmodic) and antisecretory properties. It is a quaternary compound and, unlike **hyoscine hydrobromide**, it does not cross the blood-brain barrier. Consequently, it does not have a central anti-emetic effect or cause drowsiness.

Oral bio-availability, based on urinary excretion, is < 1%.[1] Thus, any antispasmodic effect reported after PO administration probably relates to a local contact effect on the GI mucosa.[2] In an RCT, hyoscine *butylbromide* 10mg t.d.s. PO and **paracetamol** 500mg t.d.s. both significantly reduced the severity of intestinal colic by > 50%.[3] However, the difference between the benefit from these two drugs (both given in suboptimal doses) and placebo was only 0.5cm on a 10cm scale of pain intensity. This is of dubious clinical importance.[4] Thus the therapeutic value of PO hyoscine *butylbromide* for intestinal colic remains debatable.[5]

The main uses for hyoscine *butylbromide* in palliative care are as an antispasmodic and antisecretory drug in inoperable GI obstruction, and as an antisecretory drug for death rattle (noisy respiratory secretions). In an open non-randomized trial of hyoscine *butylbromide* 60mg/24h CSCI vs. **octreotide** 300microgram/24h CSCI, **octreotide** resulted in a more rapid reduction in the volume of gastric aspirate (by 75% vs. 50%) and improvement in nausea, although it was possible to remove nasogastric tubes in both groups after about 5 days.[6,7] However, higher doses of hyoscine *butylbromide*, e.g. 120–200mg/24h, have not been compared with **octreotide**.

In healthy volunteers, a bolus injection of 20mg has a maximum antisecretory duration of action of 2h.[8] On the other hand, the same dose by CSCI is often effective for 1 day in death rattle. Hyoscine *butylbromide* and **hyoscine *hydrobromide*** act faster than **glycopyrronium** for this indication,[9,10] but the overall efficacy is generally the same[11] with death rattle reduced in 1/2–2/3 of patients. However, provided that time is taken to explain the cause of the rattle to the relatives and there is ongoing support, relatives' distress is relieved in >90% of cases.[12]

Bio-availability <1% PO.[1]
Onset of action <10min SC/IM/IV; 1–2h PO.[13]
Time to peak plasma concentration 15min–2h PO.[1]
Plasma halflife 1–5h.[1]
Duration of action <2h in volunteers[8] but possibly longer in moribund patients.

Cautions

Increases the peripheral antimuscarinic effects of antihistamines, phenothiazines and TCAs (see Antimuscarinics, Box B, p.6). Use with caution in conditions predisposing to tachycardia (e.g. thyrotoxicosis, heart failure, β agonists), and bladder outflow obstruction (prostatism). Likely to exacerbate acid reflux. Narrow-angle glaucoma may be precipitated in those at risk, particularly the elderly. Use in hot weather or pyrexia may lead to heatstroke.

Drug interactions

Competitively blocks the prokinetic effect of **metoclopramide** and **domperidone**.[1,14]

Undesirable effects

Peripheral antimuscarinic effects (see Antimuscarinics, Box B, p.6).

Dose and use

For CSCI dilute with WFI, 0.9% saline or 5% glucose.

> **CSCI compatibility with other drugs**: There are 2-drug compatibility data for hyoscine *butylbromide* in WFI with **alfentanil**, **clonazepam**, **dexamethasone**, **diamorphine**, **haloperidol**, **hydromorphone**, **levomepromazine**, **midazolam**, **morphine sulfate**, **octreotide** and **oxycodone**.
>
> *Incompatibility* may occur with **cyclizine**. For more details and 3-drug compatibility data, see Appendix 3 (p.821).
>
> Compatibility charts for mixing drugs in 0.9% saline can be found in the extended appendix of the on-line PCF on www.palliativedrugs.com

Inoperable intestinal obstruction with colic[15,16]
- start with 20mg SC stat and 60mg/24h CSCI
- if necessary, increase to 120mg/24h
- maximum reported dose 300mg/24h.

Note: the maximum benefit from hyoscine *butylbromide* may be seen only after some 3 days.[6] Some centres add **octreotide** 300–500microgram/24h if hyoscine *butylbromide* 120mg/24h fails to relieve symptoms adequately.[17,18]

> For patients with obstructive symptoms without colic, **metoclopramide** (p.242) should be tried before an antimuscarinic drug because the obstruction is often more functional than organic.

Death rattle (noisy respiratory secretions)
- start with 20mg SC stat, 20–60mg/24h CSCI, and/or 20mg SC q1h p.r.n.
- some centres use higher doses, namely 60–120mg/24h CSCI[10]

For use of alternative antimuscarinics, see Quick Prescribing Guide, p.11.

Supply

Buscopan® (Boehringer Ingelheim)
Tablets 10mg, 28 days @ 20mg q.d.s. = £12. *Also available OTC as Buscopan®* IBS Relief.
Injection 20mg/mL, 1mL amp = £0.50.

1 Boehringer Ingelheim GmbH *Data on file.*
2 Tytgat GN (2007) Hyoscine butylbromide: a review of its use in the treatment of abdominal cramping and pain. *Drugs.* **67**: 1343–1357.
3 Mueller-Lissner S et al. (2006) Placebo- and paracetamol-controlled study on the efficacy and tolerability of hyoscine butylbromide in the treatment of patients with recurrent crampy abdominal pain. *Alimentary Pharmacology & Therapeutics.* **23**: 1741–1748.
4 Farrar JT et al. (2000) Defining the clinically important difference in pain outcome measures. *Pain.* **88**: 287–294.
5 Thompson DG and Wingate DL (1981) Oral hyoscine butylbromide does not alter the pattern of small intestinal motor activity. *British Journal of Pharmacology.* **72**: 685–687.
6 Mercadante S et al. (2000) Comparison of octreotide and hyoscine butylbromide in controlling gastrointestinal symptoms due to malignant inoperable bowel obstruction. *Supportive Care in Cancer.* **8**: 188–191.
7 Ripamonti C et al. (2000) Role of octreotide, scopolamine butylbromide, and hydration in symptom control of patients with inoperable bowel obstruction and nasogastric tubes: a prospective randomized trial. *Journal of Pain and Symptom Management.* **19**: 23–34.
8 Herxheimer A and Haefeli L (1966) Human pharmacology of hyoscine butylbromide. *Lancet.* **ii**: 418–421.
9 Back I et al. (2001) A study comparing hyoscine hydrobromide and glycopyrrolate in the treatment of death rattle. *Palliative Medicine.* **15**: 329–336.
10 Bennett M et al. (2002) Using anti-muscarinic drugs in the management of death rattle: evidence based guidelines for palliative care. *Palliative Medicine.* **16**: 369–374.
11 Hughes A et al. (2000) Audit of three antimuscarinic drugs for managing retained secretions. *Palliative Medicine.* **14**: 221–222.
12 Hughes A et al. (1997) Management of 'death rattle'. *Palliative Medicine.* **11**: 80–81.
13 Sanches Martinez J (1988) Clinical assessment of the tolerability and the effect of IK-19 in tablet form on pain of spastic origin. *Investigacion Medica International.* **15**: 63–65.
14 Schuurkes JAJ et al. (1986) Stimulation of gastroduodenal motor activity: dopaminergic and cholinergic modulation. *Drug Development Research.* **8**: 233–241.
15 De-Conno F et al. (1991) Continuous subcutaneous infusion of hyoscine butylbromide reduces secretions in patients with gastrointestinal obstruction. *Journal of Pain and Symptom Management.* **6**: 484–486.
16 Ripamonti C et al. (2001) Clinical-practice recommendations for the management of bowel obstruction in patients with end-stage cancer. *Supportive Care in Cancer.* **9**: 223–233.
17 Ripamonti C and Mercadante S (2004) How to use octreotide for malignant bowel obstruction. *Journal of Supportive Oncology.* **2**: 357–364.
18 Ripamonti CI et al. (2008) Management of malignant bowel obstruction. *European Journal of Cancer.* **44**: 1105–1115.

Updated April 2014

HYOSCINE HYDROBROMIDE   BNF 4.6 & 15.1.3

Class: Antimuscarinic.

Indications: Prevention of motion sickness, drying secretions (including surgical premedication, †sialorrhoea, †drooling, †death rattle (noisy respiratory secretions) and †inoperable intestinal obstruction), †paraneoplastic pyrexia and sweating, †smooth muscle spasm (e.g. intestine, bladder).

Contra-indications: Narrow-angle glaucoma (unless moribund), prostatic hyperplasia, pyloric obstruction, paralytic ileus

Pharmacology

Hyoscine *hydrobromide* is a naturally occurring belladonna alkaloid with smooth muscle relaxant (antispasmodic) and antisecretory properties. In many countries it is available as both the *hydrobromide* and *butylbromide* salts. Unlike the latter, hyoscine *hydrobromide* crosses the blood-brain barrier, and repeated administration SC q4h will result in accumulation and may lead to sedation and delirium. On the other hand, a small number of patients are stimulated rather than sedated.

Despite hyoscine *hydrobromide* having a plasma halflife of several hours, the duration of the antisecretory effect in volunteers after a single dose is only about 2h.[1] On the other hand, particularly after repeated injections in moribund patients, a duration of effect of up to 9h has been observed.[2] Hyoscine *hydrobromide* relieves death rattle in 1/2–2/3 of patients.[3] However, provided that time is taken to explain the cause of the rattle to the relatives and there is ongoing support, relatives' distress is relieved in >90% of cases.[2] Hyoscine *hydrobromide* can also be used in other situations where an antimuscarinic effect is needed.

A TD patch is available as prophylactic treatment for motion sickness:[4]
- it comprises a reservoir containing hyoscine 1.5mg
- the average amount of hyoscine absorbed over 3 days is 1mg
- because of an initial priming dose released from the patch, steady-state is reached after about 6h, and maintained for 3 days[5]
- after a single application of two patches, the average elimination half-life is 9.5h[6]
- after patch removal, because hyoscine continues to be absorbed from the skin, the plasma concentration only decreases to about one third over the next 24h
- absorption is best when the patch is applied on hairless skin behind the ear.[4]

The patch has also been used to control opioid-induced nausea.[7,8] Other off-label uses include the management of drooling and sialorrhoea in patients with disorders of the head and neck.[9,10]

Bio-availability 60–80% SL.[11]
Onset of action 3–5min IM, 10–15min SL.
Time to peak effect 20–60min SL/SC; 24h TD.
Plasma halflife 1–4h IM.[11]
Duration of action IM 15min (spasmolytic), 1–9h (antisecretory).[11]

Cautions

Increases the antimuscarinic toxicity of antihistamines, phenothiazines and TCAs (see Antimuscarinics, Box B, p.6). Likely to exacerbate acid reflux. Use in hot weather or pyrexia may lead to heatstroke. Myasthenia gravis, bladder outflow obstruction, and in conditions predisposing to tachycardia (e.g. thyrotoxicosis, heart failure and concurrent use with β agonists).

Drug interactions

Interacts competitively to block prokinetic effect of **metoclopramide** and **domperidone**.[12]

Undesirable effects

Antimuscarinic effects (see p.6), including central antimuscarinic syndrome, i.e. agitated delirium, drowsiness, ataxia.

TD patch: despite the relatively small dose, delirium has been reported;[13] local irritation ± rash occasionally occurs.

Dose and use

TD patches contain metal in the backing, and must be removed before MRI to avoid burns.[14] Wash hands after handling the TD patch (and the application site after removing it) to avoid transferring hyoscine *hydrobromide* into the eyes (may cause mydriasis and exacerbate narrow-angle glaucoma).

Drooling and sialorrhoea
- hyoscine *hydrobromide* TD 1mg/3 days; if necessary, use 2 patches concurrently.

Note: an alternative drug PO with antimuscarinic effects may be preferable in some patients because of convenience or concurrent symptom management, e.g. **amitriptyline** (see p.208).

Death rattle (noisy respiratory secretions)
With death rattle caused by excess secretions pooling in the pharynx, an antisecretory drug is best administered as soon as the rattle becomes evident because the drug cannot dry up the existing secretions:
- 400microgram SC stat
- continue with 1,200microgram/24h CSCI
- if necessary, increase to 2,000microgram/24h CSCI
- repeat 400microgram p.r.n.

For CSCI dilute with WFI, 0.9% saline or 5% glucose.

CSCI compatibility with other drugs: There are 2-drug compatibility data for hyoscine *hydrobromide* in WFI with **clonazepam, cyclizine, dexamethasone, diamorphine, haloperidol, hydromorphone, levomepromazine, midazolam, morphine sulfate** and **oxycodone.**
For more details and 3-drug compatibility data, see Appendix 3 (p.821).
Compatibility charts for mixing drugs in 0.9% saline can be found in the extended appendix of the on-line PCF on www.palliativedrugs.com

Some centres use **hyoscine butylbromide** instead (see p.15).[15] Other options include **glycopyrronium** (see p.12) and **atropine** (see p.5).

Supply
Kwells® Bayer Consumer Care
Tablets chewable 150microgram, 300microgram, 12 tablets = £2; *also available OTC.*

Scopoderm TTS® (Novartis Consumer Health)
TD (post-auricular) patch 1.5mg (releasing 1mg over 3 days), 1 patch = £2.

Hyoscine *hydrobromide* (generic)
Injection 400microgram/mL, 1mL amp = £3; 600microgram/mL, 1mL amp = £3.

1 Herxheimer A and Haefeli L (1966) Human pharmacology of hyoscine butylbromide. *Lancet.* ii: 418–421.
2 Hughes A et al. (1997) Management of 'death rattle'. *Palliative Medicine.* 11. 80–81.
3 Hughes A et al. (2000) Audit of three antimuscarinic drugs for managing retained secretions. *Palliative Medicine.* 14: 221–222.
4 Clissold S and Heel R (1985) Transdermal hyoscine (scopolamine). A preliminary review of its pharmacodynamic properties and therapeutic efficacy. *Drugs.* 29: 189–207.
5 Novartis (2014). *Personal communication.* Medical affairs.
6 Novartis (2013) Scopoderm TTS. *SPC.* www.medicines.org.uk.
7 Ferris FD et al. (1991) Transdermal scopolamine use in the control of narcotic-induced nausea. *Journal of Pain and Symptom Management.* 6: 289–393.
8 Harris SN et al. (1991) Nausea prophylaxis using transdermal scopolamine in the setting of patient-controlled analgesia. *Obstetrics and Gynecology.* 78: 673–677.
9 Gordon C et al. (1985) Effect of transdermal scopolamine on salivation. *Journal of Clinical Pharmacology.* 25: 407–412.
10 Talmi YP et al. (1990) Reduction of salivary flow with transdermal scopolamine: a four-year experience. *Otolaryngology Head and Neck Surgery.* 103: 615–618.
11 Ali-Melkkila T et al. (1993) Pharmacokinetics and related pharmacodynamics of anticholinergic drugs. *Acta Anaesthesiologica Scandinavica.* 37: 633–642.
12 Schuurkes JAJ et al. (1986) Stimulation of gastroduodenal motor activity: dopaminergic and cholinergic modulation. *Drug Development Research.* 8: 233–241.
13 Wilkinson J (1987) Side-effects of transdermal scopolamine. *Journal of Emergency Medicine.* 5: 389–392.
14 Institute for Safe Medication Practices (2004) Medication Safety Alert. Burns in MRI patients wearing transdermal patches. Available from: www.ismp.org/Newsletters/acutecare/articles/20040408.asp?ptr = y
15 Bennett M et al. (2002) Using anti-muscarinic drugs in the management of death rattle: evidence based guidelines for palliative care. *Palliative Medicine.* 16: 369–374.

Updated April 2014

PROPANTHELINE   BNF 1.2 & 7.4.2

Class: Antimuscarinic.

Indications: Smooth muscle spasm (e.g. bladder, intestine), urinary frequency and incontinence, hyperhidrosis, †gustatory sweating in diabetic neuropathy, †paraneoplastic sweating, †drooling and sialorrhoea.

Contra-indications: Narrow-angle glaucoma (unless moribund), myasthenia gravis (unless moribund), obstructive disease of GI or urinary tract, pyloric stenosis, paralytic ileus, severe ulcerative colitis, toxic megacolon, hiatus hernia associated with reflux oesophagitis, prostatic enlargement.

Pharmacology

Propantheline is a quaternary antimuscarinic (see p.5); it does not cross the blood-brain barrier and thus does *not* cause central effects. It doubles gastric emptying half-time[1] and slows GI transit generally. It has variable effects on drug absorption (see Drug interactions). Propantheline is extensively metabolized in the small intestine before absorption. *If taken with food, the effect of propantheline by mouth is almost abolished.*[2]

Bio-availability <50% PO (much reduced if taken after food).
Onset of action 30–60min.
Time to peak plasma concentration 2h.
Plasma halflife 2–3h.
Duration of action 4–6h.

Cautions

Elderly. Use with caution in conditions predisposing to tachycardia (e.g. thyrotoxicosis, heart failure, β agonists), and bladder outflow obstruction (prostatism). Likely to exacerbate acid reflux. Narrow-angle glaucoma may be precipitated in those at risk, particularly the elderly. Use in hot weather or pyrexia may lead to heatstroke.

Drug interactions

Competitively blocks the prokinetic effect of **metoclopramide** and **domperidone**.[3] May reduce the rate, but not the extent, of absorption of **paracetamol**, thereby delaying the onset of analgesia. May increase the absorption of some formulations of **digoxin** and **nitrofurantoin**.[4]

Increases the peripheral antimuscarinic toxicity of antihistamines, phenothiazines and TCAs (see Antimuscarinics, p.6).

Undesirable effects

Peripheral antimuscarinic effects (See Antimuscarinics, Box B, p.6).

Dose and use

Intestinal colic

- start with 15mg t.d.s. *1h before meals* & 30mg at bedtime
- maximum dose 30mg q.d.s.

Urinary frequency

- same as for colic, but largely replaced by **oxybutynin** (p.551), **amitriptyline** (p.208) or **imipramine**.

Sweating

One of several alternatives to reduce paraneoplastic sweating (for other options, see Antimuscarinics, Box C, p.9):
- 15–30mg b.d.–t.d.s. *on an empty stomach*.
Has also been used for hyperhydrosis associated with spinal cord injury.[5]

Drooling and sialorrhoea

Has been used in MND/ALS.
15mg t.d.s.[6] *on an empty stomach*.

Supply

Pro-Banthine® (Archimedes)
Tablets 15mg, 28 days @ 15mg t.d.s. & 30mg at bedtime = £22.

1 Hurwitz A et al. (1977) Prolongation of gastric emptying by oral propantheline. *Clin Pharmacol Ther.* **22**: 206–210.
2 Ekenved G et al. (1977) Influence of food on the effect of propantheline and L-hyoscyamine on salivation. *Scand J Gastroenterol.* **12**: 963–966.
3 Schuurkes JAJ et al. (1986) Stimulation of gastroduodenal motor activity: dopaminergic and cholinergic modulation. *Drug Development Research.* **8**: 233–241.
4 Baxter K and Preston CL. *Stockley's Drug Interactions.* London: Pharmaceutical Press www.medicinescomplete.com (accessed March 2014).
5 Canaday BR and Stanford RH (1995) Propantheline bromide in the management of hyperhidrosis associated with spinal cord injury. *Ann Pharmacother.* **29**: 489–492.
6 Norris FH et al. (1985) Motor neurone disease: towards better care. *British Medical Journal.* **291**: 259–262.

Updated April 2014

ORPHENADRINE   BNF 4.9.2

Class: Antimuscarinic antiparkinsonian.

Indications: Parkinson's disease, drug-induced parkinsonism, †sialorrhoea (drooling), †extrapyramidal dystonic reactions.

Contra-indications: Glaucoma (unless moribund), GI obstruction, prostatic hypertrophy, urinary retention, tardive dyskinesia (see Chapter 26, p.781).

Pharmacology

Orphenadrine and other antimuscarinic antiparkinsonian drugs are used primarily in Parkinson's disease.[1] They are less effective than **levodopa** in established Parkinson's disease. However, patients with mild symptoms, particularly tremor, may be treated initially with an antimuscarinic drug (alone or with **selegiline**), and **levodopa** added or substituted if symptoms progress. Antimuscarinics exert their antiparkinsonian effect by correcting the relative central cholinergic excess which occurs in parkinsonism as a result of dopamine deficiency. In most patients their effects are only moderate, reducing tremor and rigidity to some extent but without significant action on bradykinesia. They exert a synergistic effect when used with **levodopa** and are also useful in reducing sialorrhoea.

Antimuscarinics reduce the symptoms of drug-induced parkinsonism (mainly antipsychotics) but there is no justification for giving them prophylactically. *Tardive dyskinesia is not improved by the antimuscarinic drugs, and they may make it worse.* No major differences exist between antimuscarinic antiparkinsonian drugs, but orphenadrine sometimes has a mood-elevating effect. Some people tolerate one antimuscarinic better than another. **Procyclidine** may be given parenterally, and is effective emergency treatment for severe acute drug-induced dystonic reactions (see Chapter 26, p.781).
Bio-availability readily absorbed PO.
Onset of action 30–60min.
Time to peak plasma concentration 2–4h PO.
Plasma halflife 15h single dose but ≤40h with multiple doses.
Duration of action 12–24h.

Cautions

Elderly, hepatic or renal impairment, cardiovascular disease, urinary hesitancy. Avoid abrupt discontinuation. In a psychotic patient receiving a phenothiazine, the addition of orphenadrine to reverse a drug-induced acute dystonia (see Chapter 26, p.781) may precipitate a toxic confusional psychosis because of a summation of antimuscarinic effects.

Undesirable effects

Antimuscarinic effects (see p.6). Nervousness, euphoria, insomnia, confusion, hallucinations occasionally.

Dose and use
Parkinsonism
For treatment of previously unrecognized or untreated symptoms in patients with a prognosis of <6 months:

- start with 50mg b.d.–t.d.s.
- if necessary, increase by 50mg every 2–3 days
- normal dose range 150–300mg daily in divided doses
- maximum recommended daily dose 400mg.

Note: **propranolol**, a non-selective β-adrenergic receptor antagonist (β-blocker), is the treatment of choice for akathisia. Antimuscarinic antiparkinsonian drugs are *contra-indicated* in tardive dyskinesia because they may exacerbate the condition (see Chapter 26, p.781).

Supply
Orphenadrine (generic)
Tablets 50mg, 28 days @ 50mg t.d.s. = £74.
(Note: at BNF prices, this is *more expensive* than branded Disipal® tablets.)
Oral solution 50mg/5mL, 28 days @ 50mg t.d.s. = £20.

Biorphen® (Alliance)
Oral solution (sugar-free) 25mg/5mL, 28 days @ 50mg t.d.s. = £36; *anise flavour.*

Disipal® (Astellas)
Tablets 50mg, 28 days @ 50mg t.d.s. = £3. (Note: at BNF prices, this is *cheaper* than generic tablets.)

---

1 Katzenschlager R *et al.* (2003) Anticholinergics for symptomatic management of Parkinson's disease. *Cochrane Database of Systematic Reviews.* Cd003735.

Updated April 2014

PROKINETICS   BNF 1.2

Pharmacology
Prokinetics accelerate GI transit and include:
- D_2 antagonists, e.g. **domperidone** (p.246), **metoclopramide** (p.242)
- $5HT_4$ agonists, e.g. **metoclopramide, prucalopride**
- motilin agonists, e.g. **erythromycin.**

Clinical trials are underway of cholinesterase inhibitors and drugs acting at other receptors, e.g. ghrelin agonists.[1]

Drugs which enhance intestinal transit indirectly are not considered prokinetics (e.g. bulk-forming agents, other laxatives, and drugs such as **misoprostol** which cause diarrhoea by increasing GI secretions). Some drugs increase contractile motor activity but not in a co-ordinated fashion, and so do not reduce transit time, e.g. **bethanechol.** Such drugs are promotility but not prokinetic.[2]

D_2 antagonists and $5HT_4$ agonists act by triggering a cholinergic system in the wall of the GI tract (Table 1, Figure 1).[3] This action is impeded by opioids. Further, antimuscarinic drugs competitively block cholinergic receptors on the intestinal muscle fibres (and elsewhere).[4] Thus, all drugs with antimuscarinic properties reduce the impact of prokinetic drugs. The extent of this depends on several factors, including the respective doses of the interacting drugs and times of administration. Thus, the concurrent administration of prokinetics and antimuscarinic drugs is generally best avoided. On the other hand, even if the peripheral prokinetic effect is completely blocked, **domperidone** and **metoclopramide** will still exert an anti-emetic effect at the dopamine receptors in the area postrema (see p.235).

Erythromycin is reported to improve symptoms in about half of patients. A review suggested that, overall, its prokinetic effect was greater than that of **metoclopramide** (Table 1). However, the studies, mainly in diabetic gastroparesis, were small and open to bias.[7] Further, **erythromycin** can cause intestinal colic and diarrhoea. There are concerns about the possible development of bacterial resistance or tolerance to its prokinetic effects, although there are reports of **erythromycin** 250mg b.d. given for more than a year without apparent loss of efficacy.[8,9] Thus, **erythromycin** is generally used second-line when **metoclopramide** and **domperidone** have been ineffective.

Compared with **erythromycin**, **azithromycin** has a longer half-life and the potential for fewer drug interactions and undesirable effects. However, there are few trials to support its use.[10] Non-antibacterial motilin agonists are also undergoing trials, e.g. **atilmotin** and **mitemcinal**.

Use of prokinetics in palliative care

Prokinetics are used in various situations in palliative care (Box A). D_2 antagonists block the dopaminergic 'brake' on gastric emptying induced by stress, anxiety, and nausea from any cause. In contrast, $5HT_4$ agonists have a direct excitatory effect. However, when used for dysmotility dyspepsia, dual-action **metoclopramide** is no more potent than **domperidone** in standard doses.[11,12]

Doses are given in individual monographs for **metoclopramide** (p.242) and **domperidone** (p.246). For **erythromycin**:
- start with 50–100mg q.d.s PO (use suspension)
- if necessary, increase every few days by 25–50mg to a maximum dose of 250mg q.d.s.[3]

Table I Comparison of gastric prokinetic drugs[5]

Drug	Erythromycin	Domperidone	Metoclopramide
Mechanism of action			
Motilin agonist	+	−	−
D_2 antagonist	−	+	+
$5HT_4$ agonist	−	−	+
Response to treatment[a,b]			
Gastric emptying (mean % acceleration)	45	30	20
Symptom relief (mean % improvement)	50	50	40

a. all percentages rounded to nearest 5%
b. although acceleration in gastric emptying is a useful indicator of the efficacy of a prokinetic drug, it correlates poorly with symptom relief in gastroparesis.[6]

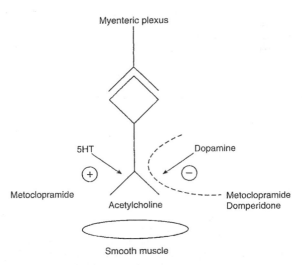

Myenteric plexus

5HT

Dopamine

Metoclopramide

Acetylcholine

Metoclopramide
Domperidone

Smooth muscle

Figure I Schematic representation of drug effects on antroduodenal co-ordination via a postganglionic effect on the cholinergic nerves from the myenteric plexus.
⊕ stimulatory effect of 5HT triggered by metoclopramide;
⊖ inhibitory effect of dopamine;
- - - blockade of dopamine inhibition by metoclopramide and domperidone.

Table 2 Drug treatment of hiccup

Class of drug	Drug	Acute relief	Maintenance regimen
Reduce gastric distension ± gastro-oesophageal reflux			
Antiflatulent (carminative)	Peppermint water[a,b]	10mL	10–20mL b.d.
Antiflatulent (defoaming agent)	Simeticone, e.g. in Altacite Plus®	10mL	10mL q.d.s.
Prokinetic	Metoclopramide[b,c]	10mg	10mg t.d.s.–q.d.s.
PPI	Lansoprazole	30mg	30mg each morning
Muscle relaxant (all of these also have central suppressant effects)			
GABA agonist	Baclofen	5mg PO	5–20mg t.d.s., occasionally more[15,16]
Calcium-channel blocker	Nifedipine	10mg PO/SL	10–20mg t.d.s., occasionally more[17,18]
Benzodiazepine	Midazolam	2mg IV, followed by 1–2mg increments every 3–5min	10–60mg/24h by CSCI if patient in last days of life[19]
Central suppression of the hiccup reflex			
Dopamine antagonist	Metoclopramide	As above	As above
	Haloperidol	5–10mg PO or IV if no response	1.5–3mg at bedtime[20,21]
	Chlorpromazine	10–25mg PO or IM; if no response 25–50mg IVI[d]	25–50mg t.d.s.
	Methylphenidate	5mg PO	5–10mg b.d.[22]
GABA agonist	Baclofen	As above	As above
	Sodium valproate	200–500mg PO	15mg/kg/24h in divided doses[23]
Anti-epileptic	Gabapentin	'Burst gabapentin', i.e. 400mg t.d.s. for 3 days, then 400mg once daily for 3 days, then stop; repeat if necessary[d,24]	400mg t.d.s.[e,25,26]

a. facilitates belching by relaxing the lower oesophageal sphincter; an old-fashioned remedy, but can cause gastro-oesophageal reflux
b. peppermint water and metoclopramide should not be used concurrently because of their opposing actions on the gastro-oesophageal sphincter
c. tightens the lower oesophageal sphincter and hastens gastric emptying
d. add to 500mL–1L 0.9% saline and administer over 1h; irritant, do not use SC
e. a smaller dose advisable in elderly frail patients and those with renal impairment, e.g. start with 100mg t.d.s.

Box A	Indications for prokinetics in palliative care

Gastro-oesophageal reflux
Hiccup
Delayed gastric emptying
Gastroparesis
   dysmotility dyspepsia
   paraneoplastic autonomic neuropathy
   spinal cord compression
   diabetic autonomic neuropathy
Functional GI obstruction
   drug-induced, e.g. opioids
   cancer of head of pancreas
   linitis plastica (locally diffuse mural infiltration by cancer)

Metoclopramide is also used to relieve hiccup associated with delayed gastric emptying and/or oesophageal reflux (Table 2).[13]

For patients with refractory symptoms, seek advice of a gastroenterologist. In some settings, patients may benefit from **clonidine** (see p.76), intrapyloric **botulinum toxin** or gastric electrical stimulation.[14] Ultimately, some patients may require a venting gastrostomy and/or a feeding jejunostomy.[1]

1 Stevens JE et al. (2013) Pathophysiology and pharmacotherapy of gastroparesis: current and future perspectives. *Expert Opinion on Pharmacotherpy.* 14: 1171–1186.

2 Rayner CK and Horowitz M (2005) New management approaches for gastroparesis. *Nature Clinical Practice Gastroenterology and Hepatology.* 2: 454–462; quiz 493.

3 Patrick A and Epstein O (2008) Review article: gastroparesis. *Alimentary Pharmacology and Therapeutics.* 27: 724–740.

4 Schuurkes JAJ et al. (1986) Stimulation of gastroduodenal motor activity: dopaminergic and cholinergic modulation. *Drug Development Research.* 8: 233–241.

5 Sturm A et al. (1999) Prokinetics in patients with gastroparesis: a systematic analysis. *Digestion.* 60: 422–427.

6 Janssen P et al. (2013) The relation between symptom improvement and gastric emptying in the treatment of diabetic and idiopathic gastroparesis. *American Journal of Gastroenterology.* 108: 1382–1391.

7 Maganti K et al. (2003) Oral erythromycin and symptomatic relief of gastroparesis: a systematic review. *American Journal of Gastroenterology.* 98: 259–263.

8 Dhir R and Richter JE (2004) Erythromycin in the short- and long-term control of dyspepsia symptoms in patients with gastroparesis. *Journal of Clinical Gastroenterology.* 38: 237–242.

9 Hunter A et al. (2005) The use of long-term, low-dose erythromycin in treating persistent gastric stasis. *Journal of Pain and Symptom Management.* 29: 430–433.

10 Potter TG and Snider KR (2013) Azithromycin for the treatment of gastroparesis. *Annals of Pharmacotherpy.* 47: 411–415.

11 Loose FD (1979) Domperidone in chronic dyspepsia: a pilot open study and a multicentre general practice crossover comparison with metoclopramide and placebo. *Pharmatheripeutica.* 2: 140–146.

12 Moriga M (1981) A multicentre double blind study of domperidone and metoclopramide in the symptomatic control of dyspepsia. In: G Towse (ed) *International congress and symposium series: Progress with Domperidone, a gastrokinetic and anti-emetic agent* (No. 36). Royal Society of Medicine, London, pp. 77–79.

13 Twycross R et al. (2009) *Symptom Management in Advanced Cancer* (4e). palliativedrugs.com, Nottingham, pp. 174–177.

14 Haans JJ and Masclee AA (2007) Review article: The diagnosis and management of gastroparesis. *Alimentary Pharmacology and Therapeutics.* 26 (Suppl 2): 37–46.

15 Ramirez FC and Graham DY (1992) Treatment of intractable hiccup with baclofen: results of a double-blind randomized, controlled, crossover study. *American Journal of Gastroenterology.* 87: 1789–1791.

16 Guelaud C et al. (1995) Baclofen therapy for chronic hiccup. *European Respiratory Journal.* 8: 235–237.

17 Lipps DC et al. (1990) Nifedipine for intractable hiccups. *Neurology.* 40: 531–532.

18 Brigham B and Bolin T (1992) High dose nifedipine and fludrocortisone for intractable hiccups. *Medical Journal of Australia.* 157: 70.

19 Wilcock A and Twycross R (1996) Case report: midazolam for intractable hiccup. *Journal of Pain and Symptom Management.* 12: 59–61.

20 Scarnati RA (1979) Intractable hiccup (singultus): report of case. *Journal of the American Osteopathic Association.* 79: 127–129.

21 Ives TJ et al. (1985) Treatment of intractable hiccups with intramuscular haloperidol. *American Journal of Psychiatry.* 142: 1368–1369.

22 Marechal R et al. (2003) Successful treatment of intractable hiccup with methylphenidate in a lung cancer patient. *Supportive Care in Cancer.* 11: 126–128.

23 Jacobson P et al. (1981) Treatment of intractable hiccups with valproic acid. *Neurology.* 31: 1458–1460.

24 Moretti R *et al.* (2004) Gabapentin as a drug therapy of intractable hiccup because of vascular lesion: a three-year follow up. *Neurologist.* **10**: 102–106.
25 Schuchmann JA and Browne BA (2007) Persistent hiccups during rehabilitation hospitalization: three case reports and review of the literature. *American Journal of Physical Medicine and Rehabilitation.* **86**: 1013–1018.
26 Tegeler ML and Baumrucker SJ (2008) Gabapentin for intractable hiccups in palliative care. *American Journal of Hospice and Palliative Care.* **25**: 52–54.

Updated March 2014

H₂-RECEPTOR ANTAGONISTS   BNF 1.3.1

Class: Gastroprotective drugs.

Indications: Chronic episodic dyspepsia, acid reflux, prevention and treatment of peptic ulceration (including NSAID-related ulceration), reduction of malabsorption and fluid loss in short bowel syndrome (**cimetidine**), prevention of degradation of pancreatin supplements (**cimetidine**).

Pharmacology

H₂-receptor antagonists (H₂ antagonists) include **cimetidine, famotidine, nizatidine** and **ranitidine**. All are equally effective at gastric acid suppression.[1] Other effects include reducing the volume of gastric secretions, and increasing lower oesophageal sphincter pressure.[2,3] **Cimetidine**, alone among H₂ antagonists, can cause serious CYP450-related drug interactions (see Table 1 and Cytochrome P450, p.771). None of the H₂ antagonists, including **cimetidine**, alters the metabolism of **morphine**.[4]

Prophylactic treatment with a standard dose of an H₂ antagonist reduces the incidence of NSAID-related *duodenal* ulcers.[5] Prevention of *gastric* erosions and ulcers is seen only with a double dose.[6,7] In patients taking NSAIDs, **ranitidine** (compared with **omeprazole**) is less effective and slower in *healing* gastroduodenal ulcers (63% vs. 80% at 8 weeks) and in *preventing* relapse (59% vs. 72% over 6 months).[5,8] **Ranitidine** is a good choice in terms of convenience and safety.
Bio-availability ranitidine 50% PO.
Onset of action < 1h.
Time to peak plasma concentration, ranitidine 2–3h PO, 15min IM.
Plasma halflife ranitidine 2–3h.
Duration of action ranitidine 8–12h.

Cautions

Hepatic impairment, renal impairment.

Drug interactions

CYP450-related drug interactions with **cimetidine** most relevant to palliative care are given in Table 1. **Cimetidine** may also increase levels of **epirubicin**, by an unknown mechanism. There are inconsistent reports of **cimetidine** and **ranitidine** increasing the plasma concentration of **midazolam**.[9]

Because H₂ antagonists increase gastric pH, they can decrease the absorption of some drugs:
• *antifungals,* e.g. **itraconazole** (capsules only), **posaconazole** (but *not* **fluconazole**)
• *antivirals,* e.g. **atazanavir, delavirdine** (not UK), **indinavir, nelfinavir** and **rilpivirine**
• *protein kinase inhibitors,* e.g. **dasatinib, erlotinib, gefitinib, lapatinib, nilotinib.**[9]
This effect varies between drugs and formulations. See the SPC and other sources[9] to determine the risk of treatment failure with concurrent use of an H₂ antagonist. When avoidance is impossible, alternative measures to reduce the interaction include increasing the dose, administering > 12h after the H₂ antagonist or giving with an acidic drink, e.g. cola.[9]

Conversely, the absorption of **saquinivir** may be *increased* and, because of the risk of QT prolongation, this could be clinically important.[9]

Table I   Cimetidine CYP450-related interactions most relevant to palliative care[9,10]

Drug group	Drug plasma levels increased
Anti-epileptics	Carbamazepine (transient), phenytoin
Benzodiazepines	Alprazolam, diazepam, chlordiazepoxide, flurazepam, nitrazepam, triazolam (midazolam reports inconsistent)
Calcium antagonists	Potentially all, including diltiazem and nifedipine
Coumarin anticoagulants	Warfarin
Local anaesthetics	Lidocaine (IV), procainamide
Opioids	Alfentanil, fentanyl, methadone
SSRIs	All
TCAs	Potentially all
Xanthines	Aminophylline, theophylline
Miscellaneous	Fluorouracil, mefloquine, mirtazapine, moclobemide, quinidine, tacrine, zolmitriptan

Undesirable effects

Cimetidine occasionally causes gynaecomastia.

Possible increased risk of pneumonia (gastric acid suppression leads to bacterial overgrowth in the upper-GI and respiratory tracts); association stronger for PPIs.[11]

Dose and use

Cochrane reviews: PPIs, H₂ antagonists and prokinetics are effective at *relieving symptoms* of non-ulcer dyspepsia and acid reflux, with PPIs having the greatest efficacy.[12,13] PPIs, **misoprostol** and double-dose H₂ antagonists are effective at *preventing* chronic NSAID-related endoscopic peptic ulcers.

Standard doses of H₂ antagonists reduce the risk of duodenal ulcers but not gastric ulcers. **Misoprostol** 400microgram/24h is less effective at preventing gastric ulcers than 800microgram/24h and is still associated with diarrhoea. Of all these treatments, only **misoprostol** 800microgram/24h has been definitely shown to reduce the overall incidence of ulcer *complications* (perforation, haemorrhage or gastric outlet obstruction).[6]

The use of PPIs following peptic ulcer-related upper-GI haemorrhage, significantly reduces rebleeding, need for surgery and rate of ulcer recurrence. In high risk patients (i.e. bleeding or blood vessel visible at endoscopy) PPIs reduce mortality.[14] Ideally, the PPI is commenced following a diagnostic/therapeutic endoscopy, except in circumstances where this is not immediately available.[15] Evidence is insufficient to determine if any differences exist between PPI given IV in high dose or IV/PO in usual doses.[16]

Adding a bedtime dose of an H₂ antagonist to a high dose PPI may improve night-time acid reflux but evidence is lacking.[17]

NICE guidance: PPIs are preferable to H₂ antagonists for the treatment of dyspepsia, gastro-oesophageal reflux disease and peptic ulcers, including NSAID-related peptic ulcers. Although PPIs are more effective in relieving uninvestigated dyspeptic symptoms, offer a trial of H₂ antagonists or a prokinetic if there has been an inadequate response to a PPI.

For patients taking an NSAID and at high risk of peptic ulcer disease, double-dose H₂ antagonists or PPIs significantly reduce endoscopically detected lesions. **Misoprostol** at low dose is less effective and has undesirable effects. When an NSAID-related ulcer is diagnosed, stop the NSAID if possible, treat *H pylori* infection if present (see p.486) and give double-dose H₂ antagonist or PPI. PPIs heal the majority of ulcers.[18]

A PPI should be offered to patients with non-variceal upper-GI haemorrhage when bleeding or stigmata of recent bleeding is confirmed at endoscopy.[19]

If it is necessary to continue with the NSAID, treatments may be less effective. The rate of healing is higher and the risk of recurrence lower with PPIs and **misoprostol** compared with H₂ antagonists.[20]

H₂ antagonists are second-line treatment for gastro-oesophageal reflux disease, non-ulcer dyspepsia and uninvestigated dyspepsia, and are available as an OTC measure for mild dyspepsia.

Cimetidine, famotidine and **nizatidine** are significantly more expensive than **ranitidine**; **cimetidine** is also intrinsically more dangerous. Thus, dose recommendations have been limited to **ranitidine**.

The dose and duration of treatment is least with duodenal ulceration and most with reflux oesophagitis and prophylaxis for NSAID-related peptic ulcer, although the dose for ulcer healing can be doubled if the initial response is poor (Table 2). **Ranitidine** is more effective if taken at bedtime rather than with the evening meal.[21]

Table 2 PO treatment regimens for ranitidine

Indication	Ranitidine
Duodenal ulcer[a,b]	150mg b.d. or 300mg at bedtime for 4–8 weeks
Gastric ulcer[a,b]	150mg b.d. or 300mg at bedtime for 4–8 weeks
Prophylaxis for NSAID-associated peptic ulcer	150mg–†300mg b.d. indefinitely
Reflux oesophagitis	150mg b.d. or 300mg at bedtime for 8–12 weeks
Short bowel syndrome	†300mg at bedtime
To reduce degradation of pancreatin supplements	†150mg 1h a.c.

a. 8 weeks for NSAID-related ulcer
b. dose can be doubled if initial response is poor.

Parenteral formulations are available for IM and IV use if treatment is considered necessary in a patient with severe nausea and vomiting (see BNF section 1.3.1). Some centres use the SC route (unauthorized), either 50mg SC b.d.–q.d.s. or CSCI 100–200mg/24h without evidence of local inflammation.

Ranitidine has a pH of 6.7–7.3 and is incompatible with **levomepromazine** and **midazolam**. Because there are limited compatibility data with other drugs, it is probably best to administer alone if giving by CSCI (see Chapter 20, p.701).

In renal impairment (creatinine clearance < 50mL/min) the dose of **ranitidine** should be reduced to 150mg at bedtime but increased to 150mg b.d. if an ulcer fails to respond at the lower dose.

Supply

Ranitidine (generic)
Tablets 150mg, 300mg, 28 days @ 150mg b.d. or 300mg at bedtime = £1.50.
Tablets effervescent 150mg, 300mg, 28 days @ 150mg b.d. = £16 or 300mg at bedtime = £15 (*Tablets may contain Na⁺*).
Oral solution 75mg/5mL, 28 days @ 150mg b.d. = £37; *may contain alcohol.*
Injection 25mg/mL, 2mL amp = £0.50.

Zantac® (GSK)
Tablets 150mg, 300mg, 28 days @ 150mg b.d. or 300mg at bedtime = £1.50.
Oral solution (sugar-free) 75mg/5mL, 28 days @ 150mg b.d. = £39; contains 8% alcohol.
Injection 25mg/mL, 2mL amp = £0.50.

Ranitidine tablets are available as an OTC measure for acid dyspepsia and heartburn.

1 Tougas G and Armstrong D (1997) Efficacy of H₂ receptor antagonists in the treatment of gastroesophageal reflux disease and its symptoms. *Canadian Journal of Gastroenterology.* **11 (Suppl B)**: 51B–54B.
2 Williams JG and Strunin L (1985) Pre-operative intramuscular ranitidine and cimetidine. Double blind comparative trial, effect on gastric pH and volume. *Anaesthesia.* **40**: 242–245.
3 Iwakiri K et al. (2011) The effects of nizatidine on transient lower esophageal sphincter relaxations (TLESRs) and acid reflux in healthy subjects. *Journal of Smooth Muscle Research.* **47**: 157–166.
4 Mojaverian P et al. (1982) Cimetidine does not alter morphine disposition in man. *British Journal of Clinical Pharmacology.* **14**: 809–813.
5 Hollander D (1994) Gastrointestinal complications of nonsteroidal anti-inflammatory drugs: prophylactic and therapeutic strategies. *American Journal of Medicine.* **96**: 274–281.
6 Rostom A et al. (2002) Prevention of NSAID-induced gastroduodenal ulcers. *Cochrane Database of Systematic Reviews.* **4**: CD002296.
7 Leontiadis GI et al. (2007) Systematic reviews of the clinical effectiveness and cost-effectiveness of proton pump inhibitors in acute upper gastrointestinal bleeding. *Health Technology Assessment.* **11**: iii–iv, 1–164.
8 Yeomans N et al. (1998) A comparison of omeprazole with ranitidine for ulcers associated with nonsteroidal anti-inflammatory drugs. Acid suppression trial. *New England Journal of Medicine.* **338**: 719–726.
9 Baxter K and Preston CL. *Stockley's Drug Interactions.* London: Pharmaceutical Press. www.medicinescomplete.com (accessed October 2012).
10 Sorkin E and Ogawa C (1983) Cimetidine potentiation of narcotic action. *Drug Intelligence and Clinical Pharmacy.* **17**: 60–61.
11 Fohl AL and Regal RE (2011) Proton pump inhibitor-associated pneumonia: Not a breath of fresh air after all? *World Journal of Gastrointestinal Pharmacology and Therapeutics.* **2**: 17–26.
12 Moayyedi P (2006) Pharmacological interventions for non-ulcer dyspepsia. *Cochrane Database of Systematic Reviews.* **4**: CD001960.
13 van Pinxteren B et al. (2010) Short-term treatment with proton pump inhibitors, H₂- receptor antagonists and prokinetics for gastro-oesophageal reflux disease-like symptoms and endoscopy negative reflux disease. *Cochrane Database of Systematic Reviews.* **11**: CD002095.
14 Leontiadis G et al. (2010) Proton pump inhibitor treatment for acute peptic ulcer bleeding. *Cochrane Database of Systematic Reviews.* **5**: CD002094.
15 Sreedharan A et al. (2010) P.Proton pump inhibitor treatment initiated prior to endoscopic diagnosis in upper gastrointestinal bleeding. *Cochrane Database of Systematic Reviews.* **7**: CD005414.
16 Neumann I et al. (2013) Comparison of different regimens of proton pump inhibitors for acute peptic ulcer bleeding. *Cochrane Database of Systematic Reviews.* **6**: CD007999.
17 Wang Y et al. (2009) Additional bedtime H₂ receptor antagonist for control of nocturnal gastirc acid breakthrough. *Cochrane Database of Systematic Reviews.* **4**: CD004275.
18 NICE (2004) Dyspepsia. Management of dyspepsia in adults in primary care. *Clinical Guideline* CG17. www.nice.org.uk
19 NICE (2012) Acute upper gastrointestinal bleeding management. *Clinical Guideline* CG141. www.nice.org.uk
20 Frech EJ and Go MF (2009) Treatment and chemoprevention of NSAID-associated gastrointestinal complications. *Therapeutics and Clinical Risk Management.* **5**: 65–73.
21 20 Johnston DA and Wormsley KG (1988) The effect of food on ranitidine-induced inhibition of nocturnal gastric secretion. *Alimentary Pharmacology and Therapeutics.* **2**: 507–511.

Updated (minor change) April 2014

MISOPROSTOL   BNF 1.3.4

Class: Prostaglandin (PG) analogue, gastroprotective drug.

Indications: Healing of gastric and duodenal ulcers, prevention and healing of NSAID-related ulcers.

Contra-indications: Women of childbearing potential should not be started on misoprostol until pregnancy is excluded (misoprostol increases uterine tone).

Pharmacology

Misoprostol is a synthetic PG analogue with gastric antisecretory and protective properties. The protective effects occur at doses lower than those required to inhibit acid secretion.[1] After oral administration, misoprostol is rapidly converted to an active free acid.

Misoprostol helps to both prevent and heal NSAID-related gastroduodenal erosions and ulcers.[2–5] For NSAID-related ulcers, the rate of healing is higher and the risk of recurrence lower with PPIs and misoprostol compared with H_2 antagonists.[6]

PPIs are more effective than misoprostol at healing and preventing the recurrence of duodenal ulcers.[6–8] Misoprostol is as effective as PPIs in preventing relapse of gastric ulcers and, in one RCT when compared with **lansoprazole**, ulcer-free intervals were longer.[9] Overall, the risk of serious GI complications are significantly reduced by misoprostol.[4,5] However, its use is limited by its tendency to cause diarrhoea and intestinal colic.

Bio-availability 90% PO.
Onset of action <30min.
Time to peak plasma concentration 30min.
Plasma halflife 1–2h for free acid.
Duration of action 2–4h.

Cautions

Women of childbearing age should use effective contraception.

Conditions where hypotension might precipitate severe complications, e.g. cerebrovascular disease, cardiovascular disease.

Undesirable effects

Diarrhoea (may necessitate stopping treatment), colic, dyspepsia, flatulence, nausea and vomiting, abnormal vaginal bleeding (intermenstrual, menorrhagia, postmenopausal), rashes, dizziness.

Dose and use

Cochrane reviews: PPIs, H_2 antagonists and prokinetics are effective at *relieving symptoms* of non-ulcer dyspepsia and acid reflux, with PPIs having the greatest efficacy.[10,11] PPIs, misoprostol and double-dose H_2 antagonists are effective at *preventing* chronic NSAID-related endoscopic peptic ulcers.

Standard doses of H_2 antagonists reduce the risk of duodenal ulcers but not gastric ulcers. Misoprostol 400microgram/24h is less effective at preventing gastric ulcers than 800microgram/ 24h, and is still associated with diarrhoea. Of all these treatments, only misoprostol 800microgram/24h has been definitely shown to reduce the overall incidence of ulcer *complications* (perforation, haemorrhage or gastric outlet obstruction).[5]

The use of PPIs following peptic ulcer-related upper-GI haemorrhage, significantly reduces rebleeding, need for surgery and rate of ulcer recurrence. In high risk patients (i.e. bleeding or blood vessel visible at endoscopy) PPIs reduce mortality.[12] Ideally, the PPI is commenced following a diagnostic/therapeutic endoscopy, except in circumstances where this is not immediately available.[13] Evidence is insufficient to determine if any differences exist between PPI given IV in high dose or IV/PO in usual doses.[14]

Adding a bedtime dose of an H_2 antagonist to a high dose PPI may improve night-time acid reflux but evidence is lacking.[15]

NICE guidance: PPIs are preferable to H_2 antagonists for the treatment of dyspepsia, gastro-oesophageal reflux disease and peptic ulcers, including NSAID-related peptic ulcers. Although PPIs are more effective in relieving uninvestigated dyspeptic symptoms, offer a trial of H_2 antagonists or prokinetic if there has been an inadequate response to a PPI.

For patients taking an NSAID and at high risk of peptic ulcer disease, double-dose H_2 antagonists or PPIs significantly reduce endoscopically detected lesions. Misoprostol at low dose is less effective and has undesirable effects. When an NSAID-related ulcer is diagnosed, stop the NSAID if possible, treat H pylori infection if present (see p.486) and give double-dose H_2 antagonist or a PPI. PPIs heal the majority of ulcers.[16]

A PPI should be offered to patients with non-variceal upper-GI haemorrhage when bleeding or stigmata of recent bleeding is confirmed at endoscopy.[17]

If it is necessary to continue with the NSAID, treatments may be less effective. The rate of healing is higher and the risk of recurrence lower with PPIs and misoprostol compared with H_2 antagonists.[6] Misoprostol 800microgram/24h is as effective as PPIs for preventing symptomatic and complicated gastric ulcers, but less effective in preventing duodenal ulcers.[7]

Prophylaxis against NSAID-related ulcers
200microgram b.d.–q.d.s. taken with the NSAID.

NSAID-related ulceration
* 200microgram t.d.s. with meals & at bedtime or
* 400microgram b.d. (breakfast and bedtime) for 4–8 weeks.[3]

If it causes diarrhoea, give 200microgram t.d.s. with meals & at bedtime and avoid **magnesium salts**.

Supply
Cytotec® (Pharmacia)
Tablets 200microgram, 28 days @ 200microgram b.d. = £10.

1 Monk JP and Clissold SP (1987) Misoprostol. A preliminary review of its pharmacodynamic and pharmacokinetic properties, and therapeutic efficacy in the treatment of peptic ulcer disease. *Drugs.* **33**: 1–30.
2 Silverstein FE et al. (1995) Misoprostol reduces serious gastrointestinal complications in patients with rheumatoid arthritis receiving nonsteroidal anti-inflammatory drugs. *Annals of internal medicine.* **123**: 241–249.
3 Bardhan KD et al. (1993) The prevention and healing of acute NSAID-associated gastroduodenal mucosal damage by misoprostol. *British Journal of Rheumatology.* **32**: 990–995.
4 Hooper L et al. (2004) The effectiveness of five strategies for the prevention of gastrointestinal toxicity induced by non-steroidal anti-inflammatory drugs: systematic review. *British Medical Journal.* **329**: 948.
5 Rostom A et al. (2002) Prevention of NSAID-induced gastroduodenal ulcers. *Cochrane Database of Systematic Reviews.* **4**: CD002296.
6 Frech EJ and Go MF (2009) Treatment and chemoprevention of NSAID-associated gastrointestinal complications. *Therapeutics and Clinical Risk Management.* **5**: 65–73.
7 Leontiadis GI et al. (2007) Systematic reviews of the clinical effectiveness and cost-effectiveness of proton pump inhibitors in acute upper gastrointestinal bleeding. *Health Technology Assessment.* **11**: iii-iv, 1–164.
8 Hawkey C et al. (1998) Omeprazole compared with misoprostol for ulcers associated with nonsteroidal anti-inflammatory drugs. *New England Journal of Medicine.* **338**: 727–734.
9 Graham DY et al. (2002) Ulcer prevention in long-term users of nonsteroidal anti-inflammatory drugs: results of a double-blind, randomized, multicenter, active- and placebo-controlled study of misoprostol vs lansoprazole. *Archives of Internal Medicine.* **162**: 169–175.
10 Sigterman KE et al. (2013) Short-term treatment with proton pump inhibitors, H_2-receptor antagonists and prokinetics for gastro-oesophageal reflux disease-like symptoms and endoscopy negative reflux disease. *Cochrane Database of Systematic Reviews.* **5**: CD002095.
11 Moayyedi P (2006) Pharmacological interventions for non-ulcer dyspepsia. *Cochrane Database of Systematic Reviews.* **4**: CD001960.
12 Leontiadis G et al. (2010) Proton pump inhibitor treatment for acute peptic ulcer bleeding. *Cochrane Database of Systematic Reviews.* **5**: CD002094.
13 Sreedharan A et al. (2010) Proton pump inhibitor treatment initiated prior to endoscopic diagnosis in upper gastrointestinal bleeding *Cochrane Database of Systematic Reviews. 1*: CD005415.
14 Neumann I et al. (2013) Comparison of different regimens of proton pump inhibitors for acute peptic ulcer bleeding. *Cochrane Database of Systematic Reviews.* **6**: CD007999.
15 Wang Y et al. (2009) Additional bedtime H_2 receptor antagonist for control of nocturnal gastirc acid breakthrough. *Cochrane Database of Systematic Reviews.* **4**: CD004275.
16 NICE (2004) Dyspepsia. Management of dyspepsia in adults in primary care. *Clinical Guideline* CG17. www.nice.org.uk
17 NICE (2012) Acute upper gastrointestinal bleeding:management. *Clinical Guideline* CG141. www.nice.org.uk

Updated (minor change) April 2014

PROTON PUMP INHIBITORS   BNF 1.3.5

Class: Gastroprotective drugs.

Indications: Authorized indications vary between products; consult the manufacturers' SPCs for details; they include acid dyspepsia, acid reflux, peptic ulceration, prevention and treatment of NSAID-related ulceration and eradication of *Helicobacter pylori* (with antibacterials).

Pharmacology

Proton pump inhibitors (PPIs) reduce gastric acid output but, unlike H_2 antagonists, they do *not* reduce the volume of gastric secretions. Because they are all rapidly degraded by acid, they are formulated as e/c granules or tablets. These dissolve in the duodenum where the drug is rapidly absorbed to be selectively taken up by gastric parietal cells and converted into active metabolites. These irreversibly inhibit the proton pump (H^+/K^+-ATPase) and thereby block gastric acid secretion. Elimination is predominantly by metabolism in the liver to inactive derivatives excreted mainly in the urine. The plasma halflives of PPIs are mostly <2h but, because they irreversibly inhibit the proton pump, the antisecretory activity continues for several days until new proton pumps are synthesized.

PPIs are effective in treating acid-related disorders. They provide symptomatic relief, help prevent and heal peptic ulcers (including those associated NSAIDs), and reduce the risk of recurrent ulceration and rebleeding.[1–3]

When treating peptic ulceration **lansoprazole** 30mg daily is as effective as **omeprazole** 40mg daily, and **pantoprazole** 40mg daily is as effective as **omeprazole** 20mg daily.[4] However, **omeprazole** shows a dose-response curve above the standard dose of 20mg daily, whereas no further benefit is seen by increasing the dose of **lansoprazole** and **pantoprazole** above 30mg and 40mg daily respectively.[5,6] Thus, **omeprazole** 40mg daily is superior to **lansoprazole** 60mg daily and **pantoprazole** 80mg daily in the management of severe gastro-oesophageal reflux disease (oesophagitis and stricture).[7]

Comparative studies with newer PPIs show **esomeprazole** (the S-enantiomer of **omeprazole**) 40mg once daily and **rabeprazole** 20mg once daily cause rapid relief of reflux symptoms and suppress acid for longer periods. However, the endoscopic healing rate of ulcers and reflex oesophagitis is similar to other PPIs.[8–10] **Esomeprazole** and **rabeprazole** may be more effective in patients who have not responded to other PPIs. Whereas **omeprazole**, **lansoprazole** and **pantoprazole** are metabolized mainly via CYP2C19, this is not so with **esomeprazole** and **rabeprazole**. Thus, in CYP2C19 extensive metabolizers, the plasma concentrations of the former three PPIs are reduced, but not **esomeprazole** and **rabeprazole**.[9]

The bio-availability of **lansoprazole** is reduced by food and the manufacturer recommends that it should be given each morning 1h before breakfast. However, the reduced bio-availability appears not to reduce efficacy.[11–13] In one study comparing **lansoprazole** given either before or after food, acid suppression was comparable with both regimens after 1 week (although on day 1 it was significantly less when taken after food).[14] Pharmacokinetic data are shown in Table 1.
Onset of action <2h.
Duration of action >24h.

Table 1   Pharmacokinetic details of PPIs given PO

	Bio-availability (%)	Time to peak plasma concentration (h)	Plasma halflife (h)
Esomeprazole	68 (20mg dose) 89 (40mg dose)	1–2	1.3
Lansoprazole	80–90	1.5–2	1–2
Omeprazole	60	3–6	0.5–3
Pantoprazole	77	2–2.5	1[a]
Rabeprazole	52	1. 6–5	1[b]

a. increases to 3–6h in cirrhosis
b. increases to 2–3h in hepatic impairment.

Cautions

The dose should be reduced in severe hepatic impairment (see Dose and use). Ocular damage has been reported, mostly with IV **omeprazole**.[15,16] PPIs possibly cause vasoconstriction by blocking H^+/K^+-ATPase. Because the retinal artery is an end-artery, anterior ischaemic optic neuropathy may result. If the PPI is stopped, visual acuity may improve but some patients have become permanently blind, in some instances after only 3 days. Impaired hearing and deafness have also been reported, again mostly with IV **omeprazole**.

A similar mechanism may be responsible for the angina and hypertension included in the US manufacturer's list of undesirable effects for **omeprazole**. Concern about serious cardiac events (infarction, death) with **omeprazole** and **esomeprazole** is now considered to be groundless.[17]

PPIs are an independent risk factor for *Clostridium difficile* infection; and the association is stronger than for other acid-reducing agents. Patients are at risk of recurrent *Clostridium difficile* colitis, up to nearly 5 times more likely.[18–23] Although the spores of *Clostridium difficile* are resistant to gastric acid, reduced acidity allows bacteria to survive. Counts of *Clostridium difficile* organisms, which cannot survive at normal stomach pH, increase when the pH is >5, and go on to infect the bowel. Further, the cells can live up to 6h on moist surfaces, long enough to allow transmission between patients.[24]

The concomitant use of PPIs and antibacterials further increases the risk of *Clostridium difficile* infection.[25]

Drug interactions

Although PPIs are metabolized by CYP450 (see Chapter 25, p.771), clinically important interactions with PPIs are rare.[26,27] Sedation and gait disturbances have been reported when **omeprazole** was given with **diazepam, flurazepam** or **lorazepam**. **Omeprazole** levels are increased by some macrolides (**clarithromycin, erythromycin**) and azole antifungals (**fluconazole, voriconazole**).[28] No other significant CYP450 drug–drug interactions have been identified with **pantoprazole** or **rabeprazole**.[28,29]

A minor pharmacokinetic interaction between **omeprazole** and **warfarin**, resulting in a less than 15% rise in **R-warfarin** levels (the less active enantiomer) is of limited clinical relevance. However, isolated cases of raised INRs have been reported with all PPIs.[28] It is recommended that, in patients taking **warfarin**, the INR is monitored if **omeprazole** or **esomeprazole** is started or stopped.[30]

The antithrombotic effect of **clopidogrel** (a pro-drug activated by CYP2C19) can be reduced by the concurrent administration of **omeprazole, esomeprazole** and **rabeprazole**.[31–33] Although the evidence for the other PPIs is inconsistent,[32–34] it would seem wise to avoid concurrent prescription with any PPI, and use an H_2 antagonist (e.g. **ranitidine**) instead.

Because PPIs increase gastric pH, they can decrease the absorption of some drugs:
• *antifungals*, e.g. **itraconazole** (capsules only), **posaconazole** (but *not* **fluconazole**)
• *antivirals*, e.g. **atazanavir, delavirdine** (not UK), **indinavir, nelfinavir** and **rilpivirine**
• *protein kinase inhibitors*, e.g. **dasatinib, erlotinib, gefitinib, lapatinib, nilotinib**.[28,35]
This effect varies between drugs and formulations. See the SPC and other sources[28] to determine the risk of treatment failure with concurrent use of a PPI. When avoidance is impossible, alternative measures to reduce the interaction include increasing the dose, administering >12h after the PPI or giving with an acidic drink, e.g. cola.[36]

Conversely, the absorption of **saquinivir** may be *increased* and, because of the risk of QT prolongation, this could be clinically important.[28]

The absorption of **digoxin** may also be *increased*; however, this may only be important with high PPI doses in the elderly.[28]

Undesirable effects

Common (<10%, >1%): headache, abdominal pain, nausea, vomiting, diarrhoea or constipation, flatulence.

Severe hypomagnesaemia: rare and generally with prolonged use, i.e. >1 year. Particularly when used concurrently with **digoxin** or a drug which can cause hypomagnesaemia (see p.571), measure serum magnesium before starting PPI and periodically during use (e.g. every 3 months).[37] Observational studies suggest a modest increase in the risk of hip and vertebral fracture in the elderly with prolonged use of PPIs. Those at risk of osteoporosis should ensure an adequate intake of vitamin D and calcium, using supplements if necessary.[38]

Possible increased risk of pneumonia (gastric acid suppression leads to bacterial overgrowth in the upper-GI and respiratory tracts); association weaker for H_2 antagonists.[39]

Dose and use

Cochrane reviews: PPIs, H_2 antagonists and prokinetics are effective at *relieving symptoms* of non-ulcer dyspepsia and acid reflux, with PPIs having the greatest efficacy.[40,41] PPIs, **misoprostol** and double-dose H_2 antagonists are effective at *preventing* chronic NSAID-related endoscopic peptic ulcers.

Standard doses of H_2 antagonists reduce the risk of duodenal ulcers but not gastric ulcers. **Misoprostol** 400microgram/24h is less effective at preventing gastric ulcers than 800microgram/24h and is still associated with diarrhoea. Of all these treatments, only **misoprostol** 800microgram/24h has been definitely shown to reduce the overall incidence of ulcer *complications* (perforation, haemorrhage or gastric outlet obstruction)[42]

The use of PPIs following peptic ulcer-related upper-GI haemorrhage, significantly reduces rebleeding, need for surgery and rate of ulcer recurrence. In high risk patients (i.e. bleeding or blood vessel visible at endoscopy) PPIs reduce mortality.[43] Ideally, the PPI is commenced following a diagnostic/therapeutic endoscopy, except in circumstances where this is not immediately available.[44] Evidence is insufficient to determine if any differences exist between PPI given IV in high dose or IV/PO in usual doses.[45]

Adding a bedtime dose of an H_2 antagonist to a high dose PPI may improve night-time acid reflux but evidence is lacking.[46]

NICE guidance: PPIs are preferable to H_2 antagonists for the treatment of dyspepsia, gastro-oesophageal reflux disease and peptic ulcers, including NSAID-related peptic ulcers. Although PPIs are more effective in relieving uninvestigated dyspeptic symptoms, offer a trial of an H_2 antagonists or a prokinetic if there has been an inadequate response to a PPI.

For patients taking an NSAID and at high risk of peptic ulcer disease, double-dose H_2 antagonists or PPIs significantly reduce endoscopically detected lesions. **Misoprostol** at low dose is less effective and has undesirable effects. When an NSAID-related ulcer is diagnosed, stop the NSAID if possible, treat H pylori infection if present (see p.486) and give double-dose H_2 antagonist or PPI. PPIs heal the majority of ulcers.[47]

A PPI should be offered to patients with non-variceal upper-GI haemorrhage when bleeding or stigmata of recent bleeding is confirmed at endoscopy.[48]

PPIs are used together with antibacterials for the eradication of *Helicobacter pylori* (see p.486).

Lansoprazole

The SPC for **lansoprazole** states that administration should be 1h before breakfast each morning in order to achieve 'optimal acid inhibition'. However, this precaution is unnecessary.[11,14]
- 30mg each morning for 4–8 weeks for treatment of ulcers and reflux oesophagitis
- 15mg each morning for prophylaxis of ulcers and reflux oesophagitis, increase to 30mg daily if necessary
- 30mg b.d. when used with antibacterials to eradicate *Helicobacter pylori* (see p.487).

Omeprazole
- 20mg each morning for both treatment and prevention of ulcer recurrence
- 40mg each morning in reflux oesophagitis if poor response to standard dose
- 20mg b.d. or 40mg each morning when used with antibacterials to eradicate *Helicobacter pylori* (see p.487).

In severe hepatic impairment, the dose should be limited to **lansoprazole** 30mg/day and **omeprazole** 20mg/day.

For patients who cannot safely swallow tablets, **lansoprazole** and **omeprazole** can be given as orodispersible or dispersible tablets. Some capsules containing e/c granules can be opened and the e/c granules swallowed with water or fruit juice, or mixed with apple sauce or yoghurt; check with the specific manufacturer's SPC. *Care must be taken not to crush or chew the e/c granules.*

Specific procedures are available from the manufacturers for administration by enteral feeding tubes (see p.731). For patients with obstructive dysphagia and acid dyspepsia or with severe gastritis and vomiting, the rectal route has also been used.[49]

Omeprazole, when given for non-variceal upper-GI haemorrhage, is administered either PO or IV.[48] **Omeprazole** and **esomeprazole** have been used parenterally in palliative care to treat painful reflux oesophagitis in patients unable to take PO medication.

Although not authorized for SC administration, **omperazole** 40mg for infusion diluted as per IVI (see supply) has been given by CSCI over 3–4h for $\leqslant$4 days.[50,51]

After reconstitution, PPI injections/infusions are alkaline (pH 9–10.5) and should not be mixed with other drugs.

Supply
Lansoprazole (generic)
Capsules enclosing e/c granules 15mg, 30mg, 28 days @ 30mg each morning = £2.

Zoton® (Wyeth)
Tablets orodispersible (FasTab®) 15mg, 30mg, 28 days @ 30mg each morning = £6.

Omeprazole (generic)
Capsules enclosing e/c granules 10mg, 20mg, 40mg, 28 days @ 20mg each morning = £2.
Capsules enclosing e/c tablet 10mg, 20mg, 28 days @ 20mg each morning = £2; *do not open capsules.*
Tablets e/c 10mg, 20mg, 40mg, 28 days @ 20mg each morning = £5.
Tablets dispersible (e/c pellets) 10mg, 20mg, 40mg, 28 days @ 20mg each morning = £12.
Injection (as bolus) powder for reconstitution in 10mL of diluent provided. Give as a slow IV injection over 5min. 40mg vial with diluent = £5.
Infusion powder for reconstitution in 5mL of infusion fluid 0.9% saline or 5% glucose. Further dilute to 100mL and give IVI over at least 20–30min. 40mg vial = £5.

Losec® (AstraZeneca)
Capsules enclosing e/c granules 10mg, 20mg, 40mg, 28 days @ 20mg each morning = £12.
Tablets dispersible (multiple-unit pellet system, MUPS®) *enclosing e/c pellets* 10mg, 20mg, 40mg, 28 days @ 20mg each morning = £12.
Injection (as bolus) powder for reconstitution in 10mL of diluent provided. Give as a slow IV injection over 5min. 40mg vial with diluent = £5.
Infusion powder for reconstitution in 5mL of infusion fluid 0.9% saline or 5% glucose. Further dilute to 100mL.and give IVI over at least 20–30min. 40mg vial = £5.

Omeprazole e/c tablets are available as an OTC measure for heartburn.

For details of **esomeprazole, pantoprazole** *and* **rabeprazole**, *see BNF;* **esomeprazole** *and* **rabeprazole** *are significantly more expensive. Combination products of* **omeprazole** *with* **ketoprofen** *and* **esomeprazole** *with* **naproxen** *are also available.*

1 Frech EJ and Go MF (2009) Treatment and chemoprevention of NSAID-associated gastrointestinal complications. *Therapeutics and Clinical Risk Management.* **5**: 65–73.
2 Leontiadis GI et al. (2007) Systematic reviews of the clinical effectiveness and cost-effectiveness of proton pump inhibitors in acute upper gastrointestinal bleeding. *Health Technology Assessment.* **11**: iii–iv, 1–164.
3 Leontiadis GI et al. (2005) Systematic review and meta-analysis of proton pump inhibitor therapy in peptic ulcer bleeding. *British Medical Journal.* **330**: 568.
4 DTB (1997) Pantoprazole - a third proton pump inhibitor. *Drug and Therapeutics Bulletin.* **35**: 93–94.
5 Dammann H et al. (1993) The effects of lansoprazole, 30 or 60mg daily, on intragastric pH and on endocrine function in healthy volunteers. *Alimentary Pharmacology and Therapeutics.* **7**: 191–196.
6 Koop H et al. (1996) Intragastric pH and serum gastrin during administration of different doses of pantoprazole in healthy subjects. *European Journal of Gastroenterology and Hepatology.* **8**: 915–918.
7 Jaspersen D et al. (1998) A comparison of omeprazole, lansoprazole and pantoprazole in the maintenance treatment of severe reflux oesophagitis. *Alimentary Pharmacology and Therapeutics.* **12**: 49–52.
8 Zheng N (2009) Comparative study of omeprazole, lansoprazole, pantoprazole and esomeprazole for the system relief in patients with reflux oesophagitis. *World Journal of Gastroenterology.* **28**: 900–995.
9 Shi S and Klotz U (2008) Proton pump inhibitors: an update of their clinical use and pharmacokinetics. *European Journal of Clinical Pharmacology.* **64**: 935–951.
10 Pace F et al. (2007) A review of rabeprazole in the treatment of acid-related diseases. *Therapeutics and Clinical Risk Management.* **3**: 363–379.
11 Moules I et al. (1993) Gastric acid inhibition by the proton pump inhibitor lansoprazole is unaffected by food. *British Journal of Clinical Research.* **4**: 153–161.
12 Delhotal-Landes B et al. (1991) The effect of food and antacids on lansoprazole absorption and disposition. *European Journal of Drug Metabolism and Pharmacokinetics.* **3**: 315–320.
13 Andersson T (1990) Bioavailability of omeprazole as enteric coated (EC) granules in conjunction with food on the first and seventh days of treatment. *Drug Investigations.* **2**: 184–188.
14 Brummer RJM and Geerling BJ (1995) Acute and chronic effect of lansoprazole and omeprazole in relation to food intake. *Gut.* **37**: 127.
15 Schonhofer P (1994) Intravenous omeprazole and blindness. *Lancet.* **343**: 665.
16 Schonhofer P et al. (1997) Ocular damage associated with proton pump inhibitors. *British Medical Journal.* **314**: 1805.
17 Health Canada (2008). Available from: www.hc-sc.gc.ca/ahc-asc/media/advisories-avis/_2008/2008_34-eng.php
18 Kim JW et al. (2010) Proton pump inhibitors as a risk factor for recurrence of Clostridium difficile-associated diarrhea. *World Journal of Gastroenterology.* **16**: 3573–3577.
19 Cunningham R and Dial S (2008) Is over-use of proton pump inhibitors fuelling the current epidemic of Clostridium difficile-associated diarrhoea? *Journal of Hospital Infection.* **70**: 1–6.

20 Yearsley KA et al. (2006) Proton pump inhibitor therapy is a risk factor for Clostridium difficile-associated diarrhoea. Alimentary Pharmacology and Therapeutics. **24**: 613–619.

21 Dial S et al. (2005) Use of gastric acid suppressive agents and the risk of community acquired Clostridium difficile-associated diarrhoea. Journal of the American Medical Association. **294**: 2984–2995.

22 Cadle RM et al. (2007) Association of proton-pump inhibitors with outcomes in Clostridium difficile colitis. American Journal of Health System Pharmacy. **64**: 2359–2363.

23 Garey KW et al. (2008) Meta-analysis to assess risk factors for recurrent Clostridium difficile infection. Journal of Hospital Infection. **70**: 298–304.

24 Jump RL et al. (2007) Vegetative Clostridium difficile survives in room air on moist surfaces and in gastric contents with reduced acidity: a potential mechanism to explain the association between proton pump inhibitors and C. difficile-associated diarrhea? Antimicrobial Agents and Chemotherapy. **51**: 2883–2887.

25 Kwok CS et al. (2012) Risk of Clostridium difficile infection with acid suppressing drugs and antibiotics: meta-analysis. American Journal of Gastroenterology. **107**: 1011–1019.

26 Andersson T (1996) Pharmacokinetics, metabolism and interactions of acid pump inhibitors. Focus on omeprazole, lansoprazole and pantoprazole. Clinical Pharmacokinetics. **31**: 9–28.

27 Tucker G (1994) The interaction of proton pump inhibitors with cytochrome P450. Alimentary Pharmacology and Therapeutics. **8**: 33–38.

28 Baxter K and Preston CL Stockley's Drug Interactions. London: Pharmaceutical Press www.medicinescomplete.com (accessed October 2012).

29 Steinijans W (1996) Lack of pantoprazole drug interactions in man: an updated review. International Journal of Clinical Pharmacology and Therapeutics. **34**: S31–S50.

30 MHRA (2009) Public assessment report. Warfarin: changes to product safety information December 2009. Available from: www.mhra.gov.uk/home/groups/pl-p/documents/websiteresources/con065506.pdf

31 Kreutz RP et al. (2010) Impact of proton pump inhibitors on the effectiveness of clopidogrel after coronary stent placement: the clopidogrel Medco outcomes study. Pharmacotherapy. **30**:787–796.

32 Ho M et al. (2009) Risk of adverse outcomes associated with concomitant use of clopidogrel and proton pump inhibitors following acute coronary syndrome. Journal of the American Medical Association. **301**: 937–944.

33 Juurlink DN et al. (2009) A population-based study of the drug interaction between proton pump inhibitors and clopidogrel. Canadian Medical Association Journal. **180**: 713–718.

34 MHRA (2010) Clopidogrel and proton pump inhibitors: interaction - updated advice. Drug Safety Update **3**. www.mhra.gov.uk/safetyinformation

35 European Agency for the Evaluation of Medicinal Products (2004) Important new pharmacokinetic data demostrating that REYATAZ (atazanavir sulphate) combined with NORVIR (ritonavir) and omeprazole should not be co-administered. In: EMEA public statement. Available from: http://www.ema.europa.eu/docs/en_GB/document_library/Public_statement/2010/08/WC500095461.pdf

36 Baxter K (2012) Stockley's Drug Interactions (online edition). Pharmaceutical Press, London. Available from: www.medicinescomplete.com

37 MHRA (2012) Proton pump inhibitors in long term use: reports of hypomagnesaemia. Drug Safety Update **5**. www.mhra.gov.uk/safetyinformation

38 MHRA (2012) Proton pump inhibitors in long-term use: recent epidemiological evidence of increased risk of bone fracture. Drug Safety Update **5**. www.mhra.gov.uk/safetyinformation

39 Fohl AL and Regal RE (2011) Proton pump inhibitor-associated pneumonia: Not a breath of fresh air after all? World Journal of Gastrointestinal Pharmacology and Therapeutics. **2**: 17–26.

40 Moayyedi P (2006) Pharmacological interventions for non-ulcer dyspepsia. Cochrane Database of Systematic Reviews. **4**: CD001960.

41 Sigterman KE et al. (2013) Short-term treatment with proton pump inhibitors, H_2- receptor antagonists and prokinetics for gastro-oesophageal reflux disease-like symptoms and endoscopy negative reflux disease. Cochrane Database of Systematic Reviews. **5**: CD002095.

42 Rostom A et al. (2002) Prevention of NSAID-induced gastroduodenal ulcers. Cochrane Database of Systematic Reviews. **4**: CD002296.

43 Leontiadis G et al. (2010) Proton pump inhibitor treatment for acute peptic ulcer bleeding. Cochrane Database of Systematic Reviews. **5**: CD002094.

44 Sreedharan A et al. (2010) P.Proton pump inhibitor treatment initiated prior to endoscopic diagnosis in upper gastrointestinal bleeding. Cochrane Database of Systematic Reviews. **7**: CD005414. DOI.

45 Neumann I et al.(2013) Comparison of different regimens of proton pump inhibitors for acute peptic ulcer bleeding. Cochrane Database of Systematic Reviews. **6**: CD007999.

46 Wang Y et al. (2009) Additional bedtime H_2 receptor antagonist for control of nocturnal gastirc acid breakthrough. Cochrane Database of Systematic Reviews. **4**: CD004275.

47 NICE (2004) Dyspepsia. Management of dyspepsia in adults in primary care. Clinical Guideline CG17. www.nice.org.uk

48 NICE (2012) Acute upper gastrointestinal bleeding management. Clinical Guideline CG141. www.nice.org.uk

49 Zylicz Z and van Sorge A (1998) Rectal omeprazole in the treatment of reflux pain in esophageal cancer. Journal of Pain and Symptom Management. **15**: 144–145.

50 Desmidts T and Constans T (2009) Subcutaneous infusion of esomeprazole in elderly patients in palliative care: A report of two cases. Journal of the American Geriatrics Society. **57**: 1724–1725.

51 Agar M et al. (2004) The use of subcutaneous omeprazole in the treatment of dyspepsia in palliative care patients. Journal of Pain and Symptom Management. **28**: 529–531.

Updated (minor change) April 2014

LOPERAMIDE   BNF 1.4.2

Class: Antimotility drug.

Indications: Acute and chronic diarrhoea, †ileostomy (to improve faecal consistency).[1]

Contra-indications: Colitis (ulcerative, infective, or antibiotic-associated); acute dysentery; conditions where inhibition of peristalsis should be avoided because of a risk of ileus, megacolon or toxic megacolon.

Pharmacology

Loperamide is a potent μ-opioid receptor agonist (μ agonist).[2] Although well absorbed from the GI tract, loperamide is almost completely extracted and metabolized by cytochrome P450 in the liver (particularly CYP3A4) where it is conjugated, and the conjugates excreted in the bile. Because of this extensive first-pass metabolism, little loperamide reaches the systemic circulation.

The antidiarrhoeal action of loperamide results from direct absorption into the gut wall. Like **morphine** and other μ agonists, loperamide increases intestinal transit time by decreasing propulsive activity and increasing non-propulsive activity via its effect on the myenteric plexus in the longitudinal muscle layer.[3,4] Loperamide also increases anal sphincter tone and improves night-time continence in patients with ileo-anal pouches.[5]

Loperamide also modifies the intestinal transport of water and electrolytes by stimulating absorption,[6] and by an anti-secretory action mediated by calmodulin antagonism, a property not shared by other opioids.[7-9]

Paradoxically, loperamide reduces the sodium-dependent uptake of glucose and other nutrients from the small bowel.[10] The development of tolerance to the GI effects of loperamide has been demonstrated in animal studies.[11] However, loperamide has been successfully used in patients with chronic diarrhoea for several years without evidence of tolerance.[12]

Loperamide is a substrate for P-glycoprotein, the efflux membrane transporter in the blood-brain barrier; and, although highly lipophilic,[4] loperamide is actively excluded from the CNS.[13,14] Consequently, unlike **morphine** which has both central and peripheral constipating effects, loperamide generally acts only peripherally[2] (but see Drug interactions and Undesirable effects).

Loperamide has an effect on peripheral μ-opioid receptors activated by inflammation, and has been investigated as a possible *topical analgesic* for painful ulcers of the skin or mouth.[15,16] There are preliminary reports of the successful use of orodispersible tablets (Imodium® Instants) 2mg q3-2h p.r.n. as an adjuvant analgesic for oral pain from mucositis or cancer.[17] (Note: Imodium® *oral solution* contains alcohol and should *not* be used.) However, oral **morphine** solution (without alcohol) may be a better option, particularly long-term.

Unlike other drugs used for diarrhoea, e.g. **diphenoxylate** (in **co-phenotrope**) and **codeine**, loperamide has no analgesic effect in therapeutic and supratherapeutic doses. The lack of CNS effects is one reason why loperamide is a popular first-line choice for the control of diarrhoea, including when secondary to surgery, radiotherapy or chemotherapy.[18,19]

However, **octreotide** (see p.530) is recommended first-line for chemotherapy or radio-therapy-induced diarrhoea when severe (i.e. an increase of $\geqslant$7 stools/24h over baseline, hospital admission and IV fluids required for >24h), and second-line for less severe diarrhoea which does not respond to loperamide 16–24mg/24h.[18-20]

As an antidiarrhoeal, loperamide is about 3 times more potent mg for mg than **diphenoxylate** and 50 times more potent than **codeine**.[21] It is longer acting and, if used regularly, generally needs to be given only b.d. However, its maximum therapeutic impact may not manifest for 16–24h; this has implications for initial dosing.[14] The following regimens are approximately equivalent:

- loperamide 2mg b.d.
- **diphenoxylate** 2.5mg q.d.s. (in **co-phenotrope**)
- **codeine phosphate** 60mg q.d.s.

Loperamide is available in a range of formulations. Orodispersible tablets (Imodium® Instants), which melt on the tongue, are bio-equivalent to the capsules and are preferred by some patients. A combination product with **simeticone** provides more rapid relief of diarrhoea and abdominal discomfort from bloating in acute non-specific diarrhoea than either loperamide or **simeticone** alone.[22,23] One suggested explanation is that the surfactant effect of **simeticone** enhances the contact of loperamide with the gut mucosa. However, both these formulations are relatively expensive (see Supply).

Bio-availability ~0.3%.
Onset of action about 1h; maximum effect 16–24h.[24]
Time to peak plasma concentration 2.5h (oral solution); 5h (capsules).[25]
Plasma halflife 11h.[25]
Duration of action up to 3 days.[12]

Cautions

In severe diarrhoea, ensure adequate fluid and electrolyte replacement is given with loperamide, e.g. by using oral rehydration salts or, if necessary, IV fluids. Patients with AIDS are at risk of toxic megacolon if loperamide is used in viral or bacterial colitis.

A patient on **clozapine** (an atypical antipsychotic) died of toxic megacolon after taking loperamide during an episode of food poisoning. Additive inhibition of intestinal motility was considered the precipitating cause.[26]

Severe hepatic impairment can increase plasma concentrations of loperamide and the risk of undesirable effects, including depression of consciousness.[27] Depression of consciousness may also occur in children, particularly <2 years, who receive excessive doses[28,29] or after an unintentional overdose.[30] If **naloxone** is considered necessary, repeated doses may be needed because loperamide has a longer duration of action than **naloxone** (see p.455).

Imodium® *oral solution* contains Na^+ 4.85mg/5mL, which should be taken into account for patients on a sodium-controlled diet.

Drug interactions

CYP3A4 inhibitors (e.g. **erythromycin, fluconazole, quinidine** (not UK), **ritonavir**) can increase plasma concentrations of loperamide (see Chapter 25, Table 8, p.775).[27]

Inhibitors of P-glycoprotein (e.g. **ciclosporin, clarithromycin, erythromycin, itraconazole, quinidine** (not UK), **ritonavir, verapamil**) could potentially allow more loperamide to cross the blood-brain barrier and cause central opioid effects. Although one study in healthy volunteers of **quinidine** (not UK) with loperamide found a blunted respiratory response to CO_2 (indicating respiratory depression),[14] others have failed to demonstrate significant CNS effects.[31]

However, with typical doses of loperamide, it is unlikely that these interactions are clinically relevant.[31]

Undesirable effects

Common (<10%, >1%): headache, dizziness, nausea, flatulence, constipation.
Uncommon (<1%, >0.1%): drowsiness, dry mouth, dyspepsia, vomiting, abdominal pain or discomfort, rash.
Rare (<0.1%, >0.01%): fatigue, depression of consciousness, unco-ordination, hypertonia, abdominal distension, ileus, faecal impaction, megacolon, urinary retention, angioedema, pruritus, urticaria, bullous skin eruptions.

Dose and use

Ensure that the diarrhoea is not secondary to faecal impaction.

Acute diarrhoea
• start with 4mg PO stat
• continue with 2mg after each loose bowel action for up to 5 days
• maximum recommended dose 16mg/24h.

Chemotherapy- or radiotherapy-induced diarrhoea
• if mild–moderate, give 4mg stat and 2mg after each loose bowel action
• if not responding to doses of 24mg/24h, switch to **octreotide** (see p.530)
• if severe, use **octreotide** first-line (see p.530).

Chronic diarrhoea

If symptomatic treatment is appropriate, the same initial approach is used for 2–3 days, after which a prophylactic b.d. regimen is instituted based on the needs of the patient during the previous 24h, plus 2mg after each loose bowel action. The effective dose varies widely. In palliative care, it is occasionally necessary to increase the dose to as much as 32mg/24h; *this is twice the recommended maximum daily dose.*

Supply

Loperamide (generic)
Capsules 2mg, 28 days @ 2mg q.d.s. = £4.
Tablets 2mg, 28 days @2mg q.d.s. = £8.

Imodium® (Janssen)
Oral solution (sugar-free) 1mg/5mL, 28 days @ 2mg q.d.s. = £13; *contains alcohol*; also contains Na⁺ 4.85mg/5mL.

With **simeticone**

Imodium® Plus (McNeil)
Caplets (capsule-shaped tablets) containing loperamide 2mg, **simeticone** 125mg, 28 days @ 1 q.d.s. = £33 (based on 12-caplet pack); also available OTC: 12 caplets = £7.
Note: the following NHS brands can be bought OTC but are expensive: Imodium® Instant Melts, Imodium® Soft Capsules, Imodium® Plus Comfort tablets.

---

1   UK Medicines Information (2013) Can high dose loperamide be used to reduce stoma output? *Medicines Q & A.* **185.3**: www.evidence.nhs.uk

2   Shannon H and Lutz E (2002) Comparison of the peripheral and central effects of the opioid agonists loperamide and morphine in the formalin test in rats. *Neuropharmacology.* **42**: 253–261.

3   Van Nueten JM et al. (1979) Distribution of loperamide in the intestinal wall. *Biochemical Pharmacology.* **28**: 1433–1434.

4   Ooms L et al. (1984) Mechanisms of action of loperamide. *Scandinavian Journal of Gastroenterology.* **19 (Suppl 96)**: 145–155.

5   Hallgren T et al. (1994) Loperamide improves anal sphincter function and continence after restorative proctocolectomy. *Digestive Diseases and Sciences.* **39**: 2612–2618.

6   Dashwood MR et al. (1990) Autoradiographic demonstration of [3H] loperamide binding to opioid receptors in rat and human small intestine. *Progress in Clinical and Biological Research.* **328**: 165–169.

7   Merritt J et al. (1982) Loperamide and calmodulin. *Lancet.* **1**: 283.

8   Zavecz J et al. (1982) Relationship between anti-diarrheal activity and binding to calmodulin. *European Journal of Pharmacology.* **78**: 375–377.

9   Daly J and Harper J (2000) Loperamide: novel effects on capacitative calcium influx. *Celluar and Molecular Life Sciences.* **57**: 149–157.

10 Klaren P et al. (2000) Effect of loperamide on Na+/D-glucose cotransporter activity in mouse small intestine. *Journal of Pharmacy and Pharmacology.* **52**: 679–686.

11 Tan-No K et al. (2003) Development of tolerance to the inhibitory effect of loperamide on gastrointestinal transit in mice. *European Journal of Pharmaceutical Sciences.* **20**: 357–363.

12 Heel R et al. (1978) Loperamide: A review of its pharmacological properties and therapeutic efficacy in diarrhoea. *Drugs.* **15**: 33–52.

13 Heykants J et al. (1974) Loperamide (R 18553), a novel type of antidiarrheal agent. Part 5: The pharmacokinetics of loperamide in rats and man. *Arzneimittel-Forschung.* **24**: 1649–1653.

14 Sadeque A et al. (2000) Increased drug delivery to the brain by P-glycoprotein inhibition. *Clinical Pharmacology and Therapeutics.* **68**: 231–237.

15 Nozaki-Taguchi N et al. (2008) Potential utility of peripherally applied loperamide in oral chronic graft-versus-host disease related pain. *Japan Journal of Clinical Oncology.* **38**: 857–860.

16 Nozaki-Taguchi N and Yaksh TL (1999) Characterization of the antihyperalgesic action of a novel peripheral mu-opioid receptor agonist–loperamide. *Anesthesiology.* **90**: 225–234.

17 Regnard C (2011) Personal communication. St Oswald's Hospice, Newcastle.

18 Maroun JA et al. (2007) Prevention and management of chemotherapy-induced diarrhea in patients with colorectal cancer: a consensus statement by the Canadian Working Group on Chemotherapy-Induced Diarrhea. *Current Oncology.* **14**: 13–20.

19 Benson AB et al. (2004) Recommended Guidelines for the Treatment of Cancer Treatment-Induced Diarrhea *Journal of Clinical Oncology.* **22**: 2918–2926.

20 Bhattacharya S (2009) Octreotide in chemotherapy induced diarrhoea in colorectal cancer: a review article. *Acta Gastroenterologica Belgica.* **72**: 289–295.

21 Schuermans V et al. (1974) Loperamide (R18553), a novel type of antidiarrhoeal agent. Part 6: clinical pharmacology. Placebo-controlled comparison of the constipating activity and safety of loperamide, diphenoxylate and codeine in normal volunteers. *Arzneimittel-Forschung Drug Research.* **24**: 1653–1657.

22 Kaplan MA et al. (1999) Loperamide-simeticone vs loperamide alone, simeticone alone, and placebo in the treatment of acute diarrhea with gas-related abdominal discomfort. A randomized controlled trial. *Archives of Family Medicine.* **8**: 243–248.

23 Hanauer SB et al. (2007) Randomized, double-blind, placebo-controlled clinical trial of loperamide plus simethicone versus loperamide alone and simethicone alone in the treatment of acute diarrhea with gas-related abdominal discomfort. *Current Medical Research Opinion.* **23**: 1033–1043.

---

24 Dreverman JWM and van der Poel AJ (1995) Loperamide oxide in acute diarrhoea: a double-blind placebo-controlled trial. *Alimentary Pharmacology and Therapeutics.* **9**: 441–446.

25 Killinger J et al. (1979) Human pharmacokinetics and comparative bioavailability of loperamide hydrochloride. *Journal of Clinical Pharmacology.* **19**: 211–218.

26 Eronen M et al. (2003) Lethal gastroenteritis associated with clozapine and loperamide. *American Journal of Psychiatry.* **160**: 2242–2243.

27 Baker DE (2007) Loperamide: a pharmacological review. *Reviews in Gastroenterological Disorders.* **7 (Suppl 3)**: S11–18.

28 Friedli G and Haenggeli CA (1980) Loperamide overdose managed by naloxone. *Lancet.* **ii**: 1413.

29 Minton N and Smith P (1987) Loperamide toxicity in a child after a single dose. *British Medical Journal.* **294**: 1383.

30 Litovitz T et al. (1997) Surveillance of loperamide ingestions: an analysis of 216 poison center reports. *Journal of Toxicology and Clinical Toxicology.* **35**: 11–19.

31 Vandenbossche J et al. (2010) Loperamide and P-glycoprotein inhibition: assessment of the clinical relevance. *Journal of Pharmacy and Pharmacology.* **62**: 401–412.

Updated May 2014

LAXATIVES   BNF 1.6

There is limited RCT evidence about laxative use in palliative care patients.[1,2] Consequently, guidelines for the management of constipation in palliative care are based largely on consensus best practice and expert opinion.[2–5]

Constipation is common in advanced cancer,[1,6] and is generally caused by multiple factors, e.g. poor diet, weakness, the underlying disease, drugs (particularly opioids). It can be defined as the passage of small hard faeces infrequently and with difficulty,[5] and is characterized by:
- *slow GI transit*: prolonged transit time allows more absorption of water from the faeces by the GI tract, manifesting as decreased frequency of bowel movements and small hard faeces[7,8]
- *disordered rectal evacuation*: the need to strain when defaecating.[7]

The aims of drug management of constipation are:
- to restore the amount of water in the faeces by:
  ▷ reducing bowel transit time
  ▷ increasing faecal water
  ▷ increasing the ability of the faeces to retain water.
- to improve rectal evacuation by improving faecal consistency and promoting peristalsis.

There are two broad classes of laxatives: those acting predominantly as *faecal softeners* and those acting predominantly as *bowel stimulants* (Table 1).

Faecal softeners also increase faecal mass, and can thereby stimulate peristalsis. Further, **lactulose** (an osmotic laxative) is converted by colonic fermentation to organic acids which act as contact stimulants in the large bowel (see p.52).[9] Conversely, stimulant laxatives reduce water absorption from the faeces and thus have a softening action (see p.48).

Table 1 Classification of commonly used laxatives

Class of laxative	General mode of action	Common laxatives
Faecal softeners		
Surface-wetting agents	Act as a detergent, lowering surface tension, thereby allowing water and fats to penetrate hard, dry faeces	Docusate sodium Poloxamer 188 (in co-danthramer)
Osmotic laxatives	Water is retained in the gut lumen with a subsequent increase in faecal volume	Lactulose syrup Magnesium hydroxide suspension (Phillips' Milk of Magnesia®); sometimes combined with liquid paraffin (a lubricant), e.g. Mil-Par® Magnesium sulfate (Epsom Salts) Macrogols (e.g. Movicol®)

continued

Table I Continued

Class of laxative	General mode of action	Common laxatives
Stimulant laxatives	Act via direct contact with the submucosal and myenteric plexus, resulting in rhythmic muscle contractions and improved intestinal motility. Also increase water secretion into the bowel lumen	
	Acting on small and large bowel	Bisacodyl Dantron
	Acting on large bowel	Senna Sodium picosulfate
Lubricants	Coat the surface of the stool to make it more slippery and easier to pass	Liquid paraffin[a] Arachis oil
Bulk-forming agents (fibre)	Increases faecal bulk through water-binding and increasing bacterial cell mass. This causes intestinal distension and thereby stimulates peristalsis; only a limited role in palliative care	Ispaghula (psyllium) husk (e.g. Fybogel®, Regulan®) Methylcellulose (e.g. Celevac®) Sterculia (e.g. Normacol®)

a. limited role in palliative care due to potentially serious undesirable effects.

At doses commonly used, **docusate sodium** ($\leqslant$400mg/24h) acts mainly by lowering surface tension (enabling water and fats to penetrate into the substance of the faeces) but at higher doses it also acts as a stimulant laxative (see p.51).

To date, RCTs of laxatives in palliative care patients have failed to show clinically meaningful differences (Table 2). Two Cochrane reviews on the management of constipation in palliative care patients have concluded that there is inadequate experimental evidence to guide the optimal treatment of constipation with laxatives.[1,2]

Given the limited RCT evidence, the following should be noted:
- an appreciation of the pathophysiology of constipation (particularly opioid-induced),[5,16] and of how different laxatives work, and their cost will guide laxative choice
- generally, all laxatives given in sufficient quantities are capable of normalizing bowel function in constipated patients[17,18]
- compliance with laxative therapy may be limited in individual patients by palatability, undesirable effects (e.g. colic, flatulence), volume required, and polypharmacy. Patient preference and drug tolerability should be taken into account
- the concurrent prescription of several different laxatives should be avoided
- laxative doses should be titrated every 1–2 days according to response up to the maximum recommended or tolerable dose before changing to an alternative
- different laxatives from the same class may have slightly different effects/modes or action. Thus, of the stimulant laxatives, **senna** and **sodium picosulfate** act mainly in the large bowel, whereas **bisacodyl** and **dantron** act on both large and small bowel
- immobile patients with faecal incontinence are at risk of perineal skin irritation from **dantron**-containing laxatives
- anal seepage with associated irritation can be problematic with **liquid paraffin**. Absorption of **liquid paraffin** can also cause granulomatous reaction formation. Absorption is enhanced by concomitant use of **docusate sodium**
- traditionally a combination of a bowel stimulant with a faecal softener has been recommended in palliative care patients.[5,19] However, the results of the RCT which compared **senna** alone with **senna** and **docusate** in hospice patients (see Table 1)[14] and comparable results from a non-randomized non-blinded sequential cohort study in cancer inpatients[20] suggest that it is reasonable to prescribe a stimulant laxative alone, at least initially[15]

- if an adequate result is not achieved after 3–4 days using a stimulant laxative alone despite dose titration, consider adding a faecal softener
- if colic occurs, a softener should be added
- if faecal leakage occurs, the dose of the faecal softener will need to be reduced.[3,5]

Table 2 RCTs of laxatives in palliative care patients

Interventions	Sample size	Outcome
Senna and lactulose vs. co-danthramer (dantron and poloxamer)[10]	N = 51	Participants on high-dose strong opioids; those receiving senna and lactulose had more bowel evacuations compared with those receiving co-danthramer, but there was no difference in patient preference
Senna and lactulose vs. magnesium hydroxide and liquid paraffin (unpublished data)[11]	N = 118	No significant difference in efficacy outcomes between interventions
Senna vs. lactulose[12]	N = 75	No significant difference in efficacy outcomes between interventions
Senna vs. misrakasneham (Ayurvedic herbal remedy)[13]	N = 36	No significant difference in efficacy outcomes between interventions
Senna vs. senna and docusate[14]	N = 74	No significant difference between the groups, suggesting no benefit in routinely adding docusate. However, a high proportion of patients in each group required rescue rectal interventions (74% and 69%), suggesting neither treatment was very effective. Although the dose of senna could be titrated to response, the dose of docusate was fixed, and thus may not always have been optimal[15]

Rectal interventions (also see Rectal products for constipation, p.57)

About one third of patients also need rectal measures[21,22] either because of failed oral treatment or electively, e.g. in bedbound frail elderly patients, patients with paralysis (see p.46).

Rectal products available for the management of constipation include suppositories and enemas. As far as possible, rectal interventions should be avoided in patients who are neutropenic or thrombocytopenic because of the risk, respectively, of infection or bleeding.

Opioid-induced constipation

Opioids are a major contributory factor for constipation in palliative care patients, reducing quality of life, and sometimes resulting in opioid discontinuation.[23–25] Opioids cause constipation by increasing ring contractions, decreasing propulsive intestinal activity, and by enhancing the resorption of fluid and electrolytes.[26,27] Tolerance does not develop to these effects.[28] Although some strong opioids are possibly less constipating than **morphine** (e.g. **buprenorphine, fentanyl, methadone**), most patients receiving any opioid regularly will need a laxative concurrently.[1,29] Thus, as a general rule, all patients prescribed **morphine** (or other opioid) should also be prescribed a laxative (see p.44).

Methylnaltrexone, a peripherally-acting opioid antagonist, represents an additional approach to the management of opioid-induced constipation (see p.44 and p.456). A recent Cochrane review concluded that there is some evidence that, compared with placebo, **methylnaltrexone** is effective in patients taking opioids who have not had a good response with conventional laxatives.[2]

---

1 Miles CL et al. (2006) Laxatives for the management of constipation in palliative care patients. *Cochrane Database of Systematic Reviews.* **4**: CD003448.

2 Candy B et al. (2011) Laxatives or methylnaltrexone for the management of constipation in palliative care patients. *Cochrane Database of Systematic Reviews.* **19**: CD003448.

3 NICE (2013) Palliative cancer care - constipation. Clinical Knowledge Summaries http://cks.nice.org.uk

4 Librach SL et al. (2010) Consensus recommendations for the management of constipation in patients with advanced, progressive illness. *Journal of Pain and Symptom Management*. **40**: 761–773.

5 Larkin PJ et al. (2008) The management of constipation in palliative care: clinical practice recommendations. *Palliative Medicine*. **22**: 796–807.

6 Droney J et al. (2008) Constipation in cancer patients on morphine. *Supportive Care in Cancer*. **16**: 453–459.

7 Soligo M et al. (2006) Patterns of constipation in urogynecology: clinical importance and pathophysiologic insights. *American Journal of Obstetrics and Gynecology*. **195**: 50–55.

8 Lewis SJ and Heaton KW (1997) Stool form scale as a useful guide to intestinal transit time. *Scandinavian Journal of Gastroenterology*. **32**: 920–924.

9 Jouet P et al. (2008) Effects of therapeutic doses of lactulose vs. polyethylene glycol on isotopic colonic transit. *Alimentary Pharmacology and Therapeutics*. **27**: 988–993.

10 Ramesh P et al. (1998) Managing morphine-induced constipation: a controlled comparison of an Ayurvedic formulation and senna. *Journal of Pain and Symptom Management*. **16**: 240–244.

11 Tarumi Y et al. (2013) Randomized, double-blind, placebo-controlled trial of oral docusate in the management of constipation in hospice patients. *Journal of Pain and Symptom Management*. **45**: 2–13.

12 Sykes N (1991) A clinical comparison of lactulose and magnesium hydroxide and liquid paraffin emulsion in a palliative care population. [cited in Candy B et al. (2011) Laxatives or methylprednisolone for the management of constipation in palliative care patients. *Cochrane Database of Systematic Reviews*. CD003448.]

13 Agra Y et al. (1998) Efficacy of senna versus lactulose in terminal cancer patients treatment with opioids. *Journal of Pain and Symptom Management*. **15**: 1–7.

14 Sykes N (2013) Emerging evidence on docusate: commentary on Tarumi et al. *Journal of Pain and Symptom Management*. **45**: 1.

15 Clemens KE and Klaschik E (2008) Management of constipation in palliative care patients. *Current Opinion in Supportive and Palliative Care*. **2**: 22–27.

16 Fallon M and Hanks G (1999) Morphine, constipation and performace status in advanced cancer patients. *Palliative Medicine*. **13**: 159–160.

17 Sykes NP (1996) A volunteer model for the comparison of laxatives in opioid-related constipation. *Journal of Pain and Symptom Management*. **11**: 363–369.

18 Portenoy RK (1987) Constipation in the cancer patient: causes and management. *Medical Clinics of North America*. **71**: 303–311.

19 Hawley PH and Byeon JJ (2008) A comparison of sennosides-based bowel protocols with and without docusate in hospitalized patients with cancer. *Journal of Palliative Medicine*. **11**: 575–581.

20 Sykes N (1991) A clinical comparison of laxatives in a hospice. *Palliative Medicine*. **5**: 307–314.

21 Twycross RG and Lack SA (1986) *Control of Alimentary Symptoms in Far Advanced Cancer*. Churchill Livingstone, Edinburgh, pp. 173–174.

22 Twycross RG and Harcourt JMV (1991) The use of laxatives at a palliative care centre. *Palliative Medicine*. **5**: 27–33.

23 Sykes N (1998) The relationship between opioid use and laxative use in terminally ill cancer patients. *Palliative Medicine*. **12**: 375–382.

24 Bell T et al. (2009) Opioid-induced constipation negatively impacts pain management, productivity, and health-related quality of life: findings from the National Health and Wellness Survey. *Journal of Opioid Management*. **5**: 137–144.

25 Candrilli SD et al. (2009) Impact of constipation on opioid use patterns, health care resource utilization, and costs in cancer patients on opioid therapy. *Journal of Pain and Palliative Care Pharmacotherapy*. **23**: 231–241.

26 Beubler E (1983) Opiates and intestinal transport: in vivo studies. In: LA Turnberg (ed) *Intestinal secretion*. Smith Kline and French, Hertfordshire, pp. 53–55.

27 Kurz A and Sessler DI (2003) Opioid-induced bowel dysfunction: pathophysiology and potential new therapies. *Drugs*. **63**: 649–671.

28 Ross GR et al. (2008) Morphine tolerance in the mouse ileum and colon. *Journal of Pharmacology and Experimental Therapeutics*. **327**: 561–572.

29 Radbruch L et al. (2000) Constipation and the use of laxatives: a comparison between transdermal fentanyl and oral morphine. *Palliative Medicine*. **14**: 111–119.

Updated June 2014

Quick Prescribing Guide: Opioid-induced constipation

Generally, all patients prescribed an opioid should also be prescribed a stimulant laxative, with the aim of achieving a regular bowel movement, without straining, every 1–3 days. A standardized protocol aids management.

Sometimes, rather than automatically changing to the local standard laxative, it may be more appropriate to optimize a patient's existing regimen.

These guidelines can also be followed in patients who are not on opioids, although smaller doses may well suffice.

1 Ask about the patient's past and present bowel habit and use of laxatives; record the date of last bowel action.

2 Palpate for faecal masses in the line of the colon; examine the rectum digitally if the bowels have not been open for ≥3 days or if the patient reports rectal discomfort or has diarrhoea suggestive of faecal impaction with overflow.

3 For inpatients, keep a daily record of bowel actions.

4 Encourage fluids generally, and fruit juice and fruit specifically.

5 When an opioid is prescribed, prescribe senna (see below) or dantron-containing stimulant laxative (see overleaf), and titrate the dose according to response.

6 During dose titration and subsequently, if ≥3 days since last bowel action, give suppositories, e.g. bisacodyl 10mg and glycerol 4g, or a micro-enema. If these are ineffective, administer a phosphate enema and possibly repeat the next day.

7 If the maximum dose of the stimulant laxative is ineffective, halve the dose and add an osmotic laxative, then titrate as necessary, e.g.
   • macrogols (e.g. Movicol®) 1 sachet each morning or
   • lactulose 15mL once daily–b.d.

8 In a patient receiving opioids, if adequately titrated conventional laxatives fail to produce the desired response, consider SC methylnaltrexone (see below).

9 If the stimulant laxative causes bowel colic, divide the total daily dose into smaller more frequent doses or change to a faecal softener (see above), and titrate as necessary.

10 As initial treatment, a faecal softener is preferable in patients with a history of colic with stimulant laxatives.

Dose schedule for senna

• if *not* constipated:
   ▷ generally start with 15mg at bedtime
   ▷ if no response after 24–48h, increase to 15mg at bedtime and each morning
• if already constipated
   ▷ generally start with 15mg at bedtime and each morning
   ▷ if no response after 24–48h, increase to 22.5mg at bedtime and each morning
• if no response after a further 24–48h, consider adding a third daytime dose
• if necessary, consider increasing to a maximum of 30mg t.d.s.

Dose schedule for dantron-containing laxatives[a,b]				
	Co-danthramer strong capsules	Co-danthramer strong suspension	Co-danthrusate capsules	Co-danthrusate suspension
Dantron content	37.5mg/capsule	75mg/5mL	50mg/capsule	50mg/5mL
Start with:				
• prophylactic	1 at bedtime	2.5mL at bedtime	1 at bedtime	5mL at bedtime
• if constipated	2 at bedtime	5mL at bedtime	2 at bedtime	10mL at bedtime
If necessary, adjust every 2–3 days up to:				
	3 t.d.s.	10mL b.d. or 20mL at bedtime	3 b.d.	15mL b.d.
Total daily dose	337.5mg	300mg	300mg	300mg

a. because dantron has been linked with liver and bowel tumours in rodents, dantron-containing laxatives are licensed for use only in the 'terminally ill'

b. in patients with urinary or faecal incontinence, dantron-containing laxatives are best avoided because of the risk of a contact skin burn in the perineum and surrounding areas.

Methylnaltrexone

Methylnaltrexone is relatively expensive (£21 per 12mg vial) and should be considered only when the optimum use of laxatives is ineffective. Because constipation in advanced disease is generally multifactorial in origin, methylnaltrexone is likely to augment rather than replace laxatives.

• marketed as a SC injection for use in patients with 'advanced illness' and opioid-induced constipation despite treatment with laxatives
• about 1/3–1/2 of patients given methylnaltrexone have a bowel movement within 4h, without loss of analgesia or the development of opioid withdrawal symptoms
• dose recommendations:
  ▷ for patients weighing 38–61kg, start with 8mg on alternate days
  ▷ for patients weighing 62–114kg, start with 12mg on alternate days
  ▷ outside this range, give 150microgram/kg on alternate days
  ▷ the interval between administrations can be varied, either extended or reduced, but not more than once daily
• in severe renal impairment (creatinine clearance <30mL/min) reduce the dose:
  ▷ for patients weighing 62–114kg, reduce to 8mg
  ▷ outside this range, reduce to 75microgram/kg, rounding up the dose volume to the nearest 0.1mL
• methylnaltrexone is contra-indicated in cases of known or suspected bowel obstruction. It should be used with caution in patients with conditions which may predispose to perforation. Common undesirable effects include abdominal pain/colic, diarrhoea, flatulence, and nausea; these generally resolve after a bowel movement; postural hypotension can also occur.

Updated June 2014

Quick Prescribing Guide: Bowel management in paraplegia and tetraplegia

Theoretically, management is determined by the level of the spinal cord lesion:
- above T12–L1 = cauda equina intact → spastic GI tract with preserved sacral reflex; generally responds to digital stimulation of the rectum; the presence of an anal reflex suggests an intact sacral reflex
- below T12–L1 = cauda equina involved → flaccid GI tract; generally requires digital evacuation of the rectum
- a lesion at the level of the conus medullaris (the cone shaped distal end of the spinal cord, surrounded by the sacral nerves) may manifest a mixture of clinical features.

However, in practice, management tends to follow a common pathway.

Aims

1 Primary: to achieve the controlled regular evacuation of normal formed faeces:
- every day in long-term paraplegia/tetraplegia, e.g. post-traumatic
- every 1–3 days in advanced cancer.

2 Secondary: to prevent both incontinence (faeces too soft, over-treatment with laxatives) and an anal fissure (faeces too hard, under-treatment with laxatives).

Oral measures

3 In debilitated patients with a poor appetite, a bulking agent is unlikely to be helpful, and may result in a soft impaction.

4 Particularly if taking morphine or another constipating drug, an oral stimulant laxative should be prescribed, e.g. senna 15mg b.d., bisacodyl tablets 5–10mg b.d. The dose should be carefully titrated to a level which results in normal faeces *in the rectum* but without causing an uncontrolled evacuation.

5 In relatively well patients with a good appetite (probably the minority):
- maintain a high fluid intake
- encourage a high roughage diet, e.g. wholegrain cereals, wholemeal foods, greens, bran or a bulk-forming laxative, e.g. ispaghula.

6 Beware:
- the prescription of docusate sodium, a faecal softener, may result in a soft faecal impaction of the rectum, and faecal leakage through a patulous anus
- oral bisacodyl in someone not on opioids may cause multiple uncontrolled evacuations, at the wrong time and in the wrong place.

Rectal measures

7 Initially, if impacted with faeces, empty the rectum digitally. Then, develop a daily routine:
- as soon as convenient after waking up in the morning, insert 2 glycerol suppositories, or 1–2 bisacodyl suppositories (10–20mg), or an osmotic micro-enema deep into the rectum, and wait for 1.5–2 hours
- because the bisacodyl acts only after absorption and biotransformation, bisacodyl suppositories must be placed against the rectal wall, and not into faeces
- the patient should be encouraged to have a hot drink after about 1h in the hope that it will stimulate a gastro-colonic reflex
- if there is a strong sacral reflex, some faeces will be expelled as a result of the above two measures
- to ensure complete evacuation of the rectum and sigmoid colon, digitally stimulate the rectum:
  ▷ insert gloved and lubricated finger (either soap or gel)
  ▷ rotate finger 3–4 times
  ▷ withdraw and wait 5min
  ▷ if necessary, repeat 3–4 times
  ▷ check digitally that rectum is fully empty.

8 Patients who are unable to transfer to the toilet or a commode will need nursing assistance. Sometimes it is easiest for a patient to defaecate onto a pad while in bed in a lateral position.

9 If the above measures do not achieve complete evacuation of the rectum and sigmoid colon, proceed to digital evacuation (more likely with a flaccid bowel). A pattern will emerge for each patient, allowing the rectal measures to be adjusted to the individual patient's needs and response.

Updated June 2014

ISPAGHULA (PSYLLIUM) HUSK   BNF 1.6.1

Ispaghula husk is *not recommended* for patients taking constipating drugs, and in those with decreasing dietary intake and activity. However, it can be helpful in regulating the consistency of faeces (making them more formed) in a patient with a colostomy/distal ileostomy.

Class: Bulk-forming laxative.

Indications: Colostomy/ileostomy regulation, anal fissure, haemorrhoids, diverticular disease, irritable bowel syndrome, ulcerative colitis.

Contra-indications: Dysphagia, bowel obstruction, colonic atony, faecal impaction.

Pharmacology
Ispaghula (psyllium) is derived from the husks of an Asian plant, *Plantago ovata*. It has very high water-binding capacity, is partly fermented in the colon, and increases bacterial cell mass, thereby further increasing faecal bulk. Like other bulk-forming laxatives, ispaghula stimulates peristalsis by increasing faecal mass. Its water-binding capacity also helps to make loose faeces more formed in some patients with a colostomy/distal ileostomy.
Onset of action full effect obtained only after several days.
Duration of action best taken regularly to obtain a consistent ongoing effect; may continue to act for 2–3 days after the last dose.

Cautions
Adequate fluid intake should be maintained to avoid bowel obstruction.

Undesirable effects
Flatulence, abdominal distension, faecal impaction, bowel obstruction.

Dose and use
Ispaghula swells in contact with fluid and needs to be drunk quickly before it absorbs water. Stir the granules or powder briskly in 150mL of water and swallow immediately; carbonated water can be used if preferred. Alternatively, the granules can be swallowed dry, or mixed with a vehicle such as jam, but must be followed by 100–200mL of water. Give 1 sachet each morning–t.d.s., preferably after meals; not immediately before going to bed.

Supply
Fybogel® (Reckitt Benckiser)
Oral powder 3.5g/sachet, 28 days @ 1 sachet b.d. = £4; *low Na⁺; sugar- and gluten-free; plain, lemon or orange flavour.*

Regulan® (Procter & Gamble)
Oral powder 3.4g/sachet, 28 days @ 1 sachet b.d. = £ 4.50; *sugar- and gluten-free; orange or lemon-lime flavour.*

This is not a complete list; see BNF for more information.

Updated June 2014

STIMULANT LAXATIVES BNF1.6.2

Indications: Prevention and treatment of constipation.

Contra-indications: Severe dehydration, acute inflammatory bowel disease, large bowel obstruction.

Pharmacology

Stimulant laxatives vary in terms of onset times, sites of action, and undesirable effects, depending on where in the GI tract the parent drug is converted to its active metabolite. Stimulant laxatives act through direct contact with the submucosal (Meissner's) plexus and the deeper myenteric (Auerbach's) plexus, resulting in both a secretory and a motor effect in the large intestine. The motor effect precedes the secretory effect, and is the more important laxative action. There is a decrease in segmenting muscular activity and an increase in propulsive waves.

Senna (sennosides) is a naturally-occurring plant-derived anthranoid. It is an inactive glycoside which passes unabsorbed and unchanged through the small intestine and is hydrolyzed by *bacterial glycosidases* in the large intestine to yield active compounds.[1] Thus, **senna** has no effect on the small intestine but becomes active in the large intestine. Differences in bacterial flora may be partly responsible for differences in individual responses.

Dantron, a synthetic anthranoid, is not a glycoside and has a direct action on the small intestine as well as the large intestine.[2] Whereas systemic absorption of **senna** or its metabolites is small, **dantron** is absorbed to some extent from the small intestine with subsequent significant urinary excretion.

Phenolics such as **bisacodyl** and **sodium picosulfate** are also pro-drugs. They are hydrolyzed to the same active metabolite but the mode of hydrolysis differs.[1] **Bisacodyl** is hydrolyzed by *intestinal enzymes* and thus acts on both the small and large intestines. When applied directly to the intestinal mucosa in normal subjects, **bisacodyl** induces powerful propulsive motor activity within minutes.[3] **Bisacodyl** is often given by suppository. The laxative effect is the result of local direct contact with the rectal mucosa after dissolution of the suppository, and after activation by hydrolysis. Thus the minimum time for response is generally >20min.[4] In contrast, **sodium picosulfate** is hydrolyzed by *colonic bacteria* and its action is thus confined to the large intestine. Its activity is potentially more uncertain because it depends on bacterial flora.

Phenolphthalein is another stimulant laxative, and is present in some proprietary laxatives. **Phenolphthalein** exists in two forms: white and yellow. The yellow form contains several impurities produced during manufacture. These impurities enhance the laxative effect of **phenolphthalein** so that the comparable dose of the yellow form is only two thirds that of the pure white form. The active constituent of **phenolphthalein** is released in two stages: by metabolism in the liver and subsequently in the colon, and it probably undergoes enterohepatic circulation.[5] Some people respond to small doses. However, it can cause a drug rash (see Undesirable effects) and is generally not considered a first-line laxative.

To date, RCTs of stimulant laxatives in palliative care patients have failed to show clinically meaningful differences (see Laxatives, Table 2, p.42). A small non-blinded dose-ranging study in palliative care patients with opioid-induced constipation, showed that **sodium picosulfate** alone yielded a satisfactory result in 15/20 patients (normal stool consistency, no need for enemas, suppositories or manual evacuation, and no noteworthy undesirable effects).[6]

Traditionally a combination of a bowel stimulant with a stool softener has been recommended in palliative care patients.[7,8] However, the results of the RCT which compared **senna** alone with senna and docusate in hospice patients (see Laxatives, Table 2, p.42)[9] and comparable results from a non-randomized non-blinded sequential cohort study in cancer inpatients suggest that it is reasonable to prescribe a stimulant laxative alone, at least initially.[10] In countries where combined products are not available, this also reduces the patient's tablet load.[11]

If a stimulant laxative is used alone but an adequate result is not achieved despite dose titration within a week, consider adding a faecal softener. If faecal leakage occurs, the dose of the faecal softener will need to be reduced.[7,12]

Onset of action
Bisacodyl tablets 6–12h;[4] suppositories 20–60min.
Dantron 6–12h.
Senna 8–12h.
Sodium picosulfate 6–24h (median 12h).[6]

Cautions

Because very high doses in rodents revealed a carcinogenic risk,[13–15] UK marketing authorizations for laxatives containing **dantron** are limited to constipation in terminally ill patients.

Undesirable effects

Intestinal colic, diarrhoea. **Bisacodyl** suppositories may cause local rectal inflammation. **Dantron** discolours urine, typically red but sometimes green or bluish. It may also stain the peri-anal skin. Prolonged contact with skin (e.g. in urinary or faecally incontinent patients) may cause a **dantron** burn (a red erythematous rash with a definite edge); if ignored, this may cause painful excoriation.

Phenolphthalein occasionally causes a drug rash or photosensitivity. Rarely, it causes encephalitis which can be fatal.

Dose and use

The doses recommended here for opioid-induced constipation are often higher than those featured in the BNF and SPCs. For frail patients not receiving opioids or other constipating drugs, the PO starting doses of a stimulant laxative will generally be lower.

Because round-the-clock opioids constipate, b.d. or t.d.s. laxatives may well be necessary, rather than the traditional once daily dose (at bedtime or each morning). Requirements do not correlate closely with the opioid dose; individual titration is necessary.

All palliative care services should have a protocol for the management of opioid-induced constipation (see Quick Prescribing Guide, p.44).[16–19] Likewise, there is need for a protocol for patients with paraplegia and tetraplegia (see Quick Prescribing Guide, p.46).

Bisacodyl
• start with 10–20mg PO at bedtime
• if necessary, increase by stages to 20mg PO t.d.s.
• by suppository: 10–20mg PR once daily.

Dantron
Variable, according to preparation, individual need and patient acceptance (see Quick Prescribing Guide, p.44).

Senna
• if *not* constipated:
  ▷ generally start with 15mg at bedtime
  ▷ if no response after 24–48h, increase to 15mg at bedtime and each morning
• if already constipated:
  ▷ generally start with 15mg at bedtime and each morning
  ▷ if no response after 24–48h, increase to 22.5mg at bedtime and each morning
• if no response after a further 24–48h, consider adding a third daytime dose
• if necessary, consider increasing to a maximum of 30mg t.d.s.

Sodium picosulfate
- start with 5–10mg (5–10mL of oral solution) at bedtime; 10mg if taking regular opioids
- if necessary, increase daily by 5mg until a satisfactory result is achieved
- median satisfactory dose = 15mg at bedtime
- typical maximum dose = 30mg.[6]

Consider a lower dose b.d. in the frail elderly.

Supply
Bisacodyl (generic)
Tablets e/c 5mg, 28 days @ 10mg at bedtime = £2.
Suppositories 10mg, 28 days @ 10mg once daily = £8.

Dantron
Co-danthramer (dantron and **poloxamer 188)** (generic)

Co-danthramer suspension 5mL = 1 **co-danthramer** capsule.
Co-danthramer suspension 15mL = 5mL *strong* **co-danthramer** suspension.
Strong **co-danthramer** suspension 5mL = 2 *strong* **co-danthramer** capsules.

Capsules co-danthramer 25/200 (**dantron** 25mg, **poloxamer 188** 200mg), 28 days @ 2 at bedtime = £12.

Strong capsules co-danthramer 37.5/500 (**dantron** 37.5mg, **poloxamer 188** 500mg), 28 days @ 2 at bedtime = £15.

Oral suspension co-danthramer 25/200 in 5mL (**dantron** 25mg, **poloxamer 188** 200mg/5mL), 28 days @ 10mL at bedtime = £96.

Strong oral suspension co-danthramer 75/1000 in 5mL (**dantron** 75mg, **poloxamer 188** 1g/5mL), 28 days @ 5mL at bedtime = £117.

Co-danthrusate (dantron and **docusate sodium)** (generic)
Capsules co-danthrusate 50/60 (**dantron** 50mg, **docusate sodium** 60mg), 28 days @ 2 at bedtime = £29.

Oral suspension co-danthrusate 50/60 in 5mL (**dantron** 50mg, **docusate sodium** 60mg/5mL), 28 days @ 10mL at bedtime = £126.

Senna (generic)
Tablets total **sennosides**/tablet 7.5mg, 28 days @ 15mg at bedtime = £10.

Senokot® (Reckitt Benckiser)
Tablets total **sennosides**/tablet 7.5mg (NHS).
Oral solution (sugar-free) total **sennosides** 7.5mg/5mL, 28 days @ 10mL at bedtime = £1.50.

Sodium picosulfate (generic)
Oral solution (elixir) 5mg/5mL, 28 days @ 10mL at bedtime = £5; *contains alcohol.*

Note: **sodium picosulfate** oral solution 5mg/5mL is available as Dulcolax® Pico liquid. The proprietary name Dulcolax® (NHS) is also used for **bisacodyl** tablets and suppositories.

1 Jauch R et al. (1975) Bis-(p-hydroxyphenyl)-pyridyl-2-methane: the common laxative principle of bisacodyl and sodium picosulfate. *Arzneimittel-Forschung Drug Research.* **25**: 1796–1800.
2 Lennard-Jones J (1994) Clinical aspects of laxatives, enemas and suppositories. In: M Kamm and J Lennard-Jones (eds) *Constipation.* Wrightson Biomedical Publishing, Petersfield, pp. 327–341.
3 De Schryver AM et al. (2003) Effects of a meal and bisacodyl on colonic motility in healthy volunteers and patients with slow-transit constipation. *Digestive Diseases Sciences.* **48**: 1206–1212.
4 Flig E et al. (2000) Is bisacodyl absorbed at all from suppositories in man? *International Journal of Pharmaceutics.* **196**: 11–20.
5 Godding EW (1975) Constipation and allied disorders: 3. Therapeutic agents-chemical laxatives (section 2). *Pharmaceutical Journal.* **215**: 60–62.
6 Twycross RG et al. (2006) Sodium picosulfate in opioid-induced constipation: results of an open-label, prospective, dose-ranging study. *Palliative Medicine.* **20**: 419–423.

7 Larkin PJ et al. (2008) The management of constipation in palliative care: clinical practice recommendations. Palliative Medicine. **22**: 796–807.

8 Portenoy RK (1987) Constipation in the cancer patient: causes and management. Medical Clinics of North America. **71**: 303–311.

9 Tarumi Y et al. (2013) Randomized, double-blind, placebo-controlled trial of oral docusate in the management of constipation in hospice patients. Journal of Pain and Symptom Management. **45**: 2–13.

10 Sykes N (2013) Emerging evidence on docusate: commentary on Tarumi et al. Journal of Pain and Symptom Management. **45**: 1.

11 Hawley PH and Byeon JJ (2008) A comparison of sennosides-based bowel protocols with and without docusate in hospitalized patients with cancer. Journal of Palliative Medicine. **11**: 575–581.

12 NICE (2013) Palliative cancer care - constipation. Clinical Knowledge Summaries. http://cks.nice.org.uk

13 Mori H et al. (1985) Induction of intestinal tumours in rats by chrysazin. British Journal of Cancer. **52**: 781–783.

14 Mori H et al. (1986) Carcinogenicity of chrysazin in large intestine and liver of mice. Japanese Journal of Cancer Research (Gann). **77**: 871–876.

15 CSM (Committee on Safety of Medicines and Medicines Control Agency) (2000) Danthron restricted to constipation in the terminally ill. Current Problems in Pharmacovigilance. **26 (May)**: 4.

16 Levy MH (1996) Pharmacologic treatment of cancer pain. New England Journal of Medicine. **335**: 1124–1132.

17 Pappagallo M (2001) Incidence, prevalence, and management of opioid bowel dysfunction. American Journal of Surgery. **182 (Suppl 5A)**: 11s–18s.

18 Bouvy ML et al. (2002) Laxative prescribing in relation to opioid use and the influence of pharmacy-based intervention. Journal of Clinical Pharmacy and Therapeutics. **27**: 107–110.

19 Herndon CM et al. (2002) Management of opioid-induced gastrointestinal effects in patients receiving palliative care. Pharmacotherapy. **22**: 240–250.

Updated June 2014

DOCUSATE SODIUM   BNF 1.6.2

Class: Surface-wetting agent (faecal softener).

Indications: Constipation, haemorrhoids, anal fissure, bowel preparation before abdominal radiography, †partial bowel obstruction.

Pharmacology

Although sometimes classified as a stimulant laxative, docusate sodium is principally an emulsifying and wetting agent and has a relatively weak effect on GI transit. Other wetting agents include **poloxamer 188** (in **co-danthramer**). Docusate lowers surface tension, thereby allowing water and fats to penetrate hard, dry faeces. It also stimulates fluid secretion by the small and large intestines.[1,2] Docusate does not interfere with protein or fat absorption.[3] Docusate has been evaluated in several groups of elderly patients; frequency of defaecation increased and the need for enemas decreased almost to zero.[4–6] Given these clinical results, it is surprising that, in a study in normal subjects, docusate did not increase faecal weight.[7]

In palliative care, docusate is generally *not* recommended as the sole laxative except in patients with partial bowel obstruction. The routine combination of docusate (or alternative surface- wetting agent) and a stimulant laxative has been criticized because of a lack of published data supporting such a regimen.[8] A non-randomized non-blinded sequential cohort study in cancer inpatients failed to show any benefit when docusate was added to **senna**.[9] A more recent 10-day blinded RCT in hospice patients of docusate and **senna** vs **senna** alone likewise showed no significant difference.[10] However, a high proportion of patients in each group required rescue rectal interventions (around 70%), suggesting neither treatment was fully effective. The dose of **senna** could be titrated to response but the dose of docusate was fixed (200mg b.d.), and this may not have been optimal for some patients.[11] On the other hand, it is a high dose in terms of typical UK practice with stimulant-softener laxative combination regimens (e.g. **co-danthrusate**) for opioid-induced constipation.

Onset of action 1–2 days.

Cautions

Docusate enhances the absorption of **liquid paraffin**;[12] combined preparations of these substances are prohibited in some countries.

Undesirable effects

Diarrhoea, nausea, abdominal cramp, rashes. Docusate oral solution may cause a bitter aftertaste or burning sensation, minimized by drinking plenty of water after taking the solution.

Dose and use

At many centres, docusate is used in combination with a stimulant laxative, e.g. **senna, bisacodyl** or **dantron** (in **co-danthrusate**) (see Quick Prescribing Guide, p.44). Docusate is often used alone for patients with persistent partial bowel obstruction. Dose varies according to individual need:

* generally start with 100mg b.d.
* if necessary, increase to 200mg b.d.–t.d.s.; *the latter is higher than the BNF maximum dose of 500mg/day*.

Docusate can also be used as an enema (see Rectal products for constipation, p.57).

Supply

Dioctyl® (UCB Pharma)
Capsules 100mg, 28 days @ 100mg b.d. = £4 (based on 100-capsule pack).

Docusol® (Typharm)
Oral solution (sugar-free) 50mg/5mL, 28 days @ 10mL b.d. = £10.

1 Donowitz M and Binder H (1975) Effect of dioctyl sodium sulfosuccinate on colonic fluid and electrolyte movement. *Gastroenterology.* **69**: 941–950.
2 Moriarty K et al. (1985) Studies on the mechanism of action of dioctyl sodium sulphosuccinate in the human jejunum. *Gut.* **26**: 1008–1013.
3 Wilson J and Dickinson D (1955) Use of dioctyl sodium sulfosuccinate (aerosol O.T.) for severe constipation. *Journal of the American Medical Association.* **158**: 261–263.
4 Cass L and Frederik W (1956) Doxinate in the treatment of constipation. *American Journal of Gastroenterology.* **26**: 691–698.
5 Harris R (1957) Constipation in geriatrics. *American Journal of Digestive Diseases.* **2**: 487–492.
6 Hyland C and Foran J (1968) Dicotyl sodium sulphosuccinate as a laxative in the elderly. *Practitioner.* **200**: 698–699.
7 Chapman R et al. (1985) Effect of oral dioctyl sodium sulfosuccinate on intake-output studies of human small and large intestine. *Gastroenterology.* **89**: 489–493.
8 Hurdon V et al. (2000) How useful is docusate in patients at risk for constipation? A systematic review of the evidence in the chronically ill. *Journal of Pain and Symptom Management.* **19**: 130–136.
9 Hawley PH and Byeon JJ (2008) A comparison of sennosides-based bowel protocols with and without docusate in hospitalized patients with cancer. *Journal of Palliative Medicine.* **11**: 575–581.
10 Tarumi Y et al. (2013) Randomized, double-blind, placebo-controlled trial of oral docusate in the management of constipation in hospice patients. *Journal of Pain and Symptom Management.* **45**: 2–13.
11 Sykes N (2013) Emerging evidence on docusate: commentary on Tarumi et al. *Journal of Pain and Symptom Management.* **45**: 1.
12 Godfrey H (1971) Dangers of dioctyl sodium sulfosuccinate in mixtures. *Journal of the American Medical Association.* **215**: 643.

Updated June 2014

LACTULOSE   BNF 1.6.4

Class: Osmotic laxative.

Indications: Constipation, hepatic encephalopathy.

Contra-indications: Intestinal obstruction, galactosaemia.

Pharmacology

Lactulose is a synthetic disaccharide, a combination of galactose and fructose, which is not absorbed by the small intestine.[1] It is a 'small bowel flusher', i.e. through an osmotic effect lactulose deposits a large volume of fluid into the large intestine. Lactulose is fermented by colonic bacteria to organic acids which act as contact stimulants in the large bowel.

The low pH discourages the proliferation of ammonia-producing organisms and thus reduces the absorption of ammonium ions and other nitrogenous compounds; hence its use in hepatic encephalopathy.[2]

Lactulose has been shown to be more effective than increasing dietary fibre.[3] It also increases colonic bacterial flora, i.e. is prebiotic (whereas **macrogols** are not).[4] Lactulose does not affect the management of diabetes mellitus; 15mL of Duphalac® (NHS) contains 14 calories. However, because bio-availability is negligible, the number of calories absorbed is negligible. (Note: other generic products may differ.)

In a small RCT in palliative care patients receiving high-dose strong opioids, those given a combination of lactulose and **senna** had more bowel evacuations compared with those given **co-danthramer**, but there was no difference in patient preference.[5] In healthy volunteers, lactulose alone was effective in opioid-induced constipation, but the volumes required (mean 55mL b.d.) is likely to preclude widespread use.[6]

A Cochrane review of lactulose and **macrogols** for chronic constipation concluded that **macrogols** are better than lactulose in terms of bowel movements per week, faecal consistency, relief of abdominal pain, and the need for additional products.[7] This review included 10 trials, with a total of nearly 900 patients, aged 3 months to 70 years. However, the volume per dose of **macrogols** is 5–10 times greater than lactulose (see p.54), which will be unacceptable to many patients. Lactulose is also cheaper.

Bio-availability negligible.
Onset of action up to 48h.

Cautions
Lactose intolerance.

Undesirable effects
Abdominal bloating, flatulence (generally only in the first few days of treatment), nausea (may be reduced if diluted with water or fruit juice, or taken with meals), intestinal colic.

Dose and use
Lactulose can be used in patients who experience intestinal colic with stimulant laxatives, or who fail to respond to stimulant laxatives alone:
- start with 15mL b.d. and adjust according to need
- in hepatic encephalopathy, start with 30–50mL t.d.s. and adjust the dose to produce 2–3 soft evacuations per day.

Supply
Lactulose (generic)
Oral solution 10g/15mL, 28 days @ 15mL b.d. = £5.

1 Schumann C (2002) Medical, nutritional and technological properties of lactulose. An update. *European Journal of Nutrition*. **41 (Suppl 1)**: 117–25.
2 Zeng Z et al. (2006) Influence of lactulose on the cognitive level and quality of life in patients with minimal hepatic encephalopathy. *Chinese Journal of Clinical Rehabilitation*. **10**: 165–167.
3 Quah HM et al. (2006) Prospective randomized crossover trial comparing fibre with lactulose in the treatment of idiopathic chronic constipation. *Techniques in Coloproctology*. **10**: 111–114.
4 Bouhnik Y et al. (2004) Prospective, randomized, parallel-group trial to evaluate the effects of lactulose and polyethylene glycol-4000 on colonic flora in chronic idiopathic constipation. *Alimentary Pharmacology and Therapeutics*. **19**: 889–899.
5 Sykes N (1991) A clinical comparison of laxatives in a hospice. *Palliative Medicine*. **5**: 307–314.
6 Sykes NP (1996) A volunteer model for the comparison of laxatives in opioid-related constipation. *Journal of Pain and Symptom Management*. **11**: 363–369.
7 Lee-Robichaud H et al. (2011) Lactulose versus polyethylene glycol for chronic constipation. *Cochrane Database of Systematic Reviews*. **7**: CD007570.

Updated June 2014

MACROGOLS (POLYETHYLENE GLYCOLS) BNF 1.6.4

Class: Osmotic laxative.

Indications: Constipation, faecal impaction (macrogol 3350 sachets).

Contra-Indications: Severe inflammatory bowel conditions, bowel obstruction, paralytic ileus.

Pharmacology

Macrogol 3350 and 4000 are available in the UK (the numbers refer to their respective molecular weights). They act by virtue of an osmotic action in the intestines. Due to the large molecular structure of the macrogol, water is not transported across the bowel wall out of the lumen and hence the volume of the macrogol solution is retained within the lumen to soften the stool directly and stimulate peristalsis indirectly (by producing an increase in faecal volume).

Macrogols are unchanged in the GI tract, virtually unabsorbed and have no known pharmacological activity. Any absorbed macrogols are excreted via the urine; no reduction is required in renal impairment. Macrogols reduce colonic bacterial flora, whereas the use of **lactulose** causes an increase.[1]

Most studies have used isotonic solutions. Adding more water to make a hypotonic (dilute) solution of macrogols is as effective as an isotonic solution in treating constipation but causes hyponatraemia.[2] There are no data on the effect on appetite of the volume of fluid needed with macrogols.

There are no studies in chronic constipation comparing macrogols with stimulant laxatives. However, when clearing the colon before colonoscopy, macrogols are inferior to stimulant laxatives.[3,4]

In an RCT in opioid-induced constipation, macrogols were found to be no better than **lactulose**.[5] On the other hand, a Cochrane review of macrogols and **lactulose** for chronic constipation in adults and in children concluded that macrogols are better than **lactulose** in terms of bowel movements per week, faecal consistency, relief of abdominal pain (children only), and the need for additional products.[6] An earlier systematic review also favoured macrogols.[7] However, the volume per dose of macrogols is 5–10 times greater than **lactulose** (see p.52); this will be unacceptable to many seriously ill patients.

In a second systematic review limited to chronic constipation in children, macrogols were found to be little better than other treatments.[8] Further, in childhood faecal impaction, they are no better than enemas, and cause more faecal incontinence.[9] Children also find macrogols less palatable than **lactulose**.[10] Macrogols are also more expensive.

Onset of action 1–2 days for constipation; 1–3 days for faecal impaction.

Cautions

Macrogol 3350: stop treatment if symptoms of fluid and electrolyte shift occur (see Undesirable effects).

Macrogol 3350 *concentrated oral liquid* contains both benzyl alcohol and ethanol. Because the dose required for faecal impaction would exceed the maximum acceptable daily intake of benzyl alcohol, this formulation is not authorized for faecal impaction, and the manufacturer's maximum recommended dose for constipation is 25mL (diluted with 100mL of water) t.d.s.

Undesirable effects

Uncommon (<1%, >0.1%): abdominal bloating, discomfort, borborygmi, hyponatraemia (when used as a hypotonic solution), nausea.

Very rare (<0.01%): severe electrolyte shift (oedema, shortness of breath, heart failure, dehydration).

Frequency unknown: hyper- or hypokalaemia (macrogol 3350 with electrolytes).

Dose and use

Macrogols are generally supplied as powder in sachets. A concentrated oral liquid is also available, but is not authorized for faecal impaction (see Cautions). All formulations need to be dissolved or diluted in water. For adults:

- macrogol 3350 (with electrolytes), dissolve one sachet in half a glass of water (about 125mL) or dilute 25mL of the concentrated oral liquid with 100mL water (total volume 125mL)
- macrogol 4000 (without electrolytes), dissolve in a glass of water (about 250mL). Half-strength macrogol 3350 sachets (with electrolytes) are available for fine-tuning the dose. Paediatric sachets are also available for children aged ≤12 years (see *BNF for Children*).

Constipation

The solution is generally used immediately after reconstitution or dilution. However, reconstituted macrogol 3350 sachets can be kept (covered) for up to 6h in a refrigerator, and the diluted oral liquid concentrate can be kept (covered) for 24h at room temperature:

- start with 1 sachet or 125mL of *diluted* oral liquid concentrate daily
- if necessary, increase to:
  ▷ 1 sachet or 125mL of *diluted* oral liquid concentrate b.d.–t.d.s. (macrogol 3350)
  ▷ 2 sachets each morning. or 1 sachet b.d. (macrogol 4000).

Faecal impaction

Macrogol 3350:

- start with 8 sachets on day 1, each dissolved in 125mL of water, and taken in <6h (total 1L)
- *patients with cardiovascular impairment should restrict intake to 2 sachets/h, i.e. 250mL/h*
- if necessary, repeat on days 2 and 3; most patients do not need the full dose on the second day.

For convenience, all 8 sachets can be made up together in 1L of water and kept in a refrigerator for a maximum of 6h, after which any remaining solution should be discarded.

Supply

Macrogol 3350 (generic)
Oral powder macrogol 3350 13.125g, sodium bicarbonate 178.5mg, sodium chloride 350.7mg, potassium chloride 46.6mg/sachet, 28 days @ 1 sachet once daily = £6; *orange flavour (Laxido®) or lemon flavour (Molaxole®)*.

Movicol® (Norgine)
Oral powder macrogol 3350 13.125g, sodium bicarbonate 178.5mg, sodium chloride 350.7mg, potassium chloride 46.6mg/sachet, 28 days @ 1 sachet once daily = £6; *lime-lemon flavour. Also available in plain (sugar-free) and chocolate flavour.*
Concentrated oral liquid macrogol 3350 13.125g, sodium bicarbonate 178.5mg, sodium chloride 350.7mg, potassium chloride 46.6mg/25mL, 28 days @ 25mL (diluted with 100mL water) once daily = £6; *orange flavour, contains alcohol.*

Movicol-Half® (Norgine)
Oral powder (sugar-free) macrogol 3350 6.563g, sodium bicarbonate 89.3mg, sodium chloride 175.4mg, potassium chloride 23.3mg/sachet, 28 days @ 1 sachet once daily = £4; *lime-lemon flavour.*

Macrogol 4000 Dulcobalance® (Boehringer Ingelheim)
Oral powder (sugar-free) macrogol 4000 10g/sachet, 28 days @ 1 sachet once daily = £8; *orange-grapefruit flavour. Available OTC.*

1 Bouhnik Y et al. (2004) Prospective, randomized, parallel-group trial to evaluate the effects of lactulose and polyethylene glycol-4000 on colonic flora in chronic idiopathic constipation. *Alimentary Pharmacology and Therapeutics.* 19: 889–899.
2 Seinela L et al. (2009) Comparison of polyethylene glycol with and without electrolytes in the treatment of constipation in elderly institutionalized patients: a randomized, double-blind, parallel-group study. *Drugs and Aging.* 26: 703–713.
3 Radaelli F et al. (2005) High-dose senna compared with conventional PEG-ES lavage as bowel preparation for elective colonoscopy: a prospective, randomized, investigator-blinded trial. *American Journal of Gastroenterology.* 100: 2674–2680.
4 Valverde A et al. (1999) Senna vs polyethylene glycol for mechanical preparation the evening before elective colonic or rectal resection: a multicenter controlled trial. French Association for Surgical Research. *Archives of Surgery.* 134: 514–519.
5 Freedman MD et al. (1997) Tolerance and efficacy of polyethylene glycol 3350/electrolyte solution versus lactulose in relieving opiate induced constipation: a double-blinded placebo-controlled trial. *Journal of Clinical Pharmacology.* 37: 904–907.
6 Lee-Robichaud H et al. (2010) Lactulose versus polyethylene glycol for chronic constipation. *Cochrane Database of Systematic Reviews.* 7: CD007570.

7 Ramkumar D and Rao SS (2005) Efficacy and safety of traditional medical therapies for chronic constipation: systematic review. *American Journal of Gastroenterology.* **100**: 936–971.
8 Pijpers MA *et al.* (2009) Currently recommended treatments of childhood constipation are not evidence based: a systematic literature review on the effect of laxative treatment and dietary measures. *Archives of Disease in Childhood.* **94**: 117–131.
9 Bekkali NL *et al.* (2009) Rectal fecal impaction treatment in childhood constipation: enemas versus high doses oral PEG. *Pediatrics.* **124**: e1108–1115.
10 Voskuijl W *et al.* (2004) PEG 3350 (Transipeg) versus lactulose in the treatment of childhood functional constipation: a double blind, randomised, controlled, multicentre trial. *Gut.* **53**: 1590–1594.

Updated June 2014

MAGNESIUM SALTS BNF 1.6.4

Class: Osmotic laxative.

Indications: Constipation, particularly in patients who experience intestinal colic with stimulant laxatives, or who fail to respond to the latter.

Contra-indications: Severe renal impairment.

Pharmacology

Magnesium ions are poorly absorbed from the gut. Their action is mainly osmotic but other factors may be important, e.g. the release of cholecystokinin.[1,2] Magnesium ions also decrease absorption or increase secretion in the small bowel.

Magnesium salts are generally not used first line in palliative care patients as they may be unpredictably effective. Magnesium sulfate is more potent than magnesium hydroxide and tends to produce a large volume of liquid faeces. In patients with idiopathic constipation, magnesium salts often lead to a sense of distension and the sudden passage of offensive liquid faeces which is socially inconvenient; it is difficult to adjust the dose to produce a normal soft result. However, when used as an osmotic laxative in conjunction with a stimulant laxative in opioid-induced constipation, this is not generally a problem.

An RCT of magnesium hydroxide and **liquid paraffin** vs. **senna** and **lactulose** failed to differentiate between the two combination treatments.[3]

Cautions

Risk of hypermagnesaemia in patients with renal impairment.

Drug interactions

Oral magnesium salts act as antacids and the resulting increase in gastric pH may affect the absorption of several drugs if taken concurrently (see p.2).

Dose and use

Magnesium hydroxide mixture BP

For opioid-induced constipation (see Quick Prescribing Guide, p.44), as an alternative to **lactulose** when an osmotic laxative is indicated:

- if the maximum dose of a stimulant laxative (e.g. **dantron, senna**) is ineffective, halve the dose and add magnesium hydroxide 15–30mL b.d., and titrate as necessary
- alternatively, switch completely to magnesium hydroxide 15–60mL b.d.

Magnesium hydroxide (or **lactulose**) may be preferable in patients with a history of colic with stimulant laxatives (see p.48).

Magnesium sulfate

A typical dose is 5–10g of crystals (one or two 5mL spoonfuls) once daily *before breakfast*; dissolve in about 250mL of warm water.

Supply
All the preparations below are available OTC.

Magnesium Hydroxide Mixture BP
Oral suspension hydrated magnesium oxide 415mg (7.1mmol elemental magnesium)/5mL, available OTC as Phillips' Milk of Magnesia®; *do not store in a cold place.*

Magnesium sulfate
Oral powder (Epsom Salts), also Original Andrew's Salts® (magnesium sulfate, citric acid, sodium bicarbonate).
Oral solution magnesium sulfate (Epsom Salts) 5g/10mL, locally prepared.

---

1 Donowitz M (1991) Magnesium-induced diarrhea and new insights into the pathobiology of diarrhea. *New England Journal of Medicine.* **324**: 1059–1060.
2 Harvey R and Read A (1975) Mode of action of the saline purgatives. *American Heart Journal.* **89**: 810–813.
3 Sykes N (1991) A clinical comparison of lactulose and senna with magnesium hydroxide and liquid paraffin emulsion in a palliative care population. [cited in Candy B *et al.* (2011) Laxatives or methylprednisolone for the management of constipation in palliative care patients. *Cochrane Database of Systematic Reviews.* CD003448.]

Updated June 2014

RECTAL PRODUCTS FOR CONSTIPATION   BNF 1.6.2–1.6.4

Indications: Constipation and faecal impaction if oral laxatives are ineffective or not feasible.

Pharmacology
The evidence base for laxative suppositories and enemas in palliative care is generally limited to clinical experience and retrospective studies. Survey data indicate that about one third of palliative care patients receiving opioids require rectal measures (laxative suppositories, enemas and/or digital evacuation) either regularly and electively, or intermittently and p.r.n., generally in addition to laxatives PO (Table 1).[1] However, the need for enemas and digital evacuation has decreased since the introduction of **macrogols** (see p.54).[2,3]

Table 1   Rectal measures for the relief of constipation or faecal impaction[a]

Rectal laxative	Predominant mode of action	Time to effect[b]
Suppositories[c] *(place in contact with rectal mucosa)*		
Bisacodyl 10mg	Stimulates propulsive activity after hydrolysis by enteric enzymes[4]	20–45min
Glycerol 4g	Hygroscopic; softens and lubricates	15–30min
Enemas *(warm to room temperature before use)*		
Osmotic micro-enema (5mL volume)	Faecal softener and osmotic effect (see text below)	15min
Osmotic standard phosphate enema (118–128mL volume)	Osmotic effect	2–5min
Docusate sodium micro-enema	Faecal softener (surface-wetting agent), some direct stimulant action	5–20min
Arachis (peanut) oil retention enema (130mL volume)	Faecal softener	Overnight retention enema

a. PR digital examination will indicate what is the most appropriate intervention
b. as stated in SPC
c. suppositories should be administered only if there are faeces in the rectum.

There is evidence supporting the use of **bisacodyl** suppositories in postoperative ileus[5] and in pre-colonoscopy preparations,[6] and of **docusate sodium** enemas in spinal injury patients.[7] In practice, for soft faeces, a **bisacodyl** suppository is given on its own; and, for hard faeces, **glycerol** alone or **glycerol** plus **bisacodyl**.

The laxative effect of **bisacodyl** is the result of local direct contact with the rectal mucosa after dissolution of the suppository and after activation by enteric enzymes (see p.48). The minimum time for response is thus generally >20min, and may be up to 3h.[8] Defaecation a few minutes after the insertion of a **bisacodyl** suppository is the result of anorectal stimulation. Bisacodyl suppositories occasionally cause faecal leakage, even after a successful evacuation.

Osmotic *micro-enemas* contain sodium citrate and **sodium lauryl sulfoacetate** with several excipients, including **glycerol** and **sorbitol**. **Sodium lauryl sulfoacetate** is a faecal softener (surface-wetting agent) similar to docusate sodium (see p.51), whereas **sodium citrate** draws fluid into the intestine by osmosis, an action enhanced by **sorbitol**.

Osmotic standard enemas contain phosphates. These should be used with caution in elderly patients because of a risk of serious electrolyte disturbances. Fatalities have been reported.[9]

When treating a hard faecal impaction, a **docusate sodium** micro-enema will help to soften the faecal mass. This should be instilled into the rectum and retained overnight before giving a stimulant suppository (**bisacodyl**) or an osmotic enema (Table 1).

An **arachis (peanut) oil** retention enema is sometimes used in patients with a hard faecal impaction: instil and leave overnight before giving a stimulant laxative suppository or an osmotic enema. *Do not use in patients with peanut allergy.*

Digital evacuation is the ultimate approach to faecal impaction but is a distressing procedure and may need sedation. Distress can be reduced by explaining the procedure, using plenty of lubrication, and encouraging the patient to respond to any urge to defaecate.

Supply
Suppositories
Glycerol BP
Glycerol 700mg, gelatin 140mg/1g, adult suppositories 4g, 28 days @ 4g once daily = £7; available OTC.

Bisacodyl (generic) 10mg, 28 days @ 10mg once daily = £8.Dulcolax® (Boehringer Ingelheim) 10mg, 28 days @ 10mg once daily = £4.50 (NHS); available OTC.

Micro-enemas
Faecal softener, Norgala® (Norgine), **docusate sodium** 120mg in 10g single-use disposable pack, 1 enema = £0.50.

Osmotic, **sodium citrate**, **sodium lauryl sulphoacetate**, **glycerol** and **sorbitol**, supplied in 5mL single-dose disposable packs with nozzle:
Micolette® (Pinewood), Micralax® (RPH), Relaxit® (Crawford), 5mL = £0.50.

Standard enemas
Phosphate enema BP Formula B (generic), **sodium acid phosphate** 12.8g, **sodium phosphate** 10.24g in 128mL, 1 enema with standard tube = £3, 1 enema with long rectal tube = £10.

Fleet® Ready-to-use enema (De Witt), **sodium acid phosphate** 21.4g, **sodium phosphate** 9.4g in 118mL, 1 enema with standard tube = £0.50.

Oil retention enema
Arachis Oil retention enema (generic), **arachis (peanut) oil** in 130mL single-dose disposable pack, 130mL = £8; *do not use in patients with peanut allergy.*

1 Twycross RG and Harcourt JMV (1991) The use of laxatives at a palliative care centre. *Palliative Medicine.* **5**: 27–33.
2 Goldman M (1993) Hazards of phosphate enemas. *Gastroenterology Today.* **3**: 16–17.
3 Culbert P *et al.* (1998) Highly effective oral therapy (polyethylene glycol/electrolyte solution) for faecal impaction and severe constipation. *Clinical Drug Investigation.* **16**: 355–360.
4 von Roth W and von Beschke K (1988) Pharmakokinetik und laxierende wirkung von bisacodyl nach gabe verschiedener zubereitungsformen. *Arzneimittel Forschung Drug Research.* **38**: 570–574.

5 Wiriyakosol S et al. (2007) Randomized controlled trial of bisacodyl suppository versus placebo for postoperative ileus after elective colectomy for colon cancer. *Asian Journal of Surgery.* **30**: 167–172.

6 Rapier R and Houston C (2006) A prospective study to assess the efficacy and patient tolerance of three bowel preparations for colonoscopy. *Gastroenterology Nursing.* **29**: 305–308.

7 Amir I et al. (1998) Bowel care for individuals with spinal cord injury: comparison of four approaches. *Journal of Spinal Cord Medicine.* **21**: 21–24.

8 Flig E et al. (2000) Is bisacodyl absorbed at all from suppositories in man? *International Journal of Pharmaceutics.* **196**: 11–20.

9 Ori Y et al. (2012) Fatalities and severe metabolic disorders associated with the use of sodium phosphate enemas: a single center's experience. *Archives of Internal Medicine.* **172**: 263–265.

Updated (minor change) April 2014

PRODUCTS FOR HAEMORRHOIDS BNF 1.7 & 15.2

Because haemorrhoids can be more troublesome if associated with the evacuation of hard faeces, constipation must be corrected (see Laxatives, p.40).

Peri-anal pruritus, soreness and excoriation are generally best treated by the application of a bland ointment or cream. Suppositories are often not effective because they are inserted into the rectum, bypassing the anal canal where the medication is needed.

For haemorrhoids, products containing mild astringents (e.g. **bismuth subgallate, zinc oxide, hamamelis (witch hazel)**) often provide symptomatic relief. Some products, not featured here, also contain vasoconstrictors and/or antiseptics.

Lidocaine ointment is used mainly to relieve pain associated with an anal fissure, but will also relieve pruritus ani. Alternative local anaesthetics include **pramocaine (pramoxine)** and **cinchocaine (dibucaine)**. Painful spasm of the internal anal sphincter is often eased by topical glyceryl trinitrate ointment (off-label use, p.79).

Local anaesthetic ointments are absorbed through the anal mucosa but, given the amount of ointment likely to be used, there is no realistic risk of systemic toxicity.[1] However, local anaesthetic ointments should be used for only a few days because all 'caines' can cause contact dermatitis.

Corticosteroids may be helpful if local inflammation is exacerbating discomfort. Infection (bacterial, viral, e.g. *Herpes simplex* or fungal, e.g. candidosis) must first be excluded, and treatment generally limited to 7–10 days because prolonged use with excessive amounts can lead to atrophy of the anal skin. However, this is unlikely with low concentration hydrocortisone.

Dose and use
Topical products should be applied:
- t.d.s.–q.d.s. for the first 24h
- then b.d. and after defaecation for 5–7 days, or longer if necessary
- then daily for 3–5 days after symptoms have cleared.

Products containing a local anaesthetic (to ease painful defaecation) are best applied 15–20min before defaecation, and p.r.n.

Supply
The following list is highly selective. Other OTC products are also available.

Astringent
Anusol® (McNeil)
Ointment zinc oxide, bismuth subgallate, **Peru balsam, bismuth oxide** 25g. (Available OTC).

Local anaesthetic
Lidocaine (generic)
Ointment 5%, 15g = £6.

Corticosteroid plus astringent
Anusol HC® (McNeil)
Ointment hydrocortisone acetate 0.25%, **zinc oxide, benzyl benzoate, bismuth oxide, bismuth subgallate, Peru balsam** 30g = £3. (Also available OTC as Anusol Plus HC ointment).

Corticosteroid plus local anaesthetic
Scheriproct® (Bayer)
Ointment cinchocaine hydrochloride 0.5%, **prednisolone hexanoate** 0.19%, 30g = £3.

Corticosteroid plus local anaesthetic and astringent
Xyloproct® (Astra Zeneca)
Ointment (water miscible) **aluminium acetate** 3.5%, **hydrocortisone acetate** 0.275%, **lidocaine** 5%, **zinc oxide**, 20g (with applicator) = £4.

---

1 Brosh-Nissimov T et al. (2004) Central nervous system toxicity following topical skin application of lidocaine. *European Journal of Clinical Pharmacology*. **60**: 683–684.

Updated December 2013

PANCREATIN BNF 1.9.4

Class: Enzyme supplement.

Indications: †Symptomatic steatorrhoea caused by biliary and/or pancreatic obstruction.

Pharmacology
Steatorrhoea (the presence of undigested faecal fat) typically results in pale, bulky, offensive, frothy and greasy faeces which flush away with difficulty, associated with abdominal distension, increased flatus, weight loss, and mineral and vitamin deficiency (A, D, E and K).

Pancreatin is a standardized preparation of porcine lipase, protease and amylase. Pancreatin hydrolyzes fats to glycerol and fatty acids, degrades protein into amino acids, and converts starch into dextrin and sugars. Because it is inactivated by gastric acid, pancreatin is best taken with food (or immediately before or after food).

Reducing gastric acid by concurrently prescribing a PPI leads to greater efficacy.[1] With gastro-resistant (e/c) granules, acid reduction is generally unnecessary provided the granules are swallowed whole without chewing.[2] However, in patients who are not adequately controlled on high-dose gastro-resistant pancreatin (e.g. ⩾120,000 units of lipase/24h), concurrent prescription of a PPI generally leads to improvement.[3,4]

On the other hand, mixing e/c granules with alkaline foods or drinks, or crushing or chewing them before swallowing, destroys the gastro-resistant coating. This causes release of the enzymes in the mouth, possible stomatitis, and reduced efficacy.

Cautions
Fibrotic strictures of the colon have developed in children with cystic fibrosis who have used certain high-strength pancreatin products. This has not been reported in adults or in patients without cystic fibrosis; Creon® has not been implicated.

Undesirable effects
Very common (>10%): abdominal pain.
Common (<10%, >1%): nausea and vomiting, constipation or diarrhoea.

Dose and use
There are several different pancreatin products, of which Creon® is a good choice. Capsule strength denotes lipase unit content, e.g. Creon® 10,000 contains 10,000 units. The dose is adjusted upwards according to faecal size, consistency, and frequency:
- generally start with Creon® 10,000 1–2 capsules with each meal
- if a smaller dose is required, use Creon® Micro; this contains 5,000 units of lipase in 100mg of granules
- if necessary, change to a higher strength capsule.

The granules in the capsules are gastro-resistant (e/c). The capsules may be swallowed whole, or the contents sprinkled onto slightly acidic fluid or soft food, e.g. fruit juice or apple sauce, and *swallowed without chewing:*

- avoid very hot food or drinks because heat inactivates pancreatin
- do not mix the capsule contents with alkaline foods or drinks, e.g. dairy products, because this degrades the gastro-resistant coating
- take immediately after mixing because the gastro-resistant coating dissolves if left to stand.

Extra capsules may be needed if snacks are taken between meals. If the pancreatin continues to be ineffective, prescribe a PPI or H_2-receptor antagonist concurrently, and review.

Supply

Creon® (Abbott Healthcare) A standardized product obtained from pigs; *there is no non-porcine alternative.*

Capsules enclosing gastro-resistant granules Creon® 10,000, lipase 10,000 units, amylase 8,000 units, protease 600 units, 28 days @ 2 t.d.s. = £22.

Creon® 25,000, lipase 25,000 units, amylase 18,000 units, protease 1,000 units, 28 days @ 2 t.d.s. = £47.

Creon® 40,000, lipase 40,000 units, amylase 25,000 units, protease 1,600 units, 28 days @ 2 t.d.s. = £95.

If smaller doses are required:

Gastro-resistant granules Creon® Micro, lipase 5,000 units, amylase 3,600 units, protease 200 units in 100mg, (measuring scoop provided), 28 days @ 200mg t.d.s. = £26.

1 Vecht J et al. (2006) Efficacy of lower than standard doses of pancreatic enzyme supplementation therapy during acid inhibition in patients with pancreatic exocrine insufficiency. *Journal of Clinical Gastroenterology.* **40**: 721–725.

2 Stead RJ et al. (1988) Treatment of steatorrhoea in cystic fibrosis: a comparison of enteric-coated microspheres of pancreatin versus non-enteric-coated pancreatin and adjuvant cimetidine. *Alimentary Pharmacology and Therapeutics.* **2**: 471–482.

3 Proesmans M and De Boeck K (2003) Omeprazole, a proton pump inhibitor, improves residual steatorrhoea in cystic fibrosis patients treated with high dose pancreatic enzymes. *European Journal of Pediatrics.* **162**: 760–763.

4 Dominguez-Munoz JE et al. (2006) Optimising the therapy of exocrine pancreatic insufficiency by the association of a proton pump inhibitor to enteric coated pancreatic extracts. *Gut.* **55**: 1056–1057.

Updated January 2014

2: CARDIOVASCULAR SYSTEM

This chapter features cardiovascular drugs used in palliative *cancer* care. It does *not* include guidance about the drug treatment of end-stage congestive heart failure (CHF). Also see Chapter 16, p.675.

More detailed guidance about caring for patients with end-stage CHF is available from NICE[1] and various other authorities.[2–4] Additional resources include:
- *Heart Failure: From advanced disease to bereavement*[5]
- *Supportive Care in Heart Failure*[6]
- *Heart Failure and Palliative Care: a team approach.*[7]

Unlike cancer, where disease-specific treatment tends to become increasingly burdensome and futile (and possibly counterproductive), the continued disease-specific treatment of CHF continues to be essential for symptom management even when end-stage.

Note: CHF can be a concurrent cause of breathlessness in some cancer patients, which needs to be recognized and treated appropriately.

1 NICE (2010) Chronic heart failure: management of chronic heart failure in adults in primary and secondary care. *Clinical Guideline* CG108. www.nice.org.uk
2 Arnold JM et al. (2006) Canadian Cardiovascular Society consensus conference recommendations on heart failure 2006: diagnosis and management.[erratum appears in Canadian Journal of Cardiology. 2006 Mar 1;22(3):271]. *Canadian Journal of Cardiology.* 22: 23-45.
3 Swedberg K et al. (2005) Guidelines for the diagnosis and treatment of chronic heart failure: full text (update 2005). European Heart Journal. Available from: 10.1093/eurheartj/ehi205
4 Hunt SA et al. (2005) Guideline Update for the Diagnosis and Management of Chronic Heart Failure in the Adult. ACC/AHA. Available from: http://circ.ahajournals.org/cgi/content/full/112/12/e154
5 Johnson M et al. (eds) (2013) Heart Failure: From advanced disease to bereavement. Oxford University Press, Oxford.
6 Beattie J and Goodlin S (eds) (2008) *Supportive Care in Heart Failure.* Oxford University Press, Oxford.
7 Johnson MJ and Lehman R (eds) (2006) *Heart Failure and Palliative Care: a team approach.* Radcliffe Publishing Ltd., Oxford.

FUROSEMIDE   BNF 2.2.2

Class: Loop diuretic.

Indications: Oedema, hypertension (unresponsive to usual treatments), †malignant ascites associated with portal hypertension and hyperaldosteronism (with **spironolactone**), †bronchorrhoea.

Pharmacology

Furosemide inhibits Na^+ (and hence water) resorption from the ascending limb of the loop of Henlé in the renal tubule. It also increases urinary excretion of K^+, H^+, Cl^- and Mg^{2+}. Diuretics such as furosemide are used to treat fluid overload in CHF in order to improve symptoms.[1–3]

In ascites caused by a *transudate* associated with cirrhosis, extensive liver metastases and portal hypertension, furosemide alone has little effect, even when used in total daily doses of 100–200mg PO.[4,5] Thus the use of furosemide in ascites is best limited to concurrent use with **spironolactone**, when the latter alone is insufficient (see p.68).

A diuretic-induced reduction in plasma volume can activate several neurohumoral systems, e.g. renin-aldosterone-angiotensin, resulting in impaired renal perfusion and increased Na^+ and water resorption. These changes reduce the effect of the diuretic and contribute to renal impairment. **Octreotide** 300microgram SC b.d. (see p.530) can suppress this diuretic-induced activation of the renin-aldosterone-angiotensin system and its addition has improved renal function and Na^+ and water excretion in patients with cirrhosis and ascites receiving furosemide and **spironolactone.**[6,7]

There is current interest in the use of *nebulized* furosemide for the treatment of breathlessness (Box A). However, a review of 42 trials concluded that there was insufficient evidence to currently support its routine use.[8] Further, in one study,[9] 5/7 patients reported a deterioration in their breathing after furosemide. It is thus recommended that the use of nebulized furosemide is restricted to closely controlled circumstances. Anecdotally, nebulized furosemide is of benefit in bronchorrhea.[10]

Box A Nebulized furosemide for breathlessness

Experimentally-induced cough and breathlessness
Allergen-induced asthma
Nebulized furosemide 20–40mg attenuates cough and breathlessness,[11-13] possibly via an effect on vagal sensory nerve endings. The reduction in breathlessness may result from increasing sensory traffic to the brain stem from sensitized slowly adapting pulmonary stretch receptors. However, the effect:
• has not been demonstrated consistently
• shows wide interindividual variability
• is of short duration (generally <2h)
• systemic absorption can be sufficient to induce a diuresis.[14-16]

COPD
Compared with placebo in moderate–severe COPD, nebulized furosemide has reduced breathlessness ± increased exercise time during endurance testing,[17,18] but *not* incremental exercise testing.

The mechanism underlying the benefit is unclear, but improvements are seen in airway function (e.g. slow vital capacity at rest) and dynamic ventilatory mechanics (e.g. inspiratory capacity and breathing pattern).[18] Although small but significant bronchodilation was seen in one study,[17] this is unlikely to be a direct effect of nebulized furosemide.

When given alongside initial 'standard' treatment for an exacerbation of COPD, nebulized furosemide results in additional improvement in breathlessness and various respiratory parameters.[19] However, it does not have an established role in this setting.

Cancer
In patients with cancer, nebulized furosemide has been used to relieve severe breathlessness.[20,21] However, RCTs have failed to show benefit.[9,22]

In heart failure, compared with bolus IV doses, furosemide by CIVI appears to provide a greater diuresis with a similar or better safety profile.[23,24] However, the data are inconsistent and insufficiently robust to specifically recommend one approach rather than the other.[24,25]

Furosemide is effective when given by SC injection (unauthorized). However, because the concentration of the injection is 10mg/mL, volume considerations may limit feasibility. Diuresis persists for about 4h, reaching a maximum at 2–3h, and urine output is significantly increased.[26,27] Furosemide has been successfully given SC/CSCI as a means of avoiding hospital admission or of continuing its use after oral medication becomes problematic in the last days of life.[28,29] In a report of 47 episodes of the use of furosemide CSCI in 37 patients, the majority benefited (>80%), with mild or severe site reactions seen in one quarter and one episode respectively.[28]

Furosemide may also be given SL (unauthorized). The bio-availability of Lasix® (Sanofi-Aventis) 20mg tablet by this route is at least as good as PO, if not better.[30] However, this may be formulation-dependent.

Other loop diuretics include **bumetanide** and **torasemide**, with respective PO doses of 1mg and 10mg equivalent to 40mg of furosemide.[31,32] Compared with furosemide, they have a higher ($\geqslant$80%) and more consistent PO bio-availability, but are more expensive.[31,32]

Some guidelines recommend PO **torasemide** for patients in whom poor or erratic absorption may be contributing to the failure to respond to high doses of other loop diuretics.[33]

Bio-availability 60–70% PO; varies widely due to erratic absorption and can be as low as 10%.[34]
Onset of action 30–60min PO; 2–5min IV; 30min SC.[35]
Time to peak plasma concentration 1.5h PO/SL.[30]
Plasma halflife 30–120min in healthy subjects, 50min–6h in heart failure, 10h in end-stage renal disease.
Duration of action 4–6h PO; 2h IV; 4h SC.[35]

Cautions

Severe electrolyte disturbances (correct before treatment and monitor for during use); elderly (lower doses); renal impairment; hepatic impairment; diabetes, hypoproteinaemia.

Some patients receive long-term diuretic therapy for hypertension or non-heart failure ankle oedema. This often becomes inappropriate as physical deterioration progresses, and may lead to postural hypotension and prerenal failure. In such circumstances the dose of furosemide should be reduced and possibly discontinued altogether. However, the withdrawal of diuretics requires careful monitoring to prevent the subsequent insidious onset of CHF.[36]

Drug interactions

Serious drug interaction: furosemide-induced electrolyte disturbances, particularly hypokalaemia, can increase the risk of:
- cardiac arrhythmia and death with drugs known to prolong the QT interval, e.g. **ketanserin** (not UK), **methadone** (see Chapter 24, p.759)
- **digoxin** toxicity
- **lithium** toxicity (possibly).
Plasma electrolytes, drug concentrations, and the patient's clinical condition should be monitored closely.

Concurrent use of furosemide with **risperidone** is associated with an increased risk of death in elderly patients with dementia. The reason is unclear, but the manufacturer advises avoiding this combination unless the benefits clearly outweigh the risks.

Furosemide can *decrease* **vancomycin** levels (up to 50%).

Aliskiren, phenytoin (up to 50% reduction), **indometacin** and possibly other NSAIDs can reduce the diuretic effect of furosemide; a larger dose of furosemide may be required.

Additive pharmacodynamic interactions with furosemide increase the risk of:
- hypokalaemia with other K^+ depleting drugs, e.g. corticosteroids, β_2 agonists, **amphotericin**, **carbenoxolone** and **theophylline**
- hyponatraemia with other Na^+ depleting drugs, e.g. **carbamazepine**
- hypotension with other drugs that lower blood pressure, e.g. ACE inhibitors, angiotensin II receptor antagonists, TCAs
- nephrotoxicity with other renally toxic drugs, e.g. NSAIDs, aminoglycosides
- ototoxicity, e.g. aminoglycosides, polymixins, **vancomycin**.
Colestyramine, colestipol and **sucralfate** decrease absorption of furosemide; give furosemide 2–3h before these drugs.

Undesirable effects

Transient pain at the site of SC injection.[35,37]
Frequency not stated: dyspepsia, thirst, dizziness, dehydration, drowsiness, weakness, muscle cramps.
Rare: tinnitus and deafness (generally after rapid injection; may be permanent).
Biochemical disturbances: hyperglycaemia, hyperuricaemia, hypocalcaemia, hypokalaemia, hypomagnesaemia, hyponatraemia, metabolic alkalosis.

Dose and use
CHF
• start with 40mg PO each morning
• if necessary, increase the dose progressively in 40mg increments
• usual maximum dose 160mg, generally given as 80mg each morning and noon
• usual maintenance dose 40–80mg each morning.
SL use may be an option in patients with swallowing difficulties.

CSCI

Incompatibility: Furosemide injection is alkaline and there is a high risk of *incompatibility* when mixed with acidic drugs. Because of this and the lack of compatibility data, *furosemide should not be mixed in the same syringe with any other drugs* (see p.701).[38]
    If further dilution is required, 0.9% saline is recommended; do *not* mix or dilute with glucose solutions or other acidic fluids.

Some palliative care services use CSCI furosemide as a means of managing decompensated CHF in the community:[28]
• start with the same dose CSCI as the patients current PO dose
• weigh the patient daily
• after 48h, if the daily weight loss is not ≥1kg/day, consider obtaining cardiologist/heart failure nurse specialist advice; options include:
  ▷ increasing the furosemide dose by 50%
  ▷ adding a thiazide diuretic, e.g. PO **bendroflumethiazide**
  ▷ adding or increasing the dose of an aldosterone antagonist, e.g. PO **spironolactone**
• because furosemide injection is 10mg/mL, a practical dose limits for a T34 McKinley syringe driver are 200mg and 300mg for a 30mL and 50mL syringe respectively
• if CSCI furosemide fails to provide the necessary weight loss, admission to hospital/hospice for IV furosemide may be unavoidable.

Ascites
Use only as a supplement to **spironolactone** (see p.68):
• start with 40mg PO each morning
• usual maintenance dose 20–40mg each morning
• usual maximum dose 160mg each morning.

Supply
Furosemide (generic)
Tablets 20mg, 40mg, 500mg, 28 days @ 20mg, 40mg each morning = £1.
Oral solution (sugar-free) 20mg/5mL, 40mg/5mL, 50mg/5mL, 28 days @ 40mg each morning = £19.
Injection 10mg/mL, 2mL or 5mL amp = £0.50, 25mL amp = £2.50.

Bumetanide (generic)
Tablets 1mg, 5mg, 28 days @ 1mg each morning = £1.20.
Oral solution 1mg/5mL, 28 days @ 1mg each morning = £128.
Injection 500microgram/mL, 4mL amp = £2.

Torasemide (generic)
Tablets 5mg, 10mg, 28 days @ 10mg each morning = £18 (*Note: these are more expensive than the branded version*).

Torem (Meda)
Tablets 2.5mg, 5mg, 10mg, 28 days @ 10mg each morning = £8.

1 NICE (2010) Chronic heart failure: management of chronic heart failure in adults in primary and secondary care *Clinical Guideline*. CG108. www.nice.org.uk
2 Faris R et al. (2006) Diuretics for heart failure. *Cochrane Database of Systematic Reviews*. CD003838.

3 McMurray JJ et al. (2012) ESC Guidelines for the diagnosis and treatment of acute and chronic heart failure 2012: The Task Force for the Diagnosis and Treatment of Acute and Chronic Heart Failure 2012 of the European Society of Cardiology. Developed in collaboration with the Heart Failure Association (HFA) of the ESC. European Heart Journal. 33: 1787–1847.

4 Amiel S et al. (1984) Intravenous infusion of frusemide as treatment for ascites in malignant disease. British Medical Journal. 288: 1041.

5 Fogel M et al. (1981) Diuresis in the ascitic patient: a randomized controlled trial of three regimens. Journal of Clinical Gastroenterology. 3: 73–80.

6 Kalambokis G et al. (2006) The effects of treatment with octreotide, diuretics, or both on portal hemodynamics in nonazotemic cirrhotic patients with ascites. Journal of Clinical Gastroenterology. 40: 342–346.

7 Kalambokis G et al. (2005) Renal effects of treatment with diuretics, octreotide or both, in non-azotemic cirrhotic patients with ascites. Nephrology, Dialysis, Transplantation. 20: 1623–1629.

8 Newton PJ et al. (2008) Nebulized furosemide for the management of dyspnea: does the evidence support its use? Journal of Pain and Symptom Management. 36: 424–441.

9 Stone P et al. (2002) Re: nebulized furosemide for dyspnea in terminal cancer patients. Journal of Pain and Symptom Management. 24: 274–275; author reply 275–276.

10 Twycross R et al. (2009) Symptom Management in Advanced Cancer (4e). palliativedrugs.com, Nottingham, pp. 160–166.

11 Ventresca P et al. (1990) Inhaled furosemide inhibits cough induced by low-chloride solutions but not by capsaicin. American Review of Respiratory Disease. 142: 143–146.

12 Bianco S et al. (1989) Protective effect of inhaled furosemide on allergen-induced early and late asthmatic reactions. New England Journal of Medicine. 321: 1069–1073.

13 Nishino T et al. (2000) Inhaled furosemide greatly alleviates the sensation of experimentally induced dyspnea. American Journal of Respiratory and Critical Care Medicine. 161: 1963–1967.

14 Laveneziana P et al. (2008) Inhaled furosemide does not alleviate respiratory effort during flow-limited exercise in healthy subjects. Pulmonary Pharmacology and Therapeutics. 21: 196–200.

15 Newton PJ et al. (2012) The acute haemodynamic effect of nebulised frusemide in stable, advanced heart failure. Heart Lung Circulation. 21: 260–266.

16 Moosavi SH et al. (2006) Effect of inhaled furosemide on air hunger induced in healthy humans. Respiratory Physiology and Neurobiology. 156: 1–8.

17 Ong KC et al. (2004) Effects of inhaled furosemide on exertional dyspnea in chronic obstructive pulmonary disease. American Journal of Respiratory and Critical Care Medicine. 169: 1028–1033.

18 Jensen D et al. (2008) Mechanisms of dyspnoea relief and improved exercise endurance after furosemide inhalation in COPD. Thorax. 63: 606–613.

19 Sheikh Motahal Vahedi H et al. (2013) The adjunctive effect of nebulized furosemide in acute treatment of patients with chronic obstructive pulmonary disease exacerbation: A randomized controlled clinical trial. Respir Care. 58: 1073–1877.

20 Shimoyama N and Shimoyama M (2002) Nebulized furosemide as a novel treatment for dyspnea in terminal cancer patients. Journal of Pain and Symptom Management. 23: 73–76.

21 Kohara H et al. (2003) Effect of nebulized furosemide in terminally ill cancer patients with dyspnea. Journal of Pain and Symptom Management. 26: 962–967.

22 Wilcock A et al. (2008) Randomised, placebo-controlled trial of nebulised furosemide for breathlessness in patients with cancer. Thorax. 63: 872–875.

23 Salvador DR et al. (2009) Continuous infusion versus bolus injection of loop diuretics in congestive heart failure. Cochrane Database of Systematic Reviews. CD003178.

24 Amer M et al. (2012) Continuous infusion versus intermittent bolus furosemide in ADHF: an updated meta-analysis of randomized control trials. Journal of Hospital Medicine. 7: 270–275.

25 Felker GM et al. (2011) Diuretic strategies in patients with acute decompensated heart failure. New England Journal of Medicine. 364: 797–805.

26 Goenaga MA et al. (2004) Subcutaneous furosemide. Annals of Pharmacotherapy. 38: 1751.

27 Farless LB et al. (2012) Intermittent subcutaneous furosemide: parenteral diuretic rescue for hospice patients with congestive heart failure resistant to oral diuretic. American Journal of Hospice and Palliative Care. 30: 791–792.

28 Zacharias H et al. (2011) Is there a role for subcutaneous furosemide in the community and hospice management of end-stage heart failure? Palliative Medicine. 26: 658–663.

29 Galindo-Ocana J et al. (2013) Subcutaneous furosemide as palliative treatment in patients with advanced and terminal-phase heart failure. British Medical Journal Supportive and Palliative Care. 3: 7–8.

30 Haegeli L et al. (2007) Sublingual administration of furosemide: new application of an old drug. British Journal of Clinical Pharmacology. 64: 804–809.

31 Ward A and Heel RC (1984) Bumetanide. A review of its pharmacodynamic and pharmacokinetic properties and therapeutic use. Drugs. 28: 426–464.

32 Vargo DL et al. (1995) Bioavailability, pharmacokinetics, and pharmacodynamics of torsemide and furosemide in patients with congestive heart failure. Clin Pharmacol Ther. 57: 601–609.

33 Heart Failure Society of America (2010) Comprehensive heart failure practice guideline. Journal of Cardiac Failure. 16: e1–194.

34 Murray MD et al. (1997) Variable furosemide absorption and poor predictability of response in elderly patients. Pharmacotherapy. 17: 98–106.

35 Verma AK et al. (2004) Diuretic effects of subcutaneous furosemide in human volunteers: a randomized pilot study. Annals of Pharmacotherapy. 38: 544–549.

36 Walma E et al. (1997) Withdrawal of long term diuretic medication in elderly patients: a double blind randomised trial. British Medical Journal. 315: 464–468.

37 Baxter K, Preston CL Stockley's Drug Interactions. London: Pharmaceutical Press www.medicinescomplete.com (accessed October 2013).

38 Trissel LA Handbook on Injectable Drugs Maryland, USA. American Society of Health-System Pharmacists www.medicinescomplete.com (accessed October 2013).

Updated November 2013

SPIRONOLACTONE   BNF 2.2.3 & 2.5.5

Class: Potassium-sparing diuretic; aldosterone antagonist.

Indications: Ascites and peripheral oedema associated with portal hypertension and hyperaldosteronism (i.e. cirrhosis, hepatocellular cancer, massive hepatic metastases), CHF, nephrotic syndrome, primary hyperaldosteronism, †hypertension.

Contra-indications: Hyperkalaemia, Addison's disease, anuria, severe renal impairment, concurrent use with potassium supplements or potassium-sparing diuretics.

Pharmacology

Spironolactone and two metabolites (7α-thiomethyl-spironolactone and canrenone) bind to cytoplasmic mineralocorticoid receptors and function as aldosterone antagonists. In the distal tubules of the kidney, this results in a potassium-sparing diuretic effect.

Hyperaldosteronism is a concomitant of ascites associated with portal hypertension (a *transudate* with a relatively low albumin concentration, best indicated by a serum–ascites albumin difference of $\geqslant 11g/L$) as seen in cirrhosis, hepatocellular cancer, massive hepatic metastases.[1,2] Most evidence comes from cirrhosis, but spironolactone in a median daily dose of 200–300mg is successful in most patients with these conditions (90% in cirrhosis).[1–6] Spironolactone alone is the initial drug of choice, it is as safe and effective as spironolactone + **furosemide**, and requires less frequent dose adjustments.[4,5] In contrast, treatment with even large PO doses of a loop diuretic alone, e.g. **furosemide** 200mg, generally fails to reduce ascites.[7]

Note: paracentesis is used for patients failing to respond to or tolerate diuretic therapy. Paracentesis is also preferable for patients with predominantly peritoneal ascites (an *exudate* with relatively high albumin concentration, best indicated by a serum–ascites albumin gradient of $\leqslant 11g/L$) or chylous ascites as these are unlikely to respond to diuretics,[3,6] and also for patients with a tense distended abdomen in need of rapid relief.

A diuretic-induced reduction in plasma volume can increase the activity of various closely related neurohumoral systems, e.g. the renin-aldosterone-angiotensin system, sympathetic nervous system, ADH secretion, and result in impaired renal perfusion and increased Na^+ and water resorption. These changes reduce the effect of the diuretic and contribute to renal impairment. In patients with cirrhosis receiving spironolactone $\pm$ **furosemide**, improved renal function and diuresis is seen with co-administration of **octreotide** 300microgram SC b.d. (see p.530) or **clonidine** 75microgram PO b.d. (see p.76) due to inhibition of the renin-aldosterone-angiotensin (**octreotide** and **clonidine**) and sympathetic nervous (**clonidine**) systems.[8–10] Patients in the **clonidine** study were considered to have an overactive sympathetic nervous system based on a higher than normal serum noradrenaline (norepinephrine) level.[10]

Spironolactone is also added in low dose (12.5–50mg daily) to standard treatment for patients with severe symptomatic CHF.[11–13] Its aldosterone antagonist action helps reduce vascular and myocardial fibrosis, sympathetic nervous system activation, baroreceptor dysfunction and K^+ and Mg^{2+} depletion.[14] Spironolactone is also used to treat hypertension unresponsive to usual treatments.[15]

The non-specific binding of spironolactone to various steroid receptors can result in undesirable effects such as menstrual disorders and, in men, gynaecomastia, breast pain or impotence. **Eplerenone**, an aldosterone antagonist with greater selectively for the mineralocorticoid receptor, has been used as an alternative in these circumstances.[16,17]

Caution is required when using spironolactone in patients with prostate cancer. Although there are reports of cancer regression in keeping with an androgen blocking effect, disease progression has also been reported.[18] It is suggested that spironolactone acts as an androgen receptor modulator and thus can exert both anti- and pro-androgenic effects.

Spironolactone has an anti-inflammatory effect through inhibition of the nuclear factor-κB pathway involved in the production of pro-inflammatory cytokines.[19–22] The therapeutic potential of this effect remains to be determined.

Bio-availability 60–90%.
Onset of action 2–4h; maximum effect 7h (single dose), 2–3 days (multiple doses).
Time to peak plasma concentration 2–3h; active metabolites 3–4.5h PO.
Plasma halflife 1–1.5h; active metabolites 14–16.5h (multiple doses).
Duration of action >24h (single dose), 2–3 days (multiple doses).

Cautions

Prostate cancer (see Pharmacology).

Elderly; hepatic impairment, may induce reversible hyperchloraemic metabolic acidosis in patients with decompensated hepatic cirrhosis; renal impairment. Initial drowsiness and dizziness (may impair driving).

Drug interactions

Serious additive pharmacodynamic interactions with other drugs, notably *hyperkalaemia* with potassium supplements (avoid concurrent use), table salt substitutes (contain both potassium and sodium chlorides), potassium-sparing diuretics, ACE inhibitors, angiotensin II receptor antagonists, certain antibiotics (**trimethoprim, nitrofurantoin**), **ciclosporin**, LMWH and **tacrolimus**, particularly if other risk factors also present, e.g. elderly, renal impairment, diabetes.[23,24]

May induce *hyponatraemia*, particularly if used with other diuretics. Natriuretic effect reduced by **aspirin, indometacin** and possibly other NSAIDs.

Spironolactone increases the plasma concentration of digoxin by up to 25% and can interfere with digoxin plasma concentration assays; measure free digoxin levels using a chemiluminescent assay.[23]

Undesirable effects

Very common (>10%): CNS disturbances (drowsiness, lethargy, confusion, headache, fever, ataxia, fatigue), GI disturbances (anorexia, dyspepsia, nausea, vomiting, peptic ulceration, colic).
Common (<10%, >1%): gastritis, hyperkalaemia, gynaecomastia, breast pain.[25]

Dose and use

To reduce the risk of gastric irritation, advise patient to take with food. If, despite this, once daily spironolactone causes nausea and vomiting, try giving in divided doses.

For patients with swallowing difficulties, although an oral suspension is available, it is expensive. A cheaper (and authorized) alternative is to crush and disperse spironolactone tablets in food or cold drink (also see Chapter 22, p.725).

Cirrhotic or malignant ascites

Elimination of ascites may take 10–28 days:
- monitor body weight and renal function
- start with 100–200mg PO each morning
- if necessary, increase by 100mg every 3–7 days to achieve a weight loss of 0.5–1kg/24h (<0.5kg/24h when peripheral oedema absent)
- a typical maintenance dose is 200–300mg/24h; maximum dose 400–600mg/24h[1,2,5,7]
- if not achieving the desired weight loss with spironolactone 300–400mg/24h, consider adding **furosemide** 40–80mg each morning
- in cirrhosis, **furosemide** is generally increased in 40mg steps every 3 days to a maximum of 160mg/24h[4,5,26,27]
- if Na$^+$ falls to <120mmol/L, temporarily stop diuretics
- if K$^+$ falls to <3.5mmol/L, temporarily stop or decrease the dose of **furosemide**; if it rises to >5.5mmol/L, halve the dose of spironolactone; if >6mmol/L, temporarily stop spironolactone
- if creatinine rises to >150micromol/L, temporarily stop diuretics.[4]

Even if paracentesis becomes necessary, diuretics should be continued as they reduce the rate of recurrence.[4]

Severe CHF (NYHA class III or IV disease)

The following is based on several sets of published guidelines:
- do *not* prescribe spironolactone unless serum K$^+$ <5mmol/L and creatinine <200micromol/L
- start with 12.5–25mg once daily; check serum K$^+$ and creatinine after 4–7 days
- if necessary, *after 1 month*, increase to 50mg once daily; check serum K$^+$ and creatinine after 1 week
- if K$^+$ rises to >5mmol/L, halve the dose; if >5.5mmol/L, stop spironolactone completely
- it is particularly important to monitor potassium levels when spironolactone and an ACE inhibitor are prescribed concurrently.[11,14,28]

Supply

Spironolactone (generic)

Tablets 25mg, 50mg, 100mg, 28 days @ 200mg each morning = £5.

Oral suspension (sugar-free) 5mg/5mL, 10mg/5mL, 25mg/5mL, 50mg/5mL, 100mg/5mL; 28 days @ 200mg each morning = £292. (Unauthorized, available as a special order from Rosemont; see Appendix 1, p.817). *Note specials tariff applies in community.*

Spironolactone oral suspension can also be prepared locally for individual patients.[29]

Spironolactone is also available in fixed dose combinations with hydroflumethiazide or furosemide. However, these are more expensive and do not allow titration of the individual drugs.

1 Greenway B et al. (1982) Control of malignant ascites with spironolactone. British Journal of Surgery. **69**: 441–442.
2 Fernandez-Esparrach G et al. (1997) Diuretic requirements after therapeutic paracentesis in non-azotemic patients with cirrhosis. A randomized double-blind trial of spironolactone versus placebo. Journal of Hepatology. **26**: 614–620; erratum 1430.
3 Pockros P et al. (1992) Mobilization of malignant ascites with diuretics is dependent on ascitic fluid characteristics. Gastroenterology. **103**: 1302–1306.
4 Moore KP et al. (2003) The management of ascites in cirrhosis: report on the consensus conference of the International Ascites Club. Hepatology. **38**: 258–266.
5 Santos J et al. (2003) Spironolactone alone or in combination with furosemide in the treatment of moderate ascites in nonazotemic cirrhosis. A randomized comparative study of efficacy and safety. Journal of Hepatology. **39**: 187–192.
6 Becker G et al. (2006) Malignant ascites: systematic review and guideline for treatment. European Journal of Cancer. **42**: 589–597.
7 Fogel M et al. (1981) Diuresis in the ascitic patient: a randomized controlled trial of three regimens. Journal of Clinical Gastroenterology. **3**: 73–80.
8 Kalambokis G et al. (2005) Renal effects of treatment with diuretics, octreotide or both, in non-azotemic cirrhotic patients with ascites. Nephrology, Dialysis, Transplantation. **20**: 1623–1629.
9 Kalambokis G et al. (2006) The effects of treatment with octreotide, diuretics, or both on portal hemodynamics in nonazotemic cirrhotic patients with ascites. Journal of Clinical Gastroenterology. **40**: 342–346.
10 Lenaerts A et al. (2006) Effects of clonidine on diuretic response in ascitic patients with cirrhosis and activation of sympathetic nervous system. Hepatology. **44**: 844–849.
11 NICE (2010) Chronic heart failure: management of chronic heart failure in adults in primary and secondary care Clinical Guideline. CG108. www.nice.org.uk
12 McMurray JJ et al. (2012) ESC Guidelines for the diagnosis and treatment of acute and chronic heart failure 2012: The Task Force for the Diagnosis and Treatment of Acute and Chronic Heart Failure 2012 of the European Society of Cardiology. Developed in collaboration with the Heart Failure Association (HFA) of the ESC. European Heart Journal. **33**: 1787–1847.
13 Heart Failure Society of America (2010) Comprehensive heart failure practice guideline. Journal of Cardiac Failure. **16**: e1–194.
14 Swedberg K et al. (2005) Guidelines for the diagnosis and treatment of chronic heart failure: full text (update 2005). European Heart Journal. Available from: 10.1093/eurheartj/ehi205
15 NICE (2011) Hypertension. Clinical Guideline. CG127. www.nice.org.uk
16 Barnes BJ and Howard PA (2005) Eplerenone: a selective aldosterone receptor antagonist for patients with heart failure. Annals of Pharmacotherapy. **39**: 68–76.
17 Dimitriadis G et al. (2011) Eplerenone reverses spironolactone-induced painful gynaecomastia in cirrhotics. Hepatology International. **5**: 738–739.
18 Sundar S and Dickinson PD (2012) Spironolactone, a possible selective androgen receptor modulator, should be used with caution in patients with metastatic carcinoma of the prostate. BMJ Case Reports. doi:10.1136/bcr.11.11.2011.5238.
19 Chantong B et al. (2012) Mineralocorticoid and glucocorticoid receptors differentially regulate NF-kappaB activity and pro-inflammatory cytokine production in murine BV-2 microglial cells. Journal of Neuroinflammation. **9**: 260.
20 Syngle A et al. (2009) Effect of spironolactone on endothelial dysfunction in rheumatoid arthritis. Scandinavian Journal of Rheumatology. **38**: 15–22.
21 Syngle A et al. (2013) Spironolactone improves endothelial dysfunction in ankylosing spondylitis. Clinical Rheumatology. **32**: 1029–1036.
22 Sun YE et al. (2012) Intrathecal injection of spironolactone attenuates radicular pain by inhibition of spinal microglia activation in a rat model. PLoS One. **7**: e39897.
23 Baxter K, Preston CL Stockley's Drug Interactions. London: Pharmaceutical Press www.medicinescomplete.com (accessed July 2013).
24 Antoniou T et al. (2011) Trimethoprim-sulfamethoxazole induced hyperkalaemia in elderly patients receiving spironolactone: nested case-control study. British Medical Journal. **343**: d5228.
25 Williams EM et al. (2006) Use and side-effect profile of spironolactone in a private cardiologist's practice. Clinical Cardiology. **29**: 149–153.
26 Gines P et al. (1987) Comparison of paracentesis and diuretics in the treatment of cirrhotics with tense ascites. Gastroenterology. **93**: 234–241.
27 Sharma S and Walsh D (1995) Management of symptomatic malignant ascites with diuretics: two case reports and a review of the literature. Journal of Pain and Symptom Management. **10**: 237–242.

28 Arnold JM *et al.* (2006) Canadian Cardiovascular Society consensus conference recommendations on heart failure 2006: diagnosis and management.[erratum appears in Canadian Journal of Cardiology. 2006 Mar 1;22(3):271]. *Canadian Journal of Cardiology.* **22**: 23–45.

29 Allen LV Jr and Erickson MA 3rd (1996) Stability of ketoconazole, metolazone, metronidazole, procainamide hydrochloride, and spironolactone in extemporaneously compounded oral liquids. *American Journal of Health System Pharmacy.* **53**: 2073–2078.

Updated November 2013

SYSTEMIC LOCAL ANAESTHETICS   BNF 2.3.2 & 15.2

General overview

Local anaesthetics and their orally administered congeners are sometimes useful as third- or fourth-line drugs in the treatment of neuropathic pain. An analgesic effect has been reported when such drugs have been administered systemically:[1]

- **lidocaine** CSCI, IVI[2,3] (also TD)
- **flecainide** PO
- **mexiletine** PO (not UK; may be imported as a special order)
- **tocainide** PO (not UK).

The mechanism by which they provide relief is not fully understood, but probably includes blockade of sodium channels. This stabilizes the nerve membrane and thus suppresses injury-induced hyperexcitability in the peripheral and central nervous systems. Antidepressants and anti-epileptics which benefit neuropathic pain also have membrane stabilizing properties, e.g. **amitriptyline, carbamazepine.**[4]

A systematic review of 32 RCTs, mostly of IV **lidocaine** and PO **mexiletine**, for neuropathic pain of various causes concluded that systemic local anaesthetics are better than placebo and as effective as **amantadine, carbamazepine, gabapentin, morphine** (Box A).[1]

Box A   Systemic local anaesthetics and neuropathic pain[1]

Of overall benefit in:
- trigeminal neuralgia
- post-herpetic neuralgia
- diabetic neuropathy
- lumbosacral radiculopathy
- post-stroke pain
- chronic post-surgery pain
- chronic post-trauma pain
- spinal cord injury pain
- complex regional pain syndrome.

Not of benefit in:
- cancer-related neuropathy (but see main text)
- HIV-related neuropathy.

Lidocaine dose used ranged from 1mg/kg IV over 2–3min to 1–5mg/kg IVI over 30min–2h.

Mexiletine median dose 600mg/24h (range 300–1200mg/24h).

Improvement equivalent to a reduction of 10mm on a 100mm VAS, but about 50% of patients achieve an improvement of ⩾30%.

Even so, despite the occasional impressive anecdotal account, RCT evidence of benefit is not overwhelming. The overall degree of improvement is small, and some studies suggest that not all components of neuropathic pain are relieved, e.g. constant pain and touch allodynia improve but cold-induced allodynia does not.[5,6] The systematic review found benefit to be inconsistent in some types of pain, e.g. diabetic neuropathy, and absent in others, e.g. cancer-related neuropathic

---

pain.[1,7,8] Further, in a study of elderly patients (mean age 77 years), **lidocaine** 5mg/kg IVI over 2h provides no greater analgesic benefit than 1mg/kg, despite producing higher serum levels which were potentially toxic in some patients.[9]

Thus, generally in cancer-related neuropathic pain, systemic local anaesthetics should be considered for use only when the combination of a strong opioid + NSAID + TCA + anti-epileptic is ineffective or poorly tolerated. Even then, **ketamine** (see p.625) may be preferable because:
- the serum level does not need to be monitored
- it can be given PO
- it is more effective than **lidocaine** in spinal cord injury pain.[10]

*Systemic lidocaine

*The use of systemic **lidocaine** is limited to specialist palliative care or pain services.*

Lidocaine has a narrow therapeutic index, and there are important contra-indications and cautions to be observed (see manufacturer's SPC). Contra-indications include patients at greater risk of cardiac arrhythmias, e.g. any type of cardiac disease, electrolyte abnormalities, and those already taking an anti-arrhythmic drug. Cautions include factors which increase the risk of toxicity, e.g. patients who are elderly, cachectic, or have renal or hepatic impairment.

A normal 12-lead ECG is a mandatory prerequisite. When administering IV **lidocaine** as a day case for non-cancer pain, some services monitor heart rhythm continuously and blood pressure/SpO$_2$ frequently, e.g. every 8 minutes, and ensure immediate access to resuscitation equipment.

In non-cancer pain, improvement lasting 4–20 weeks following a single dose of IV **lidocaine** has been reported in patients with, e.g. central pain syndrome, diabetic neuropathy.[11,12] However, benefit is mostly limited to a few hours or days.[11,13] Ongoing relief will necessitate CIVI or CSCI **lidocaine** or the use of an oral analogue, e.g. **flecainide, mexiletine** (not UK). However, the response to IV **lidocaine** does not reliably predict subsequent benefit from **mexiletine** and undesirable effects can limit its chronic use.[5,12] For example, in a cohort of patients with non-cancer neuropathic pain treated with **mexiletine**, the median time to discontinuation (for any reason) was 6 weeks with only 20% persisting with its use > 1 year.[14]

In cancer-related neuropathic pain, subsequent to the systematic review,[1] there has been one positive RCT of IV **lidocaine**.[15] Compared with placebo, pain relief with **lidocaine** was faster (40 vs. 75min), of greater magnitude (75 vs. 25% reduction) and duration (9 vs. 4 days). Otherwise, reports of benefit are limited to case reports. Regimens include:
- IV 2mg/kg over 20min followed by 2mg/kg over 1h[15]
- IV 1–2mg/kg over 15–20min[16]
- CIVI 0.5–1mg/kg/h[16,17]
- CSCI 4 or 10% **lidocaine** hydrochloride solution, generally 10–80mg/h; 100–160mg/h reported in patients aged ~ 60 years.[17,18]

Continuous infusions have been given for up to 6 months.[18] As a minimum, some suggest monitoring serum levels 1–3 days after starting or a dose increase and when toxicity is suspected.[17]

Analgesia is generally seen with serum levels of 1.5–5microgram/mL and severe neurotoxicity with levels ⩾10microgram/mL.[2,19] However, there is large interindividual variation and the beneficial/toxic effect relates more to the amount of free **lidocaine** (unbound to protein), rather than the total serum level (bound plus unbound).[20]

With a continuous infusion, accumulation of **lidocaine** and its active metabolites, e.g. monoethylglycinexylidide and glycinexylidide, can occur and lead to toxicity. Particular caution is required in the elderly in whom clearance is already reduced.[20–22] For example, two elderly patients (⩾70 years) despite normal renal/liver function and receiving a relatively small dose of **lidocaine** (200–300mg/day), developed severe drowsiness after 10 days.[23]

Generally, developing toxicity should be clinically obvious because as serum levels rise, there is a progressive worsening of neurotoxicity:
- lightheadedness, dizziness
- circumoral numbness
- tinnitus
- visual changes
- dysarthria
- muscle spasm
- seizures
- coma
- respiratory arrest.

However, monitoring serum levels is the most effective way of maintaining a consistent and safe **lidocaine** dose.[3,19,21]

Note: prolonged toxicity has also been reported when 10mL of 2% viscous **lidocaine** (not UK) was used hourly for a painful mouth ulcer (twice the recommended daily dose), and was probably partly caused by accumulation of metabolites.[22]

Lidocaine medicated plasters

These are authorized for post-herpetic neuralgia (Box B). Sufficient high-quality data are lacking to recommend them for first-line use in this setting.[24,25] Indeed, NICE considers the data insufficient to make any recommendation on their use.[26] Thus, in post-herpetic neuralgia, the plasters are best reserved for situations where tricyclic antidepressants (e.g. **amitriptyline**) and anti-epileptics (e.g. **gabapentin**) are contra-indicated, ineffective or poorly tolerated.

Box B Use of lidocaine 5% medicated plaster

Each plaster (Versatis 5%®) contains 700mg lidocaine. *Only about 5% of the plaster dose is absorbed.* Steady-state is achieved after three days. Maximum concentrations (0.07–0.19microgram/mL) are well below systemic analgesic (1.5–5microgram/mL) and serious toxic levels (≥10microgram/mL).

A recommended maximum of three plasters are applied to the painful area on a 12h on–off basis. The plasters can be cut if required but must not be applied close to the eyes or mouth, or on inflamed/broken skin or wounds.

Similar considerations apply as for other medical transdermal products, e.g. skin hair should be clipped rather than shaved, fold plasters in half and dispose of safely (> 660mg remains in the plasters).

The 12h off periods are to help reduce the risk of skin reactions, but these still occur in about 15% of patients. The skin over the head and neck appears most susceptible.[42] The skin can be rested for longer when necessary, but up to 5% of patients have to discontinue.

Generally, high quality data are lacking. A study of post-herpetic neuralgia suggests that overall <50% of patients will obtain sufficient benefit to warrant continuing with the plasters.[43] For those who respond, sustained benefit (≥1 year) has been reported.[44] The magnitude of the benefit appears similar to that obtained with pregabalin but the plasters are better tolerated.[31]

Anaphylaxis is a very rare complication (≤1:10,000).

The analgesic effect of the **lidocaine** plasters is considered to be local via a non-selective block of peripheral sodium channels on sensory afferents in the epidermis.[27] However, in patients with painful distal sensory neuropathy, neither the density of epidermal nerve fibres nor the results of quantitative sensory testing/nerve conduction studies predict the response to the plasters.[28] Indeed, some patients with a complete loss of epidermal nerve fibres reported benefit. Thus, the exact mechanism of effect is unclear.[28,29]

There is also a strong placebo effect. In chronic back pain, active and placebo plasters provide similar reductions in pain intensity, sensory and affective scores and pain-related brain activity (functional MRI).[30]

Further, if the main effect of the **lidocaine** plasters is physical protection in patients with allodynia, they are an unnecessarily expensive form of plaster.

The **lidocaine** plasters have been used in various settings, including:
- diabetic polyneuropathy[31]
- post-surgical scar pain[3,32,33]
- post-traumatic neuropathic pain[33]
- osteoarthritis[34]
- carpal tunnel syndrome[35]
- erythromelalgia[36]
- myofascial pain[37]
- cancer-related.[38,39]

These have mostly been low-quality open studies, case series or reports, with mixed results. Despite initial reports of benefit in traumatic rib fracture, a RCT found no difference between active and placebo plasters in relation to pain relief, opioid use or length of hospital stay.[40]

A survey showed that, in palliative care, the main use of the plasters is neuropathic pain associated with invasion of the chest wall by mesothelioma, breast or lung cancer. They were considered acceptable, well tolerated and beneficial to most patients. On the other hand, there were concerns about an unpredictable or variable response and high cost.[41]

*Flecainide

*The use of **flecainide** is limited to specialist palliative care or pain services.*

Flecainide is a class 1C anti-arrhythmic authorized for use primarily in the prevention and treatment of supraventricular and ventricular arrhythmias. Rarely, it is used to treat nerve injury pain. There are important contra-indications and cautions to be observed (see manufacturer's SPC). **Flecainide** has a narrow therapeutic index, and some patients experience psychoneurological and cardiac toxicity within the recommended therapeutic range (also see **lidocaine** above).[45,46] Flecainide is both metabolized by and inhibits CYP2D6 (see CYP450).

Response rate for neuropathic pain in non-controlled studies in cancer and AIDS patients varies between 30–60%.[47–50] Generally, tricyclic antidepressants should be stopped at least 48h before starting **flecainide**. Initial doses are comparable to those used in cardiology:
- start with 50mg PO b.d.
- usual dose 100mg b.d.
- maximum dose 200mg b.d.[47,50]

Supply

Lidocaine hydrochloride (generic)
Injection 5mg/mL (0.5%), 10mg/mL (1%), 20mg/mL (2%) 2mL, 5mL, 10mL and 20mL = £1.

Versatis® (Grunenthal)
Medicated plaster 5% 30 = £73.

For topical use of **lidocaine** in oral inflammation and ulceration see Drugs for oral inflammation and ulceration, p.604.

Flecainide (generic)
Tablets 50mg, 100mg, 28 days @100mg b.d. = £12.

1 Challapalli V et al. (2005) Systemic administration of local anesthetic agents to relieve neuropathic pain. *Cochrane Database of Systematic Reviews.* CD003345.
2 Devulder J et al. (1993) Neuropathic pain in a cancer patient responding to subcutaneously administered lignocaine. *The Clinical Journal of Pain.* 9: 220–223.
3 Meier T et al. (2003) Efficacy of lidocaine patch 5% in the treatment of focal peripheral neuropathic pain syndromes: a randomized, double-blind, placebo-controlled study. *Pain.* 106: 151–158.
4 Devor M (2006) Sodium channels and mechanisms of neuropathic pain. *Journal of Pain.* 7: S3–S12.
5 Attal N et al. (2000) Intravenous lidocaine in central pain: a double-blind, placebo-controlled, psychophysical study. *Neurology.* 54: 564–574.
6 Attal N et al. (2004) Systemic lidocaine in pain due to peripheral nerve injury and predictors of response. *Neurology.* 62: 218–225.
7 Bruera E et al. (1992) A randomized double-blind crossover trial of intravenous lidocaine in the treatment of neuropathic cancer pain. *Journal of Pain and Symptom Management.* 7: 138–140.
8 Ellemann K et al. (1989) Trial of intravenous lidocaine on painful neuropathy in cancer patients. *Clinical Journal of Pain.* 5: 291–294.
9 Baranowski AP et al. (1999) A trial of intravenous lidocaine on the pain and allodynia of postherpetic neuralgia. *Journal of Pain and Symptom Management.* 17: 429–433.
10 Kvarnstrom A et al. (2004) The analgesic effect of intravenous ketamine and lidocaine on pain after spinal cord injury. *Acta anaesthesiologica Scandinavica.* 48: 498–506.
11 Backonja M and Gombar KA (1992) Response of central pain syndromes to intravenous lidocaine. *Journal of Pain and Symptom Management.* 7: 172–178.
12 Viola V et al. (2006) Treatment of intractable painful diabetic neuropathy with intravenous lignocaine. *Journalk of Diabetes and Its Complications.* 20: 34–39.
13 Kosharskyy B et al. (2013) Intravenous infusions in chronic pain management. *Pain Physician.* 16: 231–249.
14 Carroll IR et al. (2008) Mexiletine therapy for chronic pain: survival analysis identifies factors predicting clinical success. *Journal of Pain and Symptom Management.* 35: 321–326.

15 Sharma S et al. (2009) A phase II pilot study to evaluate use of intravenous lidocaine for opioid-refractory pain in cancer patients. Journal of Pain and Symptom Management. 37: 85–93.

16 Thomas J et al. (2004) Intravenous lidocaine relieves severe pain: results of an inpatient hospice chart review. Journal of Palliative Medicine. 7: 660–667.

17 Ferrini R (2000) Parenteral lidocaine for severe intractable pain in six hospice patients continued at home. Journal of Palliative Medicine. 3: 193–200.

18 Massey GV et al. (2002) Continuous lidocaine infusion for the relief of refractory malignant pain in a terminally ill pediatric cancer patient. Journal of Pediatric Hematology/Oncology. 24: 566–568.

19 Ferrante FM et al. (1996) The analgesic response to intravenous lidocaine in the treatment of neuropathic pain. Anesthesia and Analgesia. 82: 91–97.

20 Rosenberg PH et al. (2004) Maximum recommended doses of local anesthetics: a multifactorial concept. Regional Anesthesia and Pain Medicine. 29: 564–575; discussion 524.

21 Brose W and Cousins M (1991) Subcutaneous lidocaine for treatment of neuropathic pain. Pain. 45: 145–148.

22 Yamashita S et al. (2002) Lidocaine toxicity during frequent viscous lidocaine use for painful tongue ulcer. Journal of Pain and Symptom Management. 24: 543–545.

23 Tei Y et al. (2005) Lidocaine intoxication at very small doses in terminally ill cancer patients. Journal of Pain Symptom and Management. 30: 6–7.

24 Khaliq W et al. (2007) Topical lidocaine for the treatment of postherpetic neuralgia. Cochrane Database of Systematic Reviews. CD004846.

25 Scottish Medicines Consortium (2008) Lidocaine 5% medicated plaster (Versatis(R)). 334/06. Available from: www.scottish-medicines.org.uk

26 NICE (2013) Pharmacological management of neuropathic pain in adults in non-specialist setting. Clinical Guideline. CG173. www.nice.org.uk

27 Madsen CS et al. (2013) Differential Effects of a 5% lidocaine medicated patch in peripheral nerve injury. Muscle Nerve. 48: 265–271.

28 Herrmann DN et al. (2006) Skin biopsy and quantitative sensory testing do not predict response to lidocaine patch in painful neuropathies. Muscle Nerve. 33: 42–48.

29 Campbell JN (2012) How does topical lidocaine relieve pain? Pain. 153: 255–256.

30 Hashmi JA et al. (2012) Lidocaine patch (5%) is no more potent than placebo in treating chronic back pain when tested in a randomised double blind placebo controlled brain imaging study. Molecular Pain. 8: 29.

31 Baron R et al. (2009) 5% lidocaine medicated plaster versus pregabalin in post-herpetic neuralgia and diabetic polyneuropathy: an open-label, non-inferiority two-stage RCT study. Current Medical Research and Opinion. 25: 1663–1676.

32 Cheville AL et al. (2009) Use of a lidocaine patch in the management of postsurgical neuropathic pain in patients with cancer: a phase III double-blind crossover study (N01CB). Supportive Care in Cancer. 17: 451–460.

33 Delorme C et al. (2011) Treatment of neuropathic pain with 5% lidocaine-medicated plaster: Five years of clinical experience. Pain Research and Management. 16: 259–263.

34 Burch F et al. (2004) Lidocaine patch 5% improves pain, stiffness, and physical function in osteoarthritis pain patients. A prospective, multicenter, open-label effectiveness trial. Osteoarthritis and Cartilage. 12: 253–255.

35 Nalamachu S et al. (2006) A comparison of the lidocaine patch 5% vs naproxen 500 mg twice daily for the relief of pain associated with carpal tunnel syndrome: a 6-week, randomized, parallel-group study. Medscape General Medicine. 8: 33.

36 Davis MD and Sandroni P (2005) Lidocaine patch for pain of erythromelalgia: follow-up of 34 patients. Archives of Dermatology. 141: 1320–1321.

37 Affaitati G et al. (2009) A randomized, controlled study comparing a lidocaine patch, a placebo patch, and anesthetic injection for treatment of trigger points in patients with myofascial pain syndrome: evaluation of pain and somatic pain thresholds. Clinical Therapeutics. 31: 705–720.

38 Fleming JA and O'Connor BD (2009) Use of lidocaine patches for neuropathic pain in a comprehensive cancer centre. Pain Research and Management. 14: 381–388.

39 Lopez Ramirez E (2013) Treatment of acute and chronic focal neuropathic pain in cancer patients with lidocaine 5 % patches. A radiation and oncology department experience. Supportive Care Cancer. 21: 1329–1334.

40 Ingalls NK et al. (2010) Randomized, double-blind, placebo-controlled trial using lidocaine patch 5% in traumatic rib fractures. Journal of the American College of Surgeons. 210: 205–209.

41 Palliativedrugs.com (2009) Survey. Lidocaine 5% medicated plasters - What is your experience? Available from: www.palliativedrugs.com/download/090731_lidocaine_survey_sc.pdf

42 Nalamachu S et al. (2013) Influence of anatomic location of lidocaine patch 5% on effectiveness and tolerability for postherpetic neuralgia. Patient Prefer Adherence. 7: 551–557.

43 Binder A et al. (2009) Topical 5% lidocaine (lignocaine) medicated plaster treatment for post-herpetic neuralgia: results of a double-blind, placebo-controlled, multinational efficacy and safety trial. Clinical Drug Investigation. 29: 393–408.

44 Hans G et al. (2009) Efficacy and tolerability of a 5% lidocaine medicated plaster for the topical treatment of post-herpetic neuralgia: results of a long-term study. Current Medical Research Opinion. 25: 1295–1305.

45 Nestico PF et al. (1988) New antiarrhythmic drugs. Drugs. 35: 286–319.

46 Bennett M (1997) Paranoid psychosis due to flecainide toxicity in malignant neuropathic pain. Pain. 70: 93–94.

47 von Gunten CF et al. (2007) Flecainide for the treatment of chronic neuropathic pain: a Phase II trial. Palliative Medicine. 21: 667–672.

48 Chong S et al. (1997) Pilot study evaluating local anesthetics administered systemically for treatment of pain in patients with advanced cancer. Journal of Pain and Symptom Management. 13: 112–117.

49 Sinnott C et al. (1991) Flecainide in cancer nerve pain. Lancet. 337: 1347.

50 Dunlop R et al. (1988) Analgesic effects of oral flecainide. Lancet. 1: 420–421.

Updated January 2014

*CLONIDINE   BNF 2.5.2 & 4.7.4.2

Class: α-Adrenergic receptor agonist (α agonist).

Indications: Hypertension, migraine prophylaxis, menopausal flushing, ↑pain poorly responsive to epidural or intrathecal **diamorphine/morphine** and **bupivacaine**, ↑spasticity, ↑diarrhoea or ↑gastroparesis related to autonomic dysfunction in diabetes mellitus, ↑sweating, ↑ascites, ↑opioid withdrawal.

Contra-indications: Cardiac conduction defects.

Pharmacology

Clonidine is a mixed α_1 and α_2 agonist (mainly α_2). It acts centrally to inhibit the release of noradrenaline (norepinephrine) which decreases sympathetic tone. This reduces cardiac output and peripheral vascular resistance, lowering blood pressure. However, its use as an antihypertensive has been eclipsed by the development of other drugs. Clonidine has a range of other clinical effects:

Analgesia: Clonidine analgesia is probably mediated by an effect at α_2-receptors resulting in:
- peripheral and/or central suppression of sympathetic transmitter release[1,2]
- peripheral and central inhibition of nociceptive afferents[3,4]
- post-synaptic inhibition of spinal cord neurones[5,6]
- facilitation or inhibition of brain stem pain modulating systems.[7]

In postoperative pain, clonidine given by various routes (PO, IV, IT) augments the analgesic effects of opioids.[8,9] Clonidine also enhances the analgesic effects of local anaesthetics administered IT or peripherally (e.g. single nerve or plexus blocks or applied directly to the wound).[10–15] Further, treatment with high-dose ED clonidine alone (a bolus of 10microgram/kg followed by an infusion of 6microgram/kg/h) can provide effective postoperative analgesia.[16]

In neuropathic pain, clonidine provides reproducible pain relief in some patients, particularly when given via the ED or IT routes.[1,17 22] A clonidine 0.1% gel applied topically improves painful diabetic neuropathy, but only in patients with functioning cutaneous nociceptors as indicated by experiencing pain from topical capsacin.[23]

ED clonidine is effective in cancer-related neuropathic pain, generally as an 'add-on' drug (see Spinal analgesia, p.713). It is particularly useful for patients who do not respond to high-dose systemic opioids or who tolerate them poorly, and for those who fail to respond to spinal **morphine** plus **bupivacaine**.[24,25] A typical dose is 150–300microgram/24h ED, but benefit has been reported in some patients on higher IT doses, up to 1mg/24h.[22] Benefit has also been reported in patients receiving clonidine by CSCI, with increasing benefit in a few patients with doses of up to 1.5mg/24h.[26]

ED clonidine is absorbed into the systemic circulation producing significant plasma concentrations (reflected clinically by drowsiness and cardiovascular effects), reaching a peak after 20min. IT clonidine produces similar effects; sedation occurs within 15–30min and lasts 1–2h.[22,27,28] The analgesic effect of clonidine can be reversed by α antagonists but not by **naloxone**.[1] Clonidine can thus be used in the management of unexpected acute pain in addicts receiving naltrexone (see Opioid antagonists, Box A, p.454).

Spasticity: In patients with spinal cord injury, the addition of clonidine reduces muscle spasticity which has failed to respond to maximal doses of **baclofen**.[29,30] In healthy volunteers, clonidine induces muscular relaxation and reduces pain caused by distension in the stomach, colon and rectum.[31,32]

Diabetic GI autonomic neuropathy: Clonidine improves symptoms of gastroparesis and chronic diarrhoea.[33–35] The improvement in diarrhoea is due partly to the stimulation of α_2-adrenergic receptors on enterocytes, which promotes intestinal fluid and electrolyte absorption, inhibits anion secretion and may also modify intestinal motility.[34,35]

Sweats and hot flushes: There is RCT evidence that clonidine relieves sweating and hot flushes resulting from hormonal manipulation in women with breast cancer, but not in men with prostate cancer.[36,37] More recent trials in patients with breast cancer and hot flushes have overall found **venlafaxine** (p.215) to be as effective as clonidine.[38–40] **Gabapentin** is another option (see p.270). Despite the lack of data, some suggest that SSRIs, **gabapentin** or clonidine could also be tried in men with hot flushes resulting from medical or surgical castration.[41]

Ascites: In patients with cirrhosis receiving **spironolactone** ± **furosemide**, improved renal function and diuresis is seen with co-administration of clonidine 75microgram PO b.d. (see p.68) due to inhibition of the renin-aldosterone-angiotensin and sympathetic nervous systems.[42,43]

Patients were considered to have an overactive sympathetic nervous system based on higher than normal serum noradrenaline (norepinephrine) levels.[43]

Opioid withdrawal: Increased sympathetic (noradrenergic) activity has been implicated in various symptoms of opioid withdrawal, e.g. shivering, sweating, anxiety, diarrhoea. Clonidine reduces these symptoms and has been used alone to manage opioid withdrawal. However, although as effective as reducing doses of **methadone**, clonidine is associated with more undesirable effects, e.g. hypotension.[44]

Nausea and vomiting: Clonidine reduces post-operative nausea and vomiting; this may relate to a reduced sympathetic outflow or analgesic requirement, or general sedative effect.[8,45]

Other uses: Clonidine is also used improve symptoms in attention-deficit/hyperactivity disorder, and several other psychiatric conditions, e.g. post-traumatic stress disorder, autism.[46]

About half of a dose of clonidine is excreted unchanged by the kidneys, and most of the remainder is metabolized by the liver to inactive metabolites. Accumulation occurs in renal impairment, extending its halflife up to 40h.

Bio-availability 75–100% PO; 60% TD.[47]
Onset of action 30–60min IV, PO; 2–3 days TD.
Time to peak plasma concentration 1.5–5h PO; 20min ED; 2 days TD.
Plasma halflife 12–16h.
Duration of action 8–24h PO; 24h TD.

Cautions

Severe coronary insufficiency, recent myocardial infarction, stroke, peripheral vascular disease, renal impairment. May precipitate depression in susceptible patients; occasionally precipitates delirium.[48] Abrupt curtailment of long-term treatment likely to cause agitation, sympathetic overactivity, rebound hypertension (worsened if also taking a β-blocker); withdraw treatment progressively over 2–4 days (ED) or 1 week (PO). Discontinue any β-blocker several days before discontinuing clonidine.

TD patches (not UK) contain metal in the backing and must be removed before MRI to avoid burns (see, p.657).[49]

Drug interactions

Effects reduced or abolished by drugs with α antagonist activity, e.g. **mirtazapine**, TCAs (e.g. **amitriptyline, clomipramine, desipramine** (not UK), **imipramine**), and antipsychotic drugs, although the hypotensive effects of the phenothiazines can be additive. Concerns regarding serious undesirable effects with concurrent use of **methylphenidate** (see SPC) appear unfounded.[50]

Undesirable effects

Very common (>10%): sedation and dry mouth (initially), dizziness, orthostatic hypotension, transient pruritus and erythema (TD route).
Common (<10%, >1%): headache, fatigue, depression (long-term use), disturbed sleep, nausea, vomiting, constipation, erectile dysfunction, salivary gland pain, local reactions with TD route (e.g. rash, hyperpigmentation, excoriation).
Rare(≥0.01%): decreased lacrimation.

Dose and use

Clonidine can be given as a TD patch (not UK, but see Supply),[21,51] PO, by CSCI, and spinally. TD is generally better tolerated than PO, but the relationship between effective doses of PO and TD clonidine is not predictable. Start with a patch delivering 100microgram/24h applied once every 7 days and review.

Spinal analgesia

ED clonidine is generally given with **diamorphine/morphine** and **bupivacaine** (see Chapter 21, p.713). A typical ED regimen would be:
- a test bolus dose of 50–150microgram in 5mL saline injection over 5min
- if relief obtained, 150–300microgram/24h by infusion.

Clonidine is also used IT. A typical IT regimen would be:
- a test bolus dose of 50microgram in 5mL saline injection over 5min
- if relief obtained, 50–150microgram/24h by infusion.

Spasticity
Generally used as an adjunct to maximum dose of **baclofen**:
- start with 50microgram PO b.d.
- if necessary, increase by 50microgram every 3–7 days
- usual maximum dose 200microgram b.d.

Gastroparesis or diarrhoea related to autonomic dysfunction in diabetes mellitus
- start with 50microgram PO b.d.
- if necessary, increase by 50microgram every 24h
- usual maintenance dose 150microgram b.d.
- usual maximum dose for diabetic gastroparesis 300microgram b.d.
- usual maximum dose for diabetic diarrhoea 600microgram b.d.

Hormonal/menopausal sweating
- start with 50microgram PO b.d.
- after 2 weeks, if necessary, increase to 75microgram b.d.
- for some patients, the optimum dose is 100microgram b.d.

Supply
Clonidine (generic)
Tablets 25microgram, 28 days @ 50microgram b.d. = £4.

Catapres® (Boehringer Ingelheim)
Tablets (scored) 100microgram, 28 days @ 50microgram b.d. = £2.
Injection 150microgram/mL, 1mL amp = £0.50. *Available but not listed in the BNF as no longer recommended for use in hypertensive crisis.*

Catapres® TTS
Transdermal patch 2.5mg (100microgram/24h), 5mg (200microgram/24h) 7.5mg (300microgram/24hr) 1 patch (7 days treatment) = £8, £9, £248 respectively. (Unauthorized, available from IDIS, but cost can be prohibitive; see Appendix 1, p.817).

1 Quan D et al. (1993) Clonidine in pain management. *Annals of Pharmacotherapy.* **27**: 313–315.
2 Langer SZ et al. (1980) Recent developments in noradrenergic neurotransmission and its relevance to the mechanism of action of certain antihypertensive agents. *Hypertension.* **2**: 372–382.
3 Calvillo O and Ghignone M (1986) Presynaptic effect of clonidine on unmyelinated afferent fibers in the spinal cord of the cat. *Neuroscience Letters.* **64**: 335–339.
4 Riedl MS et al. (2009) Coexpression of alpha 2A-adrenergic and delta-opioid receptors in substance P-containing terminals in rat dorsal horn. *Journal of Comparative Neurology.* **513**: 385–398.
5 Yaksh T (1985) Pharmacology of spinal adrenergic systems which modulate spinal nociceptive processing. *Pharmacology, Biochemistry and Behaviour.* **22**: 845–858.
6 Michel MC and Insel PA (1989) Are there multiple imidazoline binding sites? *TIPS.* **10**: 342–344.
7 Bie B et al. (2003) Roles of alpha1- and alpha2-adrenoceptors in the nucleus raphe magnus in opioid analgesia and opioid abstinence-induced hyperalgesia. *Journal of Neuroscience.* **23**: 7950–7957.
8 Samantaray A et al. (2012) The effect on post-operative pain of intravenous clonidine given before induction of anaesthesia. *Indian Journal of Anaesthesia.* **56**: 359–364.
9 Engelman E and Marsala C (2013) Efficacy of adding clonidine to intrathecal morphine in acute postoperative pain: meta-analysis. *British Journal of Anaesthesia.* **110**: 21–27.
10 Elia N et al. (2008) Clonidine as an adjuvant to intrathecal local anesthetics for surgery: systematic review of randomized trials. *Regional Anesthesia and Pain Medicine.* **33**: 159–167.
11 Popping DM et al. (2009) Clonidine as an adjuvant to local anesthetics for peripheral nerve and plexus blocks: a meta-analysis of randomized trials. *Anesthesiology.* **111**: 406–415.
12 Ya Deau JT et al. (2008) Clonidine and analgesic duration after popliteal fossa nerve blockade: Randomized, double-blind, placebo-controlled study. *Anesthesia and Analgesia.* **106**: 1916–1920.
13 Schnabel A et al. (2011) Efficacy and safety of clonidine as additive for caudal regional anesthesia: a quantitative systematic review of randomized controlled trials. *Paediatric Anaesthesia.* **21**: 1219–1230.
14 Mohamed SA and Abdel-Ghaffar HS (2013) Effect of the addition of clonidine to locally administered bupivacaine on acute and chronic postmastectomy pain. *Journal of Clinical Anesthesia.* **25**: 20–27.
15 Bharti N et al. (2013) Postoperative analgesic effect of intravenous (i.v.) clonidine compared with clonidine administration in wound infiltration for open cholecystectomy. *British Journal of Anaesthesia.* **111**: 656–661.
16 deKock M et al. (1999) Epidural clonidine or bupivacaine as the sole analgesic agent during and after abdominal surgery. [Erratum appears in *Anesthesiology* (1999) **91**:602.]. *Anesthesiology.* **90**: 1354–1362.

17 Siddall PJ et al. (2000) The efficacy of intrathecal morphine and clonidine in the treatment of pain after spinal cord injury. Anesthesia and Analgesia. 91: 1493–1498.
18 Walters JL et al. (2012) Idiopathic peripheral neuropathy responsive to sympathetic nerve blockade and oral clonidine. Case Reports in Anesthesiology. Article ID 407539.
19 Glynn C et al. (1988) A double-blind comparison between epidural morphine and epidural clonidine in patients with chronic noncancer pain. Pain. 34: 123–128.
20 Max MB et al. (1988) Association of pain relief with drug side effects in postherpetic neuralgia: a single-dose study of clonidine, codeine, ibuprofen and placebo. Clinical Pharmacology and Therapeutics. 43: 363–371.
21 Zeigler D et al. (1992) Transdermal clonidine versus placebo in painful diabetic neuropathy. Pain. 48: 403–408.
22 Ackerman LL et al. (2003) Long-term outcomes during treatment of chronic pain with intrathecal clonidine or clonidine/opioid combinations. Journal of Pain and Symptom Management. 26: 668–677.
23 Campbell CM et al. (2012) Randomized control trial of topical clonidine for treatment of painful diabetic neuropathy. Pain. 153: 1815–1823.
24 Eisenach JC et al. (1995) Epidural clonidine analgesia for intractable cancer pain. The Epidural Clonidine Study Group. Pain. 61: 391–399.
25 Chen H et al. (2004) Contemporary management of neuropathic pain for the primary care physician. Mayo Clinic Proceedings. 79: 1533–1545.
26 Glynn C (1997) Personal communication.
27 Wells J and Hardy P (1987) Epidural clonidine. Lancet. i: 108.
28 Malinovsky JM et al. (2003) Sedation caused by clonidine in patients with spinal cord injury. British Journal of Anaesthesia. 90: 742–745.
29 Weingarden S and Belen J (1992) Clonidine transdermal system for treatment of spasticity in spinal cord injury. Archives of Physical Medicine and Rehabilitation. 73: 876–877.
30 Yablon S and Sipski M (1993) Effect of transdermal clonidine on spinal spasticity: a case series. American Journal of Physical Medicine and Rehabilitation. 72: 154–156.
31 Thumshirn M et al. (1999) Modulation of gastric sensory and motor functions by nitrergic and alpha2-adrenergic agents in humans. Gastroenterology. 116: 573–585.
32 Viramontes BE et al. (2001) Effects of an alpha(2)-adrenergic agonist on gastrointestinal transit, colonic motility, and sensation in humans. American Journal of Physiology Gastrointestinal and Liver Physiology. 281: G1468–1476.
33 Rosa-Silva L et al. (1995) Treatment of diabetic gastroparesis with oral clonidine. Alimentary Pharmacology and Therapeutics. 9: 179–183.
34 Fedorak R et al. (1985) Treatment of diabetic diarrhea with clonidine. Annals of Internal Medicine. 102: 197–199.
35 Fedorak R and Field M (1987) Antidiarrheal therapy prospects for new agents. Digestive Diseases and Science. 32: 195–205.
36 Rada G (2010) Non-hormonal interventions for hot flashes in women with a history of breast cancer. Cochrane Database of Systematic Reviews. 2: CD004923.
37 Frisk J (2010) Managing hot flushes in men after prostate cancer–a systematic review. Maturitas. 65: 15–22.
38 Buijs C et al. (2009) Venlafaxine versus clonidine for the treatment of hot flashes in breast cancer patients: a double-blind, randomized cross-over study. Breast Cancer Research and Treatment. 115: 573–580.
39 Loibl S et al. (2007) Venlafaxine is superior to clonidine as treatment of hot flashes in breast cancer patients–a double-blind, randomized study. Annals of Oncology. 18: 689–693.
40 Boekhout AH et al. (2011) Management of hot flashes in patients who have breast cancer with venlafaxine and clonidine: a randomized, double-blind, placebo-controlled trial. Journal of Clinical Oncology. 29: 3862–3868.
41 Loprinzi CL et al. (2011) Nonestrogenic management of hot flashes. Journal of Clinical Oncology. 29: 3842–3846.
42 Kalambokis G et al. (2005) Renal effects of treatment with diuretics, octreotide or both, in non-azotemic cirrhotic patients with ascites. Nephrology, Dialysis, Transplantation. 20: 1623–1629.
43 Lenaerts A et al. (2006) Effects of clonidine on diuretic response in ascitic patients with cirrhosis and activation of sympathetic nervous system. Hepatology. 44: 844–849.
44 Gowing L et al. (2009) Alpha2-adrenergic agonists for the management of opioid withdrawal. Cochrane Database of Systematic Reviews. CD002024.
45 Yadav G et al. (2013) A prospective, randomized, double blind and placebo-control study comparing the additive effect of oral midazolam and clonidine for postoperative nausea and vomiting prophylaxis in granisetron premedicated patients undergoing laparoscopic cholecystectomy. Journal of Anaesthesiology, Clinical Pharmacology. 29: 61–65.
46 Dowben JS et al. (2011) Clonidine: diverse use in pharmacologic management. Perspectives in Psychiatric Care. 47: 105–108.
47 Toon S et al. (1989) Rate and extent of absorption of clonidine from a transdermal therapeutic system. Journal of Pharmacy and Pharmacology. 41: 17–21.
48 Delaney J et al. (2006) Clonidine-induced delirium. International Journal of Cardiology. 113: 276–278.
49 Institute for Safe Medication Practices (2004) Medication Safety Alert. Burns in MRI patients wearing transdermal patches. Available from: www.ismp.org/Newsletters/acutecare/articles/20040408.asp?ptr=y
50 Baxter K, Preston CL Stockley's Drug Interactions. London: Pharmaceutical Press www.medicinescomplete.com (accessed July 2013).
51 Davis K et al. (1991) Topical application of clonidine relieves hyperalgesia in patients with sympathetically maintained pain. Pain. 47: 309–317.

Updated November 2013

GLYCERYL TRINITRATE   BNF 1.7.4 & 2.6.1

Class: Nitrate.

Indications: Angina, left ventricular failure, anal fissure, †smooth muscle spasm pain (particularly of the oesophagus, rectum and anus or cutaneous leiomyomas),[1] †biliary and †renal colic, †painful diabetic neuropathy,[2,3] †symptomatic relief of breathlessness in acute pulmonary oedema (in conjunction with opioids and diuretics)[4] or paroxysmal nocturnal dyspnoea. TD patch (selected brands): maintenance of venous patency, prevention of phlebitis, treatment of drug extravasation.

Contra-indications: Severe hypotension (systolic < 90mmHg), or severe aortic or mitral stenosis, cardiac tamponade, constrictive pericarditis, hypertrophic obstructive cardiomyopathy, marked anaemia, severe hypovolaemia, raised intracranial pressure, narrow-angle glaucoma. Concurrent use of **sildenafil**, **tadalafil** and **vardenafil** (may precipitate hypotension and myocardial infarction).[5]

Pharmacology

Glyceryl trinitrate (GTN) relaxes smooth muscle in blood vessels and the GI tract. This effect is mediated via its metabolism to nitric oxide (NO), which stimulates guanylate cyclase. This leads to an increase in cyclic guanosine monophosphate which reduces the amount of intracellular calcium available for muscle contraction.[6]

Endogenous NO is produced when the NMDA-receptor is stimulated by excitatory amino acids (see **ketamine**, p.625), and NO synthase inhibitors attenuate the development of opioid tolerance.[7] This points to a wider role of NO in pain modulation.

NO is involved in the regulation of distal oesophageal peristalsis and relaxation of the lower oesophageal sphincter. Thus, GTN can improve dysphagia and odynophagia associated with oesophagitis and oesophageal spasm.[8,9]

NO is also the major inhibitory neurotransmitter in the internal anal sphincter. In patients with acute anal fissure, GTN ointment 0.2–0.4% applied b.d. to the anal canal relieves painful spasm, improves quality of life and aids healing.[10] However, most patients experience headache which, although this may be transient, is severe in ≤25%.[11]

Diltiazem 2% cream is an alternative; it is as effective as GTN ointment, but causes less headache and less anal irritation.[12] Injections of **botulinum toxin** into the internal sphincter have also been used, but their exact role remains to be clarified. About 90% of acute anal fissures resolve with non-surgical approaches. However, for chronic fissures, i.e. those persisting > 6 weeks, surgery is the most effective approach.[10]

GTN administered systemically using a TD patch enhances pain relief in cancer patients; when applied directly as a gel or TD patch, it also reduces local pain and inflammation, e.g. from thrombophlebitis, tendinopathies.[13–18] In a placebo-controlled RCT in diabetic neuropathic pain affecting the feet, locally applied GTN spray reduced mean pain scores significantly from 7.5 to 4.6 (NNT = 4).[2] In a second RCT, the concurrent use of PO **sodium valproate** provided no additional benefit.

Nitrates cause venous then arterial dilation in a dose-related manner. Nitrates such as GTN and **isosorbide dinitrate** are thus used SL or IVI in acute heart failure to reduce pre- and after-load, which, in conjunction with opioids and diuretics, helps to relieve breathlessness. This is not suitable for patients with hypotension (systolic < 90mmHg), severe obstructive valvular disease, or long-term use (nitrate tolerance generally develops after 24–48h).[4] Also because of tolerance, the chronic use of nitrates in cardiovascular disease is best reserved for specific circumstances, such as nocturnal angina or paroxysmal nocturnal dyspnoea. In this setting, p.r.n. GTN spray SL may be helpful or, if a frequent occurrence, a regular bedtime dose of a longer-acting nitrate PO. In those unable to swallow tablets, a bedtime application of TD GTN can be used. All these approaches permit a reasonable daily nitrate-free period.

In patients with lung cancer, a TD patch for 5 days with each cycle of chemotherapy increases the frequency and duration of response. This may reflect improved perfusion of the tumour, thereby increasing drug delivery or decreasing hypoxia, which is associated with invasion, metastasis, and drug resistance.[19] Improving hypoxia alone may be sufficient to impede tumour growth;[20,21] use of a low-dose (i.e. application of one-sixth of a 5mg TD patch daily) in patients with prostate cancer and an increasing PSA after surgery or radiotherapy, increased the PSA doubling time from 13 to 32 months.[21]

Nitric oxide also plays a role in bone metabolism. Nitrates impact on the number and activity of osteoclasts (decreased) and osteoblasts (increased), resulting in both a reduction in bone resorption and an increase in bone formation. Benefit appears dose-related, and is lost with higher doses.[22] GTN ointment has been studied as a potential treatment for osteoporosis, with mixed results.[23,24]

GTN is rapidly absorbed through the buccal mucosa but orally it is inactivated by extensive first-pass metabolism in the GI mucosa and liver. Many patients on long-acting or TD nitrates develop tolerance, i.e. experience a reduced therapeutic effect. Tolerance is generally prevented if nitrate levels are allowed to fall for 4–8h in every 24h (a 'nitrate holiday'). This may not be possible for patients with persistent pain. If tolerance develops, it will be necessary to increase the dose to restore efficacy.

Bio-availability 40% SL.
Onset of action 1–3min SL; 30–60min ointment or TD patch.
Time to peak plasma concentration 3–6min SL; 2h TD.
Plasma halflife 1–3min SL; 2–4min TD.
Duration of action 30–60min SL; 8h ointment; 24h TD patch.

Cautions

Severe hepatic or renal impairment, hypothyroidism, hypovolaemia, hypoxaemia, hypothermia, recent myocardial infarction. Topically applied GTN can be absorbed in sufficient quantities to cause undesirable systemic effects.

TD patches: some contain metal in the backing, e.g. Transiderm-Nitro® and must be removed before MRI to avoid burns (see, p.657).[25]

Injection: glass, polyethylene or polypropylene apparatus should be used with parenteral GTN as loss of potency will occur if PVC is used.

Drug interactions

Serious drug interactions: Concurrent use of **sildenafil**, **tadalafil** and **vardenafil** may precipitate profound hypotension and myocardial infarction and is contra-indicated.

Exacerbates the hypotensive effect of other drugs. Drugs causing dry mouth may reduce the effect of sublingual nitrates.

Undesirable effects

Very common (>10%): headache (sometimes severe).
Common (<10%, >1%): flushing, dizziness, nausea.
Uncommon (<1%, ≥0.1%): local stinging, itching or burning sensation after SL spay, TD or rectal administration.
Rare (<0.1%, ≥0.01%): postural hypotension, tachycardia (paradoxical bradycardia also reported); may be more frequent with IV use.
These effects generally settle with continued use.

Dose and use

If necessary, paracetamol can be used for headache.
Intermittent dysphagia and/or odynophagia
• start with 400–500microgram SL 5–15min before eating
• if necessary, increase to a maximum single dose of 1mg
• instruct the patient to swallow or spit out tablet once pain relief is obtained (or if headache develops)
• repeat p.r.n.
Persistent spasm
Consider:
• GTN TD patches *or*
• orally active nitrates, e.g. **isosorbide mononitrate**.
Anal fissure pain
• use 0.2–0.4% rectal ointment
• using a covered finger, gently insert a 2.5cm length (or pea-sized quantity) of ointment about 1cm into the anal canal b.d. for 6 weeks.[26]

Painful diabetic neuropathy
- apply GTN spray locally to the painful extremity: 1 spray/sole of foot/day.

Acute pulmonary oedema in conjunction with diuretics and opioids
   Use under the guidance of a cardiologist. Give by SL tablet or spray, or in more severe cases by IVI, e.g.:
- 400–500microgram SL every 5–10min, *or*
- 10–20microgram/min IVI, titrate every 3–5min as needed in 5–10microgram/min increments, up to a maximum of 200microgram/min.

Supply

Because GTN is an explosive substance, spray formulations contain additives (e.g. medium chain partial glycerides or alcohol) to stabilize the solution and minimize the potential for explosion.

Glyceryl trinitrate (generic)
Tablets SL 300microgram, 500microgram, 600microgram, 100 = £3, £2 and £13 respectively; *store in the original glass container; because of degradation, unused tablets should be discarded after 8 weeks.*
Aerosol spray 400microgram/metered dose, 200-dose unit = £3, *contains alcohol.*

TD products
Nitro-Dur® (Schering-Plough)
TD patch 200microgram/h (approx 5mg/24h), 400microgram/h (approx 10mg/24h), 600microgram/h (approx 15mg/24h), 28 days @ 1 patch daily = £11, £12 and £13 respectively.

Topical
Ointment 0.2%, 30g = £41 (Unauthorized, available as a special order; see Appendix 1, p.817). *Note price based on specials tariff in community.*

Rectogesic® (ProStrakan)
Rectal ointment 0.4%, 30g = £40. *Discard 8 weeks after opening. Contains propylene glycol and lanolin (irritants).*

Parenteral
Injection 1mg/mL, 50mL = £16.
Injection 5mg/mL, 5mL and 10mL = £7 and £13 respectively; *must be diluted before use. Contains propylene glycol; maximum recommended use of 3 days.*

Nitrocine (UCB Pharma)
Injection 1mg/mL, 10mL = £6.

Nitronal (Merk Serono)
Injection 1mg/mL, 5mL and 50mL = £2 and £15 respectively.
This is not a complete list; see BNF for more information.

Diltiazem
Cream or ointment 2%, 30g = £84 or £133 respectively (Unauthorized, available as a special order; see Appendix 1, p.817). *Note price based on specials tariff in community.*

1 George S et al. (1997) Pain in multiple leiomyomas alleviated by nifedipine. *Pain.* **73**: 101–102.
2 Agrawal RP et al. (2007) Glyceryl trinitrate spray in the management of painful diabetic neuropathy: a randomized double blind placebo controlled cross-over study. *Diabetes Research and Clinical Practice.* **77**: 161–167.
3 Agrawal RP et al. (2009) Management of diabetic neuropathy by sodium valproate and glyceryl trinitrate spray: a prospective double-blind randomized placebo-controlled study. *Diabetes Research and Clinical Practice.* **83**: 371–378.
4 McMurray JJ et al. (2012) ESC Guidelines for the diagnosis and treatment of acute and chronic heart failure 2012: The Task Force for the Diagnosis and Treatment of Acute and Chronic Heart Failure 2012 of the European Society of Cardiology. Developed in collaboration with the Heart Failure Association (HFA) of the ESC. *European Heart Journal.* **33**: 1787–1847.
5 Baxter K and Preston CL. *Stockley's Drug Interactions.* London: Pharmaceutical Press www.medicinescomplete.com (accessed November 2013).
6 Hashimoto S and Kobayashi A (2003) Clinical pharmacokinetics and pharmacodynamics of glyceryl trinitrate and its metabolites. *Clinical Pharmacokinetics.* **42**: 205–221.
7 Elliott K et al. (1994) The NMDA receptor antagonists, LY274614 and MK-801, and the nitric oxide synthase inhibitor, NG-nitro-L-arginine, attenuate analgesic tolerance to the mu-opioid morphine but not to kappa opioids. *Pain.* **56**: 69–75.

8   McDonnell F and Walsh D (1999) Treatment of odynophagia and dysphagia in advanced cancer with sublingual glyceryl trinitrate. *Palliative Medicine.* **13**: 251–252.
9   Tutuian R and Castell DO (2006) Review article: oesophageal spasm - diagnosis and management. *Alimentary Pharmacology and Therapeutics.* **23**: 1393–1402.
10 Nelson RL et al. (2012) Non surgical therapy for anal fissure. *Cochrane Database of Systematic Reviews.* **2**: CD003431.
11 Fenton C et al. (2006) 0.4% nitroglycerin ointment : in the treatment of chronic anal fissure pain. *Drugs.* **66**: 343–349.
12 Sajid MS et al. (2013) Systematic review of the use of topical diltiazem compared with glyceryltrinitrate for the nonoperative management of chronic anal fissure. *Colorectal Disease.* **15**: 19–26.
13 Ferreira S et al. (1992) Blockade of hyperalgesia and neurogenic oedema by topical application of nitroglycerin. *Eur J Pharmacol.* **217**: 207–209.
14 Berrazueta J et al. (1994) Local transdermal glyceryl trinitrate has an antiinflammatory action on thrombophlebitis induced by sclerosis of leg varicose veins. *Angiology.* **5**: 347–351.
15 Lauretti G et al. (1999) Oral ketamine and transdermal nitroglycerin as analgesic adjuvants to oral morphine therapy and amitriptyline for cancer pain management. *Anesthesiology.* **90**: 1528–1533.
16 Lauretti GR et al. (2002) Double-blind evaluation of transdermal nitroglycerine as adjuvant to oral morphine for cancer pain management. *Journal of Clinical Anesthesia.* **14**: 83–86.
17 El-Sheikh SM and El-Kest E (2004) Transdermal nitroglycerine enhanced fentanyl patch analgesia in cancer pain management. *Egyptian Journal of Anaesthesia.* **20**: 291–294.
18 Gambito ED et al. (2010) Evidence on the effectiveness of topical nitroglycerin in the treatment of tendinopathies: a systematic review and meta-analysis. *Archives of Physical Medicine and Rehabilitation.* **91**: 1291–1305.
19 Yasuda H et al. (2006) Randomized phase II trial comparing nitroglycerin plus vinorelbine and cisplatin with vinorelbine and cisplatin alone in previously untreated stage IIIB/IV non-small-cell lung cancer. *Journal of Clinical Oncology.* **24**: 688–694.
20 Maeda H (2010) Nitroglycerin enhances vascular blood flow and drug delivery in hypoxic tumor tissues: analogy between angina pectoris and solid tumors and enhancement of the EPR effect. *Journal of Controlled Release.* **142**: 296–298.
21 Siemens DR et al. (2009) Phase II study of nitric oxide donor for men with increasing prostate-specific antigen level after surgery or radiotherapy for prostate cancer. *Urology.* **74**: 878–883.
22 Khosla S (2011) Is nitroglycerin a novel and inexpensive treatment for osteoporosis? *JAMA.* **305**: 826–827.
23 Wimalawansa SJ et al. (2009) Transdermal nitroglycerin therapy may not prevent early postmenopausal bone loss. *Journal of Clinical Endocrinology and Metabolism.* **94**: 3356–3364.
24 Jamal SA et al. (2011) Effect of nitroglycerin ointment on bone density and strength in postmenopausal women: a randomized trial. *Journal of the American Medical Association.* **305**: 800–807.
25 Institute for Safe Medication Practices (2004) Medication Safety Alert. Burns in MRI patients wearing transdermal patches. Available from: www.ismp.org/Newsletters/acutecare/articles/20040408.asp?ptr = y
26 Gagliardi G et al. (2010) Optimal treatment duration of glyceryl trinitrate for chronic anal fissure: results of a prospective randomized multicenter trial. *Techniques in Coloproctology.* **14**: 241–248.

Updated January 2014

NIFEDIPINE   BNF 2.6.2

Class: Calcium-channel blocker.

Indications: Prophylaxis of stable angina, hypertension, Raynaud's phenomenon (immediate-release only authorized formulation), †severe smooth muscle spasm pain (particularly of the oesophagus, rectum and anus, cutaneous leiomyomas),[1–5] †intractable hiccup.[6,7]

Contra-indications: Cardiogenic shock, severe aortic stenosis, acute or unstable angina (immediate-release capsules PO or SL may cause hypotension and reflex tachycardia precipitating myocardial or cerebrovascular ischaemia). *Do not use within one month of myocardial infarction.* Adalat® LA: hepatic impairment; previous or current GI obstruction or stenosis, inflammatory bowel disease.

Pharmacology

Nifedipine inhibits the influx of calcium through L-type channels into cells, thereby modifying cell function, e.g. smooth muscle contraction and neural transmission.[8] It is used to relieve dysphagia and chest pain in oesophageal spasm.[9,10] It also relieves painful spasm associated with an anal fissure,[11] although topical treatment with either **glyceryl trinitrate** or **diltiazem** are generally preferred in practice (see p.79). Nifedipine may help hiccup by relieving oesophageal spasm or by interference with nerve pathways involved in hiccup.[6,7,12]

In animal studies, nifedipine and other calcium-channel blockers augment the analgesic effects of paracetamol, morphine and anti-epileptics.[13–15] The clinical relevance of this is uncertain; inconsistent benefit has been found from the addition of calcium-channel blockers to post-operative pain regimens.[16–18]

Nifedipine has a relatively greater effect on blood vessels than the myocardium and has no anti-arrhythmic activity. It rarely precipitates heart failure because any negative inotropic effect is offset by a reduction in left ventricular work.

Nifedipine undergoes extensive first-pass metabolism in the liver to inactive metabolites which are excreted in the urine. Higher plasma concentrations are seen in slow metabolizers, which are more prevalent in South American, South Asian and black African populations.[19,20] Hepatic impairment increases bio-availability and halflife.

Bio-availability 45–75% PO (immediate-release capsules).

Onset of action 15min (immediate-release capsules); 1.5h (m/r tablets, Adalat® Retard).

Time to peak plasma concentration 30min PO (immediate-release capsules).

Plasma halflife about 2h (immediate-release capsules); 2–2.5h (m/r tablets, Adalat® Retard).

Duration of action 8h (immediate-release capsules); 12 or 24h (m/r tablets, depending on brand).

Cautions

May exacerbate angina; discontinue nifedipine if angina occurs 30–60min after the first dose. Rarely, it may precipitate or worsen heart failure; avoid in patients with significantly impaired cardiac function or heart failure. Hepatic impairment. May impair glucose tolerance and worsen diabetes mellitus.

Drug interactions

Serious drug interactions: augments the hypotensive and negative inotropic effects of other drugs, e.g. α and β antagonists, **chlorpromazine**.[21]

Nifedipine is metabolized by and inhibits CYP3A4 and CYP2D6; it also inhibits CYP1A2 and CYP2C8/9. Caution is required with concurrent use of drugs which inhibit or induce these enzymes, particularly in poor CYP2D6 metabolizers (see Chapter 25, p.767).[21] Reports of interactions where dose adjustment or close monitoring are needed are listed in Table 1.

Table 1 CYP450 interactions with nifedipine which can alter drug plasma concentrations

Nifedipine plasma concentration		Drug plasma concentration	
increased by	decreased by	increased by nifedipine	decreased by nifedipine
Azole antifungals	Carbamazepine	Digoxin	Quinidine
Cimetidine[a]	Phenobarbital	Quinidine	
Fluoxetine	Phenytoin	Sertindole (not UK)	
Grapefruit juice	Rifampicin[b]	Tacrolimus	
Imatinib	St Johns wort	Theophylline	
Macrolide antibacterials			
Protease inhibitors			
Quinupristin/dalfopristin (not UK)			

a. reduce nifedipine dose by 50%
b. manufacturer considers that rifampicin renders nifedipine ineffective.

Undesirable effects

Common (<10%, >1%): headache, dizziness, vasodilation, peripheral oedema, constipation.

Uncommon (<1%, >0.1%): asthenia, lethargy, malaise, agitation, nervousness, sleep disorder, tremor, vertigo, abnormal vision, chest pain, tachycardia, palpitations, postural hypotension, oedema, dyspnoea, dry mouth, dyspepsia, abdominal pain, nausea, rash, pruritus, sweating, transient increase in liver enzymes.

Dose and use

Patients with angina should not bite into or use an immediate-release capsule SL because of the risk of rapid-onset hypotension and reflex tachycardia, which could lead to myocardial or cerebrovascular ischaemia.

For SL administration, patients should bite into and use the liquid contents of the immediate-release capsules immediately (unauthorized use). *Modified release formulations must not be used SL or chewed.*

- start with 10mg PO/SL stat and 10–20mg t.d.s. or m/r 20mg PO b.d. or 30–60mg PO once daily
- for achalasia, start with 10–20mg SL 30min before food; usual maximum dose 60–80mg/24h
- for painful spasm associated with anal fissure, use m/r 20mg PO b.d.
- for intractable hiccup, ≤160mg/24h PO has been used with concurrent **fludrocortisone** 0.5–1mg PO to overcome associated orthostatic hypotension.[7]

Note: remains of some m/r tablets (Adalat® LA) may appear in the patient's faeces ('ghost tablets'), but these are inert residues, and do not affect the efficacy of the products.

Supply

Because of their different dosing regimens and concern over possible non-bio-equivalence, the BNF recommends that m/r formulations of nifedipine should be prescribed by brand name.[22]

Immediate-release
Nifedipine (generic)
Capsules 5mg, 10mg, 28 days @ 10mg t.d.s. = £10.
Oral Solution 10mg/5mL, 28 days @ 10mg t.d.s. = £730. (Unauthorized, available as a special order; see Appendix 1, p.817). *Note price based on specials tariff in community.*
Oral solution (drops) 20mg/mL, 30mL = £30. (Unauthorized, available as a special order imported via The Specials Laboratory; see Appendix 1, p.817).

Adalat® (Bayer)
Capsules 5mg, 10mg, 28 days @ 10mg t.d.s. = £7.

Modified-release
Adalat Retard (Bayer)
Tablets m/r 10mg, 20mg, 28 days @ 20mg b.d. = £9.

Adalat LA (Bayer)
Tablets m/r 20mg, 30mg, 60mg, 28 days @ 30mg once daily = £7.

Adipine® MR (Chiesi)
Tablets m/r 10mg, 20mg, 28 days @ 20mg b.d. = £5.

Adipine® XL (Chiesi)
Tablets m/r 30mg, 60mg, 28 days @ 30mg once daily = £5.

This is not a complete list; see BNF for more information.

1 McLoughlin R and McQuillan R (1997) Using nifedipine to treat tenesmus. *Palliative Medicine.* **11**: 419–420.
2 George S et al. (1997) Pain in multiple leiomyomas alleviated by nifedipine. *Pain.* **73**: 101–102.
3 Cargill G et al. (1982) Nifedipine for relief of esophageal chest pain. *New England Journal of Medicine.* **307**: 187–188.
4 Al-Waili N (1990) Nifedipine for intestinal colic. *Journal of the American Medical Association.* **263**: 3258.
5 Celik A et al. (1995) Hereditary proctalgia fugax and constipation: report of a second family. *Gut.* **36**: 581–584.
6 Lipps DC et al. (1990) Nifedipine for intractable hiccups. *Neurology.* **40**: 531–532.
7 Brigham B and Bolin T (1992) High dose nifedipine and fludrocortisone for intractable hiccups. *Medical Journal of Australia.* **157**: 70.
8 Castell DO (1985) Calcium-channel blocking agents for gastrointestinal disorders. *American Journal of Cardiology.* **55**: 210B–213B.
9 Achem SR and Gerson LB (2013) Distal esophageal spasm: an update. *Curr Gastroenterol Rep.* **15**: 325.
10 Cross-Adame E et al. (2013) Treatment of esophageal (non-cardiac) chest pain: Review. (epub ahead of print). *Clinical Gastroenterology and Heptology.*
11 Mustafa NA et al. (2006) Comparison of topical glyceryl trinitrate ointment and oral nifedipine in the treatment of chronic anal fissure. *Acta Chirurgica Belgica.* **106**: 55–58.
12 Williams M (2004) The management of hiccups in advanced cancer. *CME Cancer Medicine.* **2**: 68–70.
13 Koleva M and Dimova S (2000) Effects of nifedipine, verapamil, diltiazem and trifluoperazine on the antinociceptive activity of acetaminophen. *Methods Find Exp Clin Pharmacol.* **22**: 741–745.
14 Michaluk J et al. (1998) Effects of various Ca2+ channel antagonists on morphine analgesia, tolerance and dependence, and on blood pressure in the rat. *Eur J Pharmacol.* **352**: 189–197.
15 El-Azab MF and Moustafa YM (2012) Influence of calcium channel blockers on anticonvulsant and antinociceptive activities of valproic acid in pentylenetetrazole-kindled mice. *Pharmacological Reports.* **64**: 305–314.
16 Carta F et al. (1990) Effect of nifedipine on morphine-induced analgesia. *Anesth Analg.* **70**: 493–498.

17 Zarauza R et al. (2000) A comparative study with oral nifedipine, intravenous nimodipine, and magnesium sulfate in postoperative analgesia. Anesth Analg. **91**: 938–943.

18 Casey G et al. (2006) Perioperative nimodipine and postoperative analgesia. Anesth Analg. **102**: 504–508.

19 Sowunmi A et al. (1995) Ethnic differences in nifedipine kinetics: comparisons between Nigerians, Caucasians and South Asians. British Journal of Clinical Pharmacology. **40**: 489–493.

20 Castaneda-Hernandez G et al. (1996) Interethnic variability in nifedipine disposition: reduced systemic plasma clearance in Mexican subjects. British Journal of Clinical Pharmacology. **41**: 433–434.

21 Baxter K and Preston CL Stockley's Drug Interactions. London: Pharmaceutical Press www.medicinescomplete.com (accessed November 2013).

22 British National Formulary London: BMJ Group and Pharmaceutical Press www.bnf.org (accessed November 2013).

Updated December 2013

ANTICOAGULANTS   BNF 2.8

Anticoagulants are used predominantly to prevent or treat venous thrombo-embolism (VTE).[1] There is a range of drugs which act at various points in the coagulation cascade (Figure 1), but **LMWH** (see p.89) and **warfarin** are still generally the most frequently used.

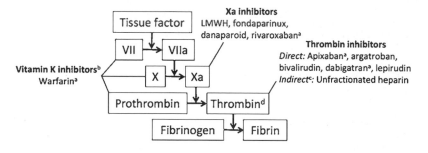

Figure 1   Sites of action of anticoagulants. Unless indicated otherwise, administration is parenteral, e.g. SC, IV, CIVI (see individual SPC). Heparins are antagonized by protamine sulfate; warfarin by vitamin K_1 (phytomenadione).[2] Novel oral anticoagulants have no antidote (see text).

a. administered PO
b. vitamin K inhibitors also reduce factor IX synthesis, inhibiting coagulation amplification pathways
c. indirect thrombin inhibitors activate antithrombin III, a regulator of coagulation
d. thrombin also triggers several amplification pathways (factors V, VIII, IX and XI) which promote further factor X activation and thus further thrombin generation.

LMWH (derived from porcine heparin) and **fondaparinux** (a synthetic heparin pentasaccharide) both inhibit factor Xa.[3] LMWH is the current gold standard anticoagulant for cancer patients. **Fondaparinux** is a useful alternative in those patients who need to avoid LMWH because of hypersensitivity, history of heparin induced thrombocytopenia, or for religious or cultural reasons.[4–6]

Warfarin is likely to be increasingly replaced by novel oral anticoagulants (NOAC), such as **apixaban** and **dabigatran etexilate** (direct thrombin inhibitors) or **rivaroxaban** (direct Xa inhibitor). Potential advantages of NOAC include standard doses and no need to monitor the patient's INR.

Rivaroxaban is non-inferior to **warfarin** in the treatment of VTE with respect to recurrent VTE and bleeding.[7,8] Currently, it is the only NOAC authorized for both treatment of VTE and prevention of recurrent VTE, and is recommended by NICE.[9] However, in cancer patients, its use requires caution because efficacy and safety data are limited in this group.[7,8,10] Indeed, some currently recommend against the use of NOAC in cancer patients for several reasons, including:[11]

- non-inferiority with LMWH has not been demonstrated
- the risk of significant drug–drug interactions with CYP3A4 inducers or inhibitors (these include several chemotherapy drugs) which could lead to clinically important changes in plasma concentrations of NOAC, and result in therapeutic failure or bleeding
- major bleeding is more likely in patients with cancer who are anticoagulated,[12] and the lack of standardized methods of monitoring NOAC and of antidotes could cause problems.

Nonetheless, **rivaroxaban** (and eventually other NOAC) is likely to be increasingly used in cancer patients unwilling to tolerate daily SC injections of LMWH. Seek advice from a haematologist about such use, and urgently if bleeding occurs during use (Box A).

Box A   Management of bleeding in patients on rivaroxaban[13,14]

There is no antidote to rivaroxaban; it is not dialysable.

Pharmacokinetic data
- maximum anticoagulant effect 2–4h after administration (T_{max} 2–3h)
- duration of action 24h (plasma halflife 5–13h)
- renal excretion 33% (deteriorating renal function → increased effect).

Minor bleeding
- document the time of the last dose
- apply local haemostatic measures, if feasible
- if bleeding continues, consider tranexamic acid (see below)
- delay next dose of rivaroxaban or stop.

Major bleeding
- apply local haemostatic measures, if feasible
- give IV fluid replacement
- *obtain advice from haematologist urgently*
- stop rivaroxaban
- document the time of the last dose; if taken < 2h ago, consider giving activated charcoal PO
- arrange laboratory tests as recommended by haematologist, e.g. FBC, prothrombin time (PT), APTT, eGFR:
  - ▷ PT is more sensitive to rivaroxaban than APTT, but both only provide a rough estimate of the degree of anticoagulation. However, when:
    - ○ one or both are raised, the degree of anticoagulation is significant
    - ○ both are normal, the degree of anticoagulation can be regarded as similar to that achieved with prophylactic LMWH
  - ▷ for small and frail elderly patients (> 60 years old) use the Cockcroft Gault formula (see p.656) to calculate creatinine clearance, as eGFR can overestimate renal function in these patients
- give tranexamic acid:
  - ▷ 15mg/kg IV t.d.s–q.d.s. (or 25mg/kg PO t.d.s.); reduce dose in renal impairment (see p.100)
  - ▷ if feasible, apply topically to bleeding point, e.g. mouthwash, nasal drops
- consider also other possible causes of raised PT/APTT
- give IV blood product support as indicated by Hb, other coagulopathy, platelets (if count < 75 x 10^9/L).

If ongoing life- or limb- threatening bleeding
- *obtain further advice from haematologist urgently*
- consider use of prothrombin complex concentrate (Octaplex®) 30 units/kg or other prohaemostatic concentrate (limited evidence-base).

General considerations

Compared with non-cancer patients, those with cancer are three times more likely to experience recurrent VTE (21% vs. 7%), *even with optimal treatment with* **warfarin**.[15] The increased risk results from a cancer-related pro-inflammatory state associated with:

- activation of the coagulation cascade by procoagulant proteins expressed by the cancer
- damage to blood vessel walls
- venous stasis
- other general risk factors (Box B).

Box B   Main risk factors for VTE in medical patients

Age ≥40 years, particularly >60 years

Immobility

Dehydration

Obesity

Cancer, particularly metastatic, especially of the pancreas, stomach, bladder, ovary, uterus, kidney or lung; also haematological

Chronic respiratory or cardiac disease

Other serious medical conditions, e.g. sepsis, lower limb weakness (including spinal cord compression), inflammatory bowel disease, collagen disorder

Varicose veins/chronic venous insufficiency

Previous VTE

Cancer chemotherapy, e.g. platinum compounds, 5-FU, mitomycin-C, thalidomide

Growth factors, e.g. granulocyte colony stimulating factor, erythropoietin

Radiation therapy, e.g. to the pelvis

Hormone therapy, e.g. oral contraceptives, hormone replacement, tamoxifen, anastrozole, and possibly progestins

Thrombophilia

Specialist guidelines recommend that thromboprophylaxis should be considered if an acute medical illness is likely to render a cancer patient bedbound for ≥3 days, particularly in the presence of one or more additional risk factors (Box B).[4,23,24] Duration of treatment is generally about 2 weeks.[21]

If anticoagulation is contra-indicated, the use of graduated compression stockings and/or intermittent pneumatic compression is recommended.[16] However, the evidence base in medical patients is limited, and in some populations there have been reports of harm.[25]

In palliative care, LMWH is preferable because haemorrhagic complications with **warfarin** may occur in up to 50% of patients, possibly related to poor performance status, drug interactions and hepatic impairment. Those patients agreeing to the indefinite use of LMWH have found it acceptable.[26-29] Compared with **warfarin**, treatment with LMWH is more straightforward: no need to check INR, and little need for dose adjustments. However, compared with warfarin, LMWH is much more expensive (Table 1).

Table 1   Cost of anticoagulants

Drug	Route	Dose	Approximate 28 day cost
Dabigatran	PO capsules	1 capsule b.d.	£76
LMWH	SC injection	1 injection daily	£84–£96
Rivaroxaban	PO tablets	1 tablet daily	£60
Warfarin	PO tablets	Based on INR, 1–2 tablets once daily (any strength)	£1–2[a]

a. does not include cost of checking INR.

1 Farge D et al. (2013) International clinical practice guidelines for the treatment and prophylaxis of venous thromboembolism in patients with cancer. Journal of Thrombosis and Haemostasis. 11: 56–70.
2 Noble S and Johnson M (2012) Management of cancer associated thrombosis in people with advanced disease. BMJ Supportive and Palliative Care. 2: 163–167.
3 Hoppensteadt D et al. (2003) Heparin, low-molecular-weight heparins, and heparin pentasaccharide: basic and clinical differentiation. Hematology Oncology Clinics of North America. 17: 313–341.
4 Baglin T et al. (2006) Guidelines on the use and monitoring of heparin. British Journal of Haematology. 133: 19–34.
5 Blann AD and Lip GY (2006) Venous thromboembolism. British Medical Journal. 332: 215–219.
6 Cohen AT et al. (2006) Efficacy and safety of fondaparinux for the prevention of venous thromboembolism in older acute medical patients: randomised placebo controlled trial. British Medical Journal. 332: 325–329.
7 Schulman S et al. (2009) Dabigatran versus warfarin in the treatment of acute venous thromboembolism. New England Journal of Medicine. 361: 2342–2352.
8 Bauersachs R et al. (2010) Oral rivaroxaban for symptomatic venous thromboembolism. New England Journal of Medicine. 363: 2499–2510.
9 NICE (2012) Rivaroxaban for the treatment of deep vein thrombosis and prevention of recurrent deep vein thrombosis and pulmonary embolism. Technology appraisal TA261www.nice.org.uk
10 Romualdi E et al. (2011) Oral rivaroxaban after symptomatic venous thromboembolism: the continued treatment study (EINSTEIN-extension study). Expert Review of Cardiovascular Therapy. 9: 841–844.
11 Carrier M et al. (2013) Management of challenging cases of patients with cancer-associated thrombosis including recurrent thrombosis and bleeding: guidance from the SSC of the ISTH. Journal of Thrombosis and Haemostasis. 12: 116–117.
12 Streiff MB (2006) Long-term therapy of venous thromboembolism in cancer patients. Journal of the National Comprehensive Cancer Network. 4: 903–910.
13 Baglin T et al. (2012) Effects on routine coagulation screens and assessment of anticoagulant intensity in patients taking oral dabigatran or rivaroxaban: guidance from the British Committee for Standards in Haematology. British Journal of Haematology. 159: 427–429.
14 Makris M et al. (2012) Guideline on the management of bleeding in patients on antithrombotic agents. British Journal of Haematology. 160: 35–46.
15 Prandoni P et al. (2002) Recurrent venous thromboembolism and bleeding complications during anticoagulant treatment in patients with cancer and venous thrombosis. Blood. 100: 3484–3488.
16 Kearon C et al. (2012) Antithrombotic therapy for VTE disease: Antithrombotic Therapy and Prevention of Thrombosis, 9th ed: American College of Chest Physicians Evidence-Based Clinical Practice Guidelines. Chest. 141: e419S–494S.
17 Samama MM et al. (1999) A comparison of enoxaparin with placebo for the prevention of venous thromboembolism in acutely ill medical patients. Prophylaxis in Medical Patients with Enoxaparin Study Group. New England Journal of Medicine. 341: 793–800.
18 De Cicco M (2004) The prothrombotic state in cancer: pathogenic mechanisms. Critical Reviews in Oncology Hematology. 50: 187–196.
19 Deitcher SR and Gomes MP (2004) The risk of venous thromboembolic disease associated with adjuvant hormone therapy for breast carcinoma: a systematic review. Cancer. 101: 439–449.
20 Leizorovicz A et al. (2004) Randomized, placebo-controlled trial of dalteparin for the prevention of venous thromboembolism in acutely ill medical patients. Circulation. 110: 874–879.
21 Leizorovicz A and Mismetti P (2004) Preventing venous thromboembolism in medical patients. Circulation. 110: 13–19.
22 Chew HK et al. (2006) Incidence of venous thromboembolism and its effect on survival among patients with common cancers. Archives of Internal Medicine. 166: 458–464.
23 NICE (2010) Reducing the risk of venous thromboembolism (deep vein thrombosis and pulmonary embolism) in patients admitted to hospital. Clinical Guideline 92. www.nice.org.uk
24 Cunningham MS et al. (2006) Prevention and management of venous thromboembolism in people with cancer: a review of the evidence. Clinical Oncology (Royal College of Radiologists). 18: 145–151.
25 Dennis M et al. (2009) Effectiveness of thigh-length graduated compression stockings to reduce the risk of deep vein thrombosis after stroke (CLOTS trial 1): a multicentre, randomised controlled trial. Lancet. 373: 1958–1965.
26 Johnson M (1997) Problems of anticoagulation within a palliative care setting: an audit of hospice patients taking warfarin. Palliative Medicine. 11: 306–312.
27 Johnson M and Sherry K (1997) How do palliative physicians manage venous thromboembolism? Palliative Medicine. 11: 462–468.
28 Noble SI and Finlay IG (2005) Is long-term low-molecular-weight heparin acceptable to palliative care patients in the treatment of cancer related venous thromboembolism? A qualitative study. Palliative Medicine. 19: 197–201.
29 Noble SI et al. (2006) Acceptability of low molecular weight heparin thromboprophylaxis for inpatients receiving palliative care: qualitative study. British Medical Journal. 332: 577–580.

Updated August 2013

LOW MOLECULAR WEIGHT HEPARIN (LMWH) BNF 2.8.1

Class: Parenteral anticoagulant.

Indications: Authorized indications vary between products; consult SPCs for details. Thromboprophylaxis, initial treatment of venous thrombo-embolism (VTE), treatment of cancer-associated thrombosis, †thrombophlebitis migrans, †disseminated intravascular coagulation (DIC).

Contra-indications: IM use (risk of injection site haematoma); active major bleeding; suspected or confirmed heparin-induced thrombocytopenia (HIT) with LMWH; known bleeding diathesis (including bleeding peptic ulcer); severe uncontrolled hypertension; haemorrhagic stroke; diabetic or haemorrhagic retinopathy; bacterial endocarditis; injury or surgery to brain, spinal cord, eyes or ears.

Note: *stated contra-indications and cautions vary; see individual SPCs.*

Pharmacology

Three low molecular weight heparins (LMWHs) are available in the UK, **dalteparin**, **enoxaparin**, **tinzaparin**, all derived from porcine heparin. Some patients need to avoid the use of LMWH because of known hypersensitivity, or for religious or cultural reasons; the most appropriate parenteral alternative is **fondaparinux**, a non-porcine synthetic heparin pentasaccharide.[1-3]

LMWH acts mainly by potentiating the inhibitory effect of antithrombin III on factor Xa. The dose of LMWH is determined by the patient's weight, and routine monitoring is not necessary. However, in cases where the patient is considered at risk of bleeding, has renal impairment (CrCl < 30mL/min) or a history of recurrent thrombosis, anti-factor Xa activity levels can be measured.

LMWH is as effective as unfractionated heparin (UFH) for the treatment of DVT and pulmonary embolism (PE) and is now considered the initial treatment of choice.[1] Advantages include a longer duration of action permitting once daily administration, and possibly a better safety profile (fewer major haemorrhages).[4,5]

In cancer patients, LMWH is more effective than **warfarin** with a similar or reduced risk of bleeding.[6-8] LMWH is the anticoagulant of choice for long-term use in patients for whom maintaining a stable INR is difficult (risking either therapeutic failure or haemorrhagic complications) or in those who have recurrent VTE despite a therapeutic INR.

LMWH has an anticancer effect, possibly by inhibiting cancer cell growth, angiogenesis and metastasis, thereby prolonging survival.[9-13] The effect is greater in those whose life expectancy is > 6 months at the start of treatment, is greater with LMWH than UFH, and is not attributable to a reduction in VTE.[14,15] However, at present LMWH is *not* recommended as routine adjunctive treatment.[1] The results of an RCT in patients with lung cancer are expected in late 2013.[16]

For pharmacokinetic details, see Table 1.

Table 1   LMWH pharmacokinetics[17-21]

	Dalteparin	Enoxaparin	Tinzaparin
Bio-availability SC[a]	87%	100%	87%
Onset of action	3min IV	5min IV	5min IV
	2–4h SC	3h SC	2–3h SC
Time to peak plasma activity[a]	4h SC	2–6h SC	4–5h SC
Plasma activity halflife[a]	2h IV	2–4.5h IV	1.5h IV
	3–5h SC	4.5–7h SC	3–4h SC
Duration of action	10–24h SC	> 24h SC	24h

a. based on anti-factor Xa activity.

Cautions

Contra-indications and cautions vary between manufacturers; see individual SPCs.

Risk factors for bleeding include serious concurrent illness, severe renal and hepatic impairment (see Dose and use below), chronic heavy consumption of alcohol, age, and possibly female gender.

Monitor closely if spinal analgesia is used in a patient receiving LMWH *thromboprophylaxis*, and, because of the risk of a spinal haematoma, spinal analgesia should be avoided in a patient receiving *therapeutic* doses of LMWH.

Drug interactions

Enhanced bleeding tendency with NSAIDs (particularly **ketorolac**) and other drugs with anticoagulant/antiplatelet effect.

Inhibition of aldosterone secretion by heparin/LMWH may cause hyperkalaemia. The risk appears to increase with duration of therapy and is higher in patients with diabetes mellitus, chronic renal failure, acidosis and those taking potassium supplements or potassium-sparing drugs. The CSM recommends measuring plasma potassium in such patients before starting heparin and regularly thereafter, particularly if heparin is to be continued for > 1 week, although a specific frequency is not stated.

Undesirable effects

Common (<10%, >1%): headache, dizziness, pain at the injection site, minor bleeding (haematoma at the injection site), major bleeding in surgical patients receiving thromboprophylaxis and patients being treated for VTE, tachycardia, chest pain, oedema, hypotension, hypertension, anaemia, nausea, constipation, reversible increases in liver transaminases, back pain, haematuria.

Uncommon (<1%, >0.1%): major bleeding in patients receiving thromboprophylaxis, immune-mediated heparin-induced thrombocytopenia (HIT, see Quick Clinical Guide, p.97), abdominal pain, diarrhoea.

Dose and use
Routine platelet count monitoring
All patients should have a baseline platelet count before starting LMWH.
Those who have received UFH in the last 3 months should have a repeat platelet count after 24h to exclude rapid-onset HIT caused by pre-existing cross-reacting antibodies. All patients should have their platelet count checked every few days for 2 weeks.[22]

Renal impairment
Clearance of **enoxaparin** is reduced by ≤65% and **tinzaparin** by ≤25%. The manufacturer recommends dose reduction for **enoxaparin** in patients with a *creatinine clearance <30mL/min*. The anti-factor Xa activity halflives of **dalteparin** and **tinzaparin** are prolonged, and specialist guidelines advise monitoring anti-factor Xa activity to guide dosing in severe renal impairment (also see SPC for Fragmin® haemodialysis/haemofiltration).[1] For example, the dose of **tinzaparin** should be reduced if anti-factor Xa activity exceeds 1.5 units/mL (usual range 1–1.2 units/mL).[23]

During haemodialysis, the IV or extracorporeal circuit dose of **dalteparin** should be reduced in patients with acute renal failure, or with chronic renal failure and an increased risk of bleeding. The dose of **tinzaparin** should be reduced in patients with severe hepatic impairment who require haemodialysis (see respective SPCs).

Specialist guidelines suggest using unfractionated heparin IV instead of LMWH in severe renal impairment but the evidence is level III, i.e. not based on an RCT.[1,8,24]

Severe hepatic impairment
Reduced synthesis of clotting factors increases the risk of bleeding. Consider dose reduction for **dalteparin, enoxaparin** (also possible risk of accumulation) and **tinzaparin**. Dose reduction is recommended for **tinzaparin** in patients with severe hepatic impairment who are also undergoing haemodialysis.

SC injections
May cause transient stinging and local bruising.[25] Long-term treatment is not acceptable to some cancer patients (about 15% in one survey).[26]

Rotate injection sites daily, e.g. between different abdominal quadrants (see SPCs for the manufacturers' recommendations). Create a skin fold by squeezing the skin between thumb and forefinger, and insert the total length of the needle vertically into the thickest part of the fold; do *not* rub the injection site.

Thromboprophylaxis in patients with cancer
Undergoing surgery
Patients with cancer undergoing major surgery are at high risk of VTE; they have twice the risk of developing a DVT and three times the risk of a fatal PE.[27] Abdominal and pelvic surgery is particularly high-risk.[28,29]

Four weeks of thromboprophylaxis is more effective than 1 week (Table 2). Standard additional mechanical measures are advisable, e.g. graduated compression stockings or intermittent pneumatic compression.[7]

Thromboprophylaxis should be continued for 2–4 weeks (and in non-cancer patients >60 years old or with a history of VTE).[8,30,31]

Table 2   Thromboprophylaxis with LMWH in patients with cancer

	Dalteparin	Enoxaparin	Tinzaparin
Undergoing surgery	5,000 units SC once daily; start evening before surgery, continue for 2–4 weeks [8,31]	40mg SC once daily; start 12h before surgery, continue for 2–4 weeks[8,30,31]	50 units/kg 2h before surgery, then once daily for 7–10 days or 4,500 units 12h before surgery, then once daily for 7–10 days
Immobile or confined to bed because of an intercurrent illness (treat latter for about 2 weeks)	5,000 units SC once daily [32,33]	40mg SC once daily [32,34]	Not authorized for medical thromboprophylaxis

Immobile or confined to bed because of an intercurrent illness

Compared with surgical patients, thromboprophylaxis is underused in medical patients, even though mortality and morbidity from VTE (major/fatal PE) and its treatment (major/fatal haemorrhage) are higher in medical patients.[35]

Hospitalized cancer patients are at high risk of VTE. Specialist guidelines recommend that thromboprophylaxis should be considered if circumstances are likely to render a patient bedbound for ⩾3 days (Table 2), particularly when there are additional risk factors (see Anticoagulants, Box B, p.88).[1,24,29] Duration of treatment is generally ⩽2 weeks.[32]

Thromboprophylaxis is generally acceptable to palliative care inpatients.[36] The decision to start should take into account the views of patients, family/informal carers and the multiprofessional team, and be kept under review. NICE guidance suggests reviewing daily, but this seems excessive and will often be impractical.[24]

If anticoagulation is contra-indicated, consider using graduated compression stockings or intermittent pneumatic compression.[8] However, the evidence base in medical patients is limited and there are reports of harm.[37] Thromboprophylaxis is less relevant for patients with a poor performance status in their last weeks-days of life, at a stage when symptom relief alone is more appropriate.[24]

Indwelling venous catheters

The presence of a central (subclavian) or peripheral indwelling venous catheter can lead to catheter-related thrombosis. It has been reported in up to two thirds of patients and is symptomatic in possibly half of these.[24] Recent figures suggest that the incidence has fallen markedly, most likely related to improved catheter materials and placement.[24]

Routine thromboprophylaxis with LMWH is not recommended because RCTs show no benefit from its use (e.g. **enoxaparin** 40mg once daily), or from low-dose **warfarin** (1mg once daily).[24,38–40]

Long-distance air travel

The evidence for an association between prolonged travel and venous VTE is controversial.[8] The risk appears greatest in journeys of >6h and in those travellers with pre-existing risk factors (see Anticoagulants, Box B, p.88).

Although there is insufficient evidence to support routine thromboprophylaxis for all travellers, it is generally advisable in patients with cancer:
- prescribe three injections (one each for the outward and return journeys, and one spare)
- provide training in the correct administration of the injection (see the information on self-administration included in the patient information leaflet)
- self-administer **dalteparin** 5,000 units SC or **enoxaparin** 40mg SC 2–4h before departure
- if there is a stop-over followed by another long flight, another injection is not necessary unless the second flight is more than 24h after the first.

In addition, patients should be advised to:
- avoid constrictive clothing around the waist and lower limbs
- avoid dehydration
- stretch the calf muscles frequently by moving the feet up and down
- wear properly fitted below-knee graduated compression stockings, providing 15–30mmHg of pressure at the ankle.

Treatment
DVT and PE in cancer patients: initial treatment
Confirm the diagnosis radiologically (e.g. ultrasound, CT pulmonary angiography). Treat with LMWH for 6 months:
- **dalteparin** 200 units/kg SC once daily for the first month, followed by 150 units/kg SC once daily for a further 2–5 months *or*
- **enoxaparin** 1.5mg/kg SC once daily *or*
- **tinzaparin** 175 units/kg SC once daily.[8,41]

Note: in the UK, only **dalteparin is authorized for extended (6 months) treatment of cancer-associated VTE.**

DVT and PE cancer patients: ongoing treatment
Indefinite anticoagulation beyond 6 months should be considered for patients who have a DVT or PE and have an ongoing major risk factor for VTE such as cancer (see Anticoagulants, Box B, p.88).[8,42]

In cancer patients, indefinite LMWH appears more effective than **warfarin**, with a similar or reduced risk of bleeding.[43–45] If a switch to **warfarin** is considered in a patient with stable or cured cancer, LMWH should be continued until a therapeutic INR has been achieved on two consecutive days.

VTE in a seemingly cured cancer patient may be an indication of occult recurrence. If truly idiopathic, a minimum of 6–12 months of anticoagulation is recommended, and indefinite anticoagulation considered.

Provided no contra-indications develop, indefinite anticoagulation is generally continued in patients with cancer until they reach the stage when symptom relief alone becomes more appropriate, e.g. in the last few weeks or days of life.

In patients at high risk of recurrent VTE for whom anticoagulation is contra-indicated or ineffective, an inferior vena caval filter is an option.[7,41,46]
An alternative fixed-dose dalteparin regimen
After an initial week of weight-adjusted **dalteparin** treatment, one centre uses a fixed-dose regimen in patients with metastatic cancer (Box A). Published data show that, although (inevitably) some patients had major bleeding (sometimes fatal) or recurrent VTE, complications were no higher in patients with liver or brain metastases, thrombocytopenia, or those undergoing surgical or invasive procedures.[42]

Box A   Fixed-dose dalteparin regimen in patients with metastatic cancer and VTE[42]

First week
Give dalteparin in a dose according to body weight.

Subsequent weeks (continue indefinitely)
Dalteparin in a fixed-dose of 10,000 units SC once daily.
- *if DVT recurs:* increase the fixed-dose of dalteparin to 12,500 units SC once daily.
- *if PE occurs/recurs:* treat with an inferior vena caval filter.

Dose modification in thrombocytopenia
- if the platelet count falls below 50×10^9/L reduce the dose of dalteparin to 5,000 units SC once daily.
- if the platelet count falls below 10×10^9/L reduce the dose of dalteparin to 2,500 units SC once daily.

Surgical procedure
Give dalteparin 5,000 units SC once daily for the first 4 days postoperatively and then return to the patient's usual dose.

Other invasive procedure (e.g. biopsy)
Give dalteparin 5,000 units SC on the day of the procedure and then return to the patient's usual dose.

Thrombophlebitis migrans

- do not use **warfarin** because it is ineffective
- generally responds rapidly to small doses of LMWH:
  - ▷ **dalteparin**: 2,500–5,000 units SC once daily; if necessary, titrate to maximum permitted dose, 200 units/kg once daily or
  - ▷ **enoxaparin**: ≤60mg once daily; if necessary, titrate to maximum permitted dose, 1.5mg/kg SC once daily
- continue treatment indefinitely.[5,47]

Disseminated intravascular coagulation (DIC)

Confirm the diagnosis:
- thrombocytopenia (platelet count $< 150 \times 10^9$/L in 95% of cases)
- decreased plasma fibrinogen concentration
- elevated plasma D-dimer concentration, a fibrin degradation product (85% of cases)
- prolonged prothrombin time and/or partial thromboplastin time.[48]

A normal plasma fibrinogen concentration (200–250mg/100mL) is also suspicious because fibrinogen levels are generally raised in cancer (e.g. 450–500mg/100mL) unless there is extensive liver disease. Infection and cancer both may be associated with an increased platelet count which likewise may mask an evolving thrombocytopenia.

Management:
- do not use **warfarin** because it is ineffective
- for chronic DIC presenting with recurrent thromboses, give LMWH as for treatment of DVT
- for acute or chronic DIC presenting with haemorrhagic manifestations (e.g. ecchymoses, haematomas), seek specialist advice.

Antifibrinolytic drugs, e.g. **tranexamic acid** and **aminocaproic acid** (not UK), should not be used in DIC because they increase the risk of end-organ damage from microvascular thromboses.

LMWH is also the anticoagulant of choice in the treatment of chronic DIC; this commonly presents as recurrent thromboses in both superficial and deep veins which do not respond to **warfarin**.

Overdose

See individual SPCs for details.
With recommended doses of LMWH, there should be no need for an antidote. However, an accidental overdose may result in haemorrhagic complications.

Protamine sulfate partially reverses the effects of LMWH on factor Xa (**dalteparin** 25%, **enoxaparin** 60%, **tinzaparin** 65–80%). Because **protamine** in excess can have an anticoagulant effect[49] and, because the effect of LMWH may outlast that of **protamine** (this will depend on the interval between the last dose of LMWH and administering **protamine**), it should be used only in an emergency and in accordance with the recommendations in the individual LMWH SPCs. However, typically:
- for each 100 units (or 1mg **enoxaparin**) of LMWH, **protamine sulfate** 1mg is given
- a maximum of 50mg by slow IV injection is given over 10min.

Decisions regarding the necessity and dose of subsequent **protamine** injections are based on clinical response.

Alternatively, recombinant **activated factor VIIa concentrate** can be used. In three patients who bled after surgery or an invasive procedure, a single IV dose of 20–30microgram/kg successfully reversed anticoagulation from LMWH. It did not precipitate thrombosis, despite the patients all having a risk factor for hypercoagulation, e.g. cancer-related surgery.[50]

Supply

Dalteparin

Fragmin® (Pharmacia)
Injection (single-dose graduated syringe for SC injection) 10,000 units/mL 1mL syringe = £6.
Injection (single-dose syringe for SC injection) 2,500 units/0.2mL = £2.
Injection (single-dose syringe for SC injection) 5,000 units/0.2mL = £3, 7,500 units/0.3mL = £4, 10,000 units/0.4mL = £6, 12,500 units/0.5mL = £7, 15,000 units/0.6mL = £9, 18,000 units/0.72mL = £10.

Injection (single-dose ampoule for SC or IV injection) 10,000 units/4mL amp = £5; 10,000 units/mL amp = £5.

Injection (multiple-dose vial for SC injection), 100,000 units/4mL = £49.

Enoxaparin
Note: enoxaparin 1mg = 100 units.
Clexane® (Sanofi-Aventis)
Injection (single-dose syringe for SC injection) 20mg/0.2mL = £3, 40mg/0.4mL = £4, 60mg/0.6mL = £5, 80mg/0.8mL = £7, 100mg/1mL = £8.

Injection (single-dose syringe for SC injection; Clexane® Forte) 120mg/0.8mL = £10, 150mg/1mL = £11.

Injection (multiple-dose vial for SC or IV injection; Clexane® Multidose) 300mg/3mL = £21.

Tinzaparin
Innohep® (Leo)
Injection (single-dose syringe for SC injection), 2,500 units/0.25mL = £2, 3,500 units/0.35mL = £3, 4,500 units/0.45mL = £4.

Injection (single-dose syringe for SC injection), 10,000 units/0.5mL = £8, 14,000 units/0.7mL = £12, 18,000 units/0.9mL = £15.

Injection (multiple-dose vial for SC injection) 20,000 units/2mL vial = £11; 40,000 units/2mL vial = £34.

Protamine sulfate (generic)
Injection 10mg/mL, 5mL and 10mL amp = £1.50 and £4 respectively.

1   Baglin T et al. (2006) Guidelines on the use and monitoring of heparin. British Journal of Haematology. 133: 19–34.
2   Blann AD and Lip GY (2006) Venous thromboembolism. British Medical Journal. 332: 215–219.
3   Cohen AT et al. (2006) Efficacy and safety of fondaparinux for the prevention of venous thromboembolism in older acute medical patients: randomised placebo controlled trial. British Medical Journal. 332: 325–329.
4   Quinlan D et al. (2004) Low-molecular weight heparin compared with intravenous unfractionated heparin for treatment of pulmonary embolism. Annals of internal medicine. 140: 175–183.
5   Van Dongen CJ et al. (2004) Fixed dose subcutaneous low molecular weight heparins versus adjusted dose unfractionated heparin for venous thromboembolism. Cochrane Database of Systematic Reviews. 4: CD001100.
6   Baglin TP et al. (2006) British Committee for Standards in Haematology. Guidelines on oral anticoagulation (warfarin): third edition-2005 update. British Journal of Haematology. 132: 277–285.
7   Noble SI et al. (2008) The management of venous thromboembolism in advanced cancer: a systematic review and meta-analysis by the thrombosis task group, on behalf of the Association for Palliative Medicine Science Committee. Lancet Oncology. 9: 577–584.
8   Kearon C et al. (2012) Antithrombotic therapy for VTE disease: Antithrombotic Therapy and Prevention of Thrombosis, 9th ed: American College of Chest Physicians Evidence-Based Clinical Practice Guidelines. Chest. 141: e419S–494S.
9   Hettiarachchi RJ et al. (1999) Do heparins do more than just treat thrombosis? The influence of heparins on cancer spread. Journal of Thrombosis and Haemostasis. 82: 947–952.
10 Khorana AA and Fine RL (2004) Pancreatic cancer and thromboembolic disease. Lancet Oncology. 5: 655–663.
11 Klerk CP et al. (2005) The effect of low molecular weight heparin on survival in patients with advanced malignancy. Journal of Clinical Oncology. 23: 2130–2135.
12 Cunningham RS (2006) The role of low-molecular-weight heparins as supportive care therapy in cancer-associated thrombosis. Seminars in Oncology. 33: S17–25; quiz S41–12.
13 Zhang J et al. (2013) Efficacy and safety of adjunctive anticoagulation in patients with lung cancer without indication for anticoagulants: a systematic review and meta-analysis. Thorax. 68: 442–450.
14 Lazo-Langner A et al. (2007) The effect of low-molecular-weight heparin on cancer survival. A systematic review and meta-analysis of randomized trials. Journal of Thrombosis and Haemostasis. 5: 729–737.
15 Akl EA et al. (2008) Parenteral anticoagulation may prolong the survival of patients with limited small cell lung cancer: a Cochrane systematic review. Journal of Experimental and Clinical Cancer Research. 27: 4.
16 Griffiths GO et al. (2009) FRAGMATIC: a randomised phase III clinical trial investigating the effect of fragmin added to standard therapy in patients with lung cancer. BMC Cancer. 9: 355.
17 Fossler MJ et al. (2001) Pharmacodynamics of intravenous and subcutaneous tinzaparin and heparin in healthy volunteers. American Journal of Health System Pharmacy. 58: 1614–1621.
18 Fareed J et al. (1990) Pharmacologic profile of a low molecular weight heparin (enoxaparin): experimental and clinical validation of the prophylactic antithrombotic effects. Acta Chirurgica Scandinavica Suppl. 556 (suppl): 75–90.
19 Dawes J (1990) Comparison of the pharmacokinetics of enoxaparin (Clexane) and unfractionated heparin. Acta Chirurgica Scandinavica Supplementum. 556 (suppl): 68–74.
20 Bara L and Samama M (1990) Pharmacokinetics of low molecular weight heparins. Acta Chirurgica Scandinavica Supplementum. 556 (suppl): 57–61.
21 Hirsh J et al. (2001) Heparin and low-molecular-weight heparin: mechanisms of action, pharmacokinetics, dosing, monitoring, efficacy, and safety. Chest. 119 (suppl): 64s–94s.
22 Keeling D et al. (2006) The management of heparin-induced thrombocytopenia. (Guidelines of the Haemostasis and Thrombosis Task Force of the British Committee for Standards in Haematology). British Journal of Haematology. 133: 259–269.

23 Leo Laboratories *Personal communication.*
24 NICE (2010) Reducing the risk of venous thromboembolism (deep vein thrombosis and pulmonary embolism) in patients admitted to hospital. *Clinical Guideline* CG92. www.nice.org.uk
25 Noble SI and Finlay IG (2005) Is long-term low-molecular-weight heparin acceptable to palliative care patients in the treatment of cancer related venous thromboembolism? A qualitative study. *Palliative Medicine.* 19: 197–201.
26 Wittkowsky AK (2006) Barriers to the long-term use of low-molecular weight heparins for treatment of cancer-associated thrombosis. *Journal of Thrombosis and Haemostasis.* 4: 2090–2091.
27 Kakkar AK and Williamson RC (1999) Prevention of venous thromboembolism in cancer patients. *Seminars in Thrombosis and Hemostasis.* 25: 239–243.
28 Negus JJ et al. (2006) Thromboprophylaxis in major abdominal surgery for cancer. *European Journal of Surgical Oncology.* 32: 911–916.
29 Cunningham MS et al. (2006) Prevention and management of venous thromboembolism in people with cancer: a review of the evidence. *Clinical Oncology (Royal College of Radiologists).* 18: 145–151.
30 Bergqvist D et al. (2002) Duration of prophylaxis against venous thromboembolism with enoxaparin after surgery for cancer. *New England Journal of Medicine.* 346: 975–980.
31 Kher A and Samama MM (2005) Primary and secondary prophylaxis of venous thromboembolism with low-molecular-weight heparins: prolonged thromboprophylaxis, an alternative to vitamin K antagonists. *Journal of Thrombosis and Haemostasis.* 3: 473–481.
32 Leizorovicz A and Mismetti P (2004) Preventing venous thromboembolism in medical patients. *Circulation.* 110: 13–19.
33 Leizorovicz A et al. (2004) Randomized, placebo-controlled trial of dalteparin for the prevention of venous thromboembolism in acutely ill medical patients. *Circulation.* 110: 874–879.
34 Samama MM et al. (1999) A comparison of enoxaparin with placebo for the prevention of venous thromboembolism in acutely ill medical patients. Prophylaxis in Medical Patients with Enoxaparin Study Group. *New England Journal of Medicine.* 341: 793–800.
35 Monreal M et al. (2004) The outcome after treatment of venous thromboembolism is different in surgical and acutely ill medical patients. Findings from the RIETE registry. *Journal of Thrombosis and Haemostasis.* 2: 1892–1898.
36 Noble SI et al. (2006) Acceptability of low molecular weight heparin thromboprophylaxis for inpatients receiving palliative care: qualitative study. *British Medical Journal.* 332: 577–580.
37 Dennis M et al. (2009) Effectiveness of thigh-length graduated compression stockings to reduce the risk of deep vein thrombosis after stroke (CLOTS trial 1): a multicentre, randomised controlled trial. *Lancet.* 373: 1958–1965.
38 Tesselaar ME et al. (2004) Risk factors for catheter-related thrombosis in cancer patients. *European Journal of Cancer.* 40: 2253–2259.
39 Couban S et al. (2005) Randomized Placebo-Controlled Study of Low-Dose Warfarin for the Prevention of Central Venous Catheter-Associated Thrombosis in Patients With Cancer. *Journal of Clinical Oncology.* 23: 4063–4069.
40 Verso M et al. (2005) Enoxaparin for the Prevention of Venous Thromboembolism Associated With Central Vein Catheter: A Double-Blind, Placebo-Controlled, Randomized Study in Cancer Patients. *Journal of Clinical Oncology.* 23: 4057–4062.
41 NICE (2012) Venous thromboembolic diseases: the management of venous thromboembolic diseases and the role of thrombophilia testing. *Clinical Guideline* CG144 www.nice.org.uk
42 Monreal M et al. (2004) Fixed-dose low-molecular-weight heparin for secondary prevention of venous thromboembolism in patients with disseminated cancer: a prospective cohort study. *Journal of Thrombosis and Haemostasis.* 2: 1311–1315.
43 Meyer G et al. (2002) Comparison of low-molecular-weight heparin and warfarin for the secondary prevention of venous thromboembolism in patients with cancer: a randomized controlled study. *Archives of Internal Medicine.* 162: 1729–1735.
44 Lee A et al. (2003) Low molecular weight heparin versus a coumarin for the prevention of recurrent venous thromboembolism in patients with cancer. *New England Journal of Medicine.* 349: 146–153.
45 Hull RD et al. (2006) Long-term low-molecular-weight heparin versus usual care in proximal-vein thrombosis patients with cancer. *American Journal of Medicine.* 119: 1062–1072.
46 Farge D et al. (2013) International clinical practice guidelines for the treatment and prophylaxis of venous thromboembolism in patients with cancer. *Journal of Thrombosis and Haemostasis.* 11: 56–70.
47 Walsh-McMonagle D and Green D (1997) Low-molecular weight heparin in the management of Trousseau's syndrome. *Cancer.* 80: 649–655.
48 Spero J et al. (1980) Disseminated intravascular coagulation: findings in 346 patients. *Journal of Thrombosis and Haemostasis.* 43: 28–33.
49 *British National Formulary* (2012) Section 2.8.3 Protamine sulfate. London: BMJ Group and Pharmaceutical Press www.bnf.org (accessed July 2012).
50 Firozvi K et al. (2006) Reversal of low-molecular-weight heparin-induced bleeding in patients with pre-existing hypercoagulable states with human recombinant activated factor VII concentrate. *American Journal of Hematology.* 81: 582–589.

Updated October 2013

Quick Clinical Guide: Heparin-Induced Thrombocytopenia (HIT)

1 Unfractionated heparin (UFH) and low molecular weight heparin (LMWH) can both cause thrombocytopenia (platelet count $< 100 \times 10^9$/L).

2 An early mild fall in platelet count is often seen after starting heparin (< 4 days), particularly postoperatively. This is asymptomatic, and corrects spontaneously despite continuing heparin.

3 In < 1% of patients, *immune* HIT develops 5–10 days after starting heparin. Can occur sooner or later; rarely several days after heparin has been stopped.

4 If a patient has had treatment with heparin within the last 3 months, HIT can manifest < 1 day after restarting treatment.

5 HIT is less common with:
- LMWH than UFH
- low-dose prophylactic regimens than higher-dose therapeutic ones.

6 Heparin-dependent IgG antibody–platelet factor 4 complexes bind to the platelet surface, causing disruption and release of procoagulant material.

7 HIT manifests as *venous* or *arterial* thrombo-embolism, and can be fatal.

8 **Clinical features**
If any of the following occur, seek urgent advice from a haematologist:
- platelet count falls below $< 100 \times 10^9$/L or by > 50%
- new thrombotic or thrombo-embolic event after starting heparin
- acute systemic reaction after injection of UFH or LMWH (e.g. flushing, tachycardia, tachypnoea)
- skin necrosis or erythematous plaques at injection sites.

9 **Treatment**
Stop heparin immediately if HIT seems probable.
While awaiting laboratory results (e.g. platelet activation assay, antibody assay):
- prescribe a synthetic heparin or a non-heparin parenteral anticoagulant (e.g. fondaparinux, danaparoid, lepirudin) whether or not there is clinical evidence of a DVT
- only when the platelet count has recovered to $\geqslant 150 \times 10^9$/L, prescribe warfarin
- continue the non-heparin anticoagulant until the INR has reached a therapeutic level, typically 5–7 days.

Do *not* use warfarin alone (risk of skin necrosis and venous limb gangrene).
Do *not* give prophylactic platelet transfusions.

10 **Preventing recurrence**
- record the diagnosis in the patient's notes as a serious allergy
- issue an antibody card (although most patients are antibody negative after 3 months)
- if possible, avoid surgery for > 3 months after HIT
- although cross-reactivity between UFH and LMWH is uncommon, advise the patient not to have injections of any type of heparin in the future
- if subsequent anticoagulation is required, a synthetic heparin or a non-heparin parenteral anticoagulant (e.g. fondaparinux, danaparoid, lepirudin) should be used.

11 For patients with a history of HIT requiring renal dialysis, seek specialist advice.

1 Keeling D et al. (2006) The management of heparin-induced thrombocytopenia. (Guidelines of the Haemostasis and Thrombosis Task Force of the British Committee for Standards in Haematology). *British Journal of Haematology.* 133: 259–269.
2 Srinivasan AF et al. (2004) Warfarin-induced skin necrosis and venous limb gangrene in the setting of heparin-induced thrombocytopenia. *Archives of Internal Medicine.* 164: 66–70.

3 Warkentin T et al. (1995) Heparin-induced thrombocytopenia in patients treated with low molecular weight heparin or unfractionated heparin. New England Journal of Medicine. 332: 1330–1335.
4 Warkentin TE and Heddle NM (2003) Laboratory diagnosis of immune heparin-induced thrombocytopenia. Current Hematology Reports. 2: 148–157.
5 Warkentin TE and Greinacher A (2008) Treatment and prevention of heparin-induced thrombocytopenia: American College of Chest Physicians Evidence-Based Clinical Practice Guidelines (8th Edition). Chest. 133 (6 Suppl): 340S–380S.

Updated October 2013

HAEMOSTATICS   BNF 2.11

Indications: Authorized indications vary between products; consult SPC for details. Prevention of bleeding after dental extraction in haemophilia or postoperatively, haemorrhagic complications after thrombolytic treatment, menorrhagia, epistaxis, hereditary angioedema, †subarachnoid haemorrhage, †surface bleeding from ulcerating tumours on the skin, in the nose, mouth, pharynx and other hollow organs (lungs, stomach, rectum, bladder, uterus).

Contra-indications: Active thrombo-embolic disease, e.g. recent thrombo-embolism, DIC, history of convulsions; severe renal impairment (**tranexamic acid**, but see below).

Pharmacology

Tranexamic acid and **aminocaproic acid** (not UK) are structurally related synthetic antifibrinolytic drugs derived from lysine. They bind to plasminogen and prevent its interaction as plasmin with fibrin, thereby preventing dissolution of haemostatic plugs.[1] **Tranexamic acid** is preferable to **aminocaproic acid** because it has a longer duration of action and causes fewer undesirable GI effects.[2]

Systemic or topical use of antifibrinolytics reduces blood loss in various circumstances, e.g. menorrhagia (PO), major injury (IV) and peri-operatively (IV, topical).[3–5] They are used in cancer patients to control surface bleeding. In patients with leukaemia and thrombocytopenia, antifibrinolytics appear to reduce bleeding and platelet transfusion requirements, but supporting data are too limited to routinely recommend such use.[6,7] Although sometimes used for haemoptysis caused by lung cancer, supporting data are lacking.[8]

The evidence that antifibrinolytics may increase the risk of thrombosis is generally limited to case reports, with many RCTs identifying no such concerns.[3] However, this has not been well evaluated in patients with cancer and other diseases associated with an underlying prothrombotic tendency. On the other hand, it is suggested that **tranexamic acid** could be antithrombotic by inhibiting the wider effects of prothrombin and plasmin which include promoting inflammation, platelet aggregation and coagulation.[9]

Antifibrinolytics are generally contra-indicated in DIC, even when haemorrhagic manifestations (ecchymoses, haematomas) are predominant, because clot formation is the trigger for further intravascular coagulation and platelet consumption, and an increased risk of end-organ damage from microvascular thromboses.[10] Rarely, they have been used in DIC when there is severe bleeding due to a marked hyperfibrinolytic state;[10]seek specialist advice.

Tranexamic acid and **aminocaproic acid** are excreted in the urine mainly unchanged. Because of accumulation, dose reduction will be necessary in renal impairment. Although the SPC gives severe renal impairment as a contra-indication to **tranexamic acid**, there are reports of its use in this circumstance in reduced doses (see Table 2 below).[11,12]

Etamsylate (not UK, see Supply) acts by increasing capillary vascular wall resistance and platelet adhesiveness in the presence of a vascular lesion. This is achieved by inhibiting the biosynthesis and actions of those PGs which cause platelet disaggregation, vasodilation and increased capillary permeability, thereby promoting platelet activation and aggregation, and also by increasing communication between platelets, leucocytes and endothelial cells via the cell adhesion molecule P-selectin.[13] Thus, **etamsylate** is of limited value in thrombocytopenia. It does not cause vasoconstriction, nor does it affect normal coagulation; it has no effect on prothrombin time, fibrinolysis, or platelet count.

Studies have mainly explored the use of **etamsylate** for menorrhagia or peri-ventricular haemorrhage in premature infants.[13] In palliative care, it is used for surface bleeding ± **tranexamic**

acid. Rarely, parenteral use may be necessary, e.g. in patients with bleeding and complete dysphagia due to oesophageal cancer. **Etamsylate** is excreted in the urine mainly unchanged.

Pharmacokinetic details are listed in Table 1.

Table 1 Pharmacokinetics of antifibrinolytic and haemostatic drugs

	Tranexamic acid	Aminocaproic acid	Etamsylate
Bio-availability PO	30–50%[a]	'complete'	'complete'
Onset of action (route-dependent)	1–3h	1–3h	30min IV
Time to peak plasma concentration	3h PO	2h	4h PO; 1h IV
Plasma halflife	2h	2h	5–17h PO; 1.7–2.5h IM; 1.8–2h IV
Duration of action	24h	12–18h	no data

a. systemic bio-availability minimal with oral rinse.

Cautions

History of thrombo-embolism, renal impairment. In both microscopic and macroscopic haematuria there is a risk of clot formation causing ureteric obstruction or urinary retention.[14] Nonetheless, **tranexamic** acid has been used successfully in patients with polycystic kidneys and severe haematuria failing to respond to usual treatment.[15]

Undesirable effects

Tranexamic acid and aminocaproic acid: hypotension, bradycardia, arrhythmia (IV; give slowly), possible increased risk of thrombosis; nausea, vomiting, abdominal pain, diarrhoea (generally settle if the dose is reduced); muscle weakness; seizures (generally following IV use in high dose, e.g. 100mg/kg).[16]

Tranexamic acid: disturbances in colour vision (discontinue drug).

Etamsylate: fever, headache, rash.

Dose and use

In countries where **aminocaproic acid** is available, it can be used instead of **tranexamic acid**. Likewise, in certain circumstances, **etamsylate** may be a useful alternative or supplement.

Surface bleeding

Box A summarizes the clinical management of surface bleeding; also see text below.

Box A Management of surface bleeding

For specific advice on haematuria, see p.101.

Physical

Gauze applied with pressure for 10min soaked in:
- tranexamic acid 500mg in 5mL *or*
- adrenaline (epinephrine) (1 in 1,000) 1mg in 1mL. } use standard undiluted ampoules.

Long-term application of adrenaline (epinephrine) is *not* recommended because of the risk of ischaemic necrosis and rebound vasodilation.

Silver nitrate sticks applied to bleeding points in the nose and mouth, and on skin nodules and fungating tumours.

Haemostatic dressings, i.e. alginate (e.g. Kaltostat®, Sorbsan®).

Specialist therapy:
- radiotherapy (e.g. skin, lung, oesophagus, rectum, bladder, uterus, vagina)[17]
- coagulation: diathermy, cryotherapy, LASER
- embolization.[18,19]

continued

Box A Continued

Drugs

Review existing medication
Discontinue aspirin and/or other platelet-impairing NSAID.
Prescribe paracetamol or an NSAID which does not impair platelet function (see NSAIDs, Table 5, p.312).

Topical
Tranexamic acid solution[20]
Sucralfate paste 2g (two 1g tablets crushed in 5mL aqueous lubricant, e.g. KY jelly).[21]
Sucralfate suspension 2g in 10mL b.d. for the mouth and rectum.[22]
Sympathomimetic vasoconstrictors have been used for posterior epistaxis, e.g. xylometazoline nasal spray;[23] they have also been applied directly onto malignant wounds,[24] but the risk of rebound vasodilation after several days of use limits long-term application.

Systemic
First-line: antifibrinolytic drug, e.g. tranexamic acid.[25]
Second-line: switch to or combine with etamsylate (not UK).
Third-line: desmopressin (see p.514).[26]
Note: etamsylate and desmopressin augment platelet function; thus of limited value in thrombocytopenia.

Tranexamic acid
The following recommendations are taken mainly from anecdotal reports.
Epistaxis (anterior)[27]
• use standard undiluted 500mg/5mL ampoule for injection (10%), soak into cotton pledget or gauze and insert into nostril and leave for 10min; remove once bleeding stopped.
As an oral rinse for local bleeding[3,28]
As a mouthwash, **tranexamic acid** can be used as a 5% (500mg/10mL) aqueous solution, 10mL q.d.s. (can swallow after use):
• dilute contents of a standard 10% (500mg/5mL) ampoule for injection with 5mL of water *or*
• use a locally prepared 5% (500mg/10mL) solution.
Surface bleeding from any site[25,29]
• 1.5g PO stat and 1g t.d.s.
• if bleeding not subsiding after 3 days, increase dose to 1.5–2g t.d.s.
• manufacturer's recommended maximum dose = 1.5g t.d.s.
• in practice, doses of ≤2g q.d.s. have been used
• discontinue 1 week after cessation of bleeding or reduce to 500mg t.d.s.
• restart if bleeding occurs, and possibly continue indefinitely.
Parenteral use may occasionally be indicated, e.g. in patients with bleeding and complete dysphagia due to oesophageal cancer:
• 15mg/kg IV over 5–10min t.d.s.–q.d.s.
Note: in renal impairment the dose should be reduced (Table 2).

Table 2 Tranexamic acid doses in renal impairment

Plasma creatinine (micromol/L)	Creatinine clearance (mL/min)	PO dose	IV dose
120–249	50–80	15mg/kg b.d.	10mg/kg b.d.
250–500	10–50	15mg/kg once daily	10mg/kg once daily
>500	<10	7.5mg/kg once daily or 15mg/kg every 2 days[4,5]	5mg/kg once daily or 10mg/kg every 2 days

Topical solution for bleeding from fungating cancer in the skin[30]
• solution: use standard undiluted 500mg/5mL ampoule for injection (10%), soak into gauze and apply with pressure for 10min, then leave *in situ* with a dressing *or*
• paste: 2g tablets crushed in 60g base, e.g. Hydrophilic Ointment USP36 applied b.d. and covered with a dressing has been used.[31]

Topical solution for bleeding from cancer in rectum, bladder or pleura[20,32]
Generally used only if PO **tranexamic acid** has failed:
• instil 50mL (10 ampoules) of undiluted 10% (500mg/5mL) injection, at body temperature PR/PV/ via urinary catheter, once daily–b.d. *or*
• use 50mL of a locally prepared 10% (500mg/5mL) solution.

Aminocaproic acid (not UK)
In oliguria or end-stage renal disease, give 15–25% of the normal dose.[12]
Acute bleeding syndromes due to elevated fibrinolytic activity[33]
• stat dose of 5g PO (or 4–5g IVI in 250mL of diluent) during the first hour of treatment, then 1.25g/h PO (or 1g/h IVI in 50mL of diluent) for 8h or until bleeding stops; suitable diluents for IVI are 0.9% saline or 5% glucose
• manufacturer's maximum recommended dose = 30g/24h PO/IV.
Chronic bleeding tendency
• 5–30g PO daily in divided doses at 3–6h intervals
• when bleeding controlled, adjust to the lowest effective dose.
Bleeding from oral cancers[34]
• 500mg PO q.d.s. until bleeding stops
• then discontinue by tapering dose frequency every 2–3 days.

Etamsylate (not UK)
Generally one part of a multimodal approach to the management of surface bleeding (see Box A):
• 500mg q.d.s. either indefinitely or until 1 week after cessation of bleeding
• if it causes nausea, vomiting or diarrhoea, take after food.

Haematuria

Haematuria in advanced cancer is generally associated with urinary tract cancer, most commonly bladder cancer. It may also be caused by chronic radiation cystitis which may not develop until several years after pelvic radiotherapy. In many cases haematuria is mild, and no intervention is necessary.
Correct the correctable
Can the cancer be modified?
If the patient is well enough, consider cystoscopy for cystodiathermy and resection. If unclear if haematuria is due to recurrence of bladder cancer or radiation cystitis, a biopsy can be taken.
Can other factors be modified?
• instead of a non-selective NSAID, prescribe **paracetamol** or an NSAID which does not impair platelet function (see NSAIDs, Table 4, p.311)
• consider checking PT, APTT and FBC
• culture urine; treat infection if present.
Drug treatment
If the haematuria is marked, **tranexamic acid** PO may be used, even though there is a risk of clot retention until the bleeding has completely stopped. Other options include bladder instillations and irrigations (Table 3).
    Daily bladder instillations of **carboprost tromethamine**, a PGE_1 analogue, are occasionally used in **cyclophosphamide**-induced haematuria, second-line to **alum**. Although no anaesthesia is required, **carboprost** is expensive and requires close monitoring.[35,36]
Non-drug treatment
Rarely, it may be necessary to consider:
• cauterization
• arterial embolization[37–39]
• urinary diversion, e.g. nephrostomy
• hyperbaric oxygen.
Hyperbaric oxygen is successful in >80% patients with radiation cystitis, but is not widely available, is expensive and time-consuming, e.g. mean requirement 30 sessions of 90min each.[40]

Table 3 Bladder instillations and irrigations for haemorrhagic cystitis[35,39,41,42]

Treatment	Administration	Duration	Comment
Preferred options			
0.9% Saline	Continuous irrigation	Until urine is clear	No undesirable effects but not effective in severe cases
Sodium citrate solution 3%	Continuous irrigation	Until urine is clear	No undesirable effects but not effective in severe cases
Tranexamic acid	Instil 50mL (10 ampoules) of undiluted 10% (500mg/5mL) injection via a urinary catheter once daily–b.d.	Until urine is clear	Alternatively use 50mL of a locally prepared 10% (500mg/5mL) solution
Sucralfate suspension	Instil 5g, follow with 10mL 0.9% saline flush	Repeat up to t.d.s if no response	Suspension must be sterile, so use sachets (not UK). If the patient is prone to UTIs, give PO antibacterial cover
If the above fail			
Alum 1%	Continuous irrigation bladder at 250–300mL/h	Until urine is clear	No anaesthesia required. Solution is acidic and may cause bladder spasms; treat with antispasmodics. Expensive, 1L costs about £24. Recurrence common; aluminium toxicity rare
Silver nitrate 0.5–1%	Instillation, retain for 10–20min	Repeat if no response	Anaesthesia required. Often successful but short duration of response
Formalin 1–3%	Instillation, retain for 20–30min	Repeat if no response	Anaesthesia required. Often successful but risk of ureteric stenosis and obstruction if formalin refluxes into the ureters

Supply

Tranexamic acid (generic)
Tablets 500mg, 28 days @ 1g t.d.s. = £20.
Oral solution or suspension 500mg/5mL (10%), 28 days @ 1g t.d.s. = £205 or £489 respectively (unauthorized products available as a special order, see Appendix 1, p.817); *price based on Specials tariffin community.*

Cyklokapron® (Pfizer)
Injection 100mg/mL (10%), 5mL amp = £1.50.

Etamsylate
Tablets 500mg, 28 days @ 500mg q.d.s. = £126 (unauthorized product, obtainable as an import from IDIS; see Appendix 1, p.817).
Injection 125mg/mL, 2mL amp = £1 (unauthorized product, obtainable as an import from IDIS; see Appendix 1, p.817).

Sucralfate Antepsin® (Chugai)
Tablets 1g, 50 = £7.
Oral suspension 1g/5mL, 250mL = £7.

1   Mannucci PM (1998) Hemostatic drugs. *New England Journal of Medicine.* **339**: 245–253.

2   Okamoto S et al. (1964) An active stereoisomer (trans form) of AMCHA and its antifibrinolytic (antiplasminic) action in vitro and in vivo. *Keio Journal of Medicine.* **13**: 177–185.

3   McCormack PL (2012) Tranexamic acid: a review of its use in the treatment of hyperfibrinolysis. *Drugs.* **72**: 585–617.

4   Ker K et al. (2012) Effect of tranexamic acid on surgical bleeding: systematic review and cumulative meta-analysis. *British Medical Journal.* **344**: e3054.

5   Roberts I et al. (2013) The CRASH-2 trial: a randomised controlled trial and economic evaluation of the effects of tranexamic acid on death, vascular occlusive events and transfusion requirement in bleeding trauma patients. *Health Technology Assessment.* **17**: 1–79.

6   Wardrop D et al. (2013) Antifibrinolytics (lysine analogues) for the prevention of bleeding in patients with haematological disorders. *Cochrane Database of Systematic Reviews.* **7**: CD009733.

7   Antun AG et al. (2013) Epsilon aminocaproic acid prevents bleeding in severely thrombocytopenic patients with hematological malignancies. *Cancer.* **119**: 3784–3787.

8   Prutsky G et al. (2012) Antifibrinolytic therapy to reduce haemoptysis from any cause. *Cochrane Database of Systematic Reviews.* **4**: CD008711.

9   Godier A et al. (2012) Tranexamic acid: less bleeding and less thrombosis? *Critical Care.* **16**: 135.

10 Wada H et al. (2013) Guidance for diagnosis and treatment of DIC from harmonization of the recommendations from three guidelines. *Journal of Thrombosis and Haemostasis.* **11**: 761–767.

11 Andersson L et al. (1978) Special considerations with regard to the dosage of tranexamic acid in patients with chronic renal diseases. *Urological Research.* **6**: 83–88.

12 Lacy C et al. (eds) (2003) Lexi-Comp's Drug Information Handbook. (11e). Lexi-Comp and the American Pharmaceutical Association, Hudson, Ohio.

13 Garay RP et al. (2006) Therapeutic efficacy and mechanism of action of ethamsylate, a long-standing hemostatic agent. *American Journal of Therapeutics.* **13**: 236–247.

14 Schultz M and van der Lelie H (1995) Microscopic haematuria as a relative contraindication for tranexamic acid. *British Journal of Haematology.* **89**: 663–664.

15 Peces R et al. (2012) Medical therapy with tranexamic acid in autosomal dominant polycystic kidney disease patients with severe haematuria. *Nefrologia.* **32**: 160–165.

16 Murkin JM et al. (2010) High-dose tranexamic Acid is associated with nonischemic clinical seizures in cardiac surgical patients. *Anesthesia and Analgesia.* **110**: 350–353.

17 Cihoric N et al. (2012) Clinically significant bleeding in incurable cancer patients: effectiveness of hemostatic radiotherapy. *Radiation Oncololgy.* **7**: 132.

18 Rankin E et al. (1988) Transcatheter embolisation to control severe bleeding in fungating breast cancer. *European Journal of Surgical Oncology.* **14**: 27–32.

19 Broadley K et al. (1995) The role of embolization in palliative care. *Palliative Medicine.* **9**: 331–335.

20 McElligott E et al. (1991) Tranexamic acid and rectal bleeding. *Lancet.* **337**: 431.

21 Regnard C and Makin W (1992) Management of bleeding in advanced cancer: a flow diagram. *Palliative Medicine.* **6**: 74–78.

22 Kochhar R et al. (1988) Rectal sucralfate in radiation proctitis. *Lancet.* **332**: 400.

23 Krempl GA and Noorily AD (1995) Use of oxymetazoline in the management of epistaxis. *Annals of Otology, Rhinology, and Laryngology.* **104**: 704–706.

24 Recka K et al. (2012) Management of bleeding associated with malignant wounds. *Journal Palliative of Medicine.* **15**: 952–954.

25 Dean A and Tuffin P (1997) Fibrinolytic inhibitors for cancer-associated bleeding problems. *Journal of Pain and Symptom Management.* **13**: 20–24.

26 Hedges SJ et al. (2006) Evidence-based treatment recommendations for uremic bleeding. *Nature Clinical Practice Oncology.* **3**: 138–153.

27 Zahed R et al. (2013) A new and rapid method for epistaxis treatment using injectable form of tranexamic acid topically: a randomized controlled trial. *American Journal of Emergency Medicine.* **31**: 1389–1392.

28 Dunn CJ and Goa KL (1999) Tranexamic acid: a review of its use in surgery and other indications. *Drugs.* **57**: 1005–1032.

29 Seto AH and Dunlap DS (1996) Tranexamic acid in oncology. *Annals of Pharmacology.* **30**: 868–870.

30 Palliativedrugs.com (2013) Topical Tranexamic Acid - What do you do? *Survey.* March-April: Available from www.palliative drugs.com

31 Kennedy B *Personal Communication.*

32 deBoer W et al. (1991) Tranexamic acid treatment of haemothorax in two patients with malignant mesothelioma. *Chest.* **100**: 847–848.

33 Roberts SB et al. (2010) Palliative use of aminocaproic acid to control upper gastrointestinal bleeding. *Journal of Pain and Symptom Management.* **40**: e1–3.

34 Setla J (2004) Duration of aminocaproic acid therapy in bleeding for malignant wounds. In: *Bulletin Board.* Palliativedrugs.com Ltd. Available from: www.palliativedrugs.com

35 West N (1997) Prevention and treatment of hemorrhagic cystitis. *Pharmacotherapy.* **17**: 696–706.

36 Denton AS et al. (2002) Non-surgical interventions for late radiation cystitis in patients who have received radical radiotherapy to the pelvis. *Cochrane Database of Systematic Reviews.* CD001773.

37 Lang E et al. (1979) Transcatheter embolization of hypogastric branch arteries in the management of intractable bladder haemorrhage. *Journal of Urology.* **121**: 30–36.

38 Appleton D et al. (1988) Internal iliac artery embolisation for the control of severe bladder and prostate haemorrhage. *British Journal of Urology.* **61**: 45–47.

39 Choong SK et al. (2000) The management of intractable haematuria. *BJU International.* **86**: 951–959.

40 Corman JM et al. (2003) Treatment of radiation induced hemorrhagic cystitis with hyperbaric oxygen. *Journal of Urology.* **169**: 2200–2202.

41 Abt D et al. (2013) Therapeutic options for intractable hematuria in advanced bladder cancer. *International Journal of Urology.* **20**: 651–660.

42 Crew JP et al. (2001) Radiation-induced haemorrhagic cystitis. *European Urology.* **40**: 111–123.

Updated May 2014

3: RESPIRATORY SYSTEM

BRONCHODILATORS   BNF 3.1

Palliative care clinicians caring for patients with end-stage COPD need to be aware of the latest management guidelines. Further, some patients with cancer also suffer from COPD or asthma, and occasionally both. Concurrent COPD can be a major cause of breathlessness, notably in lung cancer, but may be unrecognized, and so go untreated.

The guidelines provided here (Box A–Box C, Table 1) for the use of bronchodilators in patients with asthma and COPD are based on the recommendations of the British Thoracic Society/Scottish Intercollegiate Guidelines Network Guidelines on Asthma[1] and the National Institute for Health and Clinical Excellence COPD Guidelines.[2] These have much in common with international guidelines produced by the Global Initiative for Asthma (GINA) and the Global Initiative for Chronic Obstructive Lung Disease (GOLD), although there are some differences in emphasis.[3,4]

Generally, the guidelines should be followed. However, for patients in the last weeks or days of life, particularly those having difficulties with metered-dose inhalers (MDIs), the regular use of short-acting nebulized bronchodilators may be preferable. Further, if a patient is receiving long-term PO corticosteroids for another indication (see p.499), it is often possible to discontinue inhaled corticosteroids.

Inhalation delivers the drug directly to the bronchi and enables a smaller dose to work more quickly and with fewer undesirable systemic effects. β₂-Adrenergic receptor agonists (β₂ agonists), e.g. **salbutamol** (p.115) and **salmeterol** (p.117), act directly on bronchial smooth muscle to cause bronchodilation whereas antimuscarinics, e.g. **ipratropium** (p.111) and **tiotropium** (p.113), act by reducing the vagal tone to the airways. Both classes of drug improve breathlessness by airway bronchodilation and/or reducing air-trapping at rest (static hyperinflation) and on exertion (dynamic hyperinflation). A reduction in hyperinflation probably explains why clinical benefit may be seen in patients with COPD with little or no change in the FEV_1.[5]

β₂ Agonists are used in both asthma and COPD; antimuscarinic drugs in COPD and *acute* asthma. Their use is often combined in *acute* asthma and COPD (Table 1, Box B). In asthma and in severe COPD, bronchodilators are generally combined with inhaled corticosteroids (Box A, Table 1, also see p.125).

In asthma and COPD, if the optimal use of inhaled therapy provides inadequate relief, a third class of bronchodilators, the methylxanthines, are sometimes used systemically, e.g. PO m/r **theophylline** (p.122). Because of a narrow therapeutic index, their use requires careful monitoring to avoid toxicity.

β-Adrenergic receptor blocking drugs (β-blockers), both cardioselective and non-selective, are contra-indicated in patients with asthma. They should also be avoided in patients with COPD, unless there are compelling reasons for their use, e.g. severe glaucoma. In such circumstances, a cardioselective β-blocker should be used with extreme caution under specialist guidance.

Table 1 Summary of the immediate management of acute exacerbations of asthma in adults[1], [a]

	Severity of exacerbation		
	Moderate	Severe	Life-threatening[b]
Assessment			Any of the following:
PEF[c]	>50–75%	33–50%	<33%
SpO$_2$ (pulse oximeter)		≥92%	<92%; check blood gases
Speech	No features of severe asthma	Unable to complete sentence in one breath	Silent chest, poor respiratory effort, cyanosis, PaO$_2$ <8kPa, normal or raised PaCO$_2$[d], arrhythmia, hypotension, exhaustion, altered consciousness
Respiration (breaths/min)		≥25	
Heart rate (beats/min)		≥110	
Chest radiograph	When pneumothorax, pneumomediastinum or consolidation suspected, life-threatening asthma, failure to respond to treatment or ventilation required		
Place of care	Hospital for life-threatening; severe or moderate when, e.g. failure to respond to treatment or psychosocial concerns. Intensive care for life-threatening or severe when failure to respond to treatment or ventilation required		
Treatment			
Oxygen	Not applicable	via face/venturi mask or nasal cannulae at flow rate which maintains SpO$_2$ 94–98%	
Bronchodilators[e]	Salbutamol or terbutaline MDI 4 puffs via spacer (give one puff at a time), followed by 2 puffs every 2min, up to maximum of 10 puffs or	salbutamol 5mg or terbutaline 10mg via oxygen-driven nebulizer	Use nebulized β$_2$ agonist as for moderate-severe but give with ipratropium 500microgram via an oxygen-driven nebulizer; use spacer only if nebulizer unavailable
	If inadequate response after 15min, give nebulized β$_2$ agonist		Repeat above
	If inadequate response after 15min:		
		Use nebulized β$_2$ agonist + ipratropium (if not already given) or consider continuous nebulization of salbutamol 5–10mg/h (requires specific nebulizer)	
Corticosteroid[f]	Prednisolone 40–50mg PO stat & once daily for 5 days or until recovery		
Other treatments[g]	IV magnesium sulfate 1.2–2g over 20min		
	IV aminophylline 5mg/kg over 20min, followed by 500–700microgram/kg/h[h]		

a. full guidance available at www.brit-thoracic.org.uk
b. obtain senior/intensive care unit help as soon as life-threatening asthma recognized
c. % of best peak expiratory flow (PEF) within last two years or, if unavailable, predicted PEF
d. termed near-fatal asthma when PaCO$_2$ is raised and/or mechanical ventilation is required with raised inflation pressures
e. IV β$_2$ agonists are reserved for patients in whom inhaled route unreliable (see full guidance)
f. the earlier corticosteroids are given, the better the outcome; where PO not possible, give hydrocortisone 100mg IV stat & q.d.s.
g. when poor response to standard bronchodilator therapies requires therapies escalation from senior/experienced staff (see full guidance)

Box A   Summary of the management of chronic asthma in adults[1]

Start at the step most appropriate to the initial severity of asthma. The aim is to achieve control as soon as possible, defined as:
- no daytime symptoms
- no night-time awakening due to asthma
- no exacerbations
- no limitation of physical activity
- normal lung function, i.e. $FEV_1 \pm PEF > 80\%$ predicted or best.

This aim is balanced against the potential undesirable effects or inconvenience of drug treatment. Before initiating a new drug, check adherence, inhaler technique and eliminate trigger factors.

Step 1: mild intermittent asthma
Inhaled short-acting β_2-adrenergic receptor agonist (β_2 agonist) p.r.n., e.g. salbutamol.

Move to Step 2 if:
- symptomatic/inhaler needed $\geqslant 3$ times a week
- night-time symptoms $\geqslant 1$ times a week
- exacerbation of asthma requiring PO corticosteroids in the last 2 years.

Step 2: regular preventer therapy
Regular inhaled corticosteroid[a,b]
+ inhaled short-acting β_2 agonist p.r.n.

Consider a move to Step 3 if asthma not controlled on beclometasone 400–800microgram/24h or equivalent. (Note: an absolute threshold does not exist and individual patient factors are also taken into account.)

Step 3: initial add-on therapy
Regular inhaled long-acting β_2 agonist (LABA), e.g. salmeterol 50microgram b.d. or formoterol 12microgram b.d.[c]
+ regular inhaled corticosteroid[a,b]
+ inhaled short-acting β_2 agonist p.r.n.

If there is:
- *insufficient response*, continue the LABA and increase the inhaled corticosteroid to beclometasone 800microgram/24h or equivalent; *if control remains poor go to Step 4*
- *no response*, discontinue the LABA and increase inhaled corticosteroid to beclometasone 800microgram/24h or equivalent; *if control remains poor consider therapeutic trials of:*
  ▷ PO leukotriene receptor antagonist
  ▷ PO m/r theophylline
  ▷ PO m/r β_2 agonist.
If control remains poor go to Step 4.

Step 4: persistent poor control
Regular moderate-dose inhaled corticosteroid, i.e. beclometasone 800microgram/24h or equivalent
+ regular inhaled LABA (when of known benefit)[c]
+ inhaled short-acting β_2 agonist p.r.n.

If above inadequate, consider sequential therapeutic trials of the following:
- regular high-dose inhaled corticosteroid, i.e. beclometasone 2,000microgram/day or equivalent (via a spacer device with MDIs)
- PO leukotriene receptor antagonist
- PO m/r theophylline
- PO m/r β_2 agonist (use with caution if already on inhaled LABA).
If add-on drug ineffective, discontinue, except for the inhaled corticosteroid (reduce back to moderate dose)

If asthma not controlled, consider referral to asthma clinic before proceeding to Step 5.

continued

Box A Continued

Step 5: continuous or frequent use of oral corticosteroids
Regular high-dose inhaled corticosteroid, i.e. beclometasone 2,000microgram/24h or equivalent

+ one or more long-acting bronchodilator (see Step 4)
+ regular PO prednisolone at lowest effective dose once daily (monitor blood/urine glucose, blood pressure, cholesterol and bone mineral density)
+ inhaled short-acting β_2 agonist p.r.n.
Refer to asthma clinic.

Moving up or stepping down
Review treatment regularly, moving up a step if control inadequate. Conversely, if control good, consider going down a step. The most appropriate drug to reduce first may be influenced by individual patient circumstances. Reduce dose of inhaled corticosteroid slowly, e.g. ≤50% every 3 months.

---

a. typical starting doses are beclometasone or budesonide 200microgram b.d. or fluticasone 100microgram b.d., but up to double these doses can be used according to the severity of the asthma; ultimately, the dose is titrated to the lowest which provides effective control, at which point giving the total daily dose once daily can be considered
b. less well established inhaled corticosteroids include mometasone and ciclesonide (see full guidance)
c. inhaled LABAs should *not* be used without inhaled corticosteroids because of concern over an increase in severe asthma exacerbations and asthma-related deaths; combination inhalers are thus recommended to ensure the LABA is taken with an inhaled corticosteroid and to improve adherence.

Diagnosing asthma and COPD

The diagnosis of asthma or COPD is based mainly on the history and examination, supported by objective tests and, ultimately, the response to treatment.

In asthma, objective tests are recommended to try to confirm the diagnosis before long-term therapy is started, i.e. the demonstration of variable airflow obstruction over short periods of time using spirometry preferably or peak expiratory flow rate. Patients with airflow obstruction and a high probability of asthma can be given a trial of treatment. Those with an intermediate probability can be offered either a trial of treatment or reversibility testing. In those with obstruction, asthma is strongly suggested by an improvement in symptoms and FEV_1 >400mL in response to either:[1]

- inhaled **salbutamol** 400microgram *or when there is incomplete response*
- corticosteroids, either inhaled, e.g. **beclometasone** 200microgram b.d. or equivalent for 6–8 weeks, or PO, e.g. **prednisolone** 30mg once daily for 2 weeks.

Further tests are recommended for patients without obstruction and an intermediate probability of asthma, and when there is only a low probability of asthma.[1]

In suspected COPD, post-bronchodilator spirometry is generally sufficient to indicate the presence of airflow obstruction (FEV_1/FVC <0.7) and its severity. COPD is now classified as stage 1 (mild; FEV_1 ≥80% of predicted), stage 2 (moderate; FEV_1 50–79%), stage 3 (severe; FEV_1 30–49%) and stage 4 (very severe; FEV_1 <30%).[2]

In palliative care, when airflow obstruction is suspected, evaluating the impact on symptoms of a 1–2 week trial of a bronchodilator is probably the most pragmatic and relevant approach.

Delivery devices

Pressurized metered-dose inhalers (MDIs) are the most commonly prescribed delivery device and the correct inhaler technique should be carefully explained to the patient and subsequently checked.[1] The patient should be instructed to inhale slowly and then, if possible, hold their breath for 10sec. With an MDI, even with a good technique, 80% of a dose is deposited in the mouth and oropharynx.

Box B Summary of palliative drug therapy in COPD[2]

Smoking and β-blockers may cause bronchoconstriction and should be avoided.

The choice of drug(s) is informed by the degree of benefit obtained from a therapeutic trial, patient preference, undesirable effects, potential to reduce exacerbations and cost. Assess benefit in terms of improvement in symptoms, activities of daily living, exercise capacity, and rapidity of symptom relief; discontinue if ineffective.

Breathlessness and/or exercise limitation
Short-acting β_2 agonist, e.g. salbutamol, or short-acting antimuscarinic bronchodilator, e.g. ipratropium, p.r.n.

Exacerbations or persistent breathlessness
Short-acting β_2 agonist p.r.n. +
• if FEV_1 ≥50%, regular LABA *or* long-acting antimuscarinic bronchodilator, e.g. tiotropium
• if FEV_1 <50%, regular LABA + corticosteroid combination inhaler *or*, if corticosteroid declined or not tolerated, LABA + long-acting antimuscarinic bronchodilator, *or* long-acting antimuscarinic bronchodilator.

Persistent exacerbations or breathlessness (irrespective of FEV_1)
Short-acting β_2 agonist p.r.n. +
• if previously only on LABA, regular LABA + corticosteroid combination inhaler, *or*, if corticosteroid declined or not tolerated, LABA + long-acting antimuscarinic bronchodilator, *or ultimately*
• regular LABA + corticosteroid combination inhaler + long-acting antimuscarinic bronchodilator.
Patients with distressing or disabling breathlessness despite maximal use of inhalers (with spacer if appropriate) should be considered for nebulizer therapy.

Other drugs
Reserved for patients with distressing symptoms despite maximal inhaled therapy:
• oral corticosteroids; when unavoidable in advanced COPD keep dose to a minimum and in patients >65 years provide routine osteoporosis prophylaxis; in those <65 years, monitor for osteoporosis and treat if required
• theophylline; requires caution, particularly in the elderly, monitoring of serum concentration and for risk of drug-drug interaction; can be used earlier in patients unable to use inhaled therapy
• mucolytics; can be considered in patients with chronic productive cough
• for the role of oxygen in COPD, see, p.129
• for the role of opioids and benzodiazepines for breathlessness in advanced COPD and the last days of life, see p.379 and p.669.

If inhaler technique does not improve with training or in patients with poor respiratory effort, consider using an MDI plus a large-volume (650–850mL) spacer device to deliver single-dose actuations. There should be minimal delay between actuation and inhalation, but normal (tidal) breathing is as effective as taking a single breath. Build up of static on plastic and polycarbonate spacers attracts drug particles and reduces drug delivery. To reduce static, spacers should be washed once a month with detergent, rinsed and left to dry without wiping.[1] Spacers should be replaced every 6–12 months.[1]

Dry powder inhalers, e.g. Turbohalers® and breath-actuated MDIs, are other options; but they are no more effective than an MDI ± a spacer.[1,6] Patients generally prefer Turbohalers® over an MDI ± a spacer, but they are not suited to patients with poor inspiratory effort. Compared to MDIs, actuation of a dry powder inhaler causes less sensation in the oropharynx and patients should be informed of this to avoid inadvertent overuse. Breath-actuated MDIs are triggered at low inspiratory flow rates, are popular with patients and are the easiest to use correctly.[7]

Box C   Summary of the initial management of exacerbations of COPD[2]

Diagnosis
A sustained worsening of symptoms of acute onset, beyond the normal day-to-day variation experienced by the patient. Commonly reported symptoms are:
• worsening breathlessness, cough
• increased sputum volume
• change in sputum colour.

Management
Optimize bronchodilator use (see Box B); for patients with distressing or disabling breathlessness despite maximal use of inhalers:
• consider use of a nebulizer
• oral corticosteroid, e.g. prednisolone 30mg once daily for 1–2 weeks
• antibacterials if purulent sputum.

Admission to hospital should be considered if:
• rapid onset of symptoms
• acute confusion or impaired consciousness
• severe breathlessness, cyanosis, SpO_2 <90%, PaO_2 <7kPa, arterial pH <7.35
• already receiving long-term oxygen
• increasing peripheral oedema
• living alone or unable to cope at home
• poor ± deteriorating general condition and level of activity
• significant co-morbidity (particularly cardiac disease, insulin-dependent diabetes mellitus)
• changes on chest radiograph.

For those requiring hospitalization, investigations will include:
• chest radiograph, ECG
• arterial blood gases
• serum theophylline concentration, if already taking theophylline
• if sputum purulent, sputum microscopy and culture
• if pyrexial, blood cultures.

For those requiring hospitalization, management will also include:
• oxygen to keep SaO_2 within an individualized target range, according to local protocols
• consideration of the need for:
  ▷ IV aminophylline if poor response to other bronchodilators
  ▷ non-invasive ventilation (NIV)
  ▷ a respiratory stimulant, e.g. doxapram (if NIV unavailable)
  ▷ intubation.

Nebulizers are more expensive and less convenient than an MDI but may be preferable in patients with a poor inhaler technique, e.g. children, the frail, and patients with end-stage disease. Because of improved drug delivery, there may be better symptom relief in this group of patients.[8] However, the higher doses administered can increase the risk of undesirable effects and their use should be carefully monitored (also see Nebulized drugs, p.753).

However, overall, there is no evidence to suggest that a nebulizer is superior to any inhaler device for the delivery of a β_2 agonist or corticosteroid for the treatment of stable asthma, or to an MDI + spacer in the initial treatment of acute asthma, unless there are life-threatening features. In patients with COPD and a good inhaler technique, nebulized bronchodilator therapy is only indicated in severe acute exacerbations or when there is distressing or disabling breathlessness despite maximal therapy using inhalers.[2]

In patients with lung cancer, concurrent COPD can be a major cause of breathlessness but may be unrecognized and so go untreated.[9] Breathlessness can be improved in most patients with lung cancer and COPD by a combination of a β_2 agonist and an antimuscarinic bronchodilator; this is equally effective when given by an MDI + a spacer or by nebulizer (see Nebulized drugs, p.753).[9]

Propellants

In the UK, hydrofluoroalkane-134a (HFA) has now replaced chlorofluorocarbons (CFC) as the propellant in all pressurized MDIs. Compared with CFC, 'clogging' is more likely with HFA because of a reduced exit velocity, and weekly cleaning of the nozzle is recommended, particularly with drugs suspended rather than dissolved in the propellant, e.g. **salbutamol**.

Supply

Spacer devices are not interchangeable; prescribe a device that Is compatible with the pressurized MDI.

Inhaler and spacer devices
AeroChamber Plus® (GSK)
Spacer medium-volume for use with all pressurized MDIs, standard adult device = £5, with mask = £8.

Haleraid® (A&H)
Inhaler device to aid operation of manually actuated pressurized MDIs by patients with impaired strength in hands, For use with *Flixotide*®, *Seretide*®, *Serevent*®, and *Ventolin*® inhalers, available for 120 and 200-dose inhalers = £1. NHS

Volumatic® (A&H)
Spacer large-volume for use with *Flixotide*®, *Seretide*®, *Serevent*®, and *Ventolin*® inhalers, pressurized MDIs = £4, with paediatric mask = £7.

This is not a complete list; see BNF for more information including devices for paediatric use.

---

1 BTS/SIGN (2012) British Guideline on the Management of Asthma. A National Clinical Guideline. Revised edition January 2012. British Thoracic Society and Scottish Intercollegiate Guidelines Network. Available from: www.sign.ac.uk/pdf/sign101.pdf
2 NICE (2010) Chronic obstructive pulmonary disease: management of chronic obstructive pulmonary disease in adults in primary and secondary care. *Clinical Guideline.* CG101. www.nice.org.uk
3 NHLBI/WHO (2013) Global Initiative for Chronic Obstructive Lung Disease. Global strategy for the diagnosis, management and prevention of chronic obstructive pulmonary disease. Available from: www.goldcopd.com
4 NHLBI/WHO (2012) Global Initiative for Asthma (GINA). Pocket guide for asthma management and prevention. Available from:www.ginasthma.com
5 Laveneziana P et al. (2012) New physiological insights into dyspnea and exercise intolerance in chronic obstructive pulmonary disease patients. *Expert Reviews in Respiratory Medicine.* **6**: 651–662.
6 Anonymous (2003) Inhaler devices for the management of asthma and COPD. *Effective Health Care Bulletins.* **8**: 1–12.
7 Lenney J et al. (2000) Inappropriate inhaler use: assessment of use and patient preference of seven inhalation devices. *Respiratory Medicine.* **94**: 496–500.
8 Tashkin DP et al. (2007) Comparing COPD treatment: nebulizer, metered dose inhaler, and concomitant therapy. *American Journal of Medicine.***120**: 435–441.
9 Congleton J and Muers MF (1995) The incidence of airflow obstruction in bronchial carcinoma, its relation to breathlessness, and response to bronchodilator therapy. *Respiratory Medicine.* **89**: 291–296.

Updated February 2014

IPRATROPIUM BROMIDE BNF 3.1.2

Class: Quaternary ammonium antimuscarinic bronchodilator.

Indications: Reversible airways obstruction, particularly in COPD.

Contra-indications: Hypersensitivity to **atropine** or its derivatives.

Pharmacology

Ipratropium is a short-acting antimuscarinic. In patients with COPD, cholinergic vagal efferent nerves to the airways activate muscarinic receptors, resulting in increased resting bronchial tone and mucus secretion.[1] Antimuscarinics block these effects and cause bronchodilation. Short-acting antimuscarinics increase FEV_1 but have less consistent benefit on breathlessness, need for rescue medication, walking distance and quality of life.[2]

For patients with COPD-related breathlessness and exercise limitation, an inhaled short-acting antimuscarinic bronchodilator *or* a short-acting β_2 agonist are recommended as initial treatment on a p.r.n. basis. However, a short-acting β_2 agonist is generally preferred as it has a more rapid onset of action and, unlike a short-acting antimuscarinic bronchodilator, can also be prescribed concurrently with a long-acting antimuscarinic bronchodilator (e.g. **tiotropium**, p.113), which subsequently may be required (see Bronchodilators, Box B, p.109). For persistent symptoms, compared with the regular use of ipratropium, **tiotropium** is safer and more effective across a range of outcomes.[3]

In acute exacerbations of COPD when there is insufficient relief with an inhaled short-acting β_2 agonist, a short-acting antimuscarinic bronchodilator is often added despite limited evidence to support this (also see Bronchodilators, Box C, p.110).[4]

Antimuscarinic bronchodilators have no role in the management of chronic asthma, but nebulized ipratropium bromide is used in severe or life-threatening exacerbations (see Bronchodilators, Table 1, p.106).[5]

Bio-availability most of the 10–30% of the inhaled dose which reaches the lower airways is absorbed.
Onset of action 3–30min asthma; 15min COPD.
Peak response 1.5–3h asthma; 1–2h COPD.
Plasma halflife 2.3–3.8h.
Duration of action 4–8h.

Cautions

Nebulized solution reaching the eye may precipitate narrow-angle glaucoma in susceptible patients; bladder neck obstruction, prostatic hypertrophy.

Undesirable effects

A small increase in cardiovascular events (e.g. myocardial infarction, heart failure, cardiac arrhythmia, stroke) has been reported in patients with COPD using ipratropium regularly and requires further investigation.[6]

Common (<10%, >1%): headache, dizziness, dry mouth, oropharyngeal irritation, cough, bronchoconstriction, vomiting, GI motility changes.
Uncommon (<1%, >0.1%): visual accommodation changes, tachycardia.
Rare (<0.1%, >0.01%): cardiac arrhythmia, e.g. atrial fibrillation, laryngospasm, nausea, urinary retention.

Nebulized drug droplets may reach the eye and there have been uncommon reports of precipitation of narrow-angle glaucoma and rare reports of eye pain, mydriasis and increased intra-ocular pressure.

Dose and use

In most patients, administration t.d.s. is sufficient.

Aerosol inhalation
- 20–40microgram (1–2 puffs) p.r.n. up to t.d.s.–q.d.s.
- 20–40microgram (1–2 puffs) before exercise in exercise-induced bronchoconstriction.

Nebulizer solution
- use with a mouthpiece to minimize any nebulized drug entering the eye
- 250–500microgram p.r.n. up to t.d.s.–q.d.s in COPD; generally given q.d.s. in an exacerbation of COPD
- 500microgram q6h–q4h in acute exacerbation of asthma (see Bronchodilators, Table 1, p.106).[5]
Also see Chapter 23, p.753.

Supply

Ipratropium bromide (generic)
Nebulizer solution (single-dose units) 250microgram/mL, 20×1mL (250microgram) = £5, 20×2mL (500microgram) = £6; *may be diluted with sterile 0.9% saline.*

Atrovent® (Boehringer Ingelheim)
Aerosol inhalation (CFC-free) 20microgram/metered inhalation, 28 days @ 40microgram (2 puffs) t.d.s. = £5.
Nebulizer solution (single-dose units) 250microgram/ml, 20×1mL (250microgram) = £5, 20×2mL (500microgram) = £5; *may be diluted with sterile 0.9% saline.*

With **salbutamol** (generic)
Nebulizer solution (single-dose units) ipratropium bromide 500microgram, **salbutamol** 2.5mg/2.5mL, 60×2.5mL = £24.

---

1 Gross NJ et al. (1989) Cholinergic bronchomotor tone in COPD. Estimates of its amount in comparison with that in normal subjects. *Chest.* **96**: 984–987.
2 NICE (2010) Chronic obstructive pulmonary disease: management of chronic obstructive pulmonary disease in adults in primary and secondary care. *Clinical Guideline.* CG101. www.nice.org.uk
3 Cheyne L et al. (2013) Tiotropium versus ipratropium bromide for chronic obstructive pulmonary disease. *Cochrane Database Systematic Reviews.* **9**: CD009552.
4 McCrory D and Brown CD (2008) Anticholinergic bronchodilators versus beta2-sympathomimetic agents for acute exacerbations of chronic obstructive pulmonary disease. *Cochrane Database of Systematic Reviews.* **4**: CD003900.
5 BTS/SIGN (2012) British Guideline on the Management of Asthma. A National Clinical Guideline. Revised edition January 2012. British Thoracic Society and Scottish Intercollegiate Guidelines Network. Available from: www.sign.ac.uk/pdf/sign101.pdf
6 NHLBI/WHO (2013) Global initiative for chronic obstructive lung disease. Global strategy for the diagnosis, management and prevention of chronic obstructive pulmonary disease. Available from: www.goldcopd.com

Updated February 2014

TIOTROPIUM   BNF 3.1.2

Class: Quaternary ammonium antimuscarinic bronchodilator.

Indications: Maintenance treatment of airways obstruction in COPD.

Contra-indications: Hypersensitivity to **atropine** or its derivatives, including **ipratropium**, lactose intolerance (dry powder formulation).

Pharmacology

Tiotropium bromide is structurally related to **ipratropium bromide** but is longer acting and thus has the convenience of once daily administration.[1–3] Its main effect is to inhibit muscarinic M_3-receptors in airway smooth muscle and mucous glands, and M_1-receptors in parasympathetic ganglia. Because it is a quaternary compound, relatively little tiotropium is absorbed into the systemic circulation. However, a small amount of tiotropium is excreted renally unchanged and, theoretically at least, accumulation could occur in patients with moderate-severe renal impairment.

In patients with COPD, tiotropium is safer and more effective than the use of regular **ipratropium** in improving lung function, relieving breathlessness, reducing exacerbations, exacerbation-related hospitalizations, and improving quality of life.[4,5] Compared with **salmeterol**, tiotropium has similar efficacy, but appears better tolerated.[6] It is cost-effective, although not cost-saving.[4] Tiotropium can be introduced and used alone when symptoms are unrelieved by the use of p.r.n. short-acting bronchodilators, or as an add-on therapy when other regular long-acting bronchodilator approaches are insufficient (see Bronchodilators, Box B, p.109).[7]

Tiotropium has a relatively slow onset of bronchodilation and it should not be used as rescue therapy for acute bronchospasm.[8] Patients receiving tiotropium should use a short-acting β_2 agonist, e.g. **salbutamol**, as a rescue bronchodilator; **ipratropium** should *not* be used as it has a slower onset of action and the muscarinic receptors will already be occupied by tiotropium.[9]

Concerns have been expressed about an increase in mortality from cardiovascular disease and from all causes associated with the use of the Respimat® mist inhaler compared with inhalers containing placebo, tiotropium as a dry powder, LABA, or LABA + corticosteroid.[10,11] However, data are mixed and a recent large trial found no difference in mortality between patients using tiotropium mist or dry powder inhalers, even in those with previous cardiac disease.[12] However, because those with unstable cardiovascular disease or moderate-severe renal impairment were excluded, use of the Respimat® inhaler is probably best avoided in these groups (see Dose and use).

Alternative antimuscarinic bronchodilators authorized for maintenance treatment in COPD are **aclidinium** and **glycopyrronium** (p.12).

Bio-availability 20% dry powder inhalation, 33% solution for inhalation (soft mist inhaler).
Onset of action ≤30min.
Peak response 1–3h.
Plasma halflife 5–6 days.
Duration of action > 24h.

Cautions

Powder or solution accidentally sprayed into the eye may precipitate narrow-angle glaucoma in susceptible patients; cardiac arrhythmia, bladder neck obstruction, prostatic hypertrophy, moderate-severe renal impairment (creatinine clearance ≤50mL/min).

Undesirable effects

Common (<10%, >1%): dry mouth (generally mild and improves with continued use).
Uncommon (<1%, >0.1%): dizziness, headache, cardiac arrhythmia, e.g. atrial fibrillation, tachycardia, epistaxis, oropharyngeal candidosis, pharyngitis, cough, dysphagia, dysphonia, constipation, dysuria, urinary retention, pruritus, rash.
Rare (<0.1%, >0.01%): blurred vision, increased intra-ocular pressure, glaucoma, oropharyngeal irritation, bronchoconstriction, gastro-oesophageal reflux, dry skin.

Dose and use
Dry powder inhalation
- regular administration of 1 capsule once daily via the HandiHaler® inhalation device.

Solution for inhalation (soft mist inhaler)

Increased mortality from cardiovascular disease and from all causes has been reported with use of the Respimat® mist inhaler.[11] Data are mixed, with no excess deaths seen in a recent large study comparing the mist and dry powder inhalers.[12] However, because those with unstable cardiovascular disease (defined as myocardial infarction within 6 months; hospitalized for Class III or IV heart failure, or had unstable or life-threatening arrhythmia requiring new treatment within 12 months) or moderate-severe renal impairment were excluded, the Respimat® mist inhaler is best avoided in these groups.

- regular administration of 5microgram (2 puffs) once daily via the Respimat® inhalation device.

Supply
Spiriva® (Boehringer Ingelheim)
Dry powder inhalation capsules for use with the HandiHaler® device, 18microgram/capsule, 28 days @ 1 capsule once daily = £35; contains lactose.
Solution for inhalation (soft mist inhaler) cartridges for use with the Respimat® device, 2.5microgram/metered inhalation, 28 days @ 5microgram (2 puffs) once daily = £36.

1 Barnes PJ (2000) The pharmacological properties of tiotropium. Chest. 117 (suppl): 63s–66s.
2 Hvizdos KM and Goa KL (2002) Tiotropium bromide. Drugs. 62: 1195–1203; discussion 1204–1195.
3 Gross NJ (2004) Tiotropium bromide. Chest. 126: 1946–1953.
4 Barr RG et al. (2006) Tiotropium for stable chronic obstructive pulmonary disease: A meta-analysis. Thorax. 61: 854–862.

5 Cheyne L et al. (2013) Tiotropium versus ipratropium bromide for chronic obstructive pulmonary disease. *Cochrane Database Systematic Reviews.* **9**: CD009552.
6 Chong J et al. (2012) Tiotropium versus long-acting beta-agonists for stable chronic obstructive pulmonary disease. *Cochrane Database Systematic Reviews.* **9**: Cd009157.
7 NICE (2010) Chronic obstructive pulmonary disease: management of chronic obstructive pulmonary disease in adults in primary and secondary care. *Clinical Guideline.* CG101. www.nice.org.uk
8 Calverley PMA (2000) The timing and dose pattern of bronchodilation with tiotropium in stable COPD [abstract P523]. *European Respiratory Journal.* **16 (suppl 31)**: 56s.
9 Sutherland ER and Cherniack RM (2004) Management of chronic obstructive pulmonary disease. *N Engl J Med.* **350**: 2689–2697.
10 NHLBI/WHO (2013) Global initiative for chronic obstructive lung disease. Global strategy for the diagnosis, management and prevention of chronic obstructive pulmonary disease. Available from: www.goldcopd.com
11 Jenkins CR and Beasley R (2013) Tiotropium Respimat increases the risk of mortality. *Thorax.* **68**: 5–7.
12 Wise RA et al. (2013) Tiotropium Respimat inhaler and the risk of death in COPD. *New England Journal of Medicine.* **369**: 1491–1501.

Updated February 2014

SALBUTAMOL   BNF 3.1.1.1

Class: β_2-Adrenergic receptor agonist (β_2 agonist, sympathomimetic).

Indications: Asthma and other conditions associated with reversible airways obstruction.

Contra-indications: Lactose intolerance (dry powder formulation).

Pharmacology

Short-acting β_2 agonists (salbutamol, **terbutaline**) have an important role in the management of chronic asthma and COPD and acute exacerbations of both (see Bronchodilators, p.105).[1,2] At low doses, they have predominantly a β_2 agonist bronchodilator effect and no major impact on the heart. However, with increasing dose, tachycardia can occur and rarely prolongation of the QT interval, which may predispose to *torsade de pointes*, a ventricular tachyarrhythmia (see Chapter 24, p.759).

In chronic asthma, short-acting β_2 agonists should be used only p.r.n.[1] They are not recommended for regular use because little benefit has been shown in RCTs. Further, regular use has also been associated with poorer asthma control.[3] Thus, p.r.n. use ⩾3 times a week is one indication for the need for prophylactic therapy with an inhaled corticosteroid (see Bronchodilators, Box A, p.107).[1]

In chronic COPD, for breathlessness and exercise limitation, either a short-acting β_2 agonist or a short-acting antimuscarinic bronchodilator can be used p.r.n. If symptoms persist, a regular long-acting bronchodilator is recommended (see Bronchodilators, Box B, p.109).[2] Thus, for p.r.n. symptom relief, a short-acting β_2 agonist is generally preferred; it has a more rapid onset of action and, unlike a short-acting antimuscarinic bronchodilator, can also be prescribed concurrently with a long-acting antimuscarinic bronchodilator (see **Tiotropium**, p.113).

Plasma potassium concentration should be monitored in severe asthma because β_2 agonists, particularly in combination with **theophylline** and inhaled corticosteroids, can cause *hypokalaemia* which further increases the QT interval and risk of arrhythmia.

For details of the use of salbutamol in the treatment of *hyperkalaemia*, see **Potassium**, p.568.

Bio-availability 10–20% of the dose reaches the lower airways.
Onset of action 5min inhaled; 3–5min nebulized.
Peak response 0.5–2h inhaled; 1.2h nebulized.
Plasma halflife 4–6h inhaled and nebulized.
Duration of action 4–6h inhaled and nebulized.

Cautions

Hyperthyroidism, myocardial insufficiency, cardiac arrhythmia, susceptibility to QT prolongation, hypertension, diabetes mellitus (risk of keto-acidosis if given by CIVI).

Drug interactions

Serious drug interaction: increased risk of hypokalaemia with corticosteroids, diuretics, theophylline.[4]

Undesirable effects

Common (<10%, >1%): tremor, headaches, tachycardia.
Uncommon (<1%, >0.1%): mouth and throat irritation from dry powder inhalation.

Dose and use

Also see Chapter 23, p.753.

Asthma

In moderate–severe exacerbations of asthma, β_2 agonists can be given by MDI + spacer or nebulizer, and repeated until symptoms improve. In life-threatening asthma, they should be nebulized and combined with **ipratropium** (see Bronchodilators, Table 1, p.106).

Aerosol inhalation
Chronic asthma:
- 100–200microgram (1–2 puffs). p.r.n. up to q.d.s.
- 200microgram (2 puffs) before exercise in exercise-induced bronchoconstriction.

Acute asthma (see Bronchodilators, Table 1, p.106):
- 400microgram (4 puffs) via a spacer, given one at a time and inhaled separately, followed by 200microgram (2 puffs) every 2min, up to a maximum of 1mg (10 puffs).[1]

Nebulizer solution
Chronic asthma:
- 2.5–5mg p.r.n. up to q.d.s. in patients for whom inhalers are unsuitable.

Acute asthma (see Bronchodilators, Table 1, p.106):
- 5mg up to every 15–30min via an oxygen-driven nebulizer
- 5–10mg/h by continuous nebulization (requires specific nebulizer).[1]

COPD

In acute exacerbations of COPD, bronchodilator use should be optimized (see Bronchodilators, Box B, p.109); both nebulizers and inhalers can be used to administer inhaled therapy during exacerbations (see Bronchodilators, Box B, p.109; and Box C, p.110).

In stable COPD, patients with distressing or disabling breathlessness despite maximal bronchodilator therapy using inhalers should be considered for nebulizer therapy (also see Delivery devices, p.108).[2]

Aerosol inhalation
- 100–200microgram (1–2 puffs) p.r.n. up to q.d.s.

Nebulizer solution
- 2.5–5mg p.r.n. up to q.d.s. via an oxygen-driven nebulizer, unless the patient is hypercapnic or acidotic, when compressed air should be used. If oxygen therapy is required by such patients, administer simultaneously by nasal cannulae.

Supply

Salbutamol (generic)
Aerosol inhalation (CFC-free) 100microgram/metered inhalation, 28 days @ 200microgram (2 puffs) p.r.n. up to q.d.s. = £1.50.
Nebulizer solution (single-dose units) 1mg/mL, 20 × 2.5mL (2.5mg) = £2; 2mg/mL, 20 × 2.5mL (5mg) = £4; *may be diluted with sterile 0.9% saline.*

Airomir® (IVAX)
Aerosol inhalation (CFC-free) 100microgram/metered inhalation, 28 days @ 200microgram (2 puffs) p.r.n. up to q.d.s. = £2.
Breath-actuated aerosol inhalation (CFC-free) Autohaler®, 100microgram/metered inhalation, 28 days @ 200microgram (2 puffs) p.r.n. up to q.d.s. = £6.

Easyhaler Salbutamol® (Orion)
Dry powder inhalation 100microgram/metered inhalation, 200microgram/metered inhalation, 28 days @ 200microgram p.r.n. up to q.d.s. = £3.50; *contains lactose.*

Ventolin® (A&H)
Aerosol inhalation (CFC-free) Evohaler®, 100microgram/metered inhalation, 28 days @ 200microgram (2 puffs) p.r.n. up to q.d.s. = £1.50.
Dry powder inhalation blisters for use with Accuhaler® device, 200microgram/blister, 28 days @ 200microgram (1 blister) p.r.n. up to q.d.s = £3.
Nebulizer solution (single-dose units for use with nebulizer) Nebules®, 1mg/mL, 20 × 2.5mL (2.5mg) = £2; 2mg/mL, 20 × 2.5mL (5mg) = £3; *may be diluted with sterile 0.9% saline if administration time > 10min is required.*
Nebulizer solution (multiple-dose bottle for use with a nebulizer or ventilator) 5mg/mL, 20mL = £2.50; *only available for use in hospitals, may be diluted with sterile 0.9% saline.*

With **ipratropium bromide**, see p.111

For spacer devices, see p.105

---

1 BTS/SIGN (2012) British Guideline on the Management of Asthma. A National Clinical Guideline. Revised edition January 2012. British Thoracic Society and Scottish Intercollegiate Guidelines Network. Available from: www.sign.ac.uk/pdf/sign101.pdf
2 NICE (2010) Chronic obstructive pulmonary disease: management of chronic obstructive pulmonary disease in adults in primary and secondary care. *Clinical Guideline.* CG101. www.nice.org.uk.
3 Sears M (2000) Short-acting inhaled B-agonists: to be taken regularly or as needed? *Lancet.* **355**: 1658–1659.
4 Baxter K and Preston CL. *Stockley's Drug Interactions.* London: Pharmaceutical Press www.medicinescomplete.com (accessed January 2014).

Updated February 2014

INHALED LONG-ACTING β₂-AGONISTS (LABAs)   BNF 3.1.1.1

Class: β₂-Adrenergic receptor agonist (β₂ agonist, sympathomimetic).

Indications: Reversible airways obstruction in patients requiring long-term regular bronchodilator therapy. *In selected patients only* (see Pharmacology): relief of acute asthma symptoms (Fostair®, Oxis®, and Symbicort®) or prevention of exercise-induced bronchospasm (Oxis®).

Contra-indications: Salmeterol should not be used for the relief of acute asthma because of its slow onset of action.

Pharmacology

The selective LABAs **salmeterol** and **formoterol** have a bronchodilating effect which lasts for 12h.[1] **Indacaterol**, authorized only for COPD, has a duration of action of 24h but is less well established than other LABAs.[2] **Salmeterol** has a relatively slow onset of action; **formoterol** has an onset of action similar to **salbutamol** and can thus also be used as an alternative reliever inhaler in patients with asthma. However, **formoterol** should be used as a reliever inhaler *only* in patients already on regular maintenance treatment with an inhaled corticosteroid, preferably via a combination inhaler authorized for such use, i.e. Fostair® and Symbicort®. The need for ⩾1 dose for symptom relief on a daily basis should prompt a treatment review.[3] This approach has not been studied with other combination inhalers containing LABA and corticosteroids.

In patients with asthma, inhaled LABAs are added when symptoms are inadequately relieved by a regular standard-dose inhaled corticosteroid (see Bronchodilators, Box A, p.107).[3] The addition of inhaled LABAs to inhaled corticosteroids improves lung function and symptoms, and decreases exacerbations more effectively than increasing the dose of inhaled steroids alone.[4,5]

However, the findings of post-marketing studies have been generally less impressive and safety concerns have been identified when LABAs have been used *without* an inhaled corticosteroid, i.e. increased life-threatening and fatal exacerbations of asthma.[6,7] *Thus in patients with asthma inhaled LABAs should not be used without inhaled corticosteroids* (see Cautions).[8]

Inhalers which combine a LABA and a corticosteroid are recommended in asthma guidelines;[3] there is no difference in efficacy compared with the use of separate inhalers, they may aid patient adherence and ensure that inhaled LABAs are not used alone without corticosteroids.[3]

The safety of LABAs used even with an inhaled corticosteroid remains a controversial issue, with the FDA mandating a large trial to explore this further. However, doubts have been expressed that even this could fail to fully resolve the issue.[9]

LABAs can also be used *regularly* to prevent exercise-induced bronchospasm in patients whose asthma is otherwise well controlled on an inhaled corticosteroid. Although Oxis® is approved for *p.r.n.* use to prevent exercise-induced bronchospasm, a short-acting β₂ agonist is generally preferred.[3]

In patients with COPD, a LABA can be introduced and used alone when symptoms are unrelieved by the use of p.r.n. short-acting bronchodilators, or as an add-on therapy when other regular long-acting bronchodilator approaches are insufficient (see Bronchodilators, Box B, p.109).[10]

Unlike asthma, the combined use of LABAs with an inhaled corticosteroid is not essential in COPD, but is recommended for patients with exacerbations or persistent breathlessness and a predicted FEV_1 < 50%, or when other approaches are inadequate (see Bronchodilators, Box B, p.109). Inhaled LABAs and long-acting antimuscarinic bronchodilators have similar efficacy in terms of improving lung function, relieving breathlessness, reducing exacerbations and hospitalizations, and improving quality of life. Compared with **salmeterol**, **tiotropium** appears better tolerated.[10,11] For pharmacokinetic details see Table 1.

Table 1 Pharmacokinetics of inhaled LABAs

	Formoterol	Salmeterol
Bio-availability	30–50% of the delivered dose reaches the lungs (Turbohaler®)	Approximately 10% of the delivered dose reaches the lungs (aerosol)[12]
Onset of action	1–3min	10–20min
Peak response	5–10min	≤30min[12]
Plasma halflife	≤8h	≤8h (plasma concentration low or undetectable after therapeutic doses)[12]
Duration of action	About 12h	12–16h[12]

Cautions

In asthma, inhaled LABAs should *not* be used without inhaled corticosteroids because of concern over an increase in life-threatening and fatal exacerbations. To ensure safe use, the MHRA/CHM advise that in chronic asthma:[7]
- patients receiving **formoterol** or **salmeterol** should always be prescribed an inhaled corticosteroid
- adherence will be aided by the use of a combination LABA + corticosteroid inhaler.

Hyperthyroidism, cardiovascular disease, arrhythmias, susceptibility to QT prolongation or concurrent use of drugs which prolong the QT interval, (see p.759), hypertension, paradoxical bronchoconstriction (discontinue and use alternative treatment), severe liver cirrhosis (**formoterol**), diabetes mellitus (may cause hyperglycaemia; monitor blood glucose).

Drug interactions

Serious drug interaction: increased risk of hypokalaemia with corticosteroids, diuretics, **theophylline**.

Table 2 Adult doses (as puffs) of LABA

Formulation	Formoterol or Foradil® (DPI)	Atimos Modulite® (MDI)[a]	Oxis® Turbohaler® (DPI)[b]		Salmeterol or Serevent® Evohaler® (MDI)	Serevent® Accuhaler® or Serevent® Diskhaler® (DPI)
LABA Strength (microgram)	Formoterol 12	Formoterol 12[a]	Formoterol 6[b]	Formoterol 12[b]	Salmeterol 25	Salmeterol 50
Asthma						
Starting dose	1 b.d.	1 b.d.	1–2 daily–b.d.	1 daily–b.d	2 b.d.	1 b.d.
Maximum dose	2 b.d.	2 b.d.	4 b.d.[d]	2 b.d.[d]	4 b.d.	2 b.d.
Reliever dose	n/a	n/a	1–2 p.r.n.	1 p.r.n.	n/a	n/a
Prevention of exercise-induced bronchospasm	n/a	n/a	2 before exercise	1 before exercise	n/a	n/a
COPD						
Starting dose	1 b.d.	1 b.d.[c]	2 daily–b.d.	1 daily–b.d	2 b.d.	1 b.d.
Maximum dose	1 b.d.	1 b.d.[c]	2 b.d.[e]	1 b.d.[e]	2 b.d.	1 b.d.
Cost per 60 puffs	£12, £24	£18	£25	£25	£14, £15	£30, £36

DPI = dry powder inhaler; MDI = metered dose inhaler (pressurized); n/a = not authorized

a. each nominal 12microgram metered inhalation delivers 10.1microgram of formoterol fumarate
b. each nominal 6microgram or 12microgram metered inhalation delivers 4.5microgram or 9microgram of formoterol fumarate respectively
c. additional doses above those prescribed for regular therapy may be used for relief of symptoms, up to a maximum total daily dose of 4 puffs (regular plus p.r.n.)
d. occasionally higher doses are used; seek specialist advice
e. additional doses above those prescribed for regular therapy may be used for relief of symptoms, up to a maximum total daily dose of 8 puffs of Oxis® 6 or 4 puffs of Oxis® 12 (regular plus p.r.n.).

Table 3 Adult doses (as puffs) of LABA and corticosteroid combination inhalers

Formulation	Fostair® (MDI)	Symbicort® Turbohaler® (DPI)		Flutiform® (MDI)	Seretide® Evohaler® (MDI)	Seretide® Accuhaler® (DPI)
Corticosteroid	Beclometasone	Budesonide	Budesonide	Fluticasone	Fluticasone	Fluticasone
LABA	Formoterol	Formoterol	Formoterol	Formoterol	Salmeterol	Salmeterol
Strengths[a]	100/6	100/6, 200/6	400/12	50/5, 125/5, 250/10	50/25, 125/25, 250/25	100/50, 250/50, 500/50
Asthma maintenance						
Starting dose	1–2 b.d.	1–2 b.d.	1 b.d.	2 b.d.	2 b.d.	1 b.d.
Maximum dose	2 b.d.	4 b.d.	2 b.d.	2 b.d.	2 b.d.	1 b.d.
Asthma maintenance and reliever therapy						
Maintenance dose	1 b.d.	1 b.d. (or 2 daily)[b]	n/a	n/a	n/a	n/a
Reliever dose	1 p.r.n.	1 p.r.n (maximum of 6 per episode)	n/a	n/a	n/a	n/a
Maximum reliever doses/24h	8	8[c]	n/a	n/a	n/a	n/a
COPD when FEV₁ <50% predicted						
Starting dose	n/a	2 b.d.[b]	1 b.d.	n/a	n/a	1 b.d.[d]
Maximum dose	n/a	2 b.d.[b]	1 b.d.	n/a	n/a	1 b.d.[d]
Cost per 60 puffs	£15	£17, £19	£38	£9, £15, £23	£9, £17, £30	£18, £35, £41

DPI = dry powder inhaler; MDI = metered dose inhaler (pressurized); n/a = not authorized

a. inhaled corticosteroid/LABA dose in microgram/metered inhalation
b. Symbicort® Turbohaler® 200/6 only; authorized to a maximum of 2 puffs b.d.
c. up to 12 puffs/24h for a limited time
d. Seretide 500 Accuhaler® only; authorized for COPD when FEV₁ <60% predicted.

Undesirable effects

Common (<10%, >1%): headache, tremor, palpitations, muscle cramps.
Uncommon (<1%, >0.1%): tachycardia.
Rare (<0.1%) or very rare (<0.01%): arrhythmias, e.g. atrial fibrillation, supraventricular tachycardia, QT interval prolongation, paradoxical bronchoconstriction.

Dose and use

The dose varies for **formoterol** and **salmeterol** with formulation and indication (see Table 2).

Asthma

An inhaled LABA should be added *only* if p.r.n. treatment with a short-acting β₂ agonist *and* regular prophylactic therapy with an inhaled corticosteroid is insufficient to control symptoms (see Bronchodilators, Box A, Step 3, p.107). Use of a combination inhaler will help ensure the concurrent use of a LABA + a corticosteroid (see Table 3).

With certain LABA inhalers (i.e. Oxis®, or those combined with a corticosteroid, i.e. Fostair®, Symbicort®), extra doses can be used on a p.r.n. basis to relieve bronchospasm, instead of a short-acting β₂ agonist (Tables 2 and 3). However, such use ⩾1/day should prompt a treatment review.[3] In addition, Oxis® is authorized for use before exercise to prevent bronchospasm.

COPD

An inhaled LABA is one option when exacerbations or persistent symptoms occur despite short-acting bronchodilators p.r.n. Combined use with an inhaled corticosteroid is recommended for patients with exacerbations or persistent breathlessness and a predicted FEV_1 <50%, or when other approaches are inadequate (Table 3; also see Bronchodilators, Box B, p.109).

With certain LABA inhalers, i.e. Atimos Modulite®, Oxis®, extra doses can be used on a p.r.n. basis to relieve bronchospasm, instead of a short-acting β₂ agonist (Table 2). However, such use ⩾1/day should prompt a treatment review.[3]

Supply

See Table 2 and Table 3.

1 Kips JC and Pauwels RA (2001) Long-acting inhaled beta(2)-agonist therapy in asthma. *American Journal of Respiratory and Critical Care Medicine.* **164**: 923–932.
2 Anonymous (2012) Indacaterol for COPD. *Drugs and Therapeutics Bulletin.* **50**: 58-60.
3 BTS/SIGN (2012) British Guideline on the Management of Asthma. A National Clinical Guideline. Revised edition January 2012. British Thoracic Society and Scottish Intercollegiate Guidelines Network. Available from: www.sign.ac.uk/pdf/sign101.pdf
4 Pauwels RA et al. (1997) Effect of inhaled formoterol and budesonide on exacerbations of asthma. Formoterol and Corticosteroids Establishing Therapy (FACET) International Study Group. *New England Journal of Medicine.* **337**: 1405–1411.
5 Shrewsbury S et al. (2000) Meta-analysis of increased dose of inhaled steroid or addition of salmeterol in symptomatic asthma (MIASMA). *British Medical Journal.* **320**: 1368–1373.
6 Nelson HS et al. (2006) The Salmeterol Multicenter Asthma Research Trial: a comparison of usual pharmacotherapy for asthma or usual pharmacotherapy plus salmeterol. *Chest.* **129**: 15–26.
7 MHRA (2010) Long-acting B2-agonists for asthma: review. *Drug Safety Update.* **4**. www.mhra.gov.uk/safetyinformation
8 Cates CJ and Cates MJ (2010) Regular treatment with salmeterol for chronic asthma: serious adverse events. *Cochrane Database of Systematic Reviews.* **1**: CD006363.
9 Sears MR (2013) The FDA-mandated trial of safety of long-acting beta-agonists in asthma: finality or futility? *Thorax.* **68**: 195–198.
10 NICE (2010) Chronic obstructive pulmonary disease: management of chronic obstructive pulmonary disease in adults in primary and secondary care. *Clinical Guideline.* CG101. www.nice.org.uk
11 Chong J et al. (2012) Tiotropium versus long-acting beta-agonists for stable chronic obstructive pulmonary disease. *Cochrane Database Systematic Reviews.* **9**: CD009157.
12 Cazzola M et al. (2002) Clinical pharmacokinetics of salmeterol. *Clinical Pharmacokinetics.* **41**: 19–30.

Updated February 2014

THEOPHYLLINE   BNF 3.1.3

Class: Methylxanthine.

Indications: Reversible airways obstruction; given by injection as **aminophylline** for severe or life-threatening exacerbations of asthma (see below).

Contra-indications: Uncontrolled arrhythmias, seizure disorders.

Pharmacology

In patients with asthma and COPD, because of its inferior safety and efficacy, theophylline should generally be considered only after the use of an inhaled corticosteroid and one or more inhaled long-acting bronchodilators (see Bronchodilators Box A, p.107 and Box B, p.109).[1,2]

Theophylline is given by injection as **aminophylline**, a mixture containing ethylenediamine to increase the solubility of theophylline. **Aminophylline** must be given by slow IV injection over 20–30min; it is too irritant for IM use and is a potent gastric irritant PO. **Aminophylline** should be used only with guidance from senior/experienced staff. It has a limited role in patients with life-threatening or near fatal asthma or an exacerbation of COPD who are not responding to initial therapy (see Bronchodilators, Table 1, p.106 and Box C, p.110).[1,2]

Theophylline shares the actions of the other xanthine alkaloids (e.g. caffeine) on the CNS, myocardium, kidney and smooth muscle. It has a relatively weak CNS effect but a more powerful relaxant effect on bronchial smooth muscle. This is mainly by inhibiting phosphodiesterase 3 (PDE3). This leads to an accumulation of cyclic AMP which through various mechanisms, e.g. reduced intracellular calcium, leads to smooth muscle relaxation.

An anti-inflammatory effect in the airways, e.g. through inhibition of PDE4 and activation of histone deacetylase-2, has been shown at plasma concentrations as low as 5mg/L.[3] Thus, there is increasing interest in the use of low-dose theophylline alongside inhaled corticosteroids in patients with asthma and COPD, particularly as reduced histone deacetylase-2 activity is associated with corticosteroid resistance and reduced benefit.[3,4] Preliminary data suggests that this effect of theophylline could also be utilized in other inflammatory diseases where corticosteroid resistance is evident.[5]

Numerous other effects of theophylline have been described but their benefit in relation to asthma or COPD is unclear; some require plasma concentrations at the higher end of, or exceeding, the usual therapeutic range.[6] Theophylline is an adenosine receptor antagonist. Plasma adenosine levels are increased in situations where intra-abdominal pressure is pathologically increased, e.g. as a result of bowel obstruction, pancreatitis and peritonitis, resulting in tissue hypoxia. Early work suggests that infusions of theophylline improve mortality in this situation, possibly by preventing the deleterious effect of adenosine on renal perfusion.[7] This may also explain why theophylline reduces the incidence of radiological contrast-induced acute kidney injury.[8] Conversely, an adenosine antagonist effect may account for some of the more serious undesirable effects of theophylline, e.g. cardiac arrhythmia, seizure.

Although theophylline inhibits proliferation and augments apoptosis of cancer cells, the clinical relevance of this remains to be determined.[9] An anti-inflammatory effect may also explain the benefit seen in an animal model of cancer cachexia.[10]

Theophylline is metabolized by the liver. Its therapeutic index is narrow and some patients experience toxic effects even in the therapeutic range. Plasma concentrations of theophylline are influenced by infection, hypoxia, smoking, various drugs (see below), hepatic impairment, thyroid disorders, and heart failure; all these can make the use of theophylline difficult. Steady-state theophylline levels are attained within 3–4 days of adjusting the dose of a m/r preparation. Blood for theophylline levels should be taken 4–6h after the last dose.

Bio-availability ≥90%; 80% m/r.
Onset of action 40–60min PO; immunomodulation ≤3 weeks.
Plasma halflife 6–12h, but wide interindividual variation.
Duration of action 12h m/r theophylline PO; immunomodulation several days.

Cautions

Elderly, cardiac disease, hypertension, hyperthyroidism and hypothyroidism, peptic ulcer, hepatic impairment, pyrexia.

Drug interactions

Theophylline may potentiate hypokalaemia associated with β_2 agonists, corticosteroids, diuretics and hypoxia.[11,12]

Theophylline is metabolized mainly by CYP1A2, and to some extent by CYP3A4 and CYP2E1. Caution is required with concurrent use of drugs which inhibit or induce these enzymes, (see Chapter 25, p.767). Reports of interactions where closer monitoring ± dose adjustment are required are listed in Box A.

Theophylline can reduce the plasma levels of **lithium** by 20–30%.

Box A   Interactions between theophylline and other drugs involving CYP450[12]

Plasma concentrations of theophylline

Increased by	**Decreased by**
Aciclovir	Smoking
Allopurinol	Heavy alcohol intake
Cimetidine	Carbamazepine
Clarithromycin	Isoprenaline
Diltiazem	Phenobarbital and other barbiturates
Erythromycin	Phenytoin
Fluconazole	Rifampicin
Fluvoxamine[a]	Ritonavir
Mexiletine[b]	St John's wort
Oral contraceptives	Sulfinpyrazone
Quinolone antibacterials (ciprofloxacin, but not ofloxacin)	
Troleandomycin[b] (not UK)	
Verapamil	

a. avoid concurrent use; if unavoidable, reduce the dose of theophylline by 50% and monitor closely
b. reduce the dose of theophylline by 50%.

Undesirable effects

Common (<10%, >1%): headache, dyspepsia, nausea, vomiting; risk of seizures and arrhythmias increases as plasma levels increase; hyperpnoea (fast breathing) when given IV.

Dose and use

Because it is not possible to ensure bio-equivalence between different m/r theophylline products, they should be prescribed by brand name and not interchanged.

A m/r formulation should be used.[1] For patients with swallowing difficulties, Slo-phyllin® capsules containing m/r granules can be opened and the contents sprinkled onto soft food and swallowed whole. An unauthorized immediate-release oral liquid is also available for patients who may require it, e.g. those being fed by enteral feeding tube (see Chapter 22, Table 2, p.733). For m/r products:
- starting dose varies between brands; see individual SPCs
- maintain on a single brand because absorption rates vary between products
- titrate dose according to response and plasma theophylline level
- in patients whose symptoms manifest diurnal fluctuation, a larger evening or morning dose is appropriate to ensure maximum therapeutic benefit when symptoms are most severe

---

- samples for drug plasma concentration monitoring should be taken 4–6h after a PO dose of theophylline m/r, and at least 5 days after the dose was started/adjusted
- for bronchodilation, the recommended therapeutic range is 10–20mg/L (55–110micromol/L). However, some patients may experience unacceptable undesirable effects even within the recommended therapeutic range and for them a lower range may suffice, e.g. 5–15mg/L (28–83micromol/L). This is also considered an appropriate range for the anti-inflammatory effects of theophylline.[3] Ultimately, the clinical response, rather than the plasma level, will determine the need for dose adjustment.

Give IV **aminophylline** in acute severe asthma or exacerbation of COPD only with guidance from senior/experienced staff:[1,2]

- loading dose 250–500mg (maximum 5mg/kg) IV over 20–30min; omit if already on regular PO theophylline and check theophylline levels stat
- maintenance dose 500–700microgram/kg/h CIVI; check blood levels 4–6h after starting CIVI and then daily; adjust dose to achieve a level of 10–20mg/L (55–110micromol/L).

If converting a patient from IV **aminophylline** to PO theophylline, multiply the total daily dose of IVI **aminophylline** by 0.8 (salt factor) to give the total daily dose of PO theophylline; this should be halved into a practical b.d. m/r dose and plasma levels monitored as above.[13]

Supply

Modified-release
Uniphyllin Continus® (Napp)
Tablets m/r 200mg, 300mg, 400mg, 28 days @ 200mg b.d. = £3.

Slo-phyllin® (Merk Sorono)
Capsules containing m/r granules 60mg, 125mg, 250mg, 28 days @ 250mg b.d. = £4.50; *capsule contents can be opened, sprinkled on soft food and swallowed whole.*

Immediate-release
Oral liquid 60mg/5mL, 28 days @ 120mg t.d.s. = £294. (Unauthorized, available as a special order from Martindale; see Appendix 1, p.817); *3 month expiry.*

Aminophylline (generic)
Injection 25mg/mL, 10mL amp = £1.

This is not a complete list; see BNF for full details.

---

1 BTS/SIGN (2012) British Guideline on the Management of Asthma. A National Clinical Guideline. Revised edition January 2012. British Thoracic Society and Scottish Intercollegiate Guidelines Network. Available from: www.sign.ac.uk/pdf/sign101.pdf

2 NICE (2010) Chronic obstructive pulmonary disease: management of chronic obstructive pulmonary disease in adults in primary and secondary care. *Clinical Guideline*. CG101. www.nice.org.uk

3 Barnes PJ (2013) Theophylline. *American Journal of Respiratroy and Critical Care Medicine*. **188**: 901–906.

4 Ford PA et al. (2010) Treatment effects of low-dose theophylline combined with an inhaled corticosteroid in COPD. *Chest*. **137**: 1338–1344.

5 Kendrick SF et al. (2010) Theophylline improves steroid sensitivity in acute alcoholic hepatitis. *Hepatology*. **52**: 126–131.

6 Mokry J and Mokra D (2013) Immunological aspects of phosphodiesterase inhibition in the respiratory system. *Respiratory Physiology and Neurobiology*. **187**: 11–17.

7 Bodnar Z et al. (2011) Beneficial effects of theophylline infusions in surgical patients with intra-abdominal hypertension. *Langenbecks Arch Surg*. **396**: 793–800.

8 Dai B et al. (2012) Effect of theophylline on prevention of contrast-induced acute kidney injury: a meta-analysis of randomized controlled trials. *American Journal of Kidney Disease*. **60**: 360–370.

9 Kapoor S (2013) Theophylline and its direct anti-neoplastic effects. *Respiratory Medicine* Epub ahead of print.

10 Olivan M et al. (2012) Theophylline is able to partially revert cachexia in tumour-bearing rats. *Nutrition and Metabolism*. **9**: 76.

11 Sweetman S. *Martindale: The Complete Drug Reference*. London: Pharmaceutical Press, www.medicinescomplete.com (accessed January 2014).

12 Baxter K and Preston CL. *Stockley's Drug Interactions*. London: Pharmaceutical Press www.medicinescomplete.com (accessed January 2014).

13 UK Medicines Information (2013) How is an intravenous aminophylline dose converted to an oral aminophylline dose? *Medicines Q & A*. 130.4a www.evidence.nhs.uk

Updated February 2014

INHALED CORTICOSTEROIDS BNF 3.2

Indications: Reversible and irreversible airways obstruction, †stridor, †lymphangitis carcinomatosa, †radiation pneumonitis, †cough after insertion of a bronchial stent (see Nebulized drugs, p.753).

Pharmacology

Inhaled corticosteroids reduce airway inflammation. **Fluticasone** is given in a smaller dose because it is twice as potent as **beclometasone** and **budesonide**, which are considered approximately equivalent. However, variations with different formulations can occur. For example, one **beclometasone** formulation (Qvar®), delivers a greater fraction of smaller particles to the lung, approximately doubling its potency compared with other **beclometasone** formulations (see Dose and use, Table 2). This is also true for the combined **beclometasone** + **formoterol** inhaler, Fostair®.[1] **Ciclesonide** and **mometasone** are relatively new and less well-established inhaled corticosteroids.

Inhaled corticosteroids reach the systemic circulation via both the pulmonary circulation and the GI tract. Long-term high-dose inhaled corticosteroids have been associated with adrenal suppression, and deaths from Addisonian crisis (acute adrenal failure) have occurred rarely (see Cautions).[2] Daily doses of **budesonide** ≤1,500microgram or equivalent do not generally lead to adrenal suppression. However, there is significant variation amongst individuals, and formulation and duration of treatment are also important. Accordingly, systemic corticosteroids (see p.499) should be considered to cover stressful periods (e.g. infection, surgery) in patients receiving long-term high-dose inhaled corticosteroids, i.e. **budesonide** >800microgram/day or equivalent.[3]

Inhaled corticosteroids are the most effective preventer drug in asthma and there is a low threshold for their use (see Bronchodilators, Box A, p.107).[4] Improvement in symptoms generally occurs within 3–7 days, but maximal improvement in symptoms and lung function may take 1–2 months. If standard doses fail to improve symptoms, it is recommended that an inhaled long-acting β_2 agonist (LABA), e.g. **salmeterol** or **formoterol** (p.117), is added before using higher doses of an inhaled corticosteroid (see Bronchodilators, Box A, p.107).[4] If high-dose inhaled corticosteroids are subsequently used, they should be continued only if they have clear benefit over the lower dose. If there is insufficient response to higher-dose inhaled corticosteroids, alternatives include PO leukotriene-receptor antagonists (**montelukast, zafirlukast**), which complement the anti-inflammatory effect of inhaled corticosteroids (see Bronchodilators, Box A, p.107).

In COPD, inhaled corticosteroids are recommended in conjunction with an inhaled LABA for patients with exacerbations or persistent breathlessness and a predicted FEV_1 <50%, or when other approaches are inadequate (see Bronchodilators, Box B, p.109).[5] It should be noted that studies in COPD have generally used high-dose inhaled corticosteroids, e.g. **fluticasone** 1,000microgram/day. Despite this, the overall clinical benefit of inhaled corticosteroids is relatively small.[6] For example, the addition of an inhaled corticosteroid to a LABA reduces the proportion of people experiencing one or more exacerbations from 47% to 42% per annum.[6] Further, inhaled corticosteroids do not modify the long-term decline in FEV_1, nor mortality.[7] This relatively small benefit must be balanced on an individual patient basis against the undesirable effects of using inhaled corticosteroids.

Corticosteroid resistance may partly explain the poor response to inhaled corticosteroids in COPD and in some patients with asthma. This has led to renewed interest in **theophylline**, which in low-dose has anti-inflammatory effects and reverses corticosteroid resistance (see p.122).[8]

The only evidence to support the other indications for inhaled or nebulized corticosteroids listed above is clinical experience.

For pharmacokinetic details, see Table 1.

Cautions

Active or quiescent tuberculosis, mycetoma, immunosuppression.

Because of the risk of adrenal suppression, patients receiving the following should be warned not to abruptly stop treatment, and should be given a steroid card (see Systemic corticosteroids, Box G, p.506):[13]

- long-term high-dose inhaled corticosteroids (e.g. doses higher than the authorized maximum, such as **beclometasone** >2,000microgram/24h)
- inhaled corticosteroids with drugs which may inhibit their metabolism by CYP3A4 e.g. azole antifungals, protease inhibitors (see below); patients have also become Cushingoid.

Table 1 Pharmacokinetics of inhaled corticosteroids in asthma

	Beclometasone dipropionate[9–11]	Budesonide[a,12]	Fluticasone propionate[a,12]
Bio-availability	62%[b] CFC-containing and CFC-free aerosol inhalers	39% Turbohaler® 6% Respules®	30% aerosol inhaler 14% powder inhaler
Onset of action	Days to weeks	Days to weeks	Days to weeks
Time to peak plasma concentration	30–60min[b] CFC-containing and CFC-free aerosol inhalers	5–10min Turbohaler® 10–30min Respules®	1–2h powder inhaler
Plasma halflife	3h[b] CFC-containing and CFC-free aerosol inhalers	2–3h	8h

a. data from Micromedex
b. values for beclometasone 17-*monopropionate*, the form to which most of the dipropionate is converted before reaching the circulation.

Drug interactions

Increased systemic exposure can occur when co-administered with strong CYP3A4 inhibitors, e.g. **itraconazole, nelfinavir, ritonavir.**

Undesirable effects

Oropharyngeal candidosis, sore throat, hoarse voice, cough, paradoxical bronchospasm, hypersensitivity reactions (e.g. rash), skin bruising. Rarely, psychiatric effects, including psychomotor hyperactivity, sleep disorders, anxiety, depression or aggression.[14]

Inhaled corticosteroids are associated with increased risk of cataract, which is dose and duration related.[15] There is a small increased risk of glaucoma with higher doses (i.e. **beclomethasone** > 1600microgram/day).[16] Increased risk of onset and worsening of diabetes, particularly in patients receiving the equivalent of **fluticasone** ≥ 1,000microgram/day.[17]

Data on the impact of inhaled corticosteroids on bone mineral density and risk of fracture are mixed; a recent meta-analysis found a small statistically significant, but clinically questionable, increase in risk of fracture.[18]

In COPD, inhaled corticosteroids are associated with a small increase in the frequency of non-fatal pneumonia;[19] and it is recommended that patients are informed of this when inhaled corticosteroids are prescribed.[5] Data are mixed, but the risk appears higher with **fluticasone** compared with **budesonide**.[20,21] An increased risk of infection may also exist in patients with asthma taking inhaled corticosteroids.[22] However, any such risk is far outweighed by their overall benefit in asthma.

Dose and use

Because of their differing potency and doses, CFC-free aerosol inhalers containing beclometasone should be prescribed by brand name and not interchanged.[1]

Aerosol inhalation

MDIs are most commonly prescribed, alternatives include breath-actuated and dry powder inhalers.
- check the patient's inhaler technique
- use a large-volume spacer device if patient on an MDI, particularly when they:
  ▷ have a poor inhaler technique
  ▷ are using a high dose (Table 2)
  ▷ develop a hoarse voice, sore throat or oral candidosis

Table 2 Approximate equivalent doses for inhaled corticosteroids in adults with asthma[4]

Corticosteroid and examples of formulations	Equivalent dose (microgram)
Beclometasone	
Pulvinal® Beclometasone, Easyhaler®	400
Beclometasone, Asmabec Clickhaler®, Clenil Modulite®	
Qvar® a	200–300
Fostair® a	200
Budesonide	
Easyhaler® Budesonide, Budelin Novolizer®, Pulmicort Turbohaler®	400
Ciclesonide	200–300
Fluticasone	
Flixotide Evohaler®, Flixotide Accuhaler®	200
Mometasone	200

a. approximately twice as potent as other beclometasone inhalers; Fostair® is a combination inhaler with formoterol (see p.117).

- instruct patient to rinse mouth out after use to reduce systemic availability and oral candidosis
- in asthma, start with a dose appropriate to severity, e.g. **beclometasone** 100–400microgram b.d. or equivalent (Table 2), and titrate to the lowest dose effective against symptoms (see Bronchodilators, Box A, p.107); b.d. dosing is generally preferred (except for **ciclesonide** which is always given once daily);[4] however, if subsequently the asthma is controlled on a low dose, e.g. 200–400microgram/day, once daily administration could be considered[4,23]
- in COPD, inhaled corticosteroids, e.g. **fluticasone** 1,000microgram/day, are recommended in conjunction with an inhaled LABA for patients with a predicted FEV_1 <50%, or when other approaches are inadequate (see Bronchodilators, Box B, p.109).[5]

Nebulizer solution
- **budesonide** 1–2mg b.d.; occasionally more or **fluticasone** 0.5–2mg b.d.
- use a mouthpiece to limit environmental contamination and/or contact with the patient's eyes. However, a mask may be unavoidable in those incapable of using a mouthpiece, e.g. when acutely ill, fatigued or very young.

Supply
Beclometasone (generic)
Dry powder inhalation 100microgram, 200microgram, 400microgram/metered inhalation, 28 days @ 200microgram (1 puff) b.d. = £6; brands include Pulvinal® Beclometasone and Easyhaler® Beclometasone.

Asmabec® (UCB)
Dry powder inhalation Clickhaler®, 100microgram, 250microgram/metered inhalation, 28 days @ 200microgram (2 puffs) b.d. = £6, 28 days @ 250microgram (1 puff) b.d. = £6.

Clenil Modulite® (Chiesi)
Aerosol inhalation (CFC-free) 50microgram, 100microgram, 200microgram, 250microgram/ metered inhalation, 28 days @ 200microgram (1 puff) b.d. = £4.50.

Qvar® (Teva)
Aerosol inhalation (CFC-free) 50microgram, 100microgram/metered inhalation, 28 days @ 100microgram (1 puff) b.d. = £5.

Breath-actuated aerosol inhalation (CFC-free) Autohaler®, 50microgram, 100microgram/ metered inhalation, 28 days @ 100microgram (1 puff) b.d. = £5.

Breath-actuated aerosol inhalation (CFC-free) Easi-Breathe®, 50microgram, 100microgram/metered inhalation, 28 days @ 100microgram (1 puff) b.d. = £5.
Qvar® is approximately twice as potent as Clenil Modulite®

Budesonide (generic)
Dry powder inhalation 100microgram, 200microgram, 400microgram/metered inhalation, 28 days @ 200microgram (1 puff) b.d. = £5; brands include Easyhaler® Budesonide.

Budelin Novolizer® (Meda)
Dry powder inhalation cartridges for use in refillable Novolizer® device, 200microgram, 28 days @ 200microgram (1 puff) b.d. = £6.

Pulmicort® (AstraZeneca)
Dry powder inhalation Turbohaler®, 100microgram, 200microgram, 400microgram/metered inhalation, 28 days @ 200microgram (1 puff) b.d. = £6.
Nebulizer solution (single-dose units) Respules®, 250microgram/mL, 20×2mL (500microgram) = £27; 500microgram/mL, 20 x 2mL (1,000microgram) = £40.

Fluticasone
Flixotide® (A&H)
Aerosol inhalation (CFC-free) Evohaler®, 50microgram, 125microgram, 250microgram/metered inhalation, 28 days @ 100microgram (2 puffs) b.d. = £6.
Dry powder inhalation blisters for use with Accuhaler® device, 50microgram, 100microgram, 250microgram, 500microgram/blister, 28 days @ 100microgram (1 blister) b.d. = £9.
Nebulizer solution (single-dose units) Nebules®, 250microgram/mL, 10×2mL (500microgram) = £10; 1mg/mL, 10×2mL (2mg) = £38.

Ciclesonide
Alvesco® (Takeda)
Aerosol inhalation (CFC-free) 80microgram, 160microgram/metered inhalation, 28 days @ 160microgram (1 puff) once daily = £9.

Mometasone
Asmanex® (MSD)
Dry powder inhalation Twisthaler®, 200microgram, 400microgram/metered inhalation, 28 days @ 200microgram (1 puff) once daily = £11.

For combination products containing inhaled corticosteroids and LABAs, see Inhaled long-acting β_2 agonists (LABAs, p.117).

1 MHRA (2008) Inhaled products that contain corticosteroids. *Drug Safety Update.* 1. www.mhra.gov.uk/safetyinformation
2 Tattersfield AE et al. (2004) Safety of inhaled corticosteroids. *Proceedings of the American Thoracic Society.* 1: 171–175.
3 DTB (2000) The use of inhaled corticosteroids in adults with asthma. *Drug and Therapeutics Bulletin.* 38: 5–8.
4 BTS/SIGN (2012) British Guideline on the Management of Asthma. A National Clinical Guideline. Revised edition January 2012. British Thoracic Society and Scottish Intercollegiate Guidelines Network. Available from: www.sign.ac.uk/pdf/sign101.pdf
5 NICE (2010) Chronic obstructive pulmonary disease: management of chronic obstructive pulmonary disease in adults in primary and secondary care. *Clinical Guideline.* CG101. www.nice.org.uk
6 Nannini LJ et al. (2012) Combined corticosteroid and long-acting beta(2)-agonist in one inhaler versus long-acting beta(2)-agonists for chronic obstructive pulmonary disease. *Cochrane Database of Systematic Reviews.* 9: CD006829.
7 NHLBI/WHO (2013) Global initiative for chronic obstructive lung disease. Global strategy for the diagnosis, management and prevention of chronic obstructive pulmonary disease. Available from: www.goldcopd.com
8 Barnes PJ (2013) Theophylline. *American Journal of Respiratory and Critical Care Medicine.* 188: 901–906.
9 Daley-Yates PT et al. (2001) Beclomethasone dipropionate: absolute bioavailability, pharmacokinetics and metabolism following intravenous, oral, intranasal and inhaled administration in man. *British Journal of Clinical Pharmacology.* 51: 400–409.
10 Harrison LI et al. (2002) Pharmacokinetics of beclomethasone 17-monopropionate from a beclomethasone dipropionate extrafine aerosol in adults with asthma. *European Journal of Clinical Pharmacology.* 58: 197–201.
11 Woodcock A et al. (2002) Modulite technology: pharmacodynamic and pharmacokinetic implications. *Respiratory Medicine.* 96 (Suppl D): S9–15.
12 Harrison TW and Tattersfield AE (2003) Plasma concentrations of fluticasone propionate and budesonide following inhalation from dry powder inhalers by healthy and asthmatic subjects. *Thorax.* 58: 258–260.
13 CHM (2006) High dose inhaled steroids: new advice on supply of steroid treatment cards. *Current Problems in Pharmacovigilance.* 31 (May): 5.
14 MHRA (2010) Inhaled and intranasal corticosteroids: risk of psychological and behavioural side effects. *Drug Safety Update.* 4. www.mhra.gov.uk/safetyinformation

15 Smeeth L et al. (2003) A population based case-control study of cataract and inhaled corticosteroids. British Journal of Ophthalmology. **87**: 1247–1251.

16 Carnahan M and Goldstein D (2000) Ocular complications of topical, peri-ocular, and systemic corticosteroids. Current Opinion in Ophthalmology. **11**: 478–483.

17 Suissa S et al. (2010) Inhaled corticosteroids and the risks of diabetes onset and progression. American Journal of Medicine. **123**: 1001–1006.

18 Loke YK et al. (2011) Risk of fractures with inhaled corticosteroids in COPD: systematic review and meta-analysis of randomised controlled trials and observational studies. Thorax. **66**: 699–708.

19 Crim C et al. (2009) Pneumonia risk in COPD patients receiving inhaled corticosteroids alone or in combination: TORCH study results. European Respiratory Journal. **34**: 641–647.

20 Suissa S et al. (2013) Inhaled corticosteroids in COPD and the risk of serious pneumonia. Thorax. **68**: 1029–1036.

21 Janson C et al. (2013) Pneumonia and pneumonia related mortality in patients with COPD treated with fixed combinations of inhaled corticosteroid and long acting beta2 agonist: observational matched cohort study (PATHOS). British Medical Journal. **346**: f3306.

22 McKeever T et al. (2013) Inhaled corticosteroids and the risk of pneumonia in people with asthma: a case-control study. Chest. **144**: 1788–1794.

23 Chisholm S et al. (1998) Once-daily budesonide in mild asthma. Respiratory Medicine. **92**: 421–425.

Updated February 2014

OXYGEN

Note. Publication of the British Thoracic Society Guideline for Home Oxygen (due 2014) is anticipated to impact significantly on this monograph.

Oxygen is used to correct hypoxaemia. It should not be used to relieve breathlessness per se unless the patient is hypoxic and other treatment options are ineffective.[1] It should be prescribed only after careful consideration, particularly if for home use.[2,3] Used inappropriately, oxygen can have serious effects, or even be fatal (see Cautions and Box A).[4]

Indications: Acute and chronic hypoxaemia; breathlessness unrelieved by other measures in, for example, severe COPD, pulmonary fibrosis, heart failure, or cancer.

Pharmacology

Oxygen is prescribed for hypoxaemic patients to increase alveolar oxygen tension and decrease the work of breathing necessary to maintain a given arterial oxygen tension. The appropriate concentration varies with the underlying condition and the dose is generally titrated to achieve normoxaemia/near normoxaemia which is associated with better outcomes than hyperoxaemia.[5]

Medical emergencies are an exception, e.g. anaphylaxis, carbon monoxide poisoning, cardiopulmonary resuscitation, sepsis, when high concentration oxygen should initially be used. Examples of established short- and long-term uses include severe exacerbation of asthma and selected patients with COPD (see Prescribing oxygen below).

Despite the widespread use of oxygen to relieve breathlessness per se, most of the available evidence does not support this.[6] One short-term study in cancer-related breathlessness suggests that oxygen is generally better than medical air in severe hypoxaemia (SpO$_2$ <90%)[7] However, short and long-term (7 days) studies in patients mainly with lesser degrees of hypoxaemia/normoxia have found no additional benefit from oxygen over that seen with medical air delivered by nasal prongs.[8–11] This suggests that a sensation of airflow is an important determinant of benefit.[12–16] Thus, these patients should be encouraged to test the benefit of a cool draught (open window or electric table or hand-held fan).[17]

Consequently, national guidelines now recommend that home oxygen should not be prescribed simply for the relief of breathlessness, unless the patient has hypoxaemia (SpO$_2$ ≤92%) and other treatment options are ineffective.[1] Because both medical air and oxygen at 2L/min have provided similar benefit in patients who are not hypoxaemic,[11] it could be argued that when other treatment options are ineffective, a therapeutic trial of medical air may be reasonable. However, in practice, piped oxygen may be more readily accessible and cheaper to use than medical air.

Ideally, patients should undergo a formal assessment, e.g. shuttle walk test, symptom scores/diaries, to examine the benefit of oxygen, e.g. on exercise capacity, breathlessness and quality of life.[3] The assessment should be tailored to the circumstances of each patient. As a minimum, a pulse oximeter will help identify those patients who are hypoxaemic at rest for whom it appears reasonable to give sufficient oxygen to achieve a SpO_2 of 94–98% (or 88–92% for those at risk of hypercapnic respiratory failure). A trial of oxygen therapy can be given for 10–15min and the impact on any breathlessness assessed. When oxygen is being used in hypoxaemic patients for purely palliative purposes (i.e. to improve breathlessness rather than impact on long-term survival), the degree of symptom relief rather than the SpO_2 should be used to help guide the dose of oxygen given. If benefit is obtained, review again after a longer period of use, e.g. 3–4 days. If the patient has persisted in using the oxygen and has found it useful, it can be continued but, if the patient has any doubts about its benefit, it should be stopped.[11]

High-flow oxygen therapy has been compared with non-invasive ventilation (NIV) in patients with cancer and acute respiratory failure due to complications of their disease, e.g. bronchial obstruction, lymphangitis.[18] Compared with high-flow oxygen, NIV provided greater relief of breathlessness and reduced opioid requirements, particularly in patients with hypercapnia. However, about 10% of patients were unable to tolerate NIV and the wider clinical relevance of these findings remain to be determined, particularly as NIV is a specialist intervention.[18]

When death is imminent, the findings of one study suggest that in the absence of respiratory distress, even when severe hypoxaemia is present, oxygen should not be routinely given.[19] Further, in 90% of those already receiving oxygen, it was possible to discontinue it without causing distress.[19]

Helium 79%-oxygen 21% mixture (Heliox®) is less dense and viscous than air.[20] Its use helps to reduce the respiratory work required to overcome upper airway obstruction.[21–23] It can be used as a temporary measure in patients breathless at rest while more definitive therapy is arranged. A high concentration non-rebreathing mask must be used for optimal benefit, and the patient's voice will be squeaky. Mixtures containing higher concentrations of oxygen are also available, e.g. **helium** 72%-oxygen 28%. This improves exercise capacity, oxygen saturation and breathlessness in patients with lung cancer.[24] However, this approach is expensive (each cylinder lasts only 2–3h) and limited by the practical difficulties of transporting a large cylinder. Nonetheless, there is interest in the use of **helium**-oxygen mixtures in various settings, e.g. acute exacerbations of asthma or COPD, or to improve exercise capacity in patients with COPD.[25–28] However, in a study of patients with COPD undergoing pulmonary rehabilitation, there was no overall benefit from breathing **helium**-oxygen (or supplemental oxygen) during exercise training.[29]

Cautions

Patients with hypercapnic respiratory failure who are dependent upon hypoxia for their respiratory drive, e.g. some patients with COPD, cystic fibrosis, neuromuscular disease, kyphoscoliosis or morbid obesity.

Patients should be advised of the fire risks of oxygen therapy:
• no smoking in the vicinity of the cylinder
• no open flames, including candles, matches and gas stoves
• keep away from sources of heat, e.g. radiators and direct sunlight.
Patients should notify the fire brigade and their home insurer that they have oxygen at home.

Undesirable effects

Patients who benefit from oxygen under the care of a home palliative care service report that the advantages outweigh the disadvantages.[30]

Equipment

In medical emergencies a high concentration reservoir (non-rebreathe) mask is used. In other circumstances, either constant or variable performance masks are used. Constant supply masks provide an almost constant supply of 28% oxygen over a wide range of oxygen supply (generally 4L/min) irrespective of the patient's breathing pattern. The flow rate should be adjusted for optimal patient comfort and symptom relief. *Constant supply masks should be used when an accurate delivery of oxygen is necessary, i.e. in patients at risk of hypercapnic respiratory failure.* With variable performance masks, the concentration of oxygen supplied to the patient varies with the rate of flow of the oxygen (2L/min is recommended and provides 24% oxygen) and with the patient's breathing pattern.

Box A   Undesirable effects of oxygen therapy[3]

Hypercapnic respiratory failure (see Cautions)
Psychological dependence:
- increased anxiety
- increased likelihood of excessive use
- excessive restriction of normal activities
- withdrawal difficult.

Apparatus restricts activities.

Oxygen mask may cause claustrophobia.

Nasal prongs may cause dryness and soreness of the nasal mucosa.

If necessary, humidification is noisy and not always effective.

Impaired communication.

Social stigmatization.

Cost.

Nasal cannulae permit talking, eating and drinking and are thus better suited to chronic use. However, they are the least accurate, with the concentration of oxygen delivered dependent on factors other than flow rate. At 2L/min, oxygen concentrations can vary from 24–35%.[31] High flow nasal oxygen delivery devices are now available which deliver humidified oxygen at 40–70L/min and are increasingly used outside of intensive care units.[32,33]

Oxygen can be provided via a cylinder (large and small for home or ambulatory use respectively), oxygen concentrator, or liquid oxygen system. It is more economical to use an oxygen concentrator for long-term oxygen therapy, and other situations where use is likely to exceed 3 cylinders/month. Modern concentrators are compact, quiet and cheap to run (2p per hour; reimbursed to the patient). If necessary, two concentrators can be linked by tubing and a Y-connector to deliver higher flow rates (6–8L/min). A 'back up' oxygen cylinder is provided to all patients using a concentrator.

Liquid oxygen systems make use of the fact that 1L of liquid oxygen produces 860L of gaseous oxygen. Relatively compact base units can provide home oxygen, or be used to fill portable units to provide ambulatory oxygen; these are lighter and last longer than a portable cylinder, e.g. about 8h vs. 2h at 2L/min. Liquid oxygen systems are the most expensive, but are quiet, and require no electric power; the base unit is refilled as required.

Oxygen-conserving devices significantly increase the duration of use of an oxygen cylinder or liquid oxygen system. These permit gas flow during inspiration only, generally either as a fixed volume per breath (pulsed devices), or as a variable volume according to the length of inspiration (demand devices).

Prescribing oxygen

Oxygen is generally poorly prescribed and monitored.[34] Ideally, there should be a specific oxygen prescription chart which includes details of:[35–37]
- target SpO_2 range
- name of delivery device
- flow rate/oxygen concentration
- duration of use
- method for monitoring to avoid under- or over-dosing of oxygen.

For domiciliary use, the home oxygen order form (HOOF) requires the prescriber to specify:
- number of hours per day that oxygen will be used
- whether nasal cannulae or a mask
- flow rate
- oxygen concentration (if using a mask)
- need for humidification.

Completion of a home oxygen record form (HORF) is also recommended to document initial and ongoing assessments. Generally, these will be required unless home oxygen is provided on a palliative basis.

Short-term/intermittent

Emergency oxygen therapy
This is primarily used to treat hypoxaemia resulting from acute illness, e.g. acute heart failure, pneumonia, pulmonary embolism and severe exacerbation of asthma. Specialty guidelines exist.[37] In brief, for patients not at risk of hypercapnic respiratory failure, initial oxygen therapy is via:
- preferably nasal cannulae at 2–6L/min *or*
- simple face mask at 5–10L/min *or*
- when SpO_2 <85%, a high concentration reservoir (non-rebreathe) mask at 15L/min.

Subsequently the delivery device and flow rate are adjusted to maintain the SpO_2 within a specified target range, typically 94–98%. Avoid flow rates <5L/min with a simple face mask because this may result in carbon dioxide rebreathing.

Greater caution is required in patients at risk of hypercapnic respiratory failure; oxygen treatment should commence using a 24% Venturi mask (2–4L/min) or 28% Venturi mask (4L/min) with a target SpO_2 of 88–92% pending urgent blood gas results:
- if $PaCO_2$ normal:
  - ▷ + no past history of hypercapnic respiratory failure requiring ventilation, adjust oxygen therapy to achieve SpO_2 target of 94–98%
  - ▷ + past history of hypercapnic respiratory failure requiring ventilation, maintain SpO_2 target of 88–92%
- if $PaCO_2$ raised, but pH ⩾7.35, maintain SpO_2 target of 88–92%
- for all of the above, recheck blood gases after 30–60min
- if at any time $PaCO_2$ raised and pH <7.35, consider non-invasive ventilation (seek experienced help urgently).

In the emergency setting, humidification is generally reserved for patients:
- with a tracheostomy or artificial airway
- with difficulty clearing viscous airway secretions (nebulized 0.9% saline is an alternative)
- needing high-flow oxygen >24h with upper airway discomfort because of dryness.

Humidification requires the use of an oxygen cylinder and cold nebulizer; *bubble bottles should not be used because they are ineffective and pose an infection risk.*

Short-burst oxygen therapy
This is no longer recommended in the absence of hypoxaemia. When the underlying cause is irreversible, patients should be assessed for long-term/continuous oxygen ± ambulatory oxygen as below.[1]

Short-term (intermittent) home oxygen therapy may be required for patients rendered temporarily hypoxaemic, e.g. as a result of a chest infection or episode of heart failure. These patients should also undergo a specialist assessment. For those likely to continue to experience recurrent episodes of hypoxaemia, an intermittent source of home oxygen, probably in the form of cylinders, may be appropriate.[1]

When death is imminent, if severe intractable breathlessness is present, oxygen may be used when hypoxaemia cannot be confirmed without discomfort to the patient (this should be rare given the wide availability of pulse oximeters).[1]

Previously, for exercise-induced breathlessness, some patients used oxygen before the exercise and others afterwards to aid recovery. However, in patients with COPD, most studies fail to show benefit from this strategy.[38]

Ambulatory oxygen
This can be prescribed in patients who fulfil the criteria for long-term oxygen therapy who are mobile and wish to leave the home (see below).

Ambulatory oxygen can also be considered for patients who are not hypoxaemic at rest but desaturate on exertion by at least 4% to a level <90%, and whose walking distance and/or breathlessness improves when using oxygen to keep SpO_2 >90% in a formal evaluation, e.g. shuttle walk test.[1,2,3,39]

In some patients, ambulatory oxygen fails to prevent significant desaturation on exertion. Failure varied with different delivery devices, but was as high as 20% and 40% of those with COPD and interstitial lung disease respectively.[40] This emphasizes the importance of individual assessment.

A breath-activated conserver can be added into ambulatory oxygen circuits using nasal cannulae to extend the life of the cylinder. However, conservers are unsuitable for patients who mouth breathe.

Long-term/continuous

Long-term oxygen ($\geqslant$15h/day) can be considered for use in patients with cancer or other life threatening diseases who are hypoxaemic (SpO_2 <92%).[1] More specifically with:

- COPD or cystic fibrosis with PaO_2 <7.3kPa or $\leqslant$8kPa with either secondary polycythaemia or nocturnal hypoxaemia (SaO_2 <90% for at least 30% of the night) or peripheral oedema or evidence of pulmonary hypertension
- interstitial lung disease and PaO_2 $\leqslant$8kPa
- pulmonary hypertension, without parenchymal lung involvement and PaO_2 $\leqslant$8kPa
- obstructive sleep apnoea who remain hypoxic during sleep despite nasal continuous positive airway pressure (CPAP)
- heart failure and PaO_2 <7.3kPa or nocturnal hypoxaemia
- neuromuscular or skeletal disorders causing inspiratory muscle weakness, either alone or in combination with ventilatory support.

The oxygen is used overnight, and for several hours during the day. Evidence of benefit from such use relates mainly to patients with COPD, where correction of severe hypoxaemia improves survival (especially at 20h/day use), breathlessness, quality of life and possibly cognitive function.[41,42] The precise mechanism for the improved survival is unknown, but possibilities include a reduction in pulmonary vascular resistance and the subsequent load on the right side of the heart.

When long-term oxygen is considered appropriate (if necessary, obtain advice from a specialist respiratory physician), a referral should be made to a specialist home oxygen service for further assessment, provision of long-term $\pm$ ambulatory oxygen and ongoing review. For example, in patients with COPD, blood gas tensions should be measured before treatment when the patient's condition has been stable for at least 5 weeks to ensure the criteria are met (see first bullet above). Supplemental oxygen is given for $\geqslant$30min to ensure a PaO_2 of >8kPa is achieved without an unacceptable rise in $PaCO_2$. Generally, these assessments should be detailed on the home oxygen record form (see Prescribing oxygen).

A full assessment is not always appropriate when home oxygen is purely palliative as part of end of life care.[1]

Travel by air

Patients with lung conditions and certain other comorbidities who wish to travel by air should be given specific advice (Box B).

In-flight oxygen provision

- generally airlines charge for providing in-flight oxygen (fees and services vary)
- passengers may carry their own small, full oxygen cylinders with them as hand luggage for medical use, provided they have airline approval; a charge may be made for this service, in addition to a charge for in-flight oxygen
- certain types of lightweight battery-operated portable oxygen concentrators may be permitted with airline approval; sufficient batteries are required to cover the flight and possible delays
- the airline must be informed at the time of the booking, and at least one month before the flight
- the airline will issue a Medical Information Form (MEDIF) to be completed by the patient and GP/hospital specialist; the airline's Medical Officer then evaluates the patient's needs; regular flyers can obtain a Frequent Travellers Medical Card from the airline which avoids the need to complete multiple forms
- in-flight oxygen is usually prescribed at a rate of 2–4L/min through nasal cannulae and has to be used in accordance with the airline's instructions
- pulsed dose (breath-actuated) systems are increasingly used by airlines; if there is concern over the patient's suitability for such a system, e.g. the patient is frail or has an irregular or shallow breathing pattern, a trial should be undertaken, and if necessary, an alternative system arranged with the airline.

For guidance on specific diseases, patients oxygen-dependent at sea level, those requiring ventilation, and infants and children, see the full guidance.[43]

Box B Fitness to undertake air travel in adults[43]

Air travel exacerbates hypoxaemia in patients with lung disease and may cause compensatory hyperventilation and tachycardia.

Aircraft cabins are pressurized, generally to reflect an altitude of about 8,000ft. This is equivalent to breathing a PO_2 of 15% instead of 21% at sea level. Even in the healthy, blood oxygen levels (PaO_2) will fall to between 8–10kPa (60–75mmHg; SpO_2 89–94%) or more during exercise or sleep.

Contra-indications to commercial air travel
- need for >4L/min of oxygen (at sea level)
- infectious tuberculosis
- pneumothorax
- major haemoptysis.

Evaluation
Undertake a clinical history and examination, ± simple spirometry, to determine if the patient is low or high risk.

Low risk
Patients who can walk 50m on the level at a steady pace without oxygen, breathlessness or needing to stop are unlikely to experience problems with reduced cabin pressure.

High risk
Referral for a more detailed assessment by a specialist respiratory physician is advised when any of the following are present:
- previous air travel intolerance with respiratory symptoms (breathlessness, chest pain, confusion or syncope)
- use of oxygen, continuous positive airway pressure or ventilator support
- severe COPD (FEV_1 <30% predicted) or asthma
- bullous lung disease
- severe (vital capacity <1L) restrictive disease (including chest wall and respiratory muscle disease), particularly with blood gas abnormalities
- cystic fibrosis
- co-morbidity worsened by hypoxaemia (cerebrovascular disease, cardiac disease, pulmonary hypertension)
- pulmonary tuberculosis
- <6 weeks since hospital discharge for acute respiratory illness
- recent pneumothorax (avoid flights for at least 7 days (spontaneous) or 14 days (traumatic) *after* full radiographic resolution)
- risk of VTE or previous VTE (avoid flights for ≥4 weeks, unless no residual symptoms and no hypoxaemia at rest or following exercise)
- other concerns regarding the patient's fitness to fly.

Further assessment can include the hypoxic challenge test where the patient breathes 15% oxygen at sea level for 20min to mimic air cabin conditions:
- if PaO_2 ≥6.6kPa (>50mmHg) or SpO_2 ≥85%, oxygen is not required
- if PaO_2 <6.6kPa (<50mmHg) or SpO_2 <85%, in-flight oxygen required at 2L/min via nasal cannulae.

For guidance on specific diseases, patients oxygen-dependent at sea level, those requiring ventilation and infants and children, see the full guidance.[43]

General advice
- *medical insurance*, travel with a European Health Insurance Card (if visiting a European Economic Area country) and ensure fully covered for medical costs that may arise related to the lung disease, including the cost of an air ambulance
- *documentation*, have a medical letter on their person detailing condition and medication
- *medication*, take a full supply of all medication as hand luggage, e.g. well-filled reliever and preventer inhalers (also see Appendix 2, p.819)

- *equipment,* e.g. portable battery-operated nebulizers may be used at the discretion of the cabin crew, but the airline must be notified in advance (an inhaler + spacer is an alternative)
- *ground transportation,* airports can usually provide transport assistance
- *DVT prophylaxis,* see LMWH, p.92.

Free booklets/fact sheets are also available from various patient organisations, e.g.:
- 'Going on Holiday with a Lung Condition', British Lung Foundation (Tel: 0845 850 5020, www.lunguk.org)
- 'Air travel for those affected by chest heart or stroke conditions' and 'Holiday Information', Chest Heart & Stroke Scotland Advice Line (Tel: 0845 077 6000, www.chss.org.uk).

Supply

Oxygen is classified as a General Sales List (GSL) product and therefore some companies will sell or rent cylinders privately if needed e.g. for travel outside the UK (see below) or as an emergency back-up supply in a care home.[44]

England and Wales

Any registered health professional can order home oxygen from regional suppliers using a home oxygen order form (HOOF). Patient consent, using the home oxygen consent form (HOCF), must also be obtained to allow their details to be passed on to the supplier and relevant authorities e.g. the fire service. The following types of oxygen treatment can be ordered:
- short-burst (intermittent) oxygen
- long-term oxygen; unless for palliative care, patients should be referred to the hospital home oxygen service for a full assessment
- ambulatory oxygen.

Standard delivery is generally within 3 days of receipt of order, during working hours. Other delivery services can also be specified but will incur a higher charge:
- urgent response (4-hour delivery)
- next day (clinical assessment services and hospital discharges only).

HOOFs and HOCFs can be downloaded from the NHS Primary Care Commissioning website www.pcc-cic.org.uk.

The completed HOOF should be faxed to the appropriate regional supplier (Table 1) which are available 24h a day, 7 days a week. Copies should be sent to the NHS regional/CCG home oxygen service contract lead or to the patient's GP if appropriate, and placed in the patient's notes.

A breath-activated conserver can be added into ambulatory oxygen circuits using nasal cannulae to extend the life of the cylinder. However, conservers are unsuitable for patients who mouth breathe.

Table 1 Regional suppliers of home oxygen in England and Wales[45]

Supplier	Region covered	Contact details
Air Liquide South	London East Midlands North West South West	Tel: 0808 143 9991 (9999 South West) Fax: 0800 781 4610 www.uk.airliquide.com/en/home-healthcare.html
Baywater Healthcare	Yorkshire & Humberside West Midlands Wales	Tel: 0800 373 580 Fax: 0800 214 709 www.baywater.co.uk
BOC Healthcare	East of England North East	Tel: 0800 136 603 Fax: 0800 169 9989 www.bochomeoxygen.co.uk
Dolby Vivisol	South East Coast South Central	Tel: 08443 814402 Fax: 0800 781 4610 www.dolbyvivisol.com/england

The supplier will ensure that the appropriate equipment is provided (cylinder or oxygen concentrator), contact the patient to arrange its delivery, installation and maintenance, payment of patient's electricity costs in relation to use of equipment supplied and train the patient in its use. The supplier will continue the service until a revised order is received, or until notified that the patient no longer requires home oxygen. For more information contact the relevant supplier (Table 1).

Scotland[46]

The Scottish Home Oxygen Order Form (SHOOF) should be completed and faxed to Health Facilities Scotland, who work in partnership with Dolby Vivisol to provide the equipment required and arrange installation in the patient's home. The ordering/prescribing of oxygen via the NHS must be by a specialist, generally a respiratory or paediatric consultant, who is specified by the local health authority.

For palliative care patients, each health board should have a local solution developed, e.g. access by palliative care teams to portable concentrators or facilities placed in local cottage hospitals. For further details including the national guidance document see the Health Facilities Scotland website www.hfs.scot.nhs.uk. Alternatively, contact them via Tel: 0131 275 6860; Fax: 0131 314 0724; e-mail: nss.oxycon@nhs.net.

Northern Ireland

Home oxygen is supplied via the Home Oxygen Service Contractor, BOC using the Northern Ireland Health and Social Care HOOF. The prescription form can only be signed by a qualified prescriber whose name is included on the Trust register of authorised oxygen prescribers held by BOC or by a qualified GP. In primary care, community pharmacy oxygen contractors may also be used by GPs to supply oxygen using a HS21 prescription. The type of equipment available from these two routes of supply varies. For further details, the HOOF and guidelines see the Home Oxygen Services section of the Business Services Organisation website www.hscbusiness.hscni.net. Alternatively, contact them via Tel: 02890 535613; Fax: 02890 535557.

Note: Community pharmacies that have a trained Community Pharmacy Palliative Care Network (CPPCN) pharmacist all provide oxygen.

Temporary supplies at other UK addresses

Patients travelling to other parts of the UK, e.g. for holidays, can obtain a temporary supply at the alternative address through reciprocal arrangements between the various UK authorities and oxygen suppliers. This is organized as a holiday order on a HOOF, including Scottish or Northern Irish residents.[46,47] Ideally, at least 2 weeks' notice should be given, but up to 4 weeks may be needed during peak holiday periods in popular tourist destinations or remote areas such as the Scottish Isles. Permission has to be obtained from the householder/hotel to allow oxygen onto the premises.

Patients travelling outside the UK (including the Isle of Man, the Channel Islands, and on cruises which start in the UK) need to arrange a private supply with their local oxygen supplier. Some specialist travel companies can help organize this. Their details can be obtained from the Chest Heart & Stroke Scotland Holiday Information fact sheet (see above).

1 Home Oxygen Service Assessment and Review (2011). NHS. Available from: http://system.improvement.nhs.uk/ ImprovementSystem/ViewDocument.aspx?path = Cancer%2fNational%2fNational%20Project%2fhome_oxygen_service_ assessment_and_review.pdf

2 Royal College of Physicians of London (1999) Domiciliary oxygen therapy services: clinical guidelines and advice for prescribers. Royal College of Physicians, London.

3 Booth S et al. (2004) The use of oxygen in the palliation of breathlessness. A report of the expert working group of the scientific committee of the association of palliative medicine. Respiratory Medicine. 98: 66–77.

4 Lamont T et al. (2010) Improving the safety of oxygen therapy in hospitals: summary of a safety report from the National Patient Safety Agency. British Medical Journal. 340: C187.

5 Blakeman TC (2013) Evidence for oxygen use in the hospitalized patient: is more really the enemy of good? Respiratory Care. 58: 1679–1693.

6 Johnson MJ et al. (2013) The evidence base for oxygen for chronic refractory breathlessness: issues, gaps, and a future work plan. Journal of Pain and Symptom Management. 45: 763–775.

7 Bruera E et al. (1993) Effects of oxygen on dyspnoea in hypoxaemic terminal cancer patients. Lancet. 342: 13–14.

8 Booth S et al. (1996) Does oxygen help dyspnea in patients with cancer? American Journal of Respiratory and Critical Care Medicine. 153: 1515–1518.

9   Bruera E et al. (2003) A randomized controlled trial of supplemental oxygen versus air in cancer patients with dyspnea. Palliative Medicine. **17**: 659–663.

10 Philip J et al. (2006) A randomized, double-blind, crossover trial of the effect of oxygen on dyspnea in patients with advanced cancer. Journal of Pain and Symptom Management. **32**: 541–550.

11 Abernethy AP et al. (2010) Effect of palliative oxygen versus room air in relief of breathlessness in patients with refractory dyspnoea: a double-blind, randomised controlled trial. Lancet. **376**: 784–793.

12 Schwartzstein R et al. (1987) Cold facial stimulation reduces breathlessness induced in normal subjects. American Review of Respiratory Disease. **136**: 58–61.

13 Burgess K and Whitelaw W (1988) Effects of nasal cold receptors on pattern of breathing. Journal of Applied Physiology. **64**: 371–376.

14 Freedman S (1988) Cold facial stimulation reduces breathlessness induced in normal subjects. American Review of Respiratory Diseases. **137**: 492–493.

15 Kerr D (1989) A bedside fan for terminal dyspnea. American Journal of Hospice Care. **89**: 22.

16 Liss H and Grant B (1988) The effect of nasal flow on breathlessness in patients with chronic obstructive pulmonary disease. American Review of Respiratory Disease. **137**: 1285–1288.

17 Galbraith S et al. (2010) Does the use of a handheld fan improve chronic dyspnea? A randomized, controlled, crossover trial. Journal of Pain and Symptom Management. **39**: 831–838.

18 Nava S et al. (2013) Palliative use of non-invasive ventilation in end-of-life patients with solid tumours: a randomised feasibility trial. Lancet Oncol. **14**: 219–227.

19 Campbell ML et al. (2013) Oxygen is nonbeneficial for most patients who are near death. Journal of Pain and Symptom Management. **45**: 517–523.

20 Boorstein J et al. (1989) Using helium-oxygen mixtures in the emergency management of acute upper airway obstruction. Annals of Emergency Medicine. **18**: 688–690.

21 Lu T-S et al. (1976) Helium-oxygen in treatment of upper airway obstruction. Anesthesiology. **45**: 678–680.

22 Rudow M et al. (1986) Helium-oxygen mixtures in airway obstruction due to thyroid carcinoma. Canadian Anaesthesiology Society Journal. **33**: 498–501.

23 Khanlou H and Eiger G (2001) Safety and efficacy of heliox as a treatment for upper airway obstruction due to radiation-induced laryngeal dysfunction. Heart and Lung. **30**: 146–147.

24 Ahmedzai SH et al. (2004) A double-blind, randomised, controlled Phase II trial of Heliox28 gas mixture in lung cancer patients with dyspnoea on exertion. British Journal of Cancer. **90**: 366–371.

25 Laude EA and Ahmedzai SH (2007) Oxygen and helium gas mixtures for dyspnoea. Current Opinion in Supportive and Palliative Care. **1**: 91–95.

26 Chiappa GR et al. (2009) Heliox improves oxygen delivery and utilization during dynamic exercise in patients with chronic obstructive pulmonary disease. American Journal of Respiratory and Critical Care Medicine. **179**: 1004–1010.

27 Hunt T et al. (2010) Heliox, dyspnoea and exercise in COPD. Eur Respir Rev. **19**: 30–38.

28 Eves ND et al. (2009) Helium-hyperoxia: a novel intervention to improve the benefits of pulmonary rehabilitation for patients with COPD. Chest. **135**: 609–618.

29 Scorsone D et al. (2010) Does a low-density gas mixture or oxygen supplementation improve exercise training in COPD? Chest. **138**: 1133–1139.

30 Jaturapatporn D et al. (2010) Patients' experience of oxygen therapy and dyspnea: a qualitative study in home palliative care. Supportive Care in Cancer. **18**: 765–770.

31 Bazuaye E et al. (1992) Variability of inspired oxygen concentration with nasal cannulas. Thorax. **47**: 609–611.

32 Ward JJ (2013) High-flow oxygen administration by nasal cannula for adult and perinatal patients. Respiratory Care. **58**: 98–122.

33 Epstein AS et al. (2011) Humidified high-flow nasal oxygen utilization in patients with cancer at Memorial Sloan-Kettering Cancer Center. Journal of Palliative Medicine. **14**: 835–839.

34 O'Driscoll R (2012) Emergency oxygen use. British Medical Journal. **345**: e6856.

35 Bateman NT and Leach RM (1998) ABC of oxygen. Acute oxygen therapy. British Medical Journal. **317**: 798–801.

36 Dodd ME et al. (2000) Audit of oxygen prescribing before and after the introduction of a prescription chart. British Medical Journal. **321**: 864–865.

37 O'Driscoll BR et al. (2008) BTS guideline for emergency oxygen use in adult patients. Thorax. **63** (Suppl 6): vi1–68.

38 Criner GJ (2013) Ambulatory home oxygen: what is the evidence for benefit, and who does it help? Respiratory Care. **58**: 48–64.

39 Bradley J et al. (2005) Short-term ambulatory oxygen for chronic obstructive pulmonary disease. Cochrane Database of Systematic Reviews. **4**: CD004356.

40 Marti S et al. (2013) Are oxygen-conserving devices effective for correcting exercise hypoxemia? Respiratory Care. **58**: 1606–1613.

41 NICE (2010) Chronic obstructive pulmonary disease: management of chronic obstructive pulmonary disease in adults in primary and secondary care. Clinical Guideline. CG101. www.nice.org.uk

42 Thakur N et al. (2010) COPD and cognitive impairment: the role of hypoxemia and oxygen therapy. Int J Chron Obstruct Pulmon Dis. **5**: 263–269.

43 BTS Air Travel Working Group (2011) Managing passengers with stable respiratory disease planning air travel: British Thoracic Society recommends. Available from:www.brit-thoracic.org.uk

44 UKMI (2013) Do oxygen cylinders need to be prescribed on an individual patient basis in residential nursing homes? . Medicines Q&A. **335.2** www.evidence.nhs.uk

45 NHSBSA Prescirption Services (2014) The January 2014 Electronic Drug Tariff. www.nhsbsa.nhs.uk/prescriptions

46 NHS Scotland (2012) Domicillary Oxygen Therapy National Guidance. National advisory group for respiratory managed clinical networks domiciliary oxygen therapy service National guidelines/best practice. www.hfs.scot.nhs.uk

47 Health and Social Care (2013) Oxygen Services. Business Services Organisation. www.hscbusiness.hscni.net

Updated June 2014

DRUGS FOR COUGH   BNF 3.7–3.9

General strategy

Coughing helps clear the central airways of foreign matter, secretions or pus and should generally be encouraged.[1] It is pathological when:

- ineffective, e.g. dry or unproductive
- it adversely affects sleep, rest, eating, or social activities
- it causes other symptoms such as muscle strain, rib fracture, vomiting, syncope, headache, or urinary incontinence.

The primary aim is to identify and treat the cause of the distressing cough but, when this is not possible or is inappropriate, an antitussive is generally indicated (Figure 1). There is a wide range of available antitussives (Box A) but few of these are in common use (for details of the latter, see Antitussives, p.142).

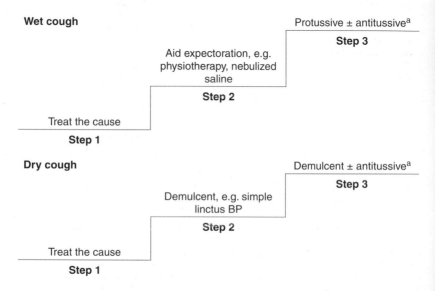

Figure 1   Treatment ladders for cough.

a. antitussives reduce the intensity and frequency of coughing; protussives make coughing more effective and less distressing.

Protussives (expectorants) make sputum less tenacious, and thus easier to expectorate. A wide range of protussives also exists (Box A). Generally, nebulized 0.9% saline is the protussive of choice but sometimes an irritant mucolytic (e.g. **guaifenesin**) or a chemical mucolytic (e.g. **carbocisteine**, p.140) may be preferable. Nebulized hypertonic 3–7% saline is used in cystic fibrosis and this is extending to other conditions, e.g. bronchiectasis (also see Chapter 23, p.753). Further specialist options are authorized for use in cystic fibrosis, e.g. **dornase alpha, mannitol**.

Generally, the evidence supporting the use of protussives or antitussives in acute or chronic cough is low-level.[5–8] However, recent advances in the understanding of cough and the mechanism of mucin production may lead to more targeted treatments.[9] For example, various transient receptor potential (TRP) receptors appear important in cough generation, and specific antagonists are being developed.[10] There is increasing interest in **menthol**, long used in OTC cough remedies, but now known to be a TRP melastin 8 receptor agonist.[11]

Box A   Examples of drugs for cough (modified from[2])

Protussives (expectorants)
Topical mucolytics
Nebulized saline (normal 09.%; hypertonic, e.g. 3–7%)
Chemical inhalations
    benzoin tincture, compound, BP (Friars' balsam)
    menthol and eucalyptus BP

Irritant mucolytics[a]
Ammonium chloride
Capsicum
Guaifenesin[b]
Ipecacuanha[b]
Potassium iodide

Chemical mucolytics
Acetylcysteine (not UK)
Carbocisteine
Erdosteine

Antitussives
Peripheral
Simple linctus BP
Benzonatate (not UK)
Levocloperastine (not UK)
Levodropizine (not UK)
Local anaesthetics (nebulized)
Mogusteine (not UK)
Sodium cromoglicate

Central
GABA agonists
    baclofen
    gabapentin
Opioids
    codeine[b]
    diamorphine
    dihydrocodeine
    hydrocodone (not UK)
    hydromorphone
    morphine
    methadone
Opioid derivatives
    dextromethorphan[b]
    pholcodine[b]

---

a. generally found as constituents in OTC cough products
b. restricted use in children;[3,4] also see Mucolytics (p.140) and Antitussives (p.142).

Sensitization of the cough reflex, resulting in cough hypersensitivity, appears important in chronic cough of various causes. Thus, there are parallels with neuropathic pain:
- paraesthesia ~ laryngeal paraesthesia, abnormal throat sensation or tickle
- hyperalgesia ~ hypertussia, increased cough sensitivity to known tussigens
- allodynia ~ allotussia, cough triggered by non-tussive stimuli, e.g. talking, cold air.[12]
This may see a greater use of drugs which target such sensitization either generally, e.g. **gabapentin** (p.270),[12] or more specifically, e.g. correction of iron deficiency.[13]

Further, some drugs are promising in specific circumstances, e.g. **thalidomide** (p.543) for cough associated with idiopathic pulmonary fibrosis.[14]

1 Twycross R et al. (2009) *Symptom Management in Advanced Cancer* (4e). palliativedrugs.com, Nottingham, pp. 160–166.
2 Homsi J et al. (2001) Important drugs for cough in advanced cancer. *Supportive Care in Cancer*. 9: 565–574.
3 MHRA (2010) Codeine-containing liquid over-the-counter medicines: should not be used for cough under 18 years. *Drug Safety Update*. 4(3): www.mhra.gov.uk/safetyinformation
4 MHRA (2009) Over-the-counter cough and cold medicines for children. *Drug Safety Update*. 2. www.mhra.gov.uk/safetyinformation
5 Smith SM et al. (2010) Over-the-counter (OTC) medications for acute cough in children and adults in ambulatory settings. *Cochrane Database of Systematic Reviews*. 9: CD001831.
6 Molassiotis M et al. (2010) Interventions for cough in cancer. *Cochrane Database of Systematic Reviews*. 9: CD007881.
7 Molassiotis A et al. (2010) Pharmacological and non-pharmacological interventions for cough in adults with respiratory and non-respiratory diseases: A systematic review of the literature. *Respiratory Medicine*.104: 934–944.
8 Wee B et al. (2012) Management of chronic cough in patients receiving palliative care: review of evidence and recommendations by a task group of the Association for Palliative Medicine of Great Britain and Ireland. *Palliative Medicine*. 26: 780–787.
9 Nadel JA (2013) Mucous hypersecretion and relationship to cough. *Pulmonary Pharmacology and Therapeutics*. 26: 510–513.
10 Grace MS et al. (2013) Pre-clinical studies in cough research: role of Transient Receptor Potential (TRP) channels. *Pulmonary Pharmacology and Therapeutics*. 26: 498–507.

11 Millqvist E *et al.* (2013) Inhalation of menthol reduces capsaicin cough sensitivity and influences inspiratory flows in chronic cough. *Respiratory Medicine.* **107**: 433–438.

12 Ryan NM *et al.* (2012) Gabapentin for refractory chronic cough: a randomised, double-blind, placebo-controlled trial. *Lancet.* **380**: 1583–1589.

13 Bucca C *et al.* (2012) Effect of iron supplementation in women with chronic cough and iron deficiency. *International Journal of Clinical Practice.* **66**: 1095–1100.

14 Horton MR *et al.* (2012) Thalidomide for the treatment of cough in idiopathic pulmonary fibrosis: a randomized trial. *Annals of Internal Medicine.* **157**: 398–406.

Updated March 2014

MUCOLYTICS   BNF 3.7

Class: Chemical mucolytic.

Indications: Reduction of sputum viscosity.

Contra-indications: Active peptic ulceration. **Erdosteine**: severe hepatic or renal impairment.

Pharmacology

Carbocisteine, **erdosteine** and **N-acetylcysteine** (not UK) are thiol compounds used as chemical mucolytics to facilitate expectoration. They reduce the viscosity of bronchial secretions by breaking links between mucin polymers. However, an anti-inflammatory effect is probably also relevant; this includes enhanced clearance of apoptotic neutrophils by alveolar macrophages (also see below).[1]

Erdosteine is only authorized up to 10 days use during an exacerbation of COPD. The long-term use of other mucolytics in COPD is controversial; they reduce the frequency of exacerbations and days of illness, but have no effect on hospitalization, lung function or quality of life.[2,3] UK guidelines recommend that they should be considered for patients with a chronic productive cough, and continued only when there is symptomatic benefit.[2] Other guidelines acknowledge that a few patients with viscous sputum benefit from mucolytics but consider the overall benefit too small to recommend widespread use.

Thiol compounds also have antioxidant, free-radical scavenging and anti-inflammatory properties. For example, IV **N-acetylcysteine** is well established in the treatment of **paracetamol** overdose when it is given to replenish glutathione, the antioxidant which neutralizes the highly reactive hepatotoxic metabolite N-acetyl-p-benzoquinoneimine (see p.299).

Although the clinical relevance remains to be determined, **N-acetylcysteine** has also shown benefit in various other conditions. These include idiopathic pulmonary fibrosis, systemic lupus erythematosis, neuropsychiatric disorders (e.g. drug addiction, Alzheimer's and Parkinson's diseases, autism, schizophrenia, depression and bipolar disorder), and animal models of ulcerative colitis.[4–6]

Benefit in such disparate neuropsychiatric disorders may be explained through a reduction in oxidative damage and inflammation. For example, in the CNS, toxic free radicals (i.e. reactive oxygen and nitrogen species) are generated as a result of neurotransmitter activity and mitochondrial metabolism, but are neutralized by antioxidants (mainly glutathione). In disease, various mechanisms increase oxidative stress to levels which overwhelm the relatively low levels of antioxidants in the CNS. The unchecked free-radicals cause damage, leading to cell dysfunction and ultimately apoptosis. **N-acetylcysteine**, in part by increasing glutathione levels, has several beneficial effects including:[6]

- decreased synaptic glutamate (thereby reducing the production of free radicals from NMDA-receptor-channel activation)
- increased neutralization of free radicals
- decreased mitochondrial dysfunction (thereby reducing the production of free radicals)
- decreased inflammation by reducing cytokine production, e.g. TNF-α and IL-6
- enhanced neurogenesis by increasing levels of neuroprotective and anti-apoptotic proteins.

Such neuroprotective effects of **N-acetylcysteine** are also evident in peripheral nerve injury, where its ability to protect against oxidative stress-related mitochondrial dysfunction appears key to preventing cell apoptosis.[7] However, any clinical role in this setting remains to be determined.

Carbocisteine, erdosteine and **N-acetylcysteine** are all metabolized in the liver and excreted in the urine as unchanged drug or metabolites. A dose reduction is advised for **erdosteine** in mild-moderate hepatic impairment.

Table I Pharmacokinetics of mucolytics

	Carbocisteine	Erdosteine	N-acetylcysteine
Bio-availability	<10%	No data	<10%
Peak plasma concentration	1–3h	1h; 1.5h (active metabolite)	0.5–1h
Plasma halflife	1.5–2.5h	1.5h	6.5h; increased by up to 80% in severe hepatic impairment

Cautions
History of peptic ulcer disease (mucolytics can disrupt the gastric mucosal barrier).
Erdosteine: limit dose to 300mg/24h in mild–moderate hepatic impairment.

Undesirable effects
Occasional dyspepsia, rash.
Rare (<0.1%, ≥0.001%): GI haemorrhage.

Dose and use
Carbocisteine
- start with 750mg t.d.s.
- reduce to 750mg b.d. once satisfactory response obtained, i.e. reduction in cough and sputum production.

Erdosteine
- 300mg b.d. for up to 10 days.

Supply
Carbocisteine (Sanofi-Aventis)
Capsules 375mg, 28 days @ 750mg t.d.s. = £27.
Oral liquid 125mg/5mL, 250mg/5mL, 28 days @ 750mg t.d.s. = £30; *cinnamon with rum flavour.*

Erdosteine
Erdotin® (Galen)
Capsules 300mg, 10 days @ 300mg b.d. = £6.

N-acetylcysteine
Capsules 600mg, 60 = £35. (Unauthorized, available to import via IDIS; see Appendix 1, p.817). Also available OTC from health food shops.

1 Inoue M et al. (2012) Carbocisteine promotes phagocytosis of apoptotic cells by alveolar macrophages. *European Journal of Pharmacology.* **677**: 173–179.
2 NICE (2010) Chronic obstructive pulmonary disease: management of chronic obstructive pulmonary disease in adults in primary and secondary care. *Clinical Guideline.* CG101. www.nice.org.uk
3 Poole P et al. (2012) Mucolytic agents for chronic bronchitis or chronic obstructive pulmonary disease. *Cochrane Database of Systematic Reviews.* **8**: CD001287.

4 Lai ZW et al. (2012) N-acetylcysteine reduces disease activity by blocking mammalian target of rapamycin in T cells from systemic lupus erythematosus patients: a randomized, double-blind, placebo-controlled trial. *Arthritis and Rheumatism.* **64**: 2937–2946.
5 Uraz S et al. (2013) N-acetylcysteine expresses powerful anti-inflammatory and antioxidant activities resulting in complete improvement of acetic acid-induced colitis in rats. *Scandinavian Journal of Clinical Laboratory Investigation.* **73**: 61–66.
6 Berk M et al. (2013) The promise of N-acetylcysteine in neuropsychiatry. *Trends in Pharmacological Sciences.* **34**: 167–177.
7 Terenghi G et al. (2011) The nerve injury and the dying neurons: diagnosis and prevention. *Journal of Hand Surgery, European Volume.* **36**: 730–734.

Updated March 2014

ANTITUSSIVES   BNF 3.9

Antitussives can be divided into peripherally-acting and centrally-acting agents. The former include local pharyngeal soothing agents (demulcents) and local anaesthetics and their derivatives.[1] Most centrally-acting antitussives are opioids or opioid derivatives. In palliative care, because the opioid antitussives are generally used in preference to local anaesthetics and other drugs they are given precedence in this section. Generally, the evidence supporting the use of antitussives in acute or chronic cough is low-level.[2–5]

Demulcents

These contain soothing substances such as syrup or **glycerol**. The high sugar content stimulates the production of saliva and soothes the oropharynx. The associated swallowing may also interfere with the cough reflex. The sweet taste itself may be antitussive by stimulating the release of endogenous opioids in the brain stem, and this may contribute to the large placebo effect seen in RCTs of demulcents.[6] Honey, a traditional remedy, presumably acts in the same way.

However, the antitussive effect of demulcents is generally short-lived and there is no evidence that combination products are better than **simple linctus BP** (5mL t.d.s.–q.d.s.). Thus, if **simple linctus BP** is ineffective, there is little point in trying combination products.

Opioids

Opioids act primarily by suppressing the cough reflex centre in the brain stem. Opioids appear less effective for cough due to upper airway disorders, e.g. upper respiratory tract infection, possibly because laryngeal cough involves opioid-insensitive central mechanisms and/or reflects a different reflex (i.e. an expiration reflex).[7]

Codeine, pholcodine and **dextromethorphan** are common ingredients in combination antitussive products but often in small and probably ineffective doses.[8] Thus, the benefit of combination products may reside mainly in the sugar content (see Demulcents above).[6] The MHRA has recently advised against the use of OTC cough products containing **codeine** for those under 18 years old, and **dextromethorphan** and **pholcodine** for those under 6 years old.[9,10]

For analgesia in palliative care, strong opioids are increasingly preferred over weak opioids. The same rationale can also be applied to cough (see Weak opioids, p.346).[5] For opioid-naïve patients, the initial dose is generally **morphine** 10–20mg/24h (see Drug treatment below). For those already receiving strong opioids, if a p.r.n. dose relieves the cough, continue to use it in this way or increase the regular dose. However, if no benefit is obtained from a p.r.n. dose, there is little point in further regular dose increments. Some patients with cough but no pain benefit from a bedtime dose of **morphine** to prevent cough disturbing sleep.

If a weak opioid is used, **codeine** is preferred to **pholcodine**, which has little analgesic effect. **Pholcodine** has been withdrawn in some countries because of concerns that it may cause IgE-sensitization to neuromuscular blocking agents;[11] however, the EMA concluded that the evidence for this is weak and that the risk:benefit ratio for **pholcodine** remains favourable.[12] If **codeine** or **hydrocodone** (not UK)[13] is ineffective, **morphine** should be prescribed. *If a patient is already receiving a strong opioid for pain relief it is a nonsense to prescribe* **codeine** *as well.*

Local anaesthetics

Nebulized local anaesthetics have been used as antitussives in patients with chronic cough and also cancer.[14-16] They probably act locally by inhibiting the sensory nerves in the airways involved in the cough reflex but there could be a central effect as well. Their use has not undergone evaluation in an RCT, and they should be considered only when other avenues have failed.

Typical doses are 5mL of either 2% **lidocaine** or 0.25% **bupivacaine** nebulized t.d.s.–q.d.s. In a case series of 100 patients with chronic cough given nebulized **lidocaine**, only about 20% considered their cough much improved and would definitely recommend it to other patients.[16] Undesirable effects include:

- unpleasant taste, irritation of the mouth or throat[16]
- oropharyngeal numbness → reduced gag/cough reflex; patients should be advised not to eat or drink for 1h after treatment to reduce risk of aspiration
- risk of bronchoconstriction → consider pretreatment with **salbutamol** in asthmatic patients[15]
- a short duration of action (10–30min).[8]

Even so, there are anecdotal reports of patients with chronic lung disease, sarcoidosis or cancer, in whom a single treatment with nebulized **lidocaine** 400mg relieved cough for 1–8 weeks.[17-19] Also see Chapter 23, p.753.

Benzonatate

Benzonatate (not UK) is chemically related to the **procaine** class of local anaesthetics. It acts peripherally by inhibiting the stretch receptors in the lower respiratory tract, lungs and pleura. It acts in 15–20min, and the effect lasts 3–8h. It is used PO at some centres in the USA when opioids such as **hydrocodone** fail to relieve a dry irritating cough, or if opioid antitussives are poorly tolerated.[20]

Management strategy
Correct the correctable

If possible, the cause of the cough should be treated specifically, e.g. antibacterials for infection. However, when the cause of the cough is not amenable to specific treatment or is unknown, measures should be taken to suppress the cough (see Drugs for cough, Figure 1, p.138).

Drug treatment

If a locally soothing demulcent (e.g. **simple linctus BP** 5mL t.d.s.–q.d.s.) is inadequate, consider a centrally-acting opioid antitussive (see also Opioids above):

- **codeine** (linctus or tablet) 15–30mg (5–10mL) t.d.s.–q.d.s.
- if not effective, switch to **morphine**, starting with:
  - ▷ an *immediate-release* formulation 5–10mg q.d.s.–q4h (but 2.5–5mg q.d.s.–q4h if not switching from **codeine**) or
  - ▷ a *modified-release* formulation 10–20mg b.d. (but 5–10mg b.d. if not switching from **codeine**)
- if necessary, increase the dose until the cough is relieved or until undesirable effects prevent further escalation (see p.372).

> If a patient is already receiving a strong opioid for pain relief it is a nonsense to prescribe **codeine** or a second strong opioid for cough suppression.

If opioid antitussives are unsatisfactory, other possible treatments include:

- **sodium cromoglicate** 10mg inhaled q.d.s. improves cough in patients with lung cancer within 36–48h[21]
- **gabapentin** 300mg PO t.d.s. increased up to 600mg PO t.d.s is more effective than placebo in idiopathic chronic cough (NNT 3.6 for a meaningful reduction in Leicester Cough Questionnaire score);[22] case reports have used smaller starting doses, e.g. 100mg PO b.d.[23]
- **diazepam** e.g. 5mg PO once daily/at bedtime is reported to have an effect in intractable cough associated with lung metastases[24]
- **baclofen** 10mg PO t.d.s. or 20mg PO once daily has an antitussive effect in healthy volunteers and in patients with ACE inhibitor cough; maximum effect is seen after 2–4 weeks.[1,25]

Baclofen, diazepam and **gabapentin** are all GABA agonists, with central inhibitory effects; they may act by interfering with the cough reflex and/or central sensitization which leads to cough hypersensitivity, present in most patients with chronic cough. **Baclofen** also inhibits relaxation of the lower oesophageal sphincter and thereby reduces gastro-oesophageal reflux, which is associated with chronic cough in some patients.[26]

Other, non-UK options include:

- **levodropropizine** 75mg PO t.d.s. (not UK) is as effective as **dihydrocodeine** 10mg PO t.d.s. in patients with lung cancer and causes less drowsiness[27]
- **benzonatate** 100mg PO t.d.s. (not UK); if necessary, increase to 200mg t.d.s.

Supply
Simple linctus BP
Oral syrup 28 days @ 5mL q.d.s. = £3.

Codeine linctus BP
Oral solution 15mg/5mL, 28 days @ 15mg q.d.s. = £4.50.
Also see **Codeine** (p.348) for other formulations.

All of the above products are available OTC.

Morphine sulfate
Oral solution 2mg/mL (10mg/5mL), 28 days @ 5mg q.d.s. = £5.
Also see **Morphine** (p.372) for other formulations.

Morphine solution is available in two strengths, 2mg/mL and a high potency concentrate of 20mg/mL supplied with a calibrated syringe. *Deaths have occurred from accidental overdose with the concentrated solution*, mostly when doses prescribed in *mg* were administered as *mL*, resulting in *20 times* the prescribed dose being given.[28]

1 Dicpinigaitis PV (2006) Current and future peripherally-acting antitussives. *Respiratory Physiology and Neurobiology.* 152: 356–362.
2 Molassiotis A et al. (2010) Pharmacological and non-pharmacological interventions for cough in adults with respiratory and non-respiratory diseases: A systematic review of the literature. *Respiratory Medicine.* 104: 934–944.
3 Molassiotis M et al. (2010) Interventions for cough in cancer. *Cochrane Database of Systematic Reviews.* 9: CD007881.
4 Smith SM et al. (2010) Over-the-counter (OTC) medications for acute cough in children and adults in ambulatory settings. *Cochrane Database of Systematic Reviews.* 9: CD001831.
5 Wee B et al. (2012) Management of chronic cough in patients receiving palliative care: review of evidence and recommendations by a task group of the Association for Palliative Medicine of Great Britain and Ireland. *Palliative Medicine.* 26: 780–787.
6 Eccles R (2006) Mechanisms of the placebo effect of sweet cough syrups. *Respiratory Physiology and Neurobiology.* 152: 340–348.
7 Eccles R (2006) Current and future centrally acting antitussives. *Respiratory Physiology and Neurobiology.* 152: 349–355.
8 Fuller R and Jackson D (1990) Physiology and treatment of cough. *Thorax.* 45: 425–430.
9 MHRA (2010) Codeine-containing liquid over-the-counter medicines: should not be used for cough under 18 years. *Drug Safety Update.* 4(3): www.mhra.gov.uk/safetyinformation
10 MHRA (2009) Over-the-counter cough and cold medicines for children. *Drug Safety Update.* 2: www.mhra.gov.uk/safetyinformation
11 Florvaag E and Johansson SG (2012) The pholcodine case. Cough medicines, IgE-sensitization, and anaphylaxis: A devious connection. *World Allergy Organ Journal.* 5: 73–78.
12 EMA (2011) Questions and answers on the review of the marketing authorisations for medicines containing pholcodine. Available from: www.ema.europa.eu
13 Homsi J et al. (2002) A phase II study of hydrocodone for cough in advanced cancer. *American Journal of Hospice and Palliative Care.* 19 (1): 49–56.
14 Truesdale K and Jurdi A (2013) Nebulized lidocaine in the treatment of intractable cough. *American Journal of Hospital Palliative Care.* 30: 587–589.
15 Slaton RM et al. (2013) Evidence for therapeutic uses of nebulized lidocaine in the treatment of intractable cough and asthma. *Annals of Pharmacotherapy.* 47: 578–585.
16 Lim KG et al. (2013) Long-term safety of nebulized lidocaine for adults with difficult-to-control chronic cough: a case series. *Chest.* 143: 1060–1065.
17 Howard P et al. (1977) Lignocaine aerosol and persistent cough. *British Journal of Diseases of the Chest.* 71: 19–24.
18 Stewart C and Coady T (1977) Suppression of intractable cough. *British Medical Journal.* 1: 1660–1661.
19 Sanders RV and Kirkpatrick MB (1984) Prolonged suppression of cough after inhalation of lidocaine in a patient with sarcoid. *Journal of the American Medical Association.* 252: 2456–2457.
20 Doona M and Walsh D (1998) Benzonatate for opioid-resistant cough in advanced cancer. *Palliative Medicine.* 12: 55–58.
21 Moroni M et al. (1996) Inhaled sodium cromoglycate to treat cough in advanced lung cancer patients. *British Journal of Cancer.* 74: 309–311.

22 Ryan NM *et al.* (2012) Gabapentin for refractory chronic cough: a randomised, double-blind, placebo-controlled trial. *Lancet.* **380**: 1583–1589.

23 Mintz S and Lee JK (2006) Gabapentin in the treatment of intractable idiopathic chronic cough: case reports. *American Journal of Medicine.* **119**: e13–15.

24 Estfan B and Walsh D (2008) The cough from hell: diazepam for intractable cough in a patient with renal cell carcinoma. *Journal of Pain and Symptom Management.* **36**: 553–558.

25 Dicpinigaitis P *et al.* (1998) Inhibition of capsaicin-induced cough by the gamma-aminobutyric acid agonist baclofen. *Journal of Clinical Pharmacology.* **38**: 364–367.

26 Lidums I *et al.* (2000) Control of transient lower esophageal sphincter relaxations and reflux by the GABA(B) agonist baclofen in normal subjects. *Gastroenterology.* **118**: 7–13.

27 Luporini G *et al.* (1998) Efficacy and safety of levodropropizine and dihydrocodeine on nonproductive cough in primary and metastatic lung cancer. *European Respiratory Journal.* **12**: 97–101.

28 FDA (2011) Medwatch safety alert. Morphine sulfate oral solution 100mg per 5mL (20mg/mL): medication use error - reports of accidental overdose. Available from: www.fda.gov/Safety/MedWatch/SafetyInformation

Updated March 2014

4: CENTRAL NERVOUS SYSTEM

PSYCHOTROPICS
BNF 4

Psychotropic drugs are primarily used to alter a patient's psychological state. Generally, smaller doses should be used in debilitated patients than in those who are physically fit, particularly if they are already receiving a strong opioid or another psychotropic drug.[1] Close supervision is essential, particularly during the first few days. Either a reduction in dose because of drug accumulation or a further increase because of a lack of response may be needed.

A few patients respond paradoxically when prescribed psychotropic drugs, e.g. **diazepam** (become more distressed) or **amitriptyline** (become wakeful and restless at night). Other patients derive little benefit from a benzodiazepine, but are helped by an antipsychotic, e.g. **haloperidol**. Tricyclic antidepressants (TCAs) are widely used to relieve neuropathic pain; dose escalation is often limited by undesirable effects.

Although prescribers will be influenced by local formularies and fashions, it is better to learn to use a small number of drugs well than to have limited experience with all possible alternatives.

---

1 Wagner B and O'Hara D (1997) Pharmacokinetics and pharmacodynamics of sedatives and analgesics in the treatment of agitated critically ill patients. *Clinical Pharmacokinetics.* **33**: 426–453.

Updated June 2014

BENZODIAZEPINES   BNF 4.1, 4.8, 10.2.2 & 15.1.4.1

Class: GABAmimetics, anxiolytic sedatives.

Benzodiazepines are useful in the management of various symptoms encountered in palliative care. Tolerance and dependence are unlikely to be a problem when used for ≤4 weeks. However, other undesirable effects include drowsiness, falls, and memory and cognitive impairment. Thus, appropriate caution and monitoring is required, particularly for those at greater risk, e.g. the elderly and frail patients.

Indications: Authorized indications vary between products; consult SPC for details; they include insomnia; anxiety and panic disorder; seizures; myoclonus; skeletal muscle spasm; alcohol withdrawal. Off-label indications include: †drug-induced movement disorders; †restless legs syndrome; †acute psychotic agitation; †terminal agitation; †neuropathic pain; †nausea and vomiting; †intractable pruritus; †intractable hiccup.

Contra-indications: Unless in the imminently dying: acute severe pulmonary insufficiency, untreated sleep apnoea syndrome, severe hepatic impairment, myasthenia gravis. Also see individual SPCs.

Pharmacology

GABA is the major inhibitory neurotransmitter of the nervous system. Several drug classes enhance its action (GABAmimetics):

- GABA$_A$ modulators: benzodiazepines, non-benzodiazepine hypnotics ('Z' drugs, e.g. **zopiclone**), barbiturates, some general anaesthetics (e.g. **propofol**), alcohol
- GABA$_B$ agonists: **baclofen**
- inhibitors of GABA transaminase (e.g. **vigabatrin**) or re-uptake (e.g. **tiagibine**).

The GABA$_A$ receptor is a chloride channel formed by 5 subunits comprising varying subtypes (Figure 1). GABA$_A$ modulators bind to sites distinct from GABA itself (allosteric modulation), increasing the receptor's affinity for GABA (benzodiazepines) or prolonging channel opening (barbiturates).[1] The α subunit of the GABA$_A$ receptor, of which there are six subtypes, is the predominant determinant of benzodiazepine affinity and function (Table 1). In an attempt to improve efficacy and/or tolerability, more selective α-modulators are under investigation, e.g. α2-selective non-sedating anxiolytics.[2]

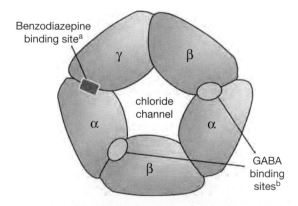

Figure 1 Structure of the GABA$_A$ receptor.

a. the binding sites for barbiturates, ethanol, neurosteroids and other allosteric modulators are less well characterized
b. the central chloride channel is opened by the concurrent binding of 2 GABA molecules.

Table 1 GABA$_A$ α-subunit subtypes and relative activity of selected GABAmimetics[2–7]

Alpha subunit subtype	1	2	3	4[a]	5	6[a]
Function	Sleep Anti-epilepsis[b]	Anxiolysis Anti-epilepsis[b]	Anti-epilepsis[b]	Anti-epilepsis[b]	Amnesia	
Clonazepam	++	++	++	−		−
Diazepam	++	++	++	−	++	−
Flunitrazepam	++	++	++	−	++	−
Midazolam	++		++	−	++	−
Zaleplon[c]	++	++/+	++/+		++/+	
Zolpidem[c]	++	++/+	++/+	−	−	−
Zopiclone	++	++	−/+[c]	−	+	−
Pentobarbital	++	++	++	++	++	
Ethanol[d]	+	+	+	++	+	

Activity: ++ high, + low, − negligible or none; blank = no data

a. benzodiazepines do not bind to α4- and α6-subunits, or to receptors lacking α and γ subunits (benzodiazepine-insensitive GABA$_A$ receptors)
b. relative importance of subunits varies with different seizure models
c. α subunit affinity varies with different β and γ subunit configurations. Prior to cloning, GABA$_A$ classifications encompassed more than one subunit configuration which may account for earlier conflicting affinity data
d. tonic α4(δ) mediated inhibition predominates at lower doses whereas synaptic (α1, 2 and 3) effects are responsible for severe intoxication. Ethanol also enhances release of GABA and GABAmimetic neurosteroids.

The sedative effects of benzodiazepines (and Z-drugs) probably result from the inhibition of the wakefulness-promoting system (see Melatonin, Figure 1, p.165).[8,9] Their anxiolytic effects result from α2-GABA$_A$ receptor agonism in the 'fear circuits' which are co-ordinated by the amygdala.[10]

Although GABA *antagonists* might be expected to improve wakefulness or memory, the use of non-selective GABA$_A$ antagonists is precluded by anxiogenic and pro-seizure properties. However, the memory-enhancing properties of α5-selective inverse agonists are being investigated.

Endogenous ligands for the benzodiazepine binding site include peptide and neurosteroid molecules, but their physiological function is not yet understood.

Most benzodiazepines are well absorbed, widely distributed and metabolized before being eliminated. Their receptor profiles are similar (Table 1) but their potency and halflives differ (Table 2). Their varied metabolic pathways affect their pharmacogenetic profiles and drug interactions (see individual SPCs for more details). **Lorazepam** is sometimes given SL, generally when a rapid onset of effect is required and/or the patient cannot reliably swallow tablets. However, ease of dissolution varies between brands (see p.162).

Cautions

Benzodiazepines with long halflives accumulate when given repeatedly and undesirable effects may manifest only after several days or weeks. Caution is required in mild-moderate hepatic impairment and renal impairment. Because their central depressant effect can depress respiration, caution is required in chronic respiratory disease.

Benzodiazepines can cause physical and psychological dependence. Patients with a history of substance abuse should be monitored closely. If long-term treatment is discontinued, taper gradually to avoid withdrawal symptoms, e.g. by one eighth of the daily dose every 2 weeks. Peak-trough variability can be sufficient to cause withdrawal symptoms when tapering short-acting benzodiazepines; consider switching to an alternative with a longer halflife.

Benzodiazepines are generally safer in overdose than barbiturates and tricyclic antidepressants. However, fatal iatrogenic overdoses of **midazolam** have occurred. Thus, regulators recommend that flumazenil is available for emergency use wherever midazolam is used clinically.[16]

Drug interactions

Most clinically relevant interactions arise from hepatic enzyme induction or inhibition or additive effects with other CNS depressants, e.g. alcohol, opioids.

Table 2 Pharmacokinetics of selected benzodiazepines and related drugs; PO unless stated otherwise[11–15]

Drug	Bio-availability PO (%)	Tmax (h)	Plasma halflife (h)	Metabolism
Alprazolam	$\geqslant 90^a$	1–2	12–15	CYP3A4
Clonazepam	>80	1–4	20–40	Multiple non-P450 pathways[b]
Clobazam	85	0.5–4	35; (80)[b]	CYP3A4[b]; metabolite inactivated by CYP2C19
Diazepam	>90	0.5–1.5	25–50; ($\leqslant$200)[b]	Multiple P450 pathways[b]
	65–85 (PR)	$\leqslant$0.5 (PR)		
Lorazepam	90	2.5	10–20	Non-P450 glucuronidation
		2.5 (SL)		
Midazolam	40	0.5–1	1–4[c]; (1)[b]	CYP3A4[b]
	95 (SC)	0.5 (SC)		
	85 (Buccal)	$\leqslant$0.5 (Buccal)		
Oxazepam	$\geqslant 90^a$	1–5	6–20	Non-P450 glucuronidation
Temazepam	$\geqslant 90^a$	1	8–15	Non-P450 glucuronidation
Zaleplon	30[d]	1.5	1	CYP3A4 and non-P450 oxidation
Zolpidem	70	1.5	2	CYP3A4 and CYP1A2
Zopiclone	75	1.5	3.5	CYP3A4[b]

a. estimated
b. active metabolite(s)
c. up to 24h when given by CIVI in critical care
d. well absorbed but undergoes extensive first pass hepatic metabolism.

The metabolism of many benzodiazepines is mostly CYP3A4 dependent (Table 2) and plasma concentrations may be decreased or increased to a clinically relevant degree by CYP3A4 inducers (e.g. **carbamazepine**) or inhibitors (e.g. **erythromycin**, protease inhibitors) respectively. For example, plasma levels of **midazolam** can be 8 times higher following the addition of a CYP3A4 inhibitor.[17]

Undesirable effects
Dose-dependent drowsiness, impaired psychomotor skills (e.g. impaired driving ability), fatigue, cognitive impairment, hypotonia (manifesting as unsteadiness/ataxia) with an increased (almost double) risk of femoral fracture in the elderly.[18]

Paradoxical arousal, agitation and aggression can occur in <10%; risk factors include high-trait anxiety, borderline personality disorder and alcohol misuse.[19–21]

Less commonly, complex actions while apparently asleep (e.g. driving, eating, cooking, conversations) occur both with benzodiazepines and Z drugs.[22]

The incidence of dementia is ~50% higher amongst users of benzodiazepines.[23] This may reflect their use for the prodromal sleep disturbance and anxiety which commonly precedes a diagnosis of dementia.[24,25] Neither a causal link nor a persistent risk beyond cessation of benzodiazepines has been established.

Dose and use
Insomnia
Initial treatment includes:
- correcting contributory factors if possible:
  - ▷ pain
  - ▷ delirium
  - ▷ depression
  - ▷ obstructive sleep apnoea
- non-drug measures.[26–29]

Where drug treatment is required, use a short-halflife benzodiazepine or a Z drug, ideally for < 4 weeks; their efficacy is comparable:
- **zopiclone** (halflife 3.5h) 7.5mg PO at bedtime (3.75mg initially if elderly or frail) *or*
- **temazepam** (halflife 8–15h) 10–20mg PO at bedtime *or*
- **midazolam** (halflife 1–4h) 2.5–5mg SC at bedtime, when PO route unavailable.

Indirect comparisons find fewer (mostly minor) undesirable effects with Z-drugs.[30] This may reflect their shorter halflives (except for **midazolam**). The clinical relevance of their greater α-subunit subtype selectivity (see above) is questionable because many undesirable effects are direct consequences of sedation.

A meta-analysis confirmed that, in people > 60 years of age, benzodiazepines and Z drugs had an NNT of 13 but an NNH of 6.[31] The undesirable effects were cognitive impairment, day-time drowsiness, ataxia and falls. Even low doses of short halflife benzodiazepines increase the risk of falls.[32] Alternatives include sedating antidepressants (e.g. **doxepin, mirtazapine, trazodone**, see p.200) and **melatonin** (see p.165).[33]

Anxiety and panic disorder

The efficacy of cognitive behavioral and drug therapy is comparable.[34] Drug treatment is tailored to the likely duration of use:
- benzodiazepine, if prognosis is < 2–4 weeks, e.g. **diazepam** 2–10mg at bedtime, **lorazepam** 0.5–1mg b.d.
- SSRI (± a benzodiazepine initially), if prognosis is > 2–4 weeks (see p.200).

Pregabalin (p.270) also acts quickly but it is generally reserved for patients not responding to antidepressants. Supporting trials are mostly confined to generalized anxiety disorder and response rates appear lower than for SSRIs and benzodiazepines.[35,36]

Depression

Benzodiazepines lack an antidepressant effect and are not routinely indicated in the management of depression.[37] However, their initial short-term use (< 4 weeks), in combination with a conventional antidepressant (see p.206), may be helpful when there is associated severe anxiety.

Acute psychotic agitation

Lorazepam is as effective as **haloperidol** 5mg every 30min in initially calming the patient:[38]
- **lorazepam** 2mg PO/IM every 30min until the patient is settled.

Terminal agitation

- start with **midazolam** 2.5–10mg SC p.r.n. and 10mg/24h CSCI
- if necessary, increase both the p.r.n. dose and CSCI until the patient is settled (commonly 10–60mg/24h CSCI, with ≤240mg/24h reported on occasion)
- however, if **midazolam** is poorly effective, or if > 30mg/24h needed, consider adding an antipsychotic (e.g. **haloperidol** or **levomepromazine**; see Chapter 16, p.672)
- if **midazolam** plus an antipsychotic are poorly effective despite titration, consider switching to **phenobarbital** or **propofol**.

Breathlessness

Benzodiazepines do not relieve breathlessness *per se*[39] but anxiolytics do have a role when *anxiety* exacerbates breathlessness. Either a benzodiazepine or an SSRI is used depending on prognosis (see above).

In the last days of life, for patients with distressing breathlessness at rest, the combined use of an opioid with a benzodiazepine is more effective than either alone.[40]

Seizures

Acute treatment[41]

Benzodiazepines are first line treatments for acute seizures, including status epilepticus:
- **lorazepam** 4mg IV over 2min *or*
- **midazolam** 10mg IV over 2min or SC/buccal; the injection can be given buccally in status epilepticus.

If necessary, repeat once after 10–20min.[42]

Particularly in children, buccal **midazolam** has mostly rendered the use of rectal **diazepam** obsolete.[43]

Chronic treatment
Long-term use is limited by the development of tolerance; thus benzodiazepines are used only for epilepsy refractory to other measures:
- start with **clonazepam** 500microgram–1mg PO at bedtime
- if necessary, increase by 500microgram every 3–5 days up to 2–4mg, occasionally more
- doses above 2mg can be divided, e.g. 2mg at bedtime and 1mg each morning.

End of life care
- **midazolam** 10mg SC p.r.n. *and* 20–30mg/24h CSCI.

Alternative SC/CSCI anti-epileptics include **phenobarbital** (p.286), **sodium valproate** (p.279) and **levetiracetam** (p.283).[44]

Myoclonus
Treat the underlying cause if possible:
- drug-related, e.g. opioids, **gabapentin** or **pregabalin**: consider dose reduction or switching to an alternative
- metabolic disturbance, e.g. hyponatraemia, uraemia.

Otherwise, a benzodiazepine should be used, e.g.:
- **clonazepam** 0.5mg PO at bedtime *or*
- **midazolam** 5mg SC stat and 10mg/24h CSCI in moribund patients.

If necessary, give as needed doses and consider increasing the regular dose.

Restless legs syndrome
Clonazepam (p.160) is an option for selected patients with restless legs syndrome when first-line options (e.g. **rotigotine**, **ropinirole**) are ineffective or inappropriate. **Gabapentin** and **pregabalin** are alternatives (see p.276). Iron supplementation may be effective in those with iron deficiency.[45,46]

Drug-induced movement disorders
Acute movement disorders. Reduce or stop the causal drug if possible. Otherwise, switch to an alternative with a lower risk of extrapyramidal reactions, e.g. **metoclopramide** → **domperidone**, **haloperidol** → **quetiapine**. If symptoms are causing distress, give an antimuscarinic, e.g. **procyclidine**; if latter ineffective or contra-indicated, RCTs indicate a *possible* role for benzodiazepines in acute akathisia and dystonia:
- **clonazepam** 0.5–1mg/24h PO, increased if necessary to 2.5mg/24h[47]*or*
- **diazepam** 5mg IV.[48]

Tardive dyskinesia. Reduce, stop or switch the causal drug as above and seek specialist advice. No symptomatic treatment has been found consistently effective. Small RCTs have found **clonazepam** (mean daily dose 5mg) of modest benefit.[49]

Neuropathic pain
Clonazepam is reported to improve both cancer-related and non-cancer neuropathic pain. Anti-hyperalgesic properties have been confirmed in healthy volunteers. Its anxiolytic and muscle-relaxant properties and the ability to administer it SC in some countries (not UK), has led to its use in selected palliative care patients despite the absence of supporting RCTs (see p.160).

Skeletal muscle spasm and spasticity
Benzodiazepines are used for the *short-term* management of pain due to skeletal muscle spasm, e.g. acute low back pain:[50]
- **diazepam** 2–5mg PO at bedtime and as required.

If the anticipated duration of use is ⩾3–4 weeks, to avoid problems associated with the long-term use of benzodiazepines (see Cautions), consider **baclofen** (p.593) as an alternative.

For the long-term management of spasticity secondary to neurological disorders, alternative skeletal muscle relaxants are also preferred, e.g. **baclofen**, **tizanidine** (see p.596).

Parenteral benzodiazepines, e.g. **midazolam** 10mg/24h CSCI, can be used to relieve muscle spasm or spasticity in the last days of life.

Nausea and vomiting
Benzodiazepines are effective for chemotherapy-related[51–53] and postoperative[54] nausea and vomiting:
- **lorazepam** 0.5mg SL p.r.n. *or*
- **midazolam** 10–20mg/24h CSCI.

Although a specific role for benzodiazepines in *anticipatory* nausea has been proposed, there is limited evidence to support this over and above their general anti-emetic effect. Alternative approaches to anticipatory nausea include relaxation, hypnosis and other psychological approaches.[55,56]

Alcohol withdrawal

Benzodiazepines reduce withdrawal symptoms, particularly seizures.[57] The choice is as for seizures (see above) with dose and route dependent on severity of withdrawal syndrome.[58,59]

Pruritus

Benzodiazepines are not consistently effective for pruritus; their role, if any, is limited to patients refractory to other measures (see Chapter 28, p.793).[60–62]

Hiccup

Midazolam is reported to improve hiccup refractory to various other approaches (see Prokinetics, Table 2, p.24), e.g. **metoclopramide, haloperidol, chlorpromazine, simeticone, baclofen**, alone or in combination.[63]

Switching between benzodiazepines

Dose conversion is not straightforward and switching is best avoided when possible. However, when necessary, use the dose equivalence table to provide a starting point (Table 3). Equivalent doses are always approximations, and appropriate caution and monitoring is required. Particularly when switching at a high dose, it is prudent to use, say, a 30–40% lower dose than predicted and to ensure that both flumazenil and additional benzodiazepine doses are available for p.r.n. use.

When converting from PO **diazepam** to SC **midazolam**, the dose should be halved (e.g. **diazepam** 5mg PO → **midazolam** 2.5mg SC).[64,65] However, PO, they are similar in potency because the bio-availability of **midazolam** is about half that of **diazepam** (Table 2).

Table 3 Approximate equivalent PO anxiolytic-sedative doses[66–69]

Drug	Dose (PO)
Alprazolam	0.25–5mg
Chlordiazepoxide	12.5mg
Clobazam	10mg
Clonazepam	250microgram
Diazepam	5mg
Lorazepam	500microgram
Midazolam	5mg
Nitrazepam	5mg
Oxazepam	10–15mg
Temazepam	10mg

1   Rudolph U and Mohler H (2006) GABA-based therapeutic approaches: GABA_A receptor subtype functions. *Current Opinion in Pharmacology.* **6**: 18–23.
2   Mohler H (2011) The rise of a new GABA pharmacology. *Neuropharmacology.* **60**: 1042–1049.
3   Graham D et al. (1996) Pharmacological profile of benzodiazepine site ligands with recombinant GABA_A receptor subtypes. *European Neuropsychopharmacology.* **6**: 119–125.
4   Pritchett DB et al. (1989) Type I and type II GABA_A-benzodiazepine receptors produced in transfected cells. *Science.* **245**: 1389–1392.
5   Smith AJ et al. (2001) Effect of alpha subunit on allosteric modulation of ion channel function in stably expressed human recombinant gamma-aminobutyric acid(A) receptors determined using (36)Cl ion flux. *Molecular Pharmacology.* **59**: 1108–1118.
6   Kumar S et al. (2009) The role of GABA(A) receptors in the acute and chronic effects of ethanol: a decade of progress. *Psychopharmacology (Berl).* **205**: 529–564.
7   Sanna E et al. (2002) Comparison of the effects of zaleplon, zolpidem, and triazolam at various GABA(A) receptor subtypes. *European Journal of Pharmacology.* **451**: 103–110.
8   Rihel J and Schier AF (2013) Sites of action of sleep and wake drugs: insights from model organisms. *Current Opinion Neurobiology.* **23**: 831–840.
9   Lazarus M et al. (2013) Role of the basal ganglia in the control of sleep and wakefulness. *Current Opinion in Neurobiology.* **23**: 780–785.
10 Dias BG et al. (2013) Towards new approaches to disorders of fear and anxiety. *Current Opinion in Neurobiology.* **23**: 346–352.
11 Riss J et al. (2008) Benzodiazepines in epilepsy: pharmacology and pharmacokinetics. *Acta Neurologica Scandinavica.* **118**: 69–86.
12 Drover DR (2004) Comparative pharmacokinetics and pharmacodynamics of short-acting hypnosedatives: zaleplon, zolpidem and zopiclone. *Clinical Pharmacokinetics.* **43**: 227–238.

13 Pecking M et al. (2002) Absolute bioavailability of midazolam after subcutaneous administration to healthy volunteers. British Journal of Clinical Pharmacology. **54**: 357–362.

14 Scott LJ et al. (2012) Oromucosal midazolam: a guide to its use in paediatric patients with prolonged acute convulsive seizures. CNS Drugs. **26**: 893–897.

15 Beigmohammadi MT et al. (2013) Pharmacokinetics Alterations of Midazolam Infusion versus Bolus Administration in Mechanically Ventilated Critically Ill Patients. Iranian Journal of Pharmaceutical Research. **12**: 483–488.

16 National Patient Safety Agency (2008) Reducing risk of overdose with midazolam injection in adults. Rapid Response Report **NPSA/2008/RRR011**. www.nrls.npsa.nhs.uk

17 Kotlinska-Lemieszek A (2013) Should Midazolam Drug-Drug Interactions be of Concern to Palliative Care Physicians? Drug Safety. **36**: 789–790.

18 Grad R (1995) Benzodiazepines for insomnia in community-dwelling elderly: a review of benefit and risk. Journal of Family Practice. **41**: 473–481.

19 Mancuso CE et al. (2004) Paradoxical reactions to benzodiazepines: literature review and treatment options. Pharmacotherapy. **24**: 1177–1185.

20 Weinbroum AA et al. (2001) The midazolam-induced paradox phenomenon is reversible by flumazenil. Epidemiology, patient characteristics and review of the literature. European Journal of Anaesthesiology. **18**: 789–797.

21 Saias T and Gallarda T (2008) Paradoxical aggressive reactions to benzodiazepine use: a review. Encephale. **34**: 330–336.

22 Dolder CR and Nelson MH (2008) Hypnosedative-induced complex behaviours : incidence, mechanisms and management. CNS Drugs. **22**: 1021–1036.

23 de Gage B (2012) Benzodiazepine use and risk of dementia: prospective population based study. British Medical Journal. **345**: e6231.

24 Bocti C (2012) Research paper most likely shows that benzodiazpeines are used to treat early symptoms of dementia. British Medical Journal. **345**: e7986.

25 Coyle-Gilchrist ITS (2012) Research paper does now show casual link between benzodiazepines use and diagnosis of dementia. British Medical Journal. **345**: e7984.

26 Morin CM et al. (1994) Nonpharmacological interventions for insomnia: a meta-analysis of treatment efficacy. American Journal of Psychiatry. **151**: 1172–1180.

27 Murtagh DR and Greenwood KM (1995) Identifying effective psychological treatments for insomnia: a meta-analysis. Journal of Consulting and Clinical Psychology. **63**: 79–89.

28 Smith MT et al. (2002) Comparative meta-analysis of pharmacotherapy and behavior therapy for persistent insomnia. American Journal of Psychiatry. **159**: 5–11.

29 Hugel H et al. (2004) The prevalence, key causes and management of insomnia in palliative care patients. Journal of Pain and Symptom Management. **27**: 316–321.

30 Buscemi N et al. (2007) The efficacy and safety of drug treatments for chronic insomnia in adults: a meta-analysis of RCTs. Journal of General Internal Medicine. **22**: 1335–1350.

31 Glass J et al. (2005) Sedative hypnotics in older people with insomnia: meta-analysis of risks and benefits. British Medical Journal. **331**: 1169.

32 Wang PS et al. (2001) Hazardous benzodiazepine regimens in the elderly: effects of half-life, dosage, and duration on risk of hip fracture. American Journal of Psychiatry. **158**: 892–898.

33 Wilson SJ et al. (2010) British Association for Psychopharmacology consensus statement on evidence-based treatment of insomnia, parasomnias and circadian rhythm disorders. Journal of Psychopharmacology. **24**: 1577–1601.

34 Bandelow B et al. (2007) Meta-analysis of randomized controlled comparisons of psychopharmacological and psychological treatments for anxiety disorders. World Journal of Biological Psychiatry. **8**: 175–187.

35 Baldwin DS et al. (2005) Evidence-based guidelines for the pharmacological treatment of anxiety disorders: recommendations from the British Association for Psychopharmacology. Journal of Psychopharmacology. **19**: 567–596.

36 Baldwin (2011) Efficacy of drug treatments for generalised anxiety disorder: systemic review and meta-analysis. British Medical Journal. **342**: 1199.

37 Furukawa TA et al. (2001) Antidepressant plus benzodiazepine for major depression. Cochrane Database Systematic Reviews. CD001026.

38 Foster S et al. (1997) Efficacy of lorazepam and haloperidol for rapid tranquilization in the psychiatric emergency room setting. International Clinical Psychopharmacology. **12**: 175–179.

39 Simon ST et al. (2010) Benzodiazepines for the relief of breathlessness in advanced malignant and non-malignant diseases in adults. Cochrane Database Systematic Reviews. CD007354.

40 Navigante AH et al. (2006) Midazolam as adjunct therapy to morphine in the alleviation of severe dyspnea perception in patients with advanced cancer. Journal of Pain and Symptom Management. **31**: 38–47.

41 Rey E et al. (1999) Pharmacokinetic optimization of benzodiazepines therapy for acute seizures. Focus on delivery routes. Clinical Pharmacokinetics. **36**: 409–424.

42 British National Formulary Section 4.8.2 Drugs used in status epilepticus. London: BMJ Group and Pharmaceutical Press www.bnf.org (accessed April 2014).

43 McIntyre J et al. (2005) Safety and efficacy of buccal midazolam versus rectal diazepam for emergency treatment of seizures in children: a randomised controlled trial. Lancet. **366**: 205–210.

44 Lopez-Saca JM et al. (2013) Repeated use of subcutaneous levetiracetam in a palliative care patient. Journal of Pain and Symptom Management. **45**: e7–8.

45 Aurora RN et al. (2012) The treatment of restless legs syndrome and periodic limb movement disorder in adults-an update for 2012: practice parameters with an evidence-based systematic review and meta-analyses: an American Academy of Sleep Medicine Clinical Practice Guideline. Sleep. **35**: 1039–1062.

46 Garcia-Borreguero D et al. (2012) European guidelines on management of restless legs syndrome: report of a joint task force by the European Federation of Neurological Societies, the European Neurological Society and the European Sleep Research Society. European Journal of Neurology. **19**: 1385–1396.

47 Lima AR et al. (2002) Benzodiazepines for neuroleptic-induced acute akathisia. Cochrane Database of Systematic Reviews. CD001950.

48 Gagrat D et al. (1978) Intravenous diazepam in the treatment of neuroleptic-induced acute dystonia and akathisia. American Journal of Psychiatry. **135**: 1232–1233.

49 Bhidayasiri R et al. (2013) Evidence-based guideline: treatment of tardive syndromes: report of the Guideline Development Subcommittee of the American Academy of Neurology. Neurology. **81**: 463–469.

50 Chou R and Huffman LH (2007) Medications for acute and chronic low back pain: a review of the evidence for an American Pain Society/American College of Physicians clinical practice guideline. *Annals of Internal Medicine*. **147**: 505–514.

51 Bishop J et al. (1984) Lorazepam: a randomized, double-blind, crossover study of a new antiemetic in patients receiving cytotoxic chemotherapy and prochlorperazine. *Journal of Clinical Oncology*. **2**: 691–695.

52 Razavi D et al. (1993) Prevention of adjustment disorders and anticipatory nausea secondary to adjuvant chemotherapy: a double-blind, placebo-controlled study assessing the usefulness of alprazolam. *Journal of Clinical Oncology*. **11**: 1384–1390.

53 Malik IA et al. (1995) Clinical efficacy of lorazepam in prophylaxis of anticipatory, acute, and delayed nausea and vomiting induced by high doses of cisplatin. A prospective randomized trial. *American Journal of Clinical Oncology*. **18**: 170–175.

54 Di Florio T and Goucke CR (1999) The effect of midazolam on persistent postoperative nausea and vomiting. *Anaesthesia and Intensive Care*. **27**: 38–40.

55 Mandala M et al. (2005) Midazolam for acute emesis refractory to dexamethasone and granisetron after highly emetogenic chemotherapy: a phase II study. *Supportive Care in Cancer*. **13**: 375–380.

56 Aapro MS et al. (2005) Anticipatory nausea and vomiting. *Supportive Care in Cancer*. **13**: 117–121.

57 Amato L et al. (2010) Benzodiazepines for alcohol withdrawal. *Cochrane Database of Systematic Reviews*. **3**: CD005063.

58 Peppers M (1996) Benzodiazepines for alcohol withdrawal in the elderly and in patients with liver disease. *Pharmacotherapy*. **16**: 49–57.

59 Chick J (1998) Review: benzodiazepines are more effective than neuroleptics in reducing delirium and seizures in alcohol withdrawal. *Evidence-Based Medicine*. **3**: 11.

60 Hagermark O (1973) Influence of antihistamines, sedatives, and aspirin on experimental itch. *Acta Dermato-Venereologica*. **53**: 363–368.

61 Muston HL et al. (1979) Differential effect of hypnotics and anxiolytics on itch and scratch. *Journal of Investigative Dermatology*. **72**: 283.

62 Ebata T et al. (1998) Effects of nitrazepam on nocturnal scratching in adults with atopic dermatitis: a double-blind placebo-controlled crossover study. *British Journal of Dermatology*. **138**: 631–634.

63 Moro C et al. (2005) Midazolam for long-term treatment of intractable hiccup. *Journal of Pain and Symptom Management*. **29**: 221–223.

64 Whitwam JG et al. (1983) Comparison of midazolam and diazepam in doses of comparable potency during gastroscopy. *British Journal of Anaesthesia*. **55**: 773–777.

65 Cole SG et al. (1983) Midazolam, a new more potent benzodiazepine, compared with diazepam: a randomized, double-blind study of preendoscopic sedatives. *Gastrointestinal Endoscopy*. **29**: 219–222.

66 British National Formulary Section 4.1 Hypnotics and anxiolytics. London: BMJ Group and Pharmaceutical Press www.bnf.org (accessed May 2014).

67 McEvoy GK *American Hospital Formulary Service* Maryland, USA: American Society of Health-System Pharmacists www.medicinescomplete.com (accessed March 2009).

68 Maudsley (2012) In: *The Maudsley Prescribing Guidelines in Psychiatry (11th edition)*. Wiley-Blackwell, pp. 307–308.

69 Bazire (2012) *Psychotropic Drug Directory*. 211.

Updated June 2014

DIAZEPAM   BNF 4.1, 4.8, 10.2.2 & 15.1.4.1

Class: Benzodiazepine.

Indications: Insomnia, anxiety and †panic disorder, acute psychotic agitation, refractory epilepsy, status epilepticus, myoclonus, skeletal muscle relaxant, alcohol withdrawal.

Contra-indications: Unless in the imminently dying: acute or severe pulmonary insufficiency, untreated sleep apnoea syndrome, severe hepatic impairment, myasthenia gravis.

Pharmacology

Diazepam is a typical benzodiazepine GABAmimetic (see p.148). In high doses, it induces hepatic metabolism. Standard parenteral products are oil-based or an oil-in-water emulsion, and absorption from muscle after IM injection is slower and more variable than after PO and PR administration. Diazepam has a long plasma halflife and several active metabolites, one of which has a plasma halflife of up to 120h in the elderly. Because of marked interindividual variation, the effects of a constant dose will vary greatly (see Chapter 25, p.767). Doses for individual patients are determined empirically.

Bio-availability > 90% PO; 65–85% PR.[1]

Onset of action 15min PO; 1–5min IV (oil-based formulation).[1]

Time to peak plasma concentration 30–90min PO; ≤30min PR (rectal solution); ≤15min IV (oil-based formulation); ≥15min IV (emulsion formulation); 1–1.5h IM (oil-based formulation), 2h IM (emulsion formulation).

Plasma halflife 25–50h; active metabolite nordiazepam ≤200h.

Duration of action 3–30h, situation dependent; may be only 15min–1h after a single IV dose.[1]

Cautions

Old age, debilitation, chronic respiratory disease, mild–moderate hepatic impairment, renal impairment. If given IV can cause hypotension and transient apnoea. Accumulation of active metabolites may necessitate a dose reduction after several days. History of alcohol or drug abuse.

Drug interactions

Diazepam is metabolized via the cytochrome P450 group of liver enzymes (see Chapter 25, p.767). Caution should be taken with concurrent use of drugs which are potent inhibitors of these enzymes, e.g. azoles, **cimetidine**, **erythromycin**, grapefruit juice, **omeprazole**, protease inhibitors, **valproate**; all inhibit the clearance of diazepam, which may result in an enhanced and more prolonged effect particularly in those who may be slow metabolizers.[2,3] Potent inducers e.g. **carbamazepine** and **rifampicin** may decrease diazepam levels.

Diazepam and **phenytoin** have unpredictable effects on each other's plasma concentrations. Diazepam may increase, decrease, or leave **phenytoin** plasma concentrations unchanged, whereas **phenytoin** can decrease the plasma concentration of diazepam. Monitor the **phenytoin** plasma concentration.[4]

Undesirable effects

Dose-dependent drowsiness, impaired psychomotor skills (e.g. impaired driving ability), daytime fatigue, cognitive impairment and hypotonia (manifesting as unsteadiness/ataxia), with an increased (almost double) risk of femoral fracture in the elderly. When given IV, the oil-based solution may cause painful thrombophlebitis.

Paradoxical arousal, agitation and aggression can occur in < 10% (see p.150).

Dose and use

Typical doses for diazepam are shown in Table 1. The initial dose will depend on the patient's age, general condition, previous use of diazepam and other benzodiazepines, the intensity of distress, and the urgency of relief. Generally, elderly and debilitated patients should be started on low doses.

Table 1   Dose recommendations for diazepam

Indication	Stat & p.r.n. doses	Common range
Anxiety[a]	2–10mg PO	2–20mg PO o.n.
Muscle spasm[b] }	2–5mg PO	2–10mg PO o.n.
Multifocal myoclonus		
Anti-epileptic[c,d]	10mg PR/IV	10–30mg o.n.
Acute akathisia or dystonia[d,e]	5mg IV	n/a

a. given as an adjunct to non-drug approaches, e.g. relaxation therapy and massage
b. if localized, consider injection of a trigger point with local anaesthetic or acupuncture
c. acute use but in the moribund can be used as a convenient substitute for long-term oral anti-epileptic therapy (also see Midazolam, p.157)
d. to reduce the risk of thrombophlebitis, inject IV diazepam slowly (rate not exceeding 5mg (1mL)/min) into a large vein, e.g. the antecubital vein and use emulsion formulation
e. only when an antimuscarinic, e.g. procyclidine, is ineffective or contra-indicated (see Chapter 26, p. 781).

Although the manufacturers of diazepam recommend giving it in divided doses, its long plasma halflife means that administration at bedtime will generally be equally effective, and easier for the patient. In an agitated moribund patient, b.d.–t.d.s. dosing is sometimes indicated so as to reduce the number of hours awake. Rectal diazepam is an alternative to buccal/SC midazolam in a crisis, or if the patient is moribund:
• rectal solution 5–10mg in 2.5mL
• suppositories 10mg (not UK)
• if the above are unavailable, the parenteral formulation can be administered with a blunt (needle-free) cannula.

Patients occasionally react paradoxically, i.e. become more distressed; if this happens, **haloperidol** (see p.177) or **olanzapine** (see p.183) should be given instead. **Midazolam** (see p.157), or **lorazepam** (*not* CSCI (see p.162)) are used if SC injections are necessary.

If using IV diazepam, the emulsion formulation is preferable because it is less irritant.

Supply

Diazepam (generic)
Tablets 2mg, 5mg, 10mg, 28 days @ 5mg at bedtime = £1.
Oral solution 2mg/5mL, 28 days @ 5mg at bedtime = £67.
Strong oral solution 5mg/5mL, 28 days @ 5mg at bedtime = £77.
Oral solution 10mg/5mL, 28 days @ 5mg at bedtime = £51 (Unauthorized product, available as a special order, see Appendix 1, p.817); *price based on specials tariff in community.*
Injection (oil-based solution) 5mg/mL, 2mL amp = £0.50; *excipients include ethanol and propylene glycol.*
Injection (emulsion) 5mg/mL, 2mL amp = £1.
Rectal solution 2mg/mL, 2.5mg or 5mg (1.25mL or 2.5mL tube) = £1; 4mg/mL, 10mg (2.5mL tube) = £2.

---

1 Mc Evoy GK. *American Hospital Formulary Service* Maryland, USA: American Society of Health-System Pharmacists www.medicinescomplete.com (accessed April 2014).
2 Klotz U and Reimann I (1980) Delayed clearance of diazepam due to cimetidine. *New England Journal of Medicine*. **302**: 1012–1014.
3 Wagner B and O'Hara D (1997) Pharmacokinetics and pharmacodynamics of sedatives and analgesics in the treatment of agitated critically ill patients. *Clinical Pharmacokinetics.* **33**: 426–453.
4 Baxter K and Preston CL. *Stockley's Drug Interactions.* London: Pharmaceutical Press www.medicinescomplete.com (accessed April 2014).

Updated June 2014

MIDAZOLAM   BNF 4.8.2 & 15.1.4.1

Class: Benzodiazepine.

Indications: Anaesthetic premedication/induction/maintenance agent, sedative for minor procedures, ICU sedation, †insomnia; †anxiety and panic disorder; †acute psychotic agitation; †terminal agitation;[1,2] †skeletal muscle relaxant; †status epilepticus (Buccolam® authorized for patients 3months–18years); †refractory epilepsy; †myoclonus; †nausea and vomiting,[3,4] †alcohol withdrawal, †intractable pruritus, †intractable hiccup.[5]

Contra-indications: Unless in the imminently dying: acute or severe pulmonary insufficiency, untreated sleep apnoea syndrome, severe hepatic impairment, myasthenia gravis.

Pharmacology

Midazolam is a short-acting, water-soluble benzodiazepine GABAmimetic. In single doses for sedation, midazolam is 3 times more potent than **diazepam**; as an anti-epileptic, it is twice as potent. With multiple doses, **diazepam** will gain in potency because of its prolonged plasma halflife, i.e. 24–120h versus 2–5h for midazolam. In the elderly, the plasma halflife of midazolam is prolonged up to 3 times and in some intensive care patients having CIVI for sedation, the plasma halflife may be prolonged up to 6 times. It also may be prolonged in hepatic impairment and heart failure. An active metabolite, α-hydroxymidazolam glucuronide, has a receptor affinity about one tenth that of midazolam. In severe renal impairment (creatinine clearance < 10mL/min) accumulation can result in prolonged sedation.[6] The main advantage of midazolam in palliative care is that it is water-soluble and is compatible with most of the drugs commonly given by CSCI. Intravenously, it does not cause thrombophlebitis, and can also be given by the buccal route as an alternative to SL **lorazepam**.[7]

When used in typical doses (see Table 2) in imminently dying patients, tolerance is not a practical problem. However, if much higher doses are used (e.g. > 10–15mg/h CSCI), then a lack of response may be seen if the dose is further escalated. This relates in part to the fact that at these doses, maximum GABA-ergic inhibition has been reached.[8]

For severe terminal breathlessness, the combination of regular **morphine** and midazolam appears more effective than either drug alone (see p.379).[9]

Benzodiazepines are not consistently effective for pruritus; their role, if any, is limited to patients refractory to other measures (see Chapter 28, p.797).

Bio-availability 95% SC; 85% buccal; 40% PO.

Onset of action 5–10min SC; 2–3min IV; 15min buccal.

Time to peak plasma concentration 30min SC; ≤30min buccal; 0.5-1h PO.

Plasma halflife 1-4h; ≤24h by CIVI in critical care.

Duration of action 5mg <4h, interindividual variation.[10]

Cautions

Fatalities from oversedation or cardiorespiratory depression have occurred after concurrent use with higher than approved doses of parenteral olanzapine (not UK) (see p.184).

Chronic respiratory disease, mild–moderate hepatic impairment, renal impairment, impaired cardiac function or low cardiac output, myasthenia gravis. If given IV can cause hypotension, reduced myocardial contractility and transient apnoea. History of alcohol or drug abuse.

Drug interactions

Midazolam is a substrate of CYP3A4 (see Chapter 25, p.767). Table 1 lists selected drugs which have clinically important drug interactions with midazolam.

Undesirable effects

Dose-dependent drowsiness, impaired psychomotor skills, daytime fatigue, cognitive impairment and hypotonia (manifesting as unsteadiness/ataxia), with an increased (almost double) risk of femoral fracture in the elderly. Paradoxical arousal, agitation and aggression can occur in < 10% (see p.150).

Dose and use

Many hospitals restrict the availability of high strength midazolam injection (2mg/mL or 5mg/mL) following fatal dose errors.[12]

Typical doses for midazolam are shown in Table 2. In practice, midazolam is mostly used in the terminal phase. If given IV rather than SC, smaller stat doses are generally used. The minimal interval between p.r.n. doses is typically 1h if SC, and 10–15min if IV.

An oromucosal solution for *buccal administration* is available (see Supply). Alternatively, the contents of an ampoule for injection can be used for *buccal administration*.

For CSCI dilute with WFI, 0.9% saline or 5% glucose.

CSCI compatibility with other drugs: There are 2-drug compatibility data for midazolam in WFI with **alfentanil, diamorphine, glycopyrronium, haloperidol, hydromorphone, hyoscine butylbromide, hyoscine hydrobromide, ketamine, levomepromazine, metoclopramide, morphine sulfate, octreotide** and **oxycodone**.
Concentration dependent *incompatibility* may occur with **cyclizine**. Midazolam is *incompatible* with **dexamethasone** and **ketorolac**. For more details and 3-drug compatibility data, see Appendix 3, (p.821).
  Compatibility charts for mixing drugs in 0.9% saline can be found in the extended appendix section of the on-line PCF on www.palliativedrugs.com

Table 1 Clinically significant cytochrome P450 interactions with midazolam resulting in changed drug plasma concentrations[11]

Midazolam plasma concentration	
Increased by	Decreased by
Aprepitant (initially, e.g. 3–5 days after starting the usual 3-day aprepitant course)[a,b]	Aprepitant (transient induction of midazolam metabolism may occur 3–5 days after the end of the usual 3-day aprepitant course)
Clarithromycin[a,c]	Carbamazepine
Diltiazem[a,d]	Phenytoin
Erythromycin[a,c]	Rifampicin
Fentanyl[e]	
Fluconazole[a,c]	
Grapefruit juice[a]	
Itraconazole[a,f]	
Nefazodone[b]	
Posaconazole[b]	
Propofol	
Protease inhibitors, e.g. lopinavir, saquinavir[a,g]	
Verapamil[a,d]	
Voriconazole[a,f]	

a. more pronounced with PO midazolam
b. monitor for excessive sedation and titrate midazolam dose accordingly (any route)
c. reduce PO midazolam dose by 50%; monitor patients on midazolam infusions for excessive sedation and titrate midazolam dose accordingly
d. reduce midazolam dose by 50% (any route)
e. reported to extend midazolam's halflife by 50%[11]
f. reduce PO midazolam dose by 75%; monitor patients on midazolam infusions for excessive sedation and titrate midazolam dose accordingly
g. avoid concurrent use with PO midazolam; reduce dose of midazolam infusion by 50%.

Table 2 Dose recommendations for SC midazolam

Indication	Stat & p.r.n. doses	Common range
Muscle tension/spasm } Multifocal myoclonus }	5mg SC	10–30mg/24h CSCI
Terminal agitation } Terminal breathlessness } Intractable hiccup }	2.5–10mg SC	10–60mg/24h CSCI[a]
Anti-epileptic	10mg IV/SC/buccal[b]	30–60mg/24h CSCI
Nausea and vomiting	2.5–5mg SC	10–20mg/24h CSCI
Insomnia	2.5–5mg SC at bedtime[c]	n/a

a. reported upper dose range 120mg for hiccup; 240mg for agitation
b. repeated after 10min if needed
c. only when the PO route is unavailable.

Nausea and vomiting

Benzodiazepines are effective for post-chemotherapeutic, postoperative, and possibly other causes of nausea and vomiting (see Benzodiazepines. p.152).

Status epilepticus

See Anti-epileptics, p.264.

Terminal agitation

Add an antipsychotic (e.g. **haloperidol**) before increasing above 30mg/24h (see Chapter 16, p.672).

Intractable hiccup

Generally limited to patients in whom persistent distressing hiccup is contributing to terminal restlessness at a time when sedation is acceptable to aid symptom relief.[5]

Supply

All products are Schedule 3 **CD**.

Midazolam (generic)
Injection 1mg/mL, 2mL amp, 5mL amp, 50mL vial = £0.50, £1 and £8 respectively; 2mg/mL, 5mL amp = £1; 5mg/mL, 2mL, 10mL amp = £1 and £2.50 respectively.

Buccolam® (Viropharma)
Oromucosal solution (prefilled oral syringe) 5mg/mL, 2.5mg, 5mg, 7.5mg and 10mg = £22.

Note: do not confuse Buccolam 5mg/mL with other *unauthorized* buccal liquids which are 10mg/mL (e.g. Epistatus®; Special products) and still available via special order (see Appendix 1, p.817).[13]

1 McNamara P et al. (1991) Use of midazolam in palliative care. *Palliative Medicine.* **5**: 244–249.
2 Bottomley DM and Hanks GW (1990) Subcutaneous midazolam infusion in palliative care. *Journal of Pain and Symptom Management.* **5**: 259–261.
3 Di Florio T and Goucke CR (1999) The effect of midazolam on persistent postoperative nausea and vomiting. *Anaesthesia and Intensive Care.* **27**: 38–40.
4 Mandala M et al. (2005) Midazolam for acute emesis refractory to dexamethasone and granisetron after highly emetogenic chemotherapy: a phase II study. *Supportive Care in Cancer.* **13**: 375–380.
5 Wilcock A and Twycross R (1996) Case report: midazolam for intractable hiccup. *Journal of Pain and Symptom Management.* **12**: 59–61.
6 Bauer T et al. (1995) Prolonged sedation due to accumulation of conjugated metabolites of midazolam. *Lancet.* **346**: 145–147.
7 McIntyre J et al. (2005) Safety and efficacy of buccal midazolam versus rectal diazepam for emergency treatment of seizures in children: a randomised controlled trial. *Lancet.* **366**: 205–210.
8 Cheng C et al. (2002) When midazolam fails. *Journal of Pain and Symptom Management.* **23**: 256–265.
9 Navigante AH et al. (2006) Midazolam as adjunct therapy to morphine in the alleviation of severe dyspnea perception in patients with advanced cancer. *Journal of Pain and Symptom Management.* **31**: 38–47.
10 Schwagmeier R et al. (1998) Midazolam pharmacokinetics following intravenous and buccal administration. *British Journal of Clinical Pharmacology.* **46**: 203–206.
11 Baxter K and Preston CL. *Stockley's Drug Interactions.* London: Pharmaceutical Press www.medicinescomplete.com (accessed March 2014).
12 DH (2013) Never events list for 2012/2013 www.gov.uk
13 MHRA (2011) Buccal midazolam (Buccolam): new authorised medicine for paediatric use—care needed when transferring from unlicensed formulations. *Drug Safety Update.* **5**. www.mhra.gov.uk/safetyinformation

Updated June 2014

CLONAZEPAM   BNF 4.8.1 & 4.8.2

Class: Benzodiazepine.

Indications: Refractory epilepsy, myoclonus, †acute akathisia, †acute dystonia, †anxiety and panic disorder,[1,2] †neuropathic pain; †restless legs syndrome.[3,4]

Contra-indications: Unless in the imminently dying: acute or severe pulmonary insufficiency, untreated sleep apnoea syndrome, severe hepatic impairment, myasthenia gravis.

Pharmacology
Clonazepam is a typical benzodiazepine GABAmimetic. It is extensively metabolized. Some metabolites are biologically active.
Bio-availability >80% PO.
Onset of action 20–60min PO; 5–10min SC.
Time to peak plasma concentration 1–4h.
Halflife 20–40h.
Duration of action 12h.

Cautions
Chronic respiratory disease, mild–moderate hepatic impairment, renal impairment, elderly or debilitated patients (may require dose reduction). Spinal or cerebellar ataxia. History of alcohol or drug abuse. Avoid abrupt withdrawal in epileptic patients (may precipitate status epilepticus). Anti-epileptic drugs are associated with suicidal thoughts or behaviour (see p.259).

Drug interactions
Clonazepam and **phenytoin** have unpredictable effects on each other's plasma concentrations, possibly because of changes in hepatic metabolism or in the volume of distribution. Clonazepam may increase, decrease, or leave **phenytoin** plasma concentrations unchanged, whereas **phenytoin** can decrease the plasma concentration of clonazepam. Monitor the **phenytoin** plasma concentration and adjust dose if necessary.[5]

Undesirable effects
Dose-dependent drowsiness, impaired psychomotor skills (e.g. impaired driving ability), daytime fatigue, cognitive impairment and hypotonia (manifesting as unsteadiness/ataxia), with an increased (almost double) risk of femoral fracture in the elderly. These effects can be minimized by starting with low doses at bedtime.
In children, clonazepam has been associated with salivary hypersecretion and drooling.

Dose and use
See Table 1. Because of the development of tolerance to its anti-epileptic effect, clonazepam is generally reserved for the treatment of refractory tonic-clonic or partial seizures.[1–3]

Table 1 Dose recommendations for clonazepam

Indication	Stat & p.r.n. doses	Common range
Epilepsy	1mg PO[a]	1mg[a] at bedtime–4mg/24h in divided doses PO, occasionally more
Acute akathisia[b] Acute dystonia[b] Myoclonus Neuropathic pain Panic disorder Restless legs	500microgram PO	500microgram at bedtime–4mg/24h in divided doses PO, occasionally more
Terminal agitation	500microgram SC[c]	2–8mg/24h CSCI[c,d]

a. because the elderly are more sensitive to central depressant effects, the manufacturer recommends a starting dose of 500microgram/24h for PO clonazepam in the elderly
b. only if an antimuscarinic, e.g. procyclidine, is ineffective or contra-indicated (see Chapter 26, p.781)
c. injection not available in the UK; for SC/IV bolus doses, dilute each 1mg/1mL amp with 1mL WFI
d. see text above about adsorption onto PVC tubing

Clonazepam is reported to improve both cancer-related and non-cancer neuropathic pain.[6-9] Anti-hyperalgesic properties have been confirmed in healthy volunteers.[10] Its anxiolytic and muscle-relaxant properties and the ability to administer it SC in some countries (not UK), has led to its use in selected palliative care patients despite the absence of supporting RCTs.[11]

In countries where a parenteral formulation is available, clonazepam can be administered by CSCI as an alternative to **midazolam** (see p.157). However, if the infusion tubing is made of PVC, up to 50% of the infused clonazepam is adsorbed onto the tubing.[12] Thus, if clonazepam is given by CSCI, non-PVC tubing should be used (e.g. IVAC®). Alternatively, because it has a long halflife, clonazepam can be administered as a bolus injection once daily, preferably at bedtime (see Chapter 20, Table 1, p.698).

Supply

Clonazepam (generic)
Tablets 500microgram, 2mg, 28 days @2mg once daily = £1.50.
Oral solution 500microgram/mL, 2mg/mL, 28 days @2mg once daily = £90; *contains ethanol and not suitable for children, do not further dilute with water.*
Injection (concentrate) 1mg/mL, 1mL amp and 1mL amp of solvent = £6 (unauthorized product, available to import via IDIS, see Appendix 1, p.817).

Rivotril® (Roche)
Tablets (scored) 500microgram, 2mg, 28 days @ 2mg once daily = £1.50.

1 Davidson J and Moroz G (1998) Pivotal studies of clonazepam in panic disorder. *Psychopharmacology Bulletin.* **34**: 169–174.
2 Wulsin L et al. (1999) Clonazepam treatment of panic disorder in patients with recurrent chest pain and normal coronary arteries. *International Journal of Psychiatry and Medicine.* **29**: 97–105.
3 Joy M (1997) Clonazepam: benzodiazepine therapy for the restless legs syndrome. *American Nephrology Nurses Association.* **24**: 686–689.
4 Vignatelli L et al. (2006) EFNS guidelines on management of restless legs syndrome and periodic limb movement disorder in sleep. *European Journal of Neurology.* **13**: 1049–1065.
5 Baxter K and Preston CL. *Stockley's Drug Interactions.* London: Pharmaceutical Press www.medicinescomplete.com (accessed March 2014).
6 Swerdlow M and Cundill J (1981) Anticonvulsant drugs used in the treatment of lancinating pain: a comparison. *Anaesthesia.* **36**: 1129–1132.
7 Bouckoms AJ and Litman RE (1985) Clonazepam in the treatment of neuralgic pain syndrome. *Psychosomatics.* **26**: 933–936.
8 Hugel H et al. (2003) Clonazepam as an adjuvant analgesic in patients with cancer-related neuropathic pain. *Journal of Pain and Symptom Management.* **26**: 1073–1074.
9 Bartusch S et al. (1996) Clonazepam for the treatment of lancinating phantom limb pain. *Clinical Journal of Pain.* **12**: 59–62.
10 Vuilleumier PH et al. (2013) Evaluation of anti-hyperalgesic and analgesic effects of two benzodiazepines in human experimental pain: a randomized placebo-controlled study. *PLoS One.* **8**: e43896.
11 Corrigan R et al. (2012) Clonazepam for neuropathic pain and fibromyalgia in adults. *Cochrane Database of Systematic Reviews.* **5**: CD009486.
12 Schneider JJ et al. (2006) Effect of tubing on loss of clonazepam administered by continuous subcutaneous infusion. *Journal of Pain and Symptom Management.* **31**: 563–567.

Updated June 2014

LORAZEPAM   BNF 4.1.2, 4.8.2 & 15.1.4.1

Class: Benzodiazepine.

Indications: Anxiety and †panic disorder; status epilepticus; †acute psychotic agitation; †alcohol withdrawal;[1] †myoclonus; †nausea and vomiting; †terminal agitation.

Contra-indications: Unless in the imminently dying: acute or severe pulmonary insufficiency, untreated sleep apnoea syndrome, severe hepatic impairment, myasthenia gravis.

Pharmacology

Lorazepam is a typical benzodiazepine GABAmimetic.[2] It is rapidly absorbed PO. Although the tablets are marketed for PO use, they are sometimes given SL, generally when a rapid onset of effect is required and/or the patient cannot reliably swallow tablets. However, although one pharmacokinetic study suggested more rapid absorption SL than PO, others have found no difference.[3–6] Thus, it is likely that the amount of lorazepam absorbed SL is variable and formulation-dependent (see Dose and use). The parenteral formulation can be used SL when the PO route is unavailable.

Despite being 85% protein-bound, lorazepam quickly reaches the CNS.[7] It is glucuronidated in the liver to an inactive compound and is excreted by the kidneys and in the bile (cytochrome P450 is *not* involved). The conjugated metabolite undergoes enterohepatic circulation. Duration of action does not correlate with plasma concentrations, and can be up to 3 days.

Bio-availability 90% PO.
Onset of action 5min SL; 10–15min PO.
Time to peak plasma concentration 2.5h SL, PO, IM.
Plasma halflife 10–20h.
Duration of action 6–72h.

Cautions

Fatalities from oversedation or cardiorespiratory depression have occurred after *concurrent use with higher than approved doses of parenteral* **olanzapine** (not UK) (see p.183).

History of alcohol or drug abuse, renal impairment, mild–moderate hepatic impairment, chronic lung disease, e.g. COPD.

Elderly and debilitated patients are more susceptible to the central depressant effects of lorazepam, e.g. on respiration, and generally require lower doses than those recommended for adults in the SPC.

Although it has been used successfully as a sole agent in acute psychotic agitation (mania),[8,9] lorazepam should not be used alone in an agitated delirium because it is likely to exacerbate the condition.[10,11] May unmask or worsen pre-existing depression.

Drug interactions

The metabolism of lorazepam is inhibited by **valproate**.[12] **Rifampicin** may decrease lorazepam levels.[13]

Undesirable effects

Dose-dependent drowsiness, impaired psychomotor skills (e.g. impaired driving ability), fatigue, cognitive impairment and hypotonia (manifesting as unsteadiness/ataxia), with an increased (almost double) risk of femoral fracture in the elderly. Paradoxical arousal, agitation and aggression can occur in < 10% (see Benzodiazepines, p.150).

Dose and use

Lorazepam can be given SL, PO, PR, SC, IM, or IV. If given by CSCI, there is a risk of precipitation.[14] Accidental intra-arterial administration or extravasation close to an artery has been associated with thrombosis and gangrene. *For IM injection, dilute with an equal volume of WFI or 0.9% saline and administer deep into muscle mass.*

SL administration

In some countries, specific SL tablets are available, *but not in the UK*. Thus, in the UK, proprietary tablets which dissolve more easily should be used SL, e.g. the generic tablets made by Genus, and the manufacturer's name should be stipulated on the prescription to ensure this.

Tablets will not dissolve SL in the absence of saliva. In patients with a dry mouth, the tablet should be dissolved in a few drops of warm water, drawn up in a 1mL oral syringe and put between the patient's cheek and gum (i.e. given buccally).[15] Alternatively, lorazepam injection can be used SL.

Buccal **midazolam**, available in prefilled buccal syringes (see p.157), may be a preferable alternative when a rapid onset of action is required but lorazepam injection formulation is impractical, e.g. in the domiciliary setting (see Chapter 17, p.681). However, it is significantly more expensive.

Acute treatment of seizures

Benzodiazepines are first line treatments for acute seizures, including Status epilepticus (see Antiepileptics, p.264).
- 4mg IV over 2min.

Anxiety and panic disorder

For short-term relief of severe anxiety (see Benzodiazepines, p.151):
- 0.5–1mg SL/PO stat and b.d.
- if necessary, increase to 2–6mg/24h.[16]

Consider starting an antidepressant concurrently if prognosis >2–4 weeks (see Antidepressants, p.200).

Acute psychotic agitation

Use with **haloperidol** or **risperidone** to control psychotic agitation,[17] although some centres use lorazepam alone:[8,9]
- give 2mg PO every 30min until the patient is settled.[8]

Terminal agitation

Used at some centres instead of **midazolam**.[14,18] Generally use with an antipsychotic (see Chapter 16, p.673):
- 1–4mg IV stat
- 4–20mg/24h CIVI or 1–2mg SC q6–8h.

Nausea and vomiting

Benzodiazepines are effective for chemotherapy-related, postoperative, and possibly other causes of nausea and vomiting (see Benzodiazepines, p.152):
- 0.5mg SL p.r.n.

Supply

Lorazepam (generic)
Tablets 1mg, 2.5mg, 28 days @ 1mg b.d. = £6; *tablets manufactured by Genus are scored.*
Injection 4mg/mL, 1mL amp = £0.50.

1 Peppers M (1996) Benzodiazepines for alcohol withdrawal in the elderly and in patients with liver disease. *Pharmacotherapy.* **16**: 49–57.
2 Ziemann U et al. (1996) The effect of lorazepam on the motor cortical excitability in man. *Experimental Brain Research.* **109**: 127–135.
3 Caille G et al. (1983) Pharmacokinetics of two lorazepam formulations, oral and sublingual, after multiple doses. *Biopharmaceutics and Drug Disposition.* **4**: 31–42.
4 Greenblatt DJ et al. (1982) Pharmacokinetic comparison of sublingual lorazepam with intravenous, intramuscular, and oral lorazepam. *Journal of Pharmaceutical Sciences.* **71**: 248–252.
5 Spenard J et al. (1988) Placebo-controlled comparative study of the anxiolytic activity and of the pharmacokinetics of oral and sublingual lorazepam in generalized anxiety. *Biopharmaceutics and Drug Disposition.* **9**: 457–464.
6 Gram-Hansen P and Schultz A (1988) Plasma concentrations following oral and sublingual administration of lorazepam. *International Journal of Clinical Pharmacology Therapy and Toxicology.* **26**: 323–324.
7 Wagner B and O'Hara D (1997) Pharmacokinetics and pharmacodynamics of sedatives and analgesics in the treatment of agitated critically ill patients. *Clinical Pharmacokinetics.* **33**: 426–453.
8 Foster S et al. (1997) Efficacy of lorazepam and haloperidol for rapid tranquilization in the psychiatric emergency room setting. *International Clinical Psychopharmacology.* **12**: 175–179.
9 Lenox R et al. (1992) Adjunctive treatment of manic agitation with lorazepam versus haloperidol: a double-blind study. *Journal of Clinical Psychiatry.* **53**: 47–52.
10 Breitbart W et al. (1996) A double-blind trial of haloperidol, chlorpromazine, and lorazepam in the treatment of delirium in hospitalized AIDS patients. *American Journal of Psychiatry.* **153**: 231–237.
11 Salzman C et al. (1991) Parenteral lorazepam versus parenteral haloperidol for the control of psychotic disruptive behavior. *Journal of Clinical Psychiatry.* **52**: 177–180.
12 Samara E et al. (1997) Effect of valproate on the pharmacokinetics and pharmacodynamics of lorazepam. *Journal of Clinical Pharmacology.* **37**: 442–450.
13 Bachmann KA and Jauregui L (1993) Use of single sample clearance estimates of cytochrome P450 substrates to characterize human hepatic CYP status in vivo. *Xenobiotica.* **23**: 307–315.
14 McCollam J et al. (1999) Continuous infusions of lorazepam, midazolam and propofol for sedation of the critically ill surgery trauma patient: a prospective, randomized comparison. *Critical Care Medicine.* **27**: 2454–2458.
15 Nicholson A (2007) Lorazepam. In: *Bulletin board.* Palliativedrugs.com Ltd. Available from: www.palliativedrugs.org
16 MacLaren R et al. (2000) A prospective evaluation of empiric versus protocol-based sedation and analgesia. *Pharmacotherapy.* **20**: 662–672.

17 Currier G and Simpson G (2001) Risperidone liquid concentrate and oral lorazepam versus intramuscular haloperidol and intramuscular lorazepam for treatment of psychotic agitation. *Journal of Clinical Psychiatry.* **62**: 153–157.
18 Fainsinger R et al. (2000) Sedation for delirium and other symptoms in terminally ill patients in Edmonton. *Journal of Palliative Care.* **16 (2)**: 5–10.

Updated June 2014

MELATONIN   BNF 4.1.1

Class: Melatonin-receptor agonist.

Indications: Primary insomnia in adults > 55yrs, †secondary insomnia, †sleep phase disorders.

Pharmacology

Melatonin acts predominantly on the suprachiasmatic nucleus, the circadian pacemaker in the hypothalamus (Figure 1). The circadian sleep-wake cycle is modified by:

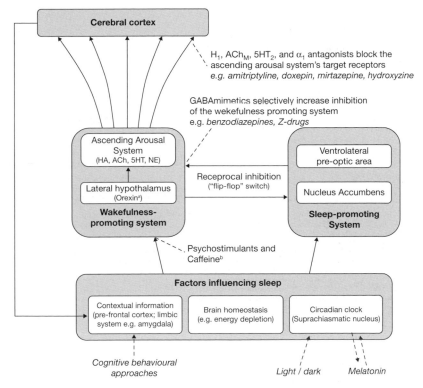

Figure 1   Putative targets of drugs influencing sleep and wakefulness.[4–7]

a. orexinergic neurons of the lateral hypothalamus stimulate the ascending activating system. They are lost in narcolepsy. Orexin receptor antagonists are currently in phase 3 RCTs for insomnia
b. the wakefulness promoting system is activated by dopamine and inhibited by adenosine. Thus both adenosine antagonists (e.g. caffeine) and dopamimetics (e.g. methylphenidate and modafinil, see p.224), have wakefulness-promoting properties.

- light (via the retinohypothalamic pathway)
- melatonin acting upon
  ▷ MT_1 receptors (suppresses wakefulness-promoting activity)
  ▷ MT_2 receptors (affects onset of sleep phase).

Melatonin is produced by the pineal gland during darkness, itself controlled by the suprachiasmatic nucleus to form a feedback loop. Its other actions include immunomodulation[1,2] and a beneficial effect on cancer survival.[3] The function of MT_3, a **quinine** reductase, is uncertain.

Oral bio-availability is limited by extensive first pass hepatic metabolism. It is 60% protein bound and is metabolised by CYP1A1 and 1A2 to an inactive sulphatoxy metabolite, which is renally excreted.

Primary insomnia

Melatonin 2mg m/r (Circadin®) has been evaluated in adults aged > 55 years using sleep diaries. The NNT for improvements of ⩾1/10 in both quality of sleep and behaviour the following morning is 5 to 9 (and NNH for any adverse event ⩾33).[8,9] The NNT for any subjective improvement in sleep quality in older adults with benzodiazepines and related hypnotics is 13 (and NNH for any adverse event 6).[10]

However, a meta-analysis of trials using objective measures of insomnia (polysomnography or actigraphy) found benefits of doubtful clinical significance (reduced sleep latency, total sleep duration and sleep efficiency of 4min, 13min and 2.2% respectively).[5] Head-to-head comparisons found no clinically significant differences between doses[11] or formulations (normal-release vs. m/r).[12,13] Reduced melatonin production does not predict response.[14] A synthetic melatonin agonist (ramelteon, not UK) was also of limited benefit.[6] Melatonin m/r is effective in patients using long-term benzodiazepine hypnotics.[15] Results of RCTs examining a possible role for melatonin in facilitating benzodiazepine discontinuation are conflicting.[16–19]

Insomnia in specific groups

Sleep-wake cycle disturbance is common in delirium and dementia. Prophylactic administration reduced the incidence of delirium from ~30% to ~10% among both medical[20] and surgical[21] patients aged ⩾65 yrs. Disordered metabolism of tryptophan, the precursor of serotonin and melatonin, is hypothesised to underlie delirium.[22] Hyperactive delirium is associated with reduced, and hypoactive delirium with increased, urinary melatonin metabolites.[23] Melatonin is reported to improve postoperative delirium refractory to **haloperidol** and **lorazepam**.[24] Evening agitation and insomnia associated with dementia improved with melatonin in several case series and 2/4 RCTs.[25]

Brain injury is associated with reduced evening melatonin production.[26] In individuals (mostly children) with various intellectual disabilities, a meta-analysis found melatonin reduced sleep latency (35min), total sleep duration (50min) and sleep efficiency. The dose, timing and preparation of melatonin varied.[27] A further RCT found similar effects on sleep latency but not sleep duration.[28]

Melatonin reduced sleep latency by 30min and improved sleep efficiency in haemodialysis patients with insomnia.[29] It is effective for jet lag,[30] shift work-related insomnia,[31] and delayed sleep phase syndrome.[32]

Bio-availability 15% (because of first-pass hepatic metabolism).
Time to peak plasma concentration 3h (with food), 45min (empty stomach).
Plasma halflife 3.5–4h.

Cautions

Despite its focused mode of action, melatonin may enhance the sedative effect of sedative drugs.

Auto-immune disease (although there are no data in humans, melatonin causes deleterious immunostimulation in animals with auto-immunity[2]); hepatic impairment (reduced clearance).

Drug interactions

Melatonin levels increased by inhibitors of CYP1A2 (e.g. **fluvoxamine**, quinolones; see Chapter 25, p.767). Melatonin can increase or decrease INR (consider increased monitoring).

Undesirable effects

No undesirable effects occurred in $>1\%$ for melatonin m/r (Circadin®). In RCTs, adverse event rates were comparable to placebo.[8,9]

Uncommon (<1%, >0.1%): Restlessness, irritability, abnormal dreams, dizziness, somnolence, constipation, dry mouth, hyperbilirubinaemia.

Rare (<0.1%, >0.01%): Laboratory changes (leukopenia, thrombocytopenia, altered LFTs), rashes, mood alteration, vertigo, blurred vision, nausea and vomiting.

Dose and use

Sleep disturbance is common in palliative care. Management involves the correction of underlying causes (sleep-disturbing symptoms, fears, concurrent depression, delirium), non-drug approaches (e.g. relaxation techniques), as well as sedative drugs. The efficacy of both conventional hypnotics and melatonin is modest.

The place of melatonin for sleep problems in palliative care remains uncertain. It could be considered when other options have failed or lack of tolerability limits the use of conventional hypnotics:

• melatonin m/r 2mg 1–2h before bedtime.

Supply

Circadin® (Flynn)
Tablets m/r 2mg, 28 days @ 2mg at night = £15.

---

1 Srinivasan V et al. (2005) Melatonin, immune function and aging. *Immunity and Ageing.* **2**: 17.
2 Carrillo-Vico A et al. (2005) A review of the multiple actions of melatonin on the immune system. *Endocrine.* **27**: 189–200.
3 Mills E et al. (2005) Melatonin in the treatment of cancer: a systematic review of randomized controlled trials and meta-analysis. *Journal of Pineal Research.* **39**: 360–366.
4 Rihel J and Schier AF (2013) Sites of action of sleep and wake drugs: insights from model organisms. *Current Opinion Neurobiology.* **23**: 831–840.
5 Brzezinski A et al. (2005) Effects of exogenous melatonin on sleep: a meta-analysis. *Sleep Medicine Reviews.* **9**: 41–50.
6 Sateia MJ et al. (2008) Efficacy and clinical safety of ramelteon: an evidence-based review. *Sleep Medicine Reviews.* **12**: 319–332.
7 Lazarus M et al. (2013) Role of the basal ganglia in the control of sleep and wakefulness. *Current Opinion in Neurobiology.* **23**: 780–785.
8 Wade AG et al. (2007) Efficacy of prolonged release melatonin in insomnia patients aged 55-80 years: quality of sleep and next-day alertness outcomes. *Current Medical Research Opinion.* **23**: 2597–2605.
9 Lemoine P et al. (2007) Prolonged-release melatonin improves sleep quality and morning alertness in insomnia patients aged 55 years and older and has no withdrawal effects. *Journal of Sleep Research.* **16**: 372–380.
10 Glass J et al. (2005) Sedative hypnotics in older people with insomnia: meta-analysis of risks and benefits. *British Medical Journal.* **331**: 1169.
11 Zhdanova IV et al. (2001) Melatonin treatment for age-related insomnia. *Journal of Clinical Endocrinology and Metabolism.* **86**: 4727–4730.
12 Haimov I et al. (1995) Melatonin replacement therapy of elderly insomniacs. *Sleep.* **18**: 598–603.
13 Hughes RJ et al. (1998) The role of melatonin and circadian phase in age-related sleep-maintenance insomnia: assessment in a clinical trial of melatonin replacement. *Sleep.* **21**: 52–68.
14 Wade AG et al. (2010) Nightly treatment of primary insomnia with prolonged release melatonin for 6 months: a randomized placebo controlled trial on age and endogenous melatonin as predictors of efficacy and safety. *BMC Medicine.* **8**: 51.
15 Garfinkel (1995) Improvement of sleep quality by controlled-release melatonin in benzodiazepine-treated elderly insomniacs. *Archives of Gerontology and Geriatrics.* **24**: 223–231.
16 Cardinali (2002) A double blind placebo controlled study of melatonin efficacy to reduce anxiolytic benzodiazepine use in the elderly. *Neuro Endocrinology Letters.* **23**: 55–60.
17 Vissers FH et al. (2007) Is melatonin helpful in stopping the long-term use of hypnotics? A discontinuation trial. *Pharmacy World and Science.* **29**: 641–646.
18 Garfinkel D et al. (1999) Facilitation of benzodiazepine discontinuation by melatonin: a new clinical approach. *Archives of Internal Medicine.* **159**: 2456–2460.
19 Lahteenmaki R et al. (2013) Melatonin for sedative withdrawal in older patients with primary insomnia: A randomised double-blind placebo-controlled trial. *British Journal of Clinical Pharmacology.*
20 Al-Aama T et al. (2011) Melatonin decreases delirium in elderly patients: a randomized, placebo-controlled trial. *International Journal of Geriatric Psychiatry.* **26**: 687–694.
21 Sultan SS (2010) Assessment of role of perioperative melatonin in prevention and treatment of postoperative delirium after hip arthroplasty under spinal anesthesia in the elderly. *Saudi Journal of Anaesthesia.* **4**: 169–173.
22 Lewis MC and Barnett SR (2004) Postoperative delirium: the tryptophan dyregulation model. *Medical Hypotheses.* **63**: 402–406.
23 Balan S et al. (2003) The relation between the clinical subtypes of delirium and the urinary level of 6-SMT. *Journal of Neuropsychiatry and Clinical Neurosciences.* **15**: 363–366.
24 Hanania M and Kitain E (2002) Melatonin for treatment and prevention of postoperative delirium. *Anesthesia and Analgesia.* **94**: 338–339.

---

25 de Jonghe A et al. (2010) Effectiveness of melatonin treatment on circadian rhythm disturbances in dementia. Are there implications for delirium? A systematic review. International Journal of Geriatric Psychiatry. **25**: 1201–1208.
26 Shekleton JA et al. (2010) Sleep disturbance and melatonin levels following traumatic brain injury. Neurology. **74**: 1732–1738.
27 Braam W et al. (2009) Exogenous melatonin for sleep problems in individuals with intellectual disability: a meta-analysis. Developmental Medicine and Child Neurology. **51**: 340–349.
28 Gringras P et al. (2012) Melatonin for sleep problems in children with neurodevelopmental disorders: randomised double masked placebo controlled trial. British Medical Journal. **345**: e6664.
29 Koch BC et al. (2009) The effects of melatonin on sleep-wake rhythm of daytime haemodialysis patients: a randomized, placebo-controlled, cross-over study (EMSCAP study). British Journal of Clinical Pharmacology. **67**: 68–75.
30 Herxheimer A (2002) Melatonin for the prevention and treatment of jet lag. Cochrane Database of Systematic Reviews. **2**: CD001520.
31 Sadeghniiat-Haghighi (2008) Efficacy and hypnotic effects of melatonin in shift-work nurses. Journal of Circadian Rhythms. **6**: 6–10.
32 Kayumov L et al. (2001) A randomized, double-blind, placebo-controlled crossover study of the effect of exogenous melatonin on delayed sleep phase syndrome. Psychosomatic Medicine. **63**: 40–48.

Updated May 2014

ANTIPSYCHOTICS   BNF 4.2.1

Indications: Psychosis, mania and bipolar disorders, †nausea and vomiting, †delirium, †terminal agitation, †intractable hiccup, †treatment-resistant depression.

Pharmacology

Antipsychotics act predominantly through D_2 receptor antagonism, countering symptoms of dopamine excess (e.g. delusions and hallucinations). However, unselective D_2 antagonism causes dopamine depletion symptoms in other pathways (e.g. parkinsonism).[1]

Antipsychotic classification reflects their varying propensity to cause such dopamine depletion symptoms (see Chapter 26, p.781). A lower risk is associated with D_2-receptor partial agonism, $5HT_{1A}$-receptor partial agonism and/or $5HT_2$-receptor antagonism (Table 1).[1–3] The risk is a spectrum (in descending order):[4]

- typical:
  ▷ butyrophenones (highest risk), e.g. **haloperidol**
  ▷ phenothiazines, e.g. **chlorpromazine, levomepromazine, prochlorperazine**
- atypical:
  ▷ less sedating, e.g. **risperidone**
  ▷ more sedating (lowest risk), e.g. **olanzapine, quetiapine**.

Table 1 Receptor affinities for selected antipsychotics[2,4–6]

	D_2	$5HT_{1A}$	$5HT_{2A}$	$5HT_{2C}$	$5HT_3$	H_1	α_1	α_2	ACh_M
Aripiprazole	+++PA	++PA	+++	+++	−	+++	+++	++	−
Chlorpromazine	+++	−	+++	++		+++	+++	+	++
Clozapine	+	++PA	+++	++	+	+++	+	+	+++
Haloperidol	+++	−	+	−	−	−	++	−	−
Levomepromazine	++		+++			+++	+++	+	++
Perphenazine	+++	−	+++	+		+++	++	+	−
Prochlorperazine	+++	−	++	+	−	++	++	−	+
Olanzapine	++	−	+++	+	+	+	++	+	++
Quetiapine	+	++PA	+	+	−	++	+	++	−
Risperidone	+++	−	+++	++	−	++	+	+++	−

Affinity: +++ high, ++ moderate, + low, − negligible or none; blank = no data. PA = partial agonist.

Dopamine and D_2 antagonism

Dopamine is central to arousal, motivation and attention (Table 2). It is released when the prefrontal/limbic cortex identifies situations requiring attention, particularly in relation to threat or pleasure. This modifies the thalamic sensory filter to allow the relevant information to pass through to the cerebral cortex. In psychosis, dopamine overactivity leads to an *exaggerated significance* becoming attached to an *excessive information* throughput (the 'salience hypothesis'). Delusions are a secondary phenomenon stemming from the information's exaggerated threatening or pleasurable significance (e.g. paranoid or grandiose delusions, respectively). D_2 antagonist antipsychotics help to correct this overactivity, and improve these 'positive' symptoms.[1,7,8]

However, other psychotic symptoms result from dopamine *depletion* (apathy, anhedonia and cognitive blunting; Table 2). Thus *unselective* D_2 antagonism worsens such 'negative' symptoms and disrupts unrelated pathways (e.g. the extrapyramidal system).[1,9]

Table 2 Dopaminergic pathways

Pathway	Function	Symptoms of dysregulation
Mesolimbic Midbrain reticular formation → limbic cortex	Pleasure, motivation and reward[a]	↑ Dopamine: 'positive' symptoms of psychosis (delusions, hallucinations)
Mesocortical system Midbrain reticular formation → prefrontal cortex	Affect, executive function, concentration	↓ Dopamine: depression; 'negative' symptoms of psychosis (apathy, anhedonia and cognitive blunting)
Nigrostriatal system Substantia nigra → corpus striatum	Extrapyramidal motor system	↓ Dopamine: Parkinson's disease, drug-induced parkinsonism, akathisia, dystonia, restless legs[a] ↑ Dopamine: dyskinesia[a]
Tubero-infundibular system	Dopaminergic inhibition of prolactin secretion	↓ Dopamine: hyperprolactinaemia
Thalamic dopamine pathway[b] Multiple origins → thalamus	Sleep and arousal through sensory gating	
Area postrema	Emetogenesis	↑ Dopamine: nausea and vomiting

a. D_2 antagonists initially cause underactivity, similar to Parkinson's disease (acute extrapyramidal symptoms). Subsequent adaptation to D_2 antagonism leads to D_2 receptor upregulation (tardive dyskinesia)
b. both the mesolimbic and thalamic dopamine pathways affect thalamic sensory gating. Mesolimbic dysregulation is best characterized in the formation of 'positive' psychotic symptoms (see text).

Some antipsychotics (e.g. **aripiprazole**) use D_2 *partial agonism* to reduce the problem of unselective D_2 antagonism. D_2 partial agonists function as D_2 antagonists in the presence of excessive dopamine, because they only partially activate the D_2 receptor. Thus they reduce overall transmission in overactive pathways. However, when there is dopamine depletion, the partial D_2 receptor activation is sufficient to increase overall transmission, and it functions as a D_2 agonist, e.g. in the nigrostriatal and mesocortical systems. Thus, a D_2 partial agonist antipsychotic can potentially improve both 'positive' and 'negative' symptoms and limit undesirable extrapyramidal effects.[3]

Non-dopaminergic actions

Dopaminergic neurones interact with many non-dopaminergic receptors. Some broadly oppose dopamine's actions (e.g. $5HT_2$, ACh_M); others synergize with it (e.g. $5HT_{1A}$). Stimulating underactive dopaminergic pathways through such receptors reduces the risks of *unselected* D_2 antagonism (e.g. extrapyramidal symptoms).

$5HT_{1A}$ receptors *stimulate*, and $5HT_2$ receptors *inhibit*, dopaminergic neurones of the nigrostriatal and mesocortical systems. Thus, both $5HT_{1A}$ partial agonist and $5HT_2$ antagonist antipsychotics increase activity in underactive pathways, countering the extrapyramidal impact of D_2 antagonism and improving 'negative' symptoms.[2,4]

Muscarinic antagonism reduces the risk of acute extrapyramidal symptoms because dopamine and acetylcholine have opposing effects within the nigrostriatal pathway; D_2 receptors inhibit cholinergic neurones.[2]

Some non-dopaminergic actions result in additional *desirable* effects. Depression and 'negative' psychotic symptoms overlap. Both relate to monoamine deficits (see p.190). 'Negative symptoms' respond to antidepressants.[9] Depression responds to some antipsychotics (e.g. **olanzapine**).[10,11] $5HT_2$ and α_2 antagonism may account for the latter. Both are important actions of some antidepressants, e.g. **mirtazapine** (see p.220). Differences in receptor profile also result in varying antiemetic properties (see p.235). **Olanzapine's** beneficial effect on cancer-related anorexia[12] may relate to $5HT_2$ and H_1 antagonism.

However, non-dopaminergic actions also result in additional *undesirable* effects: $5HT_2$ antagonism (along with α_1 and H_1 antagonism) causes sedation and metabolic effects; muscarinic antagonism causes dry mouth, cognitive impairment and constipation (see Antimuscarinics, Box B, p.6). Thus, overall, tolerability is comparable.

In an RCT, although extrapyramidal effects accounted for more discontinuations with **perphenazine** compared with several atypicals (8% vs. 2–4%), overall discontinuation rates for undesirable effects or lack of efficacy were comparable.[13] All treatment groups experienced some degree of involuntary movement (13–17%), akathisia (5–9%) or extrapyramidal signs (4–8%). Most studies are too short to evaluate the risk of tardive dyskinesia. Available data suggest a 5 times lower risk with atypicals compared with **haloperidol** in the first year of use, although **haloperidol** doses were relatively higher.[14]

Pharmacokinetic details of selected antipsychotics are summarized in Table 3. Dopamine and serotonin receptor polymorphisms effect both efficacy and the risk of undesirable effects (tardive dyskinesia and weight gain, respectively).[15,16]

Table 3 Pharmacokinetic details for selected antipsychotics[17,18]

	Oral bio-availability (%)	Time to peak plasma concentration	Halflife (h)	Metabolism (predominant P450 isoenzyme)
Chlorpromazine	10–25	2–4h (PO)	30	CYP2D6
Clozapine	50–60	2h	12	CYP1A2, CYP3A4
Haloperidol	45–75	2–6h (PO) 10–20min (SC)	13–35	Multiple
Levomepromazine	40	1–3h (PO) 30–90min (SC)	15–30	Multiple[a]
Olanzapine	60	5–8h	34^b (52^c)	CYP1A2, CYP2D6
Prochlorperazine	6 14 (buccal)	4h (PO) 4–8h (buccal); shorter with multiple doses	15–20	Multiple
Quetiapine	100	1.5h	7^d ($10–14^c$) (12^e)	CYP3A4
Risperidone	99	1–2h	$24^{f,g}$	$CYP2D6^h$

a. P450 iso-enzymes not fully characterized; some metabolites are active
b. unaffected by hepatic or renal impairment
c. in the elderly
d. clearance reduced by both renal and hepatic impairment
e. of active metabolite
f. for risperidone + active 9-hydroxy metabolite
g. clearance reduced by renal impairment
h. activity of 9-hydroxyrisperidone, the predominant CYP2D6 metabolite, is comparable to risperidone; thus overall clinical effect is not altered by CYP2D6 polymorphisms or inhibitors.

Cautions

Several pharmacodynamic interactions (additive sedation, hypotension and QT prolongation; reduced effect of antiparkinsonian drugs) can be predicted from the receptor profile of antipsychotics.

Stroke risk

Meta-analysis of RCTs in the elderly with dementia has shown that the risk of stroke with **olanzapine** and **risperidone** is 2–3 times higher compared with placebo,[19–22] with a doubling of all-cause mortality with **olanzapine**.[20] The mechanism of this association is not known, but it is regarded as a class effect. Subsequent findings indicate an increased risk in all elderly patients for both typicals and atypicals,[23–26] greatest in those with dementia,[27] within the first month of starting treatment, and with higher doses. The relative risk with individual drugs has not yet been determined.

Epilepsy

Similar to many other psychotropic medications, antipsychotics cause a dose-dependent reduction in seizure threshold. The risk for individual agents approximates to the degree of sedation: **chlorpromazine** and **clozapine** carry a higher risk and **haloperidol** a lower risk. To minimize the risk, use the lowest risk antipsychotic (e.g. **haloperidol**) at the lowest effective dose. In palliative care, depot formulations are best avoided because they cannot be withdrawn quickly if problems occur.

Parkinsonism and Parkinson's disease

All antipsychotics, through D_2 antagonism, can cause parkinsonism or worsen existing parkinsonism of any cause. The risk is lower with **clozapine** and **quetiapine**. In patients with parkinsonism, alternatives to antipsychotics should be used where possible, e.g. for agitation, consider **trazodone** (see p.222) or a benzodiazepine, for nausea and vomiting consider:
- **domperidone** (available as a suppository; not UK)
- **ondansetron**
- **hyoscine hydrobromide**, but may cause delirium.

Nonetheless, at the end of life, despite being D_2 antagonists, it may be necessary to prescribe small doses of **levomepromazine, olanzapine** or **quetiapine** if all else fails.

Where delirium or psychotic symptoms occur in the context of Parkinson's disease or Lewy Body dementia:
- look for potentially reversible causes of delirium, e.g. sepsis
- consider a trial reduction of antiparkinsonian medication:
  ▷ reduce D_2 agonists and antimuscarinic agents initially
  ▷ dopamine precursors, e.g. **levodopa**, are less likely to cause psychosis.[28]

If the above measures are unhelpful, commence **quetiapine** 12.5–25mg/24h; if not tolerated, seek specialist advice. Options include switching to **clozapine**.[28]

Drug interactions

Potentially serious interactions may result from induction or inhibition of hepatic metabolism (see Chapter 25, p.767). CYP3A4 inhibitors (e.g. **aprepitant, cimetidine,** macrolide antibiotics) can significantly increase plasma levels of **aripiprazole, pimozide** and **quetiapine**. **Carbamazepine** and protease inhibitors exhibit varied interactions.

Antipsychotics are one of several classes of drugs which can prolong the QT interval, and at least theoretically increase the risk of cardiac tachyarrthymias, including potentially fatal *torsade de pointes*. Generally, concurrent prescribing of two drugs which can significantly prolong the QT interval should be avoided (see Chapter 24, p.759).

Undesirable effects

A summary is given in Box A.

Neuroleptic (antipsychotic) malignant syndrome

Neuroleptic (antipsychotic) malignant syndrome (NMS) is a potentially life-threatening reaction which occurs in < 1% of those prescribed an antipsychotic (Box B).[35,36] This idiosyncratic syndrome is associated with all antipsychotics.[37]

Most cases of NMS occur within 2 weeks of starting treatment or a dose increase. It is a hypodopaminergic state; bradykinesia progresses to immobilization, akinesia and stupor, accompanied by lead-pipe rigidity, fever, and autonomic instability.

Symptoms indistinguishable from NMS have been reported in patients with Parkinson's disease when long-term treatment with **levodopa** and **bromocriptine** (a D_2 agonist) has been abruptly

---

Box A Undesirable effects of antipsychotics

Extrapyramidal syndromes
Parkinsonism, akathisia, dystonia, tardive dyskinesia (see Chapter 26, p.781).

Metabolic effects[25,29]
More common with typicals and risperidone
Hyperprolactinemia resulting in amenorrhoea, galactorrhoea, gynaecomastia, sexual dysfunction, osteoporosis.

More common with atypicals, particularly olanzapine, quetiapine and clozapine
Weight gain.

Dyslipidaemia

Type 2 diabetes mellitus.

Cardiovascular effects[a]
QT prolongation: dose-related, affected by presence of other risk factors, highest risk with sertindole, thioridazine (withdrawn) and ziprasidone.[25,30,31]

Venous thrombo-embolism.[32]

Stroke and increased risk of death in elderly patients (see Cautions).

Postural hypotension (α-adrenergic antagonism), particularly clozapine, phenothiazines and quetiapine.[33]

Miscellaneous[25]
Reduced seizure threshold (see Cautions).

Antimuscarinic effects; more with phenothiazines and clozapine.

Neuroleptic (antipsychotic) malignant syndrome (see below).

Agranulocytosis is seen in about 1% of patients taking clozapine, generally after 3–6 months.

a. an association with myocardial infarction is reported. This may be due to confounding life style factors and co-morbidities, rather than a causal association.[34]

Box B Clinical features of neuroleptic (antipsychotic) malignant syndrome

Essential
Severe muscle rigidity
Pyrexia ± sweating

Additional
Muteness → stupor
Tachycardia and elevated/labile blood pressure
Leukocytosis
Raised plasma creatine phosphokinase ± other evidence of muscle injury, e.g. myoglobinuria

---

discontinued.[38–40] This has led to the suggestion that the syndrome would be better called *acute dopamine depletion syndrome*.[38]

Death occurs in up to 20% of cases, mostly as a result of respiratory failure. The use of a dopamine agonist, e.g. **bromocriptine**, halves the mortality.[41] Subsequent prescription of an antipsychotic carries a 30–50% risk of recurrence.[42]

NMS is self-limiting if the causal antipsychotic drug is discontinued (and an alternative antipsychotic *not* prescribed). Generally it resolves in 1–2 weeks unless caused by a depot

antipsychotic, when it takes 4–6 weeks. Antipsychotics are *not* removed by haemodialysis. Specific measures include:
• discontinuation of the causal drug
• prescription of a muscle relaxant, e.g. a benzodiazepine
• in severe cases, prescription of **bromocriptine**.[41]
General supportive measures may need to extend to artificial hydration and nutrition. Complications such as hypoxia, acidosis and renal failure require appropriate acute management.

Use of antipsychotics in palliative care

When long term (>months) use of **olanzapine, quetiapine** or phenothiazines is anticipated, consider monitoring weight, glucose and lipids at baseline and 3-monthly thereafter.

Doses are described in individual monographs: **haloperidol** (p.177), **levomepromazine** (p.181), **prochlorperazine** (p.180), **olanzapine** (p.183), **risperidone** (p.186) and **quetiapine** (p.188). For terminal agitation, also see Chapter 16, p.672.

Nausea and vomiting
The D_2 antagonism of all antipsychotics is likely to provide anti-emetic activity in the area postrema (chemoreceptor trigger zone; see p.235). Where specific action at this site is required (e.g. most chemical causes of nausea), a selective dopaminergic agent such as **haloperidol** is used,[43] although studies in palliative care patients are open-label.[44,45]

However, many antipsychotics bind to other receptors involved in the transduction of emetic signals and, to a variable extent, are broad-spectrum anti-emetics (see p.235). **Levomepromazine** and **olanzapine** are the most widely used.[46,47] **Olanzapine** is more effective than placebo[48] and **metoclopramide**[49] for chemotherapy-related vomiting refractory to **dexamethasone, palonosetron** and **fosaprepitant**. Anti-emetic benefit is reported in advanced cancer and neurodegenerative disease.[50–53]

Delirium
Delirium is common, distressing and associated with higher mortality, reduced performance status and increased admission to nursing homes.[54,55] Management guidelines emphasise the importance of treating underlying causes, non-drug management (e.g. orientation strategies, correction of sensory deprivation) and prevention of complications.[56] Because of limited evidence and safety concerns, medication is often advocated only when non-drug measures are insufficient (particularly in patients with dementia; see below).[57]
More recent evidence suggests that antipsychotics (e.g. **haloperidol, olanzapine** or **quetiapine**) should be considered alongside non-drug measures in all forms of delirium (agitated, hypo-active and mixed). In 3 RCTs, antipsychotics not only reduced distressing symptoms but shortened the duration of the delirium[58,59] and improved outcomes (e.g. the proportion of patients discharged home).[60] Hypo-active delirium was not excluded and benefit was observed in all symptom domains, not just agitation.[59] Further, prophylactic use reduced the incidence of delirium and shortened Intensive Therapy Unit and overall hospital stay compared with use after delirium has occurred.[61,62] It is uncertain whether outcomes improve as a direct consequence of treating delirium and/or because patients are better able to co-operate with other treatments.
The efficacy and tolerability of **haloperidol, olanzapine, risperidone** and **quetiapine** are comparable.[63,64] Comparative studies with other psychotropics are lacking.[65–67] When antipsychotics alone are insufficient, or when sedation is also required, e.g. for the initial management of a hyperactive, frightened patient, benzodiazepines (see p.148) or **trazodone** (see p.222) can be added. Although benzodiazepines can paradoxically worsen agitation, they are preferred for delirium related to alcohol withdrawal, neuroleptic malignant syndrome or Parkinson's disease. Prophylactic **melatonin** reduced the incidence of delirium amongst hospital patients aged ≥65 yrs (see p.165). The use of cholinergics has been reported, but **rivastigmine** increased mortality in an RCT.[68] Hallucinations in delirium respond to antipsychotics in hours–days, whereas seemingly identical phenomena in a psychosis may not resolve for 1–2 weeks.

Challenging behaviours in dementia
Patients with dementia may become agitated for many reasons, including an appropriate response to a distressing situation. Possible precipitants should be treated or modified:

- intercurrent infections
- pain and/or other distressing symptoms
- environmental factors.

If carers or the care setting changes, seek information about the patient's daily routine. Consider the use of 'This is me' or a similar tool.[69]

If no cause is found, consider an empirical trial of **paracetamol**. Pain can be difficult to identify.[70] In an RCT, an empirical stepwise trial of analgesia (**paracetamol** → opioid → **pregabalin**) reduced agitation in unselected patients (i.e. without any specific indicator of pain).[71]

If unsuccessful, seek specialist advice. Training in non-drug management of behavioural disturbances reduces the need for psychotropic medication.[72] The first-line use of antipsychotics for behavioural disturbance in dementia is inappropriate and actively discouraged.[73–76] In addition to safety concerns (increased risk of stroke and overall mortality), a large RCT for agitation or psychosis in patients with dementia found both atypicals and typicals to be no better than placebo in all but a few secondary outcomes.[77] Taken together with other studies, the efficacy of antipsychotics in dementia is at best modest, and should be used only where other measures have failed.[78,79]

The use of antidepressants, benzodiazepines or anti-epileptics has been proposed. However, evidence is more limited than for antipsychotics, and insufficient to justify their routine use.[79–81] Larger studies have not replicated the earlier benefit reported for **trazodone** (see p.222).[79]

Even so, the serious consequences of not treating severe agitation or psychosis in dementia are also recognized.[79] Where drug treatment is required, clinicians should be guided by the individual patient's symptoms and co-morbidities, and their familiarity with the agents available. Options include:
- **haloperidol**
- atypicals, e.g. **olanzapine**, **quetiapine**, **risperidone**
- cholinesterase inhibitors (benefit is marginal, but may be better tolerated).[80]

Whichever drug is selected, use the lowest effective dose for the shortest possible time; attempt dose reduction every 2–3 months; many patients do not deteriorate when medication is withdrawn.[78,80,82]

Intractable hiccup

Chlorpromazine or **haloperidol** are used when more specific treatment, e.g. **simeticone** (an antifoaming agent; see p.4) ± **metoclopramide** (see p.242) for gastric distension, or **baclofen** are ineffective (see Prokinetics, Table 2, p.24).[72]

Refractory depression

Certain antipsychotics have been used as adjuncts for depression refractory to conventional antidepressants, particularly when switching antidepressants has been unsuccessful. Generally, either **quetiapine** or **olanzapine** is added to an SSRI (see p.199).[10,11,83]

Pain

Dopamine is implicated in pain processing[84] and, in the past, antipsychotics were sometimes used as part of an analgesic cocktail. However, RCTs yield conflicting results.[85] Although no longer used as analgesics themselves, antipsychotics are helpful for treating the undesirable effects of analgesics, particularly nausea and delirium.[86]

Switching antipsychotics

Equivalent doses of typicals have been estimated, predominantly from surveys of psychiatric practice, and provide a starting point if switching from one to another (Table 4).[87] However, doses of atypicals are less variable, and thus starting doses are unaffected by the dose of a previous antipsychotic.

Table 4 Equivalent doses of typical antipsychotics[87]

Drug	Dose (mg)
Chlorpromazine	100
Promazine	100
Perphenazine	8
Trifluoperazine	5
Haloperidol	3

1 Stahl SM (2013) Chapter 4: Psychosis and schizophrenia. In: Essential Psychopharmacology: Neuroscientific Basis and Practical Applications (4e). Cambridge University Press, USA. 79–128.

2 Stahl SM (2013) Chapter 5: Antipsychotic agents. In: Essential Psychopharmacology: Neuroscientific Basis and Practical Applications (4e). Cambridge University Press, USA. 129–236.

3 Lieberman JA (2004) Dopamine partial agonists: a new class of antipsychotic. CNS Drugs. 18: 251–267.

4 Jindal RD and Keshavan MS (2008) Classifying antipsychotic agents : need for new terminology. CNS Drugs. 22: 1047–1059.

5 Lal S et al. (1993) Levomepromazine receptor binding profile in human brain–implications for treatment-resistant schizophrenia. Acta Psychiatrica Scandinavica. 87: 380–383.

6 NIMH (National Institute of Mental Health) (2006) Psychoactive Drug Screening Program. University of North Carolina. Available from: http://pdsp.med.unc.edu

7 Boutrel B and Koob GF (2004) What keeps us awake: the neuropharmacology of stimulants and wakefulness-promoting medications. Sleep. 27: 1181–1194.

8 Alves Fda S et al. (2008) The revised dopamine hypothesis of schizophrenia: evidence from pharmacological MRI studies with atypical antipsychotic medication. Psychopharmacology Bulletin. 41: 121–132.

9 Barnes TR (2011) Evidence-based guidelines for the pharmacological treatment of schizophrenia: recommendations from the British Association for Psychopharmacology. Journal of Psychopharmacology. 25: 567–620.

10 NICE (2009) Depression. Clinical Guidelines. CG90 and CG91. www.nice.org.uk

11 Kato M and Chang CM (2013) Augmentation treatments with second-generation antipsychotics to antidepressants in treatment-resistant depression. CNS Drugs. 27 Suppl 1: S11–19.

12 Navari RM and Brenner MC (2010) Treatment of cancer-related anorexia with olanzapine and megestrol acetate: a randomized trial. Supportive Care in Cancer. 18: 951–956.

13 Lieberman JA et al. (2005) Effectiveness of antipsychotic drugs in patients with chronic schizophrenia. N Engl J Med. 353: 1209–1223.

14 Correll CU et al. (2004) Lower risk for tardive dyskinesia associated with second-generation antipsychotics: a systematic review of 1-year studies. American Journal of Psychiatry. 161: 414–425.

15 Muller DJ et al. (2013) The pharmacogenetics of antipsychotic-induced adverse events. Current Opinion in Psychiatry. 26: 144–150.

16 Arranz MJ et al. (2011) Pharmacogenetics of response to antipsychotics in patients with schizophrenia. CNS Drugs. 25: 933–969.

17 Eiermann B et al. (1997) The involvement of CYP1A2 and CYP3A4 in the metabolism of clozapine. British Journal of Clinical Pharmacology. 44: 439–446.

18 Finn A et al. (2005) Bioavailability and metabolism of prochlorperazine administered via the buccal and oral delivery route. Journal of Clinical Pharmacology. 45: 1383–1390.

19 Woolterton E (2002) Risperidone (Risperdal): increased rate of cerebrovascular events in dementia trials. Canadian Medical Association Journal. 167: 1269–1270.

20 Woolterton F (2004) Olanzapine (Zyprexa): increased incidence of cerebrovascular events in dementia trials. Canadian Medical Association Journal. 170: 1395.

21 Bullock R (2005) Treatment of behavioural and psychiatric symptoms in dementia: implications of recent safety warnings. Current Medical Research and Opinion. 21: 1–10.

22 Schneider LS et al. (2005) Risk of death with atypical antipsychotic drug treatment for dementia: meta-analysis of randomized placebo-controlled trials. Journal of the American Medical Association. 294: 1934–1943.

23 Wang PS et al. (2005) Risk of death in elderly users of conventional vs. atypical antipsychotic medications. New England Journal of Medicine. 353: 2335–2341.

24 Gill SS et al. (2007) Antipsychotic drug use and mortality in older adults with dementia. Annals of Internal Medicine. 146: 775–786.

25 Haddad PM and Sharma SG (2007) Adverse effects of atypical antipsychotics : differential risk and clinical implications. CNS Drugs. 21: 911–936.

26 Ray WA et al. (2009) Atypical antipsychotic drugs and the risk of sudden cardiac death. New England Journal of Medicine. 360: 225–235.

27 Douglas IJ and Smeeth L (2008) Exposure to antipsychotics and risk of stroke: self controlled case series study. British Medical Journal. 337: a1227.

28 Weintraub D and Hurtig HI (2007) Presentation and management of psychosis in Parkinson's disease and dementia with Lewy bodies. American Journal of Psychiatry. 164: 1491–1498.

29 Yood MU et al. (2009) The incidence of diabetes in atypical antipsychotic users differs according to agent - results from a multisite epidemiologic study. Pharmacoepidemiology and Drug Safety. 18: 791–799.

30 Twycross R and Wilcock A (2008) Prolongation of the QT interval in palliative care. In: Hospice and Palliative Care Formulary USA (2e). palliativedrugs.com, Nottingham, pp. 531–536.

31 Nielsen J et al. (2011) Assessing QT interval prolongation and its associated risks with antipsychotics. CNS Drugs. 25: 473–490.

32 Jonsson AK et al. (2012) Venous thromboembolism in recipients of antipsychotics: incidence, mechanisms and management. CNS Drugs. 26: 649–662.

33 Gugger JJ (2011) Antipsychotic pharmacotherapy and orthostatic hypotension: identification and management. CNS Drugs. 25: 659–671.

34 Brauer R et al. (2011) The association between antipsychotic agents and the risk of myocardial infarction: a systematic review. British Journal of Clinical Pharmacology. 72: 871–878.

35 Caroff S and Mann S (1993) Neuroleptic malignant syndrome. Medical Clinics of North America. 77: 185–202.

36 Adnet P et al. (2000) Neuroleptic malignant syndrome. British Journal of Anaesthesia. 85: 129–135.

37 Isbister GK et al. (2002) Comment: neuroleptic malignant syndrome associated with risperidone and fluvoxamine. Annals of Pharmacotherapy. 36: 1293; author reply 1294.

38 Keyser DL and Rodnitzky RL (1991) Neuroleptic malignant syndrome in Parkinson's disease after withdrawal or alteration of dopaminergic therapy. Archives of Internal Medicine. 151: 794–796.

39 Mann S et al. (1991) Pathogenesis of neuroleptic malignant syndrome. Psychiatry Annals. 21: 175–180.

40 Ong K et al. (2001) Neuroleptic malignant syndrome without neuroleptics. Singapore Medical Journal. 42: 85–88.

41 Sakkas P et al. (1991) Pharmacotherapy of neuroleptic malignant syndrome. Psychiatry Annals. 21: 157–164.

42 Wells A et al. (1988) Neuroleptic rechallenges after neuroleptic malignant syndrome: case report and literature review. Drug Intelligence and Clinical Pharmacy. 22: 475–479.

43 Buttner M et al. (2004) Is low-dose haloperidol a useful antiemetic?: A meta-analysis of published and unpublished randomized trials. Anesthesiology. 101: 1454–1463.

44 Hardy JR et al. (2010) The efficacy of haloperidol in the management of nausea and vomiting in patients with cancer. Journal of Pain and Symptom Management. 40: 111–116.

45 Perkins (2009) Haloperidol for the treatment of nausea and vomiting in palliative care patients. Cochrane Database of Systematic Reviews. CD006271.

46 Passik SD et al. (2004) A phase I trial of olanzapine (Zyprexa) for the prevention of delayed emesis in cancer patients: a Hoosier Oncology Group study. Cancer Investigation. 22: 383–388.

47 Navari RM et al. (2005) A phase II trial of olanzapine for the prevention of chemotherapy-induced nausea and vomiting: a Hoosier Oncology Group study. Supportive Care in Cancer. 13: 529–534.

48 Mizukami N et al. (2014) Olanzapine for the prevention of chemotherapy-induced nausea and vomiting in patients receiving highly or moderately emetogenic chemotherapy: a randomized, double-blind, placebo-controlled study. Journal of Pain and Symptom Management. 47: 542–550.

49 Navari RM et al. (2013) The use of olanzapine versus metoclopramide for the treatment of breakthrough chemotherapy-induced nausea and vomiting in patients receiving highly emetogenic chemotherapy. Supportive Care in Cancer. 21: 1655–1663.

50 Kaneishi K et al. (2012) Olanzapine for the relief of nausea in patients with advanced cancer and incomplete bowel obstruction. Journal of Pain and Symptom Management. 44: 604–607.

51 Passik SD et al. (2002) A pilot exploration of the antiemetic activity of olanzapine for the relief of nausea in patients with advanced cancer and pain. Journal of Pain and Symptom Management. 23: 526–532.

52 Jackson WC and Tavernier L (2003) Olanzapine for intractable nausea in palliative care patients. Journal of Palliative Medicine. 6: 251–255.

53 Dietz I et al. (2013) Evidence for the use of Levomepromazine for symptom control in the palliative care setting: a systematic review. BMC Palliative Care. 12: 2.

54 LeGrand SB (2012) Delirium in palliative medicine: a review. Journal of Pain and Symptom Management. 44: 583–594.

55 Hosie A et al. (2013) Delirium prevalence, incidence, and implications for screening in specialist palliative care inpatient settings: a systematic review. Palliative Medicine. 27: 486–498.

56 Bush SH et al. (2014) Treating an established episode of delirium in palliative care: expert opinion and review of the current evidence base with recommendations for future development. Journal of Pain and Symptom Management [Epub ahead of print].

57 NICE (2010) Clinical Guideline CG103. www.nice.org.uk.

58 Hu (2006) Olanzapine and haloperidol for senile delirium: a randomised controlled observation. Chinese Journal of Clinical Rehabilitation. 10: 188–190.

59 Tahir TA et al. (2010) A randomized controlled trial of quetiapine versus placebo in the treatment of delirium. Journal of Psychosomatic Research. 69: 485–490.

60 Devlin JW et al. (2010) Efficacy and safety of quetiapine in critically ill patients with delirium: a prospective, multicenter, randomized, double-blind, placebo-controlled pilot study. Critical Care Medicine. 38: 419–427.

61 Kalisvaart KJ et al. (2005) Haloperidol prophylaxis for elderly hip-surgery patients at risk for delirium: a randomized placebo-controlled study. Journal of the American Geriatrics Society. 53: 1658–1666.

62 Wang W et al. (2012) Haloperidol prophylaxis decreases delirium incidence in elderly patients after noncardiac surgery: a randomized controlled trial. Critical Care Medicine. 40: 731–739.

63 Grover S et al. (2011) Comparative efficacy study of haloperidol, olanzapine and risperidone in delirium. Journal of Psychosomatic Research. 71: 277–281.

64 Maneeton B et al. (2013) Quetiapine versus haloperidol in the treatment of delirium: a double-blind, randomized, controlled trial. Drug Design, Development Therapy. 7: 657–667.

65 Attard A et al. (2008) Delirium and its treatment. CNS Drugs. 22: 631–644.

66 Caraceni A and Simonetti F (2009) Palliating delirium in patients with cancer. Lancet Oncology. 10: 164–172.

67 Fong TG et al. (2009) Delirium in elderly adults: diagnosis, prevention and treatment. Nature Reviews Neurology. 5: 210–220.

68 van Eijk MM et al. (2010) Effect of rivastigmine as an adjunct to usual care with haloperidol on duration of delirium and mortality in critically ill patients: a multicentre, double-blind, placebo-controlled randomised trial. Lancet. 376: 1829–1837.

69 Royal College of Nursing and Alzheimer's Society This is me tool. Available from: http://www.alzheimers.org.uk

70 Achterberg WP et al. (2013) Pain management in patients with dementia. Clinical Interventions in Aging. 8: 1471–1482.

71 Husebo BS et al. (2011) Efficacy of treating pain to reduce behavioural disturbances in residents of nursing homes with dementia: cluster randomised clinical trial. British Medical Journal. 343: d4065.

72 Fossey J et al. (2006) Effect of enhanced psychosocial care on antipsychotic use in nursing home residents with severe dementia: cluster randomised trial. British Medical Journal. 332: 756–761.

73 MHRA (2004) Atypical antipsychotic drugs and stroke. Safety warnings and messages for medicines (9 March 2004). www.mhra.gov.uk/Safetyinformation

74 Mowat D et al. (2004) CSM warning on atypical psychotics and stroke may be detrimental for dementia. British Medical Journal. 328: 1262.

75 Health Canada (2005) Increased mortality associated with the use of atypical antipsychotic drugs in elderly patients with dementia. Notice to healthcare professionals. www.hc-sc.gc.ca

76 FDA (2008) Information on conventioanl antipsychotics. Postmarket drug safety information for patients and providers. FDA Alert. (16 June 2008). www.fda.gov/Drugs

77 Schneider LS et al. (2006) Effectiveness of atypical antipsychotic drugs in patients with Alzheimer's disease. New England Journal of Medicine. 355: 1525–1538.

78 Ballard C and Corbett A (2010) Management of neuropsychiatric symptoms in people with dementia. CNS Drugs. 24: 729–739.

79 Jeste DV et al. (2008) ACNP White Paper: update on use of antipsychotic drugs in elderly persons with dementia. Neuropsychopharmacology. 33: 957–970.

80 Sink KM et al. (2005) Pharmacological treatment of neuropsychiatric symptoms of dementia: a review of the evidence. Journal of the American Medical Association. 293: 596–608.

81 Herrmann N et al. (2013) Pharmacological recommendations for the symptomatic treatment of dementia: the Canadian Consensus Conference on the Diagnosis and Treatment of Dementia 2012. Alzheimer's Research and Therapy. 5: S5.

82 Lee PE et al. (2004) Atypical antipsychotic drugs in the treatment of behavioural and psychological symptoms of dementia: systematic review. British Medical Journal. 329: 75.

83 Anderson IM et al. (2008) Evidence-based guidelines for treating depressive disorders with antidepressants: a revision of the 2000 British Association for Psychopharmacology guidelines. Journal of Psychopharmacology. 22: 343–396.

84 Wood PB (2006) Mesolimbic dopaminergic mechanisms and pain control. *Pain.* **120**: 230–234.
85 Seidel (2008) Antipsychotics for acute and chronic pain in adults. *Cochrane Database of Systematic Reviews.* CD004844.
86 Coyle N et al. (1994) Delirium as a contributing factor to 'crescendo' pain: three case reports. *Journal of Pain and Symptom Management.* **9**: 44–47.
87 Foster P (1989) Neuroleptic equivalence. *Pharmaceutical Journal.* **243**: 431–432.

Updated June 2014

HALOPERIDOL   BNF 4.2.1

Class: Butyrophenone antipsychotic, anti-emetic.

Indications: Psychosis, Gilles de la Tourette's syndrome, †terminal agitation, †delirium, †nausea and vomiting, intractable hiccup.

Pharmacology

Haloperidol is a typical antipsychotic D_2 antagonist. Steady-state plasma concentrations do not vary greatly between patients after injection but they vary considerably after PO administration. The metabolism of haloperidol is not as complex as that of the phenothiazines but, even so, there are many metabolites and some may contribute to its extrapyramidal effects.[1] It is not possible to relate clinical response to plasma haloperidol concentrations. Haloperidol in solution is odourless, colourless and tasteless and can be administered clandestinely in extreme situations.

Compared with **chlorpromazine**, haloperidol has less effect on the cardiovascular system and causes less drowsiness. It has no antimuscarinic properties,[2] but causes *more* extrapyramidal reactions (see Chapter 26, p.781). In one study, haloperidol caused akathisia in >50% of schizophrenics.[3] The incidence in palliative care appears to be low, possibly because generally lower doses are used and the duration of treatment is relatively short.

Haloperidol is widely used in palliative care for delirium and as an anti-emetic. For delirium, it is as effective as **risperidone, olanzapine** and **quetiapine**.[4,5] For nausea and vomiting, it is effective postoperatively and in patients referred to specialist gastro-enterological clinics with multifactorial nausea.[6] By virtue of its D_2 antagonism, it has a profound inhibitory effect on the area postrema (chemoreceptor trigger zone). Long-standing clinical experience in palliative care indicates that haloperidol is a good anti-emetic for many chemical causes of vomiting,[7] e.g. **morphine, digoxin**, renal failure, hypercalcaemia;[8,9] and also after radiotherapy.[10] However, no RCTs have been conducted in palliative care patients.[11] Haloperidol has also been used for obstructive vomiting in relatively small doses, e.g. 2–5mg SC.[12,13] Its benefit in this circumstance is difficult to understand. However, the affinity of haloperidol for D_2-receptors is 10 times that of **domperidone** (see p.246).[14] Thus, haloperidol might have a gastric prokinetic effect.

Bio-availability 45–75% PO.[1]
Onset of action 10–15min SC; >1h PO.
Time to peak plasma concentration 2–6h PO; 10–20min SC.
Plasma halflife 13–35h.
Duration of action up to 24h, sometimes longer.

Cautions

Increased mortality in patients with dementia. Where possible, avoid. Where necessary, use the lowest effective dose for the shortest possible duration; also see stroke risk (p.171) and use for challenging behaviours in dementia (p.173).

Haloperidol can cause potentially fatal prolongation of the QT interval and *torsade de pointes*, particularly if given IV (off-label route) or at higher-than-recommended doses. Caution is required if any formulation of haloperidol is given to patients with an underlying predisposition, e.g. those with cardiac abnormalities, hypothyroidism, familial long QT syndrome, electrolyte imbalance (particularly hypokalaemia or hypomagnesaemia), or taking drugs which prolong the QT interval (see Chapter 24, p.759). If IV haloperidol is essential, ECG monitoring during administration is recommended.[15,16]

Parkinson's disease; epilepsy (lowered seizure threshold).[17]

Drug interactions

Potentiation of CNS depression caused by other CNS depressants, e.g. anxiolytics, alcohol. Increased risk of extrapyramidal effects and possible neurotoxicity with **lithium**. Plasma concentration of haloperidol is approximately halved by concurrent use of **carbamazepine**.

Undesirable effects

Extrapyramidal effects (see Chapter 26, p.781), hypothermia, sedation, hypotension, endocrine effects, blood disorders, altered LFTs, neuroleptic (antipsychotic) malignant syndrome (see p.171).

Dose and use

Haloperidol exacerbates Parkinson's disease: use alternatives where possible (see p.171).

As a general rule, the dose of haloperidol is halved when switching from PO to SC. For CSCI dilute with WFI, or 5% glucose. High concentrations of haloperidol (> 1mg/mL after mixing) are incompatible if diluted with 0.9% saline (see Chapter 20, p.699).

CSCI compatibility with other drugs: There are 2-drug compatibility data for haloperidol in WFI with **alfentanil, clonazepam, cyclizine, glycopyrronium, hyoscine** *butylbromide*, **hyoscine** *hydrobromide*, **metoclopramide, midazolam** and **oxycodone**.
   Haloperidol is *incompatible* with **ketorolac**. Concentration-dependent *incompatibility* occurs with **dexamethasone, diamorphine, hydromorphone** and **morphine sulfate**. For more details and 3-drug compatibility data, see Appendix 3 charts and tables (p.821).
   Compatibility charts for mixing drugs in 0.9% saline can be found in the extended appendix section of the on-line PCF on www.palliativedrugs.com

Anti-emetic

For chemical/toxic causes of vomiting, including **morphine**-induced vomiting:
- start with 500microgram–1.5mg PO stat & at bedtime
- typical maintenance dose 1.5–3mg at bedtime (or 500microgram–1.5mg b.d.)
- if necessary, increase the total daily dose progressively to 5–10mg
- if 10mg at bedtime (or 5mg b.d.) is ineffective, review the cause of the vomiting; consider switching to **levomepromazine** (see p.181).

Delirium

If possible, correct underlying causes, and use non-drug measures (e.g. orientation strategies, correction of sensory deprivation).[18] When symptomatic drug treatment is required:
- patient distress mild–moderate and not an immediate danger to self or others:
  ▷ start with 500microgram stat and q2h p.r.n.
  ▷ if necessary, increase the dose progressively (e.g. →1mg→1.5mg etc.)[19]
- patient distress severe and/or an immediate danger to self or others:
  ▷ start with 1.5–3mg stat, possibly combined with a benzodiazepine, and q2h p.r.n.
  ▷ if necessary, increase the dose further, e.g. 5mg.

The maintenance dose is based on the initial cumulative dose needed to settle the patient; usual maximum ≤5mg/24h. Review daily, particularly if the underlying cause can be resolved. Other strategies include:
- prescribing a more sedating antipsychotic (e.g. **olanzapine** (see p.183), **quetiapine** (see p.188)) *or*
- the concurrent use of **trazodone** (see p.222) or a benzodiazepine (see p.148).

If necessary, seek advice from a psychogeriatrician. Note: for the management of terminal agitation, see Chapter 16 (see p.673).

Behavioural problems in dementia

The management of delirium or psychosis should be distinguished from the long-term treatment of behavioural disturbance in dementia. Antipsychotics are generally not indicated in the latter (see p.173). Training in the non-drug management of behavioural disturbances reduces the need for psychotropic medication; medication is a last resort.[20] When used, dose reduction should be attempted every 2–3 months; many patients do not deteriorate when medication is withdrawn.[21–23]

Intractable hiccup

Haloperidol is generally used only when sequential therapeutic trials of **metoclopramide** (see p.242) ± an anti-foaming agent (see **Simeticone**, p.4) and **baclofen** (see p.593) have both failed (see Prokinetics, Table 2, p.24):

- give haloperidol 1.5mg PO t.d.s.
- if no response, consider giving 5mg IV
- maintenance dose 1–3mg at bedtime.[24,25]

Another option is **gabapentin** (see p.270).

Supply

Haloperidol (generic)
Tablets 500microgram, 1.5mg, 5mg, 10mg, 20mg, 28 days @ 1.5mg at bedtime = £2.50.
Oral liquid 5mg/5mL, and 10mg/5mL 28 days @ 1.5mg at bedtime = £3.
Injection 5mg/mL, 1mL amp = £0.50.

Serenace® (Ivax)
Capsules 500microgram, 28 days @ 1.5mg at bedtime = £3.50.

1 Vella-Brincat J and Macleod AD (2004) Haloperidol in palliative care. *Palliative Medicine.* **18**: 195–201.
2 de Leon J (2005) Benztropine equivalents for antimuscarinic medication. *American Journal of Psychiatry.* **162**: 627.
3 Wirshing D et al. (1999) Novel antipsychotics: comparison of weight gain liabilities. *Journal of Clinical Psychiatry.* **60**: 358–363.
4 Grover S et al. (2011) Comparative efficacy study of haloperidol, olanzapine and risperidone in delirium. *Journal of Psychosomatic Research.* **71**: 277–281.
5 Maneeton B et al. (2013) Quetiapine versus haloperidol in the treatment of delirium: a double-blind, randomized, controlled trial. *Drug Design, Development Therapy.* **7**: 657–667.
6 Buttner M et al. (2004) Is low-dose haloperidol a useful antiemetic?: A meta-analysis of published and unpublished randomized trials. *Anesthesiology.* **101**: 1454–1463.
7 Hardy JR et al. (2010) The efficacy of haloperidol in the management of nausea and vomiting in patients with cancer. *Journal of Pain and Symptom Management.* **40**: 111–116.
8 Bentley A and Boyd K (2001) Use of clinical pictures in the management of nausea and vomiting: a prospective audit. *Palliative Medicine.* **15**: 247–253.
9 Stephenson J and Davies A (2006) An assessment of aetiology-based guidelines for the management of nausea and vomiting in patients with advanced cancer. *Supportive Care in Cancer.* **14**: 348–353.
10 Stoll BA (1962) Radiation sickness. *British Medical Journal.* **2**: 507–510.
11 Perkins P and Dorman S (2009) Haloperidol for the treatment of nausea and vomiting in palliative care patients. *Cochrane Database of Systematic Reviews.* **2**: CD006271.
12 Ventafridda V et al. (1990) The management of inoperable gastrointestinal obstruction in terminal cancer patients. *Tumori.* **76**: 389–393.
13 Mercadante S (1995) Bowel obstruction in home-care cancer patients: 4 years experience. *Supportive Care in Cancer.* **3**: 190–193.
14 Sanger G (1993) The pharmacology of anti-emetic agents. In: P Andrews and G Sanger (eds) *Emesis in anti-cancer therapy: mechanisms and treatment.* Chapman and Hall, London, pp. 179–210.
15 FDA (2007) Haloperidol (marketed as Haldol, Haldol decanoate and Haldol lactate). *Postmarket Drug Safety Information for Patients and Providers: Information for heathcare professionals:* www.fda.gov/Drugs/DrugSafety
16 Canadian Pharmacists Association (2009) Haloperidol. Compendium of pharmaceuticals and specialities (eCPS). Available from: www.pharmacists.ca
17 Hedges JR et al. (2003) Antipsychotic medication and seizures: a review. *Drugs Today (Barc).* **39**: 551–557.
18 Twycross R et al. (2009) *Symptom Management in Advanced Cancer* (4e). palliativedrugs.com, Nottingham, pp. 207–211.
19 British Geriatrics Society and Royal College of Physicians (2006) The prevention, diagnosis and management of delirium in older people. National Guidelines. Available from: www.rcplondon.ac.uk
20 Fossey J et al. (2006) Effect of enhanced psychosocial care on antipsychotic use in nursing home residents with severe dementia: cluster randomised trial. *British Medical Journal.* **332**: 756–761.
21 Howard R et al. (2001) Guidelines for the management of agitation in dementia. *International Journal of Geriatric Psychiatry.* **16**: 714–717.
22 Lee PE et al. (2004) Atypical antipsychotic drugs in the treatment of behavioural and psychological symptoms of dementia: systematic review. *British Medical Journal.* **329**: 75.
23 Sink KM et al. (2005) Pharmacological treatment of neuropsychiatric symptoms of dementia: a review of the evidence. *Journal of the American Medical Association.* **293**: 596–608.
24 Ives TJ et al. (1985) Treatment of intractable hiccups with intramuscular haloperidol. *American Journal of Psychiatry.* **142**: 1368–1369.
25 Scarnati RA (1979) Intractable hiccup (singultus): report of case. *Journal of the American Osteopathic Association.* **79**: 127–129.

Updated June 2014

PROCHLORPERAZINE   BNF 4.2.1

Class: Phenothiazine antipsychotic, anti-emetic.

Indications: Nausea and vomiting, †vertigo in labyrinthine disorders.

Contra-indications: Bone marrow depression.

Pharmacology

Prochlorperazine is a D_2, $5HT_2$, H_1, α_1 and ACh_M antagonist. It has been a popular anti-emetic for many years, particularly for nausea and vomiting caused by chemical stimulation of the chemoreceptor zone. It is too irritant for SC administration, but a buccal formulation is a convenient alternative for patients at home. Although not recommended for motion sickness, prochlorperazine is used for the short-term relief of vertigo in Meniere's disease.

Oral bio-availability is low because of high first-pass hepatic metabolism.[1] Buccal prochlorperazine is about 2.5 times more bio-available and the variance is much less. Prochlorperazine is rapidly metabolized via eight isoforms of cytochrome P450; most extensively by CYP3A4, 2C19 and 2D6.[2,3] The multiple metabolic pathways suggest that clinically important drug interactions are unlikely. Undesirable effects are generally less severe than with **chlorpromazine** but, like all antipsychotics, there is still a risk of extrapyramidal effects.[4]
Bio-availability 6% PO, 14% buccal.[3]
Onset of action 30–40min PO, 10–20min IM, 1h PR.
Time to peak plasma concentration 4h PO, 8h buccal; 4h buccal when given regularly.[3]
Plasma halflife 15–20h.[3]
Duration of action 6–8h PO, PR (possibly longer when taken regularly); 12h buccal, IM.[3,5]

Cautions

Increased mortality in patients with dementia. Where possible, avoid. Where necessary, use the lowest effective dose for the shortest possible duration (also see stroke risk (p.171) and use for challenging behaviours in dementia (p.173)).

Epilepsy, hepatic impairment, severe renal impairment.

Drug interactions

Extrapyramidal effects and neurotoxicity have occurred when given concurrently with **lithium**.[6] Prochlorperazine increases the plasma concentration of **phenytoin** (mechanism unknown); if given concurrently, **phenytoin** levels must be monitored.

Undesirable effects

Very common (>10%): antimuscarinic effects (see p.249).
Frequency not stated: photosensitivity, slate-grey skin pigmentation, extrapyramidal reactions (see Chapter 26, p.781), parkinsonism, drowsiness, confusion, paradoxical psychotic behaviour and agitation, seizures, neuroleptic malignant syndrome (see p.171), postural hypotension, blood dyscrasias.

Dose and use

Prochlorperazine is a potent irritant. Avoid direct contact of the oral solution or injection with the skin; do not give by CSCI.

Because of the risk of photosensitivity, patients should be advised to use high-factor (25–30) sun screen cream and a wide-brimmed hat if going outdoors in sunny weather.

Anti-emetic

Recommended maximum 40mg/24h (except for PR route; not UK):
- 3–6mg buccally b.d. *or*
- 5–10mg PO t.d.s.–q.d.s. *or*

- 5–10mg IM q3h–q4h *or*
- 2.5–10mg IV q3h–q4h p.r.n.
- 10mg PR t.d.s.–q.d.s. (not UK).

Labyrinthine disorders
The following regimen is sometimes used:
- start with 5mg PO t.d.s.
- if necessary, increase to 10mg t.d.s.
- reduce gradually to 5mg once daily–b.d. after several weeks.

Supply

Prochlorperazine (generic)
Tablets *(as maleate)* 5mg, 28 days @ 5mg q.d.s. = £3.
Injection *(as mesilate)* 12.5mg/mL, 1mL amp = £0.50.

Stemetil® (Sanofi-Aventis)
Tablets *(as maleate)* 5mg, 28 days @ 5mg q.d.s. = £8.
Oral liquid (syrup) *(as mesilate)* 5mg/5mL, 28 days @ 5mg q.d.s. = £19.
Injection *(as mesilate)* 12.5mg/mL, 1mL amp = £0.50.

Buccastem® (Alliance)
Tablets (buccal) *(as maleate)* 3mg, 28 days @ 3mg b.d. = £7; *place tablet high between upper lip and gum and leave to dissolve.*

1 Taylor WB and Bateman DN (1987) Preliminary studies of the pharmacokinetics and pharmacodynamics of prochlorperazine in healthy volunteers. *British Journal of Clinical Pharmacology.* **23**: 137–142.
2 Collins JM et al. (2004) In-vitro characterization of the metabolism of prochlorperazine. *Clinical Pharmacology and Therapeutics.* **75**: 85.
3 Finn A et al. (2005) Bioavailability and metabolism of prochlorperazine administered via the buccal and oral delivery route. *Journal of Clinical Pharmacology.* **45**: 1383–1390.
4 Kawanishi C et al. (2007) Unexpectedly high prevalence of akathisia in cancer patients. *Palliative and Supportive Care.* **5**: 351–354.
5 Lacy C et al. (eds) (2003) *Lexi-Comp's Drug Information Handbook* (11e). Lexi-Comp and the American Pharmaceutical Association, Hudson, Ohio.
6 Baxter K and Preston CL *Stockley's Drug Interactions.* London: Pharmaceutical Press www.medicinescomplete.com (accessed 2011).

Updated June 2014

LEVOMEPROMAZINE   BNF 4.2.1

Class: Phenothiazine antipsychotic, anti-emetic.

Indications: Acute psychotic symptoms, schizophrenia, pain and accompanying distress in the terminally ill, †agitation, nausea and vomiting.

Pharmacology

Levomepromazine is a D_2, $5HT_{2A}$, α_1- and α_2-adrenergic, H_1 and muscarinic antagonist.[1] It is structurally and functionally similar to **chlorpromazine**, but is more widely used in palliative care, in part because it can be administered SC/CSCI.

Despite the absence of RCT evidence,[2,3] levomepromazine is widely used in palliative care in the UK for terminal agitation and for nausea and vomiting (see p.235).[4] Although traditionally used as a second- or third-line anti-emetic, it can be used first-line (unless a prokinetic anti-emetic is indicated, e.g. **metoclopramide**; see p.468). Doses ⩾25mg/24h tend to cause drowsiness and postural hypotension. **Olanzapine** (see p.183) is an alternative broad-spectrum anti-emetic for those unable to tolerate levomepromazine.

Although authorized for pain and accompanying distress in the terminally ill, the evidence on which this is based is relatively limited, involved higher doses (e.g. 25mg by injection) and sedation was common.[5–10] Thus, other adjuvant analgesics which have more supporting evidence and are better tolerated should generally be used in preference. Any such use of levompromazine should be in conjunction with specialist palliative care or pain teams, and will probably be reserved for use alongside other analgesics, e.g. opioids, in patients in severe pain, at the end of life, when sedation is acceptable and when all usual options have been exhausted, or are inappropriate.

Levomepromazine is metabolized by sulphoxidation, N-demethylation and 3- and 7-hydroxylation.[11,12]

Bio-availability 20–40% PO.[13]
Onset of action 30min.
Time to peak plasma concentration 2–3h PO; 30–90min SC.
Plasma halflife 15–30h, sometimes longer.[14]
Duration of action 12–24h.

Cautions

Antipsychotics increase mortality in patients with dementia. Where possible, avoid. Where necessary, use the lowest effective dose for the shortest possible duration, also see stroke risk (p.171) and use for challenging behaviours in dementia (p.173).

Parkinsonism, postural hypotension, antihypertensive medication, epilepsy (lowered seizure threshold), hypothyroidism, myasthenia gravis.

Undesirable effects

Drowsiness, postural hypotension, antimuscarinic effects (see p.249).

Dose and use

When long term (>months) use is anticipated, consider monitoring weight, glucose and lipids at baseline and 3-monthly thereafter.

Levomepromazine is often given by CSCI. Infusions must be protected from light to prevent degradation of the drug and must be discarded if a yellow/pink/purple colour occurs, see Chapter 20, Box B, p.701. To reduce the likelihood of inflammatory reactions at the skin infusion site, dilute to the largest practical volume and consider the use of 0.9% saline as the diluent (see Chapter 20, p.699). However, given its long plasma halflife, most patients can be maintained satisfactorily on intermittent injections, 1–3 times/24h.

Terminal agitation ± delirium

Generally a second-line treatment (see Chapter 16, Box A, p.673), given only if it is intended to reduce a patient's level of consciousness:
• start with 25mg SC stat and q1h p.r.n. (12.5mg in the elderly)
• if necessary, titrate dose according to response
• maintain with 50–300mg/24h CSCI.
Although high-dose levomepromazine (≥100mg/24h) is generally best given by CSCI, smaller doses can be conveniently given as an SC bolus at bedtime–b.d., and p.r.n. (see Chapter 20, Table 1, p.698) . Some centres use smaller doses first-line, e.g. 6.25–12.5mg SC stat and q1h p.r.n.[3]

Anti-emetic

• start with 6–6.25mg PO/SC stat, at bedtime & p.r.n. (use a 6mg tablet or quarter a 25mg tablet)
• some centres report benefit with even lower starting doses, e.g. 2.5–5mg PO/SC[3,4,15]
• if necessary, progressively increase to 12.5–25mg b.d.
Drowsiness generally limits dose titration. In these circumstances consider either switching to **olanzapine** (see p.183) or reducing the dose and combining with an anti-emetic of a different profile of action (e.g. **ondansetron**; see Table 2, p.238).

Analgesic

Seek advice from specialist palliative care or pain teams before such use (see Pharmacology):
* stat dose 25mg PO/SC and at bedtime
* titrate dose according to response; usual maximum daily dose 100mg SC/200mg PO.

CSCI compatibility with other drugs: There are 2-drug compatibility data for levomepromazine in WFI with **alfentanil, diamorphine, glycopyrronium, hydromorphone, hyoscine** *butylbromide,* **hyoscine** *hydrobromide,* **midazolam, morphine sulfate** and **oxycodone.**

Levomepromazine is *incompatible* with **ketorolac.** Concentration-dependent *incompatibility* occurs with **dexamethasone,** and **octreotide.** For more details and 3-drug compatibility data, see Appendix 3 charts and tables (p.821).

Compatibility charts for mixing drugs in 0.9% saline can be found in the extended appendix section of the on-line PCF on www.palliativedrugs.com

Supply

Nozinan® (Sanofi-Aventis)
Tablets (scored) 25mg , 28 days @ 12.5mg at bedtime = £3.50.
Tablets 6mg, 28 days @ 12mg at bedtime = £85. (Unauthorized, available as a special order via IDIS, see Appendix 1, p.817) Cost of a 6mg tablet is £1.50, the equivalent cost of one quarter of a 25mg tablet is £0.06.
Injection 25mg/mL, 1mL amp = £2.

1 Lal S *et al.* (1993) Levomepromazine receptor binding profile in human brain–implications for treatment-resistant schizophrenia. *Acta Psychiatrica Scandinavica.* **87**: 380–383.
2 Darvill E *et al.* (2013) Levomepromazine for nausea and vomiting in palliative care. *Cochrane Database of Systematic Reviews.* **4**: Cd009420.
3 Dietz I *et al.* (2013) Evidence for the use of Levomepromazine for symptom control in the palliative care setting: a systematic review. *BMC Palliative Care.* **12**: 2.
4 palliativedrugs.com (2006) The use of s/c levomepromazine as an antiemetic and for terminal agitation. Bulletin board: www.palliativedrugs.com (posted 7 September 2006).
5 Montilla E *et al.* (1963) Analgesic effect of methotrimeprazine and morphine: a clinical comparison. *Archives of Internal Medicine.* **111**: 725–731.
6 Bloomfield S *et al.* (1964) Comparative analgesic activity of levomepromazine and morphine in patients with chronic pain. *Canadian Medical Association Journal.* **40**: 1156–1162.
7 Beaver W *et al.* (1966) A comparison of the analgesic effects of methotrimeprazine and morphine in patients with cancer. *Clinical Pharmacology and Therapeutics.* **5**: 436–446.
8 Davidsen O *et al.* (1979) Analgesic treatment with levomepromazine in acute myocardial infarction: A randomized clinical trial. *Acta Medica Scandinavica.* **205**: 191–195.
9 Bellens J *et al.* (1981) Analgesic treatment with levopromazine (Nozinan) and methadone in patients with acute myocardial infarction. *Ugeskrift nand Laeger.* **143**: 1313–1316.
10 Minuck H (1972) Postoperative analgesia - comparison of methotrimeprazine and meperidine as postoperative analgesic agents. *Canadian Anesthetists Society Journal.* **19**: 87–96.
11 Dahl SG *et al.* (1987) Nuclear magnetic resonance analysis of methotrimeprazine (levomepromazine) hydroxylation in humans. *Journal of Pharmceutical Science.* **76**: 541–544.
12 Dahl SG and Garle M (1977) Identification of nonpolar methotrimeprazine metabolites in plasma and urine by GLC-mass spectrometry. *Journal of Pharmaceutical Science.* **66**: 190–193.
13 Bagli M *et al.* (1995) Bioequivalence and absolute bioavailability of oblong and coated levomepromazine tablets in CYP2D6 phenotyped subjects. *International Journal of Clinical Pharmacology and Therapeutics.* **33**: 646–652.
14 Dahl SG *et al.* (1977) Pharmacokinetics and relative bioavailability of levomepromazine after repeated administration of tablets and syrup. *European Journal of Clinical Pharmacology.* **11**: 305–310.
15 palliativedrugs.com (2010) Olanzapine for nausea, insomnia, anorexia, anxiety. Bulletin board: www.palliativedrugs.com (posted 10 October 2010).

Updated June 2014

OLANZAPINE   BNF 4.2.1

Class: Atypical antipsychotic.

Indications: Psychosis, mania and bipolar disorders, †delirium, †nausea and vomiting, †treatment-resistant depression.

Pharmacology

Olanzapine is a potent D_1, D_2, D_3, D_4, $5HT_{2A}$, $5HT_{2C}$, $5HT_3$ and $5HT_6$ antagonist. It also binds to other receptors, including α_1 and a_2-adrenergic, H_1 and muscarinic receptors.[1] It is metabolized in the liver by glucuronidation and, to a lesser extent, oxidation via the cytochrome P450 system (see p.767), primarily via CYP1A2 with a minor contribution via CYP2D6. The major metabolite is the 10-N-glucuronide which does not pass the blood-brain barrier. Elimination of metabolites is both renal (60%) and faecal (30%).[2] Clearance varies 4 times among patients.[3]

Olanzapine, **quetiapine** and **clozapine** cause fewer drug induced movement disorders than other antipsychotics.[4,5] However, other undesirable effects are more common (e.g. drowsiness, weight gain). Thus, overall, tolerability is comparable.[6]

In delirium, a single-blinded RCT found olanzapine, **risperidone** and **haloperidol** were equally effective.[7] For chemotherapy-related nausea and vomiting refractory to **dexamethasone**, **palonosetron** and **fosaprepitant**, olanzapine is more effective than placebo[8] and **metoclopramide**.[9] Benefit is also reported for nausea and vomiting in advanced cancer and neurodegenerative disorders.[10–12] Benefit is reported in paraneoplastic sweating.[13]

Bio-availability 60%, sometimes >80% PO.
Onset of action hours–days in delirium; days–weeks in psychoses.
Time to peak plasma concentration 5–8h, not affected by food.
Plasma halflife 34h; 52h in the elderly; shorter in smokers; unchanged in hepatic and renal impairment.
Duration of action 12–48h, situation dependent.

Cautions

Increased mortality in patients with dementia; avoid if possible. Where necessary, use the lowest effective dose for the shortest possible duration; also see stroke risk (p.171) and use for challenging behaviours in dementia (p.173).

Injections (not UK): fatalities from oversedation or cardiorespiratory depression have occurred after higher than approved doses or *concurrent use with benzodiazepines*. Monitor blood pressure, heart rate, respiratory rate and level of consciousness for ≥4h after IM olanzapine, and do not give parenteral benzodiazepines within 1h of IM olanzapine.

Elderly patients and those with renal or hepatic impairment. Parkinson's disease (exacerbation). Epilepsy (lowers seizure threshold).[14] May cause or adversely affect diabetes mellitus; rare reports of keto-acidosis. Olanzapine potentiates the sedative effects of alcohol and other CNS depressants.

Drug interactions

Omeprazole, **carbamazepine**, **rifampicin** and tobacco exposure stimulate CYP1A2 and decrease the plasma concentration of olanzapine; in contrast, **fluvoxamine**, an inhibitor of CYP1A2, increases the plasma concentration.

Undesirable effects

Common (<10%, >1%): drowsiness, weight gain.
Uncommon (<1%, >0.1%): dry mouth, constipation, orthostatic hypotension,[15–17] agitation, nervousness, dizziness, peripheral oedema.

The incidence and severity of drug-induced movement disorders are significantly less than with **haloperidol**.[3,18] Acute disorders are generally mild and are reversible if the dose is reduced and/or an antimuscarinic antiparkinsonian drug prescribed.

Dose and use

When long term (>months) use is anticipated, consider monitoring weight, glucose and lipids at baseline and 3-monthly thereafter.

Subcutaneous use of parenteral olanzapine (not UK) is reported without evidence of site reactions.[19]

Psychosis or mania
- Start with 10–15mg PO at bedtime
- if necessary, increase to 20mg at bedtime.

Agitation and/or delirium
Used as an alternative to **haloperidol**:
- start with 2.5mg PO stat, p.r.n. & at bedtime
- if necessary, increase to 5–10mg at bedtime.[20,21]

Anti-emetic
- start with 1.25–2.5mg PO stat, q2h p.r.n. & at bedtime
- if necessary, increase to 5mg at bedtime, occasionally to 5mg b.d.[11,22]

Supply
Olanzapine (generic)
Tablets 2.5mg, 5mg, 7.5mg, 10mg, 15mg, 20mg, 28 days @ 5mg at bedtime = £1.50.
Tablets orodispersible 5mg, 10mg, 15mg, 20mg, 28 days @ 5mg at bedtime = £3; *may be placed on the tongue and allowed to dissolve or dispersed in water, orange juice, apple juice, milk or coffee immediately before administration.*

1 Stahl SM (2013) Chapter 5: Antipsychotic agents. In: Essential Psychopharmacology: Neuroscientific Basis and Practical Applications (4e). Cambridge University Press, USA. 129–236.
2 Callaghan J et al. (1999) Olanzapine. Pharmacokinetic and pharmacodynamic profile. Clinical Pharmacokinetics. 37: 177–193.
3 Beasley C et al. (1997) Efficacy of olanzapine: an overview of pivotal clinical trials. Journal of Clinical Psychiatry. 58 (Suppl 10): 7–12.
4 Komossa K et al. (2010) Olanzapine versus other atypical antipsychotics for schizophrenia. Cochrane Database of Systematic Reviews. 3: CD006654.
5 Duggan L et al. (2005) Olanzapine for schizophrenia. Cochrane Database of Systematic Reviews. 2: CD001359.
6 Lieberman JA et al. (2005) Effectiveness of antipsychotic drugs in patients with chronic schizophrenia. New England Journal of Medicine. 353: 1209–1223.
7 Grover S et al. (2011) Comparative efficacy study of haloperidol, olanzapine and risperidone in delirium. Journal of Psychosomatic Research. 71: 277–281.
8 Mizukami N et al. (2014) Olanzapine for the prevention of chemotherapy-induced nausea and vomiting in patients receiving highly or moderately emetogenic chemotherapy: a randomized, double-blind, placebo-controlled study. Journal of Pain and Symptom Management. 47: 542–550.
9 Navari RM et al. (2013) The use of olanzapine versus metoclopramide for the treatment of breakthrough chemotherapy-induced nausea and vomiting in patients receiving highly emetogenic chemotherapy. Supportive Care in Cancer. 21: 1655–1663.
10 Kaneishi K et al. (2012) Olanzapine for the relief of nausea in patients with advanced cancer and incomplete bowel obstruction. Journal of Pain and Symptom Management. 44: 604–607.
11 Passik SD et al. (2002) A pilot exploration of the antiemetic activity of olanzapine for the relief of nausea in patients with advanced cancer and pain. Journal of Pain and Symptom Management. 23: 526–532.
12 Jackson WC and Tavernier L (2003) Olanzapine for intractable nausea in palliative care patients. Journal of Palliative Medicine. 6: 251–255.
13 Zylicz Z and Krajnik M (2003) Flushing and sweating in an advanced breast cancer patient relieved by olanzapine. Journal of Pain and Symptom Management. 25: 494–495.
14 Hedges D et al. (2003) Antipsychotic medication and seizures: a review. Drugs Today (Barc). 39: 551–557.
15 Tollefson G et al. (1997) Olanzapine versus haloperidol in the treatment of schizophrenia and schizoaffective and schizophreniform disorders: results of an international collaborative trial. American Journal of Psychiatry. 154: 457–465.
16 Conley R and Meltzer H (2000) Adverse events related to olanzapine. Journal of Clinical Psychiatry. 61: 26–29.
17 Worrel J et al. (2000) Atypical antipsychotic agents: a critical review. American Journal of Health-System Pharmacy. 57: 238–358.
18 Geddes J et al. (2000) Atypical antipsychotics in the treatment of schizophrenia: systematic overview and meta-regression analysis. British Medical Journal. 321: 1371–1376.
19 Elsayem (2010) Subcutaneous olanzapine for hyperactive or mixed delirium in patients with advanced cancer: a preliminary study. Journal of Pain and Symptom Management. 40: 774–782.
20 Passik S and Cooper M (1999) Complicated delirium in a cancer patient successfully treated with olanzapine. Journal of Pain and Symptom Management. 17: 191–223.
21 Meehan K et al. (2002) Comparison of rapidly acting intramuscular olanzapine, lorazepam, and placebo: A double-blind, randomized study in acutely agitated patients with dementia. Neuropsychopharmacology. 26: 494–504.
22 Srivastava M et al. (2003) Olanzapine as an antiemetic in refractory nausea and vomiting in advanced cancer. Journal of Pain and Symptom Management. 25: 578–582.

Updated June 2014

RISPERIDONE   BNF 4.2.1

Class Atypical antipsychotic.

Indications: Psychosis, mania and bipolar disorders, †agitation, †delirium.

Pharmacology

Risperidone is a potent D_2 and $5HT_{2A}$ antagonist.[1] It also binds to α_1-adrenergic receptors and with lower affinity to H_1- and α_2-receptors. Unlike **olanzapine**, risperidone does *not* bind to muscarinic receptors. The incidence of drug-induced movement disorders is less than with **haloperidol** and phenothiazines but greater than with more sedating atypical antipsychotics (e.g. **olanzapine**, **quetiapine**; see p.171). A retrospective survey reported that > 25% of patients developed akathisia or parkinsonism.[2]

In delirium, hallucinations respond to risperidone within hours but generally only after 1–2 weeks in a psychotic illness; this is true of all antipsychotics.

The major metabolite of risperidone is 9-hydroxyrisperidone. This hydroxylation is subject to **debrisoquine**-type genetic CYP2D6-related polymorphism but, because both risperidone and its major metabolite are equally active, the efficacy of risperidone is unaffected.[3] Risperidone is more slowly eliminated in the elderly and in patients with renal impairment. Doses of risperidone should be decreased in patients with hepatic impairment because the mean free fraction of risperidone is increased by up to 35% as a result of decreased levels of albumin and α_1-acid glycoprotein.[4]

Risperidone is as effective as **haloperidol** in treating delirium.[5] Its efficacy as an anti-emetic has not been fully evaluated. A retrospective review of 20 cancer patients given risperidone 1mg at bedtime for refractory opioid-induced nausea and vomiting reported complete resolution of nausea in half and a partial response in the other half, with cessation of vomiting in two thirds.[6]

Risperidone can cause a weight gain of several kg particularly over the first 2 months; this is generally less than with other atypical antipsychotics but may be more marked if it is given together with **valproate** or **lithium**.[2,7]

Bio-availability 99%.

Time to peak plasma concentration 1–2h, not affected by food.

Onset of action hours–days in delirium; days–weeks in psychoses.

Plasma halflife of active fraction (risperidone +9-hydroxyrisperidone) 24h.

Duration of action 12–48h, situation dependent.

Cautions

Increased mortality in patients with dementia. Where possible, avoid. Where necessary, use the lowest effective dose for the shortest possible duration; also see stroke risk (p.171) and use for challenging behaviours in dementia (p.173).

Elderly patients and those with renal or hepatic impairment.[4] Can cause orthostatic hypotension, particularly initially, because of α-adrenergic receptor antagonism. Parkinson's disease (deterioration). Epilepsy (lowers seizure threshold, although the risk is lower than with more sedating atypical antipsychotics).[8]

Drug interactions

Carbamazepine has been shown to decrease the combined plasma concentration of risperidone and 9-hydroxyrisperidone. A similar effect might be anticipated with other drugs which stimulate metabolizing enzymes in the liver. On initiation of **carbamazepine** or other hepatic enzyme-inducing drugs, the dose of risperidone should be re-evaluated and increased as necessary. Conversely, on discontinuation of such drugs, the dose of risperidone should be re-evaluated and decreased as necessary.

Phenothiazines, TCAs and some β-blockers may increase the plasma concentrations of risperidone but not the combined concentration of risperidone and its active metabolite. **Fluoxetine** may increase the plasma concentration of risperidone but the impact on the combined concentration is less. A dose reduction of risperidone should be considered when **fluoxetine** is added to risperidone therapy. Based on *in vitro* studies, the same interaction may occur with **haloperidol**.

Undesirable effects

Common (<10%, >1%): insomnia, agitation, anxiety, headache, movement disorders (see below), drowsiness, weight gain.

Uncommon (<1%, >0.1%): drowsiness, fatigue, dizziness, impaired concentration, seizures, blurred vision, syncope, dyspepsia, nausea and vomiting, constipation, sexual dysfunction (including priapism and erectile dysfunction), urinary incontinence, rhinitis.

The incidence and severity of drug-induced movement disorders are less than with haloperidol.[9–11] Acute disorders are generally mild and are reversible if the dose is reduced and/or an antimuscarinic antiparkinsonian drug prescribed (see Chapter 26, p.781).

Dose and use

Despite being commonly given b.d. there is no advantage in dividing the total daily dose, which can conveniently be given at bedtime.[12] Doses above 10mg/24h generally do not provide added benefit and may increase the risk of drug-induced movement disorders.

Psychosis
- start with 2mg PO at bedtime
- if necessary, increase to 4mg and 6mg at bedtime on successive days
- in elderly patients and those with severe hepatic or renal impairment, the starting dose should be halved to 1mg at bedtime and titration extended over 6 days.[13]

Delirium
- start with 1mg PO at bedtime & p.r.n.
- if necessary, increase by 1mg every other day
- median maintenance dose is 1mg/24h
- usual maximum 4mg/24h.[14]

Supply

Risperidone (generic)
Tablets 500microgram, 1mg, 2mg, 3mg, 4mg, 6mg, 28 days @ 1mg at bedtime = £1.
Tablets orodispersible 500microgram, 1mg, 2mg, 3mg, 4mg, 28 days @ 1mg at bedtime = £20; *tablets should be placed on the tongue, allowed to dissolve, then swallowed.*
Oral solution 1mg/mL, 28 days @ 1mg at bedtime = £13; *may be diluted with any non-alcoholic drink except tea.*

1 Stahl SM (2013) Chapter 5: Antipsychotic agents. In: Essential Psychopharmacology: Neuroscientific Basis and Practical Applications (4e). Cambridge University Press, USA. 129–236.

2 Guille C et al. (2000) A naturalistic comparison of clozapine, risperidone and olanzapine in the treatment of bipolar disorder. Journal of Clinical Psychiatry. 61: 638–642.

3 Bork J et al. (1999) A pilot study on risperidone metabolism: the role of cytochromes P450 2D6 and 3A. Journal of Clinical Psychiatry. 60: 469–476.

4 Snoecke E et al. (1995) Influence of age, renal and liver impairment on the pharmacokinetics of risperidone in man. Psychopharmacology (Berl). 122: 223–229.

5 Grover S et al. (2011) Comparative efficacy study of haloperidol, olanzapine and risperidone in delirium. Journal of Psychosomatic Research. 71: 277–281.

6 Okamoto Y et al. (2007) A retrospective chart review of the antiemetic effectiveness of risperidone in refractory opioid-induced nausea and vomiting in advanced cancer patients. Journal of Pain and Symptom Management. 34: 217–222.

7 Wirshing D et al. (1999) Risperidone in treatment-refractory schizophrenia. American Journal of Psychiatry. 156: 1374–1379.

8 Hedges D et al. (2003) Antipsychotic medication and seizures: a review. Drugs Today (Barc). 39: 551–557.

9 Jeste D et al. (1999) Lower incidence of tardive dyskinesia with risperidone compared with haloperidol in older patients. Journal of the American Geriatric Society. 47: 716–719.

10 Geddes J et al. (2000) Atypical antipsychotics in the treatment of schizophrenia: systematic overview and meta-regression analysis. British Medical Journal. 321: 1371–1376.

11 Umbricht D and Kane J (1995) Risperidone: efficacy and safety. Schizophrenia Bulletin. 21: 593–606.

12 Nair N (1998) Therapeutic equivalence of risperidone given once daily and twice daily in patients with schizophrenia. The Risperidone Study. Journal of Clinical Psychopharmacology. 18: 10–110.

13 Luchins D et al. (1998) Alteration in the recommended dosing schedule for risperidone. American Journal of Psychiatry. 155: 365–366.

14 Taylor D (2012) Delirium. In: The Maudsley Prescribing Guidelines in Psychiatry (11e). Wiley-Blackwell, UK. 547–554.

Updated June 2014

QUETIAPINE   BNF 4.2.1

Class: Atypical antipsychotic.

Indications: Psychosis mania and bipolar disorders, †agitation, †delirium, †treatment-resistant depression.

Pharmacology

Quetiapine is a D_2, D_3, $5HT_{2A}$ and $5HT_{2C}$ antagonist and a $5HT_{1A}$ partial agonist. It also binds to other receptors including α_1, α_2-adrenergic, H_1, and muscarinic receptors.[1-3] Quetiapine is used primarily in the treatment of schizophrenia and other psychoses. In off-label use for delirium, its efficacy and tolerability is comparable to **haloperidol**.[4]

It is rapidly absorbed after oral administration. Although not known precisely, bio-availability is at least 75% (the proportion of radio-labelled quetiapine excreted in urine).[5] Metabolism is predominantly by CYP3A4. The plasma concentration of active metabolites is $\leqslant 10\%$ that of quetiapine and thus unlikely to contribute significantly to overall activity. Elimination is both renal (75%) and faecal (25%); $< 1\%$ of quetiapine is excreted unchanged.[5]

Quetiapine and **clozapine** have the lowest risk of extrapyramidal effects of all the atypical antipsychotics (see Chapter 26, p.781).[6] The haematological monitoring required for **clozapine** makes quetiapine the drug of choice when an antipsychotic is indicated in someone with Parkinson's disease (see p.171).[7] Quetiapine shares the undesirable metabolic effects, and the increased mortality in patients with dementia, of the other atypicals.[6,8] Compared with **olanzapine** and **risperidone**, it causes more antimuscarinic effects.[2] Like **olanzapine**, it is more sedating than **risperidone**.

Bio-availability $\geqslant 75\%$.[5]
Onset of action hours–days in delirium; 1–2 weeks in psychoses.
Time to peak plasma concentration 1.5h.
Plasma halflife 7h (10–14h in the elderly).
Duration of action 12h (although serotoninergic activity may persist for much longer).[5]

Cautions

Increased mortality in patients with dementia. Where possible, avoid. Where necessary, use the lowest effective dose for the shortest possible duration; also see stroke risk (p.171) and use for challenging behaviours in dementia (p.173).

Elderly patients and those with renal or hepatic impairment. Possibly an increased risk of neutropenia. May cause or adversely affect diabetes mellitus. Parkinson's disease (deterioration) but the risk is lower than for other atypicals (see p.171). Epilepsy (lowers seizure threshold).[9,10]

Drug interactions

Plasma quetiapine concentrations can be significantly increased by CYP3A4 inhibitors (e.g. azole antifungals, macrolide antibiotics) and reduced by enzyme inducers (e.g. **carbamazepine**, **phenytoin**).

Undesirable effects

Very common (>10%): drowsiness, dizziness.
Common (<10%, >1%): dry mouth, constipation, leukopenia, tachycardia, orthostatic hypotension, peripheral oedema, altered liver transaminases.

Dose and use

When long term (> months) use is anticipated, consider monitoring weight, glucose and lipids at baseline and 3-monthly thereafter.

Reduce starting dose and rate of titration in the elderly and those with renal or hepatic impairment or Parkinson's disease.

Delirium
- start with 12.5mg PO b.d.
- if necessary, increase in 12.5–25mg increments
- mean effective dose = 40–100mg/24h.[4,10–13]

Schizophrenia
- start with 25mg PO b.d.
- increase to 50mg b.d. (day 2), 100mg b.d. (day 3), 150mg b.d. (day 4)
- then titrate according to response, up to 750mg/24h
- typical effective dose = 300–450mg/24h.

Bipolar mania
As monotherapy or as adjunct therapy to mood stabilizers:
- start with 50mg PO b.d.
- increase to 100mg b.d. (day 2), 150mg b.d. (day 3), 200mg b.d. (day 4)
- then titrate according to response, ≤200mg/24h, up to 800mg/24h
- typical effective dose = 400–800mg/24h.

Supply
Immediate-release
Quetiapine (generic)
Tablets 25mg, 100mg, 150mg, 200mg, 300mg, 28 days @ 100mg b.d. = £113.
Oral solution 12.5mg/5mL, 25mg/5mL, 50mg/5mL and 100mg/5mL 28 days @ 100mg b.d. = £149 (unauthorized, available as a special order, see Appendix 1, p.817); *price based on community specials tariff.*

Modified-release
Quetiapine (generic)
Tablets m/r 50mg, 150mg, 200mg, 300mg, 400mg, 28 days @ 200mg once daily = £57.

1 NIMH (National Institute of Mental Health) (2006) Psychoactive Drug Screening Program. University of North Carolina. Available from: http://pdsp.med.unc.edu
2 Lieberman JA et al. (2005) Effectiveness of antipsychotic drugs in patients with chronic schizophrenia. N Engl J Med. **353**: 1209–1223.
3 Stahl SM (2013) Chapter 5: Antipsychotic agents. In: Essential Psychopharmacology: Neuroscientific Basis and Practical Applications (4e). Cambridge University Press, USA. 129–236.
4 Maneeton B et al. (2013) Quetiapine versus haloperidol in the treatment of delirium: a double-blind, randomized, controlled trial. Drug Design, Development Therapy. **7**: 657–667.
5 DeVane CL and Nemeroff CB (2001) Clinical pharmacokinetics of quetiapine: an atypical antipsychotic. Clinical Pharmacokinetics. **40**: 509–522.
6 Haddad PM and Sharma SG (2007) Adverse effects of atypical antipsychotics : differential risk and clinical implications. CNS Drugs. **21**: 911–936.
7 Weintraub D and Hurtig HI (2007) Presentation and management of psychosis in Parkinson's disease and dementia with Lewy bodies. American Journal of Psychiatry. **164**: 1491–1498.
8 Schneider LS et al. (2005) Risk of death with atypical antipsychotic drug treatment for dementia: meta-analysis of randomized placebo-controlled trials. Journal of the American Medical Association. **294**: 1934–1943.
9 Hedges D et al. (2003) Antipsychotic medication and seizures: a review. Drugs Today (Barc). **39**: 551–557.
10 Yalug I et al. (2007) Quetiapine may be associated with new-onset seizures in patients with seizurogenic conditions. Journal of Neuropsychiatry and Clinical Neurosciences. **19**: 341–342.
11 Tahir TA et al. (2010) A randomized controlled trial of quetiapine versus placebo in the treatment of delirium. Journal of Psychosomatic Research. **69**: 485–490.
12 Maneeton B et al. (2007) An open-label study of quetiapine for delirium. Journal of the Medical Association of Thailand. **90**: 2158–2163.
13 Kim KY et al. (2003) Treatment of delirium in older adults with quetiapine. Journal of Geriatric Psychiatry and Neurology. **16**: 29–31.
14 Lee KU et al. (2005) Amisulpride versus quetiapine for the treatment of delirium: a randomized, open prospective study. International Clinical Psychopharmacology. **20**: 311–314.

Updated June 2014

ANTIDEPRESSANTS   BNF 4.3

Indications: Depression, anxiety and panic disorders, stress incontinence and urgency, †neuropathic pain, †agitated delirium, †sweating, †hot flushes, †insomnia, †pruritus, †bladder spasm, †pathological laughing and crying, †drooling.

Pharmacology

Antidepressants enhance transmission by one or more mono-amines by:
• inhibiting mono-amine re-uptake transporters, and/or
• inhibiting mono-amine breakdown and/or
• blocking regulatory receptors which inhibit mono-amine release (Box A, Figure 1).
Some have additional actions of relevance to both beneficial and undesirable effects (Table 1).

Box A   Classification of antidepressants according to principal actions[a]

Mono-amine re-uptake inhibitors (MARIs)
Serotonin and noradrenaline (norepinephrine) (SNRIs[b] or dual inhibitors[c])
Amitriptyline[d], venlafaxine, duloxetine

Serotonin (selective serotonin re-uptake inhibitors, SSRIs)
Sertraline, citalopram, paroxetine, fluoxetine

Noradrenaline (norepinephrine) (NRIs)
Nortriptyline[d], lofepramine[d], desipramine[d], reboxetine

Noradrenaline (norepinephrine) and dopamine (NDRIs)
Bupropion

Psychostimulant-antidepressants[e]
Dexamfetamine, methylphenidate, modafinil

Receptor antagonists
Trazodone (α_1, $5HT_2$)
Mirtazapine (central α_2, $5HT_2$, $5HT_3$)

Mono-amine oxidase inhibitors (MAOIs)[f]
Phenelzine, tranylcypromine

---

a. abbreviated names broadly reflect those found elsewhere;[1] confusion is inevitable because S is used for *Selective*, *Specific*, and *Serotonin*
b. SNRI is sometimes reserved for dual inhibitors without additional receptor binding affinities (e.g. venlafaxine and duloxetine)
c. 'dual' refers to serotonin and noradrenaline (norepinephrine), the two mono-amines traditionally associated with the pathophysiology of depression. Dopamine's significance has been recognised more recently leading to attempts to modulate all three mono-amines in refractory depression ('*tri-mono-aminergic* modulators')
d. TCAs differ in their modes of action, and do not comprise a single discrete drug class
e. reverse dopamine re-uptake transporters
f. MAOIs are included for completeness; their use by non-psychiatrists is *not* recommended.

The beneficial and undesirable effects of antidepressants vary for multiple reasons including differing:
• mono-amines affected (Box A)
• mechanisms of action (Figure 1)
• effects on other receptors (Table 1)
• pharmacokinetic profiles (Table 2).
The clearance of many antidepressants is significantly affected by CYP2D6 metabolizer phenotype, and to a lesser extent by CYP2C19. Further, serotonin re-uptake transporter polymorphisms may influence SSRI efficacy.[6] However, clinical benefit from genotyping has yet to be demonstrated.[7]

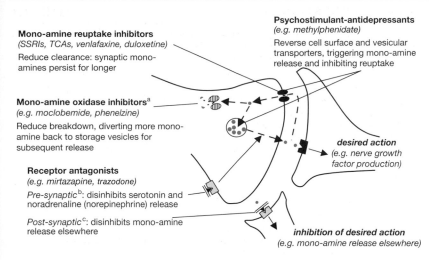

Mono-amine reuptake inhibitors
(SSRIs, TCAs, venlafaxine, duloxetine)
Reduce clearance: synaptic mono-amines persist for longer

Psychostimulant-antidepressants
(e.g. methylphenidate)
Reverse cell surface and vesicular transporters, triggering mono-amine release and inhibiting reuptake

Mono-amine oxidase inhibitors[a]
(e.g. moclobemide, phenelzine)
Reduce breakdown, diverting more mono-amine back to storage vesicles for subsequent release

desired action
(e.g. nerve growth factor production)

Receptor antagonists
(e.g. mirtazapine, trazodone)
Pre-synaptic[b]: disinhibits serotonin and noradrenaline (norepinephrine) release

Post-synaptic[c]: disinhibits mono-amine release elsewhere

inhibition of desired action
(e.g. mono-amine release elsewhere)

Figure I Predominant mechanism of action of antidepressants

a. mono-amine oxidase type A breaks down serotonin, noradrenaline (norepinephrine) and dopamine. Type B breaks down dopamine. Antidepressant-MAOIs are either non-selective (e.g. phenelzine) or type A selective (e.g. moclobemide). Antiparkinsonian MAOIs (e.g. selegiline) are Type B selective
b. blockade of pre-synaptic α-adrenergic receptors removes inhibition of serotonin and noradrenaline (norepinephrine) release
c. blockade of post-synaptic $5HT_{2A}$ and $5HT_{2C}$-receptors removes inhibition of dopamine and noradrenaline (norepinephrine) release from the post-synaptic neurone.

Depression

Although an increase in the synaptic concentration of mono-amines occurs within hours, the antidepressant effect is slower in onset because this requires normalization of receptor sensitivity *and* neuroplasticity.

Many of the early-onset undesirable effects from antidepressant drugs are a consequence of enhanced mono-amine transmission in the presence of receptors which have been unregulated to compensate for a relative mono-amine deficit. As receptor sensitivity returns to normal, these undesirable effects generally resolve and beneficial effects emerge.

Neuroplasticity is the ability of the CNS to adapt structurally and functionally in response to external stimuli and is mediated by nerve growth factors (e.g. brain-derived neurotrophic factor). In depression, neuroplasticity is impaired in the limbic and prefrontal cortex circuits which regulate mood, attention, energy, appetite and sleep. By enhancing mono-amine transmission, antidepressants help increase the production of nerve growth factors and restore neuroplasticity.[8]

Such circuits are affected to different degrees by various antidepressants. This may explain why refractory depression sometimes responds to a second-line antidepressant or combination treatment (see below) affecting different or multiple mono-amines.[9,10]

St John's wort (hypericum extract) is as effective as conventional antidepressants in treating mild–moderate depression and causes fewer undesirable effects.[11] However, NICE discourages its use because of:
- uncertainty about appropriate doses
- variation in the nature of products
- potential serious interactions with other drugs (including oral contraceptives, anticoagulants and anti-epileptics).[12]

Table 1 Transporter and receptor affinities for selected antidepressants[2-5]

	Re-uptake Transporters			Receptor affinities					
	5HT	NE[a]	DA	5HT$_{2A}$	5HT$_{2C}$	H$_I$	α$_I$	α$_2$	ACh$_M$
Agomelatine[b]				−	+	−	−	−	−
Amitriptyline	+++	++	−	+++	+++	+++	+++	+	+++
Bupropion	−	+	++	−	−	−	−	−	−
Citalopram	+++	−	−	−	−	−	−	−	−
Desipramine	+	+++	−	+	−	++	++	−	+
Duloxetine	+++	+++	+	−	−	−	−	−	−
Fluoxetine	+++	−	−	+	+	−	−	−	−
Imipramine	+++	+	−	+	+	+++	++	−	+/+++[c]
Lofepramine	+	+++	−	−	−	+	+	−	−/++[c]
Methylphenidate	−	−	++	−	−	−	−	−	−
Mirtazapine	−	−	−	++	++	+++	−	+++	−
Nortriptyline	+	+++	−	+++	+++	+++	++	−	++
Paroxetine	+++	+	−	−	−	−	−	−	+
Reboxetine	−	+++	−	−	−	−	−		−
Sertraline	+++	−	+	−	−	−	+	−	−
Trazodone	−	−	−	++	+	−	++	+	−
Venlafaxine	+	+[d]	−	−	−	−	−	−	−

Affinity: +++ high, ++ moderate, + low, − negligible or none; blank = no data.

a. the noradrenaline (norepinephrine) re-uptake transporter also clears dopamine in the prefrontal cortex where dopamine re-uptake transporters are absent. Reduced dopamine in the prefrontal cortex is related to anhedonia and inattention
b. agomelatine is also a melatonin (type 1 and 2) receptor agonist. Although animal models raise this as a target of possible interest, the contribution which this makes towards its clinical effects in humans is unclear
c. varies with different ACh$_m$ receptor subtypes
d. despite in vitro studies suggesting a relatively low affinity for serotonin and noradrenaline (norepinephrine) re-uptake transporters, in vivo studies suggest venlafaxine is a dual inhibitor. In vitro assays measure the ability of a drug to displace another compound of known affinity; it may be that venlafaxine binds to a different site on mono-amine re-uptake transporters and so cannot displace the reference compounds.[4]

Anxiety and panic disorder

Antidepressants and benzodiazepines inhibit the amygdala's 'fear circuits' through 5HT$_{1A}$ and GABA$_A$ receptors, respectively.[13,14] The amygdala is a threat sensor which integrates sensory information with contextual information (e.g. interpretations, memories). If a fear response is required, the amygdala's effector pathway activates the relevant circuits (respiratory and cardiovascular centres, pituitary-adrenal axis, sympathetic autonomic nervous system, and fear-related areas of the cerebral cortex).

Pain

The analgesic effects of antidepressants are due to enhanced mono-amine transmission in descending pain modulation pathways.[15,16] These pathways can induce both analgesia (noradrenergic/norepinephrinergic and serotoninergic activity) and hyperalgesia (serotoninergic activity).[17,18] The latter may explain both the inconsistent analgesic effect of SSRIs and why SNRIs appear no more effective than NRIs.[19] Sodium-channel blockade and NMDA-glutamate-receptor antagonism may also contribute to the analgesic efficacy of some antidepressants,[16] including the modest effect of topical doxepin.[20,21]

Urological symptoms

Antidepressants act through parasympatholytic and sympathomimetic mechanisms. Antimuscarinic-antidepressants (e.g. **amitriptyline**) inhibit detrusor stimulation and thus overactive bladder symptoms. Mono-amine re-uptake inhibitors (e.g. **duloxetine**, and possibly **amitriptyline**) enhance mono-amine transmission in descending bladder control pathways, thus stimulating the sympathetic fibres that control sphincter tone. This explains their (modest) effect on urinary incontinence.[22]

Table 2 Pharmacokinetic details for selected antidepressants[23–31]

	Bio-availability PO (%)	T_{max} (h)	Plasma halflife (h)	Metabolism
Agomelatine	>80	1–2	1–2	CYP1A2[a]
Amitriptyline	45	4	13–36	Multiple pathways[b] (nortriptyline[b])
Bupropion	>87	1.5	21	CYP2B6[b]
Citalopram	80[c]	3	36	Multiple pathways[b]
Desipramine	30–50	4–6	7–77	CYP2D6[a,b]
Duloxetine	90	6	12	CYP1A2, CYP2D6
Fluoxetine	90	4–8	1–4 days 7–15 days[b]	Multiple pathways[b]
Imipramine	45	3	21	Multiple pathways[b] (desipramine[b])
Lofepramine		1–2	1.6	Multiple pathways[b] (desipramine[b])
Methylphenidate	30	1–3	2	Non-CYP hepatic carboxylesterase[a]
Mirtazapine	50	2	20–40	CYP1A2, CYP2D6, CYP3A4
Nortriptyline	60	7–8.5	15–39	CYP2D6[a,b]
Paroxetine	50[d]	5	15–20	Multiple pathways
Reboxetine	95	2–4	12	CYP3A4
Sertraline	>44	6–8	26	CYP3A4
Trazodone	65	1	7	CYP2D6, CYP3A4[b]
Venlafaxine	13	2.5	5	CYP2D6, CYP3A4[b]
	45[e]	4.5–7.5[e]	11[b]	

Blank = no data.

a. significant first pass metabolism
b. active metabolite(s); listed in table if can be administered separately
c. tablet product: bio-availability of drops 25% higher
d. increases with multiple dosing
e. m/r product.

Cautions

In patients with a history of mania, antidepressants may precipitate a recurrent episode, particularly if administered without a mood stabilizer.

Suicide risk

The risk of antidepressant-related suicidal ideation needs to be balanced against the greater risk of non-fatal self harm and completed suicide from untreated depression.[32]

1 in 1,000 patients attempt suicide in the 6 months after starting antidepressants: one third are successful.[33] In those aged ≤25 years, antidepressants are associated with suicidal ideation and non-fatal self harm (NNH 143).[34,35] The risk is greater with SSRIs than TCAs,[36] and is present even when an antidepressant is used for non-depressive illnesses.[35] In adults ≥25 years old, there is a smaller increase in the risk of non-fatal self harm (NNH circa 700), no increase in suicidal thoughts or suicide, and no difference between SSRIs and TCAs.[36–38]

Suicidal ideation should be evaluated when treating depression in all age groups. Consider the safety in overdose of both the antidepressant and concomitant medicines. In both Europe and the USA, regulators have emphasized the need for close monitoring of adherence to treatment, treatment response, and emergence of thoughts of self harm, particularly during the first month after starting an antidepressant, and to encourage patients to report to their doctor any deterioration in mood or behaviour.[39,40]

Epilepsy

Antidepressants cause a dose-dependent reduction in seizure threshold. The risk is lowest for SSRIs, higher with TCAs, and highest with **clomipramine**, **bupropion** and **maprotiline**. There are fewer data and less experience with **mirtazapine** and **venlafaxine**. In patients with epilepsy, antidepressants may also cause seizures by altering anti-epileptic drug concentrations as a result of a drug–drug interaction.[41,42] Thus, **citalopram** is widely favoured for use in patients with epilepsy because of the low risk of reduction in seizure threshold and lack of significant interactions with anti-epileptic drugs. Antidepressants can also cause seizures through hyponatraemia.

It is hard to quantify the risk of using low-dose TCAs for neuropathic pain in patients with previous seizures because the risk is dose-related and animal studies even suggest a possible *anti*-epileptic action at low doses.[43]

Epilepsy is associated with both mood disorders and psychosis. Symptoms may occur in between (inter-ictal), during (ictal), or in the days or weeks after (post-ictal) seizures. Optimization of anti-epileptic medication should be considered alongside antidepressant treatment, particularly for ictal and post-ictal mood-related symptoms.[44] Further, anti-epileptic drugs can cause (and treat) mood disorders: seek specialist advice if negative mood changes occur after anti-epileptics are started.

Parkinson's disease

SSRIs can worsen extrapyramidal symptoms because serotonin reduces nigrostriatal dopamine release via inhibitory $5HT_2$ receptors. However, the risk appears small; few RCTs report any worsening.[45] SSRIs are thus still often used in preference to TCAs which can worsen autonomic dysfunction (α blockade) and cognitive impairment (ACh_M blockade).

$5HT_2$ antagonist antidepressants might be expected to avoid serotonin-mediated exacerbations. In small pilot RCTs, Parkinsonian symptoms improved with **nefazodone**[46] but not **mirtazapine**.[47] Antiparkinsonian D_2 agonists can themselves improve mood. In RCTs evaluating **pramipexole** for motor symptoms, mood and motivation also improved.[48] Further, in an RCT, **pramipexole** was more effective than **sertraline** for depression in patients with Parkinson's disease.[49]

Mono-amine oxidase inhibitors (MAOIs)

Included for general information. MAOIs are *not recommended* in palliative care. They can cause serious adverse events when prescribed concurrently with various other drugs. Seek advice from a psychiatrist if caring for a patient already receiving an MAOI; their previous mental illness is likely to have been difficult to treat and switching or adding other psychotropics is difficult and risky.

MAOIs are potentially dangerous because of the risk of serious dietary and drug interactions. Hypertensive crises are mainly associated with the consumption of tyramine-containing foods (Table 3). Typically, the patient experiences severe headache, and may suffer an intracranial haemorrhage. Drug interactions occur with sympathomimetics (e.g. **ephedrine, pseudoephedrine, dexamfetamine, nefopam**), serotoninergics (see below) and **levodopa**.

Table 3 Tyramine-containing foods associated with MAOI-related syndrome

Alcohol	Fava beans
red wine (white wine is safe)	Meat (smoked or pickled)
beer	Meat or yeast extracts
Broad bean pods	Pickled herring
Cheese (old)	

Toxicity has been reported with serotoninergic opioids (e.g. fentanils, **pethidine, tramadol**). However, although companies marketing **morphine** and **oxycodone** also advise against concurrent use, their affinity for the serotonin re-uptake transporter is negligible,[50] and toxicity has not been reported.[51] Insisting on a 2-week washout before treating pain is both unacceptable and unnecessary.

Drug interactions

MAOIs have numerous clinically significant drug interactions, which may result in hypertensive crises and serotonin toxicity.

Several pharmacodynamic interactions (e.g. serotonin toxicity, bleeding risk, antimuscarinic effects, QT prolongation with **citalopram** and **escitalopram**) can be predicted from the mode of action of antidepressants (see Box A and Table 1).

In addition, potentially serious interactions may result from induction or inhibition of hepatic metabolism. Some antidepressants inhibit cytochrome P450 enzymes:
- CYP1A2 inhibition by **fluvoxamine**, e.g. **tizanidine** levels increased ≤33 times
- CYP2D6 inhibition by **fluoxetine** and **paroxetine**, e.g. TCA levels increased ≤10 times; **paroxetine** may reduce the efficacy of **tamoxifen** (a pro-drug).[52]

The metabolism of some antidepressants is affected by P450 inhibitors and inducers:
- CYP2D6, most TCAs
- CYP3A4, **mirtazapine** (see Chapter 25, p.767).

Serotonin toxicity ('serotonin syndrome')

Serotonin toxicity results from the ingestion of drug(s) which increase brain serotonin to levels sufficient to cause severe symptoms necessitating hospital admission and medical intervention (see Box B and Box C).[53] It has been characterized as a triad of neuro-excitatory features:
- *autonomic hyperactivity*; sweating, fever, mydriasis, tachycardia, hypertension, tachypnoea, sialorrhoea, diarrhoea
- *neuromuscular hyperactivity*; tremor, clonus, myoclonus, hyperreflexia, and hypertonia (advanced stage)
- *altered mental status*; agitation, hypomania, and delirium (advanced stage).

The onset of toxicity is generally rapid and progressive, typically as a second serotoninergic drug reaches effective blood levels (e.g. after one or two doses). Occasionally, recurrent mild symptoms may occur for weeks before the development of severe toxicity. Clonus (inducible, spontaneous or ocular), agitation, sweating, tremor and hyperreflexia are essential features. Spontaneous clonus, in the presence of a serotoninergic drug, is the most reliable indicator of serotonin toxicity.[54] Neuromuscular signs are initially greater in the lower limbs, then become more generalized as toxicity increases. Other symptoms include shaking, shivering (and chattering of the teeth), and sometimes trismus. It can be distinguished from neuroleptic (antipsychotic) malignant syndrome by its faster onset and pyramidal rather than extrapyramidal neuromuscular findings.

Box B   Drugs with clinically relevant serotoninergic potency[50,53,55,56]

Antidepressants
Mono-amine oxidase inhibitors
Serotonin re-uptake inhibitors
  Selective (SSRIs)
  Dual (SNRIs; i.e. venlafaxine; duloxetine; TCAs, particularly clomipramine and imipramine)

Opioids
Dextromethorphan, dextropropoxyphene, fentanils, methadone, pentazocine, pethidine, tramadol (but *not* other opioids)

Other psychotropic drugs
Anti-emetic $5HT_3$ antagonists (including metoclopramide)
Psychostimulants
Selegiline (antiparkinsonian)
Sibutramine (anorectic)
Triptans ($5HT_1$ agonists e.g. sumatriptan)

Miscellaneous
Chlorphenamine, brompheniramine (but not reported with other H_1 antihistamines)
Furazolidone, linezolid (antibacterials)
Lithium
Methylene blue
Procarbazine (antineoplastic)

Box C   Treatment of serotonin toxicity[56]

In severe cases (e.g. rigidity, haemodynamic instability, temperature > 38.5° C, deteriorating blood gases) seek urgent advice from a critical care specialist: ventilation and paralysis ± inotropic support may be required.

Discontinue causal medication (toxicity generally resolves within 24h).

Provide supportive care, e.g. IV fluids, oxygen.

Symptomatic measures in mild–moderate cases:

• benzodiazepines for agitation, myoclonus and seizures, e.g. midazolam 5–10mg SC p.r.n.

• 5HT$_{2A}$ antagonist[a], e.g.:

   ▷ chlorpromazine 50–100mg IM *or*

   ▷ olanzapine 10mg IM (not UK) *or*

   ▷ cyproheptadine 12mg PO stat followed by 8mg q6h and 2mg q2h p.r.n. until symptoms resolve; tablets can be dispersed (or crushed if necessary) and given by enteral feeding tube (see Chapter 22, p.725).

---

a. prevents deaths from hyperpyrexia in animals and probably in humans. Generally give IM; the PO route is suitable only for mild toxicity and, in the case of overdose, in patients who have *not* received oral activated charcoal.[60,61]

Different drugs increase serotonin levels to differing degrees. An overdose of the older irreversible MAOI **tranylcypromine** alone will produce hyperpyrexia, and even death,[57] whereas overdoses of reversible MAOIs or SSRIs alone will cause serotoninergic effects but rarely (if ever) life-threatening serotonin toxicity.[58,59] Thus death from serotonin toxicity is generally associated with the combination of two different types of drug which elevate serotonin levels via different mechanisms of action (an MAOI combined with either an SSRI or a serotonin releaser).[58]

Opioids are relatively weak serotonin re-uptake inhibitors and may only cause symptoms in higher doses or susceptible individuals. Fatalities from serotonin toxicity involving opioids have been seen with **dextromethorphan, pethidine, tramadol**, and possibly **fentanyl**.[50]

Undesirable effects
A synopsis is contained in Table 4. Overall, discontinuation rates are marginally lower with SSRIs than with TCAs (NNT = 33, i.e. 1 less discontinuation for every 33 patients treated with an SSRI rather than a TCA).[62]

GI bleeding and platelet function
SSRIs and SNRIs (e.g. **amitriptyline, duloxetine, imipramine, venlafaxine**) decrease serotonin uptake from the blood by platelets. Because platelets do not synthesize serotonin, the amount of serotonin in platelets is reduced.[66] This reduces platelet aggregation.[67] After confounding factors have been controlled for, serotonin re-uptake inhibitors triple the risk of GI bleeding.[68,69] This may be important in already high-risk patients. If an antidepressant is indicated in such patients, safer alternatives would include an NRI (e.g. **nortriptyline**) or **mirtazapine**.

QT prolongation
Citalopram and **escitalopram** exhibit dose-related QT prolongation. Drug Regulatory Authorities recommend specific precautions and dose limits (see p.211). Other SSRIs appear less affected.[70,71]

Fracture risk
A number of observational studies found an increased fracture risk with SSRIs and TCAs.[72] The mechanism is uncertain; data regarding both the risk of falls and bone density is conflicting.

Table 4 Relative frequency and putative mechanisms of undesirable effects of antidepressants[63-65]

| Undesirable effect | mechanism | Relative frequency | | | | | | | | | | | | | |
| | | SNRI | | | | | NRI | | | SSRI | | | | RA | |
		Amitriptyline	Clomipramine	Duloxetine	Imipramine	Venlafaxine	Desipramine	Lofepramine	Nortriptyline	Citalopram	Fluoxetine	Paroxetine	Sertraline	Mirtazapine	Trazodone
GI (nausea, diarrhoea)	↑ Serotonin (acting on $5HT_3$)	–	+	++	–	++	–	–	–	++	++	++	++	–	–
CNS (agitation, restlessness, anxiety, insomnia)	↑ Serotonin (acting on $5HT_2$)	–	+	+	+	+	+	+	+	+	+	+	+	–	–
Weight gain	$5HT_2$ and H_1 antagonism	++	+	–	+	–	–	–	–	–	–	–	–	++	+
Sedation	H_1, ACh_M and α_1-adrenergic antagonism	++	+	–	+	–	+	–	+	–	–	–	–	++	++
Postural hypotension	α_1-adrenergic antagonism	++	++	–	++	–	+	+	+	–	–	–	–	–	++
Sexual dysfunction	↑ Serotonin (acting on $5HT_2$)	+	++	++	+	++	+	+	+	++	++	++	++	–	–
Dry mouth, constipation	ACh_M antagonism	++	++	–	++	–	+	+	+	–	–	–	–	–	–
SIADH	↑ Serotonin (acting on $5HT_2$); ↑ noradrenaline (norepinephrine) (acting on α_1)	+	+	+	+	+	+	+	+	++	++	++	++	+	+

++ = relatively common or strong; + = may occur or moderately strong; – = absent or rare/weak.

NRI = noradrenaline (norepinephrine) re-uptake inhibitor; SNRI = serotonin and noradrenaline (norepinephrine) re-uptake inhibitor; SSRI = selective serotonin re-uptake inhibitor; RA = receptor antagonist.

Dose and use

See individual monographs for doses and titration.

Neuropathic pain

Amitriptyline and **nortriptyline** are commonly used for neuropathic pain.[73,74–76] Most RCTs have been of **amitriptyline**, although **nortriptyline** was better tolerated when compared with **amitriptyline**.[19] **Bupropion, duloxetine, venlafaxine** and most other TCAs are also superior to placebo. In head to head comparisons, both **duloxetine** vs. **amitriptyline**,[77,78] and **venlafaxine** vs. **imipramine**[79] were comparable.[80]

SSRIs are modestly effective (3 of 4 RCTs),[81–84] but inferior to **imipramine**.[84] The benefit reported with **mirtazapine**[85] has *not* been confirmed in RCTs.

Alternatives to antidepressants include anti-epileptics[86] and opioids. Both direct comparisons[78,87–90] and a large network analysis[91] found the efficacy and tolerability of antidepressants (**amitriptyline, duloxetine** or **nortriptyline**) to be comparable with **gabapentin** or **pregabalin**.

When used together, **nortriptyline** and **gabapentin** were more effective than either drug alone.[92] **Nortriptyline** was as effective as **morphine**.[93]

Other pain syndromes

Antidepressants are of benefit for various other pain syndromes including migraine and tension headache (TCAs),[94] chronic low back pain (TCAs),[95] fibromyalgia (**amitriptyline, duloxetine, milnacipran**),[96] and osteo-arthritis (**duloxetine**).[97]

Depression

Treatment is tailored to the severity of symptoms, their functional impact and patient preference (Figure 2; also see Quick Prescribing Guide: Depression, p.206). First-line drug treatment is generally with **sertraline** or **citalopram**. They have fewer drug interactions, lower risk in overdose, and are marginally better tolerated than alternatives.[12] Efficacy has been confirmed in palliative populations.[98] Frequent re-evaluation of response, adherence, and alternative and concurrent sources of distress is required throughout.

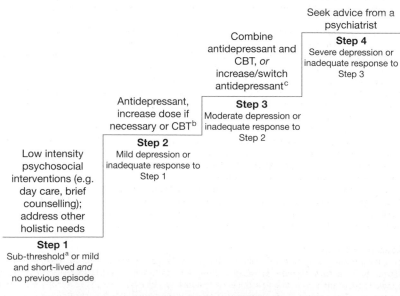

Figure 2 Overview of the management of depression.[12,105]

a. sub-threshold symptoms = patients with <5 DSM IV symptoms required for a diagnosis of depression
b. CBT = cognitive-behavioural therapy
c. see below, managing an inadequate initial response.

Methylphenidate, with its rapid onset, may be preferable in patients with a very short prognosis, e.g. 2–4 weeks. This is shorter than suggested by consensus guidance[99] because of the recognition that conventional antidepressants act faster than previously thought.[100] However, trials of psychostimulants have been limited by their short duration, use of outcome measures of uncertain clinical significance and inclusion of patients that did not meet the diagnostic criteria for depression.[99,101–104] Thus, conventional antidepressants should be used if the patient has a sufficient prognosis for a response to manifest. Concurrent use with a conventional antidepressant may hasten the response compared with the latter alone, particularly in relation to fatigue.[104] **Modafinil** can be used if methylphenidate is poorly tolerated. A rapid but temporary antidepressant effect (i.e. onset within 1h, duration 1–2 weeks) is also seen following a single dose of **ketamine** (see p.625); studies of various NMDA-receptor antagonists are ongoing.

Although an SNRI or NRI may be considered if depression and neuropathic pain co-exist, slower titration is required to avoid higher rates of discontinuation[12] They are therefore often treated separately (e.g. with an SSRI plus either **gabapentin** or **nortriptyline**).

Titrating, switching and combining antidepressants
If there is no response after 4 weeks, or only a partial response after 6–8 weeks:
- increase the dose, particularly if there has been a partial response and minimal undesirable effects or
- switch antidepressants, particularly if there has been minimal improvement or bothersome undesirable effects or
- combine with a second antidepressant or adjuvant psychotropic drug, particularly if a previous switch was unhelpful.[12]

Dose titration is straightforward but, for SSRIs, of uncertain value. A systematic review found dose titration in patients not responding to SSRIs taken for 3–6 weeks no more effective than continuing the dose unaltered.[106] Nonetheless, many guidelines highlight individual variation in effective doses and therefore recommend dose titration if the existing drug is well tolerated.[12,64] A dose-response effect is more clearly established with some TCAs and venlafaxine.

The efficacy of second-line antidepressants appears comparable regardless of mode of action.[64,107,108] Options include an alternative SSRI or **mirtazapine**. One SSRI can be directly substituted for another without cross-tapering or a washout period.[64,108] **Mirtazapine** 15mg can be directly substituted for SSRIs at usual doses (**fluoxetine, citalopram** or **paroxetine** 20mg; **sertraline** 50mg).[64,109]

Opinion varies on the need to taper higher SSRI doses before switching.[107,109] Switching SSRIs is most effective when the first SSRI is poorly tolerated but benefit is also seen in non-responders,[108] perhaps because of differing additional actions (see Table 1, p.212). The effect of **mirtazapine** on additional mono-amines is theoretically advantageous; its onset may be faster.[110]

Venlafaxine has a marginally higher response rate (NNT = 10) compared with switching to a second SSRI[108] but is less well tolerated. Switching to or from TCAs and MAOIs requires additional care because of the potential for clinically significant pharmacokinetic or pharmacodynamic drug interactions, respectively (see above).[111]

A partial response to an antidepressant can be increased ('augmented') by adding a second psychotropic drug. This avoids potential loss of the initial improvement but is generally less well tolerated than monotherapy.[12] Options include:
- an antipsychotic (e.g. **aripiprazole, quetiapine** or **olanzapine** added to an SSRI)
- **mirtazapine** (added to an SSRI or **venlafaxine**)
- a range of options used only by psychiatrists (e.g. **lithium, tri-iodothyronine**).

NICE suggests primary care clinicians seek advice before adding a second drug.[12] Palliative care specialists using some of the above for other indications should be aware of their potential benefit when concurrent depression has only partially responded to an antidepressant.[64,112]

Duration of treatment
Consider stopping treatment 6 months after full remission in those without risk factors for relapse. Risk factors include previous depression and the severity, duration, degree of treatment resistance, and the presence of residual symptoms. Treatment is tapered slowly (see below). Treat those with risk factors for longer: 1 year if full remission but one risk factor; and ≥2 years if ≥2 risk factors.[12,64] In palliative care, the latter is likely to mean lifelong/indefinitely.

Anxiety and panic disorders

The efficacy of cognitive behavioural and drug therapy is comparable.[113] Drug treatment is tailored to the likely duration of use:
• benzodiazepine, if prognosis is days to weeks
• SSRI (± a benzodiazepine initially), if prognosis is months.

Supporting evidence (and market authorization) for SSRIs varies for different anxiety disorders.[114] **Citalopram** and **sertraline** are authorized for panic disorder, well tolerated, have fewer drug interactions, and are generally more familiar to prescribers. All SSRIs can initially exacerbate anxiety: start low and consider a concurrent benzodiazepine for the first few weeks.

If response is inadequate, combine with cognitive behavioural therapy (evidence best for panic disorder)[113] or switch to an alternative SSRI or SNRI.[114,115] In general psychiatry, switching is not advocated within 3 months because benefit can take longer to manifest than in depression.[114,115] However, in patients with a short prognosis, consider adding a benzodiazepine to obtain more rapid benefit. **Pregabalin** also acts quickly but is reserved for patients not responding to antidepressants; supporting trials are fewer, mainly confined to generalized anxiety disorder and response rates appear lower than for SSRIs and benzodiazepines.[114,116]

Agitated delirium

The benefit reported with **trazodone**[117] remains unconfirmed in clinical trials. Treatment of underlying causes, non-drug management (e.g. orientation strategies, correction of sensory deprivation) and prevention of complications are central to delirium management. Antipsychotics are generally used first-line when medication is needed.[118]

Agitation and challenging behaviours in dementia

Evidence for antidepressants is even more limited than for antipsychotics, and insufficient to justify routine use.[119,120] Larger studies have not replicated the earlier benefit reported for **trazodone**.[119,121]

Sweating

Like other antimuscarinics, **amitriptyline** is used for paraneoplastic sweating unresponsive to NSAIDs.[122] However, like all mono-amine reuptake inhibitors, it can also *cause* sweating.[123]

Hot flushes

Venlafaxine and SSRIs are of benefit in hot flushes associated with the menopause, hormone therapy and androgen ablation therapy for prostate cancer.[124,125]

Insomnia

When insomnia co-exists with other indications, sedating antidepressants are often selected (e.g. TCAs, **mirtazapine**, **trazodone**). **Doxepin** 3–6mg at bedtime PO improves both sleep latency and fragmentation in primary insomnia. Benefit is sustained for ≥12 weeks without rebound insomnia after discontinuation.[126] **Trazodone** is commonly used, although evidence is limited.[127]

Pruritus

Two small RCTs suggest benefit within a few days from **sertraline** (cholestatic pruritus)[128] and **paroxetine** (pruritus of mixed cause in cancer patients).[129] Benefit is also reported in pruritus in polycythemia vera.[130] **Mirtazapine** is reported to improve pruritus of mixed cause in advanced disease.[131] Like other H₁ antagonists, **doxepin** can be used for histamine-mediated pruritus and/ or for night sedation.

Bladder spasm, stress incontinence and urgency

Antimuscarinic antidepressants (e.g. **amitriptyline**) reduce detrusor contractions associated with urgency, although licensed alternatives have additional direct effects on the detrusor muscle.[132] **Duloxetine** has a limited role in stress incontinence.[133]

Pathological laughter and crying

Frequent brief uncontrollable laughter and/or crying incongruent with external events can complicate numerous neurological disorders, including strokes, Parkinson's disease, cerebral tumours, multiple sclerosis, MND/ALS, and dementia. It can be socially disabling. Functional

imaging suggests dysregulation of serotoninergic and other mono-aminergic pathways. The differential diagnosis includes:
- seizures: generally complex partial seizures and thus an alteration of consciousness during/after episodes
- depression or other mood disorders: mood alteration is persistent whereas the emotion that may accompany pathological laughter and crying is short-lived.

Validated assessment tools are available to aid diagnosis.[134] First-line treatment is with **citalopram** or **sertraline**; doses can be lower than those required for depression. Benefit is often seen within days. Second-line options include **amitriptyline, imipramine, nortriptyline** and **levodopa**.[135]

Drooling
Like other antimuscarinics, **amitriptyline** reduces salivation.[136]

Stopping antidepressants
Abrupt cessation of antidepressant therapy (particularly an MAOI) after regular administration for >8 weeks may result in a discontinuation reaction (withdrawal syndrome).[137] Discontinuation reactions depend on the class of antidepressant, and are more common with drugs with shorter half-lives (Box D). Thus, with SSRIs, they are most common with **paroxetine** and least common with **fluoxetine**.

Box D   Antidepressant discontinuation reactions[137]

SSRIs and venlafaxine: 'FINISH'[138]
Flu-like symptoms (fatigue, lethargy, myalgia, chills)
Insomnia (including vivid dreams)
Nausea
Imbalance (ataxia, vertigo, dizziness)
Sensory disturbances (paraesthesia, sensations of electric shock)
Hyperarousal (restlessness, anxiety, agitation)

TCAs
Flu-like symptoms (fatigue, lethargy, myalgia, chills)
Insomnia (including vivid dreams)
GI disorders (nausea, diarrhoea)
Mood disorders (depression or mania)
Movement disorders (rare: akathisia, parkinsonism)

Trazodone
Flu-like symptoms (fatigue, lethargy, myalgia, chills)
GI disorders (nausea, diarrhoea)
Restlessness
Tremor
Headache

Mirtazapine
Nausea
Dizziness
Hyperarousal (anxiety, agitation)
Headache

MAOIs
Insomnia
Movement disorders (ataxia, athetosis, catatonia, myoclonus)
Mood disorders (lability, depression, agitation, aggression)
Paranoia
Hallucinations
Seizures
Altered speech (pressured, slow)

Discontinuation reactions differ from a depressive relapse or a panic disorder. They generally start abruptly within a few days of stopping the antidepressant (*or reducing its dose*). In contrast, a depressive relapse is uncommon in the first week after stopping an antidepressant, and symptoms tend to build up gradually and persist. Discontinuation reactions generally resolve within 24h of re-instating antidepressant therapy, whereas the response is slower with a depressive relapse.

Ideally, antidepressants taken for >8 weeks should be progressively reduced over 4 weeks. If a mild discontinuation reaction is suspected, re-assurance alone may be adequate. If distressing, restart the antidepressant and reduce more gradually.

Some patients experience discontinuation symptoms even during tapering. When this happens, increase the dose and, before continuing with tapering, consider:
- using a liquid formulation and reducing the dose in smaller steps *or*
- switching from **venlafaxine** or a short half-life SSRI to **fluoxetine**.[137]

1 Stahl SM (2008) Psychosis and schizophrenia. In: *Essential Psychopharmacology: Neuroscientific Basis and Practical Applications* (3e). Cambridge University Press, USA, pp. 247–325.
2 NIMH (National Institute of Mental Health) (2006) Psychoactive Drug Screening Program. University of North Carolina. Available from: http://pdsp.med.unc.edu
3 Stahl SM et al. (2004) A Review of the Neuropharmacology of Bupropion, a Dual Norepinephrine and Dopamine Reuptake Inhibitor. *Primary Care Companion Journal of Clinical Psychiatry.* 6: 159–166.
4 Beique JC et al. (1998) Affinities of venlafaxine and various reuptake inhibitors for the serotonin and norepinephrine transporters. *European Journal of Pharmacology.* 349: 129–132.
5 Hamon M and Bourgoin S (2006) Pharmacological profile of antidepressants: a likely basis for their efficacy and side effects? *European Neuropsychopharmacology.* 16(Suppl 5): s625–s632.
6 Porcelli S et al. (2012) Meta-analysis of serotonin transporter gene promoter polymorphism (5-HTTLPR) association with antidepressant efficacy. *European Neuropsychopharmacology.* 22: 239–258.
7 Kirchheiner J and Rodriguez-Antona C (2009) Cytochrome P450 2D6 genotyping: potential role in improving treatment outcomes in psychiatric disorders. *CNS Drugs.* 23: 181–191.
8 Masi G and Brovedani P (2011) The hippocampus, neurotrophic factors and depression: possible implications for the pharmacotherapy of depression. *CNS Drugs.* 25: 913–931.
9 Belmaker RH and Agam G (2008) Major depressive disorder. *New England Journal of Medicine.* 358: 55–68.
10 Tran PV et al. (2003) Dual monoamine modulation for improved treatment of major depressive disorder. *Journal of Clinical Psychopharmacology.* 23: 78–86.
11 Linde (2008) St John's wort for major depression. *Cochrane Database of Systematic Reviews.* 4: CD000448.
12 NICE (2009) Depression. *Clinical Guidelines.* CG90 and CG91. www.nice.org.uk
13 Akimova E et al. (2009) The serotonin-1A receptor in anxiety disorders. *Biological Psychiatry.* 66: 627–635.
14 Maron E and Shlik J (2006) Serotonin function in panic disorder: important, but why? *Neuropsychopharmacology.* 31: 1–11.
15 Nickel FT et al. (2012) Mechanisms of neuropathic pain. *European Neuropsychopharmacology.* 22: 81–91.
16 McCleane G (2008) Antidepressants as analgesics. *CNS Drugs.* 22: 139–156.
17 Heinricher MM et al. (2009) Descending control of nociception: Specificity, recruitment and plasticity. *Brain Research Reviews.* 60: 214–225.
18 Dogrul A et al. (2009) Differential mediation of descending pain facilitation and inhibition by spinal 5HT-3 and 5HT-7 receptors. *Brain Research Molecular Brain Research.* 1280: 52–59.
19 Watson CP et al. (1998) Nortriptyline versus amitriptyline in postherpetic neuralgia: a randomized trial. *Neurology.* 51: 1166–1171.
20 McCleane G (2000) Topical application of doxepin hydrochloride, capsaicin and a combination of both produces analgesia in chronic human neuropathic pain: a randomized, double-blind, placebo-controlled study. *British Journal of Clinical Pharmacology.* 49: 574–579.
21 McCleane (1999) Topical doxepin hydrochloride reduces neuropathic pain: a randomised, double-blind, placebo-controlled study. *Pain Clinic.* 12: 47–50.
22 Deepak P and Kumar TN (2011) Duloexetine - pharmacological aspects. *International Journal of Biological and Medical Research.* 2: 589–592.
23 Wen B et al. (2008) Detection of novel reactive metabolites of trazodone: evidence for CYP2D6-mediated bioactivation of m-chlorophenylpiperazine. *Drug Metabolism and Disposition.* 36: 841–850.
24 Jefferson JW et al. (2005) Bupropion for major depressive disorder: Pharmacokinetic and formulation considerations. *Clinical Therapeutics.* 27: 1685–1695.
25 Hiemke (2000) Pharmacokinetics of selective serotonin reuptake inhibitors. *Pharmacology and Therapeutics.* 85: 11–28.
26 Fleishaker JC (2000) Clinical pharmacokinetics of reboxetine, a selective norepinephrine reuptake inhibitor for the treatment of patients with depression. *Clinical Pharmacokinetics.* 39: 413–427.
27 Venkatakrishnan K et al. (1998) Five distinct human cytochromes mediate amitriptyline N-demethylation in vitro: dominance of CYP 2C19 and 3A4. *Journal of Clinical Pharmacology.* 38: 112–121.
28 Richelson E (1997) Pharmacokinetic drug interactions of new antidepressants: A review of the effects on the metabolism of other drugs. *Mayo Clinic Proceedings.* 72: 835–847.
29 Kaye CM et al. (1989) A review of the metabolism and pharmacokinetics of paroxetine in man. *Acta Psychiatrica Scandinavica Supplementum.* 350: 60–75.
30 Schulz P et al. (1985) Discrepancies between pharmacokinetic studies of amitriptyline. *Clinical Pharmacokinetics.* 10: 257–268.
31 Abernethyl DR et al. (1984) Absolute bioavailability of imipramine: influence of food. *Psychopharmacology (Berl).* 83: 104–106.
32 Freeman SA (2009) Suicide risk and psychopharmacology: assessment and management of acute and chronic risk factors. *Journal of Clinical Psychiatry.* 70: 1052–1053.
33 Simon GE et al. (2006) Suicide risk during antidepressant treatment. *American Journal of Psychiatry.* 163: 41–47.

34 Stone M et al. (2009) Risk of suicidality in clinical trials of antidepressants in adults: analysis of proprietary data submitted to US Food and Drug Administration. British Medical Journal. 339: b2880.

35 Bridge JA et al. (2007) Clinical response and risk for reported suicidal ideation and suicide attempts in pediatric antidepressant treatment: a meta-analysis of randomized controlled trials. Journal of the American Medical Association. 297: 1683–1696.

36 Martinez C et al. (2005) Antidepressant treatment and the risk of fatal and non-fatal self harm in first episode depression: nested case-control study. British Medical Journal. 330: 389.

37 Gunnell D et al. (2005) Selective serotonin reuptake inhibitors (SSRIs) and suicide in adults: meta-analysis of drug company data from placebo controlled, randomised controlled trials submitted to the MHRA's safety review, British Medical Journal. 330: 385.

38 Fergusson D et al. (2005) Association between suicide attempts and selective serotonin reuptake inhibitors: systematic review of randomised controlled trials. British Medical Journal. 330: 396.

39 MHRA (2007) Antidepressants: suicidal behaviour. Drug Safety Update. 1. www.mhra.gov.uk/safetyinformation

40 Reeves RR and Ladner ME (2010) Antidepressant-induced suicidality: an update. CNS Neuroscience and Therapeutics. 16: 227–234.

41 Kerr MP et al. (2011) International consensus clinical practice statements for the treatment of neuropsychiatric conditions associated with epilepsy. Epilepsia. 52: 2133–2138.

42 Harden CL et al. (2002) Mood disorders in patients with epilepsy: epidemiology and management. CNS Drugs. 16: 291–302.

43 Dailey JW and Naritoku DK (1996) Antidepressants and seizures: clinical anecdotes overshadow neuroscience. Biochemical Pharmacology. 52: 1323–1329.

44 Blumer D et al. (2004) The interictal dysphoric disorder: recognition, pathogenesis, and treatment of the major psychiatric disorder of epilepsy. Epilepsy and Behaviour. 5: 826–840.

45 Skapinakis P et al. (2010) Efficacy and acceptability of selective serotonin reuptake inhibitors for the treatment of depression in Parkinson's disease: a systematic review and meta-analysis of randomized controlled trials. BMC Neurology. 10: 49.

46 Avila A et al. (2003) Does nefazodone improve both depression and Parkinson disease? A pilot randomized trial. Journal of Clinical Psychopharmacology. 23: 509–513.

47 Zhang LS et al. (2006) Mirtazapine vs fluoxetine in treatng Parkinson's disease with depression and anxiety. Medical Journal of Chinese People's Health. DOI: CNKI:SUN:ZMYX.0.2006-2023-2001.

48 Leentjens AF et al. (2009) The effect of pramipexole on mood and motivational symptoms in Parkinson's disease: a meta-analysis of placebo-controlled studies. Clinical Therapeutics. 31: 89–98.

49 Barone P et al. (2006) Pramipexole versus sertraline in the treatment of depression in Parkinson's disease: a national multicenter parallel-group randomized study. Journal of Neurology. 253: 601–607.

50 Gillman PK (2005) Monoamine oxidase inhibitors, opioid analgesics and serotonin toxicity. British Journal of Anaesthesia. 95: 434–441.

51 Baxter K and Preston CL (2011). Stockley's Drug Interactions. London:- Pharmaceutical Press www.medicinescomplete.com (accessed June 2013).

52 Kelly CM et al. (2010) Selective serotonin reuptake inhibitors and breast cancer mortality in women receiving tamoxifen: a population based cohort study. British Medical Journal. 340: c693.

53 Gillman K (2006) Serotonin toxicity, serotonin syndrome. Psycho Tropical Research. www.psychotropical.com (accessed April 2013).

54 Dunkley EJ et al. (2003) The Hunter Serotonin Toxicity Criteria: simple and accurate diagnostic decision rules for serotonin toxicity. Quarterly Journal of Medicine. 96: 635–642.

55 Gillman PK (2006) A review of serotonin toxicity data: implications for the mechanisms of antidepressant drug action. Biological Psychiatry. 59: 1046–1051.

56 Boyer EW and Shannon M (2005) The serotonin syndrome. New England Journal of Medicine. 352: 1112–1120.

57 Whyte I (2004) Monoamine oxidase inhibitors. In: RC Dart (ed) Medical Toxicology. Lippincott Williams & Wilkins, Baltimore, pp. 823–834.

58 Isbister GK et al. (2003) Moclobemide poisoning: toxicokinetics and occurrence of serotonin toxicity. British Journal of Clinical Pharmacology. 56: 441–450.

59 Isbister GK et al. (2004) Relative toxicity of selective serotonin reuptake inhibitors (SSRIs) in overdose. Journal of Toxicology and Clinical Toxicology. 42: 277–285.

60 Gillman PK (1999) The serotonin syndrome and its treatment. Journal of Psychopharmacology. 13: 100–109.

61 Gillman PK (1998) Serotonin syndrome: history and risk. Fundamental and Clinical Pharmacology. 12: 482–491.

62 Anderson IM (2000) Selective serotonin reuptake inhibitors versus tricyclic antidepressants: a meta-analysis of efficacy and tolerability. Journal of Affective Disorders. 58: 19–36.

63 Bhuvaneswar CG et al. (2009) Adverse endocrine and metabolic effects of psychotropic drugs: selective clinical review. CNS Drugs. 23: 1003–1021.

64 Anderson IM et al. (2008) Evidence-based guidelines for treating depressive disorders with antidepressants: a revision of the 2000 British Association for Psychopharmacology guidelines. Journal of Psychopharmacology. 22: 343–396.

65 Jacob S and Spinler SA (2006) Hyponatremia associated with selective serotonin-reuptake inhibitors in older adults. Annals of Pharmacotherapy. 40: 1618–1622.

66 Ross S et al. (1980) Inhibition of 5-hydroxytryptamine uptake in human platelets by antidepressant agents in vivo. Psychopharmacology. 67: 1–7.

67 Li N et al. (1997) Effects of serotonin on platelet activation in whole blood. Blood Coagulation Fibrinolysis. 8: 517–523.

68 vanWalraven C et al. (2001) Inhibition of serotonin reuptake by antidepressants and upper gastrointestinal bleeding in elderly patients: retrospective cohort study. British Medical Journal. 323: 655–657.

69 Paton C and Ferrier IN (2005) SSRIs and gastrointestinal bleeding. British Medical Journal. 331: 529–530.

70 Isbister GK et al. (2004) Relative toxicity of selective serotonin reuptake inhibitors (SSRIs) in overdose. Clinical Toxicology. 42: 277–285.

71 Castro VM et al. (2013) QT interval and antidepressant use: a cross sectional study of electronic health records. British Medical Journal. 346: f288.

72 European Medicines Agency (2010) Pharmacovigilance working party March 2010 plenary meeting report. Available from: http://www.emea.europa.eu/docs/en_GB/document_library/Report/2010/04/WC500088721.pdf

73 Palliativedrugs.com (2009) Survey Jan-Feb 2009. Available from: www.palliativedrugs.com

74 Saarto T and Wiffen PJ (2007) Antidepressants for neuropathic pain. Cochrane Database of Systematic Reviews. CD005454.

75 Dworkin RH et al. (2007) Pharmacologic management of neuropathic pain: evidence-based recommendations. [see comment]. Pain. 132: 237–251.
76 Finnerup NB et al. (2005) Algorithm for neuropathic pain treatment: an evidence based proposal. [see comment]. Pain. 118: 289–305.
77 Kaur H et al. (2011) A comparative evaluation of amitriptyline and duloxetine in painful diabetic neuropathy: a randomized, double-blind, cross-over clinical trial. Diabetes Care. 34: 818–822.
78 Boyle J et al. (2012) Randomized, placebo-controlled comparison of amitriptyline, duloxetine, and pregabalin in patients with chronic diabetic peripheral neuropathic pain: impact on pain, polysomnographic sleep, daytime functioning, and quality of life. Diabetes Care. 35: 2451–2458.
79 Sindrup SH et al. (2003) Venlafaxine versus imipramine in painful polyneuropathy: a randomized, controlled trial. Neurology. 60: 1284–1289.
80 Watson CP et al. (2011) Nontricyclic antidepressant analgesics and pain: are serotonin norepinephrine reuptake inhibitors (SNRIs) any better? Pain. 152: 2206–2210.
81 Otto M et al. (2008) Escitalopram in painful polyneuropathy: a randomized, placebo-controlled, cross-over trial. Pain. 139: 275–283.
82 Sindrup SH et al. (1992) The selective serotonin reuptake inhibitor citalopram relieves the symptoms of diabetic neuropathy. Clinical Pharmacology and Therapeutics. 52: 547–552.
83 Max M et al. (1992) Effects of desipramine, amitriptyline, and fluoxetine on pain in diabetic neuropathy. New England Journal of Medicine. 326: 1287–1288.
84 Sindrup S et al. (1990) The selective serotonin re-uptake inhibitor paroxetine is effective in the treatment of diabetic neuropathy symptoms. Pain. 42: 135–144.
85 Christodoulou C et al. (2010) Effectiveness of mirtazapine in the treatment of postherpetic neuralgia. Journal of Pain and Symptom Management. 39: e3–6.
86 Howard P et al. (2011) Anti-epileptic drugs. Journal of Pain and Symptom Management. 42: 788–804.
87 Bansal D et al. (2009) Amitriptyline vs. pregabalin in painful diabetic neuropathy: a randomized double blind clinical trial. Diabetic Medicine. 26: 1019–1026.
88 Morello C et al. (1999) Randomized double-blind study comparing the efficacy of gabapentin with amitriptyline on diabetic peripheral neuropathy pain. Archives of Internal Medicine. 159: 1931–1937.
89 Chandra K et al. (2006) Gabapentin versus nortriptyline in post-herpetic neuralgia patients: a randomized, double-blind clinical trial–the GONIP Trial. International Journal of Clinical Pharmacology and Therapeutics. 44: 358–363.
90 Mishra S et al. (2012) A comparative efficacy of amitriptyline, gabapentin, and pregabalin in neuropathic cancer pain: a prospective randomized double-blind placebo-controlled study. American Journal of Hospice and Palliative Care. 29: 177–182.
91 NICE (2013) Neuropathic pain update consultation - appendix G. www.nice.org.uk
92 Gilron I et al. (2009) Nortriptyline and gabapentin, alone and in combination for neuropathic pain: a double-blind, randomised controlled crossover trial. Lancet. 374: 1252–1261.
93 Raja SN et al. (2002) Opioids versus antidepressants in postherpetic neuralgia: a randomized, placebo-controlled trial. [see comment]. Neurology. 59: 1015–1021.
94 Jackson JL et al. (2010) Tricyclic antidepressants and headaches: systematic review and meta-analysis. British Medical Journal. 341: c5222.
95 Staiger TO et al. (2003) Systematic review of antidepressants in the treatment of chronic low back pain. Spine (Phila Pa 1976). 28: 2540–2545.
96 Hauser W et al. (2012) The role of antidepressants in the management of fibromyalgia syndrome: a systematic review and meta-analysis. CNS Drugs. 26: 297–307.
97 Chappell AS et al. (2009) Duloxetine, a centrally acting analgesic, in the treatment of patients with osteoarthritis knee pain: a 13-week, randomized, placebo-controlled trial. Pain. 146: 253–260.
98 Rayner L et al. (2011) Antidepressants for the treatment of depression in palliative care: systematic review and meta-analysis. Palliative Medicine. 25: 36–51.
99 Block SD (2000) Assessing and managing depression in the terminally ill patient. ACP-ASIM End-of-Life Care Consensus Panel. American College of Physicians - American Society of Internal Medicine. Annals of internal medicine. 132: 209–218.
100 Tylee A and Walters P (2007) Onset of action of antidepressants. British Medical Journal. 334: 911–912.
101 Rayner L and Hotopf. M (2012) Better - but good enough? the first randomised controlled trial of psychostimulants for depressive symptoms in advanced cancer. BMJ Supportive and Palliative Care. 2: 290–291.
102 Centeno C et al. (2012) Multi-centre, double-blind, randomised placebo-controlled clinical trial on the efficacy of methylphenidate on depressive symptoms in advanced cancer patients. BMJ Supportive and Palliative Care. 2: 328–333.
103 Candy M et al. (2008) Psychostimulants for depression. Cochrane Database of Systematic Reviews. 2: CD006722.
104 Orr K and Taylor D (2007) Psychostimulants in the treatment of depression : a review of the evidence. CNS Drugs. 21: 239–257.
105 Rayner L et al. (2011) The development of evidence-based European guidelines on the management of depression in palliative cancer care. European Journal of Cancer. 47: 702–712.
106 dli M et al. (2005) Is dose escalation of antidepressants a rational strategy after a medium-dose treatment has failed? A systematic review. European Archives of Psychiatry and Clinical Neuroscience. 255: 387–400.
107 Rush AJ et al. (2009) STAR*D: revising conventional wisdom. CNS Drugs. 23: 627–647.
108 Ruhe HG et al. (2006) Switching antidepressants after a first selective serotonin reuptake inhibitor in major depressive disorder: a systematic review. Journal of Clinical Psychiatry. 67: 1836–1855.
109 Fava GA and Mangelli L (2001) Assessment of subclinical symptoms and psychological well-being in depression. European Archives of Psychiatry and Clinical Neuroscience. 251(Suppl 2): II47–52.
110 Watanabe N et al. (2011) Mirtazapine versus other antidepressive agents for depression. Cochrane Database of Systematic Reviews. 12: CD006528.
111 Taylor (2007) The Maudsley Prescribing Guidelines (9e). Informa Healthcare, London.
112 Shelton RC et al. (2010) Therapeutic options for treatment-resistant depression. CNS Drugs. 24: 131–161.
113 Bandelow B et al. (2007) Meta-analysis of randomized controlled comparisons of psychopharmacological and psychological treatments for anxiety disorders. World Journal of Biological Psychiatry. 8: 175–187.
114 Baldwin DS et al. (2005) Evidence-based guidelines for the pharmacological treatment of anxiety disorders: recommendations from the British Association for Psychopharmacology. Journal of Psychopharmacology. 19: 567–596.

115 NICE (2011) Generalised anxiety disorder and panic disorder (with or without agoraphobia) in adults: Management in primary, secondary and community care *Clinical Guideline*. CG113. www.nice.org.uk

116 Baldwin (2011) Efficacy of drug treatments for generalised anxiety disorder: systemic review and meta-analysis. *British Medical Journal*. **342**: 1199.

117 Okamoto Y et al. (1999) Trazodone in the treatment of delirium. *Journal of Clinical Psychopharmacology*. **19**: 280–282.

118 Howard P et al. (2011) Antipsychotics. *Journal of Pain and Symptom Management*. **41**: 956–965.

119 Jeste DV et al. (2008) ACNP White Paper: Update on Use of Antipsychotic Drugs in Elderly Persons with Dementia. *Neuropsychopharmacology*. **33**: 957 970.

120 Sink KM et al. (2005) Pharmacological treatment of neuropsychiatric symptoms of dementia: a review of the evidence. *Journal of the American Medical Association*. **293**: 596–608.

121 Seitz D et al. (2011) Antidepressants for agitation and psychosis in dementia. *Cochrane Database of Systematic Reviews*. CD008191.

122 Twycross R et al. (2009) *Symptom Management in Advanced Cancer* (4e). palliativedrugs.com, Nottingham, pp. 331–334.

123 Marcy TR and Britton ML (2005) Antidepressant-induced sweating. *Annals of Pharmacotherapy*. **39**: 748–752.

124 Rada G (2010) Non-hormonal interventions for hot flashes in women with a history of breast cancer. *Cochrane Database of Systematic Reviews*. **2**: CD004923.

125 Quella S et al. (1999) Pilot evaluation of venlafaxine for the treatment of hot flashes in men undergoing androgen ablation therapy for prostate cancer. *Journal of Urology*. **162**: 98–102.

126 Weber J et al. (2010) Low-dose doxepin: in the treatment of insomnia. *CNS Drugs*. **24**: 713–720.

127 Mendelson WB (2005) A review of the evidence for the efficacy and safety of trazodone in insomnia. *Journal of Clinical Psychiatry*. **66**: 469–476.

128 Mayo MJ et al. (2007) Sertraline as a first-line treatment for cholestatic pruritus. *Hepatology*. **45**: 666–674.

129 Zylicz Z et al. (2003) Paroxetine in the treatment of severe non-dermatological pruritus: a randomized, controlled trial. *Journal of Pain and Symptom Management*. **26**: 1105–1112.

130 Tefferi A and Fonseca R (2002) Selective serotonin reuptake inhibitors are effective in the treatment of polycythemia vera-associated pruritus. *Blood*. **99**: 2627.

131 Zylicz Z et al. (eds) (2004) *Pruritus in Advanced Disease*. Oxford University Press, Oxford.

132 Twycross R et al. (2009) *Symptom Management in Advanced Cancer* (4e). palliativdrugs.com, Nottingham, pp. 289-296.

133 NICE (2006) Urinary incontinence: the management of urinary incontinence in women. *Clinical Guideline*. CG40. www.nice.org.uk

134 Robinson RG et al. (1993) Pathological laughing and crying following stroke: validation of a measurement scale and a double-blind treatment study. *American Journal of Psychiatry*. **150**: 286–293.

135 Wortzel HS et al. (2008) Pathological laughing and crying : epidemiology, pathophysiology and treatment. *CNS Drugs*. **22**: 531–545.

136 Twycross R et al. (2009) *Symptom Management in Advanced Cancer* (4e). palliativedrugs.com, Nottingham, pp. 61–133.

137 Haddad PM (2001) Antidepressant discontinuation syndromes: Clinical relevance, prevention and management. *Drug Safety*. **24**: 183–197.

138 Berber MJ (1998) FINISH: remembering the discontinuation syndrome. Flu-like symptoms, Insomnia, Nausea, Imbalance, Sensory disturbances, and Hyperarousal (anxiety/agitation). *Journal of Clinical Psychiatry*. **59**: 255.

Updated October 2013

Quick Prescribing Guide: Depression

Sadness and tears, even if associated with transient suicidal thoughts, do not justify the diagnosis of depression or the prescription of an antidepressant. Often they are part of an adjustment reaction, and improve with time. Other patients are demoralized rather than medically depressed and respond to symptom management and psychosocial support.

Evaluation

1 Screening: about 5–10% of patients with advanced cancer develop a major depression. Cases will be missed unless specific enquiry is made of all patients:
'What has your mood been like lately?... Are you depressed?'
'Have you had serious depression before? Are things like that now?'

2 Assessment interview: if depression is suspected, explore the patient's mood more fully by encouraging the patient to talk further with appropriate prompts. Symptoms suggesting clinical depression include:
   - sustained low mood (i.e. most of every day for several weeks) ⎫
   - sustained loss of pleasure/interest in life (anhedonia) ⎬ core symptoms
   - diurnal variation (worse in mornings and better in evenings) ⎭
   - waking significantly earlier than usual (e.g. 1–2h) and feeling 'awful'
   - feelings of hopelessness/worthlessness
   - excessive guilt
   - withdrawal from family and friends
   - persistent suicidal thoughts and/or suicidal acts
   - requests for euthanasia.

3 Differential diagnosis: the symptoms of depression and cancer, and of depression and sadness overlap. If in doubt whether the patient is suffering from depression, an adjustment reaction or sadness, review after 1–2 weeks of general support and improved symptom management. If still undecided, seek advice from a psychologist/psychiatrist.

4 Medical causes of depression: depression may be the consequence of:
   - a medical condition, e.g. hypercalcaemia, cerebral metastases
   - a reaction to severe uncontrolled physical symptoms
   - drugs, e.g. antineoplastics, benzodiazepines, antipsychotics, corticosteroids, antihypertensives.

Management

5 Correct the correctable: treat medical causes, particularly severe pain and other distressing symptoms.

6 Non-drug treatment:
   - explanation and assurance that symptoms can be treated
   - depressed patients often benefit from the ambience of a Palliative Care Day Centre
   - specific psychological treatments (via a clinical psychologist, etc.)
   - other psychosocial professionals, e.g. chaplain and creative therapists, have a therapeutic role, but avoid overwhelming the patient with simultaneous multiple referrals.

7 Drug treatment:
   - if the patient is expected to live for >4 weeks, prescribe a conventional antidepressant; if <4 weeks, consider a psychostimulant
   - the starting and continuing doses of antidepressants are generally lower in debilitated patients than in the physically fit
   - all antidepressants can cause withdrawal symptoms if stopped abruptly; generally withdraw gradually over 4 weeks
   - at usual doses, one SSRI can be directly substituted for another without cross-tapering or a washout period. Mirtazapine 15mg can be directly substituted for SSRIs (fluoxetine, citalopram or paroxetine 20mg; sertraline 50mg)
   - taper higher SSRI doses before switching
   - switching to or from TCAs and MAOIs requires additional care — seek advice or see reference texts.[111]

PCF preferred antidepressants

First-line
Psychostimulant, e.g. methylphenidate
Particularly if prognosis <2–4 weeks:
- start with 2.5–5mg b.d. (on waking/breakfast time and noon/lunchtime)
- if necessary, increase by daily increments of 2.5mg b.d. to 20mg b.d.
- occasionally higher doses are necessary, e.g. 30mg b.d. or 20mg t.d.s.

SSRI, e.g. sertraline or citalopram
Particularly if prognosis >2–4 weeks, and if associated anxiety:
- no antimuscarinic effects, but may cause an initial increase in anxiety
- if necessary prescribe diazepam at bedtime
- start with sertraline 50mg or citalopram 10mg once daily, increasing the latter to 20mg after 1 week
- if no improvement after 4 weeks, or only a partial improvement after 6–8 weeks, either:
  ▷ increase dose by sertraline 50mg or citalopram 10mg *or*
  ▷ switch to a second-line antidepressant
- maximum daily dose sertraline 200mg or citalopram 40mg (20mg in patients >60 years, those with hepatic impairment, and consider with patients also taking cimetidine, omeprazole or other inhibitors of CYP2C19)
- low likelihood of a withdrawal (discontinuation) syndrome.

Second-line
Alternative SSRI, e.g. sertraline or citalopram
Dose as above.

Mirtazapine
Acts on receptors; it is not a MARI. A good choice for patients with anxiety/agitation:
- start with 15mg at bedtime
- if little or no improvement after 2 weeks, increase to 30mg at bedtime
- concurrent H_1-receptor antagonism leads to sedation but this decreases at the higher dose because of noradrenergic effects
- fewer undesirable effects than TCAs.
If no response after 4 weeks, consider third-line options.

Third-line options
- seek advice from a psychiatrist
- dose escalation
- switch antidepressant
- combine an SSRI with mirtazapine, olanzapine or quetiapine.

AMITRIPTYLINE   BNF 4.3.1

Class: Serotonin and noradrenaline (norepinephrine) re-uptake inhibitor (SNRI), tricyclic antidepressant (TCA).

Indications: Depression, anxiety and panic disorders, nocturnal enuresis, †neuropathic pain, †urgency and urge incontinence, †sweating, †bladder spasm, †pathological laughing and crying, †drooling.

Contra-indications: Concurrent use with an MAOI or within 2 weeks of its cessation (see Serotonin toxicity, p.195), CHF, coronary artery insufficiency, recent myocardial infarction, arrhythmias (particularly any degree of heart block), mania, severe hepatic impairment.

Pharmacology

Amitriptyline is a serotonin and noradrenaline (norepinephrine) re-uptake inhibitor and a muscarinic, $5HT_{2A}$, $5HT_{2C}$, H_1, and α_1-adrenergic receptor antagonist.[1] The combination of mono-amine re-uptake inhibition with $5HT_2$ antagonism may explain why amitriptyline is marginally more effective than other antidepressants (cf. combining **venlafaxine** and **mirtazapine**, see p.199). However, it is less well tolerated and more dangerous in overdose, and is generally reserved for severe unresponsive depression.[2]

Mono-amine re-uptake inhibition is the predominant action in neuropathic pain and tension headaches. Sodium channel blockade and NMDA-glutamate receptor antagonism may also contribute.[3] Its efficacy and tolerability are comparable with alternatives (see p.198).

Generally, a dose-response effect is evident with patients benefitting from higher doses. However, for some patients benefit is *lost* at higher doses.[4] One potential explanation for this is that at higher doses pro-nociceptive effects (e.g. serotonin re-uptake inhibition, α_1 antagonism) predominate over anti-nociceptive effects.

Bio-availability 45%.[5]
Onset of action 2–4 weeks; < 1 week in neuropathic pain.[6]
Time to peak plasma concentration 4h PO; 24–48h IM.
Plasma halflife 13–36h; active metabolite nortriptyline 15–39h.
Duration of action 24h, situation dependent.

Cautions

Suicide risk: the possibility of a suicide attempt is inherent in major depression and persists until remission. Antidepressants may themselves cause suicidal ideation, particularly in those aged ≤25 years (see p.193). For patients with risk factors for suicide, consider alternatives that are safer in overdose (e.g. an SSRI).

Bipolar disorder (can transform into manic phase); epilepsy (lowers seizure threshold); cardiac disease (risk of arrhythmia); hepatic impairment (reduce dose or avoid); urinary hesitancy and narrow-angle glaucoma (antimuscarinic).

Drug interactions

Additive pharmacodynamic interactions with other drugs (see p.194), notably serotonin toxicity (see p.195). Concurrent administration with an MAOI or within 2 weeks of its cessation is contra-indicated (see above).

Amitriptyline is metabolized mainly by CYP2D6, and to a lesser degree by CYP1A2 and possibly other hepatic enzymes. Caution should be taken with concurrent use of drugs which inhibit or induce these enzymes, particularly in those who are poor CYP2D6 metabolizers (see Chapter 25, p.767).

Specific significant interactions[7]

- TCAs and SSRIs: **fluoxetine**, **paroxetine** (strong CYP2D6 inhibitors) and **fluvoxamine** (strong CYP1A2 inhibitor) have the greatest effect, *increasing* plasma concentrations of TCAs from *20% to 10 times*. In addition, the plasma concentration of the SSRI may also *increase*. If an SSRI and a TCA are prescribed concurrently, use an alternative SSRI (e.g. **citalopram** or

sertraline) or reduce the dose of the TCA to 25–33% of the previous dose (and possibly prescribe a relatively low SSRI dose)
- other drugs shown to *increase* the plasma concentrations of amitriptyline are **cimetidine, fluconazole, quinidine** (strong CYP2D6 inhibitor) and **terbinafine**
- concurrent prescription of **carbamazepine** *decreases* the plasma concentrations of amitriptyline by up to 60%.

Undesirable effects

Antimuscarinic effects (see p.6), sedation, delirium, postural hypotension, hyponatraemia. The use of amitriptyline in the elderly is associated with a doubling of the incidence of femoral fractures.[8]

Dose and use

Because of the potential for undesirable effects, low doses should be used initially, particularly in the frail elderly.
Amitriptyline can be given as a single dose at bedtime for all indications. If a patient experiences early morning drowsiness, or takes a long time to settle at night, amitriptyline should be taken 2h before bedtime.
Avoid abrupt withdrawal after prolonged use (see Stopping antidepressants, p.201).

A small number of patients are stimulated by amitriptyline and experience insomnia, unpleasant vivid dreams, myoclonus and physical restlessness. In these patients, administer in the morning or change to an alternative.

Neuropathic pain
- start with 10mg PO at bedtime
- if tolerated, increase to 25mg after 3–7 days
- if necessary, increase by 25mg every 1–2 weeks
- if successive increases are well tolerated *and bring additional benefit*, increase up to a maximum of 150mg at bedtime (seldom required)
- if helpful but poorly tolerated, consider switching to **nortriptyline**; if dose ≤100mg give the same dose without cross-tapering or a washout period (see p.210)
- if no response, switch to an anti-epileptic (see p.254).

Urgency and urge incontinence, sweating, bladder spasm, drooling
Dose as for neuropathic pain. Benefit is from the antimuscarinic action of amitriptyline (and switching to **nortriptyline** would be unhelpful).

Depression, anxiety and panic disorders, †pathological laughing and crying
Amitriptyline is no longer used first-line for depression, panic or anxiety disorders, but might retain a place for depression refractory to other treatments or with co-existent neuropathic pain (see p.198).
Titrate the dose as for neuropathic pain; 75–100mg PO at bedtime is generally as effective as higher doses, and better tolerated.[9] Occasionally, it is necessary to increase the dose to 150–225mg/24h.

Supply

Amitriptyline (generic)
Tablets 10mg, 25mg, 50mg, 28 days @ 50mg at bedtime = £1.
Oral solution 25mg/5mL, 50mg/5mL, 28 days @ 50mg at bedtime = £17.

1 NIMH (National Institute of Mental Health) (2006) Psychoactive Drug Screening Program. University of North Carolina. University of North Carolina. Available from: http://pdsp.med.unc.edu
2 Guaiana G et al. (2007) Amitriptyline for depression. Cochrane Database Systematic Reviews. CD004186.
3 McCleane G (2008) Antidepressants as analgesics. CNS Drugs. 22: 139–156.
4 Watson C (1984) Therapeutic window for amitriptyline analgesia. Canadian Medical Association Journal. 130: 105–106.
5 Schulz P et al. (1985) Discrepancies between pharmacokinetic studies of amitriptyline. Clinical Pharmacokinetics. 10: 257–268.
6 Sindrup SH et al. (2005) Antidepressants in the treatment of neuropathic pain. Basic and Clinical Pharmacology and Toxicology. 96: 399–409.

7 Baxter K and Preston CL (2011). *Stockley's Drug Interactions.* London:- Pharmaceutical Press www.medicinescomplete.com
   (accessed June 2013).
8 Ray WA *et al.* (1987) Psychotropic drug use and the risk of hip fracture. *New England Journal of Medicine.* **316**: 363–369.
9 Furukawa (2009) Low dosage tricyclic antidepressants for depression. *Cochrane Database of Systematic Reviews.* CD003197.

Updated October 2013

NORTRIPTYLINE   BNF 4.3.1

Class: Noradrenaline (norepinephrine) re-uptake inhibitor (NRI), tricyclic antidepressant (TCA).

Indications: Depression, nocturnal enuresis, †neuropathic pain, †pathological laughing and crying.

Contra-indications: Concurrent use with an MAOI or within 2 weeks of its cessation (see Serotonin toxicity, p.195) recent myocardial infarction, arrhythmias (particularly any degree of heart block), mania, severe hepatic impairment.

Pharmacology

Nortriptyline is a noradrenaline (norepinephrine) re-uptake inhibitor and a $5HT_{2A}$, $5HT_{2C}$, H_1, and α_1-adrenergic antagonist.[1] It is the principal active metabolite of **amitriptyline** (see p.208) but lacks its serotonin re-uptake inhibition, is less antimuscarinic and not so sedating. Nortriptyline undergoes extensive first-pass metabolism to 10-hydroxynortriptyline, which is active.[2]

Nortriptyline is as effective as **amitriptyline** for depression[3] and neuropathic pain.[4] Like **amitriptyline**, it generally takes several weeks for the antidepressant effect to manifest. Given the long plasma halflife of nortriptyline, once daily administration is possible, generally at bedtime. However, nortriptyline has both stimulant and sedative properties and, if it disturbs sleep, it should be taken in the morning.

Bio-availability 60%.

Onset of action 2–6 weeks.

Time to peak plasma concentration 7–8.5h.

Plasma halflife 15–39h.

Duration of action variable, possibly several days.

Cautions

Suicide risk: the possibility of a suicide attempt is inherent in major depression and persists until remission. Antidepressants may themselves cause suicidal ideation, particularly in those aged ≤25 years (see p.193). For patients with risk factors for suicide, consider alternatives that are safer in overdose (e.g. an SSRI).

Bipolar disorder (can transform into manic phase); epilepsy (lowers seizure threshold); cardiac disease (risk of arrhythmia); hepatic impairment (reduce dose or avoid); urinary hesitancy and narrow-angle glaucoma (antimuscarinic).

Drug interactions

Additive pharmacodynamic interactions with other drugs (see p.194), notably serotonin toxicity (see p.195, Box B). Concurrent administration with an MAOI or within 2 weeks of its cessation is contra-indicated (see above).

Nortriptyline is metabolized by CYP2D6. Caution should be taken with concurrent use of drugs which inhibit or induce these enzymes, particularly in those who are poor CYP2D6 metabolizers (see Chapter 25, p.767).

Specific significant interactions[5]

- TCAs and the SSRIs: **fluoxetine, paroxetine** (strong CYP2D6 inhibitors) and **fluvoxamine** (strong CYP1A2 inhibitor) have the greatest effect, *increasing* plasma concentrations of TCAs from 20% to 10 times. In addition, the plasma concentration of the SSRI may also *increase*. If an SSRI and a TCA are prescribed concurrently, use an alternative SSRI (e.g. **citalopram** or

sertraline) or reduce the dose of the TCA to 25–33% of the previous dose (and possibly prescribe a relatively low SSRI dose)

- other drugs shown to *increase* the plasma concentrations of nortriptyline are **cimetidine, fluconazole, quinidine** (strong CYP2D6 inhibitor) and **terbinafine**
- concurrent prescription of **carbamazepine** *decreases* the plasma concentrations of nortriptyline by up to 60%.

Undesirable effects

Very common (>10%): antimuscarinic effects (see p.6), anorexia, nausea, drowsiness, fatigue, weight gain.

Very rare (<0.01%): arrhythmias, AV conduction changes, heart block.

Dose and use

See general advice for **amitriptyline**, p.208. If stimulation exceeds sedation and sleep is disturbed, administer in the morning. Avoid abrupt withdrawal after prolonged use (see Stopping antidepressants, p.201).

If the daily dose is ⩾100mg, the manufacturer advises monitoring the plasma concentration, and adjusting the dose to maintain it between 50–150nanogram/mL (a convenient though inevitably approximate 'therapeutic window').[6,7]

Depression

- start with 25mg at bedtime
- if necessary, increase the dose by 25mg every 2–4 weeks up to 150mg/day
- if no response with 150mg after 4 weeks, switch to an alternative antidepressant
- if effective, continue on the same dose until the patient has been symptom-free for 6–12 months; after this, discontinue over 2–8 weeks.

†Neuropathic pain

- start with 10–25mg at bedtime
- increase by 10mg/day every 3–5 days up to 50mg, or double dose from 25mg to 50mg after 2 weeks[4]
- if successive increases are well tolerated *and result in additional benefit*, increase further to a maximum of 150mg daily (seldom required).

Supply

Allegron® (King)

Tablets 10mg, 25mg, 28 days @ 50mg at bedtime = £14.

1. NIMH (National Institute of Mental Health) (2006) Psychoactive Drug Screening Program. University of North Carolina. University of North Carolina. Available from: http://pdsp.med.unc.edu
2. Nordin C and Bertilsson L (1995) Active hydroxymetabolites of antidepressants. Emphasis on E-10-hydroxy-nortriptyline. *Clinical Pharmacokinetics.* **28**: 26–40.
3. Barbui C and Hotopf M (2001) Amitriptyline v. the rest: still the leading antidepressant after 40 years of randomised controlled trials. *British Journal of Psychiatry.* **178**: 129–144.
4. Watson CP et al. (1998) Nortriptyline versus amitriptyline in postherpetic neuralgia: a randomized trial. *Neurology.* **51**: 1166–1171.
5. Baxter K and Preston CL (2011). *Stockley's Drug Interactions.* London:- Pharmaceutical Press www.medicinescomplete.com (accessed June 2013).
6. APA (American Psychiatric Association) (1985) Task Force on the Use of Laboratory Tests in Psychiatry: Tricyclic antidepressants-blood level measurements and clinical outcome. *American Journal of Psychiatry.* **142**: 155–162.
7. Perry PJ (1984) The relationship of free nortriptyline levels to antidepressant response. *Drug Intelligence and Clinical Pharmacy.* **18**: 510.

Updated October 2013

SELECTIVE SEROTONIN RE-UPTAKE INHIBITORS
BNF 4.3.3

Class: Antidepressant.

Indications: Depression, anxiety and panic disorders, †pruritus, †pathological laughing and crying.

Contra-indications: Concurrent use with an MAOI or within 2 weeks of its cessation (see Serotonin toxicity, p.195); known prolonged QT interval or concurrent use with other drugs which prolong the QT interval (**citalopram, escitalopram**), concurrent use with **pimozide**; mania.

Pharmacology

SSRIs inhibit the serotonin re-uptake transporter. They differ in their propensity for drug interactions, discontinuation reactions and cost. They also have varying additional actions which may partly explain why some individuals respond when switched to an alternative SSRI (Table 1).

Table 1 Differences between SSRIs

Drug	Additional actions	Hepatic enzyme inhibition					Discontinuation reaction risk[a]
		CYP1A2	CYP2C9	CYP2C19	CYP2D6	CYP3A4	
Citalopram	H_1 antagonist (R-enantiomer)				+		Low
Escitalopram	None				+		Low
Fluoxetine	$5HT_{2C}$ antagonist[b]	++	++	+++	+		Minimal
Fluvoxamine	Sigma-1 agonist[c]	+++		+++		++	Moderate
Paroxetine	Noradrenaline (norepinephrine) re-uptake inhibitor[b]				+++		High
Sertraline	Dopamine re-uptake inhibitor[b]				+		Low

+ = weak inhibition; ++ = moderate inhibition; +++ = marked inhibition (also see Chapter 25 p.767).

a. approximates to halflife (see Table 2 below)

b. these actions theoretically contribute to their antidepressant effects (see p.190) but the affinity, and overall contribution of these additional actions is much less than the predominant serotonin re-uptake inhibition.

c. the action of sigma-1 receptors is poorly defined, but sigma-1 receptor agonists may have antidepressant, pro-seizure, euphoric and/or dysphoric effects.

In palliative care, **citalopram** or **sertraline** are generally the SSRIs of choice; they combine a low risk of drug interactions and discontinuation reactions. They are first-line treatments for depression (see p.191), anxiety and panic disorders (see p.192), and pathological laughter and crying (see p.200). **Sertraline** is preferred in patients with risk factors for QT interval prolongation (see below).

Two small RCTs suggest benefit in pruritus within a few days from **sertraline** (cholestatic pruritus)[6] and **paroxetine** (pruritus of mixed cause in cancer patients).[7] Benefit is also reported in pruritus associated with polycythaemia vera.[8]

Although SSRIs are moderately effective for neuropathic pain (3 of 4 RCTs),[9-12] they are inferior to **imipramine**.[9] A TCA (e.g. **amitriptyline, imipramine, nortriptyline**) or an anti-epileptic is preferable (see p.198).

Escitalopram is the S-enantiomer of **citalopram**. **R-citalopram** does not inhibit the serotonin re-uptake transporter but may hinder the binding of **S-citalopram**. Some fixed-dose comparisons do find a marginally higher response rate with **escitalopram** 10mg vs. **citalopram** 20mg,[13] but titrating **citalopram** might be expected to achieve the same result at lower cost.

For pharmacokinetic details, see Table 2.

Cautions

Suicide risk: the possibility of a suicide attempt is inherent in major depression and persists until remission. Antidepressants may themselves cause suicidal ideation, particularly in those aged ≤25 years (see p.193).

Table 2 Pharmacokinetic details for selected SSRIs[13-15]

Drug	Bio-availability PO (%)	T_{max} (h)	Plasma halflife	Metabolism
Citalopram	80[a]	3	36h	Multiple pathways[b]
Escitalopram	80[c]	4	30h	Multiple pathways[b]
Fluoxetine	90	4–8	1–4 days; 1–2 weeks[b]	Multiple pathways[b]
Paroxetine	50[d]	5	15–20h	Multiple pathways
Sertraline	>44	6–8	26h	CYP3A4

a. for tablets; bio-availability of drops is nearly 100%
b. active metabolite(s)
c. the bio-availability of tablets and oral solution is comparable
d. increases with multiple dosing.

Bipolar disorder (can transform into manic phase). Epilepsy (may lower seizure threshold but less than other antidepressants; **citalopram** *generally preferred because it lacks significant interactions with anti-epileptics*).

QT prolongation risk factors (see below and p.759); hepatic impairment (reduce dose or avoid); renal impairment; diabetes mellitus (reduced hypoglycaemic awareness); peptic ulceration or bleeding disorders (SSRIs increase the risk of GI bleeding,[16] particularly in those aged >80 years).[17]

Drug interactions

Fluoxetine, fluvoxamine and **paroxetine** are strong hepatic enzyme inhibitors (see Chapter 25, p.767) and potentially serious interactions can result when used with other drugs that are metabolized by these enzymes.[18]
Citalopram, escitalopram and **sertraline** are only weak hepatic enzyme inhibitors and are less likely to affect the metabolism of other drugs.[4,5]

Additive pharmacodynamic interactions with other drugs (see p.194) notably bleeding risk, QT prolongation (**citalopram** and **escitalopram**) and serotonin toxicity (see p.195). Concurrent administration with an MAOI or within 2 weeks of its cessation is contra-indicated (see above).
Sertraline is metabolized mainly by CYP3A4, and to a minor degree by CYP2D6. Caution should be taken with concurrent use of drugs which inhibit or induce these enzymes particularly in those who are poor CYP2D6 metabolizers (see Chapter 25, p.767). However, generally **sertraline** rarely requires dose reduction with other enzyme inhibitors; consider only if symptoms of toxicity occur.
Citalopram (and **escitalopram**) are metabolized by CYP2C19, CYP2D6 and CYP3A4. Although the FDA recommends a reduced dose of **citalopram** when used with **cimetidine, omeprazole** or other drugs which inhibit CYP2C19, the effect on plasma citalopram levels is likely to be small.[19]

Undesirable effects
Frequencies based on **sertaline** and **citalopram**.
Very common (>10%): somnolence, insomnia, dizziness, headache, dry mouth, nausea, diarrhoea, sweating.
Common (<10%, >1%): agitation, anxiety, nervousness, confusion, tremor, tinnitus, yawning, fatigue, dizziness, paraesthesia, bruxism (teeth grinding), palpitations, altered taste, decreased appetite, vomiting, sexual dysfunction, myalgia, arthralgia, pruritus.
Uncommon (<1%, >0.1%): aggression, depersonalization, hallucinations, mania.
Rare (<0.01%) or unknown incidence: psychosis, hyponatraemia, seizures, movement disorders (e.g. dyskinesia), hepatitis, suicidal ideation (see above), haemorrhage, fracture risk (see p.196).

Myocardial infarction
The manufacturer reports myocardial infarction as a rare consequence of taking **sertraline**. However, this would be expected in antidepressant RCTs because depression is an independent

risk factor for myocardial infarction. Further, case control studies suggest that SSRIs confer a protective effect,[20] possibly because they impact negatively on platelet aggregation (see p.196). **Sertraline** has been used safely in patients with unstable angina, and after myocardial infarction.[21]

QT prolongation

Citalopram and **escitalopram** exhibit dose-related QT prolongation. Regulators recommend correction of hypokalaemia and hypomagnaesemia, advise ECG monitoring in those with cardiac disease, and contra-indication in patients receiving other QT prolonging drugs (see Box B, p.761).[22] Other SSRIs appear safer in this respect.[23] Also see Prolongation of the QT interval in palliative care, p.759.

Dose and use
Treatment should not be discontinued abruptly (see p.201).

Sertraline (depression, anxiety and panic)
- if anxiety/panic symptoms are prominent, start with 25mg each morning and increase to 50mg each morning after 1 week
- otherwise, start with 50mg each morning, if necessary, increase the dose to 100mg after 2–4 weeks
- if no response after 4 weeks, or only a partial response after 6–8 weeks, consider further increases to a maximum of 200mg or an alternative (see p.199)
- if effective, continue until the patient has been symptom-free for ⩾6 months (see, p.199); after this, discontinue over 2–4 weeks.

Citalopram (depression, anxiety and panic)
Because of concerns regarding QT prolongation, do not exceed the maximum dose (see also comments above).[22]
- start with 10mg each morning and increase to 20mg each morning after 1 week
- if no response after 4 weeks, or only a partial response after 6–8 weeks, consider further increases to a maximum of 40mg or switch to an alternative (see p.199)
- restrict maximum dose to 20mg in those over 60, hepatic impairment, and consider with patients also taking **cimetidine, omeprazole** or other inhibitors of CYP2C19[19,22]
- if effective, continue until the patient has been symptom-free for ⩾6 months (see p.199); after this, discontinue over 2–4 weeks.

Other indications
- **cholestatic pruritus**
  ▷ start with **sertraline** 25mg each morning, if necessary, increase in 25mg increments
  ▷ doses above 100mg rarely give additional relief.[6]
- **pathological laughter and crying**
  ▷ often responds to lower doses than required for depression[24]
  ▷ start with **citalopram** 5mg each morning; if necessary, increase in 5–10mg increments to a maximum of 40mg each morning (20mg in those with risk factors, see above) or
  ▷ start with **sertraline** 12.5mg each morning; if necessary, increase in 12.5–25mg increments to a maximum of 200mg each morning.

Supply
Citalopram (generic)
Tablets (as hydrobromide) 10mg, 20mg, 40mg, 28 days @ 20mg each morning = £3.50.
Oral liquid drops (as hydrochloride) 40mg/mL, 28 days @ 16mg (8 drops) each morning = £13; 16mg as drops is equivalent to 20mg as tablets. Mix with water, orange juice or apple juice before taking.

Sertraline (generic)
Tablets 50mg, 100mg, 28 days @ 50mg each morning = £2.
Oral solution 50mg/5mL, 28 days @ 50mg each morning = £95; unauthorized, available as a special order from Rosemont (see Appendix 1, p.817). Note specials tariff applies in community.

1   Hashimoto K (2009) Sigma-1 receptors and selective serotonin reuptake inhibitors: clinical implications of their relationship. *Central Nervous System Agents in Medicinal Chemistry*. **9**: 197–204.

2   Carrasco JL and Sandner C (2005) Clinical effects of pharmacological variations in selective serotonin reuptake inhibitors: an overview. *International Journal of Clinical Practice*. **59**: 1428–1434.

3   Haddad PM (2001) Antidepressant discontinuation syndromes: Clinical relevance, prevention and management. *Drug Safety*. **24**: 183–197.

4   Preskorn SH (1997) Clinically relevant pharmacology of selective serotonin reuptake inhibitors. An overview with emphasis on pharmacokinetics and effects on oxidative drug metabolism. *Clinical Pharmacokinetics*. **32(Suppl 1)**: 1–21.

5   Rao N (2007) The clinical pharmacokinetics of escitalopram. *Clinical Pharmacokinetics*. **46**: 281–290.

6   Mayo MJ et al. (2007) Sertraline as a first-line treatment for cholestatic pruritus. *Hepatology*. **45**: 666–674.

7   Zylicz Z et al. (2003) Paroxetine in the treatment of severe non-dermatological pruritus: a randomized, controlled trial. *Journal of Pain and Symptom Management*. **26**: 1105–1112.

8   Tefferi A and Fonseca R (2002) Selective serotonin reuptake inhibitors are effective in the treatment of polycythemia vera-associated pruritus. *Blood*. **99**: 2627.

9   Sindrup S et al. (1990) The selective serotonin re-uptake inhibitor paroxetine is effective in the treatment of diabetic neuropathy symptoms. *Pain*. **42**: 135–144.

10 Otto M et al. (2008) Escitalopram in painful polyneuropathy: a randomized, placebo-controlled, cross-over trial. *Pain*. **139**: 275–283.

11 Max M et al. (1992) Effects of desipramine, amitriptyline, and fluoxetine on pain in diabetic neuropathy. *New England Journal of Medicine*. **326**: 1287–1288.

12 Sindrup SH et al. (1992) The selective serotonin reuptake inhibitor citalopram relieves the symptoms of diabetic neuropathy. *Clinical Pharmacology and Therapeutics*. **52**: 547–552.

13 Garnock-Jones KP and McCormack PL (2010) Escitalopram: a review of its use in the management of major depressive disorder in adults. *CNS Drugs*. **24**: 769–796.

14 Hiemke (2000) Pharmacokinetics of selective serotonin reuptake inhibitors. *Pharmacology and Therapeutics*. **85**: 11–28.

15 Kaye CM et al. (1989) A review of the metabolism and pharmacokinetics of paroxetine in man. *Acta Psychiatrica Scandinavica Supplementum*. **350**: 60–75.

16 Paton C and Ferrier IN (2005) SSRIs and gastrointestinal bleeding. *British Medical Journal*. **331**: 529–530.

17 vanWalraven C et al. (2001) Inhibition of serotonin reuptake by antidepressants and upper gastrointestinal bleeding in elderly patients: retrospective cohort study. *British Medical Journal*. **323**: 655–657.

18 Baxter K and Preston CL (2011). *Stockley's Drug Interactions*. London:- Pharmaceutical Press www.medicinescomplete.com (accessed June 2013).

19 FDA (2012) Celexa (citalopram hydrobromide) Revised recommendations, potential risk of abnormal heart rhythms. *Drug safety communication*. http://www.fda.gov/Safety/MedWatch/

20 Sauer WH et al. (2001) Selective serotonin reuptake inhibitors and myocardial infarction. *Circulation*. **104**: 1894–1898.

21 Glassman AH et al. (2002) Sertraline treatment of major depression in patients with acute MI or unstable angina. *Journal of the American Medical Association*. **288**: 701–709.

22 MHRA (2011) Citalopram and escitalopram: QT interval prolongation - new maximum daily dose restrictions (including in elderly patients), contraindications, and warnings. *Drug Safety Update*. **5**. www.mhra.gov.uk/safetyinformation

23 Isbister GK et al. (2004) Relative toxicity of selective serotonin reuptake inhibitors (SSRIs) in overdose. *Clinical Toxicology*. **42**: 277–285.

24 Wortzel HS et al. (2008) Pathological laughing and crying : epidemiology, pathophysiology and treatment. *CNS Drugs*. **22**: 531–545.

Updated October 2013

*VENLAFAXINE   BNF 4.3.4

Class: Antidepressant; serotonin and noradrenaline (norepinephrine) re-uptake inhibitor (SNRI).

Indications: Depression, anxiety and panic disorders, †neuropathic pain, hot flushes.

Contra-indications: Concurrent use with an MAOI or within 2 weeks of its cessation (see Serotonin toxicity, p.195). Uncontrolled hypertension, high risk of ventricular arrhythmia.[1]

Pharmacology

Venlafaxine inhibits both serotonin and noradrenaline (norepinephrine) re-uptake transporters.[2,3] Inhibition of noradrenaline (norepinephrine) re-uptake increases with higher doses.[4] Venlafaxine also inhibits dopamine re-uptake in the prefrontal cortex. Venlafaxine has little or no post-synaptic antagonistic effects at muscarinic, α-adrenergic, $5HT_{2A}$, $5HT_{2C}$ or H_1-receptors.

Venlafaxine is generally reserved for the treatment of depression refractory to SSRIs. As a second-line treatment, it is marginally more effective than switching to an alternative SSRI, but less well tolerated (see p.191).[5–7]

Venlafaxine has been shown to have an antinociceptive effect in animals.[8,9] Case reports and case series suggest that venlafaxine relieves several types of chronic pain, e.g. headache, fibromyalgia and neuropathic pain.[10] Benefit in diabetic neuropathy and in a mixed group of patients has been confirmed in RCTs.[11,12] In another RCT (n = 13), benefit appeared to be positively correlated with the plasma concentration of venlafaxine.[13] In an RCT of **imipramine** 75mg daily vs. venlafaxine 112.5mg daily, both were equally effective and both were significantly better than placebo.[14] Dry mouth was more common with **imipramine**, and tiredness more common with venlafaxine.

Venlafaxine is also of benefit in hot flushes associated with the menopause or hormone therapy,[15,16] including androgen ablation therapy for prostate cancer.[17] This is not a specific effect of venlafaxine; SSRIs seem to share this property, e.g. **paroxetine** and **fluoxetine**.[18,19] Venlafaxine is metabolized to a pharmacologically active metabolite, O-desmethylvenlafaxine (ODV), which has a similar pharmacodynamic profile.

Bio-availability 13%; 45% m/r.
Onset of action >2 weeks for depression.
Time to peak plasma concentration about 2.5h; 4.5–7.5h m/r and 6.5–11h ODV m/r.
Plasma halflife 5h; 11h for ODV.
Duration of effect 12–24h, situation dependent.

Cautions

Suicide risk: the possibility of a suicide attempt is inherent in major depression and persists until remission. Antidepressants may themselves cause suicidal ideation, particularly in those aged ≤25 years (see p.193). The risk appears to be greater with venlafaxine than with SSRIs and TCAs, but this may be because patients prescribed venlafaxine (generally not a first-line antidepressant) may already be at greater risk of suicide.[1,20,21]

For patients with risk factors for suicide, the MHRA advises that a maximum of 2 week's supply should be dispensed at a time to reduce the risk from overdose.[1]

Bipolar disorder (can transform into manic phase); epilepsy (lowers seizure threshold); cardiac disease (risk of hypertension and arrhythmia); mild–moderate hepatic impairment (reduce dose); renal impairment (reduce dose); narrow-angle glaucoma (mydriasis reported).

Drug interactions

Additive pharmacodynamic interactions with other drugs (see p.194) notably QT prolongation and serotonin toxicity (see Box B, p.195). Concurrent administration with an MAOI or within 2 weeks of its cessation is contra-indicated (see above).

Venlafaxine is metabolized by CYP2D6 and CYP3A4. Concurrent use with drugs which inhibit these enzymes may result in higher plasma concentrations (see Chapter 25, p.767), and should generally be avoided in order to prevent clinically important interactions in poor metabolizers.[1]

Venlafaxine may increase concurrent **haloperidol** plasma concentrations (up to 70% increase in AUC).[22] The mechanism is unknown and the dose of haloperidol may need to be reduced. The dose of **warfarin** may need to be reduced when used concurrently with venlafaxine (reports of increased prothrombin times; unknown mechanism).[22]

Undesirable effects

Very common (>10%): dizziness, dry mouth, insomnia, nervousness, drowsiness, constipation, nausea, abnormal ejaculation/orgasm, asthenia, headache, sweating.

Common (<10%, >1%): agitation, confusion, hypertonia, paraesthesia, tremor, dyspnoea, hypertension, palpitations, postural hypotension, vasodilation, anorexia, diarrhoea, dyspepsia, vomiting, urinary frequency, ecchymosis, decreased libido, impotence, menstrual disorders, arthralgia, myalgia, weight gain/loss, abdominal pain, abnormal dreams, chills, pyrexia, pruritus, rash, abnormal vision/accommodation, mydriasis, tinnitus.

Uncommon (<1%): hallucinations, urinary retention, muscle spasm, hyponatraemia, increased liver enzymes, angioedema, maculopapular eruptions, urticaria.

Dose and use

Because of concerns about its tolerability and safety in overdose, venlafaxine should not be used as a first-line antidepressant.[1,5,23] Specialist supervision required if a dose of ⩾300mg is necessary in severely depressed or hospitalized patients.[1]

May be taken with or after food to improve tolerability (see Chapter 14, p.639). If moderate renal or mild–moderate hepatic impairment, reduce the dose by 50% and give once daily.

Monitor blood pressure; consider dose reduction or discontinuation in those who show a sustained increase.[1]

Avoid abrupt withdrawal after prolonged use (see Stopping antidepressants, p.201). If ⩾75mg/day have been taken for > 1 week, taper over at least 1 week; if ⩾150mg/day have been taken for > 6 weeks, taper over at least 2 weeks.

Note: remains of m/r tablets may appear in the patient's faeces ('ghost tablets'), but these are inert residues, and do not affect the efficacy of the products.

Depression
Venlafaxine is reserved for depression refractory to other antidepressants (see p.191).
- generally start with 37.5mg b.d.
- in frail or elderly patients, start with 37.5mg once daily for 4–7 days
- if necessary, increase by 37.5mg b.d. every 2 weeks
- maximum recommended dose 375mg daily
- if effective, continue until the patient has been symptom-free for ⩾6 months (see p.199); after this, discontinue over 2–4 weeks.

Anxiety and panic
Venlafaxine is reserved for anxiety or panic disorders refractory to other antidepressants (see p.200).
- as for depression
- maximum recommended dose 225mg daily.

Neuropathic pain and hot flushes
Venlafaxine is not a first-line treatment for neuropathic pain (see p.198).
- start with 37.5mg m/r once daily
- increase to 37.5mg b.d. after 1 week
- if necessary, increase to 75mg b.d. after a further 2 weeks.

Supply
Venlafaxine (generic)
Tablets 37.5mg, 75mg, 28 days @ 75mg b.d. = £4.
Capsules m/r 75mg, 150mg, 28 days @ 150mg once daily = £37.
Tablets m/r 37.5mg, 75mg, 150mg, 225mg, 28 days @ 150mg once daily = £19.
Oral solution 37.5mg/5mL, 75mg/5ml 28 days @ 150mg once daily = £150; unauthorized, available as a special order from Rosemont (see Appendix 1, p.817). *Note specials tariff applies in community.*

1 MHRA (2006) Updated prescribing advice for venlafaxine (Efexor/Effexor XL). Letter from the chairman of the Commission on Human Medicines, 31st May 2006. Available from: http://www.mhra.gov.uk/Safetyinformation/
2 Bymaster FP et al. (2001) Comparative affinity of duloxetine and venlafaxine for serotonin and norepinephrine transporters in vitro and in vivo, human serotonin receptor subtypes, and other neuronal receptors. Neuropsychopharmacology. 25: 871–880.
3 Beique JC et al. (1998) Affinities of venlafaxine and various reuptake inhibitors for the serotonin and norepinephrine transporters. European Journal of Pharmacology. 349: 129–132.
4 Melichar J et al. (2001) Venlafaxine occupation at the noradrenaline reuptake site: in-vivo determination in healthy volunteers. Journal of Psychopharmacology. 15: 9–12.
5 NICE (2009) Depression. Clinical Guidelines. CG90 and CG91. www.nice.org.uk.
6 Ruhe HG et al. (2006) Switching antidepressants after a first selective serotonin reuptake inhibitor in major depressive disorder: a systematic review. Journal of Clinical Psychiatry. 67: 1836–1855.
7 Anderson IM et al. (2008) Evidence-based guidelines for treating depressive disorders with antidepressants: a revision of the 2000 British Association for Psychopharmacology guidelines. Journal of Psychopharmacology. 22: 343–396.

8 Lang E *et al.* (1996) Venlafaxine hydrochloride (Effexor) relieves thermal hyperalgesia in rats with an experimental mononeuropathy. *Pain.* **68**: 151–155.

9 Schreiber S *et al.* (1999) The antinociceptive effect of venlafaxine in mice is mediated through opioid and adrenergic mechanisms. *Neuroscience Letters.* **273**: 85–88.

10 Grothe DR *et al.* (2004) Treatment of pain syndromes with venlafaxine. *Pharmacotherapy.* **24**: 621–629.

11 Kunz N *et al.* (2000) Diabetic neuropathic pain management with venlafaxine XR. In: *CINP* July.

12 Yucel A *et al.* (2005) The effect of venlafaxine on ongoing and experimentally induced pain in neuropathic pain patients: a double blind, placebo controlled study. *European Journal of Pain.* **9**: 407–416.

13 Tasmuth T *et al.* (2002) Venlafaxine in neuropathic pain following treatment of breast cancer. *European Journal of Pain.* **6**: 17–24.

14 Sindrup SH *et al.* (2003) Venlafaxine versus imipramine in painful polyneuropathy: a randomized, controlled trial. *Neurology.* **60**: 1284–1289.

15 Barlow D (2000) Venlafaxine for hot flushes. *Lancet.* **356**: 2025–2026.

16 Loprinzi C *et al.* (2000) Venlafaxine in management of hot flashes in survivors of breast cancer: a randomised controlled trial. *Lancet.* **356**: 2059–2063.

17 Quella S *et al.* (1999) Pilot evaluation of venlafaxine for the treatment of hot flashes in men undergoing androgen ablation therapy for prostate cancer. *Journal of Urology.* **162**: 98–102.

18 Stearns V *et al.* (1997) A pilot trial assessing the efficacy of paroxetine hydrochloride (Paxil) in controlling hot flashes. *Breast Cancer Research Treatment.* **46**: 23–33.

19 Loprinzi C *et al.* (1999) Preliminary data from a randomized evaluation of fluoxetine (Prozac) for treating hot flashes in breast cancer survivors. *Breast Cancer Research Treatment.* **57**: 34.

20 Cipriani A *et al.* (2007) Venlafaxine for major depression. *British Medical Journal.* **334**: 215–216.

21 Rubino A *et al.* (2007) Risk of suicide during treatment with venlafaxine, citalopram, fluoxetine, and dothiepin: retrospective cohort study. *British Medical Journal.* **334**: 242.

22 Baxter K and Preston CL (2011). *Stockley's Drug Interactions.* London:- Pharmaceutical Press www.medicinescomplete.com (accessed June 2013).

23 Buckley NA and McManus PR (2002) Fatal toxicity of serotoninergic and other antidepressant drugs: analysis of United Kingdom mortality data. *British Medical Journal.* **325**: 1332–1333.

Updated October 2013

DULOXETINE   BNF 4.3.4 & 7.4.2

Class: Antidepressant, serotonin and noradrenaline (norepinephrine) re-uptake inhibitor (SNRI).

Indications: Depression, diabetic neuropathic pain, generalised anxiety disorder (Cymbalta®); moderate–severe stress incontinence in women (Yentreve®).

Contra-indications: Concurrent use with an MAOI or within 2 weeks of its cessation (see Serotonin toxicity, p.195). Concurrent use with strong CYP1A2 inhibitors, e.g. **fluvoxamine**, **ciprofloxacin**.[1] Uncontrolled hypertension, hepatic impairment, end-stage renal failure requiring dialysis or creatinine clearance <30mL/min.

Pharmacology

Like **venlafaxine**, duloxetine inhibits serotonin and noradrenaline (norepinephrine) re-uptake transporters, but lacks the muscarinic, α-adrenergic and H_1-receptor antagonism of **amitriptyline** and other tricyclic SNRIs.[2] Its place relative to other options for depression is unclear. In an RCT, duloxetine was less well tolerated than **venlafaxine**.[3] A meta-analysis found it to be less effective than **escitalopram**, **mirtazapine**, **sertraline** and **venlafaxine**.[4]

Duloxetine is of benefit in painful peripheral neuropathy (diabetic and platinum chemotherapy related), fibromyalgia and osteo-arthitic knee pain (NNTs range 4.8–8 for 50% reduction in pain scores).[5–7] A small RCT in central pain gave an NNT of 3.4 for 30% pain reduction, of borderline statistical significance (p = 0.056).[8,9] In two head to head comparisons with **amitriptyline**, efficacy was comparable; undesirable effects were also similar, although in one dry mouth occurred less commonly and constipation more commonly with duloxetine.[10,11]

Duloxetine has a limited role in stress incontinence.[12] Serotonin and noradrenaline (norepinephrine) increase urethral sphincter tone (see p.198).

The incidence of initial nausea with duloxetine is comparable with that seen with **fluoxetine** and **paroxetine**.[13]

Bio-availability 90%.

Onset of action 2–3 weeks in depression.[14]

Time to peak plasma concentration 6h.

Plasma halflife 12h.

Duration of action >24h, situation dependent.

Cautions

Suicide risk: the possibility of a suicide attempt is inherent in major depression and persists until remission. Antidepressants may themselves cause suicidal ideation, particularly in those aged ≤25 years (see p.193).

Bipolar disorder (can transform into manic phase); epilepsy (lowers seizure threshold); cardiac disease (risk of hypertension and arrhythmia); hepatic impairment (reduce dose); renal impairment (reduce dose); urinary hesitancy and narrow-angle glaucoma (may exacerbate).

Drug interactions

Additive pharmacodynamic interactions with other drugs (see p.194), notably serotonin toxicity (see Box B, p.195). Concurrent administration with an MAOI or within 2 weeks of its cessation is contra-indicated (see above).

Duloxetine is metabolized by CYP1A2 and CYP2D6, and also *inhibits* CYP2D6. Caution should be taken with concurrent use of drugs which inhibit or induce these enzymes, particularly in those who are poor CYP2D6 metabolizers (see Chapter 25, p.767).

Specific significant interactions[1]

- **fluvoxamine** (strong CYP1A2 inhibitor) *significantly increases* duloxetine plasma concentrations, and **ciprofloxacin** probably does the same; concurrent use of these drugs with duloxetine is contra-indicated
- **fluoxetine**, **paroxetine** and **quinidine** (strong CYP2D6 inhibitors) can increase plasma concentrations
- smoking (CYP1A2 inducer) can *decrease* duloxetine plasma concentration by ≤50%; however, a routine dose increase in smokers is not recommended.

Undesirable effects

Very common (>10%): sexual dysfunction (about 30%), nausea (20%), insomnia (20%), drowsiness (15%), dry mouth (15%), constipation (10%), sweating (10%).

Common (<10%, 1%): lightheadedness, dizziness, blurred vision, headache, altered taste, anorexia, diarrhoea.[15]

Dose and use

The timing of once daily doses is immaterial, although it should be constant for an individual.

Monitor blood pressure: consider dose reduction or discontinuation in those who show a sustained increase.

Avoid abrupt withdrawal after prolonged use (see Stopping antidepressants, p.201).

Diabetic peripheral neuropathy

- start with 60mg PO once daily
- if necessary, increase to 60mg b.d.
- no dose reduction is required in mild–moderate renal impairment; use is contra-indicated in severe renal impairment (creatinine clearance <30mL/min).

Depression

Duloxetine is less effective and less well tolerated than alternatives (see above). It may have a role in depression with concurrent neuropathic pain.

- 60mg PO once daily
- no extra benefit likely with higher doses.[16–18]

Stress incontinence in women

Moderate–severe stress incontinence is defined as ≥14 episodes per week. In physically fit women, management is primarily non-drug, e.g. pelvic floor muscle training (sometimes followed by surgery).[12,19] If prescribing duloxetine:

- start with 20mg PO b.d.
- if necessary, increase to 40mg b.d. after 2 weeks.

Supply

Cymbalta® (Lilly)

Capsules enclosing e/c pellets 30mg, 60mg, 28 days @ 60mg once daily = £28.

Yentreve® (Lilly)

Capsules enclosing e/c pellets 20mg, 40mg, 28 days @ 20mg b.d. = £31.

1 Baxter K and Preston CL (2011). *Stockley's Drug Interactions*. London:- Pharmaceutical Press www.medicinescomplete.com (accessed June 2013).

2 Bymaster FP et al. (2001) Comparative affinity of duloxetine and venlafaxine for serotonin and norepinephrine transporters in vitro and in vivo, human serotonin receptor subtypes, and other neuronal receptors. *Neuropsychopharmacology*. **25**: 871–880.

3 Perahia D et al. Comparing duloxetine and venlafaxine in the treatment of major depressive disorder using a global benefit-risk approach. Florida, USA: New Clinical Drug Evaluation Unit; 2005.

4 Cipriani A et al. (2009) Comparative efficacy and acceptability of 12 new-generation antidepressants: a multiple-treatments meta-analysis. *Lancet*. **373**: 746–758.

5 Chappell AS et al. (2009) Duloxetine, a centrally acting analgesic, in the treatment of patients with osteoarthritis knee pain: a 13-week, randomized, placebo-controlled trial. *Pain*. **146**: 253–260.

6 Lunn (2009) Duloxetine for treating painful neuropathy or chronic pain. *Cochrane Database of Systematic Reviews*. **4**: CD007115.

7 Smith EM et al. (2013) Effect of duloxetine on pain, function, and quality of life among patients with chemotherapy-induced painful peripheral neuropathy: a randomized clinical trial. *JAMA*. **309**: 1359–1367.

8 Finnerup NB (2011) Is duloxetine useful for central neuropathic pain? *Pain*. **152**: 243–244.

9 Vranken JH et al. (2011) Duloxetine in patients with central neuropathic pain caused by spinal cord injury or stroke: a randomized, double-blind, placebo-controlled trial. *Pain*. **152**: 267–273.

10 Kaur H et al. (2011) A comparative evaluation of amitriptyline and duloxetine in painful diabetic neuropathy: a randomized, double-blind, cross-over clinical trial. *Diabetes Care*. **34**: 818–822.

11 Boyle J et al. (2012) Randomized, placebo-controlled comparison of amitriptyline, duloxetine, and pregabalin in patients with chronic diabetic peripheral neuropathic pain: impact on pain, polysomnographic sleep, daytime functioning, and quality of life. *Diabetes Care*. **35**: 2451–2458.

12 NICE (2006) Urinary incontinence: the management of urinary incontinence in women. *Clinical Guideline*. CG40. www.nice.org.uk

13 Greist J et al. (2004) Incidence and duration of antidepressant-induced nausea: duloxetine compared with paroxetine and fluoxetine. *Clinical Therapeutics*. **26**: 1446–1455.

14 Brannan SK et al. (2005) Onset of action for duloxetine 60 mg once daily: double-blind, placebo-controlled studies. *Journal of Psychiatric Research*. **39**: 161–172.

15 Goldstein DJ et al. (2004) Duloxetine in the treatment of depression: a double-blind placebo-controlled comparison with paroxetine. *Journal of Clinical Psychopharmacology*. **24**: 389–399.

16 Detke MJ et al. (2004) Duloxetine in the acute and long-term treatment of major depressive disorder: a placebo- and paroxetine-controlled trial. *European Neuropsychopharmacology*. **14**: 457–470.

17 Mallinckrodt CH et al. (2003) Duloxetine: A New Treatment for the Emotional and Physical Symptoms of Depression. *Primary Care Companion Journal of Clinical Psychiatry*. **5**: 19–28.

18 Nemeroff CB et al. (2002) Duloxetine for the treatment of major depressive disorder. *Psychopharmacology Bulletin*. **36**: 106–132.

19 DTB (2003) Managing postpartum stress urinary incontinence. *Drug and Therapeutics Bulletin*. **41**: 46–48.

Updated October 2013

MIRTAZAPINE   BNF 4.3.4

Class: α_2 Adrenergic and $5HT_{2A/C}$ antagonist antidepressant.

Indications: Depression, †anxiety and panic disorders, †pruritus, †serotonin toxicity.

Contra-indications: Concurrent use with an MAOI or within 2 weeks of its cessation (see Serotonin toxicity, p.195).

Pharmacology

Mirtazapine antagonises receptors which inhibit mono-amine release:[1,2]

- pre-synaptic α_2-adrenergic antagonism disinhibits serotonin and noradrenaline (norepinephrine) release
- post-synaptic $5HT_{2A}$ and $5HT_{2C}$ antagonism disinhibits noradrenaline (norepinephrine) and dopamine release.

In addition, it antagonizes H_1- and $5HT_3$-receptors. The H_1 antagonistic activity of mirtazapine is responsible for its sedative properties. At lower doses, the antihistaminic effect of mirtazapine predominates, producing sedation. With higher doses, sedation is reduced as noradrenergic and dopaminergic neural transmission increases. It has no significant antimuscarinic activity.

The antidepressant effects of mirtazapine manifest faster than with SSRIs.[3] There are also fewer relapses compared with **amitriptyline**.[4] For refractory depression, mirtazapine can be combined with an SSRI or **venlafaxine**, particularly if a previous switch of antidepressant monotherapy was unhelpful (see p.198).

Mirtazapine is not associated with cardiovascular toxicity or sexual dysfunction.[4] A blockade of $5HT_2$ leads to appetite stimulation. Its anti-emetic properties may be due to $5HT_2$ and/or $5HT_3$ antagonism.[5,6]

Benefit reported for neuropathic pain,[7,8] intractable pruritus,[9] and serotonin toxicity[10] has not been confirmed in RCTs.

Mirtazapine displays linear pharmacokinetics at usual doses. Food does not affect absorption, binding to plasma proteins is about 85% and steady-state is reached after 5 days. Mirtazapine is extensively metabolised and eliminated via the urine and faeces. It is a racemic mixture of two active enantiomers: the R-enantiomer is metabolized by CYP3A4 to the active metabolite demethylmirtazapine, whereas the S-enantiomer is metabolized by CYP2D6 and CYP1A2.[4] Clearance in the elderly may be reduced by ≤40%.

Bio-availability 50% PO.
Onset of action hours–days (off-label indications); 1–2 weeks (antidepressant).
Time to peak plasma concentration 2h.
Plasma halflife 20–40h; often shorter in men (26h) than women (37h) but can extend up to 65h.
Duration of action variable; up to several days.

Cautions

Suicide risk: the possibility of a suicide attempt is inherent in major depression and persists until remission. Antidepressants may themselves cause suicidal ideation, particularly in those aged ≤25 years (see p.193).

Bipolar disorder (can transform into manic phase); epilepsy (seizures occur rarely; risk relative to other antidepressants is uncertain); cardiac disease (manufacturer advises increased monitoring with ischaemic heart disease or risk of arrhythmia); hepatic impairment (reduce dose); renal impairment (reduce dose; clearance of a single oral dose halved when creatinine clearance < 10mL/min); diabetes mellitus (may alter glycaemic control); narrow-angle glaucoma (mydriasis reported).

Drug interactions

Additive pharmacodynamic interactions with other drugs (see p.194), notably serotonin toxicity (see Box B, p.195). Concurrent administration with an MAOI or within 2 weeks of its cessation is contra-indicated (see above).

Mirtazapine is metabolized by CYP1A2, CYP2D6, and CYP3A4. Caution should be taken with concurrent use of drugs which inhibit or induce these enzymes, particularly in those who are poor CYP2D6 metabolizers (see Chapter 25, p.767).

Specific significant interactions[11]
- **ketoconazole** (strong CYP3A4 inhibitor) can *increase* the plasma concentrations of mirtazapine by ≤40%; other strong CYP3A4 inhibitors (e.g. azole antifungals, HIV-protease inhibitors, and macrolides) will probably have a similar effect; a dose reduction of mirtazapine may be necessary
- **fluvoxamine** (strong CYP1A2 inhibitor can *increase* the plasma concentrations of mirtazapine up to four times and **cimetidine** by 50%
- **carbamazepine and phenytoin** (hepatic enzyme inducers) *decrease* mirtazapine plasma concentrations by up to 40%; other enzyme-inducing drugs (e.g. other anti-epileptic drugs and **rifampicin**) probably have a similar effect.

Undesirable effects

Very common (>10%): increase in appetite and weight gain;[12] drowsiness during the first few weeks of treatment. *Dose reduction reduces the likelihood of an antidepressant effect and does not necessarily alleviate drowsiness.*
Uncommon (<1%, >0.1%): hepatic impairment.
Very rare (<0.01%): agranulocytosis.

Dose and use
Depression, panic and anxiety disorders[4]
- start with 15mg at bedtime
- if necessary, increase the dose by 15mg every 2 weeks up to 45mg
- if no response after 4 weeks on 45mg, switch to an alternative antidepressant
- if effective, continue until the patient has been symptom-free for ≥6 months (see p.199); then discontinue over 2–4 weeks.

Intractable itch
Use as for depression; continue indefinitely.[7,9]

Supply
Mirtazapine (generic)
Tablets 15mg, 30mg, 45mg, 28 days @ 30mg at bedtime = £2.
Tablets orodispersible 15mg, 30mg, 45mg, 28 days @ 30mg at bedtime = £3; *tablets should be placed on the tongue, allowed to disperse, then swallowed.*
Oral solution 15mg/mL, 28 days @ 30mg at bedtime = £40.

1 Stahl SM (2008) *Essential Psychopharmacology. Neuroscientific basis and practical applications* (3e). Cambridge University Press, Cambridge.
2 Devoto P et al. (2004) Mirtazapine-induced corelease of dopamine and noradrenaline from noradrenergic neurons in the medial prefrontal and occipital cortex. *European Journal of Pharmacology.* **487**: 105–111.
3 Watanabe N et al. (2011) Mirtazapine versus other antidepressive agents for depression. *Cochrane Database of Systematic Reviews.* **12**: CD006528.
4 Croom KF et al. (2009) Mirtazapine: a review of its use in major depression and other psychiatric disorders. *CNS Drugs.* **23**: 427–452.
5 Kim SW et al. (2008) Effectiveness of mirtazapine for nausea and insomnia in cancer patients with depression. *Psychiatry and Clinical Neurosciences.* **62**: 75–83.
6 Chen CC et al. (2008) Premedication with mirtazapine reduces preoperative anxiety and postoperative nausea and vomiting. *Anesthesia and Analgesia.* **106**: 109–113.
7 Brannon G and Stone K (1999) The use of mirtazapine in a patient with chronic pain. *Journal of Pain and Symptom Management.* **18**: 382–385.
8 Ritzenthaler B and Pearson D (2000) Efficacy and tolerability of mirtazapine in neuropathic pain. *Palliative Medicine.* **14**: 346.
9 Krajnik M and Zylicz Z (2001) Understanding pruritus in systemic disease. *Journal of Pain and Symptom Management.* **21**: 151–168.
10 Hoes M and Zeijpveld J (1996) Mirtazapine as treatment for serotonin syndrome. *Pharmacopsychiatry.* **29**: 81.
11 Baxter K and Preston CL (2011). *Stockley's Drug Interactions.* London:- Pharmaceutical Press www.medicinescomplete.com (accessed June 2013).
12 Abed R and Cooper M (1999) Mirtazapine causing hyperphagia. *British Journal of Psychiatry.* **174**: 181–182.

Updated October 2013

TRAZODONE   BNF 4.3.1

Class: α-Adrenergic and $5HT_{2A/C}$ antagonist antidepressant; serotonin re-uptake inhibitor.

Indications: Depression, †anxiety and panic disorders, ††agitated delirium, insomnia.

Contra-indications: Concurrent use with an MAOI or within 2 weeks of its cessation (see Serotonin toxicity, p.195). Avoid use in the initial recovery period after an acute myocardial infarction.

Pharmacology
Trazodone is an α_1-adenergic, a_2-adrenergic, $5HT_{2A}$- and $5HT_{2C}$-receptor antagonist and, at higher doses, a serotonin reuptake inhibitor.[1] Its receptor profile accounts for its sedative effect and contributes to its antidepressant action by disinhibiting mono-amine release. It is devoid of antimuscarinic activity.

Although generally as effective as other antidepressants,[2] trazodone is not often used to treat depression in palliative care because of unacceptable daytime drowsiness. Thus, when used, it is generally for unlabelled indications.

Trazodone has an active metabolite, m-chlorophenylpiperazine. Excretion is almost entirely as free or conjugated metabolites. Although trazodone has less effect on cardiac function than TCAs, arrhythmias have been reported, ranging from heart block to ventricular tachycardia.[3,4]

Trazodone has been used for behavioural problems in patients with dementia (agitation, restlessness, wandering, physical aggression, inappropriate sexual activity, culturally inappropriate behaviours, hoarding, cursing, shadowing, screaming, sleep disorders).[5,6] However, larger studies have not replicated promising earlier results.[7] Such behaviours occur for many reasons, including an appropriate response to a distressing situation. Possible precipitants should be treated or modified. Medication should only be used as a last resort where non-drug measures have failed (see Antipsychotics, p.173).

Trazodone is sometimes used as a night sedative despite the absence of RCT evidence confirming its efficacy in non-depressed patients. In a dose of 25–50mg at bedtime, it is reported to be effective and well tolerated.[8]

An RCT found no benefit for spinal cord injury pain, although it may have been underpowered (n = 19).[9]

Bio-availability 65%.

Onset of action 30–60min for insomnia or agitation; 1–4 weeks as an antidepressant.

Time to peak plasma concentration 1h if taken fasting; 2h if taken after food.

Plasma halflife 7h; may be doubled in the elderly.

Duration of action variable, situation dependent.

Cautions

Suicide risk: the possibility of a suicide attempt is inherent in major depression and persists until remission. Antidepressants may themselves cause suicidal ideation, particularly in those aged ≤25 years (see p.193).

Bipolar disorder (can transform into manic phase); epilepsy (lowers seizure threshold); cardiac disease (risk of arrhythmia); severe hepatic impairment (increased drowsiness); renal impairment.

Drug interactions

Additive pharmacodynamic interactions with other drugs (see p.194) notably serotonin toxicity (see Box B, p.195). Concurrent administration with an MAOI or within 2 weeks of its cessation is contra-indicated (see above).

Trazodone is metabolized by CYP3A4, and possibly CYP2D6. Caution should be taken with concurrent use of drugs which inhibit or induce these enzymes particularly in those who are poor CYP2D6 metabolizers (see Chapter 25, p.767).

Specific significant interactions[10]
- **clarithromycin**, and **ritonavir** (strong CYP3A4 inhibitors) can *increase* plasma concentrations of trazodone by one third and double the elimination half-life; thus, strong CYP3A4 inhibitors should be avoided where possible or a lower dose of trazodone used
- **carbamazepine** can *decrease* plasma concentrations of trazodone by ≤75%.

If trazodone is prescribed concurrently, the dose of **warfarin** may need to be *increased*[11] and, because of reports of toxicity, the dose of **digoxin** and **phenytoin** *decreased*; the mechanism for these interactions is unknown.

Undesirable effects

Common (<10%, >1%): daytime drowsiness, lethargy, dizziness (orthostatic hypotension), psychomotor impairment.

Uncommon (<1%, >0.1%): nausea, vomiting, sweating.

Rare (<0.1%, >0.01%): increased libido[12,13] and priapism (in 0.01%).[14,15] These have not been reported with low-dose (25–50mg) night sedation.

Dose and use
Depression

Trazodone is not a first-line treatment for depression (see p.191). It is more commonly used as an adjunct for concurrent insomnia or anxiety.

- start with 150mg at bedtime (100mg at bedtime in frail elderly patients)
- if necessary, increase dose by 50mg weekly up to 300mg (either as a single night-time dose or in divided doses)
- maximum daily dose 600mg in divided doses (generally inpatients only).

Anxiety
- start with 75mg PO at bedtime
- if necessary, increase dose gradually up to 300mg daily (as either a single night-time dose or in divided doses).

Insomnia
- start with 50mg PO at bedtime (25mg at bedtime in frail or elderly patients)
- if necessary, increase to 100mg
- occasionally may need 150–200mg.

Agitated delirium, and challenging behaviours in those with dementia
Note: Trazodone is not a first-line choice for either indication (see Antipsychotics, p.173).
- start with 50mg PO at bedtime
- if necessary, increase the dose
- unlikely to need > 300mg/24h.[5,6]

Supply
Trazodone (generic)
Capsules 50mg, 100mg, 28 days @ 100mg at bedtime = £2.50.
Tablets (scored) 150mg, 28 days @ 150mg at bedtime = £4.50.
Oral solution (sugar-free) 50mg/5mL, 28 days @ 100mg at bedtime = £45.

---

1 Stahl SM (2008) Essential Psychopharmacology. Neuroscientific basis and practical applications (3e). Cambridge University Press, Cambridge.
2 Haria M et al. (1994) Trazodone. A review of its pharmacology, therapeutic use in depression and therapeutic potential in other disorders. Drugs Aging. 4: 331–355.
3 Vlay SC and Friedling S (1983) Trazodone exacerbation of VT. American Heart Journal. 106: 604.
4 Johnson BA (1985) Trazodone toxicity. British Journal of Hospital Medicine. 33: 298.
5 Lebert F et al. (1994) Behavioral effects of trazodone in Alzheimer's disease. Journal of Clinical Psychiatry. 55: 536–538.
6 Sultzer DL et al. (1997) A double-blind comparison of trazodone and haloperidol for treatment of agitation in patients with dementia. American Journal of Geriatric Psychiatry. 5: 60–69.
7 Jeste DV et al. (2008) ACNP White Paper: update on use of antipsychotic drugs in elderly persons with dementia. Neuropsychopharmacology. 33: 957–970.
8 Mendelson WB (2005) A review of the evidence for the efficacy and safety of trazodone in insomnia. Journal of Clinical Psychiatry. 66: 469–476.
9 Davidoff G et al. (1987) Trazodone hydrochloride in the treatment of dysesthetic pain in traumatic myelopathy: a radomized double-blind, placebo controlled study. Pain. 29: 151–161.
10 Baxter K and Preston CL (2011). Stockley's Drug Interactions. London:- Pharmaceutical Press www.medicinescomplete.com (accessed June 2013).
11 Small NL and Giamonna KA (2000) Interaction between warfarin and trazodone. Annals of Pharmacotherapy. 34: 734–736.
12 Gartrell N (1986) Increased libido in women receiving trazodone. American Journal of Psychiatry. 143: 781–782.
13 Sullivan G (1988) Increased libido in three men treated with trazodone. Journal of Clinical Psychiatry. 49: 202–203.
14 Patel AG et al. (1996) Priapism associated with psychotropic drugs. British Journal of Hospital Medicine. 55: 315–319.
15 Pescatori ES et al. (1993) Priapism of the clitoris: a case report following trazodone use. Journal of Urology. 149: 1557–1559.

Updated October 2013

---

*PSYCHOSTIMULANTS   BNF 4.4

Indications: Attention deficit hyperactivity disorder (**methylphenidate, dexamfetamine**); daytime drowsiness due to narcolepsy (**modafinil, dexamfetamine**), †obstructive sleep apnoea or chronic shift work-related sleep disorder (discouraged by regulators);[1] †depression when prognosis limited (i.e. 2–4 weeks); †opioid-related drowsiness; †fatigue refractory to correction of underlying contributory factors.

Contra-indications: Severe cardiovascular disease (e.g. uncontrolled hypertension or angina, arrhythmias; also see Cautions), use within the last 2 weeks of a monoamine oxidase inhibitor (MAOI) see p.194, including **procarbazine** (an antineoplastic drug and a weak MAOI).

Manufacturers of **methylphenidate** and **dexamfetamine** also recommend avoiding in glaucoma, phaechromocytoma, thyrotoxicosis and history of severe psychiatric illness.

Pharmacology

The psychostimulants, **dexamfetamine**, **methylphenidate** and **modafinil**, inhibit or reverse dopamine re-uptake transporters thereby increasing synaptic dopamine.[2-6] Dopamine has a central role in attention, arousal and motivation. It is released in response to stimuli and thoughts perceived as relevant, particularly with regard to 'threat' or 'reward'. Thus, psychostimulants can improve alertness, motivation and mood.[2,4-8]

Dopaminergic dysfunction in the mesolimbic and mesocortical systems is implicated in several disorders. In attention-deficit hyperactivity disorder, psychostimulants may improve attention by correcting a deficit in dopamine release in response to relevant stimuli.[9] Conversely, in psychoses, dopamine excess increases the importance attached to thoughts and perceptions, e.g. the actions of others gain an enhanced relevance, and are interpreted as evidence of threat (paranoid delusions) or importance (grandiose delusions). This explains the beneficial effects of D_2 antagonists in patients experiencing hallucinations and delusions (see p.168).[3]

Dexamfetamine, **methylphenidate** and **modafinil** have the best evidence base to support use in palliative care,[10] with **methylphenidate** probably the most widely used.[11,12] Although m/r formulations of **dexamfetamine** or **methylphenidate** are available (both generally given once daily), they have more risk of insomnia, particularly if taken later in the day.[13]

Modafinil is sometimes suggested as an alternative where **methylphenidate** is poorly tolerated. However, its undesirable cardiovascular and psychotropic effects appear similar and it is more expensive. Further, regulators have recommended withdrawing Marketing Authorizations for all Indications except narcolepsy because of concerns about undesirable skin and neuropsychiatric effects and abuse potential.[1]

The milder psychostimulant, **caffeine**, also acts indirectly via dopamine. Adenosine receptors are co-localised with and inhibit D_1 and D_2 receptors and as adenosine accumulates during the daytime, dopamine-mediated arousal is reduced; **caffeine**, which acts as an adenosine receptor antagonist, helps prevent this.[2,14] Present in some OTC combination analgesics, **caffeine** appears beneficial for headache, but not other pains.[15]

Table 1 contains selected pharmacokinetic data. About half or less of a dose of **dexamfetamine** is excreted renally and largely unchanged; thus there is a theoretical risk of increased toxicity in renal impairment.[11]

Table 1 Pharmacokinetic details for selected psychostimulants[16-19]

	Oral bio-availability (%)	Time to peak plasma concentration (h)	Halflife (h)	Metabolism
Dexamfetamine	No data	2–4	6–12	Multiple routes; 50% renally excreted unchanged
Methylphenidate	30[a]	1–3	2	Non-CYP carboxylesterase[b]
Modafinil	40–65[c]	1.5–3	d-modafinil[d] 3; l-modafinil[d] 10–16	CYP3A4; non-CYP esterase[b]

a. almost completely absorbed but undergoes extensive first-pass hepatic metabolism
b. metabolites are inactive
c. estimated from urinary recovery of radiolabelled doses; absolute bio-availability unknown because of the lack of an IV preparation
d. enantiomers are equipotent.

Cautions

Psychostimulants may exacerbate cardiovascular disease (e.g. severe hypertension, angina, arrhythmia) and are not recommended in patients with known cardiac disease without further specialist cardiac evaluation (see also Contra-indications). SPCs recommend that heart rate, BP and an ECG (**modafanil**) are assessed at baseline, and subsequently heart rate and BP are monitored at regular intervals (e.g. every 6 months) or after an increase in dose.

Psychostimulants may also exacerbate psychiatric illness (e.g. anxiety, agitation, psychosis, addiction disorders), epilepsy (possible lowering of seizure threshold), hyperthyroidism and closed-angle glaucoma (not **modafinil**).

Although rare in adults, serious skin reactions occur with **modafinil** in 1% of children; consider alternatives where possible (e.g. **methylphenidate**).

Drug interactions

Pharmacodynamic interactions include those with sympathomimetics (e.g. MAOIs, see contra-indications) and antipsychotics (reduced stimulant effect).

Methylphenidate and **modafinil** may increase plasma concentrations of TCAs, **phenytoin** and **warfarin** (check INR at least weekly until stabilized). **Modafinil** may also increase the plasma concentrations of **diazepam**.

Modafinil induces CYP3A4/5 resulting in reduced efficacy of **ciclosporin**, HIV-protease inhibitors, **midazolam**, L-type calcium-channel blockers, statins and hormonal contraception. **Modafinil** also inhibits CYP2C19 and thus may decrease the plasma concentrations of the active metabolites of **clopidogrel**.

Undesirable effects

Undesirable effects have been reported in up to 30% of patients.

Neuropsychiatric: insomnia, agitation and anorexia (generally settle after 2–3 weeks if the drug is continued or resolve after 2–3 days if the drug is discontinued), psychosis, movement disorders.

Cardiovascular: tachyarrhythmias, hypertension, angina (rare).

Other: headache, common and responds to slower dose titration; nausea; *very rarely cerebral arteritis occurs with* **methylphenidate**. Mild rashes are common with **modafinil**; serious skin reactions occur in 1% of children.

Use of psychostimulants in palliative care

Depression

Psychostimulants are used where prognosis is anticipated to be only about 2–4 weeks (see p.206). This is shorter than suggested by previous consensus guidance[20] because of the recognition that conventional antidepressants act faster than previously thought.[21] Further, although trials generally show psychostimulants to be well tolerated in the short term, methodological limitations preclude firm conclusions about their efficacy as antidepressants.[10,22,23] Thus, conventional antidepressants should be used if the patient has a prognosis sufficient for a response to manifest.[10,20,22] Concurrent use of a psychostimulant with a conventional antidepressant may hasten the response compared with the latter alone, particularly in relation to fatigue.[22]

Methylphenidate is probably the most commonly used psychostimulant for depression in palliative care. Although undesirable effects are similar for all psychostimulants, some patients may benefit by switching to an alternative (e.g. **modafinil**) if the first choice is ineffective or poorly tolerated.

Fatigue

RCTs yield conflicting results, and the use of psychostimulants for fatigue remains controversial (Table 2). Most RCTs in cancer patients used **methylphenidate**, whereas **modafinil** has been mainly examined in neurodegenerative conditions. Many trials found large placebo responses, including a recent RCT of **modafinil** for cancer-related fatigue where no difference was found between treatment groups.[24] Thus, psychostimulants should only be used when other measures are insufficient.[25–27] For example:

- when feasible, correction of underlying causal factors, e.g. anaemia, depression, electrolyte disturbance
- modification of daily routine, e.g. encourage exercise, energy conservation, practical help to aid adjustment to changing circumstances.[26,28]

Modafinil is an alternative, particularly if **methylphenidate** is poorly tolerated.

Table 2 RCTs of psychostimulants in fatigue

Patient population	Psychostimulant	Trial size (n)	Duration (weeks)	Outcome
Cancer[29]	Methylphenidate	112	1	No difference
Cancer[30]	Dexamfetamine	50	1	No difference
Cancer[31]	Methylphenidate	148	4	No overall difference. Beneficial in a subgroup with more severe fatigue (p=0.02)
Prostate cancer[32]	Methylphenidate	32	6	No difference
Mixed (predominantly cancer)[33]	Methylphenidate	30	2	Beneficial (p<0.05)
Chemotherapy[34]	D-methylphenidate	154	8	Beneficial (p<0.05)
Chemotherapy[35]	Modafinil	877	4 cycles	No overall difference. Beneficial in a subgroup with more severe fatigue
Chemotherapy[36]	D-methylphenidate	57	End of therapy	No difference
Cranial radiotherapy[37]	Methylphenidate[a]	68	8	No difference
Parkinson's disease[38]	Modafinil	19	8	No difference
Multiple sclerosis[39]	Modafinil	21	8	Beneficial (p<0.05)
Multiple sclerosis[40]	Modafinil	115	5	No difference
MND/ALS[41]	Modafinil	32	4	Beneficial (p<0.01)
HIV+[42]	Modafinil	115	4	Beneficial (NNT 2.3; p<0.001)

a. examined prophylactic use.

Opioid-related drowsiness
Drowsiness is common when opioids are commenced or the dose is increased; it is generally transient, lasting about 1 week. Persistent drowsiness may indicate opioid toxicity; a trial dose reduction should be made and other drug and non-drug approaches considered to provide adequate analgesia (see p.295). However, some patients experience persistent drowsiness despite adjusting the opioid dose. In this circumstance, switching to an alternative opioid may be of benefit (see Opioid dose conversion ratios, p.661).

Psychostimulants are occasionally used for opioid-related drowsiness refractory to these measures. They may improve psychomotor performance and allow opioid dose escalation to a higher level than would otherwise be possible, including in some instances of difficult to manage break-through (episodic) pain.[43] However, these reports predated the availability of other potential options, e.g. transmucosal **fentanyl** (see p.413).

Dose
Methylphenidate
- start with 2.5–5mg b.d. (on waking/breakfast time and noon/lunchtime)
- if necessary, increase by *daily* increments of 2.5–5mg b.d.
- usual maximum 20–40mg/24h
- up to 60mg/24h has been used for depression.[22]

Modafinil
Dose titration is slower:
- start with 100mg each morning
- if necessary after 1 week, increase to 200mg each morning
- maximum dose 400mg/24h.

The manufacturer recommends either a single morning dose or divided doses in the morning and at noon. However, given the relatively long halflife of **modafinil**, the latter may increase the risk of sleep disturbance.

Dexamfetamine
* start with 2.5–5mg each morning
* if necessary, increase progressively every 1–2 days to 40mg each morning.

Supply
All products are **CD**.

Dexamfetamine sulfate (generic)
Tablets (scored) 5mg, 28 days @ 5mg once daily = £16.
Oral solution 5mg/5mL, 28 days @ 5mg once daily = £11 (unauthorized, available as a special order product from Rosemont or Martindale Pharma, see p.817).

Methylphenidate
M/r products are available, but are not appropriate as daytime stimulants in palliative care.
Methylphenidate hydrochloride (generic)
Tablets (scored) 5mg, 10mg, 20mg, 28 days @ 10mg b.d. = £13 (note: based on BNF pricing, this is *more expensive* than branded Ritalin® tablets).

Ritalin® (Novartis)
Tablets (scored) 10mg, 28 days @ 10mg b.d. = £11 (note: based on BNF pricing, this is *cheaper* than generic tablets).

Modafinil
Provigil® (Cephalon)
Tablets (scored) 100mg, 200mg, 28 days @ 200mg each morning = £105.

---

1 MHRA (2010) European Medicines Agency recommends restricting the use of modafinil. *Drug Safety Update*. **4**. www.mhra.gov.uk/Safetyinformation
2 Boutrel B and Koob GF (2004) What keeps us awake: the neuropharmacology of stimulants and wakefulness-promoting medications. *Sleep*. **27**: 1181–1194.
3 Kapur S et al. (2005) From dopamine to salience to psychosis–linking biology, pharmacology and phenomenology of psychosis. *Schizophrenia Research*. **79**: 59–68.
4 Qu WM et al. (2008) Dopaminergic D1 and D_2 receptors are essential for the arousal effect of modafinil. *Journal of Neuroscience*. **28**: 8462–8469.
5 Volkow ND et al. (2009) Effects of modafinil on dopamine and dopamine transporters in the male human brain: clinical implications. *Journal of the American Medical Association*. **301**: 1148–1154.
6 Kumar R (2008) Approved and investigational uses of modafinil: an evidence-based review. *Drugs*. **68**: 1803–1839.
7 Fleckenstein AE et al. (2007) New insights into the mechanism of action of amphetamines. *Annual Review of Pharmacology and Toxicology*. **47**: 681–698.
8 Sulzer D et al. (2005) Mechanisms of neurotransmitter release by amphetamines: a review. *Progress in Neurobiology*. **75**: 406–433.
9 Volkow ND et al. (2005) Imaging the effects of methylphenidate on brain dopamine: new model on its therapeutic actions for attention-deficit/hyperactivity disorder. *Biological Psychiatry*. **57**: 1410–1415.
10 Candy et al. (2008) Psychostimulants for depression. *Cochrane Database of Systematic Reviews*. **2**: CD006722.
11 Dein S and George R (2002) A place for psychostimulants in palliative care? *Journal of Palliative Care*. **18**: 196–199.
12 Masand PS and Tesar GE (1996) Use of stimulants in the medically ill. *Psychiatric Clinics of North America*. **19**: 515–547.
13 Burns MM and Eisendrath SJ (1994) Dextroamphetamine treatment for depression in terminally ill patients. *Psychosomatics*. **35**: 80–83.
14 Canals M et al. (2003) Adenosine A2A-dopamine D_2 receptor-receptor heteromerization: qualitative and quantitative assessment by fluorescence and bioluminescence energy transfer. *Journal of Biological Chemistry*. **278**: 46741–46749.
15 Sawynok J (2011) Caffeine and pain. *Pain*. **152**: 726–729.
16 Challman TD and Lipsky JJ (2000) Methylphenidate: its pharmacology and uses. *Mayo Clinic Proceedings*. **75**: 711–721.
17 de la Torre R et al. (2004) Clinical pharmacokinetics of amfetamine and related substances: monitoring in conventional and non-conventional matrices. *Clinical Pharmacokinetics*. **43**: 157–185.
18 Connor DF and Steingard RJ (2004) New formulations of stimulants for attention-deficit hyperactivity disorder: therapeutic potential. *CNS Drugs*. **18**: 1011–1030.
19 Robertson P, Jr. and Hellriegel ET (2003) Clinical pharmacokinetic profile of modafinil. *Clinical Pharmacokinetics*. **42**: 123–137.
20 Block SD (2000) Assessing and managing depression in the terminally ill patient. ACP-ASIM End-of-Life Care Consensus Panel. American College of Physicians - American Society of Internal Medicine. *Annals of internal medicine*. **132**: 209–218.
21 Tylee A and Walters P (2007) Onset of action of antidepressants. *British Medical Journal*. **334**: 911–912.
22 Orr K and Taylor D (2007) Psychostimulants in the treatment of depression : a review of the evidence. *CNS Drugs*. **21**: 239–257.
23 Centeno C et al. (2012) Multi-centre, double-blind, randomised placebo-controlled clinical trial on the efficacy of methylphenidate on depressive symptoms in advanced cancer patients. *BMJ Supportive and Palliative Care*. **2**: 328–333.
24 Wee B (2012) Personal communication.

---

25 National Comprehensive Care Network (2012): Cancer related fatigue. *Clinical practice guidelines in oncology*. Available from: www.nccn.org

26 Radbruch L et al. (2008) Fatigue in palliative care patients – an EAPC approach. *Palliative Medicine*. **22**: 13–32.

27 Minton O et al. (2008) A systematic review and meta-analysis of the pharmacological treatment of cancer-related fatigue. *Journal of the National Cancer Institute*. **100**: 1155–1166.

28 Cramp F and Daniel J (2008) Exercise for the management of cancer-related fatigue in adults. *Cochrane Database of Systematic Reviews*. **2**: CD006145.

29 Bruera E et al. (2006) Patient-controlled methylphenidate for cancer fatigue: a double-blind, randomized, placebo-controlled trial. *Journal of Clinical Oncology*. **24**: 2073–2078.

30 Auret KA et al. (2009) A randomized, double-blind, placebo-controlled trial assessing the impact of dexamphetamine on fatigue in patients with advanced cancer. *Journal of Pain and Symptom Management*. **37**: 613–621.

31 Moraska AR et al. (2010) Phase III, randomized, double-blind, placebo-controlled study of long-acting methylphenidate for cancer-related fatigue: North Central Cancer Treatment Group NCCTG-N05C7 trial. *Journal of Clinical Oncology*. **28**: 3673–3679.

32 Roth AJ et al. (2010) Methylphenidate for fatigue in ambulatory men with prostate cancer. *Cancer*. **116**: 5102–5110.

33 Kerr CW et al. (2012) Effects of methylphenidate on fatigue and depression: a randomized, double-blind, placebo-controlled trial. *Journal of Pain and Symptom Management*. **43**: 68–77.

34 Lower EE et al. (2009) Efficacy of dexmethylphenidate for the treatment of fatigue after cancer chemotherapy: a randomized clinical trial. *Journal of Pain and Symptom Management*. **38**: 650–662.

35 Jean-Pierre P et al. (2010) A phase 3 randomized, placebo-controlled, double-blind, clinical trial of the effect of modafinil on cancer-related fatigue among 631 patients receiving chemotherapy: a University of Rochester Cancer Center Community Clinical Oncology Program Research base study. *Cancer*. **116**: 3513–3520.

36 Mar Fan HG et al. (2008) A randomised, placebo-controlled, double-blind trial of the effects of d-methylphenidate on fatigue and cognitive dysfunction in women undergoing adjuvant chemotherapy for breast cancer. *Supportive Care in Cancer*. **16**: 577–583.

37 Butler JM, Jr. et al. (2007) A phase III, double-blind, placebo-controlled prospective randomized clinical trial of d-threo-methylphenidate HCl in brain tumor patients receiving radiation therapy. *International Journal of Radiation Oncology, Biology, Physics*. **69**: 1496–1501.

38 Lou JS et al. (2009) Using modafinil to treat fatigue in Parkinson disease: a double-blind, placebo-controlled pilot study. *Clinical Neuropharmacology*. **32**: 305–310.

39 Lange R et al. (2009) Modafinil effects in multiple sclerosis patients with fatigue. *Journal of Neurology*. **256**: 645–650.

40 Stankoff B et al. (2005) Modafinil for fatigue in MS: a randomized placebo-controlled double-blind study. *Neurology*. **64**: 1139–1143.

41 Rabkin JG et al. (2009) Modafinil treatment of fatigue in patients with ALS: a placebo-controlled study. *Muscle and Nerve*. **39**: 297–303.

42 Rabkin JG et al. (2010) Modafinil treatment for fatigue in HIV/AIDS: a randomized placebo-controlled study. *Journal of Clinical Psychiatry*. **71**: 707–715.

43 Stone P and Minton O (2011) European Palliative Care Research collaborative pain guidelines. Central side-effects management: what is the evidence to support best practice in the management of sedation, cognitive impairment and myoclonus? *Palliative Medicine*. **25**: 431–441.

Updated October 2013

*CANNABINOIDS   BNF 4.6 & 10.2.2

Indications: Chemotherapy-induced nausea and vomiting (nabilone); refractory spasticity in multiple sclerosis (Sativex®); †pain unresponsive to standard treatments.

Contra-indications: History (including family history) of psychosis.

Pharmacology

Endocannabinoids have important regulatory roles throughout the nervous system, immune system, and elsewhere, making them a potential therapeutic target for a wide range of disorders, including nausea, pain, cancer, cardiovascular disease, spasticity, epilepsy and immunomodulation.[1–7]

Currently available cannabinoids all contain the psycho-active constituent of *Cannabis sativa*, Δ^9-tetrahydrocannabinol (Δ^9-THC) or a synthetic analogue. They are generally less effective or less well tolerated than alternative drugs and are relatively expensive. Their use as anti-emetics was rapidly eclipsed by the advent of $5HT_3$ antagonists. Although **dronabinol** (not UK) reduced AIDS-related anorexia and weight loss, there was a trend towards more rapid deterioration in performance status.[8] In cancer-related anorexia, cannabinoids were inferior to **megestrol** and no more effective than placebo.[9,10] Their analgesic effect is modest.[11] Further, despite interest in their respiratory effects,[12,13] benefit in breathlessness has *not* been confirmed by RCT.

An improved understanding of the endocannabinoid system and *Cannabis sativa*'s many non-psycho-active compounds[1,14] has led to several developments in an attempt to improve effectiveness and tolerability:

- CB$_2$-selective agonists[15,16]
- peripherally-acting cannabinoids[17]
- inhibitors of endocannabinoid breakdown[18,19]
- combining cannabinoids with different properties, e.g. Δ^9-THC with cannabidiol (CBD; see below).[20]

Endocannabinoid system

The endocannabinoid system comprises:[21]
- two known receptors
  ▷ CB$_1$, expressed mainly by central and peripheral neurones
  ▷ CB$_2$, expressed mainly by immune cells
- endogenous cannabinoids (endocannabinoids), mainly fatty acids derived from arachidonic acid, produced *de novo* as required, and then rapidly removed by hydrolysis. Several have been identified, notably:
  ▷ anandamide (arachidonylethanolamide)
  ▷ 2-arachidonyl glycerin (2-AG)[22]
- enzymes and uptake systems involved in endocannabinoid metabolism, including COX-2 and fatty acid amide hydrolase-1.[18,19]

CB$_1$ (an inhibitory receptor) reduces neuronal excitability and neurotransmitter release by opening potassium channels and blocking N/P/Q-type calcium channels respectively. It is part of a negative feedback loop which regulates neurotransmitter release and thereby the function of various CNS circuits (Figure 1). This partly explains some of the antispasticity, analgesic and other effects of cannabinoids.[21,23]

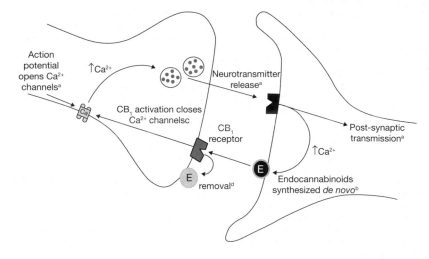

Figure 1 Cannabinoids and neurotransmission. Endocannabinoids are retrograde neurotransmitters, travelling from the post- to the pre-synaptic neurone as part of a negative feedback loop that regulates neurotransmitter release.

a. arriving action potential opens voltage gated calcium channels; increasing *pre-synaptic* intracellular calcium triggers the release of stored neurotransmitter. Post-synaptic events depend on the neurotransmitter but include an increase in intracellular calcium
b. increasing *post-synaptic* intracellular calcium triggers the *de novo* synthesis of endocannabinoids from arachidonic acid
c. activation of CB$_1$ closes *pre-synaptic* calcium channels preventing further calcium influx, thereby terminating neurotransmitter release. These channels are also targeted by other drugs of analgesic relevance, e.g. **gabapentin, pregabalin, ziconotide**
d. endocannabinoids removed by hydrolysis, e.g. fatty acid amide hydrolase-1.

Central and peripheral CB$_1$ receptors also modulate appetite and energy metabolism, respectively. CNS receptors are expressed on hypothalamic and limbic neurones; those in the periphery exist on adipocytes, skeletal muscle cells and hepatocytes. Activation of peripheral CB_1 receptors promotes fat deposition and insulin resistance.[24]

Animal studies suggest that central and peripheral CB_1 receptors also impact on the cardiorespiratory system. In the brainstem, CB_1 stimulation elicits respiratory depression, bradycardia and hypertension.[25] In the lung, the effect is variable, with CB_1 stimulation able to attenuate capsaicin-induced bronchoconstriction but also induce bronchoconstriction in vagotomized animals.[26]

CB_2 is implicated in immune regulation. Located on antigen-presenting cells, it influences their cytokine profile and thus that of T-helper cells[4] This may partly explain its anti-inflammatory and antihyperalgesic effects. Its expression on microglia is upregulated in the dorsal root ganglia and spinal cord following sciatic nerve injury. It may also be expressed on neurones.[27]

The antihyperalgesic effects of CB_1 and CB_2 activation are distinct and additive, and include:[28]
- peripheral immunomodulation (antigen-presenting cell CB_2; interactions between immune cells and neurones contributes to peripheral sensitization and neuropathic pain)[29]
- central immunomodulation (CB_2 on microglia within the dorsal columns)
- disinhibition of antinociceptive neurones of a descending pain modulatory pathway (CB_1 on the pathway's GABAergic 'brake'; cf. opioids)[15,16,30,31]
- central dissociative effects.[32]

Further, unlike opioid receptors, CB_1 persists in the spinal cord after peripheral nerve injury.[33,34]

Endocannabinoids also act at other receptors, including the capsaicin receptor (TRPV1, involved in pain signalling), and perhaps also G protein-coupled receptors 55 and 119.[35]

Exogenous cannabinoids

Δ^9-THC is a CB_1 and CB_2 partial agonist. Its effects include muscle relaxation, analgesia, anti-emesis, but it can also cause sedation, anxiety, and psychosis. **Dronabinol** (not UK) is a synthetic preparation of its (-)-trans isomer, the best studied of several isomers present in Cannabis sativa; **nabilone** is a synthetic analogue.

The effects of Δ^9-THC are modified by other cannabinoids present in Cannabis sativa. For example, cannabidiol (CBD) reduces Δ^9-THC-induced anxiety in healthy volunteers, perhaps by inhibiting the metabolism of Δ^9-THC to a more psycho-active metabolite, 11-hydroxyTHC. CBD is also a CB_1/CB_2 antagonist; its apparently low affinity for both receptors suggesting non-competitive antagonism through a separate binding site. Although a less potent analgesic and anti-emetic, CBD is anxiolytic, antipsychotic and non-sedating.[36,37]

In an attempt to improve the efficacy/tolerability profile of Δ^9-THC, a combined formulation of Δ^9-THC with CBD (**Sativex®**) has been developed; each oral spray contains Δ^9-THC 2.7mg and CBD 2.5mg. It is authorized for refractory spasticity in multiple sclerosis and, in some countries, for pain (e.g. Canada, but not UK). However, results of RCTs in patients with pain comparing Δ^9-THC and CBD in combination with Δ^9-THC alone have been mixed; two RCTs found modest improvements in tolerability and patient preference,[38,39] one found modest improvements in efficacy, but not tolerability,[40] and one found no difference.[41]

The non-psycho-active constituents of Cannabis sativa are poorly understood but they may interact with non-CB_1/CB_2 cannabinoid receptors and/or the metabolism of endocannabinoids.[14] However, an RCT examining an inhibitor of endocannabinoid breakdown found no benefit for osteoarthritic pain.[19]

The therapeutic potential of cannabinoid antagonists and inverse agonists has also been investigated. Rimonabant, a CB_1 inverse agonist (i.e. results in a reduction in basal activity of the receptor), was approved for appetite suppression in obesity. However, it also caused depression, anxiety and aggression, and has been withdrawn.

The pharmacokinetic profiles of selected cannabinoids are summarized in Table 1. Food increases the absorption of Δ^9-THC and CBD oral spray, suggesting a proportion of the dose is swallowed before absorption.

Cautions

Psychiatric history (mood, cognitive and behavioral changes can occur); severe ischemic heart disease, heart failure or arrhythmias (risk of postural hypotension or reflex tachycardia); renal or hepatic impairment (no data, but active hepatic metabolites undergo biliary and renal clearance); epilepsy (cannabinoids can either lower or raise seizure threshold).

Table I Pharmacokinetic profiles of selected cannabinoids[20,42]

	Oral bio-availability (%)	Time to peak plasma concentration (h)	Halflife (h)	Metabolism
Cannabidiol (CBD)	Not known	1–4	5–9	Multiple pathways[a,b]
Nabilone	85	1–4	2 5–10[a]	Multiple pathways[a,b]
Tetrahydrocannabinol(Δ^9-THC)	⩾50	1–4	2–5	CYP2C9[c]

a. has active metabolite(s)
b. eliminated by both biliary and renal pathways
c. affected by combined use: cannabidiol reduces Δ^9-THC-induced anxiety in healthy volunteers, perhaps by inhibiting the metabolism of Δ^9-THC to a more psycho-active metabolite, 11-hydroxyTHC.

Drug interactions

Additive CNS depressant effects with other psychotropics.

The metabolism of **Sativex**® is marginally inhibited by CYP3A4 inhibitors (e.g. **clarithromycin, ritonavir**) and may be induced by CYP3A4 inducers, (e.g. **carbamazepine, rifampicin**).

Cannabinoids inhibit numerous CYP450 enzymes, although generally not at typical therapeutic concentrations. Caution is advised when substrates for CYP2C19, 2D6 (e.g. **amitriptyline**) and 3A4 (e.g. **alfentanil, fentanyl, sufentanil**) are used concurrently with **Sativex**®.

Undesirable effects

Box A Undesirable effects of cannabinoids

Psychological[a]
Common (< 10%, > 1%): depression, euphoria, disorientation, dissociation
Uncommon (< 1%, > 0.1%): hallucinations, paranoia, delusions, suicidal ideation

Neurological[b]
Very common (> 10%): dizziness (**Sativex**®, particularly during titration)
Common: ataxia, amnesia, drowsiness, blurred vision

Gastro-intestinal[c]
Common: appetite (↑ or ↓), nausea
Uncommon: abdominal pain

Cardiovascular
Uncommon: palpitations, tachycardia, syncope, hyper/hypotension

Buccal irritation[d] (**Sativex**® only)
Common: ulceration, pain
Uncommon: discoloration

---

a. illicit use is a risk factor for schizophrenia[43]
b. tolerance to CNS depressant effects generally develops after a few days
c. delayed onset nausea and vomiting ('cannabinoid hyperemesis') are described with illicit use of *Cannabis sativa*. Symptoms are generally worst in the morning (70%), associated with abdominal colic (86%), and resolve when the cannabinoid is discontinued. Although most patients have used cannabis weekly for at least 2 years before symptom onset, a third have symptoms within one year[44]
d. **Sativex**® contains 50% v/v ethanol and propylene glycol. Two reports of suspected leukoplakia occurred in RCTs.

Use of cannabinoids in palliative care

Food increases the absorption of **Sativex**®, resulting in both an increased C_{max} (some 2–3 times) and AUC (3–5 times). Consistent timing of administration with regard to mealtimes may be important in some patients.

The spray should only be directed beneath the tongue or inside the cheeks. The site of application should be varied and the buccal mucosa inspected regularly for signs of irritation caused by the excipients (ethanol (50%v/v), propylene glycol).

Chemotherapy-induced nausea and vomiting (nabilone)
Although cannabinoids have some anti-emetic efficacy in moderately emetogenic chemotherapy regimens, $5HT_3$ antagonists are more effective and better tolerated and should be generally used instead.[45] The manufacturer advises against the use of **nabilone** for non-chemotherapy related nausea.

Nabilone should be given immediately before, during and for 2 days after each pulse of chemotherapy:
• start with 1mg PO b.d.
• if necessary, increase to 2mg b.d.
• maximum recommended dose 2mg t.d.s.

Refractory spasticity in multiple sclerosis (Sativex®)
The place, if any, of cannabinoids is uncertain. RCTs do not show consistent benefit.[11]
• start with 1 oromucosal spray at bedtime (see precautions above)
• increase over 2 weeks to a maximum of 12 sprays/24h given in divided doses, e.g. 1–2 sprays b.d.–3 sprays q.d.s.

Refractory pain (Sativex®, nabilone)
A systematic review found moderate benefit for a variety of non-cancer pains (NNT 3.5–9 for 30% pain reduction). Smoked cannabis, oromucosal cannabis extracts (including **Sativex®**), **nabilone**, and **dronabinol** (not UK) were effective for neuropathic pain, fibromyalgia, and painful spasticity. Undesirable effects were generally mild.[46–48] Most trials were short (<6 weeks) but open-label extension studies found that analgesia was maintained without dose escalation for up to 1.5 years.[49–51]

Two RCTs have examined **Sativex®** for intractable cancer pain with mixed results. In one, it was more effective than placebo or Δ^9-THC alone (NNT 4.5 for 30% pain reduction) but withdrawal due to undesirable effects was three-times higher with **Sativex®** than placebo (17% vs. 5%).[40] The other study found no difference between **Sativex®** and placebo in the primary endpoint of the proportion of patients reporting ⩾30% reduction in pain. However, this was a graded dose study, which did not include titration to an optimal effect.[52]

For chemotherapy-related neuropathic pain, a small cross-over study found **Sativex®** no better than placebo.[53]

Sativex® (adapted from the Canadian Product Monograph)
• start with 1 oromucosal spray up to q4h (maximum 4 sprays in the first 24h); see precautions above
• titrate up on a daily basis (but more slowly if dizziness occurs)
• most patients require ⩽12 sprays/24h (median dose = 5–8 sprays/24h).
Nabilone
• start with 0.25mg to 0.5mg PO b.d.
• titrate in 0.5mg increments on a weekly basis
• maximum dose 1mg b.d.[54]

Supply
Nabilone (generic) is a Schedule 2 **CD**
Capsules 250microgram, 20 = £96. (Unauthorized, available on an individual patient basis from Creo Pharma; see Appendix 1, p.817.)
Capsules 1mg, 20 = £126. A lower dose capsule can be locally prepared by diluting with lactose powder.

Sativex ® (Bayer Healthcare and GW Pharmaceuticals) is a Schedule 4 (part 1) **CD**
Oromucosal spray Cannabis sativa extract (dronabinol) 27mg and CBD 25mg/mL each spray = 0.1mL, pack of 3 x 10mL (approx. 90 sprays/bottle) = £375; the unopened pack should be stored in a refrigerator. Once opened, store at room temperature and use within 6 weeks.

Records must be kept for 2 years for cannabis-based medicines (1961 UN Convention on Narcotic Drugs); this includes the quantities possessed or destroyed by those authorized to do so (patients and their representatives are exempt). The Home Office strongly recommends using a standard **CD** register for this.

1 Hill AJ et al. (2012) Cannabidivarin is anticonvulsant in mouse and rat in vitro and in seizure models. British Journal of Pharmacology. 167: 1629–1642.
2 Preet A et al. (2011) Cannabinoid receptors, CB_1 and CB_2, as novel targets for inhibition of non-small cell lung cancer growth and metastasis. Cancer Prevention Research. 4: 65–75.
3 Torres S et al. (2011) A combined preclinical therapy of cannabinoids and temozolomide against glioma. Molecular Cancer Therapeutics. 10: 90–103.
4 Tanasescu R and Constantinescu CS (2010) Cannabinoids and the immune system: an overview. Immunobiology. 215: 588–597.
5 Stanley CP et al. (2013) Is the cardiovascular system a therapeutic target for cannabidiol? British Journal of Clinical Pharmacology. 75: 313–322.
6 Scotter EL et al. (2010) The endocannabinoid system as a target for the treatment of neurodegenerative disease. British Journal of Pharmacology. 160: 480–498.
7 Castillo PE et al. (2012) Endocannabinoid signaling and synaptic function. Neuron. 76: 70–81.
8 Beal JE et al. (1995) Dronabinol as a treatment for anorexia associated with weight loss in patients with AIDS. Journal of Pain and Symptom Management. 10: 89–97.
9 Strasser F et al. (2006) Comparison of orally administered cannabis extract and delta-9-tetrahydrocannabinol in treating patients with cancer-related anorexia-cachexia syndrome: a multicenter, phase III, randomized, double-blind, placebo-controlled clinical trial from the Cannabis-In-Cachexia-Study-Group. Journal of Clinical Oncology. 24: 3394–3400.
10 Jatoi A et al. (2002) Dronabinol versus megestrol acetate versus combination therapy for cancer-associated anorexia: a North Central Cancer Treatment Group study. Journal of Clinical Oncology. 20: 567–573.
11 Farrell M et al. (2014) Should doctors prescribe cannabinoids? British Medical Journal. 348: 2737.
12 Ahmedzai S (1988) Respiratory distress in the terminally ill patient. Respiratory Disease in Practice. 5: 21–29.
13 Pickering EE et al. (2011) Cannabinoid effects on ventilation and breathlessness: a pilot study of efficacy and safety. Chronic Respiratory Disease. 8: 109–118.
14 Izzo AA et al. (2009) Non-psychotropic plant cannabinoids: new therapeutic opportunities from an ancient herb. Trends in Pharmacological Sciences. 30: 515–527.
15 Wilkerson JL et al. (2012) Intrathecal cannabilactone CB(2)R agonist, AM1710, controls pathological pain and restores basal cytokine levels. Pain. 153: 1091–1106.
16 Gu X et al. (2011) Intrathecal administration of the cannabinoid 2 receptor agonist JWH015 can attenuate cancer pain and decrease mRNA expression of the 2B subunit of N-methyl-D-aspartic acid. Anesthesia and Analgesia. 113: 405–411.
17 Yu XH et al. (2010) A peripherally restricted cannabinoid receptor agonist produces robust anti-nociceptive effects in rodent models of inflammatory and neuropathic pain. Pain. 151: 337–344.
18 Roques BP et al. (2012) Inhibiting the breakdown of endogenous opioids and cannabinoids to alleviate pain. Nature Reviews Drug Discovery. 11: 292–310.
19 Huggins JP et al. (2012) An efficient randomised, placebo-controlled clinical trial with the irreversible fatty acid amide hydrolase-1 inhibitor PF-04457845, which modulates endocannabinoids but fails to induce effective analgesia in patients with pain due to osteoarthritis of the knee. Pain. 153: 1837–1846.
20 Barnes MP (2006) Sativex: clinical efficacy and tolerability in the treatment of symptoms of multiple sclerosis and neuropathic pain. Expert Opinion on Pharmacotherpy. 7: 607–615.
21 Rea K et al. (2007) Supraspinal modulation of pain by cannabinoids: the role of GABA and glutamate. British Journal of Pharmacology. 152: 633–648.
22 Mechoulam R et al. (1998) Endocannabinoids. European Journal of Pharmacology. 359: 1–18.
23 Pryce G and Baker D (2007) Control of spasticity in a multiple sclerosis model is mediated by CB_1, not CB_2, cannabinoid receptors. British Journal of Pharmacology. 150: 519–525.
24 Tibirica E (2010) The multiple functions of the endocannabinoid system: a focus on the regulation of food intake. Diabetology and Metabolic Syndrome. 2: 5.
25 Pfitzer T et al. (2004) Central effects of the cannabinoid receptor agonist WIN55212-2 on respiratory and cardiovascular regulation in anaesthetised rats. British Journal of Pharmacology. 142: 943–952.
26 Calignano A et al. (2000) Bidirectional control of airway responsiveness by endogenous cannabinoids. Nature. 408: 96–101.
27 Atwood BK and Mackie K (2010) CB_2: a cannabinoid receptor with an identity crisis. British Journal of Pharmacology. 160: 467–479.
28 Gutierrez T et al. (2007) Activation of peripheral cannabinoid CB_1 and CB_2 receptors suppresses the maintenance of inflammatory nociception: a comparative analysis. British Journal of Pharmacology. 150: 153–163.
29 Scholz J and Woolf CJ (2007) The neuropathic pain triad: neurons, immune cells and glia. Nature Neuroscience. 10: 1361–1368.
30 Meng ID et al. (1998) An analgesia circuit activated by cannabinoids. Nature. 395: 381–383.
31 Welch SP (2009) Interaction of the cannabinoid and opioid systems in the modulation of nociception. International Reviews on Psychiatry. 21: 143–151.
32 Lee MC et al. (2013) Amygdala activity contributes to the dissociative effect of cannabis on pain perception. Pain. 154: 124–134.
33 Farquhar-Smith WP and Rice AS (2001) Administration of endocannabinoids prevents a referred hyperalgesia associated with inflammation of the urinary bladder. Anesthesiology. 94: 507–513; discussion 506A.
34 Hohmann AG and Herkenham M (1998) Regulation of cannabinoid and mu opioid receptors in rat lumbar spinal cord following neonatal capsaicin treatment. Neuroscience Letters. 252: 13–16.
35 Brown AJ (2007) Novel cannabinoid receptors. British Journal of Pharmacology. 152: 567–575.
36 Russo E and Guy GW (2006) A tale of two cannabinoids: the therapeutic rationale for combining tetrahydrocannabinol and cannabidiol. Medical Hypotheses. 66: 234–246.

37 Fusar-Poli P et al. (2009) Distinct effects of Δ9-tetrahydrocannabinol and cannabidiol on neural activation during emotional processing. Archives of General Psychiatry. **66**: 95–105.

38 Wade DT et al. (2003) A preliminary controlled study to determine whether whole-plant cannabis extracts can improve intractable neurogenic symptoms. Clinical Rehabilitation. **17**: 21–29.

39 Notcutt W et al. (2004) Initial experiences with medicinal extracts of cannabis for chronic pain: results from 34 'N of I' studies. Anaesthesia. **59**: 440–452.

40 Johnson JR et al. (2010) Multicenter, double-blind, randomized, placebo-controlled, parallel-group study of the efficacy, safety, and tolerability of THC:CBD extract and THC extract in patients with intractable cancer-related pain. Journal of Pain and Symptom Management. **39**: 167–179.

41 Berman JS et al. (2004) Efficacy of two cannabis based medicinal extracts for relief of central neuropathic pain from brachial plexus avulsion: results of a randomised controlled trial. Pain. **112**: 299–306.

42 Grotenhermen F (2003) Pharmacokinetics and pharmacodynamics of cannabinoids. Clinical Pharmacokinetics. **42**: 327–360.

43 Malone DT et al. (2010) Adolescent cannabis use and psychosis: epidemiology and neurodevelopmental models. British Journal of Pharmacology. **160**: 511–522.

44 Simonetto DA et al. (2012) Cannabinoid hyperemesis: a case series of 98 patients. Mayo Clinic Proceedings. **87**: 114–119.

45 Davis MP (2008) Oral nabilone capsules in the treatment of chemotherapy-induced nausea and vomiting and pain. Expert Opinion Investigational Drugs. **17**: 85–95.

46 Lynch ME and Campbell F (2011) Cannabinoids for treatment of chronic non-cancer pain; a systematic review of randomized trials. British Journal of Clinical Pharmacology. **72**: 735–744.

47 Toth C et al. (2012) An enriched-enrolment, randomized withdrawal, flexible-dose, double-blind, placebo-controlled, parallel assignment efficacy study of nabilone as adjuvant in the treatment of diabetic peripheral neuropathic pain. Pain. **153**: 2073–2082.

48 Langford RM et al. (2013) A double-blind, randomized, placebo-controlled, parallel-group study of THC/CBD oromucosal spray in combination with the existing treatment regimen, in the relief of central neuropathic pain in patients with multiple sclerosis. Journal of Neurology. **260**: 984–997.

49 Wade DT et al. (2006) Long-term use of a cannabis-based medicine in the treatment of spasticity and other symptoms in multiple sclerosis. Multiple Sclerosis. **12**: 639–645.

50 Nurmikko TJ et al. (2007) Sativex successfully treats neuropathic pain characterised by allodynia: a randomised, double-blind, placebo-controlled clinical trial. Pain. **133**: 210–220.

51 Johnson JR et al. (2013) An open-label extension study to investigate the long-term safety and tolerability of thc/cbd oromucosal spray and oromucosal THC spray in patients with terminal cancer-related pain refractory to strong opioid analgesics. Journal of Pain and Symptom Management **46**: 207–218.

52 Portenoy RK et al. (2012) Nabiximols for opioid-treated cancer patients with poorly-controlled chronic pain: a randomized, placebo-controlled, graded-dose trial. Journal of Pain. **13**: 438–449.

53 Lynch ME et al. (2014) A double-blind, placebo-controlled, crossover pilot trial with extension using an oral mucosal cannabinoid extract for treatment of chemotherapy-induced neuropathic pain. Journal of Pain and Symptom Management. **47**: 166–173.

54 CADTH (2011) Nabilone for chronic pain management: a review of clinical efectiveness, safety and guidelines. In: Canadian Agency for Drugs and Technologies in Health; Rapid Response Report: summary with critical appraisal Available from: www.cadth.ca

Updated June 2014

ANTI-EMETICS   BNF 4.6

For a summary of the management of nausea and vomiting in palliative care, see the Quick Prescribing Guide (p.241).

Anti-emetic RCTs in palliative care are relatively sparse,[1–3] and some reliance on extrapolation from experimental data and RCTs in postoperative and chemotherapy-related nausea and vomiting is necessary. In practice, the choice of an anti-emetic in palliative care is guided by the probable cause of the nausea and vomiting and the mechanism by which the drug acts (Table 1, Figure 1, Table 2). This 'mechanistic approach' is successful in most patients.[4,5] Other factors to consider include:

- response to anti-emetics already given
- relative merits of alternatives:
  ▷ effects on GI motility (i.e. prokinetic (**domperidone, metoclopramide**) or antikinetic (antimuscarinics))
  ▷ appropriate route or formulation
  ▷ undesirable effects (e.g. drug-induced movement disorders (**haloperidol, metoclopramide**), prolongation of the QT interval (**domperidone, haloperidol**))
  ▷ recent recommendations to limit **metoclopramide** and **domperidone** to short-term use; nonetheless there is likely to be a greater use of **domperidone** when a long-term prokinetic is required[6,7]
  ▷ cost (5HT$_3$ antagonists, **aprepitant** and **octreotide** are expensive)

Table I Classification of drugs used to control nausea and vomiting

Putative site of action	Class	Example
Central nervous system		
Vomiting centre	Antimuscarinic	Hyoscine *hydrobromide*[a]
	Antihistaminic antimuscarinic[b]	Cyclizine
	Broad-spectrum antipsychotic	Levomepromazine, olanzapine
	NK_1 antagonist	Aprepitant
Area postrema (chemoreceptor trigger zone)	D_2 antagonist	Haloperidol, metoclopramide, domperidone
	$5HT_3$ antagonist	Granisetron, ondansetron
	NK_1 antagonist	Aprepitant
Cerebral cortex	Benzodiazepine	Lorazepam
	Cannabinoid	Nabilone
	Corticosteroid	Dexamethasone
	NK_1 antagonist	Aprepitant
GI tract		
Prokinetic	$5HT_4$ agonist	Metoclopramide
	D_2 antagonist	Metoclopramide, domperidone
	Motilin agonist	Erythromycin
Antisecretory	Antimuscarinic	Hyoscine *butylbromide*, glycopyrronium
	Somatostatin analogue	Octreotide, lanreotide
Vagal $5HT_3$-receptor blockade	$5HT_3$ antagonist	Granisetron, ondansetron, (metoclopramide at high doses)
Anti-inflammatory	Corticosteroid	Dexamethasone

a. although also has a GI tract antisecretory effect, higher doses risk undesirable CNS effects (unlike hyoscine *butylbromide* or glycopyrronium which do not cross the blood brain barrier)
b. antihistamines and phenothiazines both have H_1 antagonistic and antimuscarinic properties (see Table 2).

- when more than one anti-emetic drug is considered:
  - ▷ use combinations with different receptor affinities (e.g. **cyclizine** and **haloperidol**)
  - ▷ avoid combinations with antagonistic actions (e.g. **cyclizine** and **metoclopramide**)[8]
  - ▷ consider a single broader spectrum drug; **levomepromazine**[9] and **olanzapine**[10] have affinity at many receptors and may well be as effective as, and easier for patients to handle than, two or more different anti-emetics simultaneously
- adjuvant use of:
  - ▷ antisecretory drugs (e.g. **hyoscine** *butylbromide*, **glycopyrronium**, **octreotide**)
  - ▷ corticosteroids (e.g. **dexamethasone**)
  - ▷ benzodiazepines (e.g. **lorazepam, midazolam**), also see p.152[11]
- non-drug treatments.

Generally, in palliative care, the initial choice of an anti-emetic lies between:
- a prokinetic anti-emetic, e.g. **domperidone** (p.246) or **metoclopramide** (p.242)
- **haloperidol** (p.177)
- **cyclizine** (p.249).

The most appropriate anti-emetic should be prescribed both regularly and as needed (see Quick Prescribing Guide, p.241).

The extent to which the underlying cause is correctable (e.g. constipation, drug-induced, hypercalcemia) will determine if an anti-emetic is required short- or long-term. Drug-induced nausea and vomiting can be problematic. They may be caused by several different mechanisms (Table 3), each of which requires a distinct therapeutic response.

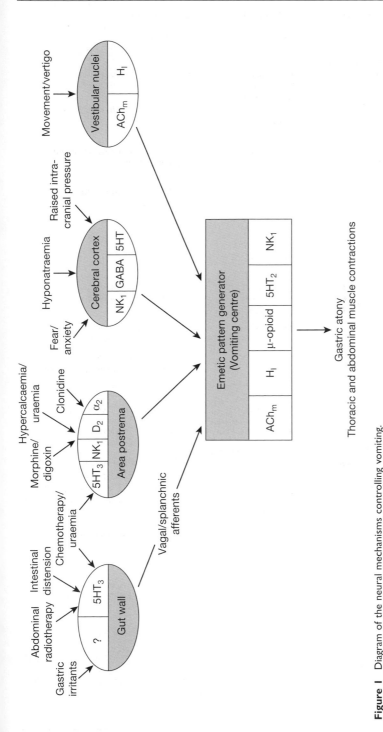

Figure 1 Diagram of the neural mechanisms controlling vomiting.
Abbreviations refer to receptor types: ACh_m = muscarinic cholinergic; α_2 = α_2-adrenergic; D_2 = dopamine type 2; GABA = gamma-aminobutyric acid; 5HT, $5HT_2$, $5HT_3$ = 5-hydroxytryptamine (serotonin) type undefined, type 2, type 3; H_1 = histamine type 1; NK_1 = neurokinin 1. Anti-emetics act as antagonists at these receptors, whereas the central anti-emetic effects of clonidine and opioids are agonistic.

Table 2 Receptor site affinities of selected anti-emetics [10,11,13,16,17]

	D_2 antagonist	H_1 antagonist	Muscarinic antagonist	$5HT_2$ antagonist	$5HT_3$ antagonist	NK_1 antagonist	$5HT_4$ agonist	CB_1 agonist	GABA mimetic
Aprepitant	–	–	–	–	–	+++	–	–	–
Chlorpromazine	+++	+++	++	++	–	–	–	–	–
Cyclizine	–	++	++	–	–	–	–	–	–
Domperidone	++[a]	–	–	–	+/–	–	–	–	–
Haloperidol	+++	–	–	–	+/–	–	–	–	–
Hyoscine hydrobromide	–	–	+++	–	–	–	–	–	–
Levomepromazine	++	+++	++	+++	–	–	–	–	–
Lorazepam	–	–	–	–	–	–	–	–	+++
Metoclopramide	++	–	–	–	+	–	++	–	–
Nabilone	–	–	–	–	–	–	–	+++	+++
Ondansetron, granisetron	–	–	–	–	+++	–	–	–	–
Olanzapine	++	+	++	++	+	–	–	–	–
Prochlorperazine	+++	++	+	+/++	–	–	–	–	–
Promethazine	+/++	++	++	–	–	–	–	–	–

Pharmacological activity: – = none or insignificant; + = slight; ++ = moderate; +++ = marked.

a. domperidone does not normally cross the blood-brain barrier; thus the risk of extrapyramidal effects is negligible (see p.246).

Table 3 Causes of drug-induced nausea and vomiting

Mechanism	Drugs
Gastric irritation	Antibacterials Baclofen Corticosteroids Iron supplements Misoprostol NSAIDs Potassium Spironolactone Tranexamic acid Venlaxafine
Gastric stasis	Antimuscarinics Opioids Phenothiazines TCAs
Area postrema stimulation (chemoreceptor trigger zone)	Antibacterials Cytotoxics Digoxin Imidazoles Opioids
$5HT_3$-receptor stimulation	Antibacterials Cytotoxics SSRIs

In bowel obstruction with large-volume vomiting or associated colic, an antisecretory agent (which acts partly by reducing the volume of GI secretions), e.g. **hyoscine butylbromide** 60–200mg/24h CSCI is combined with **levomepromazine** 6.25–25mg/24h CSCI. If *vomiting* persists, review the patient's oral intake; antisecretory drugs cannot fully alleviate the vomiting of ingested fluid and food. Consider nasogastric aspiration or a trial of **octreotide** (see p.530). If *nausea* persists, a $5HT_3$ antagonist, e.g. **ondansetron** 16–24mg/24h CSCI can be added to **levomepromazine**.

Corticosteroids and **levomepromazine** and **olanzapine** are useful options when first-line anti-emetics fail to relieve nausea and vomiting. **Dexamethasone** is generally added to an existing regimen, whereas **levomepromazine** and **olanzapine** are generally substituted. Sometimes it is necessary to use **dexamethasone** and **levomepromazine** or **olanzapine** concurrently.

$5HT_3$ antagonists were developed primarily for use alongside chemotherapy. They are used in combination with **dexamethasone** to control *acute* nausea and vomiting caused by highly or moderately emetogenic chemotherapy regimens.[12] $5HT_3$ antagonists have a definite but limited role in palliative care (see p.251).

Aprepitant, a neurokinin 1 (NK₁) antagonist,[13] is increasingly given in combination with a $5HT_3$ antagonist and **dexamethasone** to prevent *acute* and *delayed* nausea and vomiting associated with highly emetogenic **cisplatin**-based chemotherapy and moderately emetogenic anthracycline-**cyclophosphamide**-based chemotherapy.[14] Postoperatively, **aprepitant** was more effective than **ondansetron** for vomiting but not nausea.[15] A parenteral pro-drug, **fosaprepitant**, is available for IV use. Both are expensive. Their place, if any, in the palliative care setting is unclear.

1 Davis MP et al. (2010) A systematic review of the treatment of nausea and/or vomiting in cancer unrelated to chemotherapy or radiation. *Journal of Pain and Symptom Management.* **39**: 756–767.

2 Glare P et al. (2011) Treating nausea and vomiting in palliative care: a review. *Clinical Interventions in Aging.* **6**: 243–259.

3 Glare P et al. (2004) Systematic review of the efficacy of antiemetics in the treatment of nausea in patients with far-advanced cancer. *Supportive Care in Cancer.* **12**: 432–440.

4   Bentley A and Boyd K (2001) Use of clinical pictures in the management of nausea and vomiting: a prospective audit. *Palliative Medicine.* **15**: 247–253.
5   Stephenson J and Davies A (2006) An assessment of aetiology-based guidelines for the management of nausea and vomiting in patients with advanced cancer. *Supportive Care in Cancer.* **14**: 348–353.
6   MHRA (2013) Metoclopramide: risk of neurological adverse effects - restricted dose and duration of use. *Drug Safety Update.* **7**. www.mhra.gov.uk/safetyinformation
7   MHRA (2014) Domperidone: risks of cardiac side effects–indication restricted to nausea and vomiting, new contraindications, and reduced dose and duration of use. *Drug Safety Update.* **7**. www.mhra.gov.uk/safetyinformation
8   Twycross RG and Back I (1998) Nausea and vomiting in advanced cancer. *European Journal of Palliative Care.* **5**: 39–45.
9   Twycross RG et al. (1997) The use of low dose levomepromazine (methotrimeprazine) in the management of nausea and vomiting. *Progress in Palliative Care.* **5**: 49–53.
10 Fleming M and Hawkins C (2005) Use of atypical antipsychotic olanzapine as an anti-emetic. *European Journal of Palliative Care.* **12**: 144–146.
11 Aapro MS et al. (2005) Anticipatory nausea and vomiting. *Supportive Care in Cancer.* **13**: 117–121.
12 Hesketh PJ et al. (2003) Differential involvement of neurotransmitters through the time course of cisplatin-induced emesis as revealed by therapy with specific receptor antagonists. *European Journal of Cancer.* **39**: 1074–1080.
13 Saito R et al. (2003) Roles of substance P and NK(1) receptor in the brainstem in the development of emesis. *Journal of Pharmacology Science.* **91**: 87–94.
14 Roila F et al. (2010) Guideline update for MASCC and ESMO in the prevention of chemotherapy- and radiotherapy-induced nausea and vomiting: results of the Perugia consensus conference. *Annals of Oncology.* **21(Suppl 5)**: v232–243.
15 Gan TJ et al. (2007) A randomized, double-blind comparison of the NK_1 antagonist, aprepitant, versus ondansetron for the prevention of postoperative nausea and vomiting. *Anesthesia and Analgesia.* **104**: 1082–1089.
16 Peroutka SJ and Snyder SH (1982) Antiemetics: neurotransmitter receptor binding predicts therapeutic actions. *Lancet.* **1**: 658–659.
17 Davis M et al. (2007) The emerging role of cannabinoid neuromodulators in symptom management. *Supportive Care in Cancer.* **15**: 63–71.

Updated June 2014

Quick Prescribing Guide: Management of nausea and vomiting

1 From the patient's history and physical examination, decide what is the most likely cause (or causes) of the nausea and vomiting. Take a blood sample if biochemical derangement is suspected.

2 Correct correctable causes/exacerbating factors, e.g. drugs, severe pain, cough, infection, hypercalcaemia. *(Remember: antibacterial treatment and correction of hypercalcaemia are not always appropriate in a dying patient.)* Anxiety exacerbates nausea and vomiting from any cause and may need specific treatment.

3 Prescribe the most appropriate anti-emetic stat, regularly and p.r.n. (see below). Give by SC injection or CSCI if continuous nausea or frequent vomiting.

Commonly used anti-emetics

Prokinetic anti-emetic (about 50% of prescriptions)
For gastritis, gastric stasis, functional bowel obstruction (peristaltic failure):
metoclopramide 10mg PO stat & q.d.s. or 10mg SC stat & 40–100mg/24h CSCI, & 10mg p.r.n. up to q.d.s.

Anti-emetic acting principally in chemoreceptor trigger zone (about 25% of prescriptions)
For most chemical causes of vomiting, e.g. morphine, hypercalcaemia, renal failure:
haloperidol 1.5–3mg PO stat & at bedtime, or 2.5–5mg SC stat & 2.5–10mg/24h CSCI, & 2.5–5mg p.r.n. up to q.d.s.
Metoclopramide also has a central action.

Antispasmodic and antisecretory anti-emetic
If bowel colic and/or need to reduce GI secretions:
hyoscine *butylbromide* 20mg SC stat, 60–120mg/24h CSCI (occasionally as high as 300mg/24h), & 20mg SC hourly p.r.n.

Anti-emetic acting principally in the vomiting centre
For raised intracranial pressure (in conjunction with dexamethasone), motion sickness and in mechanical bowel obstruction:
cyclizine 50mg PO stat & b.d.–t.d.s. or 50mg SC stat & 150mg/24h CSCI, & 50mg p.r.n. up to b.d.

Broad-spectrum anti-emetic
For mechanical obstruction and when other anti-emetics are unsatisfactory:
levomepromazine 6–12.5mg PO/SC stat, at bedtime & p.r.n. up to q.d.s.

---

4 Initially, review anti-emetic dose each day; take note of p.r.n. use, and adjust the regular dose accordingly.

5 If little benefit despite upward titration of the dose, reconsider the likely cause(s), and review the route of administration and the choice of anti-emetic.

6 Some patients with nausea and vomiting need more than one anti-emetic.

7 Prokinetics act through a cholinergic system which is competitively antagonized by antimuscarinics; concurrent use is best avoided.

8 A $5HT_3$ antagonist, e.g. granisetron 1–2mg stat & once daily, or ondansetron 8mg stat & b.d.–t.d.s PO/SC should be considered when there is a massive release of 5HT/serotonin from enterochromaffin cells or platelets, e.g. with chemotherapy, abdominal radiation, bowel

distension, renal failure. Also consider with chemical causes of nausea and vomiting refractory to haloperidol and levomepromazine.

9 When all else fails, consider adding dexamethasone 8–16mg PO/SC stat & once daily for 7 days, and then review.

10 Continue the anti-emetic(s) unless the cause is self-limiting. Except in mechanical bowel obstruction (see below), consider changing to PO after 3 days of good control with CSCI.

More about bowel obstruction

11 Anti-emetics for inoperable bowel obstruction are best given by CSCI (for typical doses, see above), but levomepromazine can be given as a single SC dose at bedtime:

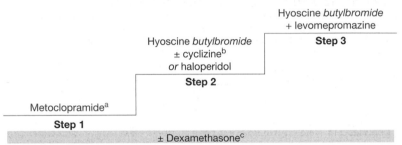

a. if colic, omit step 1
b. reports of incompatibility when cyclizine mixed with Hyoscine *butylbromide* ± haloperidol
c. the place of dexamethasone in inoperable bowel obstruction is controversial.

12 If levomepromazine is too sedative, consider reverting to step 2 but give both cyclizine and haloperidol; or use olanzapine 1.25–2.5mg SC (not UK) at bedtime instead.

13 If hyoscine butylbromide is inadequate or to obtain more rapid relief, prescribe a somatostatin analogue (= an antisecretory agent without antispasmodic effects), e.g. octreotide 100microgram stat, 250–500microgram/24h CSCI, & 100microgram p.r.n. up to q.d.s.

METOCLOPRAMIDE   BNF 4.6

Class: Prokinetic anti-emetic.

Indications: Nausea and vomiting caused by surgery, chemotherapy (delayed, not acute), radiation therapy or migraine. All other uses are unauthorized, e.g. †delayed gastric emptying, †dysmotility dyspepsia, †gastric irritation, †heartburn, †hiccups.

Contra-indications: Children <1 year old. Phaeochromocytoma (may induce an acute hypertensive response). GI haemorrhage or perforation. Use within <4 days of GI surgery (vigorous contractions may impair healing).

Pharmacology

Metoclopramide is a D_2 antagonist which acts both peripherally in the upper GI tract and centrally in the area postrema (chemoreceptor trigger zone). It is also a $5HT_4$ agonist in the upper GI tract and, in higher dose (e.g. 2–4mg/kg IV), a $5HT_3$ antagonist. Although the use of high-dose metoclopramide for chemotherapy-related *acute* nausea and vomiting has been superseded by specific $5HT_3$-receptor antagonists (see p.251), it is used in normal doses for *delayed* nausea and vomiting. As with other central dopamine receptors antagonists, there is a risk of developing extrapyramidal effects (see Undesirable effects).

Prokinetics act by triggering a cholinergic system in the wall of the GI tract (see Prokinetics p.22). Opioids impede this action, and antimuscarinics block it competitively.[1] *Thus, the concurrent use of a prokinetic and an antimuscarinic should be discouraged*; although metoclopramide will still act as D_2-antagonist in the area postrema even if its GI prokinetic effect is blocked. However, if D_2-antagonism alone is needed, **haloperidol** is generally a better choice because of the advantage of once daily administration (see p.177).

D_2 antagonists block the 'dopamine brake' on gastric emptying induced by stress, anxiety and nausea from any cause. In contrast, $5HT_4$ agonists have a direct excitatory effect. However, when used for dysmotility dyspepsia, dual-action metoclopramide is no more potent than **domperidone** in standard doses.[2]

Metoclopramide is metabolized in the liver, with CYP2D6 the main CYP450 enzyme involved. It is eliminated mainly via the kidney, either as conjugated metabolites or unchanged (20–30%). Both hepatic and renal impairment reduce the clearance of metoclopramide, resulting in higher plasma levels and a prolonged halflife and the SPC advises a reduced dose. Thus, in patients with severe cirrhosis, moderate–severe renal impairment or renal failure halve the usual starting dose and monitor carefully.[3]

Metoclopramide is a commonly used anti-emetic in palliative care, with moderate (level B) evidence supporting its first-line use in cancer-related nausea and vomiting, with respective response rates for complete control of about $\leq 33\%$ and $\leq 50\%$ seen in RCTs.[4,5] However, doses and outcomes used have varied and the results are mixed, e.g. in opioid-induced nausea and vomiting.[4,6] The use of metoclopramide to treat chemotherapy-induced nausea and vomiting is not considered here.

Although metoclopramide often has immediate effect, benefit may increase throughout the first week of use.[7–9]

Bio-availability 50–80% PO.
Onset of action 10–15min IM; 15–60min PO.
Time to peak plasma concentration 1–2.5h PO.
Plasma halflife 2.5–5h.
Duration of action 1–2h (data for single dose and relating to gastric emptying).

Cautions

Cardiac disease; enhanced effects of catecholamines in patients with essential hypertension[10,11] (also see Undesirable effects). Epilepsy (lowers seizure threshold); Parkinson's disease; mechanical GI obstruction (but is commonly used in palliative care to restore peristalsis in functional GI obstruction).[12,13]

Severe hepatic impairment, moderate–severe renal impairment or failure; halve the usual starting dose and monitor carefully (see Pharmacology).

Drug interactions

Serious drug interaction: a combination of IV metoclopramide and IV **ondansetron** occasionally causes cardiac arrhythmias.[14] $5HT_3$-receptors influence various aspects of cardiac function, including inotropy, chronotropy and coronary arterial tone,[15] effects which are mediated by both the parasympathetic and the sympathetic nervous systems. Thus, in any given patient, blockade of $5HT_3$-receptors will produce effects dependent on the pre-existing serotoninergic activity in both arms of the autonomic nervous system.

Risk of serotonin toxicity when used in combination with other serotoninergic drugs, e.g. SSRIs, see Antidepressants, Box B, p.195.

Because antimuscarinics competitively block the final common (cholinergic) pathway through which prokinetics act, concurrent prescription with metoclopramide should be avoided if possible. Opioids may also impede this action.

Undesirable effects

In 2009, in response to concerns about metoclopramide-related tardive dyskinesia, the FDA issued a black box warning recommending a maximum duration of use of ≤ 12 weeks, except for rare circumstances where the benefit of prolonged use outweighed the risks.[16] Use of metoclopramide has subsequently declined.[17]

In 2013, because of similar concerns, the EMA recommended a reduction in the number of Authorized indications, a maximum daily dose of 30mg (0.5mg/kg), a maximum duration of use of 5 days and the withdrawal of high dose formulations.[18]

The rationale behind these decisions is that the long-term use of metoclopramide for a medically non-serious disorder, e.g. dysmotility dyspepsia or heartburn, is not warranted given the risk of a potentially irreversible movement disorder.

However, the EMA recognizes that the risk:benefit ratio may be different in populations where metoclopramide is used off-label. Further, when such use is accepted practice within a specialty, this need not change as a consequence of their recommendations.[19]

Also see Drug-induced movement disorders. The risk of extrapyramidal effects is dose-related and increased by the co-administration of other drugs known to cause extrapyramidal effects, e.g. antipsychotics, $5HT_3$ antagonists and antidepressants. Other risk factors include female gender, age (<20 and >80 years), past psychiatric history, Parkinson's disease, diabetes mellitus and renal or hepatic failure.[20]

Acute dystonic reactions occur in <5% of patients receiving metoclopramide, and are more common in the young, particularly girls and young women. They generally occur ≤5 days of starting treatment, and subside within 24h of stopping the drug. When possible, use alternatives in patients 1–20 years old.

Acute akathisia occurs in 10–15% of patients receiving a single dose of metoclopramide 20mg IV, and is severe enough to require treatment in 1–3%.[21] In a small series of palliative care patients, 10% exhibited acute akathisia after two weeks of metoclopramide, median dose 30mg/24h (range 10–60mg).[22] Acute akathisia is easily missed; patients may not spontaneously volunteer the symptoms, or clinicians misinterpret them as anxiety-related or another psychiatric condition.[23] Paradoxically, this can result in the use of neuroleptic drugs which, via their dopamine antagonist effects, exacerbates the situation.

Drug-induced parkinsonism generally develops <3 months after starting metoclopramide. The exact incidence is unknown. In one series, 30% of patients had signs of parkinsonism after ≥3 months of use.[20] In another series, tremor was present in 5% after two weeks of use.[22]

The overall incidence of tardive dyskinesia is probably <1%.[24] The risk increases with duration of treatment and total cumulative dose. Onset is generally after months of use; in one series after a median of 14 months (range 4–44 months).[25] However, about 20% of palliative care clinicians report seeing tardive dyskinesia in their patients, sometimes after only 2 weeks of use.[26] Further, it has occurred in a 16 year old male after only two days of 30mg/24h PO.[27] A possible mechanism is a direct neurotoxic effect of metoclopramide.[28] The likelihood of recovery is inversely related to age, probably reflecting capacity for CNS repair.

Patients experiencing extrapyramidal effects should be counselled against future use and the reaction clearly documented in their medical records.

Other undesirable effects include neuroleptic (antipsychotic) malignant syndrome (see p.172), drowsiness, depression, diarrhoea. Very rarely: hypotension, cardiac arrhythmia and cardiac arrest; mainly with IV use in at risk patients.

Dose and use

Avoid metoclopramide in patients in whom it has previously caused extrapyramidal effects.

If a long-term prokinetic is necessary, consider **domperidone** instead (see p.246). When this is not possible (e.g. because of contra-indications or the need for parenteral administration), review the use of metoclopramide frequently (e.g. at least every week) and discontinue if an optimal dose fails to provide benefit.

With long-term use, continue to monitor the patient regularly, particularly when higher than usual doses are being used, and discontinue metoclopramide if extrapyramidal signs or symptoms develop.

Gastric irritation
- 10mg PO t.d.s.–q.d.s. or 30–40mg/24h CSCI and 10mg PO/SC p.r.n.; prescribe appropriate gastroprotective drug and, if possible, discontinue causal drug/substance.

Delayed gastric emptying
• as above, consider increasing to a maximum of 100mg/24h CSCI.

Nausea and vomiting
• as for gastric inrritation, but **haloperidol** is generally more convenient if the cause is stimulation of the chemoreceptor trigger zone/area postrema (see p.235).

For nausea and vomiting associated with serotonin release (e.g. abdominal irradiation), a selective $5HT_3$ antagonist should be used rather than high-dose metoclopramide (see p.251).

Hiccup
If caused by delayed gastric emptying, gastric distension, or acid reflux:
• 10mg PO t.d.s.–q.d.s. and p.r.n. ± an antifoaming agent (see Prokinetics, Table 2, p.24)
• if no response to PO treatment, consider stat dose of 10–20mg IV; give over ≥3min.[18]
Note: increasing IV administration time to 15min reduced the incidence of acute akathisia in one study, but not another.[21,29]
For CSCI, dilute with WFI or 0.9% saline.

CSCI compatibility with other drugs: There are 2-drug compatibility data for metoclopramide in WFI with **alfentanil, diamorphine, glycopyrronium, haloperidol, hydromorphone, ketamine, midazolam, morphine sulfate, octreotide** and **oxycodone**. For more details, and 3-drug compatibility compatibility charts see Appendix 3, p.821.

Compatibility charts for mixing drugs in 0.9% saline can be found in the extended appendix section of the on-line PCF on www.palliativedrugs.com

Supply
Metoclopramide (generic)
Tablets 10mg, 28 days @ 10mg q.d.s. − £4.
Oral solution 5mg/5mL, 28 days @ 10mg q.d.s. = £115.
Injection 5mg/mL, 2mL amp = £0.50.

1 Schuurkes JAJ et al. (1986) Stimulation of gastroduodenal motor activity: dopaminergic and cholinergic modulation. *Drug Development Research*. **8**: 233–241.
2 Barone J (1999) Domperidone: a peripherally acting dopamine$_2$-receptor antagonist. *Annals of Pharmacotherapy*. **33**: 429–440.
3 Magueur E et al. (1991) Pharmacokinetics of metoclopramide in patients with liver cirrhosis. *British Journal of Clinical Pharmacology*. **31**: 185–187.
4 Davis MP et al. (2010) A systematic review of the treatment of nausea and/or vomiting in cancer unrelated to chemotherapy or radiation. *Journal of Pain and Symptom Management*. **39**: 756–767.
5 Glare P et al. (2004) Systematic review of the efficacy of antiemetics in the treatment of nausea in patients with far-advanced cancer. *Supportive Care in Cancer*. **12**: 432–440.
6 Glare P et al. (2011) Treating nausea and vomiting in palliative care: a review. *Clinical Interventions in Aging*. **6**: 243–259.
7 Bruera E et al. (2004) Dexamethasone in addition to metoclopramide for chronic nausea in patients with advanced cancer: a randomized controlled trial. *Journal of Pain and Symptom Management*. **28**: 381–388.
8 Bruera E et al. (1996) Chronic nausea in advanced cancer patients: a retrospective assessment of a metoclopramide-based antiemetic regimen. *Journal of Pain and Symptom Management*. **11**: 147–153.
9 Bruera E et al. (2000) A double-blind, crossover study of controlled-release metoclopramide and placebo for the chronic nausea and dyspepsia of advanced cancer. *Journal of Pain and Symptom Management*. **19**: 427–435.
10 Kuchel O et al. (1985) Effect of metoclopramide on plasma catecholamine release in essential hypertension. *Clinical Pharmacology and Therapeutics*. **37**: 372–375.
11 Agabiti-Rosei E (1995) Hypertensive crises in patients with phaeochromocytoma given metoclopramide. *Annals of Pharmacology*. **29**: 381–383.
12 Twycross RG and Back I (1998) Nausea and vomiting in advanced cancer. *European Journal of Palliative Care*. **5**: 39–45.
13 Ripamonti C et al. (2001) Clinical-practice recommendations for the management of bowel obstruction in patients with end-stage cancer. *Supportive Care in Cancer*. **9**: 223–233.
14 Baguley W et al. (1997) Cardiac dysrhythmias associated with the intravenous administration of ondansetron and metoclopramide. *Anesthesia and Analgesia*. **84**: 1380–1381.
15 Saxena P and Villalon C (1991) 5-Hydroxytryptamine: a chameleon in the heart. *Trends in Pharmacological Sciences*. **12**: 223–227.
16 FDA (2009) Summary of warnings for metoclopramide containing products. *Medwatch*. www.fda.gov/Safety/MedWatch/SafetyInformation/
17 Ehrenpreis ED et al. (2013) The metoclopramide black box warning for tardive dyskinesia: effect on clinical practice, adverse event reporting, and prescription drug lawsuits. *American Journal of Gastroenterology*. **108**: 866–872.
18 MHRA (2013) Metoclopramide: risk of neurological adverse effects - restricted dose and duration of use. *Drug Safety Update*. **7**. www.mhra.gov.uk/safetyinformation
19 EMA (2013) Personal communication.

20 Ganzini L et al. (1993) The prevalence of metoclopramide-induced tardive dyskinesia and acute extrapyramidal movement disorders. Archives of Internal Medicine. **153**: 1469–1475.

21 Egerton-Warburton D and Povey K (2013) Administration of metoclopramide by infusion or bolus does not affect the incidence of drug-induced akathisia. Emergency Medicine Australasia. **25**: 207–212.

22 Currow DC et al. (2012) Pharmacovigilance in hospice/palliative care: rapid report of net clinical effect of metoclopramide. Journal of Palliative Medicine. **15**: 1071–1075.

23 Akagi H and Kumar TM (2002) Lesson of the week: Akathisia: overlooked at a cost. British Medical Journal. **324**: 1506–1507.

24 Rao A and Camilleri M (2009) Review article: metoclopramide and tardive dyskinesia. Alimentary Pharmacology and Therapeutics. **31**: 11–19.

25 Wiholm BE et al. (1984) Tardive dyskinesia associated with metoclopramide. British Medical Journal. **288**: 545–547.

26 Palliativedrugs.com (2014) Metoclopramide - What is your experience? Survey November-December 2013. www.palliativedrugs.com

27 Karimi Khaledi M et al. (2012) Tardive dyskinesia after short-term treatment with oral metoclopramide in an adolescent. International Journal of Clinical Pharmacy. **34**: 822–824.

28 Lai TK et al. (2012) Cell membrane lytic action of metoclopramide and its relation to tardive dyskinesia. Synapse. **66**: 273–276.

29 Tura P et al. (2012) Slow infusion metoclopramide does not affect the improvement rate of nausea while reducing akathisia and sedation incidence. Emergency Medical Journal. **29**: 108–112.

Updated June 2014

DOMPERIDONE   BNF 4.6

Class: Prokinetic anti-emetic.

Indications: Nausea and vomiting. All other uses are unauthorized, e.g. †symptoms associated with upper GI dysmotility (post-prandial epigastric discomfort, bloating and belching); †gastro-oesophageal reflux.

Contra-indications: Prolactinoma; conditions where cardiac conduction is, or could be, impaired, e.g. prolonged QT interval (congenital or acquired); underlying cardiac disease, e.g. CHF; concurrent use with potent CYP3A4 inhibitors or other drugs known to prolong QT interval; GI haemorrhage or perforation, mechanical GI obstruction; severe hepatic impairment.

Pharmacology

Domperidone is a D_2 antagonist. It is structurally related to the butyrophenones, but does not normally cross the blood-brain barrier.[1] Domperidone has a dual anti-emetic effect. First, it acts on D_2-receptors in the chemoreceptor trigger zone (CTZ) in the area postrema. (Although situated on the surface of the brain stem, the CTZ is outside the physiological blood-brain barrier.) Second, it acts on D_2-receptors at the gastro-oesophageal and gastroduodenal junctions, and thereby counteracts the gastric 'dopamine brake' associated with nausea from any cause.

Because negligible amounts of domperidone penetrate the blood-brain barrier, there is negligible risk of extrapyramidal effects (mediated via the basal ganglia). Domperidone is the prokinetic and anti-emetic of choice in Parkinson's disease; it counteracts the emetic effect of **levodopa** and **bromocriptine** without adversely affecting the antiparkinsonian (dopaminergic) effect of these drugs.[2]

Prokinetics act by triggering a cholinergic system in the wall of the GI tract (see Prokinetics, p.22). Opioids impede this action, and antimuscarinics block it competitively.[3] Thus, the concurrent use of aprokinetics and an antimuscarinic should be discouraged; although domperidone will still act as D_2-antagonist in the area postrema even if its GI prokinetic effect is blocked. However, if D_2-antagonism alone is needed, **haloperidol** is generally a better choice because of the advantage of once daily administration (see p.177).

Because domperidone, unlike **metoclopramide**, does not have any $5HT_4$ agonist action, it might be anticipated that domperidone would be less effective in treating gastroparesis. However, the results of a systematic review indicate otherwise (see also Prokinetics, Table 1, p.23).[4] Domperidone may be effective even when there is no response to **metoclopramide**.[3,5]

However, a lack of robustness in the evidence supporting the efficacy of domperidone has been highlighted, particularly in relation to methodological limitations and inconsistent benefit, with doses of 30mg/24h often no better than placebo.[6] Thus, many studies reporting benefit used doses of 40–80mg/24h or more, which are now considered to be associated with a greater risk of sudden cardiac death (see Undesirable effects).[6,7]

Domperidone 20mg q.d.s. causes less frequent and less severe undesirable effects than **metoclopramide** 10mg q.d.s., e.g. less drowsiness and loss of mental acuity.[8] In diabetic patients, the prokinetic effect for solids attenuates after 1–2 months, although the effect on liquid emptying persists.[9,10]

Although almost completely absorbed from the GI tract, bio-availability is relatively poor because of extensive first-pass metabolism in the wall of the GI tract and the liver. Bio-availability in healthy volunteers is nearly doubled if taken *after* a meal.[11] Maximal absorption requires an acid environment; H_2 antagonists, PPIs and antacids all reduce absorption, and bio-availability. Under standard conditions, absorption is linear up to a 40mg single dose.

Domperidone is metabolized in the liver to inactive compounds, principally via CYP3A4. Because of safety concerns regarding high plasma levels of domperidone (see Undesirable effects), severe hepatic impairment is a contra-indication to its use. However, domperidone has previously been used in this setting; nonetheless, if it is considered necessary, a reduction in dose and careful monitoring would be prudent.

Renal clearance is a minor route of elimination (< 1% unchanged). In renal failure although the plasma halflife is increased by up to three times, plasma concentration does not increase (possibly because of an altered volume of distribution).[12] Thus, although the SPC recommends reducing the dosing frequency in severe renal impairment/failure to once or twice daily, and possibly also the dose, other drug information sources do not.[13]

Although rectal bio-availability is almost the same as by mouth, the recommended rectal dose is three times the oral dose. This stems from pharmacodynamic studies, and possibly relates to slower absorption from the rectum. Suppositories were discontinued in the UK in 2012.

The usefulness of domperidone is limited by the absence of a parenteral formulation. It was withdrawn in the early 1980s, after several patients died from ventricular arrhythmia (*torsade de pointes*) when given IV domperidone.[14] The pro-arrhythmic potential of domperidone via prolongation of the QT interval remains a concern (see Undesirable effects). Transmucosal and transdermal products are in development.

Bio-availability 12–18% PO (fasting), 24% PO (after food).
Onset of action 30min.
Time to peak plasma concentration 0.5–2h PO.
Plasma halflife 7–16h; increasing up to 21h in severe renal impairment.[3]
Duration of action 12–24h (estimate based on halflife).

Cautions

Underlying cardiac disease and other risk factors for prolonged QT, e.g. electrolyte disturbances (also see p.759). Hepatic impairment and severe renal impairment/failure (see Pharmacology).

Drug interactions

Serious drug interactions: Avoid concurrent use with drugs known to:
• increase the QT interval (see Chapter 24, p.759)
• inhibit the metabolism of domperidone, i.e. CYP3A4 inhibitors. These may increase the domperidone plasma concentration, increasing the risk of QT prolongation and thus *torsade de pointes*.
Examples of strong CYP3A4 inhibitors include **aprepitant**, azoles (**fluconazole, itraconazole**) grapefruit juice, macrolide antibiotics (**clarithromycin, erythromycin**), protease inhibitors (**ritonavir**), SSRIs (**fluvoxamine, fluoxetine**). Also see Chapter 25, p.767.

Because antimuscarinics competitively block the final common (cholinergic) pathway through which prokinetics act, concurrent prescription with domperidone should be avoided if possible. Opioids may also impede this action.

H_2 antagonists, PPIs and antacids reduce absorption and bio-availability.

Undesirable effects

Several epidemiological studies have explored the relationship between serious ventricular arrhythmia/ sudden cardiac death and the use of domperidone.[15–18] The two larger and more robust studies found that current domperidone use was associated with an overall increase in risk of ≤60%,[18] and possibly higher in those >60 years old or receiving higher doses (>30mg/24h).[16,18] In many instances, there was concurrent use of a CYP3A4 inhibitor or drug known to cause QT prolongation.

In 2014, following a Europe-wide review, because of this small increased risk of serious ventricular arrhythmia or sudden cardiac death, the EMA concluded that the risk:benefit ratio was only acceptable for nausea and vomiting, and recommended several restrictions.[19] As a consequence, the MHRA advised clinicians to:

- use domepridone *only* for nausea and vomiting, at the lowest effective dose, for the shortest possible time (generally ≤1 week)
- limit it to a maximum dose of 10mg t.d.s.
- avoid it in patients:
  ▷ where cardiac conduction is, or could be, impaired
  ▷ with underlying cardiac disease, e.g. CHF
  ▷ with severe hepatic impairment
  ▷ concurrently receiving drugs known to be CYP3A4 inhibitors and/or cause QT prolongation.
- advise patients to seek prompt medical attention should symptoms such as syncope or cardiac arrhythmias occur
- advise patients with contra-indications not to use OTC domperidone products.[20]

Such concerns have led some to call for the withdrawal of domperidone.[6] However, the risk:benefit balance should be determined on an individual patient basis, taking circumstances and other options into account. For example, if a patient with end-stage CHF requires a long-term anti-emetic, domperidone may be preferable to **cyclizine** (also pro-arrhythmic) or **metoclopramide** (risk of extrapyramidal effects).

Very rare (<0.01%): transient colic, gynaecomastia, galactorrhoea, amenorrhoea (secondary to increased prolactin secretion), reduced libido, cramp, pruritus, rash;[3] headache, extrapyramidal effects (acute dystonias), which resolve rapidly and completely once domperidone is stopped.[21] In two women with polycystic ovaries, hyperoestrogenism may have been a predisposing factor.[3]

Paradoxical vomiting has been reported in children with severe brain injury requiring tube feeding. Inhibition of pyloric relaxation was considered the likely cause, due to the D_2 antagonist effect of domperidone in the presence of a severe reduction in vagal tone.[22]

Dose and use

The manufacturer recommends giving domperidone t.d.s. (previously up to q.d.s. 15–30min before meals in patients with upper GI dysmotility). However, given its halflife, b.d. may suffice and its bio-availability is higher if taken after food:

- start with 10mg PO b.d
- increase to 10mg t.d.s., the new recommended maximum dose.

Also see MHRA advice in Undesirable effects. Previously, doses were increased to 20mg b.d. or 10mg q.d.s., with 20mg q.d.s. the old maximum recommended dose.

Supply

Domperidone (generic)
Tablets 10mg, 28 days @ 10mg q.d.s. = £4.50.
Oral suspension 5mg/5mL, 28 days @ 10mg q.d.s. = £70.

1 Barone J (1999) Domperidone: a peripherally acting dopamine$_2$-receptor antagonist. *Annals of Pharmacotherapy.* **33**: 429–440.
2 Langdon N et al. (1986) Comparison of levodopa with carbidopa, and levodopa with domperidone in Parkinson's disease. *Clin Neuropharmacol.* **9**: 440–447.
3 Prakash A and Wagstaff AJ (1998) Domperidone. A review of its use in diabetic gastropathy. *Drugs.* **56**: 429–445.
4 Sturm A et al. (1999) Prokinetics in patients with gastroparesis: a systematic analysis. *Digestion.* **60**: 422–427.
5 Dumitrascu D and Weinbeck M (2000) Domperidone versus metoclopramide in the treatment of diabetic gastroparesis. *American Journal of Gastroenterology.* **95**: 316–317.
6 Hondeghem LM (2013) Domperidone: limited benefits with significant risk for sudden cardiac death. *Journal of Cardiovascular Pharmacology.* **61**: 218–225.
7 Reddymasu SC et al. (2007) Domperidone: review of pharmacology and clinical applications in gastroenterology. *American Journal of Gastroenterology.* **102**: 2036–2045.
8 Patterson D et al. (1999) A double-blind multicenter comparison of domperidone and metoclopramide in the treatment of diabetic patients with symptoms of gastroparesis. *American Journal of Gastroenterology.* **94**: 1230–1234.

9   Horowitz M et al. (1985) Acute and chronic effects of domperidone on gastric emptying in diabetic autonomic neuropathy. Dig Dis Sci. 30: 1–9.

10 Koch KL et al. (1989) Gastric emptying and gastric myoelectrical activity in patients with diabetic gastroparesis: effect of long-term domperidone treatment. American Journal of Gastroenterology. 84: 1069–1075.

11 Heykants J et al. (1981) On the pharmacokinetics of domperidone in animals and man. IV. The pharmacokinetics of intravenous domperidone and its bioavailability in man following intramuscular, oral and rectal administration. European Journal of Drug Metabolism and Pharmacokinetics. 6: 61–70.

12 Brogden RN et al. (1982) Domperidone. A review of its pharmacological activity, pharmacokinetics and therapeutic efficacy in the symptomatic treatment of chronic dyspepsia and as an antiemetic. Drugs. 24: 360–400.

13 Ashley C and Currie A (2009) The Renal Drug Handbook (3e). Radcliffe Publishing Ltd, Oxford.

14 Osborne R et al. (1985) Cardiotoxicity of intravenous domperidone. Lancet. 2: 385–385.

15 Straus SM et al. (2005) Non-cardiac QTc-prolonging drugs and the risk of sudden cardiac death. European Heart Journal. 26: 2007–2012.

16 van Noord C et al. (2010) Domperidone and ventricular arrhythmia or sudden cardiac death: a population-based case-control study in the Netherlands. Drug Safety. 33: 1003–1014.

17 De Bruin ML et al. (2007) In-hospital cardiac arrest is associated with use of non-antiarrhythmic QTc-prolonging drugs. British Journal of Clinical Pharmacology. 63: 216–223.

18 Johannes CB et al. (2010) Risk of serious ventricular arrhythmia and sudden cardiac death in a cohort of users of domperidone: a nested case-control study. Pharmacoepidemiology and Drug Safety. 19: 881–888.

19 EMEA (2014) CMDh confirms recommendations on restricting use of domperidone-containing medicines. Press release (April). EMA/236452/2014: www.ema.europa.eu

20 MHRA (2014) Domperidone: risks of cardiac side effects - indicatiion restricted to nausea and vomiting, new contraindications, and reduced dose and duration of use. Drug Safety Update. 7. www.mhra.gov.uk/safetyinformation

21 Casteels-Van Daele M et al. (1984) Refusal of further cancer chemotherapy due to antiemetic drug. Lancet. 1: 57.

22 Pozzi M et al. (2013) Case series: paradoxical action of domperidone leads to increased vomiting. European Journal of Clinical Pharmacology. 69: 289–290.

Updated June 2014

ANTIHISTAMINIC ANTIMUSCARINIC ANTI-EMETICS   BNF 3.4 & 4.6

Indications: Prevention of motion sickness, nausea and vomiting, vertigo and labyrinthine disorders (**cyclizine, promethazine**), pruritus, sedation (**promethazine, hydroxyzine**).

Contra-indications: *Promethazine:* intra-arterial or SC injection (is a chemical irritant and may cause local necrosis).

Pharmacology

Antihistaminic antimuscarinic anti-emetics embrace several chemical classes including some phenothiazines (e.g. **promethazine**), piperazines (e.g. **buclizine, cyclizine, meclozine, hydroxyzine**) and mono-ethanolamines (e.g. **diphenhydramine, dimenhydrinate**). The piperazines and mono-ethanolamines were first marketed as H_1 antihistamines, and are often classed separately as antihistaminic anti-emetics. They decrease excitability of the inner ear labyrinth and block conduction in the vestibular-cerebellar pathways, as well as acting directly on the vomiting centre in the brain stem. However, there is considerable overlap between their receptor site affinity and that of the antipsychotic phenothiazines (see Antipsychotics, Table 1, p.168).

The piperazines and mono-ethanolamines began to be used for the prevention of motion sickness after a patient with urticaria reported relief from car sickness when taking **dimenhydrinate** (available only in a combination product in the UK).[1] After the Second World War, studies were conducted in American servicemen crossing the Atlantic Ocean in the General Ballou, a modified freight ship without stabilizers. Although the drugs differ in antihistaminic potency, they were equally effective,[1,2] suggesting that their anti-emetic effect is the result of multiple receptor site activity.

Antihistaminic anti-emetics are effective in many causes of vomiting, including opioid-induced.[3,4] However, in practice **metoclopramide** (see p.468) and **haloperidol** (see p.177) are often used in preference, sometimes because of more specific indications or to avoid drowsiness and antimuscarinic effects. Drowsiness is increased if used with other CNS depressants, e.g. benzodiazepines, barbiturates, antipsychotics, and alcohol. Metabolism is mainly hepatic, and the inactive metabolites are excreted in the urine.

Hydroxyzine is a later addition to this group of drugs, and is principally used as an anxiolytic-sedative and antipruritic. Unlike other antihistaminic drugs, **hydroxyzine** inhibits apomorphine-induced vomiting, suggesting that some of its anti-emetic effect is mediated via the chemoreceptor trigger zone. In postoperative patients, **hydroxyzine** 100mg IM (not UK) has analgesic activity approaching that of **morphine** 8mg,[5] and **morphine** 5mg and **hydroxyzine** 100mg gave comparable relief to **morphine** 10mg alone.[6] The sedative effect of the combination was not significantly different from **morphine** alone. For pharmacokinetic details, see Table 1.

Table 1   Pharmacokinetic details[7]

	Cyclizine	Hydroxyzine	Promethazine
Bio-availability	No data	No data	25% PO
Onset of action	30–60min	15–30min	~20min IM, 3–5min IV
Time to peak plasma concentration	2h PO	~2h	4.5h PO (syrup), 6–9h PR
Plasma halflife	13h	3–7h	7–14h
Duration of effect	4–6h	4–6h	2–6h

Cautions

Hepatic and renal impairment; epilepsy; can precipitate or exacerbate narrow-angle glaucoma; urinary tract obstruction (see Antimuscarinics, p.5). Elderly patients are more susceptible to sedative and central antimuscarinic effects, e.g. postural hypotension, memory impairment, extrapyramidal reactions.

Cyclizine: severe heart failure (antimuscarinic effect → tachycardia).

Hydroxyzine: asthma, COPD, hepatic impairment (restrict to once daily), moderate–severe renal impairment (reduce dose by 50%). When injected IV (not UK), if there is extravasation into the SC tissues, can cause a sterile abscess and tissue induration. Give well diluted as a 15–30min IVI only if strictly necessary.

Undesirable effects

Dry mouth and other antimuscarinic effects (see Antimuscarinics, p.6), drowsiness, headache, fatigue, nervousness, dizziness, thickening of bronchial secretions.

Severe movement disorders are reported (e.g. 'locked in syndrome'; also see Chapter 26, p.781).[8]

Dose and use

Because of their antimuscarinic properties, the use of this group of drugs tends to be restricted to situations where **metoclopramide** and/or other more specific anti-emetics (e.g. **haloperidol**, $5HT_3$ antagonists) have failed to relieve, e.g. some patients with mechanical bowel obstruction, or as the anti-emetic of choice for raised intracranial pressure.

In the UK, **cyclizine** is generally the antihistaminic antimuscarinic anti-emetic of choice. Depending on circumstances, **cyclizine** is generally given PO or SC:

• 50–100mg PO b.d.–t.d.s. & p.r.n.
• 100–150mg/24h CSCI & 50mg SC p.r.n.
• usual maximum daily dose 200mg PO and CSCI.

For CSCI dilute **cyclizine** with WFI or 5% glucose; **cyclizine** is *incompatible* with 0.9% saline and will precipitate, see Chapter 20, p.697.

CSCI compatibility with other drugs: There are 2-drug compatibility data for **cyclizine** in WFI with **haloperidol**, **hyoscine** *hydrobromide*, **morphine sulfate**, and **morphine tartrate** (not UK).

Concentration-dependent *incompatibility* occurs with **alfentanil**, **dexamethasone**, **diamorphine** and **oxycodone**. *Incompatibility* has also been reported with **clonazepam**, **hydromorphone**, **hyoscine** *butylbromide*, **ketorolac**, **midazolam** and **octreotide**. For more details and 3-drug compatibility data, see Appendix 3, p.821.

Doses of **promethazine** are 25mg PO t.d.s–q.d.s. **Promethazine** is generally not recommended CSCI due to its irritant properties and must *not* be given SC, see Chapter 20, Box F, p.705.

Supply

Oral products
Cyclizine *hydrochloride* (generic)
Tablets 50mg, 28 days @ 50mg t.d.s. = £9.

Promethazine *hydrochloride*
Phenergan® (Sanofi-Aventis)
Tablets 10mg, 25mg, 28 days @ 50mg t.d.s. = £14.
Oral solution 5mg/5mL, 28 days @ 50mg t.d.s. = £120.

Promethazine *teoclate*
Avomine® (Manx)
Tablets 25mg, 28 days @ 50mg t.d.s. = £20.

Parenteral products
Cyclizine *lactate* Valoid® (Amdipharm)
Injection 50mg/mL, 1mL amp = £1.

Promethazine *hydrochloride* (generic)
Injection 25mg/mL, 1mL amp = £1, 2mL amp = £1.50.

1 Gay L and Carliner P (1949) The prevention and treatment of motion sickness. *Bulletin of John Hopkins Hospital.* **49**: 470–491.
2 Gutner B et al. (1952) The effects of potent analgesics upon vestibular function. *Journal of Clinical Investigations.* **31**: 259–266.
3 Dundee J and Jones P (1968) The prevention of analgesic-induced nausea and vomiting by cyclizine. *British Journal of Clinical Practice.* **22**: 379–382.
4 Walder A and Aitkenhead A (1995) A comparison of droperidol and cyclizine in the prevention of postoperative nausea and vomiting associated with patient-controlled analgesia. *Anaesthesia.* **50**: 654–656.
5 Beaver WT and Feise G (1976) Comparison of analgesic effects of morphine sulphate, hydroxyzine and their combination in patients with postoperative pain. In: JJ Bonica and D Albe-Fessard (eds) *Advances in Pain Research and Therapy* Vol 1. Raven Press, New York, pp. 553–557.
6 Hupert C et al. (1980) Effect of hydroxyzine on morphine analgesia for the treatment of postoperative pain. *Anesthesia and Analgesia.* **59**: 690–696.
7 Vella-Brincat JW et al. (2012) The pharmacokinetics and pharmacogenetics of the antiemetic cyclizine in palliative care patients. *Journal of Pain and Symptom Management.* **43**: 540–548.
8 Lee P (2013) Locked-in syndrome as a result of cyclizine administration. *Journal of Pain and Symptom Management.* **45**: e5–7.

Updated June 2014

5HT₃ ANTAGONISTS   BNF 4.6

Indications: Nausea and vomiting after surgery, chemotherapy and radiotherapy, †intractable vomiting due to chemical, abdominal and cerebral causes when usual approaches have failed, †diarrhoea associated with carcinoid syndrome,[1] †opioid-induced pruritus.[2,3]

Contra-indications: Congenital long QT syndrome (**ondansetron**).

Pharmacology

5HT₃ antagonists were developed specifically to control emesis associated with highly emetogenic chemotherapy, e.g. **cisplatin**. They block the effect of excess 5HT on vagal nerve fibres, and are thus of particular value in situations when excessive amounts of 5HT are released from the body's stores, i.e. from enterochromaffin cells after chemotherapy or radiation-induced damage of the GI mucosa, or because of intestinal distension, or from leaky platelets when there is severe renal impairment.

A TD **granisetron** patch is authorized for the *prevention* of nausea and vomiting associated with moderately or highly emetogenic chemotherapy. It has a slow onset of action and must be applied 24–48h before chemotherapy. It can be worn ⩽7 days if required and is removed ⩾24h after completion of chemotherapy. Because it is no more effective than PO **granisetron**, its use is limited to situations where the PO route is not available.[4]

In an open RCT, **tropisetron** (not UK) was shown to be of benefit in patients with far-advanced cancer and nausea and vomiting of indeterminate cause when given either as a sole agent or with a second anti-emetic, particularly **dexamethasone**.[5] 5HT₃ antagonists also relieve nausea and vomiting after head injury, brain stem radiotherapy,[6,7] and in multiple sclerosis with brain stem disease;[8] leakage of 5HT from the raphe nucleus probably accounts for the benefit seen in these circumstances. $5HT_3$ antagonists are also effective in nausea and vomiting associated with acute gastro-enteritis.[9] In one patient who experienced persistent nausea after the insertion of an endo-oesophageal tube, a $5HT_3$ antagonist brought about relief after failure with **metoclopramide** and **cyclizine**.[10]

IV **ondansetron** 4–8mg relieves pruritus induced by spinal opioids in 3–30min (also see Chapter 21, p.720).[2,11,12] Although trials have not been conducted with other $5HT_3$ antagonists, it is likely that the benefit shown with **ondansetron** is a class effect. In contrast, **ondansetron** does *not* relieve cholestatic or uraemic pruritus (also see Chapter 28, p.797).[13]

Ondansetron can improve diarrhoea in carcinoid syndrome. In a small case series, where diarrhoea persisted despite **octreotide, ondansetron** 8mg b.d. provided satisfactory control within 2–3 days. Subsequently, the dose was reduced to the minimum effective maintenance dose (4–8mg daily).[1]

For pharmacokinetic details see Table 1.

Table 1 Pharmacokinetic details of 5HT antagonists

		Ondansetron	Granisetron	Palonosetron
Bio-availability	PO	56–71% (60% PR)	60%	n/a
Onset of action	PO	<30min	<30min	n/a
	IV	<5min	<15min	n/a
Plasma halflife		3–5h (6h PR)	10–11h	40h
Time to peak plasma concentration	PO	1.5h	No data	n/a
	IM	10min		n/a
	PR	6h		n/a
Duration of action		12h	24h	>24h[14]

Cautions

Risk factors for QT prolongation (particularly ondansetron, see Chapter 24, p.759); moderate-severe hepatic impairment (ondansetron; reduce dose); reduced colonic motility (can cause or worsen constipation).

Drug interactions

Serious drug interaction: a combination of IV **metoclopramide** and IV **ondansetron** occasionally causes cardiac arrhythmias (p.243).

Additive effects with other drugs that cause QT interval prolongation (see Chapter 24, p.759) and serotonin toxicity (e.g. SSRIs, see Antidepressants, Box B, p.195).

There are mixed reports of the analgesic effect of **tramadol** (p.352) and **paracetamol** (p.299) being reduced by $5HT_3$ antagonists, possibly by blocking the action of serotonin at presynaptic $5HT_3$-receptors on primary afferent nociceptive neurones in the spinal dorsal horn.

Undesirable effects

Very common (>10%): headache.[15]

Common (<10%, >1%): lightheadedness, dizziness, nervousness, tremor, ataxia, asthenia, drowsiness, fever, sensation of warmth or flushing (particularly when given IV), thirst, constipation or diarrhoea.

*Uncommon (<1%, >0.1%):***ondansetron**: dystonic reactions, arrhythmia, hypotension, raised LFTs.

Rare (<0.1%, >0.01%): hiccup.

Very rare (<0.01%): **ondansetron**: transient blindness during IV administration (sight generally returns within 20min).

Dose and use

In palliative care, first-line use of 5HT$_3$ antagonistsfor nausea and vomiting is rarely appropriate (see p.235). When used for intractable nausea and vomiting in advanced cancer, 5HT$_3$ antagonists are often more effective when combined with other anti-emetics.[5] They are typically used in combination with an antipsychotic with affinity for multiple receptors (e.g. **levomepromazine, olanzapine**) ± **dexamethasone**.

Granisetron can be given once daily whereas **ondansetron** is given b.d.–t.d.s. 5HT$_3$ antagonists are equally effective PO, by injection or TD.[4,16–18]

Regimens include:
* **granisetron** 1–2mg PO/SC once daily for 3 days *or*
* **ondansetron** 8mg PO/SC b.d.–t.d.s. (or 16–24mg/24h CSCI) for 3 days
* if clearly of benefit, continue indefinitely unless the cause is self-limiting
* some patients benefit from higher doses, occasionally as high as **granisetron** 9mg daily[19]
* in patients with moderate–severe hepatic impairment, the dose of **ondansetron** should be limited to 8mg daily, whereas no dose reduction is necessary for **granisetron** (in renal impairment, no dose reduction is necessary with either drug).

For CSCI dilute with WFI, 0.9% saline or 5% glucose.

CSCI compatibility with other drugs: There are 2-drug compatibility data for **ondansetron** in WFI with **alfentanil, diamorphine**, and **octreotide**. For more details and 3-drug compatibility data, see Appendix 3 (p.821).

Compatibility charts for mixing drugs in 0.9% saline can be found in the extended appendix of the on-line PCF on www.palliativedrugs.com

Note: to control nausea and vomiting caused by severely emetogenic chemotherapy, **granisetron** (or other 5HT$_3$ antagonist) is used with other anti-emetics, typically **dexamethasone** and **metoclopramide**.[20]

For IV **ondansetron** in chemotherapy-induced nausea and vomiting only, MHRA has placed restrictions on the maximum single IV dose and administration details for patients >65years, based on the risk of dose dependent QT interval prolongation.[21]

For use in pruritus associated with spinally administered opioids or for diarrhoea in carcinoid syndrome, see Pharmacology.

Supply

Granisetron (generic)
Tablets 1mg, 28 days @ 1mg once daily = £141.
Injection 1mg/mL, for dilution and use as an injection or infusion, 1mL amp = £2, 3mL amp = £2.50.

Kytril® (Roche)
Tablets 1mg, 2mg, 28 days @ 1mg daily = £147.

Sancuso® (ProStrakan)
Transdermal Patches (for up to 7 days) 3.1 mg/24h, 1 = £56.

Ondansetron (generic)
Tablets 4mg, 8mg, 28 days @ 8mg b.d. = £20; *based on using 4mg tablets, note the 8mg tablets are 8 times the cost.*
Orodispersible film 4mg, 8mg, 28 days @ 8mg b.d. = £320.
Oral solution 4mg/5mL, 28 days @ 8mg b.d. = £403.
Injection 2mg/mL, 2mL amp = £1, 4mL amp = £11.

Zofran® (GlaxoSmithKline)
Tablets 4mg, 8mg, 28 days @ 8mg b.d. = £403.
Tablets orodispersible (Zofran Melt®) 4mg, 8mg, 28 days @ 8mg b.d. = £403.
Oral solution (sugar-free) 4mg/5mL, 28 days @ 8mg b.d. = £403; *strawberry flavour.*
Injection 2mg/mL, 2mL amp = £6, 4mL amp = £12.
Suppositories 16mg, 1 = £14.

1   Kiesewetter B and Raderer M (2013) Ondansetron for diarrhea associated with neuroendocrine tumors. *New England Journal of Medicine*. **368**: 1947–1948.
2   Borgeat A and Stimemann H-R (1999) Ondansetron is effective to treat spinal or epidural morphine-induced pruritus. *Anesthesiology*. **90**: 432–436.
3   Kyriakides K et al. (1999) Management of opioid-induced pruritus: a role for 5HT antagonists? *British Journal of Anaesthesia*. **82**: 439–441.
4   Boccia RV et al. (2011) Efficacy and tolerability of transdermal granisetron for the control of chemotherapy-induced nausea and vomiting associated with moderately and highly emetogenic multi-day chemotherapy: a randomized, double-blind, phase III study. *Supportive Care in Cancer*. **19**: 1609–1617.
5   Mystakidou K et al. (1998) Comparison of the efficacy and safety of tropisetron, metoclopramide, and chlorpromazine in the treatment of emesis associated with far advanced cancer. *Cancer*. **83**: 1214–1223.
6   Kleinerman K et al. (1993) Use of ondansetron for control of projectile vomiting in patients with neurosurgical trauma: two case reports. *Annals of Pharmacotherapy*. **27**: 566–568.
7   Bodis S et al. (1994) The prevention of radiosurgery-induced nausea and vomiting by ondansetron: evidence of a direct effect on the central nervous system chemoreceptor trigger zone. *Surgery and Neurology*. **42**: 249–252.
8   Rice G and Ebers G (1995) Ondansetron for intractable vertigo complicating acute brainstem disorders. *Lancet*. **345**: 1182–1183.
9   Cubeddu L et al. (1997) Antiemetic activity of ondansetron in acute gastroenteritis. *Alimentary Pharmacology and Therapeutics*. **11**: 185–191.
10 Fair R (1990) Ondansetron in nausea. *Pharmaceutical Journal*. **245**: 514.
11 Arai L et al. (1996) The use of ondansetron to treat pruritus associated with intrathecal morphine in two paediatric patients. *Paediatric Anaesthesia*. **6**: 337–339.
12 Larijani G et al. (1996) Treatment of opioid-induced pruritus with ondansetron: report of four patients. *Pharmacotherapy*. **16**: 958–960.
13 To TH et al. (2012) The role of ondansetron in the management of cholestatic or uremic pruritus–a systematic review. *Journal of Pain and Symptom Management*. **44**: 725–730.
14 Saito M et al. (2009) Palonosetron plus dexamethasone versus granisetron plus dexamethasone for prevention of nausea and vomiting during chemotherapy: a double-blind, double-dummy, randomised, comparative phase III trial. *Lancet Oncology*. **10**: 115–124.
15 Goodin S and Cunningham R (2002) 5-HT3-receptor antagonists for the treatment of nausea and vomiting: a reappraisal of their side-effect profile. *The Oncologist*. **7**: 424–436.
16 Perez EA et al. (1997) Efficacy and safety of different doses of granisetron for the prophylaxis of cisplatin-induced emesis. *Support Care Cancer*. **5**: 31–37.
17 Perez E et al. (1997) Efficacy and safety of oral granisetron versus IV ondansetron in prevention of moderately emetogenic chemotherapy-induced nausea and vomiting. *Proceedings of the American Society of Clinical Oncology*. **16**: 149.
18 Gralla R et al. (1997) Can an oral antiemetic regimen be as effective as intravenous treatment against cisplatin: results of a 1054 patient randomized study of oral granisetron versus IV ondansetron. *Proceedings of the American Society of Clinical Oncology*. **16**: 178.
19 Minami M (2003) Granisetron: is there a dose-response effect on nausea and vomiting? *Cancer Chemotherapy and Pharmacology*. **52**: 89–98.
20 Kris MG et al. (2006) American Society of Clinical Oncology guideline for antiemetics in oncology: update 2006. *Journal of Clinical Oncology*. **24**: 2932–2947.
21 MHRA (2013) Ondansetron for intravenous use: dose-dependent QT interval prolongation - new posology. *Drug Safety update*. **6**. www.mhra.gov.uk/safetyinformation

Updated June 2014

ANTI-EPILEPTICS   BNF 4.8.1

Indications: (Authorized indications vary; see individual drug monographs for details) Neuropathic pain, epilepsy, mania, anxiety, †terminal agitation, †sweats and hot flushes, †refractory hiccup, †restless legs syndrome, †refractory cough, †nausea and vomiting, †uraemic itch.

Pharmacology

Anti-epileptic drugs inhibit rapidly firing neurones and can thereby impact on symptoms arising from excessive neuronal activity in any part of the nervous system. They are structurally and functionally diverse. Some influence action potential generation or consequent neurotransmitter release or action. Others act indirectly, increasing the GABA-mediated inhibition of rapidly firing neurones (see Table 1 and Figure 1).

The relationship between clinical activity and mode of action is not fully understood. Further, clinically relevant differences exist between anti-epileptics acting in similar ways, and additional actions contribute to the beneficial and/or undesirable effects of some. Choice of drug thus remains partly empirical.[1]

Membrane stabilizers reduce excitability by blocking sodium channels and/or opening potassium channels. The normal transport of sodium channels is disrupted by nerve injury; they accumulate creating foci of ectopic action potential generation. Several classes of drug bind to sodium

Table 1 Mechanisms of action of anti-epileptics[1–9]

	Membrane stabilizers		↓ Neurotransmitter release		Neurotransmitter receptor antagonist		GABAmimetics		↓Thalamic burst firing
	Na channel blocker	K channel activator	Ca channel blocker (N, P and Q type)	↓vesicle release (SV2A)	AMPA	NMDA	GABA$_A$ receptor modulation	Altered GABA synthesis and reuptake	Ca channel blocker (T type)
Benzodiazepines							++		
Carbamazepine	++								
Eslicarbazepine	++								
Ethosuximide									++
Gabapentin		+	++						
Lacosamide	++								
Lamotrigine	++		++		+				
Levetiracetam				++					
Oxcarbazepine	++	+							
Perampanel					++				
Phenobarbital							++		
Phenytoin	++								
Pregabalin			++				+		
Retigabine		++							
Rufinamide	++								
Tiagabine								++[a]	
Topiramate	++						++		
Valproate	+[b]					+[b]		+[a,b]	+[b]
Vigabatrin								++[a]	
Zonisamide	++		++						++

++ = predominant action, + = putative or non-predominant action.

a. tiagabine and vigabatrin inhibit GABA reuptake and breakdown (via GABA transaminase) respectively. Valproate affects both synthesis and re-uptake/breakdown of GABA in selected brain regions

b. although many anti-epileptics have more than one mode of action, valproate in particular is thought to have no predominant mode of action, helping to explain its broad spectrum of activity (see valproate, p.279).

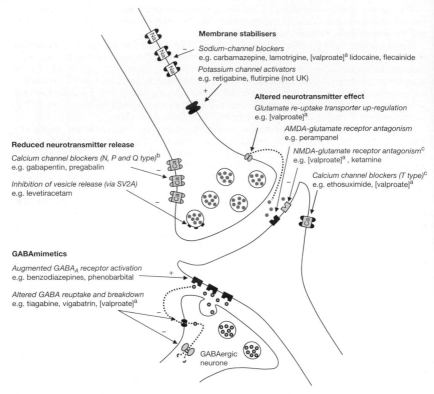

Membrane stabilisers

Sodium-channel blockers
e.g. carbamazepine, lamotrigine, [valproate][a] lidocaine, flecainide
Potassium channel activators
e.g. retigabine, flutirpine (not UK)

Altered neurotransmitter effect

Glutamate re-uptake transporter up-regulation
e.g. [valproate][a]

AMDA-glutamate receptor antagonism
e.g. perampanel

Reduced neurotransmitter release

Calcium channel blockers (N, P and Q type)[b]
e.g. gabapentin, pregabalin

Inhibition of vesicle release (via SV2A)
e.g. levetiracetam

NMDA-glutamate receptor antagonism[c]
e.g. [valproate][a] , ketamine

Calcium channel blockers (T type)[c]
e.g. ethosuximide, [valproate][a]

GABAmimetics

Augmented GABA$_A$ receptor activation
e.g. benzodiazepines, phenobarbital

Altered GABA reuptake and breakdown
e.g. tiagabine, vigabatrin, [valproate][a]

GABAergic
neurone

Figure I Mechanisms of action of anti-epileptics and related drugs.[1-7,10,11] Squared parentheses indicate a contributory, but not predominant, action of the anti-epileptic.

a. although many anti-epileptics have more than one mode of action, valproate in particular is thought to have no single predominant action (see p.279)
b. arriving action potentials open pre-synaptic N, P, Q type calcium channels. The resulting calcium influx triggers neurotransmitter release (see p.270)
c. both NMDA-glutamate receptors and T-type calcium channels affect neuronal excitability and threshold setting. T-type calcium channels also affect neuronal firing patterns, e.g. tonic or burst firing, with thalamic burst firing implicated in absence seizures.

channels during or after opening; repetitive firing thus results in an increasing proportion of blocked channels ('use-dependent block'):[12]
• some anti-epileptics, e.g. **carbamazepine** (see p.275), **oxcarbazepine** (see p.278), **phenytoin**, **lamotrigine** and **lacosamide**
• local anaesthetics, e.g. **lidocaine** (see p.71)
• class I anti-arrhythmics, e.g. **flecainide** (see p.71).
All have been shown to have antinociceptive and/or anti-neuropathic pain effects.[13-16] However, the duration of blockade before the drug dissociates from the channel varies. This, and effects on targets other than sodium channels, creates important clinical differences between such drugs.

Potential future directions for sodium channel blockers in pain management include reduced blood-brain barrier penetration (reducing undesirable central effects by targeting ectopic foci on damaged peripheral neurones)[12] or subtype-selective blockers (inherited abnormalities of one subtype, Na$_v$1.7, cause congenital insensitivity to pain while leaving other senses unaffected).[17]

The opening of potassium channels also has a membrane-stabilizing effect by hyperpolarizing the cell membrane, and is thought to account for the effect of the analgesic **flupirtine** (not UK)[18] and the anti-epileptic, **retigabine**.[9]

Neurotransmitter release is affected by both $\alpha 2\delta$ and SV2A ligands. The $\alpha 2\delta$ ligands, **gabapentin** and **pregabalin**, block N, P and Q-type calcium-channels. This reduces the calcium influx required to trigger neurotransmitter release (see p.270).[18] Neuropathic pain results in the upregulation of calcium channel $\alpha 2\delta$ subunits in the dorsal horn of the spinal cord, which **gabapentin** and **pregabalin** help counteract.[19] They also influence descending pain inhibitory pathways and pain processing. Spinal calcium channels are also targeted by **ziconotide**. **Levetiracetam** binds SV2A, a protein involved in modulating neurotransmitter vesicle release. (see p.283).[20]

GABAmimetics affect GABA metabolism or $GABA_A$ receptors. **Tiagabine** and **vigabatrin** inhibit GABA re-uptake transporters and GABA transaminase, the enzyme responsible for GABA breakdown, respectively. **Valproate** probably also affects GABA metabolism. Barbiturates and benzodiazepines affect $GABA_A$ receptors, binding at sites distinct from GABA itself (allosteric modulation). Benzodiazepines increase the receptors affinity for GABA; barbiturates prolong channel opening (see p.148, p.286 and Table 1).[21]

The broad spectrum of efficacy of **valproate** is explained by its multiple actions including blockade of sodium channels and T-type calcium channels. The latter are implicated in neuropathic pain,[22] the burst firing responsible for absence seizures and perhaps also in regulating pain excitation thresholds in a 'T-rich' subset of peripheral nociceptors.[3,23]

The endocannabinoid system is another important inhibitory neurotransmitter system; cannabinoids have been proposed as potential future anti-epileptics.[24]

Genetic variations in anti-epileptic targets have been identified (e.g. sodium and potassium channels, the $GABA_A$ receptor complex). Some cause inherited epilepsy, but there is no straightforward link between the affected channel/receptor and either the epilepsy type or optimal choice of anti-epileptic.[25,26] A polymorphism in the gene (SCN1A) encoding the sodium channel α-subunit has been linked to **carbamazepine**-resistant epilepsy.[27]

Genetic factors also affect both pharmacokinetics and the risk of undesirable effects. Two poor metabolizer CYP2C9 alleles (which occur in 10–20% of Caucasians, 10% of Japanese, and 1–5% of Asians and Africans) reduce the mean effective daily **phenytoin** dose by 20–40%.[26] Human leukocyte antigen (HLA) genes are associated with the risk of Stevens-Johnson syndrome in patients taking **carbamazepine, eslicarbazepine, oxcarbazepine** or **phenytoin** (see p.275).[28,29] The UK MHRA recommends testing HLA B*1502 status before **carbamazepine** is started in people of Han Chinese, Hong Kong Chinese or Thai origin.[30]

The pharmacokinetics of anti-epileptics are summarized in Table 2. Whereas absorption is generally unaffected by increasing age, the volume of distribution may change (reduced albumin, total body water and lean:fat mass ratio) and elimination rates slow (altered metabolism, renal function and volume of distribution).[30,31]

Cautions

Safety concerns with **vigabatrin** (visual field deficits) and **felbamate** (not UK; aplastic anaemia and hepatic failure) limit their use to refractory epilepsy under specialist supervision when all other measures have failed.

Driving

In the UK, patients suffering from epilepsy must notify the DVLA. Generally, a seizure-free period of one year is required before driving can resume (longer for heavy goods vehicles), although this varies (e.g. where a seizure was due to a transient illness).[41] Patients affected by drowsiness should not drive or operate machinery.

Skin rashes and cross-reactive hypersensitivity

In relation to skin rashes, cross-reactive hypersensitivity may occur with various anti-epileptics:[42]
- **carbamazepine**: increased risk if rash occurred with a previous anti-epileptic (particularly **phenytoin, phenobarbital** or **oxcarbazepine**) or TCA; use alternative if possible
- **phenytoin**: increased risk of skin rash if rash has occurred with a previous anti-epileptic (particularly **carbamazepine** or **phenobarbital**); use alternative if possible
- **oxcarbazepine**: 25–30% risk of cross-reactivity if previous reaction to **carbamazepine**

Table 2 Pharmacokinetic details of anti-epileptics[9,31–40]

Drug	Bio-availability PO (%)	T_{max} (h)	Plasma binding (%)	Plasma halflife (h)	Fate
Carbamazepine	80	4–8	75	8–24	CYP3A4, CYP2C8[a]
Clonazepam	≥80	1–4	80–90	30–40	CYP3A
Diazepam	≥80	1–3	95–98	24–48, 48–120[b]	CYP2C19, CYP3A4[a]
Gabapentin	30–75[c]	2–3	0	5–7	Excreted unchanged
Lamotrigine	98	1–4	55	15–30, 8–20[d], 30–90[e]	Glucuronidation
Levetiracetam	≥95	1–2	<10	6–8	Non-hepatic hydrolysis (70% excreted unchanged)
Oxcarbazepine[f]	≥95	1–3, 3–8[f]	65, 40[f]	1–5, 7–20[f]	Cytosolic keto-reduction to MHD[f], which then undergoes glucuronidation[a]
Perampanel		1	95	53–136	CYP3A4, CYP3A5
Phenobarbital	≥90	2–12	50	72–144	CYP2C9 (25% excreted unchanged)
Phenytoin	90–95	4–8	90	10–70[c]	CYP2C9
Pregabalin	>90	1	0	5–9[g]	Excreted unchanged
Retigabine	60	1–1.5	80	8	Glucuronidation and N-acetylation[a]
Rufinamide	85	5–6	25–35	8–12	Hepatic hydrolysis and oxidation
Tiagabine	≥90	1–2	96	4–13, 2–5[d]	CYP3A4
Topiramate	≥80	1–4	13	20–30, 8–15[d]	Multiple pathways (>60% excreted unchanged)
Valproate	95	1–2[h]	90	9–18, 5–12[d]	Multiple pathways[a] (see p.279)
Vigabatrin	80–90	1–2	0	6	Excreted unchanged
Zonisamide	≥50	1–4	50	50–70, 25–35[d]	CYP3A4 (15–30% excreted unchanged)

a. biologically active metabolites
b. nordiazepam, active metabolite
c. dose or plasma concentration dependent
d. with concurrent enzyme-inducers
e. with concurrent valproate
f. monohydroxycarbazepine, active metabolite of oxcarbazepine (a pro-drug)
g. >2 days in severe renal impairment and haemodialysis patients
h. 3–5h for e/c tablets, 5–10h for m/r tablets.

- **zonisamide:** avoid if hypersensitive to sulfonamides
- **lamotrigine:** increased risk of rash if rash has occurred with a previous anti-epileptic, rapidly titrated and/or receiving concurrent **valproate.**

Hepatic impairment
With the exception of **gabapentin, pregabalin,** and **vigabatrin,** the manufacturers advise caution with all the anti-epileptics listed in Table 2 (i.e. lower initial doses, slower titration and careful monitoring). Specific advice is given for **levetiracetam** (halve the dose in severe hepatic impairment because of probable concurrent renal impairment), **lamotrigine** (see SPC), **oxcarbazepine** (usual dose with mild–moderate impairment, no data with severe impairment), **phenytoin** (monitor plasma concentration), **tiagabine** (reduce dose if mild, avoid if severe), and **zonisamide** (avoid if possible).

Further, previous or concurrent hepatic disease increases the risk of **valproate** and **carbamazepine**-related hepatic failure. However, no specific information is available about the risks with hepatic metastases. They do not generally affect the hepatic metabolism of drugs unless there is concurrent cirrhosis.[43,44]

Renal impairment
With the exception of **phenytoin** and **tiagabine,** the manufacturers advise caution with all the anti-epileptics listed in Table 2 (i.e. lower initial doses, slower titration and careful monitoring). Specific advice on dose adjustment is available for **gabapentin** and **pregabalin** (p.270). Further, there are occasional reports of renal failure with **pregabalin** which improved when it was stopped.

Females of child-bearing age
Consider teratogenicity when choosing an anti-epileptic. Enquire about oral contraceptive if using an enzyme-inducing anti-epileptic.

Suicide
Overall, anti-epileptic drugs are associated with suicidal thoughts or behaviour in 1/500 patients from the start of treatment onwards. The effect appears to differ between drugs, with some even conferring a small protective effect. Nonetheless, all patients should be monitored for suicidal ideation, and advised to report any mood disturbance or suicidal thoughts to a health professional.[45–47]

Additional cautions with specific anti-epileptics
- atrioventricular block (**carbamazepine** and **oxcarbazepine** may cause complete block)
- previous bone marrow suppression (**carbamazepine,** possible increased risk)
- heart failure (**oxcarbazepine** and **pregabalin,** fluid retention can cause exacerbation; monitor weight and plasma sodium).

Drug interactions
Interactions are described in individual drug monographs:
- **gabapentin** (p.270), **pregabalin** (p.270) and **levetiracetam** have no clinically significant pharmacokinetic interactions
- **phenobarbital** (p.286), **carbamazepine** (p.275) and **phenytoin** (see Table 3) cause numerous interactions through hepatic enzyme induction.

Table 3 Clinically significant cytochrome P450 interactions with phenytoin resulting in changed drug plasma concentrations

Phenytoin plasma concentration		Drug plasma concentration	
increased by	decreased by	increased by phenytoin	decreased by phenytoin
Amiodarone	Antiretrovirals[a]	Phenobarbital	Amiodarone
Antifungal azoles[a]	Benzodiazepines[a]		Antifungal and anthelmintic azoles[a]
Azapropazone	Carbamazepine		Antiretrovirals[a]
Benzodiazepines[a]	Chlorpromazine		Aprepitant
Carbamazepine	Dexamethasone		Benzodiazepines[a]
Celecoxib	Phenobarbital		Calcium-channel blockers[a]

continued

Table 3 Continued

Phenytoin plasma concentration		Drug plasma concentration
Chlorpromazine	Rifampicin	Carbamazepine
Cimetidine	St John's wort	Clozapine
Dexamethasone	Thioridazine	Corticosteroids
Diltiazem	Valproate	Disopyramide
Ethosuximide	Vigabatrin	Doxycycline
Fluoxetine		Ethosuximide
Fluvoxamine		Fentanyl
Oxcarbazepine		Haloperidol
Phenobarbital		Hormonal contraceptives
Prochlorperazine		Lamotrigine
Stiripentol		Methadone
Thioridazine		Mexiletine
Ticlopidine		Mirtazapine
Topiramate		Primidone
Valproate		Sertindole
		Theophylline
		Tiagabine
		Topiramate
		Tramadol
		Valproate

a. effect not seen with all drug class members.

Undesirable effects

Despite their diverse actions and structures, anti-epileptics share many undesirable effects. Their relative incidence is often similar.[48,49]

All anti-epileptics cause psychotropic and CNS depressant effects including drowsiness, ataxia, cognitive impairment, agitation, diplopia and dizziness. Psychiatric effects (e.g. depression, psychosis, irritability, or lability) are commonest with **levetiracetam, phenobarbital, tiagabine, topiramate, vigabatrin** and **zonisamide**.[47] Cognitive impairment is worst with **phenobarbital** and least with newer anti-epileptics and **valproate**.[35,50] Anti-epileptics cause suicidal ideation in 1/500 patients (see Cautions).

Most cause haematological derangements. These are often asymptomatic and may not require stopping the drug (see SPCs for advice). Severe derangement (e.g. aplastic anaemia, agranulocytosis) is reported particularly with **felbamate** (limiting use) and **carbamazepine** (monitor blood counts), and with many newer anti-epileptics. Folate deficiency occurs with enzyme-inducers, e.g. **phenytoin**.

Biochemical derangements (particularly of LFTs) are also common but are generally asymptomatic. Albeit rarely, hepatic failure is seen with many anti-epileptics, again particularly with **felbamate** (not UK; also limiting its use) and **carbamazepine** (where symptoms of hepatic disease and LFTs should be monitored), as well as with newer anti-epileptics. The incidence compared with **carbamazepine** is unknown. Pancreatitis affects 1:3,000 users of **valproate**.[51] It also occurs with many newer anti-epileptics but the incidence compared with **valproate** is unknown.

Transient rashes are particularly associated with **lamotrigine, carbamazepine** and **oxcarbazepine**. Risk factors include rashes with previous anti-epileptics, higher starting doses and rapid titration (and, with **lamotrigine**, childhood and concurrent **valproate**). Severe rashes such as Stevens-Johnson syndrome are reported with all anti-epileptics, but most commonly with **lamotrigine** (affecting 1:1,000 adults). An HLA type is known to predispose specific groups to **carbamazepine**- and **phenytoin**-related Stevens-Johnson syndrome (see above).

Undesirable effects seen with particular anti-epileptics include: urolithiasis (**topiramate** and **zonisamide**); and coarse facies, acne, hirsutism and gingival hypertrophy (**phenytoin**). **Phenytoin** also exhibits distinct undesirable effects at supra-therapeutic levels (Box A).

Box A Phenytoin toxicity

Clinical features
Phenytoin toxicity generally manifests as a syndrome of cerebellar, vestibular and ocular effects, including some or all of the following:
- nystagmus:
  - ▷ on lateral gaze only (early sign)
  - ▷ spontaneous (more severe toxicity)
- blurred vision/diplopia
- slurred speech
- ataxia.

These may be accompanied by lethargy and/or delirium. Some patients experience break-through seizures (or an increase in the frequency of seizures) when the free phenytoin plasma concentration increases to toxic levels.

Evaluation
If phenytoin toxicity is suspected, check the plasma phenytoin concentration just before the next dose is due and, because phenytoin is highly protein-bound, the plasma albumin (see Chapter 14, p.650). The normal therapeutic range is 40–80micromol/L (10–20microgram/mL). In patients with a low albumin, it is important to correct the observed concentration using the equation:

$$\text{Corrected total phenytoin concentration} = \frac{\text{observed concentration}}{(0.02 \times \text{albumin}) + 0.1}$$

Note: phenytoin toxicity can be present despite being within the therapeutic range; if necessary, make the diagnosis on clinical features alone and act accordingly.

Management
There is no specific antidote to phenytoin. If the patient has clinical features suggestive of toxicity, reduce the dose of phenytoin to a known previous non-toxic level. If severe, omit a dose and reduce subsequent doses. Generally, symptoms resolve when the plasma phenytoin concentration falls.[52]

Treat breakthrough seizures with benzodiazepines (see p.148) because other anti-epileptic drugs may exacerbate the toxicity. If the frequency of seizures increases as the phenytoin toxicity resolves, obtain advice from a neurologist.

Use of anti-epileptics in palliative care

Particularly when prescribing more than one anti-epileptic, it is important to consider:
- pharmacokinetic drug–drug interactions
- seizure type (generalized seizures may be precipitated by **carbamazepine, oxcarbazepine, gabapentin, tiagabine** and **vigabatrin**)
- additive cognitive impairment.

Switching between formulations

The MHRA recommends avoiding switching between formulations of anti-epileptic drugs when used for epilepsy, except for **ethosuximide, gabapentin, lacosamide, levetiracetam, pregabalin, tiagabine** and **vigabatrin**.[53]

Switching formulation should be avoided where possible because:
- changes in packaging or appearance can cause confusion
- doses may be labelled differently, e.g. phenytoin liquid vs. capsules
- bio-availability or duration of action may differ.

Both loss of effect and new undesirable effects have been reported after switching.[53] However, if there is a delay in obtaining the patients usual brand, *it is better to give a different brand than to omit the medicine.*

Neuropathic pain

Gabapentin is a first-line choice because benefit has been confirmed for a range of causes of neuropathic pain;[54,55] it has few drug interactions; and peripheral neuropathic pain is included in its marketing authorization. **Gabapentin** is effective for cancer-related neuropathic pain, although the benefit in a RCT was small (see p.270).[56]

Pregabalin is more expensive. Its twice daily administration is an advantage for selected patients. Its marketing authorization also includes central neuropathic pain and a liquid preparation. **Gabapentin** can also be administered twice daily for some patients, particularly the elderly and those with renal impairment (see p.270).

Valproate is used in some centres when a smaller tablet load or once daily regimen is required. Benefit is reported for cancer-related neuropathic pain,[57,58] but the results of RCTs in non-cancer pain are conflicting (see p.279); thus international guidelines do not recommend its use first-line.[59,60] It appears to be well tolerated with lower rates of discontinuation because of undesirable effects (< 5%)[61–65] compared with **gabapentin** (10%)[54] and **pregabalin** (20–30%)[55] in similar populations.

Carbamazepine is an authorized first-line treatment for trigeminal neuralgia. It has long been used off-label for other neuropathic pains despite few supporting RCTs.[66] It requires slow titration and particular care with regard to drug interactions (see p.275). **Phenytoin** is also effective, at least in the short-term.[67] Of other membrane stabilizers trialled, **lamotrigine** appears ineffective[66] and **lacosamide** less effective than alternatives (in diabetic neuropathy NNT 8–11 vs. 6 for gabapentin/pregabalin).[54,55,68–71] Results of RCTs of **oxcarbazepine** in diabetic neuropathy show inconsistent benefit (see p.278).

Clonazepam is reported to improve both cancer-related and non-cancer neuropathic pain (see p.160). It has anxiolytic and muscle-relaxant properties and can be given SC (not UK), leading to its use in selected palliative care patients despite the absence of supporting RCTs.

Topiramate is reported to improve cancer-related neuropathic pain.[72] However, results of RCTs in non-cancer neuropathic pain (diabetic neuropathy, lumbar radicular pain)[73–75] do not show consistent benefit. Slow titration is required to minimise undesirable CNS effects.

Levetiracetam is ineffective for neuropathic pain (see p.283).

Alternatives to anti-epileptics include antidepressants p.190 and opioids p.357. They are also often used in combination (see p.295). Despite some methodological limitations in the head-to-head studies of **gabapentin/pregabalin** vs. antidepressants, overall, they appear to have similar efficacy and tolerability (see also **gabapentin** and **pregabalin** p.270).[76–81] When used together, **gabapentin** and **nortriptyline** were superior to either treatment alone.[82] **Morphine** was as effective as TCAs,[83] whereas the combination of **morphine** and **gabapentin** was superior to either treatment alone.[84] An open-label trial in cancer pain with a neuropathic component also found this combination to be superior to **morphine** alone.[85]

Combinations of ≥2 anti-epileptics are used less commonly. Undesirable effects may be increased and alternative options (e.g. antidepressants, opioids, **ketamine** and interventional anaesthesia, also see p.295) are often more appropriate. Where a second anti-epileptic drug is added, the first is generally withdrawn, although examples of combined use are reported. Improvements in efficacy and tolerability have been described in 11 patients with multiple sclerosis whose trigeminal neuralgia had been unsatisfactorily controlled by **carbamazepine** or **lamotrigine**. The addition of **gabapentin** brought relief in 10 patients. The former were reduced to the minimal effective dose, with improved overall tolerability, but could not be withdrawn completely in any patient, suggesting that both anti-epileptics were contributing to overall relief.[86]

Although generally not used for *nociceptive* pain, **phenytoin**, **gabapentin** and **pregabalin** have an antinociceptive/analgesic effect.[87–90]

Doses are described in individual monographs: **carbamazepine** (p.275); **clonazepam** (p.160); **gabapentin** and **pregabalin** (p.270); **oxcarbazepine**; and **valproate** (p.279).

Epilepsy

Overtreatment with anti-epileptic drugs is common. Seek specialist advice where the diagnosis of seizures or the dose or choice of anti-epileptic drug is in doubt.

Initiating treatment

A maintenance anti-epileptic is generally commenced after a first seizure when there is an irreversible underlying focal lesion, e.g. cerebral tumour, multiple sclerosis, which makes further seizures probable. In the absence of a focal lesion, the risk is lower and an anti-epileptic is generally withheld unless a second seizure occurs.[91]

Although seizure classification is an important factor in the choice of anti-epileptic in primary epilepsy, seizures caused by focal brain lesions are, by definition, focal onset, even if this is obscured by rapid secondary generalization. Thus, generally in palliative care, other factors have a greater influence on the choice of anti-epileptic, e.g. the potential for drug interactions, co-morbidities, and the simplicity of the regimen (Box B). Case series report mostly the use of **valproate, levetiracetam, gabapentin, carbamazepine** and **phenytoin** for seizures secondary to cerebral tumours.[92–95] Enzyme-inducing anti-epileptics can interfere with chemotherapy. Because of the risk of teratogenicity with some anti-epileptics, obtain specialist advice when treating women of childbearing age.

Box B   Anti-epileptics for seizures in palliative care[93,94]

First-line alternatives[a]
Valproate[b]
Can be titrated rapidly, IV or SC if necessary (see p.279)

Oxcarbazepine
Fewer drug interactions than carbamazepine and phenytoin; effective doses achieved more quickly than with lamotrigine and carbamazepine (see p.278)

Second-line
Switch to another first-line choice, or prescribe
Levetiracetam
Can be titrated rapidly, IV or SC if necessary (see p.283)

Last days of life
Midazolam
Generally first-line because of familiarity, availability, benefit in concurrent symptoms and compatibility with other drugs CSCI (see p.157)

Phenobarbital
Generally second-line where seizures are unresponsive to midazolam (see p.286)

---

a. NICE recommend carbamazepine or lamotrigine as usual first-line options for focal seizures.[98] However, both require gradual titration over many weeks. Thus, in the palliative care setting, the recommended first-line alternatives, levetiracetam, oxcarbazepine and valproate are generally preferable
b. despite abnormal in vitro haemostasis, valproate has not been shown to increase neurosurgical bleeding complications,[99,100] but some surgeons advise caution; discuss with surgeons before starting if neurosurgery is planned.

Anti-epileptics are better tolerated if commenced at lower than recommended doses.[96] Doses can be increased if seizures persist. However, less additional benefit is seen when increasing higher doses. In one observational study, 90% of those responding to a first-line anti-epileptic required:
• **valproate** ≤1,500mg/24h
• **lamotrigine** ≤300mg/24h
• **carbamazepine** ≤800mg/24h.[97]
Few patients responded to increases above these doses.[97] In non-responders, a change of anti-epileptic is indicated.

For doses, see individual monographs for **valproate** (p.279), **carbamazepine** (p.275), **oxcarbazepine** (p.278), **gabapentin** and **pregabalin** (p.270) or **levetiracetam** (p.283), or the manufacturer's SPC.

Switching vs. combining anti-epileptics for epilepsy
If the first choice treatment fails, add a second anti-epileptic (Box B). When the second one is at an adequate or maximally tolerated dose, the first one is slowly withdrawn (see below).[98] Long-term combination therapy is generally avoided unless two trials of monotherapy have proved ineffective because:
• there is an increased likelihood of drug interactions
• toxicity may be enhanced
• evidence of benefit compared with monotherapy is limited.[96,101]
Combinations are guided by the same considerations as those for choosing first- and second-line anti-epileptics. Many successful combinations have been reported,[101,102] but the relative benefits of such combinations have not been established. Studies of older anti-epileptics indicate probable benefit in combining GABAmimetics with sodium channel blockers or possibly with other GABAmimetics, but not in using two sodium channel blockers together.[103] Despite this, combinations of sodium channel blockers are among those used by epileptologists.[101] Combining **valproate** and **lamotrigine** increases the risk of skin reactions.

Do not combine three or more anti-epileptics except on specialist advice; additional benefit is rare.[96]

Prophylaxis in patients with cerebral tumours
Although about 20% of patients diagnosed with cerebral tumours will experience seizures, the risk is not reduced by prophylactic anti-epileptics. Sub-therapeutic levels, a potential explanation in some trials, does not adequately account for this lack of effect. Thus anti-epileptics should not generally be commenced in the absence of a history of seizures.[91,104]

Peri-neurosurgical use is a possible exception, but results are conflicting.[105] If used, anti-epileptics should generally be slowly tapered after one week.[104]

Convulsive status epilepticus
Figure 2 is modified from NICE guidance.[98] Hypoglycaemia should be excluded in all patients. If alcoholism or severely impaired nutrition is suspected, give thiamine 250mg IV. **Phenobarbital** has been given preference over **phenytoin** because it is more likely to be immediately available in many palliative care units.

Although IV **lorazepam** is generally recommended for the control of status epilepticus (see p.162),[106] IM **midazolam** is as effective (see p.157).[107] **Midazolam** 10mg †buccally or **diazepam** 10–20mg PR (see p.155) are alternatives.

Phenobarbital injection is diluted 1 in 10 with WFI (see p.286). **Fosphenytoin** is a pro-drug of **phenytoin** (1.5mg of the former is equivalent to 1mg of the latter). The dose is expressed as **phenytoin sodium** equivalent (PE). It can be given more rapidly than **phenytoin**. Ideally, heart rate, blood pressure and respiratory function should be monitored during and for 30min after the administration of **fosphenytoin** 15–20mg(PE)/kg (50–100mg (PE)/min), diluted with 0.9% saline to 25mgPE/mL. IV **phenytoin sodium** 15mg/kg up to a maximum total dose of 1g (≤50mg/min; dilute 500mg with 50mL 0.9% saline) can be used instead, preferably with ECG monitoring. See SPCs for full details.

Non-convulsive status epilepticus (NCSE)
NCSE is characterised by seizure activity on an EEG but without associated tonic-clonic activity. Presentations include delirium or coma.[108] In one report, NCSE was diagnosed in 5% of patients admitted to a palliative care unit; of these, half responded to treatment with anti-epileptics.[109] Treatment is less urgent than for convulsive status epilepticus (see Box B).

Mania
Valproate is generally added only when the response to an antipsychotic and a benzodiazepine is inadequate, but is an alternative first-line therapy particularly when it has been effective previously. **Carbamazepine** and **lamotrigine** can also be used.[110]

Anxiety
Despite benefit in various anxiety disorders,[111] anti-epileptics are not commonly used. In the UK, **pregabalin** (see p.270) is authorized for generalized anxiety disorder. Its efficacy is similar to **lorazepam**, **alprazolam** and **venlafaxine**. It has a faster rate of onset than **venlafaxine**, and

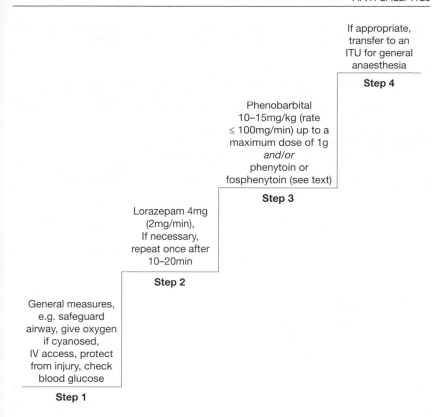

If appropriate,
transfer to an
ITU for general
anaesthesia

Step 4

Phenobarbital
10–15mg/kg (rate
≤ 100mg/min) up to a
maximum dose of 1g
and/or
phenytoin or
fosphenytoin (see text)

Step 3

Lorazepam 4mg
(2mg/min),
If necessary,
repeat once after
10–20min

Step 2

General measures,
e.g. safeguard
airway, give oxygen
if cyanosed,
IV access, protect
from injury, check
blood glucose

Step 1

Figure 2   Management of status epilepticus in adults. See text for more detail.

causes less nausea. It has a similar rate of onset to **lorazepam** and **alprazolam**, and causes less drowsiness but more dizziness.[112] It is also effective for social phobia.[113] RCTs also show some benefit with **gabapentin**,[114–116] **tiagabine**[117] and **lamotrigine**.[118]

Terminal agitation
Phenobarbital is sometimes used in the management of intractable agitation in patients who are imminently dying (see p.286).[119]

Sweats and hot flushes
Gabapentin is effective for hot flushes associated with prostate cancer, breast cancer or the menopause.[120–122] Benefit is also reported in idiopathic sweating in cancer (see p.270).[123]

Refractory hiccup
Gabapentin is reported to be effective for hiccup (see p.270).

Restless legs syndrome
Gabapentin and **pregabalin** are options for restless legs syndrome when first-line options (e.g. **rotigotine, ropinirole**) are ineffective or inappropriate.[124,125] **Clonazepam** may have a place in selected patients (e.g. where there is a concurrent indication for a benzodiazepine, and tolerance with prolonged use is less of a concern because of a limited prognosis, i.e. <4 weeks). Iron supplementation may be effective in those with iron deficiency.[124]

Refractory cough
There is RCT evidence that **gabapentin** is effective for 'idiopathic' chronic cough (i.e. persisting >8 weeks despite resolution of the initial cause).[126] Benefit probably relates to the inhibitory

effect of gabapentin on the CNS interfering with the cough reflex and/or reducing cough hypersensitivity, which is generally present in this group of patients (see p.138).

Nausea and vomiting

Nausea and vomiting are reported to respond to **carbamazepine**, **valproate** or **levetiracetam** in those with CNS lesions (e.g. meningeal carcinomatosis)[127,128] or focal seizures.[129]

Given prophylactically, **gabapentin** reduces both post-operative and chemotherapy-induced nausea and vomiting.[130,131]

Uraemic itch

Gabapentin is effective for uraemic itch. **Pregabalin** is reported to be beneficial (see p.270).

Stopping anti-epileptics

Abrupt cessation of long-term anti-epileptic therapy should be avoided because rebound seizures may be precipitated, even if use is for indications other than epilepsy. If treatment is to be discontinued, particularly barbiturates and benzodiazepines, this is best done *slowly over several months* (Table 3). However, both **gabapentin** and **pregabalin** can be stopped progressively over 1–2 weeks.

Table 3 Recommended monthly reductions of selected anti-epileptics[132]

Drug[a]	Reduction
Carbamazepine	100mg
Clobazam	10mg
Clonazepam	0.5mg
Ethosuximide	250mg
Lamotrigine	25mg
Levetiracetam	1,000mg[b]
Phenobarbital	15mg
Phenytoin	50mg
Topiramate	25mg
Valproate	250mg
Vigabatrin	500mg

a. gabapentin and pregabalin can be stopped progressively over 1–2 weeks
b. data from SPC.

In adults, the risk of relapse of pre-existing epilepsy on stopping treatment is 40–50%.[133] Caution should also be exercised when switching to an alternative anti-epileptic drug. In contrast to switching opioids (see p.365), the first drug should *not* be withdrawn until the new drug has been titrated up to an anticipated effective dose.

For patients who are unable to swallow PO medication, consider substituting a SC alternative. In the last days of life, generally **midazolam** is used (see Box B). However, remember that some anti-epileptics have a long halflife (see Table 2) and, in a moribund patient, might continue to be effective for 2–3 days after the last PO dose. When patients are not imminently dying, a less sedative alternative to **midazolam** is more appropriate, e.g. **levetiracetam**, **valproate** (see Box B).

1 Perucca E (2011) The pharmacology of new antiepileptic drugs: does a novel mechanism of action really matter? *CNS Drugs.* **25**: 907–912.
2 Lynch BA (2004) The synaptic vesicle protein SV2A is the binding site for the antiepileptic drug levetiracetam. *Proceedings of the National Academy of Sciences of the United States of America.* **101**: 9861–9866.
3 Jevtovic-Todorovic V et al. (2006) The role of peripheral T-type calcium channels in pain transmission. *Cell Calcium.* **40**: 197–203.
4 Kochegarov AA (2003) Pharmacological modulators of voltage-gated calcium channels and their therapeutical application. *Cell Calcium.* **33**: 145–162.
5 Shin HS (2006) T-type Ca2+ channels and absence epilepsy. *Cell Calcium.* **40**: 191–196.
6 Loscher W (2002) Basic pharmacology of valproate: a review after 35 years of clinical use for the treatment of epilepsy. *CNS Drugs.* **16**: 669–694.
7 Lee CH et al. (2008) Gabapentin activates ROMK1 channels by a protein kinase A (PKA)-dependent mechanism. *British Journal of Pharmacology.* **154**: 216–225.

8 Sheets PL et al. (2008) Differential block of sensory neuronal voltage-gated sodium channels by lacosamide [(2R)-2-(acetylamino)-N-benzyl-3-methoxypropanamide], lidocaine, and carbamazepine. Journal of Pharmacology and Experimental Therapeutics. 326: 89–99.

9 Stephen LJ and Brodie MJ (2011) Pharmacotherapy of epilepsy: newly approved and developmental agents. CNS Drugs. 25: 89–107.

10 Devulder J (2010) Flupirtine in pain management: pharmacological properties and clinical use. CNS Drugs. 24: 867–881.

11 Hobo (2012) Valproate upregulates glutamate transporters in rat spinal cord after peripheral nerve injury. Journal of Pain. 13(Suppl. 1): s62.

12 Devor M (2006) Sodium channels and mechanisms of neuropathic pain. Journal of Pain. 7: S3–S12.

13 Wiffen PJ et al. (2011) Carbamazepine for acute and chronic pain in adults. Cochrane Database of Systematic Reviews. 1: CD005451.

14 Wiffen PJ et al. (2010) Anitconvulsant drugs for acute and chronic pain. Cochrane Database of Systematic Reviews. 1: CD011133.

15 von Gunten CF et al. (2007) Flecainide for the treatment of chronic neuropathic pain: a Phase II trial. Palliative Medicine. 21: 667–672.

16 Challapalli V et al. (2005) Systemic administration of local anesthetic agents to relieve neuropathic pain. Cochrane Database of Systematic Reviews. CD003345.

17 Goldberg YP et al. (2012) Treatment of Na(v)1.7-mediated pain in inherited erythromelalgia using a novel sodium channel blocker. Pain. 153: 80–85.

18 Taylor CP (2009) Mechanisms of analgesia by gabapentin and pregabalin–calcium channel alpha2-delta [Cavalpha2-delta] ligands. Pain. 142: 13–16.

19 Boroujerdi A et al. (2011) Calcium channel alpha-2-delta-1 protein upregulation in dorsal spinal cord mediates spinal cord injury-induced neuropathic pain states. Pain. 149: 649–655.

20 Lynch BA (2004) The synaptic vesicle protein SV2A is the binding site for the antiepileptic drug levetiracetam. Proceedings of the National Academy of Sciences of the United States of America. 101: 9861–9866.

21 Rudolph U and Mohler H (2006) GABA-based therapeutic approaches: GABA_A receptor subtype functions. Current Opinion in Pharmacology. 6: 18–23.

22 Takahashi T et al. (2010) Upregulation of Ca(v)3.2 T-type calcium channels targeted by endogenous hydrogen sulfide contributes to maintenance of neuropathic pain. Pain. 150: 183–191.

23 Francois A et al. (2013) State-dependent properties of a new T-type calcium channel blocker enhance Ca(V)3.2 selectivity and support analgesic effects. Pain. 154: 283–293.

24 Hill AJ et al. (2012) Cannabidivarin is anticonvulsant in mouse and rat. British Journal of Pharmacology. 167: 1629–1642.

25 Mann MW and Pons G (2007) Various pharmacogenetic aspects of antiepileptic drug therapy: a review. CNS Drugs. 21: 143–164.

26 Loscher W et al. (2009) The clinical impact of pharmacogenetics on the treatment of epilepsy. Epilepsia. 50: 1–23.

27 Abe T et al. (2008) Association between SCN1A polymorphism and carbamazepine-resistant epilepsy. British Journal of Clinical Pharmacology. 66: 304–307.

28 Chung WH et al. (2004) Medical genetics: a marker for Stevens-Johnson syndrome. Nature. 428: 486.

29 Locharernkul C et al. (2008) Carbamazepine and phenytoin induced Stevens-Johnson syndrome is associated with HLA-B*1502 allele in Thai population. Epilepsia. 49: 2087–2091.

30 MHRA (2008) Carbamazepine:genetic testing in some Asian populations. Drug safety update: 1. www.mhra.gov.uk/safety information

31 Perucca E (2006) Clinical pharmacokinetics of new-generation antiepileptic drugs at the extremes of age. Clinical Pharmacokinetics. 45: 351–363.

32 Perucca E (1999) The clinical pharmacokinetics of the new antiepileptic drugs. Epilepsia. 40(Suppl 9): S7–13.

33 Garnett WR (2000) Clinical pharmacology of topiramate: a review. Epilepsia. 41(Suppl 1): S61–65.

34 Anderson et al. (2002) Handbook of clinical drug data. (10e). McGraw Hill.

35 Perucca E (2002) Pharmacological and therapeutic properties of valproate: a summary after 35 years of clinical experience. CNS Drugs. 16: 695–714.

36 May TW et al. (2003) Clinical pharmacokinetics of oxcarbazepine. Clinical Pharmacokinetics. 42: 1023–1042.

37 Bang LM and Goa KL (2004) Spotlight on oxcarbazepine in epilepsy. CNS Drugs. 18: 57–61.

38 Kwan P and Brodie MJ (2004) Phenobarbital for the treatment of epilepsy in the 21st century: a critical review. Epilepsia. 45: 1141–1149.

39 Patsalos PN and Patsalos PN (2004) Clinical pharmacokinetics of levetiracetam. Clinical Pharmacokinetics. 43: 707–724.

40 Rogawski MA and Hanada T (2013) Preclinical pharmacology of perampanel, a selective non-competitive AMPA receptor antagonist. Acta Neurologica Scandinavica. 197: 19–24.

41 Carter T (2006) Fitness to Drive: A Guide for Health Professionals. Royal Society of Medicine Press, London.

42 Hirsch LJ et al. (2008) Cross-sensitivity of skin rashes with antiepileptic drug use. Neurology. 71: 1527–1534.

43 Morgan DJ and McLean AJ (1995) Clinical pharmacokinetic and pharmacodynamic considerations in patients with liver disease. An update. Clinical Pharmacokinetics. 29: 370–391.

44 Ford-Dunn S (2005) Managing patients with cancer and advanced liver disease. Palliative Medicine. 19: 563–565.

45 FDA (2008) Antiepileptic drugs. Safety Alerts for Human Medicinal products.www.fda.gov/Safety/MedWatch/SafetyInformation

46 MHRA (2008) Antiepileptics: risk of suicidal thoughts and behaviour. Drug safety update: 2. www.mhra.gov.uk/safety information

47 Mula M et al. (2013) Antiepileptic drugs and suicidality: an expert consensus statement from the Task Force on Therapeutic Strategies of the ILAE Commission on Neuropsychobiology. Epilepsia. 54: 199–203.

48 Marson AG et al. (2007) The SANAD study of effectiveness of valproate, lamotrigine, or topiramate for generalised and unclassifiable epilepsy: an unblinded randomised controlled trial. Lancet. 369: 1016–1026.

49 Marson AG et al. (2007) The SANAD study of effectiveness of carbamazepine, gabapentin, lamotrigine, oxcarbazepine, or topiramate for treatment of partial epilepsy: an unblinded randomised controlled trial. Lancet. 369: 1000–1015.

50 Kwan P and Brodie MJ (2001) Neuropsychological effects of epilepsy and antiepileptic drugs. Lancet. 357: 216–222.

51 French JA (2007) First-choice drug for newly diagnosed epilepsy. Lancet. 369: 970–971.

52 Perkin GD (2004) Ch. 24:53. Epilepsy in later childhood and adults. In: DA Warrell et al. (eds) Oxford Textbook of Medicine (5e). Oxford University Press, Oxford.

53 MHRA (2013) Antiepileptic drugs: new advice on switching between different manufacturers' products for a particular drug. *Drug Safety Update.* **7**. A1.

54 Moore RA *et al.* (2011) Gabapentin for chronic neuropathic pain and fibromyalgia in adults. *Cochrane Database of Systematic Reviews* **3**: CD007938.

55 Moore RA *et al.* (2009) Pregabalin for acute and chronic pain in adults. *Cochrane Database of Systematic Reviews* **3**: CD007076.

56 Caraceni A *et al.* (2004) Gabapentin for neuropathic cancer pain: a randomized controlled trial from the Gabapentin Cancer Pain Study Group. *Journal of Clinical Oncology.* **22**: 2909–2917.

57 Hardy J *et al.* (2001) A phase II study to establish the efficacy and toxicity of sodium valproate in patients with cancer-related neuropathic pain. *Journal of Pain and Symptom Management.* **21**: 204–209.

58 Snare AJ (1993) Sodium Valproate. Retrospective analysis of neuropathic pain control in patients with advanced cancer. *Journal of Pharmacy Technology.* **9**: 114–117.

59 Dworkin RH *et al.* (2010) Recommendations for the pharmacological management of neuropathic pain: an overview and literature update. *Mayo Clinic Proceedings.* **85**: S3–14.

60 Attal N *et al.* (2010) EFNS guidelines on the pharmacological treatment of neuropathic pain: 2010 revision. *European Journal of Neurology.* **17**: 1113-e1188.

61 Kochar DK *et al.* (2002) Sodium valproate in the management of painful neuropathy in type 2 diabetes - a randomized placebo controlled study. *Acta Neurologica Scandinavica.* **106**: 248–252.

62 Kochar DK *et al.* (2004) Sodium valproate for painful diabetic neuropathy: a randomized double-blind placebo-controlled study. *Quarterly Journal of Medicine.* **97**: 33–38.

63 Kochar DK *et al.* (2005) Divalproex sodium in the management of post-herpetic neuralgia: a randomized double-blind placebo-controlled study. *Quarterly Journal of Medicine.* **98**: 29–34.

64 Otto M *et al.* (2004) Valproic acid has no effect on pain in polyneuropathy: a randomized, controlled trial. *Neurology.* **62**: 285–288.

65 Agrawal RP *et al.* (2009) Management of diabetic neuropathy by sodium valproate and glyceryl trinitrate spray: a prospective double-blind randomized placebo-controlled study. *Diabetes Research and Clinical Practice.* **83**: 371–378.

66 Wiffen PJ *et al.* (2011) Lamotrigine for acute and chronic pain. *Cochrane Database of Systematic Reviews.* **2**: CD006044.

67 McCleane G (1999) Intravenous infusion of phenytoin relieves neuropathic pain: a randomized, double-blinded, placebo-controlled, crossover study. *Anesthesia and Analgesia.* **89**: 985–988.

68 Rauck RL *et al.* (2007) Lacosamide in painful diabetic peripheral neuropathy: a phase 2 double-blind placebo-controlled study. *Clinical Journal of Pain.* **23**: 150–158.

69 Shaibani A (2009) Lacosamide in painful diabetic neuropathy: an 18 week double blind placebo controlled trial. *Journal of Pain.* **10**: 818–828.

70 Wymer JP *et al.* (2009) Efficacy and safety of lacosamide in diabetic neuropathic pain: an 18-week double-blind placebo-controlled trial of fixed-dose regimens. *Clinical Journal of Pain.* **25**: 376–385.

71 Ziegler D *et al.* (2010) Efficacy and safety of lacosamide in painful diabetic neuropathy. *Diabetes Care.* **33**: 839–841.

72 Bendaly EA *et al.* (2007) Topiramate in the treatment of neuropathic pain in patients with cancer. *Supportive Cancer Therapy.* **4**: 241–246.

73 Raskin P *et al.* (2004) Topiramate vs placebo in painful diabetic neuropathy: analgesic and metabolic effects. *Neurology.* **63**: 865–873.

74 Thienel U *et al.* (2004) Topiramate in painful diabetic polyneuropathy: findings from three double-blind placebo-controlled trials. *Acta Neurologica Scandinavica.* **110**: 221–231.

75 Khoromi S *et al.* (2005) Topiramate in chronic lumbar radicular pain. *Journal of Pain.* **6**: 829–836.

76 Bansal D *et al.* (2009) Amitriptyline vs. pregabalin in painful diabetic neuropathy: a randomized double blind clinical trial. *Diabetic Medicine.* **26**: 1019–1026.

77 Boyle J *et al.* (2012) Randomized, placebo-controlled comparison of amitriptyline, duloxetine, and pregabalin in patients with chronic diabetic peripheral neuropathic pain: impact on pain, polysomnographic sleep, daytime functioning, and quality of life. *Diabetes Care.* **35**: 2451–2458.

78 Morello C *et al.* (1999) Randomized double-blind study comparing the efficacy of gabapentin with amitriptyline on diabetic peripheral neuropathy pain. *Archives of Internal Medicine.* **159**: 1931–1937.

79 Chandra K *et al.* (2006) Gabapentin versus nortriptyline in post-herpetic neuralgia patients: a randomized, double-blind clinical trial–the GONIP Trial. *International Journal of Clinical Pharmacology and Therapeutics.* **44**: 358–363.

80 Mishra S *et al.* (2012) A comparative efficacy of amitriptyline, gabapentin, and pregabalin in neuropathic cancer pain: a prospective randomized double-blind placebo-controlled study. *American Journal of Hospice and Palliative Care.* **29**: 177–182.

81 Banerjee M *et al.* (2013) A comparative study of efficacy and safety of gabapentin versus amitriptyline as coanalgesics in patients receiving opioid analgesics for neuropathic pain in malignancy. *Indian Journal of Pharmacology.* **45**: 334–338.

82 Gilron I *et al.* (2009) Nortriptyline and gabapentin, alone and in combination for neuropathic pain: a double-blind, randomised controlled crossover trial. *Lancet.* **374**: 1252–1261.

83 Raja SN *et al.* (2002) Opioids versus antidepressants in postherpetic neuralgia: a randomized, placebo-controlled trial. [see comment]. *Neurology.* **59**: 1015–1021.

84 Gilron I *et al.* (2005) Morphine, gabapentin, or their combination for neuropathic pain. *New England Journal of Medicine.* **352**: 1324–1334.

85 Keskinbora K *et al.* (2007) Gabapentin and an opioid combination versus opioid alone for the management of neuropathic cancer pain: a randomized open trial. *Journal of Pain and Symptom Management.* **34**: 183–189.

86 Solaro C *et al.* (2000) Low-dose gabapentin combined with either lamotrigine or carbamazepine can be useful therapies for trigeminal neuralgia in multiple sclerosis. *European Neurology.* **44**: 45–48.

87 Webb J and Kamali F (1998) Analgesic effects of lamotrigine and phenytoin on cold-induced pain: a crossover placebo-controlled study in healthy volunteers. *Pain.* **76**: 357–363.

88 Hill CM *et al.* (2001) Pregabalin in patients with postoperative dental pain. *Eur J Pain.* **5**: 119–124.

89 Ho KY *et al.* (2006) Gabapentin and postoperative pain–a systematic review of randomized controlled trials. *Pain.* **126**: 91–101.

90 Jokela R *et al.* (2008) A randomized controlled trial of perioperative administration of pregabalin for pain after laparoscopic hysterectomy. *Pain.* **134**: 106–112.

91 Miller LC and Drislane FW (2007) Treatment strategies after a single seizure : rationale for immediate versus deferred treatment. *CNS Drugs.* **21**: 89–99.

92 Schaller B (2006) Brain tumor and seizures: pathophysiology and its implications for treatment revisited (epilepsia 2003; 44:1223-1232). *Epilepsia.* **47**: 661; author reply 661.

93 Vecht C (2006) Otimizing therapy of seizures in patients with brain tumours. *Neurology.* **67**: S10-S13.

94 van Breemen MS *et al.* (2007) Epilepsy in patients with brain tumours: epidemiology, mechanisms, and management. *Lancet Neurology.* **6**: 421–430.

95 Kerrigan S and Grant R (2011) Antiepileptic drugs for treating seizures in adults with brain tumours. *Cochrane Database of Systematic Reviews.* **8**: CD008586.

96 Perucca E and Kwan P (2005) Overtreatment in epilepsy: how it occurs and how it can be avoided. *CNS Drugs.* **19**: 897–908.

97 Kwan P and Brodie MJ (2001) Effectiveness of first antiepileptic drug. *Epilepsia.* **42**: 1255–1260.

98 NICE (2012) Clinical Guideline 137. The epilepsies: the diagnosis and management of the epilepsies in adults and children in primary and secondary care.

99 Ward MM *et al.* (1996) Preoperative valproate administration does not increase blood loss during temporal lobectomy. *Epilepsia.* **37**: 98–101.

100 Anderson GD *et al.* (1997) Absence of bleeding complications in patients undergoing cortical surgery while receiving valproate treatment. *Journal of Neurosurgery.* **87**: 252–256.

101 Karceski S *et al.* (2005) Treatment of epilepsy in adults: expert opinion. *Epilepsy & Behavior.* **7(Suppl 1)**: S1–64.

102 Stephen LJ and Brodie MJ (2002) Seizure freedom with more than one antiepileptic drug. *Seizure.* **11**: 349–351.

103 Deckers CL *et al.* (2000) Selection of antiepileptic drug polytherapy based on mechanisms of action: the evidence reviewed. *Epilepsia.* **41**: 1364–1374.

104 Glantz MJ *et al.* (2000) Practice parameter: anticonvulsant prophylaxis in patients with newly diagnosed brain tumors. Report of the Quality Standards Subcommittee of the American Academy of Neurology. *Neurology.* **54**: 1886–1893.

105 Pulman J *et al.* (2013) Antiepileptic drugs as prophylaxis for post-craniotomy seizures. *Cochrane Database of Systematic Reviews.* **2**: CD007286.

106 Prasad K *et al.* (2005) Anticonvulsant therapy for status epilepticus. *Cochrane Database of Systematic Reviews.* **4**: CD003723.

107 Silbergleit R *et al.* (2012) Intramuscular versus intravenous therapy for prehospital status epilepticus. *New England Journal of Medicine.* **366**: 591–600.

108 Twycross R *et al.* (2009) *Symptom Management in Advanced Cancer* (4e). palliativedrugs.com, Nottingham, pp. 283–284.

109 Lorenzl S *et al.* (2010) Nonconvulsive status epilepticus in palliative care patients. *Journal of Pain and Symptom Management.* **40**: 460–465.

110 NICE (2006) The management of bipolar disorder in adults, children and adolescents, in primary and secondary care. *Clinical Guideline* CG38. www.nice.org.uk

111 Van Ameringen M *et al.* (2004) Antiepileptic drugs in the treatment of anxiety disorders: role in therapy. *Drugs.* **64**: 2199–2220.

112 Frampton JE and Foster RH (2006) Pregabalin: in the treatment of generalised anxiety disorder .[erratum appears in CNS Drugs 2007;21:481]. *CNS Drugs.* **20**: 685–695.

113 Pande AC *et al.* (2004) Efficacy of the novel anxiolytic pregabalin in social anxiety disorder: a placebo-controlled, multicenter study. *Journal of Clinical Psychopharmacology.* **24**: 141–149.

114 Pande AC *et al.* (1999) Treatment of social phobia with gabapentin: a placebo-controlled study. *Journal of Clinical Psychopharmacology.* **19**: 341–348.

115 Pande AC *et al.* (2000) Placebo-controlled study of gabapentin treatment of panic disorder. *Journal of Clinical Psychopharmacology.* **20**: 467–471.

116 Lavigne JE *et al.* (2012) A randomized, controlled, double-blinded clinical trial of gabapentin 300 versus 900 mg versus placebo for anxiety symptoms in breast cancer survivors. *Breast Cancer Research and Treatment.* **136**: 479–486.

117 Pollack MH *et al.* (2005) The selective GABA reuptake inhibitor tiagabine for the treatment of generalized anxiety disorder: results of a placebo-controlled study. *Journal of Clinical Psychiatry.* **66**: 1401–1408.

118 Hertzberg MA *et al.* (1999) A preliminary study of lamotrigine for the treatment of posttraumatic stress disorder. *Biological Psychiatry.* **45**: 1226–1229.

119 Twycross R *et al.* (2009) *Symptom Management in Advanced Cancer.* palliativedrugs.com, Nottingham, pp. 430–433.

120 Pandya KJ *et al.* (2005) Gabapentin for hot flashes in 420 women with breast cancer: a randomised double-blind placebo-controlled trial. *Lancet.* **366**: 818–824.

121 Nelson HD *et al.* (2006) Nonhormonal therapies for menopausal hot flashes: systematic review and meta-analysis. *Journal of the American Medical Association.* **295**: 2057–2071.

122 Loprinzi CL *et al.* (2009) A phase III randomized, double-blind, placebo-controlled trial of gabapentin in the management of hot flashes in men (N00CB). *Annals of Oncology.* **20**: 542–549.

123 Porzio G *et al.* (2006) Gabapentin in the treatment of severe sweating experienced by advanced cancer patients. *Supportive Care in Cancer.* **14**: 389–391.

124 Aurora RN *et al.* (2012) The treatment of restless legs syndrome and periodic limb movement disorder in adults-an update for 2012: practice parameters with an evidence-based systematic review and meta-analyses: an American Academy of Sleep Medicine Clinical Practice Guideline. *Sleep.* **35**: 1039–1062.

125 Garcia-Borreguero D *et al.* (2012) European guidelines on management of restless legs syndrome: report of a joint task force by the European Federation of Neurological Societies, the European Neurological Society and the European Sleep Research Society. *European Journal of Neurology.* **19**: 1385–1396.

126 Ryan NM *et al.* (2012) Gabapentin for refractory chronic cough: a randomised, double-blind, placebo-controlled trial. *Lancet.* **380**: 1583–1589.

127 Lee JW *et al.* (2008) Emesis responsive to levetiracetam. *Journal of Neurology, Neurosurgery, and Psychiatry.* **79**: 847–849.

128 Strohscheer I and Borasio GD (2006) Carbamazepine-responsive paroxysmal nausea and vomiting in a patient with meningeal carcinomatosis. *Palliative Medicine.* **20**: 549–550.

129 Yukselen V *et al.* (2003) Partial seizure: an unusual cause of recurrent vomiting. *International Journal of Clinical Practice.* **57**: 742–743.

130 Pandey CK *et al.* (2006) Prophylactic gabapentin for prevention of postoperative nausea and vomiting in patients undergoing laparoscopic cholecystectomy: a randomized, double-blind, placebo-controlled study. *Journal of Postgraduate Medicine.* **52**: 97–100.

131 Cruz FM *et al.* (2012) Gabapentin for the prevention of chemotherapy- induced nausea and vomiting: a pilot study. *Supportive Care in Cancer.* **20**: 601–606.

132 Chadwick D (1995) The withdrawal of antiepileptic drugs. In: A Hopkins *et al.* (eds) *Epilepsy* (2e). Chapman and Hall, London, pp. 215–220.

133 Hopkins A and Shorvon S (1995) Definitions and epidemiology of epilepsy. In: A Hopkins *et al.* (eds) *Epilepsy* (2e). Chapman and Hall, London, pp. 1–24.

Updated May 2014

GABAPENTIN AND PREGABALIN   BNF 4.8.1

Class: Anti-epileptic (pre-synaptic calcium channel blocker).

Indications: Adjunctive use in epilepsy when conventional treatment is unsatisfactory, neuropathic pain, anxiety, †intractable itch, †hot flushes, †sweating, †refractory hiccup, †restless legs syndrome, †refractory cough.

Pharmacology

Gabapentin and pregabalin reduce the calcium influx responsible for triggering neurotransmitter release by binding to the $\alpha 2\delta$ type I regulatory subunit of pre-synaptic (N, P/Q-type) voltage-gated calcium channels.[1] Both the spinal dorsal horn and brainstem/forebrain are important sites of action. Calcium channel $\alpha 2\delta$ subunits are upregulated in the spinal dorsal horn by inflammation and neuropathic pain;[2,3] gabapentin and pregabalin counteract this. Brainstem/forebrain actions influence descending pain inhibitory pathways and pain processing.[1,4,5] Spinal calcium channels are also targeted by **ziconotide**.

Both gabapentin and pregabalin cause redistribution of calcium channels away from the cell surface, rather than blocking them directly. Effects on sodium and potassium channels have also been shown.[6,7] Despite being GABA analogues, neither gabapentin nor pregabalin is GABAmimetic.[1] They are unrelated to the L-type calcium channel blockers, **nifedipine**, **diltiazem** and **verapamil** (Table 1). L-type channels are also found on neurones, but the significance of anti-epileptics blocking these neuronal L-type channels (e.g. **carbamazepine**) is unclear.

Table 1 Classification of calcium channels

Type	Location (function)	Blocked by
L-type ($Ca_v 1.1–1.4$)	Cardiovascular and GI tissues (smooth muscle tone, conductivity)	Verapamil, diltiazem, nifedipine (see p.83)
N, P/Q-type ($Ca_v 2.1–2.2$)	Pre-synaptic neurones (calcium influx triggers neurotransmitter release; over-expressed in neuropathic pain)	Gabapentin and pregabalin (N and P/Q-type), ziconotide (N-type)[1]
T-type ($Ca_v 3.1–3.3$)	Thalamic and nociceptive neurones (excitability, threshold setting, pacemaker activity, firing pattern. Thalamic T-type channel dysregulation responsible for absence seizures)	Ethosuximide, valproate (see p.279)
R-type ($Ca_v 2.3$)	Cerebellum (function unknown)	

For pharmacokinetic details, see Table 2.

Gabapentin is a first-line choice for neuropathic pain because benefit has been confirmed for a range of causes;[8,9] it has few drug interactions and peripheral neuropathic pain is included in its Marketing Authorization. Pregabalin is more expensive, though it's twice daily administration is an advantage for selected patients. Its Marketing Authorization includes peripheral and central neuropathic pain.

Table 2   Pharmacokinetic details

Drug	Gabapentin	Pregabalin
Bioavailability PO (%)	Dose-dependent[a]	≥90%[a]
T_{max} (h)	2–3	1
Protein-bound	No	No
Plasma halflife (h)	5–7	5–9
Elimination	Renally excreted unchanged	Renally excreted unchanged

a. both gabapentin and pregabalin are absorbed through amino acid transporters. At higher doses, gabapentin saturates the available transporters causing a dose-dependent reduction in bio-availability, i.e.: 100mg (74%), 300mg (60%), 600mg (49%), 1200mg (33%). The absorption of pregabalin is unaffected by dose.

A large network analysis found the efficacy and tolerability of gabapentin and pregabalin to be comparable across a range of measures.[10] A small (n = 30) head to head comparison in peripheral nerve injury also found similar outcomes.[11] Pain relief was similar in a larger (n = 120) head to head RCT in cancer-related neuropathic pain; the greater reduction in **morphine** use with pregabalin compared with gabapentin may reflect the relatively higher doses used (600mg/day and 1800mg/day, respectively).[12]

It is unclear whether those with an inadequate response should be switched *between* gabapentin and pregabalin or to a drug with a *distinct action* (e.g. **valproate** or an antidepressant). A difference in response to gabapentin and pregabalin is possible because of their varied absorption at higher doses and binding affinity. Such switching has been reported,[13] but benefit has *not* been confirmed in an RCT.

Gabapentin and pregabalin are effective for other pains with suspected neuropathic and/or central sensitization mechanisms including burn injury pain,[14] fibromyalgia,[15] chronic masticatory myalgia,[16] and possibly also breakthrough pain due to bone metastases.[17] Further, perioperative use may reduce the risk of chronic postoperative pain.[18]

Pregabalin is authorized for generalized anxiety disorder. It is as effective as **lorazepam**, **alprazolam** and **venlafaxine**. Compared with **venlafaxine**, pregabalin has a faster rate of onset and causes less nausea; it has a similar rate of onset to **lorazepam** and **alprazolam** and causes less drowsiness but more dizziness.[19–22] Gabapentin is also effective.[23–25]

Neuronal dysregulation (e.g. CNS sensitization as in neuropathic pain) is implicated in a number of other symptoms. This may part explain the benefit of gabapentin in a wide range of settings, including chronic refractory cough due to cough reflex hyperexcitability;[26] idiopathic[27,28] and uraemic pruritus (also pregabablin);[29–31] idiopathic sweating in cancer;[32] hot flushes associated with prostate cancer, breast cancer or the menopause;[33–35] chemotherapy-related nausea and vomiting[36] and refractory hiccup.[37,38] In one series, 'burst gabapentin' relieved persistent hiccup in patients with a history of brain stem stroke. Patients received 400mg t.d.s. for 3 days, 400mg once daily for 3 days, and then stopped. Only 1/15 patients needed a second treatment.[38]

Gabapentin has also been used in spasticity.[39,40] Gabapentin and pregabalin are alternative options for restless legs syndrome where first-line options (e.g. **rotigotine**, **ropinirole**) are ineffective or inappropriate.[41,42]

Cautions

Absence seizures (may worsen); psychotic illness (may precipitate or exacerbate psychotic episodes); patients at high risk of drug abuse (limited evidence of possible misuse[43,44]); renal impairment (dose adjustment required; renal failure reported with pregabalin which resolved on discontinuation), CHF (exacerbation reported).

Gabapentin is reported to cause false positive readings for urinary protein with Ames N-Multistix SG®.

Drug interactions

Clinically significant pharmacokinetic interactions are unlikely.

Aluminium and **magnesium**-containing compounds reduce gabapentin's bio-availability by ≤24%; **morphine** and **naproxen** may increase gabapentin levels. High doses of gabapentin may decrease **hydrocodone** (not UK) levels; mechanism unknown.

Undesirable effects

Undesirable effects are generally similar:

Very common (>10%): drowsiness, dizziness, ataxia.

Common (<10%, >1%): amnesia, confusion, visual disturbance, dysarthria, tremor, arthralgia, myalgia, peripheral oedema, dry mouth, vomiting, constipation.

Uncommon (<1%, >0.1%): suicidal ideation 0.2% (1/500; advise patients to report mood or thought disturbance), impotence, gynaecomastia.

Possible causal association with acute pancreatitis and Stevens Johnson Syndrome.

The frequencies of some symptoms differ between SPCs. It is uncertain whether this reflects a difference in incidence or detection. For example, leukopenia and arthralgia occur commonly with gabapentin, but not pregabalin.[45] Similarly, pregabalin is associated with cardiac conduction disturbance, QT prolongation and exacerbation of CHF, but gabapentin less so.[46,47]

Dose and use

Gabapentin

- start with 300mg PO at night
- if necessary, increase by 300mg/24h every 2–3 days, e.g.:
  ▷ Day 3 300mg b.d.
  ▷ Day 5 300mg t.d.s.
  ▷ Day 8 300mg, 300mg, 600mg
  ▷ Day 11 600mg, 300mg, 600mg
  ▷ Day 14 600mg t.d.s.
- in elderly and frail patients, slower titration is advisable, e.g. 100mg at night, increased if necessary by 100mg/24h every 2–3 days
- typical doses
  ▷ neuropathic pain: 600mg t.d.s.[48]
  ▷ hot flushes: 300mg t.d.s.[35]
  ▷ uraemic itch: note the dose adjustment required in renal impairment (below)
  ▷ hiccup: consider short term use (below)
- maximum recommended dose 1,200mg t.d.s.

The starting and maximum doses of gabapentin should be reduced in adults with renal impairment and those on haemodialysis. Recommendations are shown in Table 3. However, although these may be appropriate in physically robust individuals, in palliative care the starting doses will generally be lower, as indicated above.

Table 3 Gabapentin dose adjustments in renal impairment modified from the SPC

Creatinine clearance (mL/min)	Starting dose[a]	Maximum dose
50–79	200mg t.d.s.	600mg t.d.s.
30–49	100mg t.d.s.	300mg t.d.s.
15–29	300mg alternate days	300mg b.d.[b]
<15	300mg alternate days	300mg at bedtime[b]
After every 4h of haemodialysis	Supplementary single dose of 200–300mg[c]	

a. smaller starting dose is advisable in elderly patients and those receiving other CNS-depressant drugs (see text)
b. the SPC recommends the daily dose be administered in three divided doses, but the prolonged halflife in renal impairment permits b.d. or once daily dosing as indicated
c. for anuric patients on dialysis, no regular dose is required, just a 'supplementary' dose after dialysis.

Gabapentin (short term use in hiccup)

- in relatively robust patients, consider a 6-day 'burst' of gabapentin' PO, e.g.:
  ▷ 300–400mg t.d.s. for 3 days
  ▷ 300–400mg once daily for 3 days
  ▷ if necessary, re-treat long-term if hiccup recurs after a 'burst'

- in frail elderly patients, proceed slowly as for neuropathic pain:
  ▷ start with a low dose, e.g. 100mg t.d.s.
  ▷ if necessary, titrate upwards
  ▷ if successful, consider reducing/stopping gabapentin
  ▷ if necessary, re-treat long-term if hiccup recurs after a 'burst'.[37,38]

Pregabalin
- start with 75mg PO b.d.
- if necessary, at intervals of 3–7 days, increase to 150mg b.d. → 225mg b.d. → 300mg b.d. (maximum recommended dose)
- in debilitated patients, start with 25–50mg b.d.
- if necessary, increase the dose correspondingly cautiously.

The intervals between dose increases are pragmatic rather than pharmacokinetic. In one RCT, the effective doses were:[49]
- 150mg b.d. in about a quarter of patients
- 225mg b.d. in about a third
- 300mg b.d. in another third.

Dose reduction is necessary in renal impairment (Table 4). For patients on haemodialysis, the regular dose should be adjusted according to the creatinine clearance and a supplementary single dose given after each dialysis (Table 5).

Table 4 Pregabalin dose adjustments in renal impairment modified from the SPC

Creatinine clearance (mL/min)	Starting dose	Maximum dose
>60	75mg b.d.	300mg b.d.
31–60	25mg t.d.s.[a]	150mg b.d.
15–30	25–50mg once daily	150mg once daily
<15	25mg once daily	75mg once daily

a. 37.5mg capsules not available, necessitating t.d.s. regimen.

Table 5 Post-haemodialysis supplementary doses of pregabalin

Daily dose	Supplementary single dose after every 4h of haemodialysis
25mg	25–50mg
50mg	50–75mg
75mg	100–150mg

Stopping gabapentin and pregabalin
To avoid precipitating pain or seizures, withdraw gradually over several weeks.

Supply
Gabapentin
Gabapentin (generic)
Capsules 100mg, 300mg, 400mg, 28 days @ 300mg t.d.s. = £3.
Tablets 600mg, 800mg, 28 days @ 600mg t.d.s. = £8.
Oral solution 50mg/mL, 28 days @ 300mg t.d.s. = £195.

Neurontin® (Pfizer)
Capsules 100mg, 300mg, 400mg, 28 days @ 300mg t.d.s. = £36.
Tablets 600mg, 800mg, 28 days @ 600mg t.d.s. = £71.

The authorized gabapentin oral solution available (Rosemont) contains propylene glycol and other excipients which, in high doses, may exceed WHO daily intake limits. Alternatively, for patients with swallowing difficulties, gabapentin capsules can be opened and the contents mixed with water, fruit juice or apple sauce.[50]

Pregabalin

Lyrica® (Pfizer)

Capsules 25mg, 50mg, 75mg, 100mg, 150mg, 200mg, 225mg, 300mg, 28 days @ any strength of single capsule b.d. or t.d.s = £65 or £97 respectively.

Oral solution 20mg/mL, 28 days@ 225mg b.d. = £133.

1 Taylor CP (2009) Mechanisms of analgesia by gabapentin and pregabalin–calcium channel alpha2-delta [Cavalpha2-delta] ligands. *Pain.* **142**: 13–16.
2 Boroujerdi A et al. (2008) Injury discharges regulate calcium channel alpha-2-delta-1 subunit upregulation in the dorsal horn that contributes to initiation of neuropathic pain. *Pain.* **139**: 358–366.
3 Lu (2010) Persistent inflammation alters the density and distribution of voltage activated calcium channels in subpopulations of rat cutaneous DRG neurons. *Pain.* **151**: 633-643.
4 Bee LA and Dickenson AH (2008) Descending facilitation from the brainstem determines behavioural and neuronal hypersensitivity following nerve injury and efficacy of pregabalin. *Pain.* **140**: 209–223.
5 Hayashida K et al. (2008) Gabapentin acts within the locus coeruleus to alleviate neuropathic pain. *Anesthesiology.* **109**: 1077–1084.
6 Lee CH et al. (2008) Gabapentin activates ROMK1 channels by a protein kinase A (PKA)-dependent mechanism. *British Journal of Pharmacology.* **154**: 216–225.
7 Yang RH et al. (2009) Gabapentin selectively reduces persistent sodium current in injured type-A dorsal root ganglion neurons. *Pain.* **143**: 48–55.
8 Moore RA et al. (2011) Gabapentin for chronic neuropathic pain and fibromyalgia in adults. *Cochrane Database of Systematic Reviews.* **3**: CD007938.
9 Moore RA et al. (2009) Pregabalin for acute and chronic pain in adults. *Cochrane Database of Systematic Reviews.* **3**: CD007076.
10 NICE (2013) Neuropathic pain – pharmacological management. *Clinical Guideline.* CG173 www.nice.org.uk
11 Kelle B (2012) The efficacy of gabapentin and pregabalin in the treatment of neuropathic pain due to peripheral nerve injury. *Journal of Musculoskeletal Pain.* **20**: 300–305.
12 Mishra S et al. (2012) A comparative efficacy of amitriptyline, gabapentin, and pregabalin in neuropathic cancer pain: a prospective randomized double-blind placebo-controlled study. *American Journal of Hospice and Palliative Care.* **29**: 177–182.
13 Saldana MT et al. (2012) Pain alleviation and patient-reported health outcomes following switching to pregabalin in individuals with gabapentin-refractory neuropathic pain in routine medical practice. *Clinical Drug Investigation.* **32**: 401–412.
14 Gray P et al. (2011) Pregabalin in severe burn injury pain: a double-blind, randomised placebo-controlled trial. *Pain.* **152**: 1279–1288.
15 Hauser W et al. (2009) Treatment of fibromyalgia syndrome with gabapentin and pregabalin–a meta-analysis of randomized controlled trials. *Pain.* **145**: 69–81.
16 Kimos P et al. (2007) Analgesic action of gabapentin on chronic pain in the masticatory muscles: a randomized controlled trial. *Pain.* **127**: 151–160.
17 Caraceni A et al. (2008) Gabapentin for breakthrough pain due to bone metastases. *Palliative Medicine.* **22**: 392–393.
18 Clarke H et al. (2012) The prevention of chronic postsurgical pain using gabapentin and pregabalin: a combined systematic review and meta-analysis. *Anesthesia and Analgesia.* **115**: 428–442.
19 Feltner DE et al. (2003) A randomized, double-blind, placebo-controlled, fixed-dose, multicenter study of pregabalin in patients with generalized anxiety disorder. *Journal of Clinical Psychopharmacology.* **23**: 240–249.
20 Pande AC et al. (2003) Pregabalin in generalized anxiety disorder: a placebo-controlled trial. *American Journal of Psychiatry.* **160**: 533–540.
21 Rickels K et al. (2005) Pregabalin for treatment of generalized anxiety disorder: a 4-week, multicenter, double-blind, placebo-controlled trial of pregabalin and alprazolam. *Archives of General Psychiatry.* **62**: 1022–1030.
22 Montgomery SA et al. (2006) Efficacy and safety of pregabalin in the treatment of generalized anxiety disorder: a 6-week, multicenter, randomized, double-blind, placebo-controlled comparison of pregabalin and venlafaxine. *Journal of Clinical Psychiatry.* **67**: 771–782.
23 Lavigne JE et al. (2012) A randomized, controlled, double-blinded clinical trial of gabapentin 300 versus 900 mg versus placebo for anxiety symptoms in breast cancer survivors. *Breast Cancer Research and Treatment.* **136**: 479–486.
24 Pande AC et al. (1999) Treatment of social phobia with gabapentin: a placebo-controlled study. *Journal of Clinical Psychopharmacology.* **19**: 341–348.
25 Pande AC et al. (2000) Placebo-controlled study of gabapentin treatment of panic disorder. *Journal of Clinical Psychopharmacology.* **20**: 467–471.
26 Ryan NM et al. (2012) Gabapentin for refractory chronic cough: a randomised, double-blind, placebo-controlled trial. *Lancet.* **380**: 1583–1589.
27 Kanitakis J (2006) Brachioradial pruritus: report of a new case responding to gabapentin. *European Journal of Dermatology.* **16**: 311–312.
28 Yesudian PD and Wilson NJ (2005) Efficacy of gabapentin in the management of pruritus of unknown origin. *Archives of Dermatology.* **141**: 1507–1509.
29 Gunal AI et al. (2004) Gabapentin therapy for pruritus in haemodialysis patients: a randomized, placebo-controlled, double-blind trial. *Nephrology, Dialysis, Transplantation.* **19**: 3137–3139.
30 Naini AE et al. (2007) Gabapentin: a promising drug for the treatment of uremic pruritus. *Saudi J of Kidney Diseases and Translanation.* **18**: 378–381.
31 Shavit L et al. (2013) Use of pregabalin in the management of chronic uremic pruritus. *Journal of Pain and Symptom Management.* **45**: 776–781.
32 Porzio G et al. (2006) Gabapentin in the treatment of severe sweating experienced by advanced cancer patients. *Supportive Care in Cancer.* **14**: 389–391.
33 Loprinzi CL et al. (2009) A phase III randomized, double-blind, placebo-controlled trial of gabapentin in the management of hot flashes in men (N00CB). *Annals of Oncology.* **20**: 542–549.

34 Nelson HD et al. (2006) Nonhormonal therapies for menopausal hot flashes: systematic review and meta-analysis. Journal of the American Medical Association. **295**: 2057–2071.

35 Pandya KJ et al. (2005) Gabapentin for hot flashes in 420 women with breast cancer: a randomised double-blind placebo-controlled trial. Lancet. **366**: 818–824.

36 Cruz FM et al. (2012) Gabapentin for the prevention of chemotherapy- induced nausea and vomiting: a pilot study. Supportive Care in Cancer. **20**: 601–606.

37 Alonso-Navarro H et al. (2007) Refractory hiccup: successful treatment with gabapentin. Clinical Neuropharmacology. **30**: 186–187.

38 Moretti R et al. (2004) Gabapentin as a drug therapy of intractable hiccup because of vascular lesion: a three-year follow up. Neurologist. **10**: 102–106.

39 Paisley S et al. (2002) Clinical effectiveness of oral treatments for spasticity in multiple sclerosis: a systematic review. Multiple Sclerosis. **8**: 319–329.

40 Cutter NC et al. (2000) Gabapentin effect on spasticity in multiple sclerosis: a placebo-controlled, randomized trial. Archives of Physical Medicine and Rehabilitation. **81**: 164–169.

41 Aurora RN et al. (2012) The treatment of restless legs syndrome and periodic limb movement disorder in adults-an update for 2012: practice parameters with an evidence-based systematic review and meta-analyses: an American Academy of Sleep Medicine Clinical Practice Guideline. Sleep. **35**: 1039–1062.

42 Garcia-Borreguero D et al. (2012) European guidelines on management of restless legs syndrome: report of a joint task force by the European Federation of Neurological Societies, the European Neurological Society and the European Sleep Research Society. European Journal of Neurology. **19**: 1385–1396.

43 Gahr M et al. (2013) Pregabalin abuse and dependence in Germany: results from a database query. European Journal of Clinical Pharmacology. **69**: 1335–1342.

44 CADTH (2012) Abuse and misuse potential of pregabalin: A review of the clinical evidence. Rapid Response Report. www.cadth.ca

45 Zaccara G et al. (2011) The adverse event profile of pregabalin: a systematic review and meta-analysis of randomized controlled trials. Epilepsia. **52**: 826–836.

46 MHRA Yellow card reports for gabapentin and pregabalin. Drug Analysis Prints.www.mhra.gov.uk/Safetyinformation (accessed May 2013).

47 Feldman AE and Gidal BE (2013) QTc prolongation by antiepileptic drugs and the risk of torsade de pointes in patients with epilepsy. Epilepsy and Behavior. **26**: 421–426.

48 Tremont-Lukats IW et al. (2000) Anticonvulsants for neuropathic pain syndromes: mechanisms of action and place in therapy. Drugs. **60**: 1029–1052.

49 Freynhagen R et al. (2005) Efficacy of pregabalin in neuropathic pain evaluated in a 12-week, randomised, double-blind, multicentre, placebo-controlled trial of flexible- and fixed-dose regimens. Pain. **115**: 254–263.

50 Gidal B et al. (1998) Gabapentin absorption: effect of mixing with foods of varying macronutrient composition. Annals of Pharmacotherapy. **32**: 405–409.

Updated May 2014

CARBAMAZEPINE   BNF 4.8.1

Class: Anti-epileptic (sodium channel blocker).

Indications: Focal seizures, trigeminal neuralgia, †neuropathic pain, mania.

Contra-indications: AV block, previous bone marrow depression, concurrent MAOI, hypersensitivity to TCAs (structurally related).

Pharmacology

Carbamazepine is a sodium channel blocker. These channels accumulate at sites of neuronal injury creating ectopic foci of action potential generation (see p.254). Additional actions of uncertain significance include potassium channel activation, L-type calcium-channel blockade, and antagonism of NMDA-receptor-channel complex.[1]

Absorption is affected by formulation; slower rates reduce the incidence of undesirable CNS effects.[2] Carbamazepine is mainly metabolized by CYP3A4 to a pharmacologically active epoxide metabolite; this is subsequently inactivated to several renally excreted metabolites. The halflife decreases over the first 1–2 weeks as a result of hepatic enzyme auto-induction.

Carbamazepine is a first-line drug for focal seizures and trigeminal neuralgia. Generally, because it requires slow titration, particular care with regard to drug interactions (see Table 1) and has few supporting RCTs,[3] its use in other neuropathic pains is limited to those failing to respond to authorized alternatives (see p.270). In painful diabetic neuropathy it is superior to placebo (n = 30) and comparable to **nortriptyline** (n = 16).[4] Benefit is also reported for paroxysmal nausea associated with meningeal carcinomatosis[5] and itch associated with haematological malignancy.[6]

A polymorphism in the gene (SCN1A) encoding the sodium channel α-subunit has been linked to carbamazepine-resistant epilepsy.[7] Human leukocyte antigen (HLA) genes, known to influence susceptibility to various infections and auto-immune diseases, are closely associated with the risk

Table 1 Clinically significant cytochrome P450 interactions with carbamazepine resulting in changed drug plasma concentrations

Carbamazepine[a] plasma concentration		Drug plasma concentration	
increased by	decreased by	increased by carbamazepine	decreased by carbamazepine
Antipsychotics[b]	Efavirenz	Phenytoin	Antipsychotics[b]
Antiretrovirals[b]	Phenobarbital[c]		Antiretrovirals[b]
Azole antifungals[b]	Phenytoin[c]		Azole antifungals[b]
Clarithromycin	Valproate[c]		Benzodiazepines[b]
Dextropropoxyphene			Calcium-channel blockers[b]
Diltiazem			Clozapine
Erythromycin			Corticosteroids[b]
Fluoxetine			Coumarin anticoagulants
Fluvoxamine			Ethosuximide
Haloperidol			Fentanyl
Isoniazid			Haloperidol
Lamotrigine			Indinavir
Valproate			Lamotrigine
Verapamil			Levothyroxine
			Methadone
			Oestrogens, progestogens
			Phenytoin
			Primidone
			SSRIs[b]
			TCAs[b]
			Tiagabine
			Topiramate
			Tramadol
			Valproate

a. or active metabolite
b. effect not seen with all drug class members
c. increase in active metabolite of carbamazepine.

of carbamazepine-induced skin reactions. In Han Chinese, HLA B*1502 was found in 100% of 44 individuals with Stevens-Johnson syndrome compared with 3% of unaffected carbamazepine-treated individuals.[8] The MHRA recommends testing HLA B*1502 status before carbamazepine is started in people of Han Chinese, Hong Kong Chinese or Thai origin. In Europeans, HLA-A*3101 increased the risk of less severe skin reactions from 5% to 26%.[9,10]

Bio-availability ≥85%.

Onset of action generally delayed by the need for slow titration, but anti-epileptic response is sometimes seen as early as 2 days.

Peak plasma concentration 4–8h (immediate-release tablets), 12–26h (m/r tablets), 0.5–3h (oral liquid).

Plasma halflife 36h initially, 8–24h after multiple dosing (hepatic auto-induction).

Duration of action No specific data.

Cautions

Agranulocytosis and aplastic anaemia affect about 5 and 2 patients/million/year respectively. Severe hepatic reactions are rare. Mild leukopenia, thrombocytopenia, or cholestatic abnormalities in LFTs should be monitored, and carbamazepine should be discontinued if severe or symptomatic derangement occurs.

Mild skin reactions are common and transient; monitor closely and discontinue carbamazepine if reactions worsen, or if features of Stevens-Johnson syndrome or toxic epidermal necrolysis develop.

Renal, cardiac or hepatic disease; absence seizures (may worsen); previous skin reaction to other anti-epileptic drugs or TCAs.

Drug interactions

Carbamazepine is a hepatic enzyme inducer with numerous drug interactions (see Table 1).

Undesirable effects

Very common (>10%): dizziness, ataxia, drowsiness, fatigue, nausea, mild LFT derangement (see above), urticaria, leukopenia.

Common (<10%, >1%): headache, diplopia, blurred vision, oedema, dry mouth, thrombocytopenia, eosinophilia, hyponatraemia, rectal irritation (with suppositories).

Uncommon (<1%, >0.1%): %): include suicidal ideation 0.2% (1/500; advise patients to report mood or thought disturbance).

Rare (<0.1%): aseptic meningitis, movement disorders, neuroleptic (antipsychotic) malignant syndrome, arrhythmias and cardiac conduction disorders, pancreatitis, hepatitis, jaundice, renal failure, interstitial nephritis, a delayed-onset multi-organ vasculitic hypersensitivity disorder, severe skin reactions (see above).

Dose and use

Note: the MHRA advises that the products available in the UK may differ in bio-availability, and that to avoid changes in effectiveness or increased risk of undesirable effects, it is best to avoid switching between formulations (see also p.261).

Starting dose and titration rate will depend on seizure or pain severity. Undesirable effects are minimized by a low starting dose, slow upward titration, and the use of m/r products.
- check:
  ▷ baseline FBC, U+E, LFTs, and repeat every 2–3 months
  ▷ HLA B*1502 status in people of Han Chinese, Hong Kong Chinese or Thai origin[9]
- start with 50–100mg PO b.d. (use m/r product for doses ⩾100mg)
- if necessary, increase in 50–100mg increments every 1–2 weeks
- in epilepsy, 90% require ⩽800mg/24h[11]
- maximum daily dose 2g.

Supply

Immediate-release products *(m/r products are generally preferred, see dose and use)*
Carbamazepine (generic)
Tablets 100mg, 200mg, 400mg, 28 days @ 200mg b.d. = £10.

Tegretol® (Novartis)
Tablets *(scored)* 100mg, 200mg, 400mg, 28 days @ 200mg b.d. = £2.50.
Tablets chewable (Chewtabs®) 100mg, 200mg, 28 days @ 200mg b.d. = £6.
Oral liquid (sugar-free) 100mg/5mL, 28 days @ 200mg b.d. = £12.
Suppositories 125mg, pack of 5 = £8; 250mg, pack of 5 = £11.

Modified-release products

M/r carbamazepine tablets in the UK are scored to permit splitting into halves; however they should not be crushed or chewed, see Chapter 22, Box B, p.728.

Carbagen SR® (Generics)
Tablets *m/r(scored)* 200mg, 400mg, 28 days @ 200mg b.d. = £5.

Tegretol® Prolonged Release (Novartis)
Tablets *m/r(scored)* 200mg, 400mg, 28 days @ 200mg b.d. = £5.

1 Schmidt D and Elger CE (2004) What is the evidence that oxcarbazepine and carbamazepine are distinctly different antiepileptic drugs? *Epilepsy and Behaviour.* **5**: 627–635.
2 Tothfalusi L et al. (2008) Exposure-response analysis reveals that clinically important toxicity difference can exist between bioequivalent carbamazepine tablets. *British Journal of Clinical Pharmacology.* **65**: 110–122.

3 Wiffen PJ et al. (2011) Carbamazepine for acute and chronic pain in adults. Cochrane Database of Systematic Reviews. 1: CD005451.
4 Wiffen PJ et al. (2005) Carbamazepine for acute and chronic pain. Cochrane Database of Systematic Reviews. 3: CD005451.
5 Strohscheer I and Borasio GD (2006) Carbamazepine-responsive paroxysmal nausea and vomiting in a patient with meningeal carcinomatosis. Palliative Medicine. 20: 549–550.
6 Korfitis C and Trafalis DT (2008) Carbamazepine can be effective in alleviating tormenting pruritus in patients with hematologic malignancy. Journal of Pain and Symptom Management. 35: 571–572.
7 Abe T et al. (2008) Association between SCN1A polymorphism and carbamazepine-resistant epilepsy. British Journal of Clinical Pharmacology. 66: 304–307.
8 Chung WH et al. (2004) Medical genetics: a marker for Stevens-Johnson syndrome. Nature. 428: 486.
9 MHRA (2008) Carbamazepine: genetic testing recommended in some Asian populations Drug Safety Update. 1. www.mhra.gov.uk/safetyinformation
10 MHRA (2012). Carbamazepine, oxcarbazepine and eslicarbazepine: potential risk of serious skin reactions associated with the HLA-A∗ 3101 allele. Drug Safety Update. 6. www.mhra.gov.uk/safetyinformation
11 Kwan P and Brodie MJ (2001) Effectiveness of first antiepileptic drug. Epilepsia. 42: 1255–1260.

Updated May 2014

OXCARBAZEPINE BNF 4.8.1

Class: Anti-epileptic (sodium channel blocker).

Indications: Monotherapy or adjunctive therapy for focal seizures, †neuropathic pain.

Pharmacology

Oxcarbazepine is structurally related to **carbamazepine**. Both act through sodium channel blockade (see p.275 and p.254) but differ in tolerability and propensity for drug interactions. Additional actions of uncertain significance include potassium channel activation, N, P and R- type calcium channel blockade and antagonism of the NMDA-receptor-channel complex.[1]

Oxcarbazepine is a pro-drug which is activated by reduction to its monohydroxy derivative. This is inactivated by glucuronidation and oxidation, and the metabolites are renally excreted.[2] Oxcarbazepine has fewer drug interactions than **carbamazepine** because it is a weaker inducer of hepatic enzymes.

In an RCT for epilepsy, oxcarbazepine was as effective as, but better tolerated than, **carbamazepine**; 14% vs. 25% of patients withdrew because of undesirable effects.[3]

Oxcarbazepine is reported to improve trigeminal neuralgia and post-herpetic neuralgia unresponsive to **carbamazepine** and **carbamazepine** + **gabapentin** respectively.[4,5] However, the results of 3 RCTs in painful diabetic neuropathy are conflicting. The only positive study titrated the dose to a maximum of 1,800mg daily (mean 1,450mg daily) and found a reduction in mean pain 0–10 VAS score of 1 (NNT = 6 for >50% reduction in pain).[6] A study exploring both 1,200mg and 1,800mg daily found equivocal results.[7] A dose of 1,200mg daily was ineffective.[8]

Bio-availability ≥95%.
Onset of action pain improved ≤1 week, maximum response ≤4 weeks.[6]
Peak plasma concentration 1–3h.
Plasma halflife 1–5h; 7–20h monohydroxy derivative.
Duration of action no specific data.

Cautions

HLA predisposition or previous hypersensitivity to **carbamazepine** (25–30% cross-reactivity, also see p.275), predisposition to hyponatraemia, cardiac insufficiency (fluid retention), abnormal cardiac conduction (arrhythmias and AV block occur rarely).

Drug interactions

Oxcarbazepine can induce CYP3A4 and inhibit CYP2C19 but not often to a clinically significant extent. Oral hormonal contraception may become ineffective. **Lamotrigine** and **phenytoin** may require dose adjustment.

Undesirable effects

Very common (>10%): drowsiness, dizziness, fatigue, headache, diplopia, nausea and vomiting.

Common (<10%, >1%): confusion, agitation, amnesia, altered mood, vertigo, ataxia, tremor, nystagmus, reduced attention, diarrhoea, constipation, abdominal pain, rash, alopecia, acne, asymptomatic hyponatraemia.

Uncommon (<1%, >0.1%): include suicidal ideation 0.2% (1/500; advise patients to report mood or thought disturbance).

Rare (<0.1%): AV block, arrhythmia, pancreatitis, hepatitis, multi-organ hypersensitivity, systemic lupus erythematosus, angioedema, Stevens-Johnson syndrome, toxic epidermal necrolysis, bone marrow depression.

Dose and use

Note: the MHRA advises that the products available in the UK may differ in bio-availability, and that to avoid changes in effectiveness or increased risk of undesirable effects, it is best to avoid switching between formulations (see also p.261).

Many palliative care patients have risk factors for hyponatraemia; monitor sodium at baseline, after 2 weeks, then monthly for 3 months. Doses lower than recommended by the manufacturer have been proposed:[2]

• start with 150mg b.d. (75mg b.d. in elderly and frail patients)
• increase the dose in 75–150mg increments weekly
• if necessary, increase to a maximum of 1,200mg b.d.
• halve the initial dose if creatinine clearance is ≤30mL/min.

Supply

Oxcarbazepine (generic)
Tablets 150mg, 300mg, 600mg, 28 days @ 300mg b.d. = £27.

Trileptal® (Novartis)
Tablets *(scored)* 150mg, 300mg, 600mg, 28 days @ 300mg b.d. = £23.
Oral suspension (sugar-free) 300mg/5mL, 28 days @ 300mg b.d. = £38.

---

1 Schmidt D and Elger CE (2004) What is the evidence that oxcarbazepine and carbamazepine are distinctly different antiepileptic drugs? *Epilepsy and Behaviour.* **5**: 627–635.
2 May TW et al. (2003) Clinical pharmacokinetics of oxcarbazepine. *Clinical Pharmacokinetics.* **42**: 1023–1042.
3 Dam M et al. (1989) A double-blind study comparing oxcarbazepine and carbamazepine in patients with newly diagnosed, previously untreated epilepsy. *Epilepsy Research.* **3**: 70–76.
4 Gomez-Arguelles JM et al. (2008) Oxcarbazepine monotherapy in carbamazepine-unresponsive trigeminal neuralgia. *Journal of Clinical Neuroscience.* **15**: 516–519.
5 Criscuolo S et al. (2005) Oxcarbazepine monotherapy in postherpetic neuralgia unresponsive to carbamazepine and gabapentin. *Acta Neurologica Scandinavica.* **111**: 229–232.
6 Dogra S et al. (2005) Oxcarbazepine in painful diabetic neuropathy: a randomized, placebo-controlled study. *Eur J Pain.* **9**: 543–554.
7 Beydoun A et al. (2006) Oxcarbazepine in painful diabetic neuropathy: results of a dose-ranging study. *Acta Neurologica Scandinavica.* **113**: 395–404.
8 Grosskopf J et al. (2006) A randomized, placebo-controlled study of oxcarbazepine in painful diabetic neuropathy. *Acta Neurologica Scandinavica.* **114**: 177–180.

Updated May 2014

VALPROATE   BNF 4.8.1

Class: Anti-epileptic (multimodal action).

Indications: Epilepsy (see SPC for details), mania associated with bipolar disorder, †neuropathic pain, †migraine prophylaxis.

Contra-indications: Active hepatic disease (see text), past or family history of severe hepatic impairment (particularly drug-related).

Pharmacology

Valproate is a sodium and T-type calcium channel blocker, an NMDA-receptor-channel blocker, it increases potassium conductance and alters glutamate, GABA, dopamine and serotonin transmission. The relative significance of these actions in epilepsy is unclear. Actions of possible relevance in neuropathic pain include correcting the down-regulation of glutamate re-uptake transporters[1,2] and T-type calcium channel blockade;[3] these channels may be involved in regulating pain excitation thresholds in a 'T-rich' subset of peripheral nociceptors.[4,5]

Valproate is well absorbed orally. It is ⩾90% plasma protein-bound, and crosses the blood-brain barrier and neuronal membranes via active transporters. It is metabolized by direct microsomal UDP-mediated glucuronidation (50%), mitochondrial ß-oxidation (40%) and cytochrome P450-mediated oxidation (10%: CYP2A6, 2B6, 2C9 and 2C19). Some metabolites are active, but their cerebral concentrations are too low to contribute to valproate's overall effect. Metabolites may be responsible for idiosyncratic hepatic toxicity. CYP enzyme inducers, inhibitors and polymorphisms affect the proportion of cytochrome P450 metabolites, perhaps altering this risk.[6,7]

Compared with immediate-release and enteric coated preparations, modified-release preparations halve the initial peak plasma level without reducing overall bio-availability. Further, plasma levels at 24h are 50% higher and thus peak to trough variability is significantly decreased.[8,9]

Valproate remains a first-line treatment for generalized seizures, its efficacy and tolerability comparing favourably to those of newer anti-epileptics.[10,11] Its main safety concerns are idiosyncratic hepatic damage, affecting 1:3,000–1:20,000 people, and teratogenicity.[7,12] However, the incidence of serious idiosyncratic reactions reported with newer anti-epileptics is unknown.

A beneficial effect has been reported for cancer-related neuropathic pain.[13,14] However, results of several small RCTs in non-cancer pain are mixed,[15–20] and international guidelines do not recommend it for first-line use.[21,22] Valproate was well tolerated in all 6 studies, with fewer patients (⩽5%) discontinuing because of undesirable effects compared with **gabapentin** (8–19%) and **pregabalin** (8–32%; see p.261).

Bio-availability 95% PO.
Onset of action often within 24h (for neuropathic pain).[13]
Peak plasma concentration 1–2h (3–5h for e/c, 5–10h for m/r).
Plasma halflife 9–18h (5–12h with concurrent enzyme inducers).
Duration of action 12–24h.[7]

Cautions

Idiosyncratic, potentially fatal, hepatic failure occurs in 1:3,000–1:20,000 patients, usually within the first 6 months of treatment. Risk factors include age < 3 years, pre-existing liver disease and deranged LFTs. Chronic hepatitis was the commonest reported liver disease;[23,24] it is unclear whether hepatic metastases affect the risk. Symptoms (drowsiness, fatigue, vomiting, and increased seizure frequency) may precede altered LFTs,[7] but both are common in palliative care populations. Mildly deranged LFTs do not require discontinuation but should prompt increased monitoring. Valproate should be stopped if co-existent coagulopathy, severely deranged LFTs or rapidly evolving symptoms occur in the absence of an alternative explanation. Treatment with IV **carnitine** has been proposed; seek specialist advice.

Lower initial doses and slower titration may be required in patients with renal impairment. Alternatives may be preferred in women trying to conceive; seek specialist advice. Harmless ketone metabolites, detected by bedside urinalysis, may cause diagnostic confusion in diabetic patients.

Drug interactions

The clearance of valproate is increased by hepatic enzyme inducers such as **carbamazepine**, **phenytoin**, **phenobarbital** and **rifampicin**.[7] Its clearance is inhibited by **isoniazid**.

Valproate inhibits the metabolism of **carbamazepine**'s active/epoxide metabolite (increasing undesirable effects), **ethosuximide**, **phenytoin**, **phenobarbital**, **lamotrigine** and some antiretrovirals.

Concurrent administration with carbapenem antibacterials can decrease the plasma concentration of valproate dramatically by 85–90% through the combined impact on intestinal absorption, distribution and metabolism, with consequential loss of therapeutic effect.[25] Because increasing the dose may not overcome this drug–drug interaction, alternative antibacterials should be considered for patients taking valproate.

Undesirable effects

Hepatic failure (see above) and pancreatitis are the most important idiosyncratic effects. Other rare effects include severe skin reactions (e.g. Stevens-Johnson syndrome) and reversible encephalopathy, parkinsonism, and dementia.

Common problems include gastric intolerance (particularly nausea: reduced by e/c formulations or taking with food), hair loss (transient; dose-related), drowsiness and postural tremor (a rarer flapping tremor is seen with hyperammonaemia), although the incidence varies markedly between individual studies. Hyperammonaemia is usually asymptomatic but can cause nausea, ataxia or encephalopathy.

Dose and use

The manufacturer recommends that LFTs, prothrombin time (PT) and FBC be checked before and during the first 6 months of treatment, although this may not improve the early detection of hepatotoxicity.

Epilepsy

Note: the MHRA advises that the products available in the UK may differ in bio-availability, and that to avoid changes in effectiveness or increased risk of undesirable effects, it is best to avoid switching between formulations (see also p.261).

Valproate is a commonly used first or second-line treatment in palliative care. In the last days of life, midazolam is generally preferred (see Anti-epileptics Box B, p.263)
• start with valproate 150–200mg m/r b.d.
• if necessary, increase by 150–200mg b.d. every 3 days
• 90% require ≤1.5g/24h[26]
• maximum recommended dose 2.5g/24h.

IV valproate is used when the oral route cannot be used. Patients already receiving oral treatment are given the same daily dose in continuous or intermittent (over 3–5 min) infusions. Patients starting valproate are given 500–800mg (max 10mg/kg) followed by continuous or intermittent infusions of up to 2.5g/24h.

Neuropathic pain
• start with valproate 150–200mg m/r at bedtime
• if necessary, increase by 150–200mg/24h every 2–3 days; give as a b.d. dose
• response likely at doses lower than those used in epilepsy (see above)
• some patients need 2g/24h.[13,14]

Mania

Note: not all marketed products are authorized for mania. However, they appear to be clinically equivalent; thus, in practice it is reasonable to use whatever is to hand:
• start with valproate 300mg m/r b.d.
• increase as rapidly as possible to achieve the optimal response, to a maximum of 60mg/kg/24h
• most patients respond to doses <2g/24h.[27,28]

Migraine prophylaxis
• start with valproate 150–200mg m/r b.d.[29]
• if necessary, increase progressively to a total daily dose of 1g.[30]

Subcutaneous use

Although unauthorized, sodium valproate has been used successfully via CSCI, using a PO:SC dose ratio of 1:1. In a case series of 6 patients with seizures and one with neuropathic pain, a median (range) dose of 1000mg (400–1800mg)/24h was given using the IV preparation diluted with 30mL of WFI. Duration of use ranged 3–39 days, with only one patient experiencing mild erythema at the infusion site.[31]

Supply

Note: valproate is the UK generic term for valproic acid and its salts and esters, including sodium valproate. The pharmacokinetics, efficacy, and tolerability of valproic acid and sodium valproate are similar; sodium valproate 579mg is equivalent to valproic acid 500mg,[32] and the manufacturer of valproic acid (Convulex®) advises that it is equipotent with products containing sodium valproate.

Immediate-release oral products (*m/r products are generally preferred,* see Pharmacology)
Sodium valproate (generic)
Tablets crushable*(scored)* 100mg, 28 days @ 200mg b.d. = £7.
Tablets e/c 200mg, 500mg, 28 days @ 200mg b.d. = £2.50.
Oral solution 200mg/5mL, 28 days @ 200mg b.d. = £9.

Epilim® (Sanofi-Aventis)
Tablets crushable*(scored)* 100mg, 28 days @ 200mg b.d. = £7.
Tablets e/c 250mg, 500mg, 28 days @ 200mg b.d. = £4.50.
Oral solution (sugar-free) 200mg/5mL, 28 days @ 200mg b.d. = £8.
Oral syrup 200mg/5mL, 28 days @ 200mg b.d. = £9.

Modified-release oral products
Epilim Chrono® (Sanofi-Aventis)
Tablets m/r (*sodium valproate and valproic acid*) equivalent to sodium valproate 200mg, 300mg, 500mg, 28 days @ 200mg b.d. = £7.
Oral granules m/r Epilim Chronosphere® (*sodium valproate and valproic acid*) equivalent to sodium valproate 50mg, 100mg, 250mg, 500mg, 750mg, 1g/sachet, 28 days @ 500mg at bedtime = £28; *the granules may be mixed with soft food or a drink which is cold or at room temperature, and swallowed immediately without chewing.*

Episenta® (Desitin)
Capsules enclosing m/r granules sodium valproate 150mg, 300mg, 28 days @ 150mg b.d. = £4.
Oral granules m/r sodium valproate 500mg, 1g/sachet, 28 days @ 500mg at bedtime = £6. The *granules or contents of the capsules may be mixed with cold food or drink, and swallowed immediately without chewing.*

Epival® (Chanelle Medical)
Tablets m/r*(scored)* 300mg, 500mg, 28 days @ 150mg b.d. = £3.50; *the tablets may be halved but not crushed or chewed.*

Parenteral products
Sodium valproate (generic)
Injection 100mg/mL, 3mL amp = £7, 4mL amp = £12.

Epilim Intravenous® (Sanofi-Aventis)
Injection (powder for reconstitution) 400mg vial = £14; supplied with a 4mL amp of WFI for reconstitution.

Valproic acid
Convulex® (Pharmacia)
Capsules e/c 150mg, 300mg, 500mg, 28 days @ 150mg b.d. = £4.

Depakote® (Sanofi-Aventis)
Tablets e/c (semisodium valproate) equivalent to valproic acid 250mg, 500mg, 28 days @ 250mg t.d.s. = £15; *semisodium valproate is a mixture of equimolar amounts of valproic acid and sodium valproate, and is authorized for mania.*

1 Hobo (2012) Valproate upregulates glutamate transporters in rat spinal cord after peripheral nerve injury. *Journal of Pain.* 13(Suppl 1): s62.

2 Inquimbert P *et al.* (2012) Peripheral nerve injury produces a sustained shift in the balance between glutamate release and uptake in the dorsal horn of the spinal cord. *Pain.* 153: 2422–2431.

3 Takahashi T *et al.* (2010) Upregulation of Ca(v)3.2 T-type calcium channels targeted by endogenous hydrogen sulfide contributes to maintenance of neuropathic pain. *Pain.* 150: 183–191.

4   Jevtovic-Todorovic V et al. (2006) The role of peripheral T-type calcium channels in pain transmission. *Cell Calcium.* **40**: 197–203.
5   Francois A et al. (2013) State-dependent properties of a new T-type calcium channel blocker enhance Ca(V)3.2 selectivity and support analgesic effects. *Pain.* **154**: 283–293.
6   Mann MW and Pons G (2007) Various pharmacogenetic aspects of antiepileptic drug therapy: a review. *CNS Drugs.* **21**: 143–164.
7   Perucca E (2002) Pharmacological and therapeutic properties of valproate: a summary after 35 years of clinical experience. *CNS Drugs.* **16**: 695–714.
8   Wangemann M et al. (1999) Pharmacokinetic characteristics of a new multiple unit sustained release formulation of sodium valproate. *International Journal of Clinical Pharmacology and Therapeutics.* **37**: 100–108.
9   Genton P (2005) Progress in pharmaceutical development presentation with improved pharmacokinetics: a new formulation for valproate. *Acta Neurologica Scandinavica Supplementum.* **182**: 26–32.
10 Marson AG et al. (2007) The SANAD study of effectiveness of valproate, lamotrigine, or topiramate for generalised and unclassifiable epilepsy: an unblinded randomised controlled trial. *Lancet.* **369**: 1016–1026.
11 Karceski S et al. (2005) Treatment of epilepsy in adults: expert opinion. *Epilepsy & Behavior.* **7(Suppl 1)**: S1–64.
12 French JA (2007) First-choice drug for newly diagnosed epilepsy. *Lancet.* **369**: 970–971.
13 Snare AJ (1993) Sodium Valproate. Retrospective analysis of neuropathic pain control in patients with advanced cancer. *Journal of Pharmacy Technology.* **9**: 114–117.
14 Hardy J et al. (2001) A phase II study to establish the efficacy and toxicity of sodium valproate in patients with cancer-related neuropathic pain. *Journal of Pain and Symptom Management.* **21**: 204–209.
15 Kochar DK et al. (2002) Sodium valproate in the management of painful neuropathy in type 2 diabetes - a randomized placebo controlled study. *Acta Neurologica Scandinavica.* **106**: 248–252.
16 Kochar DK et al. (2004) Sodium valproate for painful diabetic neuropathy: a randomized double-blind placebo-controlled study. *Quarterly Journal of Medicine.* **97**: 33–38.
17 Kochar DK et al. (2005) Divalproex sodium in the management of post-herpetic neuralgia: a randomized double-blind placebo-controlled study. *Quarterly Journal of Medicine.* **98**: 29–34.
18 Otto M et al. (2004) Valproic acid has no effect on pain in polyneuropathy: a randomized, controlled trial. *Neurology.* **62**: 285–288.
19 Drewes AM et al. (1994) Valproate for treatment of chronic central pain after spinal cord injury. A double-blind cross-over study. *Paraplegia.* **32**: 565–569.
20 Agrawal RP et al. (2009) Management of diabetic neuropathy by sodium valproate and glyceryl trinitrate spray: a prospective double-blind randomized placebo-controlled study. *Diabetes Research and Clinical Practice.* **83**: 371–378.
21 Attal N et al. (2010) EFNS guidelines on the pharmacological treatment of neuropathic pain: 2010 revision. *European Journal of Neurology.* **17**: 1113–e1188.
22 Dworkin RH et al. (2010) Recommendations for the pharmacological management of neuropathic pain: an overview and literature update. *Mayo Clinic Proceedings.* **85**: S3–14.
23 Konig SA et al. (1994) Severe hepatotoxicity during valproate therapy: an update and report of eight new fatalities. *Epilepsia.* **35**: 1005–1015.
24 Koenig SA et al. (2006) Valproic acid-induced hepatopathy: nine new fatalities in Germany from 1994 to 2003. *Epilepsia.* **47**: 2027–2031.
25 Mancl EE and Gidal BE (2009) The effect of carbapenem antibiotics on plasma concentrations of valproic acid. *Annals of Pharmacotherapy.* **43**: 2082–2087.
26 Kwan P and Brodie MJ (2001) Effectiveness of first antiepileptic drug. *Epilepsia.* **42**: 1255–1260.
27 Keck PE, Jr. et al. (1993) Valproate oral loading in the treatment of acute mania. *Journal of Clinical Psychiatry.* **54**: 305–308.
28 Macritchie K et al. (2003) Valproate for acute mood episodes in bipolar disorder. *Cochrane Database of Systematic Reviews.* **1**: CD004052.
29 Kinze S et al. (2001) Valproic acid is effective in migraine prophylaxis at low serum levels: a prospective open-label study. *Headache.* **41**: 774–778.
30 Freitag FG (2003) Divalproex in the treatment of migraine. *Psychopharmacol Bull.* **37(Suppl 2)**: 98–115.
31 McKenna M (2013) *Personal communication.*
32 Fisher (2003) Sodium valproate or valproate semisodium: is there a difference in the treatment of bipolar disorder? *Psychiatric Bulletin.* **27**: 446–448.

Updated May 2014

LEVETIRACETAM   BNF 4.8.1

Class: Anti-epileptic (SV2A ligand).

Indications: Mono or adjunctive therapy of focal seizures, adjunctive therapy of generalized myoclonic and tonic-clonic seizures, †monotherapy of generalized seizures (see text).

Pharmacology

Levetiracetam binds to synaptic vesicle protein SV2A, and is presumed to interfere with the release of the neurotransmitter stored within the vesicle.[1] Food affects the rate but not the extent of its absorption. It does not bind to plasma proteins. It readily crosses the blood-brain barrier and its CSF halflife is 3 times longer than that for plasma.[2] A third is metabolized predominantly by non-hepatic hydrolysis; the remainder is excreted by the kidneys unchanged.

Levetiracetam is effective for a broad range of seizure types. Its efficacy and tolerability compare favourably to other newer anti-epileptic drugs.[3] It is commonly used second-line (see p.263), or first-line when the seizure type is unclear (also see **valproate**, p.279) or when other anti-epileptics are contra-indicated because of co-morbidities.[4] Prophylactic levetiracetam is more effective than **phenytoin** at reducing the incidence of seizures following craniotomy (0% vs. 16%).[5]

Benefit for bipolar disorder and hot flushes is reported.[3,6,7] A single-blind RCT found it to be effective for multiple sclerosis-related central neuropathic pain[8] but five double-blind placebo-controlled RCTs found no benefit for post-mastectomy, multiple sclerosis, central post-stroke, mixed polyneuropathy or spinal cord injury pain.[9–13]

Bio-availability ≥95% PO.
Onset of action antiepileptic effect generally evident <3 days of starting treatment.
Peak plasma concentration 1–2h.
Plasma halflife 6–8h.
Duration of action 24h.

Cautions

Dose reduction may be required with renal impairment, look for secondary renal impairment in those with hepatic impairment.

Drug interactions

Although caution is advised when **carbamazepine** or **phenytoin** are used in combination with levetiracetam, a clinically significant interaction is unlikely.[14]

Undesirable effects

Very common (>10%): fatigue, drowsiness.
Common (<10%, >1%): ataxia, hyperkinesis, tremor, dizziness, headache, diplopia, blurred vision, amnesia, abnormal thinking, attention disturbance, behavioural disturbances (emotional lability, irritability, agitation, hostility/aggression, personality disorders), depression, insomnia, anorexia, abdominal pain, diarrhoea, dyspepsia, nausea, vomiting, myalgia, rash, pruritus, thrombocytopenia.

Behavioural disturbances occur in 3–4% of patients with epilepsy but only 0.5% of those being treated for other conditions. Risk factors include a history of aggression or psychiatric disturbance.[15,16]
Uncommon (<1%, >0.1%): include suicidal ideation 0.2% (1/500; advise patients to report mood or thought disturbance).
Rare (<0.1%): psychosis, pancreatitis, hepatic failure, bone marrow suppression, hyponatraemia.

Dose and use

In epilepsy, the PO and IV dose are identical:
• start with 250–500mg b.d.
• if starting with 250mg b.d., increase automatically after 2 weeks to 500mg b.d. (the minimum effective dose in most people)
• if necessary, increase by 250–500mg b.d. every 2 weeks
• maximum dose 1.5g b.d.
For IV use, dilute the dose in ≥100mL 0.9% saline and infuse over 15min.

SC administration

Although unauthorized, a case report and case series (n = 15) respectively suggest that administration SC and CSCI are well tolerated. Using a PO:SC dose ratio of 1:1 the required dose was givn either:
• SC b.d., with the IV preparation diluted in 100mL sodium chloride 0.9% and infused SC over 30min[17] or
• CSCI, with the IV preparation infused over 24h, using WFI as diluent when necessary; higher doses required two syringe drivers.[18]

Renal impairment

For patients with renal impairment, the doses in Table 1 should generally be adhered to.
If on dialysis:
• start with 750mg loading dose followed by 500mg–1,000mg *once daily* PO/IV
• give 250–500mg supplementary doses after dialysis.

Table I Dose adjustment for levetiracetam in renal impairment

Creatinine clearance (mL/min/1.73m²)[a]	Usual maintenance dose (mg)
>80	500–1,500 b.d.
50–79	500–1,000 b.d.
30–49	250–750 b.d.
<30	250–500 b.d.

a. based on the Cockroft-Gault formula adjusted for body surface area (see Chapter 14).

Hepatic impairment
Dose is unaffected by mild–moderate hepatic impairment. With severe hepatic impairment, creatinine clearance may underestimate the severity of renal impairment. Halve the dose if creatinine clearance <60mL/min/1.73m².

Stopping levetiracetam
Reduce by a maximum of 500mg b.d. every 2–4 weeks to avoid rebound seizures.

Supply
Levetiracetam (generic)
Tablets 250mg, 500mg, 750mg, 1g, 28 days @ 750mg or 1g b.d. = £4 and £6 respectively.
Granules 250mg, 500mg and 1g sachet, 28 days @ 750mg or 1g b.d. = £62 and £76 respectively.
Oral solution (sugar-free) 100mg/mL, 28 days @ 750mg or 1g b.d. = £91 and £121 respectively.

Keppra® (UCB Pharma)
Tablets 250mg, 500mg, 750mg, 1g, 28 days @ 750mg or 1g b.d. = £84 and £96 respectively.
Oral solution (sugar-free) 100mg/mL, 28 days @ 750mg or 1g b.d. = £94 and £125 respectively.
Injection (concentrate for dilution and use as an Intravenous infusion) 100mg/mL, 5mL vial = £13.

1 Lynch BA (2004) The synaptic vesicle protein SV2A is the binding site for the antiepileptic drug levetiracetam. *Proceedings of the National Academy of Sciences of the United States of America.* **101**: 9861–9866.
2 Patsalos PN and Patsalos PN (2004) Clinical pharmacokinetics of levetiracetam. *Clinical Pharmacokinetics.* **43**: 707–724.
3 Zaccara G et al. (2006) Comparison of the efficacy and tolerability of new antiepileptic drugs: what can we learn from long-term studies? *Acta Neurologica Scandinavica.* **114**: 157–168.
4 Karceski S et al. (2005) Treatment of epilepsy in adults: expert opinion. *Epilepsy & Behavior.* **7(Suppl 1)**: S1–64.
5 Fuller KL et al. (2013) Tolerability, safety, and side effects of levetiracetam versus phenytoin in intravenous and total prophylactic regimen among craniotomy patients: a prospective randomized study. *Epilepsia.* **54**: 45–57.
6 Dunteman ED (2005) Levetiracetam as an adjunctive analgesic in neoplastic plexopathies: case series and commentary. *Journal of Pain and Palliative Care Pharmacotherapy.* **19**: 35–43.
7 Thompson S et al. (2008) Levetiracetam for the treatment of hot flashes: a phase II study. *Supportive Care in Cancer.* **16**: 75–82.
8 Rossi S et al. (2009) Effects of levetiracetam on chronic pain in multiple sclerosis: results of a pilot, randomized, placebo-controlled study. *European Journal of Neurology.* **16**: 360–366.
9 Finnerup NB et al. (2009) Levetiracetam in spinal cord injury pain: a randomized controlled trial. *Spinal Cord.* **47**: 861–867.
10 Vilholm OJ et al. (2008) Effect of levetiracetam on the postmastectomy pain syndrome. *European Journal of Neurology.* **15**: 851–857.
11 Holbech JV et al. (2011) The anticonvulsant levetiracetam for the treatment of pain in polyneuropathy: a randomized, placebo-controlled, cross-over trial. *European Journal of Pain.* **15**: 608–614.
12 Jungehulsing GJ et al. (2013) Levetiracetam in patients with central neuropathic post-stroke pain–a randomized, double-blind, placebo-controlled trial. *European Journal of Neurology.* **20**: 331–337.
13 Falah M et al. (2012) A randomized, placebo-controlled trial of levetiracetam in central pain in multiple sclerosis. *European Journal of Pain.* **16**: 860–869.
14 Baxter K and Preston CL *Stockley's Drug Interactions.* London: Pharmaceutical Press www.medicinescomplete.com (accessed May 2014).
15 Dinkelacker V et al. (2003) Aggressive behavior of epilepsy patients in the course of levetiracetam add-on therapy: report of 33 mild to severe cases. *Epilepsy Behaviour.* **4**: 537–547.
16 Cramer JA et al. (2003) A systematic review of the behavioral effects of levetiracetam in adults with epilepsy, cognitive disorders, or an anxiety disorder during clinical trials. *Epilepsy Behaviour.* **4**: 124–132.
17 Lopez-Saca JM et al. (2013) Repeated use of subcutaneous levetiracetam in a palliative care patient. *Journal of Pain and Symptom Management.* **45**: e7–8.
18 Freiherr von Hornstein W et al. (2014) Levetiracetam continuous subcutaneous infusion in the management of seizures. First experience. Poster presentation IAPC Education & Research Seminar 2014. Available from: http://www.palliativecare.ie/download.php?id=113.

Updated (minor change) August 2014

PHENOBARBITAL　　　　　　　　BNF 4.8.1 & 4.8.2

Class: Anti-epileptic (GABAmimetic).

Indications: Epilepsy (except absence seizures), status epilepticus, †terminal agitation.

Pharmacology

Phenobarbital enhances the post-synaptic inhibitory action of GABA by prolonging the opening of the chloride channel in the GABA receptor-channel complex (see Anti-epileptics, Figure 1, p.256).[1] Phenobarbital is also an AMPA-glutamate receptor antagonist. These actions depress CNS activity, and high doses result in general anaesthesia.

There is considerable interindividual variation in the pharmacokinetics of phenobarbital. Peak CNS concentrations occur some 15–20min after peak plasma concentrations. About 25% is excreted unchanged by the kidney; the rest is converted in the liver, mainly to inactive oxidative metabolites via several enzymes including CYP2C9. Phenobarbital is a strong inducer of CYP3A and glucuronidation, thus reducing plasma concentrations of many concurrently administered drugs.[1,2]

Phenobarbital's efficacy in epilepsy is comparable to alternatives but concerns about its cognitive and behavioural effects have led to a decline in its use, other than for status epilepticus (see p.263).[1]

Phenobarbital is used at some centres for agitation in the imminently dying which fails to respond to the combined use of **midazolam** and an antipsychotic.[3,4]

Bio-availability > 90% PO; no data IM.[2]

Onset of action 5min IV, maximum effect achieved within 30min, onset after SC or IM administration is slightly slower; 2–3 *weeks* PO (= the time to achieve a therapeutic anti-seizure plasma concentration with a once daily dose of 100–200mg).[5]

Time to peak plasma concentration 2–4h IM,[6] 2h PO (some authorities report up to 12h).[5–8]

Plasma halflife 2–6 *days*; 1–3 *days* in children.

Duration of action situation dependent; chronic administration > 24h.

Cautions

Elderly, children, debilitated, hepatic impairment, renal impairment, respiratory depression. Avoid sudden withdrawal.

Drug interactions

Phenobarbital induces various enzymes involved in drug metabolism, including CYP1A2, CYP2C9, CYP2C19 and CYP3A4 (manufacturer's data), and thus reduces plasma concentrations of many drugs.[9] Table 1 lists selected drugs which have clinically important interactions with phenobarbital.

Undesirable effects

Respiratory depression (high doses), drowsiness, lethargy, ataxia, skin reactions (< 3%). Paradoxical excitement, irritability, restlessness/hyperactivity and delirium, particularly in the elderly and children.

Long-term treatment is occasionally complicated by folate-responsive megaloblastic anaemia or by osteomalacia.

Dose and use

Phenobarbital sodium injection is very alkaline and formulated in a mixture of propylene glycol and alcohol. Local necrosis has been reported after SC bolus injection or IV extravasation (manufacturer's data on file).

Undiluted, it is suitable for IM use only. If *diluted* to 10 times its own volume with WFI, it can generally be given safely *on its own* by IV injection or CSCI, but it should *never* be mixed with another drug (see Chapter 20, p.701).

Note: an alternative formulation (not UK) has been given SC without any problems, thereby highlighting the need to know which product has been used when interpreting reports of SC use.[10]

Table I   Clinically significant cytochrome P450 interactions with phenobarbital resulting in changed drug plasma concentrations

Phenobarbital plasma concentration		Drug plasma concentration	
increased by	*decreased by*	*increased by phenobarbital*	*decreased by phenobarbital*
Felbamate (not UK)	Carbamazepine[a]	Hepatotoxic metabolites of paracetamol (possibly)	Some azole antifungals (itraconazole)
Influenza vaccine	Chlorpromazine		Some calcium-channel blockers (felodipine, nifedipine, nimodipine, verapamil)
Phenytoin[a]	Folic acid	Phenytoin (sometimes)[a]	
Stiripentol (not UK)	St John's wort		Carbamazepine[a]
Valproate[a]			Chlorpromazine
			Clonazepam
			Corticosteroids (dexamethasone, methylprednisolone, prednisolone)
			Coumarins (oral anticoagulants)
			Ciclosporin
			Disopyramide
			Doxycycline
			Ethosuximide (sometimes)[a]
			IV fentanyl (significance not known for TD)
			Haloperidol
			Lamotrigine
			Methadone
			Metronidazole
			Oral contraceptives
			Paracetamol
			Phenytoin (generally)[a]
			Quinidine (not UK)
			Rifampicin
			TCAs
			Theophylline
			Tiagabine
			Valproate

a. interactions between anti-epileptic drugs are complex and unpredictable; plasma concentrations may be increased, decreased or unchanged.

Epilepsy

Note: the MHRA advises that the oral products available in the UK may differ in bio-availability, and that to avoid changes in effectiveness or increased risk of undesirable effects, it is best to avoid switching between formulations (see also p.261).

Status epilepticus
Phenobarbital is used for the emergency treatment of seizures refractory to benzodiazepines (see Anti-epileptics, Figure 2, p.265):
- give a single 10–15mg/kg bolus up to a maximum dose of 1g:[11]
  ▷ *diluted* IV bolus (each 1mL ampoule diluted to 10mL with WFI; rate 100mg/min) *or*
  ▷ *undiluted* IM injection (if the IV route is not available). Larger doses may be split between ⩾2 sites. IM absorption is significantly slower than IV.

- if seizures persist:
  - ▷ if ITU is appropriate, transfer for general anaesthesia
  - ▷ if imminently dying, give further p.r.n. doses and commence a CSCI (dose as for terminal agitation).

Maintenance anti-epileptic in patients unable to swallow
Phenobarbital is a second-line alternative to **midazolam, valproate** or **levetiracetam** (see p.263).
Because of the irritant nature of the injection (see above) a loading or stat dose is generally given IM or IV but can be followed by CSCI:
- start with loading dose of 100mg (0.5mL of a 200mg/1mL ampoule) as:
  - ▷ *undiluted* IM injection *or*
  - ▷ *diluted* IV bolus given over 2min (0.5mL of a 200mg/1mL ampoule diluted to 5mL with WFI)
- then 100mg/24h CSCI (= total volume 5mL)
- if seizures occur, give a second loading dose of 100mg IM/IV and titrate the maintenance dose up to a maximum of 400mg/24h CSCI (= total volume 20mL)
- if seizures persist, treat as for status epileptics (see above; taking account of the phenobarbital already given) or, in the imminently dying, terminal agitation (see below).

Terminal agitation
Phenobarbital is one of several sedative drugs used to treat refractory agitation in the imminently dying. It is generally third-line treatment for patients who fail to respond to **midazolam** 60–120mg/24h together with either **haloperidol** 30mg/24h or **levomepromazine** 200mg/24h (see Chapter 16, Box A, p.673).
Because of the irritant nature of the injection (see above) a loading or stat dose is generally given IM or IV but can be followed by CSCI:
- start with loading dose of 200mg (1mL ampoule) as:
  - ▷ *undiluted* IM injection *or*
  - ▷ *diluted* IV bolus given over 2min (1mL ampoule diluted to 10mL with WFI)
- if the patient remains unsettled, give 1 or 2 further doses p.r.n. of 200mg IM/IV 30min apart
- if still unsettled or agitation recurs, give further doses of 200mg IM/IV q1h p.r.n.
- maintain with 800mg/24h CSCI (= total volume 40mL); or more if total initial 'settling' dose was ≥600mg
- if necessary, increase the dose progressively to 1,600mg/24h, i.e. 800mg → 1,200mg → 1,600mg (= total volume 80mL)
- a typical dose is 800–1,200mg/24h but can range 200–3,800mg/24h.[3,12–14]
Some centres use **propofol** (see p.634) or **dexmedetomidine** instead.[15–17]

Stopping phenobarbital
Abrupt cessation of long-term PO anti-epileptic therapy, particularly barbiturates and benzodiazepines, should be avoided because rebound seizures may be precipitated. If it is decided to discontinue anti-epileptic therapy, it should be done *slowly over 6 months or more*. For phenobarbital, the recommended monthly reduction in dose is *15mg*.[18]
In adults the risk of relapse on stopping treatment is 40–50%.[19] Substituting one anti-epileptic drug regimen for another should also be done cautiously, withdrawing the first drug only when the new regimen has been introduced.

Supply
All products are Schedule 3 **CD**.

Phenobarbital sodium (generic)
Injection 15mg/mL, 30mg/mL, 60mg/mL and 200mg/mL, 1mL amp = £7; *vehicle contains propylene glycol 90%. Must be diluted to ten times it's volume before IV use.*

1 Kwan P and Brodie MJ (2004) Phenobarbital for the treatment of epilepsy in the 21st century: a critical review. *Epilepsia.* **45**: 1141–1149.
2 Dollery C (1999) Phenobarbital. In: C Dollery (ed) *Therapeutic Drugs Release 1.* Harcourt Brace Company.
3 de Graeff A and Dean M (2007) Palliative sedation therapy in the last weeks of life: a literature review and recommendations for standards. *Journal of Palliative Medicine.* **10**: 67–85.
4 Twycross R et al. (2009) *Symptom Management in Advanced Cancer.* palliativedrugs.com, Nottingham, pp. 430–433.

5 McEvoy GK *American Hospital Formulary Service*. Maryland , USA: American Society of Health-System Pharmacists www.medicinescomplete.com (accessed 2009).
6 Sweetman SC *Martindale: The Complete Drug Reference*. London: Pharmaceutical Press www.medicinescomplete.com (accessed 2009).
7 Stirling LC et al. (1999) The use of phenobarbitone in the management of agitation and seizures at the end of life. *Journal of Pain and Symptom Management*. **17**: 363–368.
8 Holford N (ed) (1998) Clinical pharmacokinetics: drug data handbook. (3e). Adis International, Auckland.
9 Baxter K and Preston CL *Stockley's Drug Interactions*. London: Pharmaceutical Press www.medicinescomplete.com (accessed 2011).
10 palliativedrugs.com (2007) Phenobarbital infusion. *Bulletin Board* Available from: www.palliativedrugs.com (posted 08-10-2007).
11 NICE (2012) The epilepsies: the diagnosis and management of the epilepsies in adults and children in primary and secondary care. *Clinical Guideline* CG137. www.nice.org.uk
12 Gillon S et al. (2010) Review of phenobarbitone use for deep terminal sedation in a UK hospice. *Palliative Medicine*. **24**: 100–101.
13 Chater S et al. (1998) Sedation for intractable distress in the dying - a survey of experts. *Palliative Medicine*. **12**: 255–269.
14 Cowan J and Walsh D (2001) Terminal sedation in palliative medicine - definition and review of the literature. *Supportive Care in Cancer*. **9**: 403–407.
15 Gertler R et al. (2001) Dexmedetomidine: a novel sedative-analgesic agent. *Proceedings (Baylor University Medical Center)*. **14**: 13–21.
16 Soares L et al. (2002) Dexmedetomidine: a new option for intractable distress in the dying. *Journal of Pain and Symptom Management*. **24**: 6–8.
17 Jackson KC, 3rd et al. (2006) Dexmedetomidine: a novel analgesic with palliative medicine potential. *Journal of Pain and Palliative Care Pharmacotherapy*. **20**: 23–27.
18 Chadwick D (1995) The withdrawal of antiepileptic drugs. In: A Hopkins et al. (eds) *Epilepsy* (2e). Chapman and Hall, London, pp. 215–220.
19 Hopkins A and Shorvon S (1995) Definitions and epidemiology of epilepsy. In: A Hopkins et al. (eds) *Epilepsy* (2e). Chapman and Hall, London, pp. 1–24.

Updated June 2014

5: ANALGESICS

PRINCIPLES OF USE OF ANALGESICS

Analgesics can be divided into three classes:
- non-opioid
- opioid
- adjuvant (Figure 1).

The principles governing their use are summarized in the WHO Method for Relief of Cancer Pain:[1,2]
- 'By the mouth'
- 'By the clock'
- 'By the ladder' (Figure 2)
- 'Individual dose titration'
- 'Use adjuvant drugs'
- 'Attention to detail'.

Drugs from different classes are used alone or in combination according to the type of pain and response to treatment (Figure 1). Because cancer pain typically has an inflammatory component, it is generally appropriate to optimize treatment with an NSAID and an opioid before introducing adjuvant analgesics. However, with treatment-related pains (e.g. chemotherapy-induced neuropathic pain, chronic postoperative scar pain) and pains unrelated to cancer (e.g. post-herpetic neuralgia, muscle spasm pain), an adjuvant may be an appropriate first-line treatment. For example, an antidepressant or an anti-epileptic for neuropathic pain, or a benzodiazepine or **baclofen** for muscle spasm. Generally, pain management in children is comparable with adults; however, because **codeine** is no longer recommended in children, the WHO analgesic ladder has been reduced to only two steps (see p.348).

In adults, there is also continuing debate about the need for Step 2 of the WHO analgesic ladder.[3,4] There is no absolute pharmacological need for using a weak opioid before progressing to a strong opioid and some palliative care services move directly from Step 1 to Step 3. However,

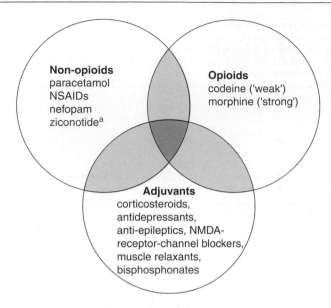

Figure I Broad-spectrum analgesia; drugs from different categories are used alone or in combination according to the type of pain and response to treatment.

a. ziconotide is an N-type calcium-channel blocker, the first of a new type of non-opioid. Its place in palliative care remains to be determined.[6,7]

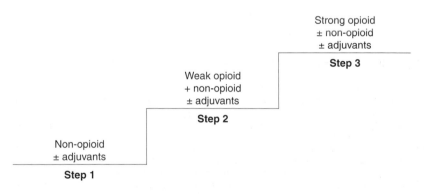

Figure 2 The World Health Organization 3-step analgesic ladder.

in some circumstances, Step 2 is effectively/practically essential. For example, there is a stigma attached to strong opioids and a patient may prefer to try alternatives first. Further, in many countries, access to strong opioids remains difficult (e.g. only as a hospital inpatient, and then sparingly by injection) and sometimes impossible.

When Step 2 is omitted, patients will start on a lower dose of **morphine** than patients who have been taking a weak opioid, e.g. **morphine** 20–30mg/24h (or the equivalent dose of an alternative strong opioid) rather than, say, **morphine** 60mg/24h. Several RCTs indicate that the latter is generally too high a starting dose if Step 2 is omitted.[5]

Break-through (episodic) pain

Break-through (episodic) pain is a term used to describe a transient exacerbation of pain which occurs either spontaneously or in relation to a specific trigger despite relatively stable and adequately controlled background pain. It may or may not be at the same location as the background (controlled) pain.[8,9]

Patients with poorly relieved background pain are excluded because this suggests overall poor pain relief which requires an increase in regular analgesia. Similarly, pain recurring shortly before the next dose of a regular analgesic is due ('end-of-dose-interval pain') is not true break-through pain.

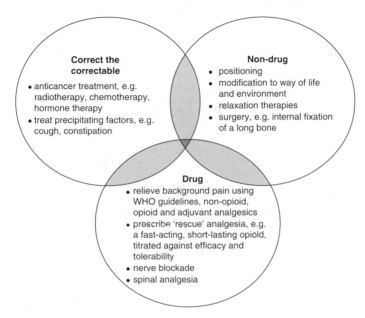

Figure 3 A multimodal approach to managing break-through (episodic) pain.

There are two main types of break-through pain:
- *predictable (incident) pain*, an exacerbation of pain caused by weight-bearing and/or activity (including swallowing, defaecation, coughing, nursing/medical procedures)
- *unpredictable (spontaneous) pain*, unrelated to movement or activity, e.g. colic, stabbing pain associated with nerve injury.

Break-through pain is common in both cancer patients (up to 90%) and non-cancer patients (up to 75%) receiving opioid medication for persistent pain.[10,11] It is often a resurgence of the background pain, and may be either functional (e.g. tension headache) or pathological, and either nociceptive (associated with tissue distortion or injury) or neuropathic (associated with nerve compression or injury). Patients may experience more than one break-through pain, and these may have different causes. Various strategies reduce the impact of break-through pain (Figure 3).[12]

A widespread drug treatment is to give an extra dose of the regular analgesic, e.g. a p.r.n. dose of immediate-release **morphine** for patients taking **morphine** regularly round-the-clock. A traditional practice, dating from before m/r opioid products were available, was to give an extra dose of the regular q4h dose of oral **morphine** (i.e. one sixth of the total daily dose). However, many break-through pains are short-lived and this approach effectively doubles the patient's opioid intake for the next 4h.

Accordingly, many centres now recommend that the patient initially takes, as an immediate-release formulation, 10% of the total daily regular dose as the p.r.n. dose.[13,14] However, a standard fixed-dose is unlikely to suit all patients and all pains, particularly because the intensity and the impact of break-through pain vary considerably. Thus, when patients have been encouraged to optimize their rescue dose, the chosen dose varies from 5–20% of the total daily dose.[15,16]

Generally, break-through pain has a relatively rapid onset and short duration (e.g. 20–30min, ranging from < 1min to > 3h), whereas oral **morphine** has a relatively slow onset of action (30 min) and long duration of effect (3–6h).[17] This helps to explain why many patients choose *not* to take a rescue dose of PO opioid with every episode of break-through pain, particularly when predictable, mild in intensity, and of relatively short duration.[18,19]

Strategies to circumvent the mismatch between break-through pain duration and drug effect latency include:

- timing a predictable painful activity or procedure to coincide with the peak plasma concentration after a regular or rescue PO dose of **morphine** (1–2h) or other strong opioid
- using routes of administration, e.g. buccal, intranasal, SL, which permit more rapid absorption of some (lipophilic) opioids, e.g. **fentanyl**.[20,21]

Transmucosal **fentanyl** (p.413) products cost substantially more than PO opioids; experience with them indicates:[22]

- there is little or no correlation between the dose of the regularly administered strong opioid and the satisfactory rescue dose
- that the rescue dose needs to be individually titrated
- that different products will not be bio-equivalent and can not be substituted for one another (the formulation and route of administration differ)
- serious adverse events and deaths can occur with inappropriate:
  - ▷ patient selection, e.g. opioid non-tolerant, transient pain (postoperative, migraine)
  - ▷ product use, e.g. exceeding recommended frequency of administration, dose-for-dose substitution of one product with another, e.g. Actiq® for Effentora®.

Other options include SL **alfentanil** (see p.385), and PO/SC **ketamine** (see p.625).

---

1 WHO (1986) *Cancer Pain Relief.* World Health Organization, Geneva.

2 WHO (1996) *Cancer Pain Relief: with a guide to opioid availability* (2e). World Health Organisation, Geneva.

3 Tassinari D et al. (2011) The second step of the analgesic ladder and oral tramadol in the treatment of mild to moderate cancer pain: a systematic review. *Palliative Medicine.* 25: 410-423.

4 Caraceni A et al. (2012) Use of opioid analgesics in the treatment of cancer pain: evidence-based recommendations from the EAPC. *Lancet Oncology.* 13: e58–68.

5 Mercadante S (2007) Opioid titration in cancer pain: a critical review. *European Journal of Pain.* 11: 823–830.

6 Prommer EE (2005) Ziconotide: can we use it in palliative care? *American Journal of Hospice and Palliative Care.* 22: 369–374.

7 Narayana AK (2005) Elan: ziconotide review focused on off-label uses. *American Journal of Hospice and Palliative Care.* 22: 408.

8 Davies AN et al. (2009) The management of cancer-related breakthrough pain: recommendations of a task group of the Science Committee of the Association for Palliative Medicine of Great Britain and Ireland. *European Journal of Pain.* 13: 331–338.

9 Douglas I et al. (2000) Central issues in the management of temporal variation in cancer pain. In: R Hillier et al. (eds) *The Effective Management of Cancer Pain.* Aesculapius Medical Press, London, pp. 93–106.

10 Davies A (ed) (2006) Cancer-related breakthrough pain. Oxford University Press, Oxford. UK.

11 Portenoy RK et al. (2006) Prevalence and characteristics of breakthrough pain in opioid-treated patients with chronic noncancer pain. *Journal of Pain.* 7: 583–591.

12 Zeppetella G and Ribeiro MD (2002) Episodic pain in patients with advanced cancer. *American Journal of Hospice and Palliative Care.* 19: 267–276.

13 Davis MP et al. (2005) Controversies in pharmacotherapy of pain management. *Lancet Oncology.* 6: 696–704.

14 Davis MP (2003) Guidelines for breakthrough pain dosing. *American Journal of Hospice and Palliative Care.* 20: 334.

15 Portenoy K and Hagen N (1990) Breakthrough pain: definition, prevalence and characteristics. *Pain.* 41: 273–281.

16 Mercadante S et al. (2002) Episodic (breakthrough) pain: consensus conference of an expert working group of the EAPC. *Cancer.* 94: 832–839.

17 Zeppetella G (2008) Opioids for cancer breakthrough pain: a pilot study reporting patient assessment of time to meaningful pain relief. *Journal of Pain and Symptom Management.* 35: 563–567.

18 Gomez-Batiste X et al. (2002) Breakthrough cancer pain: prevalence and characteristics in Catalonia. *Journal of Pain and Symptom Management.* 24: 45–52.

19 Davies AN et al. (2008) The management of cancer-related breakthrough pain: Recommendations of a task group of the Science Committee of the Association for Palliative Medicine of Great Britain and Ireland. *European Journal of Pain.* 13: 331–338.

20 Davies A et al. (2011) Multi-centre European study of breakthrough cancer pain: Pain characteristics and patient perceptions of current and potential management strategies. *European Journal of Pain.* 15: 756–763.

21 Zeppetella G and Ribeiro MD (2006) Opioids for the management of breakthrough (episodic) pain in cancer patients. *Cochrane Database of Systematic Reviews.* CD004311.

22 Christie J et al. (1998) Dose-titration, multicenter study of oral transmucosal fentanyl citrate for the treatment of breakthrough pain in cancer patients using transdermal fentanyl for persistent pain. *Journal of Clinical Oncology.* 16: 3238–3248.

Updated June 2014

ADJUVANT ANALGESICS

Adjuvant analgesics are drugs whose effect on pain is *circumstance-specific*. Some reduce the painful stimulus directly:
- cancer-related bone pain (bisphosphonates)
- skeletal muscle spasm (skeletal muscle relaxants)
- smooth muscle spasm (antispasmodics)
- cancer-related oedema (corticosteroids).

Others correct changes in pain transmission caused by persistent severe pain and/or damage to the nervous system:
- peripheral sensitization (NSAIDs, corticosteroids)
- ectopic foci caused by nerve damage (some anti-epileptics)
- central sensitization (NMDA-receptor-channel blockers, some anti-epileptics)
- altered descending pain modulation (some antidepressants).

Many act in more than one way (Figure 1). Most are marketed for indications other than pain.

Some adjuvant analgesics take longer to act than standard analgesics, and complete pain relief is not always possible. Undesirable effects are often a limiting factor, particularly in frail patients.[1] As with any analgesic, it is important to discuss with the patient desired outcomes, potential problems and the likely timing of benefits.

Low-dose combined treatment may be preferable if a single drug (appropriately titrated) does not provide adequate relief. For example, when used together for neuropathic pain, **nortriptyline** and **gabapentin** were more effective than either drug alone.[2]

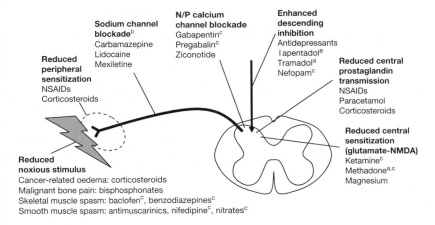

Figure 1   Overview of the peripheral and spinal non-opioid sites of action of analgesics.

a. also act as µ-opioid receptor agonists
b. reduces ectopic nerve signal transmission by damaged neurones (see p.254); the higher concentrations of lidocaine used in local/regional anaesthesia completely inhibit nerve signal transmission
c. additional actions (see individual monographs).

Use relative to other measures

Because cancer pain typically has an inflammatory component, it is generally appropriate to optimize treatment with an NSAID and an opioid before introducing adjuvant analgesics. Subsequently, adjuvant analgesics are added to:
- relieve those pains which fail to respond *and/or*
- reduce undesirable effects, e.g. by reducing opioid dose requirements.

However, with treatment-related pains (e.g. chemotherapy-induced neuropathic pain, chronic postoperative scar pain) and pains unrelated to cancer (e.g. post-herpetic neuralgia, muscle spasm pain), an adjuvant may be an appropriate first-line treatment.

Table 1 Some considerations when selecting an adjuvant analgesic for neuropathic pain[13–17]

Drug	Supporting evidence[a]	Ease of administration				Propensity for drug interactions	Cautions (also see individual monographs)			Approximate typical monthly cost	Examples of concurrent indications in palliative care
		Once daily	Syrup or dispersible	Parenteral	Topical		Cardiac disease	Renal impairment	Seizure threshold		
First line treatments for neuropathic pain											
†Amitriptyline	High	Yes	Yes	No		Moderate	Arrhythmias, CHF, HB, IHD		↓	+ (tablets) ++ (syrup)	Depression, anxiety, bladder spasms, urgency
Duloxetine	Moderate	Yes	No	No		Moderate	Arrhythmias, CHF, HT, IHD	Avoid if GFR < 30	↓	+++	Depression, anxiety, stress incontinence
Gabapentin	High	No	Yes[b]	No		Low		↓ Dose		++	Spasticity, seizures
†Nortriptyline	Moderate	Yes	No	No		Moderate	Arrhythmias, CHF, HB, IHD		↓	++	Depression
Pregabalin	High	No	Yes	No		Low	CHF	↓ Dose		++++	Anxiety, seizures
Treatments generally reserved for use second-line or in specific situations											
Lidocaine 5% plaster[c]	Moderate	Yes		No	Yes	Low	Limited systemic absorption	MAC		++++	
Carbamazepine[d]	Low	No	Yes[e]	No		High	HB			++	Seizures
†Clonazepam	Very low	Yes	Yes[e]	No		Moderate		↓ Dose		+	Spasticity, seizures, anxiety
†Oxcarbazepine	Low	No	Yes	No		Moderate	CCF, HB	↓ Dose		++	Seizures
†Valproate	Low	Yes (m/r)	Yes	Yes (↑SC)		Moderate		↓ Dose		++	Seizures
†Venlafaxine	High	Yes (m/r)	Yes[e]	No		Moderate	Arrhythmias, CHF, HT, IHD	↓ Reduce dose if GFR < 30	↓	+	Depression, anxiety

HB = heart block; CHF = congestive heart failure; HT = hypertension; IHD = ischaemic heart disease; MAC = manufacturer advises caution, but no specific dose alteration. Monthly cost; + = ≤£5, ++ = £5–20, +++ = £20–60, ++++ = ≥£60.

a. based on RCTs vs. case reports, methodological quality, consistency within and between studies, and applicability to palliative care population. Although few RCTs have been conducted in palliative care patients, generalizability was considered more likely if benefit demonstrated in ≥2 neuropathic pain types in palliative care population; also see Chapter 22, Table 2, p.733.
b. capsules can be opened and sprinkled on food (unlicensed use), also see Chapter 22, Table 2, p.733.
c. authorized for post-herpetic neuralgia only
d. first-line choice (and authorized) for trigeminal neuralgia
e. disperses in 5min (unauthorized use), also see Chapter 22, Table 2, p.733.

Antidepressants and anti-epileptics

First-line choices for neuropathic pain include **amitriptyline** (p.208) and **gabapentin** (p.270). Both direct comparisons[3-9] and a large network analysis[10] found their efficacy and tolerability to be comparable with alternatives: **pregabalin** (p.270), **duloxetine** (p.218) and **nortriptyline** (p.210). Choice is thus influenced by cost and individual circumstances (Table 1).

Drugs which act via different mechanisms can be combined if patients do not respond to a single drug (Figure 2).[2] Opioids have been shown in RCTs to at least partly relieve neuropathic pain.[11,12]

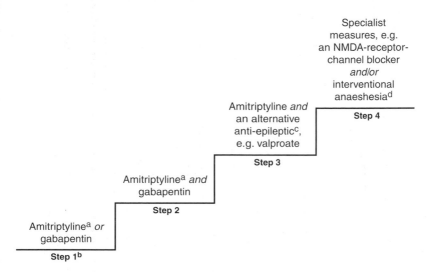

Figure 2 Suggested adjuvant analgesics for neuropathic pain.

a. consider nortriptyline or duloxetine if amitriptyline is poorly tolerated, but *not* if it is ineffective because their mechanism of action are similar (see p.198)
b. systemic corticosteroids are an alternative for *cancer-related* neuropathic pain, particularly if pain is associated with limb weakness or awaiting benefit from another treatment, e.g. radiotherapy
c. it is unknown if patients with an inadequate response to gabapentin are best switched to pregabalin (p.270) or to an anti-epileptic which differs in its mechanism of action, e.g. valproate (p.279). Gabapentin can be switched directly to pregabalin; for all others, generally, the gabapentin is withdrawn once the new anti-epileptic has been titrated to an effective dose (see p.262)
d. e.g. spinal analgesia, nerve block.

Bisphosphonates

Bisphosphonates (see p.489) are osteoclast inhibitors and are used to relieve metastatic bone pain which persists despite analgesics and radiation therapy ± orthopaedic surgery. Although published data relate mainly to breast cancer and myeloma, benefit is also seen with other cancers. About 50% of patients benefit, typically in 1–2 weeks, and this may last for 2–3 months. Benefit may be seen only after a second treatment but, if there is no response after two treatments, nothing is gained by further use.[18,19] In those who respond, continue to treat p.r.n. for as long as there is benefit.

Corticosteroids

Systemic corticosteroids are used for various types of pain (see Systemic corticosteroids, Box A, p.500) particularly for those associated with:
• nerve root/nerve trunk compression
• spinal cord compression
• raised intracranial pressure.

Systemic corticosteroids do not help in pure non-cancer nerve injury pain, e.g. chronic postoperative scar pain, post-herpetic neuralgia. However, in cancer-related nerve injury pain, a 5–7 day trial of **dexamethasone** may be beneficial.

Epidural depot corticosteroids are sometimes used to relieve radicular pain associated with a spinal metastasis (see p.583).

NMDA-receptor-channel blockers

NMDA-receptor-channel blockers are most commonly used when neuropathic pain does not respond well to standard analgesics together with an antidepressant and an anti-epileptic. They have also been used in ischaemic pain,[20] bone pain,[21] and severe mucositis.[22] NMDA-receptor-channel blockers include:

- ketamine (see p.625)
- methadone (see p.433)
- **magnesium** (see p.571).

Despite promising case reports, **amantadine** and **memantine** are *not* consistently beneficial in RCTs.[23]

Skeletal muscle relaxants

These include **baclofen, diazepam**, and **tizanidine** (see p.589). Although non-drug treatment is generally preferable for painful skeletal muscle spasm (cramp) and myofascial pain, e.g. physical therapy (local heat, massage),[24] some patients also benefit from relaxation therapy ± **diazepam** (see p.155). Myofascial trigger points often benefit from acupuncture or direct injection of local anaesthetic.[25] *However severe,* **morphine** *is ineffective for the relief of cramp and trigger point pains.*

Smooth muscle relaxants (antispasmodics)

This is a heterogeneous group of drugs encompassing antimuscarinics, **glyceryl trinitrate** (see p.79), and L-type calcium-channel blockers (e.g. **nifedipine**, see p.83). Antimuscarinics are used to relieve visceral distension pain and colic. In advanced cancer, there is little place for 'weak' antispasmodics, e.g. **dicycloverine**.

Hyoscine *butylbromide* (see p.15) and **glycopyrronium** (see p.12) are quaternary drugs which do not cross the blood–brain barrier, and are widely regarded as the antispasmodics of choice. Although **atropine** and **hyoscine** *hydrobromide* have comparable peripheral effects, they also have central effects, either stimulatory or sedative, and may precipitate delirium (see p.5).

Glyceryl trinitrate and calcium-channel blockers can be used for the same range of indications, but tend to be reserved for painful spasm of the oesophagus, rectum and anus (see p.79).

1 Bennett MI (2011) Effectiveness of antiepileptic or antidepressant drugs when added to opioids for cancer pain: systematic review. *Palliative Medicine.* **25**: 553–559

2 Gilron I et al. (2009) Nortriptyline and gabapentin, alone and in combination for neuropathic pain: a double-blind, randomised controlled crossover trial. *Lancet.* **374**: 1252–1261.

3 Boyle J et al. (2012) Randomized, placebo-controlled comparison of amitriptyline, duloxetine, and pregabalin in patients with chronic diabetic peripheral neuropathic pain: impact on pain, polysomnographic sleep, daytime functioning, and quality of life. *Diabetes Care.* **35**: 2451–2458.

4 Bansal D et al. (2009) Amitriptyline vs. pregabalin in painful diabetic neuropathy: a randomized double blind clinical trial. *Diabetic Medicine.* **26**: 1019–1026.

5 Morello CM et al. (1999) Randomized double-blind study comparing the efficacy of gabapentin with amitriptyline on diabetic peripheral neuropathy pain. *Archives of Internal Medicine.* **159**: 1931–1937.

6 Chandra K et al. (2006) Gabapentin versus nortriptyline in post-herpetic neuralgia patients: a randomized, double-blind clinical trial–the GONIP Trial. *International Journal of Clinical Pharmacology and Therapeutics.* **44**: 358–363.

7 Mishra S et al. (2012) A comparative efficacy of amitriptyline, gabapentin, and pregabalin in neuropathic cancer pain: a prospective randomized double-blind placebo-controlled study. *American Journal of Hospice and Palliative Care.* **29**: 177–182.

8 Banerjee M et al. (2013) A comparative study of efficacy and safety of gabapentin versus amitriptyline as coanalgesics in patients receiving opioid analgesics for neuropathic pain in malignancy. *Indian Journal of Pharmacology.* **45**: 334–338.

9 Kelle B (2012) The efficacy of gabapentin and pregabalin in the treatment of neuropathic pain due to peripheral nerve injury. *Journal of Musculoskeletal Pain.* **20**: 300–305.

10 NICE (2013) Neuropathic pain - pharmacological management. *Clinical Guideline.* CG173. (appendix G) www.nice.org.uk

11 Eisenberg E et al. (2006) Efficacy of mu-opioid agonists in the treatment of evoked neuropathic pain: Systematic review of randomized controlled trials. *European Journal of Pain.* **10**: 667–676.

12 Eisenberg E et al. (2005) Efficacy and safety of opioid agonists in the treatment of neuropathic pain of nonmalignant origin: systematic review and meta-analysis of randomized controlled trials. *Journal of the American Medical Association.* **293**: 3043–3052.

13 Wiffen PJ et al. (2010) Anitconvulsant drugs for acute and chronic pain. *Cochrane Database of Systematic Reviews.* **1**: CD0011133.

14 Saarto T and Wiffen PJ (2007) Antidepressants for neuropathic pain. *Cochrane Database of Systematic Reviews.* CD005454.

15 Finnerup (2010) The evidence for pharmaceutical treatment of neuropathic pain. *Pain.* **150**: 573–581.

16 Attal N et al. (2010) EFNS guidelines on the pharmacological treatment of neuropathic pain: 2010 revision. *European Journal of Neurology.* **17**: 1113–e1188.

17 Dworkin RH et al. (2010) Recommendations for the pharmacological management of neuropathic pain: an overview and literature update. *Mayo Clinic Proceedings.* **85**: S3–14.

18 Mannix K et al. (2000) Using bisphosphonates to control the pain of bone metastases: evidence-based guidelines for palliative care. *Palliative Medicine.* **14**: 455–461.

19 Wong R and Wiffen PJ (2002) Bisphosphonates for the relief of pain secondary to bone metastases. *Cochrane Database Systematic Reviews.* **2**: CD002068.

20 Mitchell AC and Fallon MT (2002) A single infusion of intravenous ketamine improves pain relief in patients with critical limb ischaemia: results of a double blind randomised controlled trial. *Pain.* **97**: 275–281.

21 Mercadante S et al. (2009) Opioid switching and burst ketamine to improve the opioid response in patients with movement-related pain due to bone metastases. *Clinical Journal of Pain.* **25**: 648–649.

22 Jackson K et al. (2001) 'Burst' ketamine for refractory cancer pain: an open-label audit of 39 patients. *Journal of Pain and Symptom Management.* **22**: 834–842.

23 Collins S et al. (2010) NMDA receptor antagonists for the treatment of neuropathic pain. *Pain Medicine.* **11**: 1726–1742.

24 Twycross R et al. (2009) *Symptom Management in Advanced Cancer* (4e). palliativedrugs.com, Nottingham.

25 Sola A and Bonica J (1990) Myofascial pain syndromes. In: J Bonica (ed) *The Management of Pain* (2e). Lea and Febiger, Philadelphia, pp. 352–367.

Updated June 2014

PARACETAMOL   BNF 4.7.1

There are increasing reports of unintentional overdose of paracetamol (acetaminophen USAN) resulting in hepatotoxicity. To reduce this risk, the dose of paracetamol should never exceed the maximum recommended dose, be appropriate for the weight of the patient, and be reduced when risk factors for hepatotoxicity exist, e.g. old age, poor nutritional status, fasting/anorexia, concurrent use of drugs which interact with paracetamol metabolism, and chronic alcohol use.

Class: Non-opioid analgesic.

Indications: *PO* mild–moderate pain, migraine and tension headache, fever.
IV short-term treatment of mild–moderate pain, moderate–severe pain (in combination with an opioid) and fever when PO or PR routes not possible.

Contra-indications: *IV* severe hepatic impairment or severe active liver disease.

Pharmacology

Paracetamol is a synthetic non-opioid analgesic and antipyretic.[1,2] It acts mainly in the CNS, where it has several effects. It is a weak inhibitor of cyclo-oxygenase (COX)-2, an effect that lasts a short time ($\leq$2h) after a dose,[3,4] but can also be anti-inflammatory through inhibition of peroxidase regeneration. The latter action, which prevents the oxidation of inactive COX to active COX, can be significant when peroxidase levels are low, e.g. in intact cells in the CNS, but not when peroxidase levels are much higher, e.g. with tissue damage and/or inflammation in the periphery.[5] In addition, paracetamol has been shown to:

- interact with L-arginine-nitric oxide, opioid and cannabinoid systems[6,7]
- activate descending serotoninergic inhibitory pain pathways.[8,9]

It is possible that the analgesic effect of paracetamol is dependent on synergy between some or all these mechanisms.[10] Evidence of synergy between paracetamol and NSAIDs suggests differing analgesic mechanisms.[11,12]

Paracetamol is widely used for acute musculoskeletal pains and acute headache. When used in combination with an opioid to treat *postoperative pain*, IV paracetamol has an 'opioid-sparing' effect and improves overall analgesia.[13] Postoperative nausea and vomiting is also reduced, but only when the paracetamol is administered before, during or immediately after surgery. The improvement correlated with the degree of pain relief (but not opioid use), suggesting a possible indirect or direct anti-emetic effect of paracetamol.[14]

Evidence of the efficacy of paracetamol in combination with an opioid in the treatment of *cancer pain* is mixed. However, the RCTs that suggested no benefit[15,16] were underpowered,[17] and another RCT showed a small but clinically important additive effect in about one-third of patients despite the fact that half were already taking an NSAID or a corticosteroid.[18] Given that a paracetamol regimen of 500mg–1g q.d.s. may pose a considerable pill burden to some patients with cancer, a pragmatic solution might be:

- to limit the long-term use of paracetamol to patients in whom definite benefit is seen within 2 days of starting it
- if already taking paracetamol with definite past benefit and increasing pain necessitates the *addition* of an opioid, the ongoing need for paracetamol should be determined by stopping it after 3–4 days of satisfactory pain relief with both drugs; the paracetamol is restarted only if the pain returns.

Single doses of IV paracetamol provide dose-dependent analgesia in doses up to 2g.[19] Increased peak plasma concentrations lead to earlier and higher concentrations of paracetamol in the CSF, which in turn lead to an earlier onset of action, a longer duration of action, and a greater overall analgesic effect.[20] In patients undergoing molar dental extraction, compared with 1g, 2g of paracetamol gave 50% more relief for 50% more time (5h vs. 3.2h).[21] Thus, there may be a place for an initial loading dose when prescribing paracetamol.

Parenteral **propacetamol**, an inactive pro-drug of paracetamol, is available in some countries (not UK), and is used particularly for orthopaedic postoperative pain management.[22] **Propacetamol** 2g yields paracetamol 1g.[23] Because of a significant risk of sensitization, the manufacturer's protocol must be adhered to.

Only 2–5% of a therapeutic dose of paracetamol is excreted unchanged in the urine; the remainder is metabolized mainly by the liver. At therapeutic doses, >80% of paracetamol is metabolized to glucuronide and sulfate conjugates. About 5–10% is converted by hepatic CYP450 enzymes to a highly reactive metabolite, N-acetyl-p-benzoquinoneimine (NAPQI; Figure 1) which is hepatotoxic. However, with typical therapeutic doses (≤1g q.d.s.), NAPQI is generally inactivated sufficiently rapidly so as not to cause liver damage.

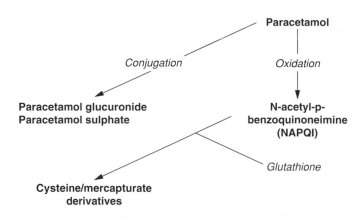

Figure 1 Metabolism of paracetamol.

The main enzyme involved is CYP2E1 which metabolizes 30–80% of a dose of paracetamol. Up to about 25% is metabolized by CYP3A4 (particularly at lower doses) and CYP2D6 (particularly at higher doses).[24] There are also genetic variations.[25] For example, those with CYP2D6 gene duplication (ultra-rapid metabolizers), have a greater susceptibility to hepatotoxicity because of the increased production of NAPQI.[26]

The metabolism of paracetamol is also gender-dependent (women eliminate the drug more slowly[27]) and age-dependent (increased risk of hepatotoxicity in the elderly[28]). An 80 year-old may be exposed to 1.5 times the NAPQI concentration as a 20 year-old when given the same dose of IV paracetamol.[28] Specific drugs also may inhibit glucuronidation or induce the oxidation of paracetamol to NAPQI (Box A).

Box A Risk factors for paracetamol hepatoxicity[24,29,30]

Old age
Poor nutritional status } lower glutathione stores
Fasting/anorexia
Concurrent use of glucuronidation inhibitors and/or CYP2E1-inducing drugs, e.g. phenobarbital, probably isoniazid, and possibly St John's wort
Chronic alcohol abuse.

Unintentional and deliberate overdose and NAPQI-induced hepatotoxicity

An overdose of paracetamol overwhelms its normal metabolism, shifting more paracetamol into the NAPQI pathway. NAPQI is normally inactivated by conjugation with glutathione but, in overdose, the body's glutathione store becomes exhausted and the accumulation of NAPQI leads to liver parenchymal cell death.

Although overdose is traditionally associated with ingestion of a large single dose of paracetamol as a deliberate suicide attempt, reports of unintentional overdose from its analgesic use are increasing.[31,32] A man aged 43 with Crohn's colitis and weighing 30kg died of hepatic failure after taking 4g/24h for only 4 days.[33] Indeed, there are numerous reports of hepatotoxicity associated with chronic use of 5–7.5g/24h.[34] Thus, the dose of paracetamol must always be appropriate for the weight and circumstances of the patient, and the maximum recommended dose not exceeded.

Repeated suprathreshold ingestion over a time period of >8h ('staggered overdose') produces a higher risk of liver and multi-organ failure, and a lower unassisted survival rate, than single time point overdose. About two-thirds of staggered overdoses relate to medicinal use rather than attempted suicide.[35] The likelihood of an unintentional/staggered overdose is greater in patients with one or more risk factors for paracetamol hepatotoxicity (see Box A).

A single time point overdose of paracetamol below 125mg/kg (7.5g or 15 tablets in a 60kg person) is unlikely to result in liver damage. At twice this dose, the probability of liver damage is around 50%, but the individual may remain well. A dose of 500mg/kg (30g or 60 tablets in a 60kg person) is almost certain to produce life-threatening liver damage. Paracetamol overdose can also lead to acute renal failure, although this is often reversible without the need for dialysis.[36]

With IV paracetamol poisoning, contact the UK National Poisons Information Service for advice (0844 892 0111).

Overdose can be treated with a glutathione precursor, e.g. IVI **acetylcysteine** (Box B)[37–39] or PO **methionine** (not UK).[40] If given within 15h of the overdose, acetylcysteine prevents NAPQI from reacting with liver cell proteins. Further, because it has a protective effect against apoptosis (programmed cell death), acetylcysteine can help to a lesser extent if given for ≤3 days after the overdose.

Box B IVI acetylcysteine[38]

Three separate consecutive IVI totalling 300mg/kg are given in 5% glucose over 21h. For those weighing 41–100kg:
* *first (loading)* IVI:150mg/kg diluted in 200mL over 1h
* *second IVI:* 50mg/kg diluted in 500mL over 4h
* *third IVI:* 100mg/kg diluted in 1000mL over 16h.
For those weighing 21–40kg, use half the volume.
For patients whose weight falls outside of these ranges, see SPC.
Saline 0.9% can be used as an alternative diluent.

Acute alcohol intake does *not* increase the risk of hepatotoxicity. Indeed, because alcohol and paracetamol compete for the same oxidative enzymes, acute alcohol consumption at the time of a paracetamol overdose may be protective. However, because alcohol consumption induces the production of the relevant enzymes, if *chronic* alcohol use suddenly stops, paracetamol will be metabolized more rapidly, and could lead to hepatotoxicity.[41] In any case, some alcoholics are more susceptible to paracetamol toxicity, possibly because of their poor nutritional status.[42]

In the USA, to reduce the chance of unintentional overdose, the FDA has recommended that:[43,44]

- the amount of paracetamol in a prescription tablet, capsule, or other dosage unit is limited to a maximum of 325mg
- the maximum single dose is lowered to 650mg
- a boxed warning is added highlighting the potential for severe liver injury
- patients should not to exceed a total daily dose of 4g.

Implementation is in process and 'extra strength' products containing 500mg/dose unit remain available. However, over-the-counter products now recommend a maximum dose of 2.6–3g/24h, which patients should not exceed unless directed by a doctor.

Bio-availability 60% after 500mg PO, 90% after 1g PO; PR is about two thirds of PO, but is higher with two 500mg suppositories than with one 1g suppository.

Onset of action 15–30min PO; 5–10min IV (pain relief), 30min IV (antipyretic effect).

Time to peak plasma concentration widely variable PO, e.g. 20min in fasting state but 1–2h if delayed gastric emptying;[45] 15min IVl (this is synchronous with the end of a 15min infusion).

Plasma halflife 1.25–3h PO;[45] 2–3h IV.

Duration of action 4–6h PO and IV.

Cautions

Severe hepatic impairment or severe active liver disease (IV use contra-indicated in this setting), particularly if associated with alcohol dependence and malnutrition. In severe renal impairment (creatinine clearance <30mL/min), the dose interval should ⩾6h.

Most dispersible or effervescent paracetamol-containing tablets (alone or combined with an opioid) have a Na^+ content of ⩾14mmol/tablet. Thus, a dose of 8 tablets/24h would exceed the recommended maximum daily dietary Na^+ intake of 100mmol (6g of sodium chloride). Dispersible or effervescent formulations should thus be avoided in patients with hypertension or renal impairment, particularly if already on a salt-restricted diet. In contrast, non-soluble formulations contain negligible Na^+.[46]

Paracetamol can be taken by at least two thirds of patients who are hypersensitive to **aspirin** or other NSAID.[47,48] In people with a history of **aspirin**/NSAID-induced asthma, give a test dose of 250mg (half a tablet) and observe for 2–3h. If no undesirable effects occur, paracetamol can safely be used in standard doses.[49]

Drug interactions

Concurrent use of glucuronidation inhibitors and/or CYP2E1-inducing drugs, e.g. **phenobarbital**, probably **isoniazid**, and possibly **St John's wort** may increase the risk of paracetamol toxicity (Box A).[24]

There are mixed reports of the analgesic effect of paracetamol being reduced by $5HT_3$ antagonists, possibly by blocking the action of serotonin at presynaptic $5HT_3$-receptors on primary afferent nociceptive neurones in the spinal dorsal horn.[10,50]

Concurrent use with **warfarin**: a regular *daily* intake of paracetamol ⩾1300mg for one week may increase the INR to >6,[51,52] but a total *weekly* dose of paracetamol of ⩽2g has no effect. The underlying mechanism is not clear, but may relate to interference with the hepatic synthesis of factors II, VII, IX and X. A recent post-mortem series found that concurrent paracetamol increases the risk of a bleed with **warfarin** 2.7 times.[53]

Undesirable effects

Very common (>10%): dyspepsia, elevated liver enzymes (Box C).

Rare (<0.1%, >0.01%): PO cholestatic jaundice,[54,55] acute pancreatitis, thrombocytopenia, agranulocytosis, serious skin reactions,[56] anaphylaxis.[57–59] **IV** malaise, hypotension.

Box C   Paracetamol and elevated liver enzymes[60,61]

The plasma concentrations of liver enzymes (alanine aminotransferase (ALT), aspartate aminotransferase, γ-glutamyl transferase) can increase with normal doses of paracetamol.

For example, ALT increased >3 times the upper limit of normal in 40% of young healthy volunteers receiving 4g/day, with the highest increase 14–16 times greater. The rise was evident after 72h, and persisted for a median of one week after discontinuation.

These changes are probably unimportant in the absence of functional or synthetic liver impairment (e.g. indicated by an increase in plasma bilirubin or a reduction in clotting factors respectively) and possibly improve with ongoing use, although this is poorly documented.

Awareness of this phenomenon may aid interpretation of abnormal LFTs, and help avoid the erroneous assumption that rapidly worsening LFTs must indicate rapidly worsening disease within the liver, e.g. from liver metastases.

Chronic paracetamol use increases the risk of renal impairment 2.5 times; and the risk is related to dose and cumulative exposure over a lifetime.[62,63] The risk is higher in diabetics, and when renal impairment is associated with systemic vasculitis.

The use of paracetamol in pregnancy and early childhood increases the risk of a child developing asthma.[64] However, there is no hard evidence that paracetamol precipitates asthma in established asthmatics.[49,65]

Dose and use

In palliative care, typical PO doses for adults generally range from 500mg–1g q.d.s.[18] However, in patients with risk factors for paracetamol hepatotoxicity (Box A), it is safer to opt for a submaximal dose. Further, despite the lower PR bio-availability, in practice the rectal dose is generally the same as the PO dose.

IV

IV paracetamol (1g in 100mL) is given by infusion over 15min. There have been case reports of massive inadvertent iatrogenic IV overdose leading to hepatic failure, sometimes fatal, particularly in children.[66] The available IV solution contains 10mg/mL. When written up just as mg, it has occasionally been misread and given as mL, with the result that the patient has received *10 times* the prescribed dose. To minimize the chance of this happening, a prescription for IV paracetamol should be written in terms of *both* mg *and* mL, not just as mg.

IV paracetamol can be used when administration PO or PR is not possible. The dose depends on body weight and the presence/absence of risk factors for paracetamol hepatotoxicity:
• adults and children >50kg, 1g up to q4h, maximum recommended dose 4g/24h
• adults and children >50kg *plus any risk factors*, restrict maximum dose to 3g/24h
• adults and children 10–50kg, 15mg/kg up to q4h, maximum recommended dose 60mg/kg/24h.

Supply

PO paracetamol is available OTC alone and in several combination products with weak opioids (see **Codeine**, p.348, **Dihydrocodeine**, p.350 and **Tramadol**, p.352).

Paracetamol (generic)
Tablets and caplets 500mg, 28 days @ 1g q.d.s. = £6.
Tablets dispersible 120mg, 500mg, 28 days @ 1g q.d.s. = £21; *may contain Na+ up to 20mmol/ tablet.*
Capsules 500mg, 28 days @ 1g q.d.s. = £9.
Oral suspension 120mg/5mL, 250mg/5mL, 28 days @ 1g q.d.s. = £19; *available sugar free.*

A *500mg/5mL oral suspension is available but is almost 10 times the cost.*
Suppositories 60mg, 125mg, 250mg, 500mg, 1g, 28 days @ 1g q.d.s. = £560.

Panadol OA® (GSK)
Tablets 1g, 28 days @ 1g q.d.s. = £4.

Perfalgan® (Bristol-Myers Squibb)
Injection (for IV infusion) 10mg/mL, 50mL (500mg) vial = £1.50, 100mL vial (1g) = £1.50.

1 Twycross RG et al. (2000) Paracetamol. *Progress in Palliative Care.* **8**: 198–202.
2 Flower RJ and Vane JR (1972) Inhibition of prostaglandin synthetase in brain explains the anti-pyretic activity of paracetamol. *Nature.* **240**: 410–411.
3 Hinz B et al. (2008) Acetaminophen (paracetamol) is a selective cyclooxygenase-2 inhibitor in man. *FASEB J.* **22**: 383–390.
4 Hinz B and Brune K (2012) Paracetamol and cyclooxygenase inhibition: is there a cause for concern? *Annals of the Rheumatic Diseases.* **71**: 20–25.
5 Mattia A and Coluzzi F (2009) What anesthesiologists should know about paracetamol (acetaminophen). *Minerva Anestesiologica.* **75**: 644–653.
6 Bjorkman R et al. (1994) Acetaminophen (paracetamol) blocks spinal hyperalgesia induced by NMDA and substance P. *Pain.* **57**: 259–264.
7 Pini L et al. (1997) Naloxone-reversible antinociception by paracetamol in the rat. *Journal of Pharmacology and Experimental Therapeutics.* **280**: 934–940.
8 Mallet C et al. (2008) Endocannabinoid and serotonergic systems are needed for acetaminophen-induced analgesia. *Pain.* **139**: 190–200.
9 Dogrul A et al. (2012) Systemic paracetamol-induced analgesic and antihyperalgesic effects through activation of descending serotonergic pathways involving spinal 5-HT(7) receptors. *European Journal of Pharmacology.* **677**: 93–101.
10 Pickering G et al. (2006) Analgesic effect of acetaminophen in humans: first evidence of a central serotonergic mechanism. *Clinical and Pharmacology and Therapeutics.* **79**: 371–378.
11 Miranda HF et al. (2006) Synergism between paracetamol and nonsteroidal anti-inflammatory drugs in experimental acute pain. *Pain.* **121**: 22–28.
12 Ong CK et al. (2010) Combining paracetamol (acetaminophen) with nonsteroidal antiinflammatory drugs: a qualitative systematic review of analgesic efficacy for acute postoperative pain. *Anesthesia and Analgesia.* **110**: 1170–1179.
13 Tzortzopoulou A et al. (2011) Single dose intravenous propacetamol or intravenous paracetamol for postoperative pain. *Cochrane Database of Systematic Reviews.* **10**: CD007126.
14 Apfel CC et al. (2013) Intravenous acetaminophen reduces postoperative nausea and vomiting: a systematic review and meta-analysis. *Pain.* **154**: 677–689.
15 Axelsson B and Christensen S (2003) Is there an additive analgesic effect of paracetamol at step 3? A double-blind randomized controlled study. *Palliative Medicine.* **17**: 724–725.
16 Israel FJ et al. (2010) Lack of benefit from paracetamol (acetaminophen) for palliative cancer patients requiring high-dose strong opioids: a randomized, double-blind, placebo-controlled, crossover trial. *Journal of Pain and Symptom Management.* **39**: 548–554.
17 Formby FT (2010) Re: lack of benefit from paracetamol (acetaminophen) for palliative cancer patients. *Journal of Pain and Symptom Management.* **40**: e6; author reply e6–7.
18 Stockler M et al. (2004) Acetaminophen (paracetamol) improves pain and well-being in people with advanced cancer already receiving a strong opioid regimen: a randomized, double-blind, placebo-controlled cross-over trial. *Journal of Clinical Oncology.* **22**: 3389–3394.
19 Piguet V et al. (1998) Lack of acetaminophen ceiling effect on R-III nociceptive flexion reflex. *European Journal of Clinical Pharmacology.* **53**: 321–324.
20 Jarde O and Boccard E (1997) Parenteral versus oral route increases paracetamol efficacy. *Clinical Drug Investigations.* **14**: 474–481.
21 Juhl GI et al. (2006) Analgesic efficacy and safety of intravenous paracetamol (acetaminophen) administered as a 2g starting dose following third molar surgery. *European Journal of Pain.* **10**: 371–377.
22 Peduto VA et al. (1998) Efficacy of propacetamol in the treatment of postoperative pain. Morphine-sparing effect in orthopedic surgery. Italian Collaborative Group on Propacetamol. *Acta anaesthesiologica Scandinavica.* **42**: 293–298.
23 Flouvat B et al. (2004) Bioequivalence study comparing a new paracetamol solution for injection and propacetamol after single intravenous infusion in healthy subjects. *International Journal of Clinical Pharmacology and Therapeutics.* **42**: 50–57.
24 Kalsi S and Wood DM (2011) Does cytochrome P450 liver isoenzyme induction increase the risk of liver toxicity after paracetamol overdose? *Open Access Emergency Medicine.* **3**: 69–76.
25 Zhao L and Pickering G (2011) Paracetamol metabolism and related genetic differences. *Drug Metabolism Reviews.* **43**: 41–52.
26 Dong H et al. (2000) Involvement of human cytochrome P450 2D6 in the bioactivation of acetaminophen. *Drug Metabolism and Disposition.* **28**: 1397–1400.
27 Liukas A et al. (2011) Pharmacokinetics of intravenous paracetamol in elderly patients. *Clinical Pharmacokinetics.* **50**: 121–129.
28 Mitchell SJ et al. (2011) Age-related changes in the hepatic pharmacology and toxicology of paracetamol. *Current Gerontology and Geriatrics Research* **624156**: www.hindawi.com/journals/cggr/2011/624156/
29 Zimmerman H and Maddrey W (1995) Acetaminophen (paracetamol) hepatotoxicity with regular intake of alcohol: analysis of instances of therapeutic misadventure. *Hepatology.* **22**: 767–773.
30 Horsmans Y et al. (1998) Paracetamol-induced liver toxicity after intravenous administration. *Liver.* **18**: 294–295.
31 MHRA (2010) Intravenous paracetamol (Perfalgan): risk of accidental overdose especially in infants and neonates. *Drug Safety Update.* **3**. www.mhra.gov.uk/Safetyinformation
32 Larson AM et al. (2005) Acetaminophen-induced acute liver failure: results of a United States multicenter, prospective study. *Hepatology.* **42**: 1364–1372.
33 Claridge LC et al. (2010) Acute liver failure after administration of paracetamol at the maximum recommended daily dose in adults. *British Medical Journal.* **341**: c6764.

34 Krenzelok EP (2009) The FDA Acetaminophen Advisory Committee Meeting - what is the future of acetaminophen in the United States? The perspective of a committee member. *Clinical Toxicology.* **47**: 784–789.

35 Craig DG et al. (2012) Staggered overdose pattern and delay to hospital presentation are associated with adverse outcomes following paracetamol-induced hepatotoxicity. *British Journal of Clinical Pharmacology.* **73**: 285–294.

36 von Mach MA et al. (2005) Experiences of a poison center network with renal insufficiency in acetaminophen overdose: an analysis of 17 cases. *Clinical Toxicology.* **43**: 31–37.

37 MHRA (2012) Paracetamol overdose: new guidance on treatment with intravenous acetylcysteine. *Drug Safety Update.* **6**. www.mhra.gov.uk//Safetyinformation

38 British National Formulary *Emergency treatment of poisoning.* London: BMJ Group and Pharmaceutical Press www.bnf.org (accessed March 2014).

39 UCB Pharma (2012) Parvolex 200mg/mL Concentrate for solution for infusion. *SPC.* www.medicines.org.uk

40 Ferner RE et al. (2011) Management of paracetamol poisoning. *British Medical Journal.* **342**: 968–972.

41 Gomez-Moreno G et al. (2008) Interaction of paracetamol in chronic alcoholic patients. Importance for odontologists. *Medicina Oral, Patologia Oral Y Cirugia Bucal.* **13**: E235–238.

42 Riordan SM and Williams R (2002) Alcohol exposure and paracetamol-induced hepatotoxicity. *Addiction Biology.* **7**: 191–206.

43 FDA (2009) Liver injury related to the use of acetaminophen in both over-the-counter and prescription products. Advisory Committee Meeting (transcript). www.fda.gov/Drugs/DrugSafety/InformationbyDrugClass/ucm165107.htm

44 FDA (2011) Prescription acetaminophen products to be limited to 325mg per dosage unit; boxed warning will highlight potential for severe liver failure. Drug Safety Communication. www.fda.gov/Drugs/DrugSafety

45 Prescott LF (1996) *Paracetamol (Acetaminophen) A Critical Bibliographic Review.* Taylor & Francis, London

46 UK Medicines Information (2012) What is the sodium content of medicines? *Q&As.* **145.4**: www.evidence.nhs.uk

47 Szczeklik A (1986) Analgesics, allergy and asthma. *Drugs.* **32**: 148–163.

48 Settipane R et al. (1995) Prevalence of cross-sensitivity with acetaminophen in aspirin-sensitive asthmatic subjects. *Journal of Allergy and Clinical Immunology.* **96**: 480–485.

49 Shin G et al. (2000) Paracetamol and asthma. *Thorax.* **55**: 882–884.

50 Jokela R et al. (2010) The influence of ondansetron on the analgesic effect of acetaminophen after laparoscopic hysterectomy. *Clinical Pharmacology and Therapeutics.* **87**: 672–678.

51 Bell W (1998) Acetaminophen and warfarin: undesirable synergy. *Journal of the American Medical Association.* **279**: 702–703.

52 Hylek E et al. (1998) Acetaminophen and other risk factors for excessive warfarin in anticoagulation. *Journal of the American Medical Association.* **279**: 657–662.

53 Launiainen T et al. (2010) Adverse interaction of warfarin and paracetamol: evidence from a post-mortem study. *European Journal of Clinical Pharmacology.* **66**: 97–103.

54 Waldum H et al. (1992) Can NSAIDs cause acute biliary pain and cholestasis? *Journal of Clinical Gastroenterology.* **14**: 328–330.

55 Wong V et al. (1993) Paracetamol and acute biliary pain with cholestasis. *Lancet.* **342**: 869.

56 FDA (2013) FDA warns of rare but serious skin reactions with the pain reliever/fever reducer acetaminophen. Drug Safety Communication 08/01/2013. www.fda.gov/drugs/drugSafety

57 Leung R et al. (1992) Paracetamol anaphylaxis. *Clinical and Experimental Allergy.* **22**: 831–833.

58 Mendizabal S and Gomez MD (1998) Paracetamol sensitivity without aspirin intolerance. *Allergy.* **53**: 457–458.

59 Morgan S and Dorman S (2004) Paracetamol (acetaminophen) allergy. *Journal of Pain and Symptom Management.* **27**: 99–101.

60 Watkins PB et al. (2006) Aminotransferase elevations in healthy adults receiving 4 grams of acetaminophen daily: a randomized controlled trial. *Journal of the American Medical Association.* **296**: 87–93.

61 Dart RC and Bailey E (2007) Does therapeutic use of acetaminophen cause acute liver failure? *Pharmacotherapy.* **27**: 1219–1230.

62 D'Arcy P (1997) Paracetamol. *Adverse Drug Reaction Toxicology Review.* **16**: 9–14.

63 Fored CM et al. (2001) Acetaminophen, aspirin, and chronic renal failure. *New England Journal of Medicine.* **345**: 1801–1808.

64 Holgate ST (2011) The acetaminophen enigma in asthma. *American Journal of Respiratory Critical Care Medicine.* **183**: 147–148.

65 Shaheen S et al. (2000) Frequent paracetamol use and asthma in adults. *Thorax.* **55**: 266–270.

66 Dart RC and Rumack BH (2012) Intravenous acetaminophen in the United States: iatrogenic dosing errors. *Pediatrics.* **129**: 349–353.

Updated (minor change) June 2014

NEFOPAM   BNF 4.7.1

Class: Non-opioid analgesic, benzoxazocine.

Indication: Pain.

Contra-indications: Concurrent use of an MAOI, epilepsy.

Pharmacology

Nefopam is a centrally acting synthetic analgesic. Its dominant mode of action is uncertain. Mono-amine re-uptake inhibition may explain its effect on the descending pain modulatory pathway.[1] However, despite being used for over 30 years, there are no reports of nefopam causing serotonin toxicity either alone or with other serotoninergic drugs.[2]

Nefopam also blocks voltage-gated sodium and calcium channels associated with glutamic acid, an excitatory neurotransmitter.[3,4] Its effects are not reversed by **naloxone**. It does not inhibit cyclo-oxygenase (COX) or affect platelet function.[5] Antimuscarinic and sympathomimetic properties may account for some of its undesirable effects.

Nefopam is metabolized in the liver to an active metabolite, desmethylnefopam. This is subsequently renally eliminated.[6] Despite this, excretion of nefopam itself is prolonged in end-stage renal failure, perhaps because of secondary hepatic impairment.[7] Post-operatively, single parenteral doses provided analgesia for ⩽5h.[8,9] However, pharmacological effects were seen for ⩽12h after oral doses in healthy volunteers,[6] possibly reflecting the longer halflife of desmethylnefopam.

Nefopam is as effective as NSAIDs in cancer pain[10] and osteo-arthritis but less well tolerated.[11] In postoperative pain, IV or IM nefopam 20mg (equivalent to 60mg PO) is:
- comparable with NSAIDs, reducing morphine requirements in the first 24h by 10–15mg[12,13]
- comparable with ketamine 10mg[14]
- superior to propacetamol 2g.[15]

Nefopam does not consistently improve analgesia or reduce opioid requirements when combined with an NSAID ± ketamine.[16–19] Nefopam is reported to control refractory hiccup.[20,21]

Bio-availability 36%.
Onset of action < 1h.
Time to peak plasma concentration 1–3h PO, 1.5h IM.
Plasma halflife 4–5h; desmethylnefopam 10–15h.[6]
Duration of action ⩽12h PO; ⩽5h IV (see text).

Cautions

Hepatic and renal impairment (reduce dose); prostatism; closed angle glaucoma (antimuscarinic). Exacerbates the undesirable effects of concurrently administered antimuscarinic (see Antimuscarinics, Box B, p.6) or sympathomimetic agents.

Undesirable effects

Most common: nausea and vomiting, drowsiness, hypotension, epigastric pain.[10] In critical care, tachycardia and sweating was reported in ⩽30% and ⩽20% of patients respectively.[22] Sweating was also common in patients with rheumatoid arthritis.[23] However, in an RCT in cancer patients, tachycardia was noted in only 3%.[10]

Less common: diarrhoea, confusion and hallucinations (particularly in the elderly), tremor, paraesthesia, dizziness, syncope, seizures, palpitations, dry mouth, urinary retention.

Infrequent: blurred vision, insomnia, headache, pink discolouration of the urine.

Dose and use

- start with 60mg PO t.d.s. (30mg PO t.d.s. in the elderly or those with end-stage renal failure)[7] or 20mg IM q6h (not UK)
- if necessary, increase to 90mg PO t.d.s.
- for patients with swallowing difficulties, the tablets will disperse in 10mL of water (see Chapter 22, p.725).

Supply

Acupan® (Meda)
Tablets 30mg, 28 days @ 60mg t.d.s. = £20.
Injection 10mg/mL, 2mL amp = £3.50. (Unauthorized, available to import via IDIS, see Appendix 1, p.817); minimum order quantity of 30 amps.

1 Hunskaar S et al. (1987) Involvement of central serotonergic pathways in nefopam-induced antinociception. European Journal of Pharmacology. **138**: 77–82.
2 Gillman K (2007) Personal communication.
3 Novelli A et al. (2005) Nefopam inhibits calcium influx, cGMP formation, and NMDA receptor-dependent neurotoxicity following activation of voltage sensitive calcium channels. Amino Acids. **28**: 183–191.
4 Verleye M et al. (2004) Nefopam blocks voltage-sensitive sodium channels and modulates glutamatergic transmission in rodents. Brain Research Reviews. **1013**: 249–255.
5 Dordoni PL et al. (1994) Effect of ketorolac, ketoprofen and nefopam on platelet function. Anaesthesia. **49**: 1046–1049.

6 Aymard G et al. (2003) Comparative pharmacokinetics and pharmacodynamics of intravenous and oral nefopam in healthy volunteers. Pharmacology and Toxicology. 92: 279–286.

7 Mimoz O et al. (2010) Nefopam pharmacokinetics in patients with end-stage renal disease. Anesthesia and Analgesia. 111: 1146–1153.

8 Beaver WT and Feise GA (1977) A comparison of the analgetic effect of intramuscular nefopam and morphine in patients with postoperative pain. Journal of Clinical Pharmacology. 17: 579–591.

9 Phillips G and Vickers MD (1979) Nefopam in postoperative pain. British Journal of Anaesthesia. 51: 961–965.

10 Minotti V et al. (1989) Double-blind evaluation of analgesic efficacy of orally administered diclofenac, nefopam, and acetylsalicylic acid (ASA) plus codeine in chronic cancer pain. Pain. 36: 177–183.

11 Stamp J et al. (1989) A comparison of nefopam and flurbiprofen in the treatment of osteoarthrosis. British Journal of Clinical Practice. 43: 24–26.

12 Evans MS et al. (2008) Nefopam for the prevention of postoperative pain: quantitative systematic review. British Journal of Anaesthesia. 101: 610–617.

13 Cindea I et al. (2012) Effect of intraoperative nefopam on acute pain management after major abdominal surgery. European Journal of Anaesthesiology. 29: 204.

14 Kapfer B et al. (2005) Nefopam and ketamine comparably enhance postoperative analgesia. Anesthesia and Analgesia. 100: 169–174.

15 Mimoz O et al. (2001) Analgesic efficacy and safety of nefopam vs. propacetamol following hepatic resection. Anaesthesia. 56: 520–525.

16 Delage N et al. (2005) Median effective dose (ED50) of nefopam and ketoprofen in postoperative patients: a study of interaction using sequential analysis and isobolographic analysis. Anesthesiology. 102: 1211–1216.

17 Remerand F et al. (2013) Nefopam after total hip arthroplasty: role in multimodal analgesia. Orthopaedics and Traumatology, Surgery and Research. 99: 169–174.

18 Moustafa F et al. (2013) Usefulness of nefopam in treating pain of severe uncomplicated renal colics in adults admitted to emergency units: a randomised double-blind controlled trial. The 'INCoNU' study. Emergency Medicine Journal. 30: 143–148.

19 Moffat AC et al. (1990) Postoperative nefopam and diclofenac. Evaluation of their morphine-sparing effect after upper abdominal surgery. Anaesthesia. 45: 302–305.

20 Bilotta F and Rosa G (2000) Nefopam for severe hiccups. N Engl J Med. 343: 1973–1974.

21 Bilotta F et al. (2001) Nefopam for refractory postoperative hiccups. Anesthesia and Analgesia. 93: 1358–1360.

22 Chanques G et al. (2011) Analgesic efficacy and haemodynamic effects of nefopam in critically ill patients. British Journal of Anaesthesia. 106: 336–343.

23 Emery P and Gibson T (1986) A double-blind study of the simple analgesic nefopam in rheumatoid arthritis. British Journal of Rheumatology. 25: 72–76.

Updated May 2014

NON-STEROIDAL ANTI-INFLAMMATORY DRUGS (NSAIDs)   BNF 10.1.1 & 15.1.4.2

Non-steroidal anti-inflammatory drugs (NSAIDs) prevent or reverse inflammation-induced hyperalgesia locally[1] and in the CNS by inhibiting the synthesis of prostaglandins (PGs).[2,3] Thus, NSAIDs are of particular benefit for pains associated with inflammation. These include most forms of cancer pain.[4–6] The efficacy of NSAIDs in pure neuropathic pain is less well established, but there is suggestive evidence of benefit from both animal and human studies.[7]

NSAIDs also have a major role in postoperative pain.[8,9] However, there is little high level evidence for benefit in some chronic non-cancer pains, e.g. low back.[10] NSAIDs are also antipyretic.[11] It is generally accepted that inhibition of cyclo-oxygenase is their main mechanism of action.[12]

Quantitatively, the most serious undesirable effects of NSAIDs are GI and cardiovascular toxicity.[13] Although quantifying the combined risk is not easy,[14,15] it is important that the dangers are kept in perspective. Based on cohort studies, in patients taking an NSAID for at least 2 months the risk of a bleeding ulcer or perforation is of the order of 1 in 500.[16] Further, on average, 1 in 1,200 patients taking NSAIDs for at least 2 months will die from gastroduodenal complications.[16]

In relation to selective COX-2 inhibitors, the number of additional thrombotic events (mainly myocardial infarctions) is 3/1,000 patients per year of use.[17] If 1/6–1/3 of these are fatal, this would give a death rate of about 1 in 1,000–2,000 patients per year of use from thrombosis. With patients with a short prognosis, the risk may be smaller, although many terminal conditions themselves predispose to thrombosis and other complications.

In end-stage disease, the benefit associated with greater physical comfort generally far outweigh the potential harm from GI or thrombotic complications. On the other hand, worsening heart failure after an infarct or disability from a stroke can be a high price to pay. Thus, in order to minimize harm as much as possible:

• select the safest drug for each patient (see p.321)[15]

- use the smallest effective dose for the shortest possible time
- prescribe appropriate gastroprotection
- consider whether there are alternative measures which carry less risk; but bear in mind that these will generally have been studied in less depth and there may thus be unidentified risks.

Cyclo-oxygenase

There are two distinct cyclo-oxygenase (COX) isoforms.[18] COX-1 is mainly 'constitutive', i.e. physiological, with near constant levels and activity in most tissues, including the CNS. COX-2 is constitutive in parts of the CNS, renal cortex, stomach, uterus, cartilage, bone and seminal vesicles (Figure 1) but is massively inducible within a few hours by inflammation, dehydration or trauma. However, COX-1 also plays an indispensable role in inflammation; and COX-2, although initially producing pro-inflammatory prostaglandins, later induces anti-inflammatory PGD2.[19] Both peptic ulcer and bone healing require COX-2.[20,21]

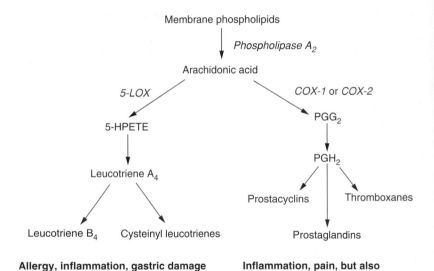

Membrane phospholipids

Phospholipase A$_2$

Arachidonic acid

5-LOX   COX-1 or COX-2

5-HPETE   PGG$_2$

PGH$_2$

Leucotriene A$_4$

Prostacyclins   Thromboxanes

Leucotriene B$_4$ Cysteinyl leucotrienes   Prostaglandins

Allergy, inflammation, gastric damage   **Inflammation, pain, but also gastroprotective PGs**

Figure 1   Products of arachidonic acid metabolism involved in inflammation.

COX = cyclo-oxygenase; 5-HPETE = hydroperoxyeicosatetrenoic acid; LOX = lipoxygenase; PG = prostaglandin.

Cyclo-oxygenase inhibition

Inflammation is associated with increased PG production both in the peripheral tissues and in the CNS.[22] The peripheral free nerve endings responsive to noxious stimuli become hypersensitive in the presence of inflammatory substances, increasing transduction and resulting in increased pain (*peripheral* sensitization). Increased production of PGs in the CNS in response to a noxious stimulus leads to *central* sensitization of neurones in the dorsal horn, with further magnification of the noxious stimulus and more severe pain.[23–25] COX-2 plays a key role in central hyperalgesia.[26]

By inhibiting the production of COX, NSAIDs block the synthesis of PGs both peripherally in the tissues and in the CNS. The relative peripheral and central contributions to the total analgesic effect depends, among other things, on the NSAID in question, its pharmacokinetic characteristics, and the route of administration.[12]

NSAIDs also modify the endocannabinoid system. Endocannabinoids, like PGs, are produced *de novo* from arachidonic acid and are broken down by COX-2 (see p.229). Further, some NSAIDs (e.g. **ibuprofen**) inhibit other enzymes involved in endocannabinoid metabolism (e.g. fatty acid amide hydroxylase). However, the relative contribution of PG[27] and endocannabinoid to the analgesic effect of NSAIDs is uncertain.[28]

Classification

NSAIDs are now generally classified on the basis of their relative ability to inhibit COX-1 and COX-2. However, the degree of COX-2 selectivity varies according to the assay used,[29,30] and whether the result is expressed in terms of 50 or 80% inhibition of the enzyme.[31,32] Although 80% inhibition is theoretically a better comparator *in vivo*, most studies use 50% (Table 1). Further, the results of *in vitro* assays may not reliably reflect *in vivo* reality.[33] This is certainly the case in relation to **celecoxib**. Despite its relatively modest ranking (Table 1), no significant COX-1 inhibition was seen in volunteers taking 400mg b.d.[34] Dose and inter-patient variation are the main determinants of COX-2 selectivity *in vivo*.[35]

Table 1 COX-2 selectivity ratio of IC_{50} COX-1/COX-2 (human whole blood assays)[32]

Drug	COX-2 selectivity ratio
Etoricoxib	106
Rofecoxib[a]	35
Valdecoxib[b]	30
Celecoxib	7.6
Nimesulide[c]	7.3
Diclofenac	3.0
Etodolac	2.4
Meloxicam	2.0
Indometacin	0.4
Ibuprofen	0.2
Piroxicam	0.08

a. withdrawn worldwide
b. withdrawn in Europe, the USA and Canada
c. not UK.

Although it is more correct to think of a spectrum of selectivity,[29,31] it is customary to divide NSAIDs into several seemingly disparate categories (Table 2). Inevitably, there will be differences of opinion as to where the cut off between categories should come, particularly because selectivity is partly dose-dependent.[29] For example, with **meloxicam** 7.5mg/day, there is 70% COX-2 and 7% COX-1 inhibition but, with 15mg/day, there is 80% COX-2 and 25% COX-1 inhibition.[36] Further, thromboxane B_2 production is reduced 66% by **meloxicam** 15mg/day, the result of COX-1 inhibition.[37]

Table 2 Classification of NSAIDs

Preferential COX-1 inhibitors	Non-selective COX inhibitors	Preferential COX-2 inhibitors	Selective COX-2 inhibitors
Flurbiprofen	Aspirin	Diclofenac	Celecoxib
Indometacin	Fenamates	Etodolac	Etoricoxib
Ketoprofen	Ibuprofen	Meloxicam	Parecoxib
Ketorolac	Nabumetone	Nimesulide (not UK)	
	Naproxen		
	Salicylates		

Additional sites of action[38]

The anti-inflammatory properties of an NSAID are not predictive of its analgesic effect, suggesting that other mechanisms must be involved.[39] Individual NSAIDs have also been shown to have effects on:

- neutrophils[40–42]
- synthesis and regulation of activity of dorsal horn neurotransmitters and modulators[41]
- modulation of pain transduction through spinal serotoninergic, adrenergic and cholinergic systems[43]
- endocannabinoids[28]
- nitric oxide production[44]
- interleukin release.[38]

NSAIDs also affect brain concentrations of kynurenic acid, an endogenous antagonist which acts on the glycine recognition site of the NMDA-receptor-channel complex.[45] **Diclofenac** (preferential COX-2 inhibitor) and **indometacin** (preferential COX-1 inhibitor) increase brain kynurenic acid concentrations, whereas **meloxicam** and **parecoxib** (preferential and selective COX-2 inhibitors respectively) cause a decrease. It is possible that at least some NSAIDs tonically modulate kynurenic acid metabolism, and thereby impact on central nociceptive mechanisms.

It is possible that non-selective NSAIDs are intrinsically more broad-spectrum in their central effects than selective COX-2 inhibitors.[46] However, clinically, selective COX-2 inhibitors appear to be equally effective when compared with non-selective NSAIDs in inflammatory, dental and postoperative pain.[47] On the other hand, in dental pain, there is a tendency for weak COX inhibitors to be superior to **aspirin** and for strong inhibitors to be inferior, emphasizing the importance of not adopting too simplistic a view of the mode of action of these drugs (Table 3).

Table 3 Analgesic efficacy of oral NSAIDs in dental pain compared with aspirin 650mg[39]

Significantly superior	Not significantly different	Significantly inferior
Azapropazone (3)[a,b]	Diclofenac (1)	Fenbufen (1)[b]
Diflunisal (3)[b]	Etodolac (1)	Nabumetone (1)
Flurbiprofen (1)	Sulindac (1)	Ketoprofen (2)
Ketorolac (3)[b]	Naproxen (3)	Tolmetin (3)[b]

a. numbers indicate capacity to inhibit PG synthesis: 1 = strong; 2 = moderate; 3 = weak
b. PO formulation no longer available in the UK.

NSAIDs and pyrexia

All NSAIDs are antipyretic.[11,48] Paraneoplastic fever responds to all NSAIDs, not just to **naproxen** as initially thought.[49] Although the antipyretic effect tends to wear off after a few months, further benefit may be obtained by switching to an alternative NSAID. However, the duration of benefit with second- and third-line drugs is generally shorter. Box A provides guidance on the drug treatment of paraneoplastic pyrexia and sweating.

There is emerging evidence that the use of antipyretics, both NSAIDs and paracetamol, doubles mortality in septic critically ill patients.[55] Although this is generally unlikely to impact on palliative care, it may lead to a re-appraisal of antipyretic use in the next few years.

NSAIDs and cachexia

Several RCTs in cancer patients with cachexia have reported additional benefit when an NSAID is combined with a progestogen (see Progestogens, p.536).[56–58] It is hypothesized that the NSAID provides benefit by reducing the chronic inflammatory response. In some studies, an NSAID has been used alone.[59,60] At present, such use remains experimental.

NSAIDs, platelet function and bleeding time

NSAIDs differ in their effect on platelet function and bleeding time (Table 4; also see p.315). However, bleeding time is affected by various technical and clinical factors, is difficult to standardize,[61] and is a poor predictor of bleeding in invasive procedures.[62] Although there are

---

Box A   Symptomatic drug treatment of paraneoplastic pyrexia and sweating

Begin by prescribing an antipyretic:
- paracetamol 500mg–1g q.d.s. or p.r.n. (generally less toxic than an NSAID)
- NSAID, e.g. ibuprofen 200–400mg t.d.s. or p.r.n. (or the locally preferred alternative).

If the sweating does not respond to an NSAID, prescribe an antimuscarinic drug:
- amitriptyline 25–50mg at bedtime (may cause sedation, dry mouth and other antimuscarinic effects)
- hyoscine *hydrobromide* 1mg/3days TD[50]
- glycopyrronium ≤2mg PO t.d.s.

If an antimuscarinic fails, other options include:
- propranolol 10–20mg b.d.–t.d.s.
- cimetidine 400–800mg b.d.[51]
- olanzapine 5mg b.d.[52]
- thalidomide 100mg at bedtime;[53,54] high response rate but last resort because it is very expensive, and can cause irreversible painful peripheral neuropathy and drowsiness (see p.543).

Table 4   NSAIDs, platelet function and bleeding time

Drug	Comment
Aspirin	Irreversible platelet dysfunction and prolonged bleeding time as a result of acetylation of platelet COX-1
Non-acetylated salicylates e.g. choline magnesium trisalicylate[a], salsalate[a]	No effect on platelet function or bleeding time at recommended doses
Classical NSAIDs (except diclofenac), e.g. flurbiprofen, ibuprofen, ketorolac, naproxen	Reversible platelet dysfunction and prolonged bleeding time
Diclofenac	Reversible inhibition of platelet aggregation in 2/3 of subjects.[62] IV diclofenac has a measurable effect on bleeding time, but most subjects remain within normal limits
Etodolac	No data
Meloxicam[64] Nabumetone Nimesulide[a,65] Coxibs[36,66]	No effect on platelet function or bleeding time

a. not UK.

other methods for measuring platelet function,[63] these have not clarified our understanding about the differing effects of NSAIDs on bleeding.

Undesirable effects

NSAIDs differ in their propensity to cause a range of undesirable effects. For convenience, these have been categorized as type A and type B. Generally, type A effects are mainly dose-dependent and partly predictable, whereas type B effects are mainly dose-independent and unpredictable (Table 5 and Table 6).

Table 5 Type A ('predictable') reactions to NSAIDs[67]

Organ/system	Clinical reaction
Blood	Decreased platelet aggregation, prolonged bleeding time (see Table 4)
GI tract	Dyspepsia
	Peptic ulceration, bleeding, perforation
	Small bowel stricture, bleeding, perforation
	Exacerbation of inflammatory bowel disease
	Protein-losing enteropathy
Kidney	Salt and water retention
Cardiovascular	Thrombosis, e.g. myocardial infarction, stroke
Lung	Bronchospasm (asthma)

Table 6 Type B ('unpredictable') reactions to NSAIDs

Organ/system	Clinical reaction	Most likely NSAIDs[67]
Immunological	Anaphylaxis	Most NSAIDs
Skin	Morbilliform rash	Fenbufen
	Angioedema	Ibuprofen
		Azapropazone
		Piroxicam
Blood	Thrombocytopenia	Diclofenac
		Ibuprofen
		Piroxicam
	Haemolytic anaemia	Mefenamic acid
		Diclofenac
GI tract	Diarrhoea	Fenamates, e.g. mefenamic acid
Kidney	Interstitial nephritis	Fenoprofen[68]
Liver	Reye's syndrome (in children)	Aspirin
	Hepatotoxicity	Diclofenac
		Sulindac
CNS	Aseptic meningitis	Ibuprofen

NSAIDs and the GI tract

NSAIDs increase the risk of upper GI complications. A meta-analysis of several hundred RCTs indicates that, compared with placebo, the risk with coxibs and **diclofenac** is almost doubled, and quadrupled with *high dose* **ibuprofen** (i.e. 2,400mg/24h) and *high dose* **naproxen** (i.e. 1,000mg/24h).[13] The risk with **nabumetone** is comparable with that of the coxibs (see p.343).[69] Note: combining thromboprotective **aspirin** with a coxib removes the lower GI risk of selective COX-2 inhibitors.

The most GI toxic NSAIDs are **azapropazone**, **ketorolac** and **piroxicam**.[70] Although prescription may be justifiable in specific limited circumstances, e.g. **ketorolac** (see p.338), they should *not* generally be used.

Stomach and duodenum

The relative risk of gastric ulcer when taking an NSAID is 5–6.[71] For duodenal ulceration, the relative risk is only 1.1, although a recent population-based nested case-control study suggested it is higher.[72] One patient in 1,200 on an NSAID for ≥ 2 months without adequate gastroprotection dies mainly as a result of complicated gastric ulceration (i.e. bleeding or perforation).[16] This translates into 2,000 excess deaths annually in the UK.

Various factors account for a lower gastroduodenal toxicity (Box B). How much of the benefit relates to COX-2 selectivity is uncertain.

Box B   Factors intrinsic to NSAIDs which result in low gastroduodenal toxicity[73]

Competitive masking of COX-1 by inactive forms, e.g. *R*-ibuprofen, *R*-etodolac.

Weak/no uncoupling of oxidative phosphorylation ⎫
Low disruption of phospholipids in protective ⎬ non-acidic compounds,
mucus and mucous membranes ⎭ e.g. nabumetone, coxibs.

High protein-binding (less available).

Weak/no inhibition of platelet aggregation, e.g. non-acetylated salicylates, coxibs, meloxicam, and diclofenac sometimes.

The situation may change when dual LOX/COX inhibitors come onto the market. Such drugs inhibit lipoxygenase (LOX) as well as both COX-1 and COX-2 and are said to have similar GI toxicity to placebo,[74] a positive cardiovascular risk profile, and to reduce cartilage damage in osteo-arthritis.[75]

The nitric oxide NSAIDs (NO-NSAIDs, also known as CINODs, COX-inhibiting NO donors) are another group of novel NSAIDs designed to provide improved GI safety, and lower rather than raise blood-pressure. However, an RCT of one NO-NSAID showed GI safety to be no better than with **naproxen**, although blood pressure was unaffected.[76] Also in development are the H_2S-donating NSAIDs, which have similar vasodilator properties.[77] Another new concept under investigation is linking an NSAID molecule with phosphatidylcholine.[78]

In patients who are *H.pylori* positive, the risk of developing an NSAID-related ulcer is almost doubled, and the risk of bleeding trebled.[79] The explanation for this lies in the *H.pylori*-associated chronic atrophic gastritis (mainly affecting the antrum) and makes the extracellular matrix in that part of the stomach wall vulnerable to the back-diffusion of acid. Ionized NSAID molecules, circulating in the plasma, are transported passively through leaky capillary walls into the inflamed matrix where they become unionized in the acidic environment. In this state, the molecules are lipid-soluble and they move freely into the mucosal cells where, at a higher pH, the molecules become ionized again and consequently trapped.

The local high concentration of NSAID leads to inhibition of the production of gastroprotective COX-1 in the stomach mucosa. Eradication of *H. pylori* infection (see p.486) will correct the atrophic gastritis and end the sequence of events initiated by acid back-diffusion. Thus, eradication of *H. pylori* makes all COX-1-inhibiting NSAIDs safer to use, reducing peptic ulcer disease by half.[79] However, when trying to prevent ulcer recurrence in patients on NSAIDs, *H.pylori* eradication is less effective than a PPI.[80]

Risk factors for an NSAID-related upper GI complication (i.e. ulceration, bleeding, perforation) are listed in Box C. For example, concurrent administration of a non-selective NSAID and

---

Box C   Risk factors for NSAID-related upper GI complications[71,82]

Age > 65 years (see text).

Peptic ulcer ± GI bleeding in the last year confirmed by endoscopy, or strong clinical suspicion, e.g. haematemesis, melaena.

Long-term use of maximum recommended doses of an NSAID.

Serious morbidity, e.g. cancer, diabetes mellitus, hypertension, cardiovascular disease, hepatic impairment, renal impairment.

Concurrent use of a corticosteroid, low-dose aspirin, or anticoagulant (warfarin or heparin).

Concurrent use of a serotonin re-uptake inhibitor (see text).

Platelets < 50 x 10^9/L.

Acid dyspepsia with an NSAID despite concurrent use of a gastroprotective drug, now or in the past.

Gastric infection with *H. pylori*.

---

warfarin increases the risk of bleeding > 10 times, nearly 4 times that of **warfarin** alone, and nearly 4 times the risk when using a coxib plus **warfarin**.[81]

In rheumatoid arthritis, the risk of hospitalization and/or death increases progressively from 50 years.[71] Thus, compared with those under 50, the risk is twice as great in patients aged 50–65 years, 6 times greater in patients aged 65–75, and some 14 times greater in the over 75s. However, in rheumatoid arthritis there may well be concurrent interacting risk factors. Thus, 65 years is widely considered to be the appropriate point for regarding age as a risk factor in other situations.

Antidepressants which inhibit presynaptic serotonin re-uptake, notably SSRIs and **clomipramine**, **amitriptyline** and **venlafaxine**, decrease serotonin uptake from the blood by platelets.[83] Because platelets do not synthesize serotonin, serotonin re-uptake inhibitors decrease the platelet serotonin concentration, and this may adversely affect platelet aggregation. Serotonin re-uptake inhibitors are an independent risk factor for GI bleeding, increasing the risk > 6 times, giving an NNH of 106 when combined with an NSAID.[84] Low-dose aspirin in addition to an NSAID and an SSRI reduces the NNH to 28, i.e. is much more dangerous.[85]

Patients with a high risk of serious gastropathy are best treated with an NSAID with a low propensity for causing gastrotoxicity, e.g. **celecoxib**, **diclofenac** (also see Box B). Concurrent prophylaxis with a gastroprotective agent also helps to prevent upper GI complications (Box D). Evidence suggests that the combination of a coxib and gastroprotection provides the best prophylaxis, and should be recommended in high risk patients.[86,87]

Box D　Gastroprotection

Cochrane reviews[88–91]

PPIs (see p.31), misoprostol (see p.29) and double-dose H_2 antagonists (see p.26) are effective at *preventing* chronic NSAID-related endoscopic peptic ulcers.

Standard doses of H_2 antagonists reduce the risk of duodenal ulcers but not gastric ulcers. Misoprostol 400microgram/24h is less effective at preventing gastric ulcers than 800microgram/24h, and is still associated with diarrhoea.

Of all these treatments, only misoprostol 800microgram/24h has been definitely shown to reduce the overall incidence of ulcer *complications* (bleeding, perforation, gastric outlet obstruction).

The use of PPIs after peptic ulcer-related upper-GI bleeding, significantly reduces rebleeding, need for surgery, and ulcer recurrence. In high risk patients, PPIs reduce mortality.

NICE guidance[92,93]

PPIs are preferable to H_2 antagonists for the treatment of dyspepsia, gastro-oesophageal reflux disease and peptic ulcers, including NSAID-related ulcers.

For patients taking an NSAID and at high risk of peptic ulcer disease, double-dose H_2 antagonists or PPIs significantly reduce endoscopically detected lesions. Low-dose misoprostol (400microgram/24h) is less effective and has undesirable effects.

When an NSAID-related ulcer is diagnosed, stop the NSAID if possible, treat *H. pylori* infection if present (see p.486) and give double-dose H_2 antagonist or a PPI. PPIs heal the majority of ulcers.

A PPI should be offered to patients with non-variceal upper-GI bleeding when bleeding or stigmata of recent bleeding are confirmed at endoscopy.

Small bowel

NSAIDs can also cause small bowel ulceration, bleeding, and perforation. In addition, they can cause protein-losing enteropathy and very thin annular strictures which may eventually reduce the bowel lumen to a pinhole.[80]

NSAID effects on the small bowel may be as important as NSAID gastropathy.[94] In a capsule endoscopy study, macroscopic changes were found in more than two thirds of volunteers on a

---

2-week course of **diclofenac**. Used long-term (> 3 months), similar numbers were seen with both non-selective COX and selective COX-2 inhibitors,[95] although the latter are probably safer in the short-term.[96,97] Other studies have given comparable results.[98–101]

The mechanisms of NSAID enteropathy are still being elucidated.[102] Changes in bowel permeability may be the root cause.[103] Prostaglandin deficiency (not achieved via COX inhibition[104]) is important.[105] NSAIDs which are recirculated in bile (enterohepatic circulation, e.g. **diclofenac, indomethacin, piroxicam**) are significantly more likely to damage the bowel than NSAIDs which are not (**aspirin, nabumetone, sulindac**).[106]

It is postulated that contact by the NSAID with the bowel wall damages the phosphatidylcholine in the mucosal cell membrane. Mitochondrial and endoplasmic reticulum damage decouples oxidative phosphorylation, leads to release of calcium, and the production of free radicals. The resulting leakiness of bowel mucosal membranes leads to an ingress of Gram negative bacteria, bile acids and proteolytic enzymes. The inflammation produced is mediated by neutrophils, and causes both local and distant damage.[103,107,108] It has been suggested that this is related to the shift in intestinal microflora seen when acid is suppressed.[109]

Accordingly, in addition to the enterohepatic recirculation of NSAIDs and age > 65 years, concurrent use of a PPI or H_2 antagonist appears to be a risk factor.[110,111] Thus, although gastric acid-reducing drugs reduce the risk of gastric damage, they may increase enteropathy. As more is learned about the balance between gastric and small bowel risk, the prophylactic use of PPIs in patients prescribed an NSAID is likely to come under scrutiny.

Prevention of bowel damage is still in its infancy. Drugs and other agents being investigated in this respect include:

- **lansoprazole**, may have a mucosal protective properties as well as PPI activity
- **metronidazole**, via reduced bowel wall permeability changes
- other non-absorbed antibacterials
- NO-NSAIDs and H_2S-NSAIDs (vasodilation, anti-inflammatory, cytoprotective)
- NSAIDs-PC (preserve muosal phosphatidylchloine barrier)
- **Rebamipide**,[111] a novel free radical scavenger
- *Lactobacillus*
- lactoferrin, a food constituent.[107,112]

Large bowel

In the large bowel, NSAIDs can re-activate Crohn's disease and ulcerative colitis.[113] Although the evidence is not high level,[114] NSAIDs should be avoided in these conditions. Women who use NSAIDs (but not aspirin) for > 15 days a month for six years have an increased risk of developing inflammatory bowel disease de novo.[115] As elsewhere in the GI tract, these NSAID-related effects are probably associated with changes in bowel wall permeability, and possibly influenced by PG-mediated aspects of GI neuromuscular control.[116] NSAIDs can also cause a colitis directly, and increase the risk of complications from diverticular disease.[117]

NSAIDs and the cardiovascular system

All NSAIDs raise blood pressure, and this needs to be monitored in patients susceptible to cardiac problems or who are already hypertensive.[118] NSAIDs increase the risk of heart failure;[119] and the use of NSAIDs in heart failure carries a dose-dependent risk of death.[120] Thus, NSAIDs should be generally be avoided in patients with chronic heart failure (CHF).[121]

In recent years, increasing concern has been expressed about NSAID-related major cardiovascular events. This has been extensively reviewed in a meta-analysis of several hundred RCTs comparing various combinations of NSAID or an individual NSAID with placebo, with particular emphasis on the coxibs, **diclofenac, ibuprofen** or **naproxen** (Box E).[13]

In short, patients with CHF or with other NSAID-related cardiovascular risk factors (age ≥80 years, rheumatoid arthritis, chronic kidney disease, and COPD[122]) generally should be prescribed **naproxen** (or *low-dose* **ibuprofen**, i.e. ≤ 1,200mg/24h), but definitely not **diclofenac** (or *high-dose* **ibuprofen**).

The thromboprotective effect of **aspirin** for stroke may be compromised in people taking a concurrent NSAID.[123] Thus, as a general rule, patients on **aspirin** for thromboprotection should *not* take another NSAID of any type. However, if a round-the-clock NSAID is considered essential, stop the **aspirin** and prescribe **naproxen** b.d. (see Box E).

Box E   NSAID-related major vascular events: a meta-analysis of >600 RCTs

'Major cardiovascular event' includes coronary artery- and stroke-related death, non-fatal myocardial infarction, and non-fatal stroke.

The traditional NSAID regimens studied were all *high-dose*, and it was not possible to examine dose dependency. However, since vascular hazard is probably related to the degree of COX-2 inhibition (which is greater at higher doses), dose dependency seems likely.

Coxibs increase the risk of major cardiovascular events by about a third. The excess risk relates mainly to an increased risk of a major coronary event.

Overall, the vascular risks of different coxib are similar, although there was a trend towards less risk with celecoxib 200mg daily (the most widely used coxib regimen).

High-dose diclofenac (150mg/24h) has similar vascular risks to a coxib. However, the absolute excess risk is small: prescription of a coxib or diclofenac causes around three additional major vascular events per 1000 participants per year, with one such event causing death.

The meta-analysis does not allow definite conclusions about how soon diclofenac increases vascular risk. Data relating to IV parecoxib and PO valdecoxib after coronary artery bypass surgery suggest that the hazard from coxibs is probably an early effect.

Although the meta-analysis also showed that high-dose ibuprofen (2,400mg/24h) significantly increased the risk of major coronary events, there were many fewer relevant events in trials of ibuprofen vs. coxib compared with placebo-controlled RCTs. Thus, the cardiovascular risk of ibuprofen is still uncertain.

High-dose naproxen (500mg b.d.) appears *not* to increase the risk of a major vascular event. This is consistent with experimental studies showing that this dose of naproxen can produce sufficient COX-1 inhibition to achieve intense and prolonged platelet inhibition in some individuals, which could attenuate any adverse vascular effects of COX-2 inhibition.

There was no evidence of an increased risk of stroke for any of the NSAIDs studied, but few strokes were recorded. However, the absence of any stroke risk for drug regimens known to increase blood pressure is implausible.

All NSAIDs doubled the risk of heart failure causing hospital admission (i.e. not just ankle oedema), consistent with this being a COX-2 dependent hazard unrelated to variable platelet inhibition.

NSAIDs and the kidneys

All NSAIDs cause an increase in Cl^- resorption from the proximal tubules, and enhance ADH activity, leading to sodium (Na^+) and water retention. Thus NSAIDs antagonize the action of diuretics, and can exacerbate existing hypertension or lead to new onset hypertension.[124] The proximal passive resorption of Na^+ leads to increased resorption of K^+ in the distal tubules; this can result in hyperkalemia.

NSAIDs can cause acute or acute-on-chronic renal failure.[125,126] Chronic NSAID use increases the risk of chronic renal failure.[127] Sporadic cases of interstitial nephritis ($\pm$ nephrotic syndrome or $\pm$ papillary necrosis) have been reported with most NSAIDs. The renal risks of different NSAIDs, including coxibs, are similar, and thus are not a factor in determining choice.[128] Less than 1% of patients given an NSAID develop renal impairment sufficient to cause discontinuation of therapy.[129]

However, the prevalence in palliative care patients might be higher, because NSAID-induced renal failure is associated with hypovolaemia and conditions of low effective circulating volume. In situations such as hypovolaemia, the plasma concentrations of vasoconstrictor substances such as angiotensin II, noradrenaline (norepinephrine) and vasopressin are increased, e.g. in heart failure, cirrhosis and nephrotic syndrome, persistent vomiting or diarrhoea, third space losses (e.g. ascites) and diuretic use. Normally, this would lead to increased vasodilator prostaglandin secretion in the kidneys to maintain renal perfusion, but the inhibition of renal PG production by NSAIDs prevents this, thereby precipitating renal failure.[126,130] Except in patients expected to die

---

in a few days, dehydrated patients should be rehydrated when starting treatment with an NSAID, or the NSAID should not be used. The acute renal failure due to NSAIDs is generally reversible if the drug is stopped promptly, but not always; it can be fatal.

Patients with multiple myeloma are at particular risk, although this is rare in the absence of Bence-Jones (light chain) proteinuria.[131–133]

NSAIDs and the liver

Patients with hepatic impairment are more susceptible to NSAID-related renal impairment. Hence most SPCs for NSAIDs include active liver disease or significant hepatic impairment as a contra-indication.

In patients with cirrhosis it is difficult to obtain an accurate measure of renal function because the plasma creatinine concentrations tends to be low. This may relate to a reduced muscle mass and reduced conversion of creatine to creatinine.[134] NSAID-related impairment of platelet function may increase the risk of bleeding from oesophageal varices.

Cholestasis may reduce the elimination of NSAIDs excreted in bile (**indometacin, sulindac**), and may reduce or delay absorption of fat-soluble NSAIDs, e.g. **ibuprofen**.[135]

Hepatotoxicity is a rare and unpredictable effect seen with most NSAIDs, including COX-2-selective ones. **Diclofenac** and **sulindac** may have the highest risk, and **ibuprofen** the least.[135]

NSAIDs and bronchospasm

Some patients, with or without a history of atopic asthma, give a history of **aspirin**- or NSAID-induced asthma. The prevalence, derived from oral provocation testing studies, is about 20% in the general adult population, and 5% in children.[136] Chronic non-aspirin NSAID users have almost double the risk of developing adult onset asthma.[137]

Genetic polymorphisms in prostanoid receptor genes[138] and leukotriene synthase genes[139] have been described in **aspirin**-induced asthmatics, suggesting that the asthma is caused by an **aspirin**-induced (COX-1 inhibitory) imbalance between bronchodilator PGE2 and bronchoconstrictor leukotrienes, and is not immunologically mediated (as in atopic asthmatics).[140–142]

Aspirin-induced asthma typically occurs 30min–3h after ingestion of **aspirin**. Half of those affected react to even low-dose **aspirin** (80mg). Cross-sensitivity with other NSAIDs is normal, e.g. **diclofenac** (93%), **ibuprofen** (98%), **naproxen** (100%).[136] A history of allergic-type reactions (asthma, acute rhinitis, nasal polyps, angioedema, urticaria) with **aspirin** or other NSAID calls for extreme caution in prescribing a further NSAID (Table 7).

Table 7 Use of NSAIDs in asthmatic patients

Patient characteristics	Recommendations
Anyone who has ever had an asthmatic reaction to aspirin or a non-coxib NSAID; or anyone with high risk features of aspirin-induced asthma (severe asthma, nasal polyps, urticaria, or chronic rhinitis)	Avoid all products containing aspirin or a non-coxib NSAID; use paracetamol instead unless also contra-indicated. However, coxibs are almost always safe, but give the first dose under medical supervision
All other asthmatic patients	Any NSAID, including aspirin, may be considered but, if any respiratory reaction occurs, stop the NSAID and manage as above

In contrast, the incidence of cross-sensitivity to **paracetamol** is only 7%, and <2% of asthmatic patients are sensitive to both **aspirin** and **paracetamol**.[143] Further, reactions to **paracetamol** are generally less severe. Thus, **paracetamol** should always be the initial non-opioid of choice for asthmatic patients.

Bronchospasm has not been observed with **choline salicylate** (available only as a dental gel and ear drops in the UK), **sodium salicylate** (not UK), or **azapropazone**; it is rare with **benzydamine** (available only as a mouthwash and throat spray in the UK).[144]

Coxibs rarely induce asthma, and the cause may well be isolated idiosyncratic allergy and not cross-reactivity with **aspirin** or other NSAID.[145,146]

Management of NSAID-induced asthma is along usual lines, but leukotriene receptor inhibitors, e.g. **montelukast**, have a particular place. Some patients may have been treated by **aspirin** desensitization. Such patients will be on daily **aspirin** and can safely take an NSAID without provoking an attack. It is essential *not* to stop the **aspirin** in such patients or sensitization may return.[146]

NSAIDs and bone healing

Some NSAIDs (**indometacin, diclofenac, tenoxicam**) delay bone healing in animals, but this has not been seen in others (**ibuprofen, ketorolac, piroxicam**).[147] The clinical impact of this is uncertain, and human data are very limited. However, there is evidence that long-term NSAID use is associated with an increased risk of non-union of fractures.[148] Further, even when used for only 2–5 days, NSAIDs decrease heterotopic (ectopic) bone formation, commonly seen after major hip surgery.[148,149]

Some orthopaedic departments prohibit the use of NSAIDs, including coxibs, for up to 6 weeks postoperatively. There is evidence for impairment in healing with high doses of both non-selective and selective NSAIDs.[147] Thus, when using NSAIDs after fracture or orthopaedic surgery, it would be sensible to use the lowest effective dose for as short a time as necessary. For example, limit the use of an NSAID to $\leqslant 10$ days, and then discontinue until healing is complete. However, in patients with other risk factors for delayed union or non-union (e.g. smoking, diabetes mellitus, corticosteroids), use **paracetamol** instead.[147] On the other hand, if pain relief is inadequate when using both **paracetamol** and an opioid, an NSAID should be prescribed (instead of the **paracetamol**) despite its potential negative impact.

Contra-indications for NSAIDs

Although the SPCs are not completely consistent in this respect, the following is a general list of contra-indications for NSAIDs:
- hypersensitivity to **aspirin** or other NSAID (urticaria, rhinitis, asthma, angioedema)
- active GI ulceration, bleeding, perforation or inflammation
- severe heart failure
- active liver disease or moderate–severe hepatic impairment
- severe renal impairment (creatinine clearance <30mL/min), deteriorating renal function, hyperkalaemia (>5mmol/L).

These contra-indications are not necessarily absolute. There may well be occasions when 'contra-indication' means 'use with great caution and in the absence of a safer alternative'. **Diclofenac** and **celecoxib** are both contra-indicated in patients with established cardiovascular disease.

Important drug-drug interactions

Pharmacodynamic

Many pharmacodynamic interactions can be predicted from the mode of action and undesirable effects of NSAIDs:
- increased risk of renal toxicity with other renally toxic drugs, e.g. aminoglycosides, **ciclosporin**
- increased risk of bleeding due to anti-platelet or anti-clotting effects, e.g. SSRIs, LMWH, **warfarin**
- increased risk of upper GI complications e.g. concurrent prescription of low-dose **aspirin**, corticosteroids or **warfarin**
- antagonistic effect of NSAIDs due to Na^+ and fluid retention, e.g. antihypertensives and diuretics
- antagonistic effect of some NSAIDs with thromboprotective effect of low-dose **aspirin** (see individual NSAID monographs)
- antagonistic effect of NSAIDs with the uricosuric drug **probenecid**.

Pharmacokinetic

Pharmacokinetic interactions are summarized in Tables 8 and 9 (also see Chapter 25, p.767). Topical NSAIDs are unlikely to reach sufficient plasma concentrations to interact with other drugs.

Drug affected	Effect of NSAIDs	Clinical implications
Aminoglycosides	May reduce renal function in susceptible individuals, thus reducing aminoglycoside clearance and increasing plasma concentration	Monitor aminoglycoside plasma concentration and renal function; adjust dose accordingly
Ciclosporin	May inhibit the renal prostacyclin synthesis needed to maintain glomerular filtration and renal blood flow. Increased and decreased ciclosporin plasma concentration reported	Monitor ciclosporin plasma concentration and renal function; adjust dose accordingly
Clofarabine	May reduce renal function, thus increasing clofarabine plasma concentration	Increased risk of clofarabine toxicity. Manufacturer of clofarabine advises against concurrent use with an NSAID
Digoxin	May precipitate renal failure, particularly in those with heart failure, thus reducing digoxin excretion and increasing digoxin plasma concentration	Increased risk of digoxin toxicity. Monitor digoxin plasma concentration and renal function; adjust dose accordingly
Lithium	May inhibit renal excretion of lithium, increasing plasma lithium concentration	Increased risk of lithium toxicity. Avoid NSAID if possible; alternatively halve dose of lithium and monitor lithium plasma concentration. *Ketorolac is contra-indicated*
Methotrexate	Competitively inhibit the tubular excretion of methotrexate and inhibit PGE₂ synthesis, reducing renal perfusion; both increase methotrexate plasma concentration. Effect varies between NSAIDs and individuals	Increased risk of methotrexate toxicity. *Fatalities have occurred* (see text). Avoid aspirin and other salicylates during chemotherapy; probably safe between pulses. Use other NSAIDs with caution. Much lower risk with low-dose chronic methotrexate therapy used in psoriasis or rheumatoid arthritis and if no pre-existing renal impairment. Monitor methotrexate dose and its haematological effects
Phenytoin	May displace phenytoin from plasma proteins. May inhibit liver enzymes responsible for phenytoin metabolism	Clinical significance uncertain because the excess free phenytoin may be metabolized by the liver. However, phenytoin toxicity can develop even when the plasma concentration is still within the therapeutic range
Sulfonylureas	May inhibit renal tubular excretion, increasing sulfonylurea plasma concentration and hypoglycaemic effect	Reduce sulfonylurea dose if necessary
Valproate	May displace valproate from plasma proteins, inhibit valproate metabolism and increase plasma concentration	Avoid aspirin. Importance of interaction with other NSAIDs unclear; reduce the dose of valproate if toxicity suspected
Warfarin	May inhibit metabolism of warfarin and increase INR	Isolated cases reported with most NSAIDs (including coxibs); check INR closely during the first week after starting an NSAID and weekly for the next 3–4 weeks, increases of up to 60% have been reported; reduce dose of warfarin if necessary; *ketorolac is contra-indicated*
Zidovudine	May increase the risk of haematological toxicity, particularly in haemophiliacs treated with ibuprofen	Monitor blood count

Table 9 Pharmacokinetic interactions: other drugs affecting NSAIDs[150,154]

Drug implicated	NSAIDs affected	Effect	Clinical implications
Antacids	All e/c NSAIDs	Destruction of enteric coating	Administer at different times
Antacids	?All NSAIDs except celecoxib and diclofenac	Variable. Aluminium-containing antacids can reduce rate and/or extent of absorption of fenamates, diflunisal, indometacin and naproxen. Magnesium hydroxide alone can increase the absorption of ibuprofen and flurbiprofen; also increases gastric toxicity of ibuprofen. Sodium bicarbonate increases naproxen absorption	Avoid aluminium-containing antacids or use an alternative NSAID
Ciclosporin	Diclofenac	Increased plasma concentration of diclofenac due to reduced first-pass metabolism	Halve the dose of diclofenac
Colestyramine	All NSAIDs	Anion exchange resin binds NSAIDs in the GI tract, reducing and/or delaying absorption. Binding in GI tract prevents enterohepatic recycling and increases faecal loss, even if NSAID administered IV (meloxicam, piroxicam, tenoxicam, sulindac)	Separate administration of PO NSAIDs by 4h. Colestyramine may be used to speed removal of NSAID after overdose
Fluconazole	Celecoxib Flurbiprofen Ibuprofen	Increased plasma concentration due to CYP2C9 inhibition by fluconazole	Halve the dose of celecoxib. Lower doses of flurbiprofen and ibuprofen may be necessary
Probenecid	?All NSAIDs	Reduced metabolism and renal clearance of NSAIDs and glucuronide metabolite which are hydrolyzed back to parent drug; NSAIDs also reduce the uricosuric effect of probenecid	Increased toxicity seen with indometacin, particularly if renal function impaired. Consider a reduction in NSAID dose but could be used therapeutically to increase the response. Ketorolac is contra-indicated with probenecid
Rifampicin	Celecoxib Diclofenac	Decreased plasma concentration due to CYP3A4 induction by rifampicin	Consider alternative NSAID if pain returns
Ritonavir	Piroxicam ?Other NSAIDs	Increased plasma concentration of piroxicam with increased risk of toxicity	Manufacturer of ritonavir advises against concurrent use with prioxicam
Voriconazole	Diclofenac Flurbiprofen Ibuprofen	Increased plasma concentration due to CYP2C9 inhibition and reduced clearance by voriconazole	Lower doses of NSAID may be necessary

NSAIDs can significantly affect the plasma concentrations of renally excreted drugs by causing reduced renal function and/or reduced tubular excretion. Of particular importance is the risk of toxic plasma concentrations of aminoglycosides, **ciclosporin, clofarabine, digoxin, lithium,** and **methotrexate** (see Table 8).

Fatalities or severe renal failure have occurred when **methotrexate** has been prescribed concurrently with an NSAID, e.g. **aspirin, ibuprofen, indomethacin, ketoprofen, naproxen,** and life-threatening neutropenia has been reported with several NSAIDs.[150,151]

NSAIDs can interact with **warfarin,** resulting in an increased INR; increases of up to 60% have been reported.[152,153] Patients should have their INR closely monitored during the first week after starting an NSAID and weekly for the next 3–4 weeks. The interaction may be due to CYP2C9 inhibition or competitive metabolism and may be more significant in those who are poor CYP2C9 metabolizers (see Chapter 25, p.770).

There are few clinically significant interactions of drugs affecting the pharmacokinetics of NSAIDs (see Table 9).

Choice of NSAID

In practice, the choice of NSAID will depend on various factors, including availability, efficacy, safety, fashion, cost, and local guidelines. The renal risks of different NSAIDs including coxibs are similar, and thus are not a factor in determining choice.[128]

It is unclear if some cancer patients obtain more benefit from one particular NSAID, as is anecdotally reported in rheumatoid arthritis, or whether apparent differences simply relate to a relative increase in inhibition of PG synthesis.

Although some centres favour other ones (see p.333 and p.343), the choice in practice is generally between four NSAIDs (Box F). In short, *low-dose* **ibuprofen** (≤1,200mg/24h) is a good all-round first choice. When this is insufficient, choice is guided by the relative GI and cardiovascular risks. **Ketorolac** SC + PPI is occasionally used in patients with severe nociceptive pain who fail to obtain good relief with other NSAIDs and a strong opioid (see p.338).

Box F Choice of NSAID[13]

First choice

Ibuprofen in *low dose* (≤1,200mg/24h) carries a low risk of GI toxicity and possibly a low risk of a major cardiovascular event.

In *high dose* (2,400mg/24h), ibuprofen's GI toxicity is comparable with naproxen and its cardiovascular toxicity is comparable with diclofenac. It is thus generally *not* advisable to use ibuprofen in *high dose* (2,400mg/24h).

Patients with a high risk of upper GI complications

Celecoxib and diclofenac (150mg/24h) have a low risk of upper GI complications, but a higher risk of major cardiovascular events. *Use in patients with cardiovascular disease is contra-indicated,* and should be discouraged in patients with cardiovascular risk factors (see p.315).

Celecoxib (200mg/24h) or diclofenac + *PPI* is the best choice for patients at *very high* risk of upper GI complications, e.g. recent bleed, and for whom the use of an NSAID is considered essential.

Celecoxib has no effect on bleeding time, and is thus also a good choice in patients with thrombocytopenia (e.g. from chemotherapy or other cause) for whom an NSAID is considered essential (see p.310).

Patients with a high risk of a major cardiovascular event

Naproxen (1g/24h) is the drug of choice for patients with cardiovascular risk factors (no increased risk; see p.315).

It is still unclear whether PPI gastroprotection completely corrects the higher risk of upper GI complications compared with diclofenac and coxibs (four times vs. two times in the absence of gastro-protection).

As far as possible, all NSAIDs should be avoided in end-stage heart failure (see Chapter 16, p.675). Patients with hypertension and/or with cardiac, hepatic or renal impairment may deteriorate, and should be monitored.

Because of the risk of upper GI complications with all NSAIDs coupled with other GI risk factors present in most palliative care patients (see Box C), a gastroprotective drug is prescribed almost routinely with NSAIDs at some centres. Tolerability favours PPIs but the evidence is more robust for **misoprostol** 800microgram/24h (a large good quality RCT vs. epidemiological studies for PPIs).[88] Further, in patients suffering from constipation, **misoprostol** could be a useful 'co-laxative'.

Although SPCs often recommend taking NSAIDs with/after food, there is no evidence that food reduces the incidence of upper GI complications. Further, food may delay the absorption of an NSAID, although this will be of importance only when treating acute pain. (See Chapter 14 for general guidance about prescribing in palliative care, and the importance of keeping multi-drug regimens as straightforward as possible, p.640).

Route of administration

Except for the relief of biliary and renal colic,[155] NSAIDs should generally be given PO in patients who can swallow. In patients who can no longer reliably take oral medication, SC **diclofenac** 150mg/24h can be given instead. Apart from **ketorolac**,[137,138] there is no evidence of greater efficacy by other routes.[156]

Alternatively, the rectal route can be used:
- **diclofenac** suppositories 50mg b.d.–t.d.s.
- **indometacin** suppositories 100mg up to b.d.

A further option is to switch to **paracetamol** (p.299) suppositories.

Piroxicam given as an orodispersible 20mg tablet (Feldene Melt®) once daily is another option. This dissolves rapidly and completely if placed on the tongue or in the mouth. However, absorption is GI, which means that Feldene Melt® tablets can be used only in patients who can swallow their saliva. However, in someone expected to die within 1–2 days, it is generally possible to discontinue the NSAID without provoking a resurgence of pain.

1 Guindon J and Beaulieu P (2006) Antihyperalgesic effects of local injections of anandamide, ibuprofen, rofecoxib and their combinations in a model of neuropathic pain. *Neuropharmacology*. **50**: 814–823.

2 Burian M et al. (2003) Peripheral and central antihyperalgesic effects of diclofenac in a model of human inflammatory pain. *Clinical Pharmacology and Therapeutics*. **74**: 113–120.

3 Koppert W et al. (2004) The cyclooxygenase isozyme inhibitors parecoxib and paracetamol reduce central hyperalgesia in humans. *Pain*. **108**: 148–153.

4 McNicol E et al. (2004) Nonsteroidal anti-inflammatory drugs, alone or combined with opioids, for cancer pain: a systematic review. *Journal of Clinical Oncology*. **22**: 1975–1992.

5 Shah S and Hardy J (2001) Non-steroidal anti-inflammatory drugs in cancer pain: a review of the literature as relevant to palliative care. *Progress in Palliative Care*. **9**: 3–7.

6 Mercadante S et al. (2002) A randomised controlled study on the use of anti-inflammatory drugs in patients with cancer pain on morphine therapy: effects on dose-escalation and a pharmacoeconomic analysis. *European Journal of Cancer*. **38**: 1358–1363.

7 Vo T et al. (2009) Non-steroidal anti-inflammatory drugs for neuropathic pain: how do we explain continued widespread use? *Pain*. **143**: 169–171.

8 Jirarattanaphochai K and Jung S (2008) Nonsteroidal anti-inflammatory drugs for postoperative pain management after lumbar spine surgery: a meta-analysis of randomized controlled trials. *Journal of Neurosurgery Spine*. **9**: 22–31.

9 Derry C et al. (2009) Single dose oral ibuprofen for acute postoperative pain in adults. *Cochrane Database of Systematic Reviews*. **3**: CD001548.

10 Roelofs PD et al. (2008) Non-steroidal anti-inflammatory drugs for low back pain. *Cochrane Database of Systematic Reviews*. CD000396.

11 Simmons DL et al. (2000) Nonsteroidal anti-inflammatory drugs, acetaminophen, cyclooxygenase 2, and fever. *Clinical Infectious Diseases*. **31 (Suppl 5)**: S211–218.

12 Burian M and Geisslinger G (2005) COX-dependent mechanisms involved in the antinociceptive action of NSAIDs at central and peripheral sites. *Pharmacology and Therepeutics*. **107**: 139–154.

13 CNT Collaboration (2013) Vascular and upper gastrointestinal effects of non-steroidal anti-inflammatory drugs: meta-analyses of individual participant data from randomised trials. *Lancet*. **382**:769–779

14 Varas-Lorenzo C et al. (2007) Quantitative assessment of the gastrointestinal and cardiovascular risk-benefit of celecoxib compared to individual NSAIDs at the population level. *Pharmacoepidemiology and Drug Safety*. **16**: 366–376.

15 Turajane T et al. (2009) Gastrointestinal and cardiovascular risk of non-selective NSAIDs and COX-2 inhibitors in elderly patients with knee osteoarthritis. *Journal of the Medical Association of Thailand*. **92 (Suppl 6)**: S19–26.

16 Tramer M et al. (2000) Quantitative estimation of rare adverse events which follow a biological progression: a new model applied to chronic NSAID use. *Pain*. **85**: 169–182.

17 Kearney PM et al. (2006) Do selective cyclo-oxygenase-2 inhibitors and traditional non-steroidal anti-inflammatory drugs increase the risk of atherothrombosis? Meta-analysis of randomised trials. *British Medical Journal*. **332**: 1302–1308.

18 Simmons DL et al. (2004) Cyclooxygenase isozymes: the biology of prostaglandin synthesis and inhibition. Pharmacological Reviews. 56: 387–437.

19 Kapoor M et al. (2005) Possible anti-inflammatory role of COX-2-derived prostaglandins: implications for inflammation research. Current Opinion in Investigational Drugs. 6: 461–466.

20 Gerstenfeld LC and Einhorn TA (2004) COX inhibitors and their effects on bone healing. Expert Opinion on Drug Safety. 3: 131–136.

21 Peskar BM (2005) Role of cyclooxygenase isoforms in gastric mucosal defense and ulcer healing. Inflammopharmacology. 13: 15–26.

22 Schwab JM and Schluesener HJ (2003) Cyclooxygenases and central nervous system inflammation: conceptual neglect of cyclooxygenase 1. Archives of Neurology. 60: 630–632.

23 Baba H et al. (2001) Direct activation of rat spinal dorsal horn neurons by prostaglandin E2. Journal of Neuroscience. 21: 1750–1756.

24 Samad T et al. (2001) Interleukin-1B-mediated induction of COX-2 in the CNS contributes to inflammatory pain hypersensitivity. Nature. 410: 471–475.

25 Farooqui M et al. (2007) COX-2 inhibitor celecoxib prevents chronic morphine-induced promotion of angiogenesis, tumour growth, metastasis and mortality, without compromising analgesia. British Journal of Cancer. 97: 1523–1531.

26 Jain NK et al. (2008) COX-2 expression and function in the hyperalgesic response to paw inflammation in mice. Prostaglandins Leukotrienes and Essential Fatty Acids. 79: 183–190.

27 Severine Vandevoorde (2008) Overview of the chemical families of fatty acid amide hydrolase and monoacylglycerol lipase inhibitors. Current Topics in Medicinal Chemistry. 8: 247–267.

28 Telleria-Diaz A et al. (2010) Spinal antinociceptive effects of cyclooxygenase inhibition during inflammation: Involvement of prostaglandins and endocannabinoids. Pain. 148: 26–35.

29 Churchill L et al. (1996) Selective inhibition of human cyclo-oxygenase-2 by meloxicam. Inflammopharmacology. 4: 125–135.

30 Brooks P et al. (1999) Interpreting the clinical significance of the differential inhibition of cyclooxygenase-1 and cyclooxygenase-2. Rheumatology. 38: 779–788.

31 Warner T et al. (1999) Nonsteroidal drug selectivities for cyclo-oxygenase-1 rather than cyclo-oxygenase-2 are associated with human gastrointestinal toxicity: a full in vitro analysis. Proceedings of the National Academy of Science USA. 96: 7563–7568.

32 Riendeau D et al. (2001) Etoricoxib (MK-0663): Preclinical profile and comparison with other agents that selectively inhibit cyclooxygenase-2. Journal of Pharmacology and Experimental Therapeutics. 296: 558–566.

33 Blain H et al. (2002) Limitation of the in vitro whole blood assay for predicting the COX selectivity of NSAIDs in clinical use. British Journal of Clinical Pharmacology. 53: 255–265.

34 Fries S et al. (2006) Marked interindividual variability in the response to selective inhibitors of cyclooxygenase-2. Gastroenterology. 130: 55–64.

35 Capone ML et al. (2007) Pharmacodynamic of cyclooxygenase inhibitors in humans. Prostaglandins Other Lipid Mediators. 82: 85–94.

36 vanHecken A et al. (2000) Comparative inhibitory activity of rofecoxib, meloxicam, diclofenac, ibuprofen and naproxen on COX-2 versus COX-1 in healthy volunteers. Journal of Clinical Pharmacology. 40: 1109–1120.

37 deMeijer A et al. (1999) Meloxicam, 15mg/day, spares platelet function in healthy volunteers. Clinical Pharmacology and Therapeutics. 66: 425–430.

38 Hamza M and Dionne RA (2009) Mechanisms of non-opioid analgesics beyond cyclooxygenase enzyme inhibition. Current Molecular Pharmacology. 2: 1–14.

39 McCormack K and Brune K (1991) Dissociation between the antinociceptive and anti-inflammatory effects of the nonsteroidal anti-inflammatory drugs: a survey of their analgesic efficacy. Drugs. 41: 533–547.

40 Abramson S et al. (1991) Non-steroidal anti-inflammatory drugs: effects on a GTP binding protein within the neutrophil plasma membrane. Biochemical Pharmacology. 41: 1567–1573.

41 McCormack K (1994) Nonsteroidal anti-inflammatory drugs and spinal nociceptive processing. Pain. 59: 9–43.

42 Svensson CI and Yaksh TL (2002) The spinal phospholipase-cyclooxygenase-prostanoid cascade in nociceptive processing. Annual Review of Pharmacology and Toxicology. 42: 553–583.

43 Miranda HF et al. (2001) An isobolographic analysis of the adrenergic modulation of diclofenac antinociception. Anesthesia and Analgesia. 93: 430–435.

44 Vandivier RW et al. (1999) Down-regulation of nitric oxide production by ibuprofen in human volunteers. Journal of Pharmacology and Experimental Therapeutics. 289: 1398–1403.

45 Schwieler L et al. (2005) Prostaglandin-mediated control of rat brain kynurenic acid synthesis - opposite actions by COX-1 and COX-2 isoforms. Journal of Neural Transmission. 112: 863–872.

46 McCormack K and Twycross RG (2001) Are COX-2 selective inhibitors effective analgesics? Pain Review. 8: 13–26.

47 Dougados M et al. (2001) Evaluation of the structure-modifying effects of diacerein in hip osteoarthritis: ECHODIAH, a three-year, placebo-controlled trial. Evaluation of the Chondromodulating Effect of Diacerein in OA of the Hip. Arthritis and Rheumatism. 44: 2539–2547.

48 Kathula SK et al. (2003) Cyclo-oxygenase II inhibitors in the treatment of neoplastic fever. Supportive Care in Cancer. 11: 258–259.

49 Tsavaris N et al. (1990) A randomized trial of the effect of three nonsteroidal anti-inflammatory agents in ameliorating cancer-induced fever. Journal of Internal Medicine. 228: 451–455.

50 Mercadante S (1998) Hyoscine in opioid-induced sweating. Journal of Pain and Symptom Management. 15: 214–215.

51 Pittelkow M and Loprinzi C (2003) Pruritus and sweating in palliative medicine. In: D Doyle et al. (eds) Oxford Textbook of Palliative Medicine (3e). Oxford University Press, Oxford, pp. 573–587.

52 Zylicz Z and Krajnik M (2003) Flushing and sweating in an advanced breast cancer patient relieved by olanzapine. Journal of Pain and Symptom Management. 25: 494–495.

53 Calder K and Bruera E (2000) Thalidomide for night sweats in patients with advanced cancer. Palliative Medicine. 14: 77–78.

54 Deaner P (2000) The use of thalidomide in the management of severe sweating in patients with advanced malignancy: trial report. Palliative Medicine. 14: 429–431.

55 Lee BH et al. (2012) Association of body temperature and antipyretic treatments with mortality of critically ill patients with and without sepsis: multi-centered prospective observational study. Critical Care. 16: R33.

56 McMillan DC et al. (1999) A prospective randomized study of megestrol acetate and ibuprofen in gastrointestinal cancer patients with weight loss. British Journal of Cancer. 79: 495–500.

57   Cerchietti LC et al. (2004) Effects of celecoxib, medroxyprogesterone, and dietary intervention on systemic syndromes in patients with advanced lung adenocarcinoma: a pilot study. Journal of Pain and Symptom Management. 27: 85–95.

58   Maccio A et al. (2012) A randomized phase III clinical trial of a combined treatment for cachexia in patients with gynecological cancers: evaluating the impact on metabolic and inflammatory profiles and quality of life. Gynecologic Oncology. 124: 417–425.

59   Bosaeus I et al. (2002) Dietary intake, resting energy expenditure, weight loss and survival in cancer patients. Journal of Nutrition. 132 (Suppl): 3465s–3466s.

60   Lai V et al. (2008) Results of a pilot study of the effects of celecoxib on cancer cachexia in patients with cancer of the head, neck, and gastrointestinal tract. Head & Neck. 30: 67–74.

61   Peterson P et al. (1998) The preoperative bleeding time test lacks clinical benefit: College of American Pathologists' and American Society of Clinical Pathologists' position article. Archives of Surgery. 133: 134–139.

62   Ng KF et al. (2008) Comprehensive preoperative evaluation of platelet function in total knee arthroplasty patients taking diclofenac. Journal of Arthroplasty. 23: 424–430.

63   Brass L (2010) Understanding and evaluating platelet function. Hematology/ the Education Program of the American Society of Hematology Education Program. 2010: 387–396.

64   Guth B et al. (1996) Therapeutic doses of meloxicam do not inhibit platelet aggregation in man. Rheumatology in Europe. 25: Abstract 443.

65   Cullen L et al. (1997) Selective suppression of cyclooxygenase-2 during chronic administration of nimesulide in man. In: Fourth International Congress on essential fatty acids and eicosanoids; Edinburgh.

66   Clemett D and Goa K (2000) Celecoxib: a review of its use in osteoarthritis, rheumatoid arthritis and acute pain. Drugs. 59: 957–980.

67   Rawlins M (1997) Non-opioid analgesics. In: D Doyle et al. (eds) Oxford Textbook of Palliative Medicine (2e). Oxford University Press, Oxford, pp. 355–361.

68   Rossert J (2001) Drug-induced acute interstitial nephritis. Kidney International. 60: 804–817.

69   Bannwarth B (2008) Safety of the nonselective NSAID nabumetone: focus on gastrointestinal tolerability. Drug Safety. 31: 485–503.

70   Castellsague J et al. (2012) Individual NSAIDs and upper gastrointestinal complications: a systematic review and meta-analysis of observational studies (the SOS project). Drug Safety. 35: 1127–1146.

71   Fries J et al. (1991) Nonsteroidal anti-inflammatory drug-associated gastropathy: incidence and risk factor models. American Journal of Medicine. 91: 213–222.

72   Garcia Rodriguez LA and Hernandez-Diaz S (2004) Risk of uncomplicated peptic ulcer among users of aspirin and nonaspirin nonsteroidal anti-inflammatory drugs. American Journal of Epidemiology. 159: 23–31.

73   Rainsford K (1999) Profile and mechanisms of gastrointestinal and other side effects of nonsteroidal anti-inflammatory drugs (NsAIDs). American Journal of Medicine. 107 (suppl 6A): 27s–36s.

74   Kulkarni SK and Singh VP (2008) Licofelone: the answer to unmet needs in osteoarthritis therapy? Current Rheumatology Reports. 10: 43–48.

75   Raynauld JP et al. (2009) Protective effects of licofelone, a 5-lipoxygenase and cyclo-oxygenase inhibitor, versus naproxen on cartilage loss in knee osteoarthritis: a first multicentre clinical trial using quantitative MRI. Annals of the Rheumatic Diseases. 68: 938–947.

76   Lohmander LS et al. (2005) A randomised, placebo controlled, comparative trial of the gastrointestinal safety and efficacy of AZD3582 versus naproxen in osteoarthritis. Annals of the Rheumatic Diseases. 64: 449–456.

77   Fiorucci S and Santucci L (2011) Hydrogen sulfide-based therapies: focus on H_2S releasing NSAIDs. Inflammation and Allergy Drug Targets. 10: 133–140.

78   Lichtenberger LM et al. (2009) Association of phosphatidylcholine and NSAIDs as a novel strategy to reduce gastrointestinal toxicity. Drugs Today (Barc). 45: 877–890.

79   Tang CL et al. (2012) Eradication of Helicobacter pylori infection reduces the incidence of peptic ulcer disease in patients using nonsteroidal anti-inflammatory drugs: a meta-analysis. Helicobacter. 17: 286–296.

80   Malfertheiner P et al. (2007) Current concepts in the management of Helicobacter pylori infection: the Maastricht III Consensus Report. Gut. 56: 772–781.

81   Cheetham TC et al. (2009) Gastrointestinal safety of nonsteroidal anti-inflammatory drugs and selective cyclooxygenase-2 inhibitors in patients on warfarin. Annals of Pharmacotherapy. 43: 1765–1773.

82   Hawkins C and Hanks G (2000) The gastroduodenal toxicity of nonsteroidal anti-inflammatory drugs. A review of the literature. Journal of Pain and Symptom Management. 20: 140–151.

83   Ross S et al. (1980) Inhibition of 5-hydroxytryptamine uptake in human platelets by antidepressant agents in vivo. Psychopharmacology. 67: 1–7.

84   Loke YK et al. (2008) Meta-analysis: gastrointestinal bleeding due to interaction between selective serotonin uptake inhibitors and non-steroidal anti-inflammatory drugs. Alimentary Pharmacology and Therapeutics. 27: 31–40.

85   Dall M et al. (2009) An association between selective serotonin reuptake inhibitor use and serious upper gastrointestinal bleeding. Clinical Gastroenterology and Hepatology. 7: 1314–1321.

86   Chan FK et al. (2007) Combination of a cyclo-oxygenase-2 inhibitor and a proton-pump inhibitor for prevention of recurrent ulcer bleeding in patients at very high risk: a double-blind, randomised trial. Lancet. 369: 1621–1626.

87   Targownik LE et al. (2008) The relative efficacies of gastroprotective strategies in chronic users of nonsteroidal anti-inflammatory drugs. Gastroenterology. 134: 937–944.

88   Rostom A et al. (2002) Prevention of NSAID-induced gastroduodenal ulcers. Cochrane Database of Systematic Reviews. 4: CD002296.

89   Moayyedi P (2006) Pharmacological interventions for non-ulcer dyspepsia. Cochrane Database of Systematic Reviews. 4: CD001960.

90   Leontiadis G et al. (2010) Proton pump inhibitor treatment for acute peptic ulcer bleeding. Cochrane Database of Systematic Reviews. 5: CD002094.

91   van Pinxteren B et al. (2010) Short-term treatment with proton pump inhibitors, H_2- receptor antagonists and prokinetics for gastro-oesophageal reflux disease-like symptoms and endoscopy negative reflux disease. Cochrane Database of Systematic Reviews. 11: CD002095.

92   NICE (2004) Dyspepsia. Management of dyspepsia in adults in primary care. Clinical Guideline. CG17. www.nice.org.uk

93   NICE (2012) Acute upper gastrointestinal bleeding management. Clinical Guideline CG141. www.nice.org.uk

94 Adebayo D and Bjarnason I (2006) Is non-steroidal anti-inflammaory drug (NSAID) enteropathy clinically more important than NSAID gastropathy? *Postgraduate Medical Journal.* **82**: 186–191.

95 Maiden L (2009) Capsule endoscopic diagnosis of nonsteroidal anti-inflammatory drug-induced enteropathy. *Journal of Gastroenterology.* **44 Suppl 19**: 64–71.

96 Smecuol E et al. (2001) Acute gastrointestinal permeability responses to different non-steroidal anti-inflammatory drugs. *Gut.* **49**: 650–655.

97 Goldstein JL et al. (2005) Video capsule endoscopy to prospectively assess small bowel injury with celecoxib, naproxen plus omeprazole, and placebo. *Clinical Gastroenterology and Hepatology.* **3**: 133–141.

98 Maiden L et al. (2005) A quantitative analysis of NSAID-induced small bowel pathology by capsule enteroscopy *Gastroenterology.* **128**: 1172–1178.

99 Matsumoto T et al. (2008) Prevalence of non-steroidal anti-inflammatory drug-induced enteropathy determined by double-balloon endoscopy: a Japanese multicenter study. *Scandinavian Journal of Gastroenterology.* **43**: 490–496.

100 Fujimori S et al. (2010) Distribution of small intestinal mucosal injuries as a result of NSAID administration. *European Journal of Clinical Investigations.* **40**: 504–510.

101 Graham DY et al. (2005) Visible small-intestinal mucosal injury in chronic NSAID users. *Clinical Gastroenterology and Hepatology.* **3**: 55–59.

102 Fortun PJ and Hawkey CJ (2007) Nonsteroidal anti-inflammatory drugs and the small intestine. *Current Opinion in Gastroenterology.* **23**: 134–141.

103 Bjarnason I and Takeuchi K (2009) Intestinal permeability in the pathogenesis of NSAID-induced enteropathy. *Journal of Gastroenterology.* **44 (Suppl 19)**: 23–29.

104 Wallace JL (2012) NSAID gastropathy and enteropathy: distinct patogenesis likely necessitates distinct prevention strategies. *British Journal of Pharmacology.* **165**: 67-74.

105 Adler DH et al. (2009) The enteropathy of prostaglandin deficiency. *Journal of Gastroenterology.* **44 (Suppl 19)**: 1–7.

106 Hedner T et al. (2004) Nabumetone: Therapeutic use and safety profile in the management of osteoarthritis and rheumatoid arthritis. *Drugs.* **64**: 2315–2343; discussion 2344–2345.

107 Park SC et al. (2011) Prevention and management of non-steroidal anti-inflammatory drugs-induced small intestinal injury. *World Journal of Gastroenterology.* **17**: 4647–4653.

108 Boelsterli UA et al. (2013) Multiple NSAID-induced hits injure the small intestine: underlying mechanisms and novel strategies. *Toxicol Sci.* **131**: 654–667.

109 Wallace JL et al. (2011) Proton pump inhibitors exacerbate NSAID-induced small intestinal injury by inducing dysbiosis. *Gastroenterology.* **141**: 1314–1322, 1322 e1311–1315.

110 Watanabe T et al. (2013) Risk factors for severe nonsteroidal anti-inflammatory drug-induced small intestinal damage. *Digestive and Liver Disease.* **45**: 390–395.

111 Zhang S et al. (2013) Rebamipide helps defend against nonsteroidal anti-inflammatory drugs induced gastroenteropathy: a systematic review and meta-analysis. *Digestive Diseases and Sciences.* **58**: 1991–2000.

112 Satoh H and Takeuchi K (2012) Management of NSAID/aspirin-induced small intestinal damage by GI-sparing NSAIDs, anti-ulcer drugs and food constituents. *Current Medicinal Chemistry.* **19**: 82–89.

113 Hawkey CJ (2006) NSAIDs, coxibs, and the intestine. *Journal of Cardiovascular Pharmacology.* **47 (Suppl 1)**: S72–75.

114 Singh S et al. (2009) Do NSAIDs, antibiotics, infections, or stress trigger flares in IBD? *American Journal of Gastroenterology.* **104**: 1298–1313.

115 Ananthakrishnan AN et al. (2012) Aspirin, nonsteroidal anti-inflammatory drug use, and risk for Crohn disease and ulcerative colitis: a cohort study. *Annals of Internal Medicine.* **156**: 350–359.

116 Fornai M et al. (2010) Emerging role of cyclooxygenase isoforms in the control of gastrointestinal neuromuscular functions. *Pharmacology and Therapeutics.* **125**: 62–78.

117 Ballinger A (2008) Adverse effects of nonsteroidal anti-inflammatory drugs on the colon. *Current Gastroenterology Reports.* **10**: 485–489.

118 White WB (2007) Cardiovascular risk, hypertension, and NSAIDs. *Current Pain and Headache Reports.* **11**: 428–435.

119 Huerta C et al. (2006) Non-steroidal anti-inflammatory drugs and risk of first hospital admission for heart failure in the general population. *Heart.* **92**: 1610–1615.

120 Gislason GH et al. (2009) Increased mortality and cardiovascular morbidity associated with use of nonsteroidal anti-inflammatory drugs in chronic heart failure. *Archives of Internal Medicine.* **169**: 141–149.

121 McGettigan P and Henry D (2006) Cardiovascular risk and inhibition of cyclooxygenase: a systematic review of the observational studies of selective and nonselective inhibitors of cyclooxygenase 2. *Journal of the American Medical Association.* **296**: 1633–1644.

122 Solomon DH et al. (2008) Subgroup analyses to determine cardiovascular risk associated with nonsteroidal anti-inflammatory drugs and coxibs in specific patient groups. *Arthritis and Rheumatism.* **59**: 1097–1104.

123 Gengo FM et al. (2008) Effects of ibuprofen on the magnitude and duration of aspirin's inhibition of platelet aggregation: clinical consequences in stroke prophylaxis. *Journal of Clinical Pharmacology.* **48**: 117–122.

124 Cheng HF and Harris RC (2004) Cyclooxygenases, the kidney, and hypertension. *Hypertension.* **43**: 525–530.

125 Griffin M et al. (2000) Nonsteroidal anti-inflammatory drugs and acute renal failure in elderly persons. *American Journal of Epidemiology.* **151**: 488–496.

126 Huerta C et al. (2005) Nonsteroidal anti-inflammatory drugs and risk of ARF in the general population. *American Journal of Kidney Disease.* **45**: 531–539.

127 Perneger TV et al. (1994) Risk of kidney failure associated with the use of acetaminophen, aspirin, and nonsteroidal anti-inflammatory drugs. *New England Journal of Medicine.* **331**: 1675–1679.

128 Schneider V et al. (2006) Association of selective and conventional nonsteroidal anti-inflammatory drugs with acute renal failure: A population-based, nested case-control analysis. *American Journal of Epidemiology.* **164**: 881–889.

129 Venturini C et al. (1998) Nonsteroidal anti-inflammatory drug-induced renal failure: a brief review of the role of cyclooxygenase isoforms. *Current Opinion in Nephrology and Hypertension.* **7**: 79–82.

130 Harirforoosh S and Jamali F (2009) Renal adverse effects of nonsteroidal anti-inflammatory drugs. *Expert Opinion on Drug Safety.* **8**: 669–681.

131 Winearls C (1995) Acute myeloma kidney. *Kidney International.* **48**: 1347–1361.

132 Iggo N et al. (1997) The development of cast nephropathy in multiple myeloma. *QJM: monthly journal of the Association of Physicians.* **90**: 653–656.

133 Irish AB et al. (1997) Presentation and survival of patients with severe renal failure and myeloma. QJM: monthly journal of the Association of Physicians. **90**: 773–780.
134 Delco F et al. (2005) Dose adjustment in patients with liver disease. Drug Safety. **28**: 529–545.
135 North-Lewis P (ed) (2008) Drugs and the Liver. Pharmaceutical Press, London, pp. 178–187.
136 Jenkins C et al. (2004) Systematic review of prevalence of aspirin induced asthma and its implications for clinical practice. British Medical Journal. **328**: 434.
137 Thomsen SF et al. (2009) Regular use of non-steroidal anti-inflammatory drugs increases the risk of adult-onset asthma: a population-based follow-up study. Clinical Respiratory Journal. **3**: 82–84.
138 Kim SH et al. (2007) Association between polymorphisms in prostanoid receptor genes and aspirin-intolerant asthma. Pharmacogenet Genomics. **17**: 295–304.
139 Sanak M and Szczeklik A (2001) Leukotriene C4 synthase polymorphism and aspirin-induced asthma. Journal of Allergy and Clinical Immunology. **107**: 561–562.
140 Simon RA (2004) Adverse respiratory reactions to aspirin and nonsteroidal anti-inflammatory drugs. Current Allergy and Asthma Reports. **4**: 17–24.
141 Mastalerz L et al. (2008) Prostaglandin E2 systemic production in patients with asthma with and without aspirin hypersensitivity. Thorax. **63**: 27–34.
142 Taniguchi M et al. (2008) Hyperleukotrieneuria in patients with allergic and inflammatory disease. Allergology International. **57**: 313–320.
143 Settipane R et al. (1995) Prevalence of cross-sensitivity with acetaminophen in aspirin-sensitive asthmatic subjects. Journal of Allergy and Clinical Immunology. **96**: 480–485.
144 Dicpinigaitis P (2001) Effect of the cyclooxygenase-2 inhibitor celecoxib on bronchial responsiveness and cough reflex sensitivity in asthmatics. Pulmonary Pharmacology and Therapeutics. **14**: 93–97.
145 Kowalski ML and Makowska J (2006) Use of nonsteroidal anti-inflammatory drugs in patients with aspirin hypersensitivity : safety of cyclo-oxygenase-2 inhibitors. Treatments in Respiratory Medicine. **5**: 399–406.
146 Stevenson DD (2009) Aspirin sensitivity and desensitization for asthma and sinusitis. Current Allergy and Asthma Reports. **9**: 155–163.
147 Boursinos LA et al. (2009) Do steroids, conventional non-steroidal anti-inflammatory drugs and selective Cox-2 inhibitors adversely affect fracture healing? Journal of Musculoskeletal Neuronal Interactions. **9**: 44–52.
148 Pountos I et al. (2008) Pharmacological agents and impairment of fracture healing: what is the evidence? Injury. **39**: 384–394.
149 Vuolteenaho K et al. (2008) Non-steroidal anti-inflammatory drugs, cyclooxygenase-2 and the bone healing process. Basic & Clinical Pharmacology and Toxicology. **102**: 10–14.
150 Baxter K and Preston CL. Stockley's Drug Interactions. London:- Pharmaceutical Press www.medicinescomplete.com
151 Patrignani P et al. (1997) Differential inhibition of human prostaglandin endoperoxide synthase-1 and -2 by nonsteroidal anti-inflammatory drugs. Journal of Physiology and Pharmacology. **48**: 623–631.
152 Brown A et al. (2003) An interaction between warfarin and COX-2 inhibitors: two case studies. The Pharmaceutical Journal. **271**: 782.
153 Verrico M et al. (2003) Adverse drug events involving COX-2 inhibitors. Annals of Pharmacotherapy. **37**: 1203–1213.
154 Tonkin A and Wing L (1988) Interactions of nonsteroidal anti-inflammatory drugs. In: P Brooks (ed) Bailliere's Clinical Rheumatology Anti-rheumatic drugs Vol 2. Bailliere Tindall, London, pp. 455–483.
155 Lundstam SOA et al. (1982) Prostaglandin-synthetase inhibition with diclofenac sodium in treatment of renal colic: comparison with use of a narcotic analgesic. Lancet. **1**: 1096–1097.
156 Tramer M et al. (1998) Comparing analgesic efficacy of non-steroidal anti-inflammatory drugs given by different routes in acute and chronic pain: a qualitative systematic review. Acta Anaesthesiologica Scandinavica. **42**: 71–79.

Updated June 2014

CELECOXIB BNF 10.1.1

Class: Non-opioid analgesic, NSAID, selective COX-2 inhibitor.

Indications: Pain and inflammation in osteoarthritis, rheumatoid arthritis, and ankylosing spondylitis, †acute pain, †cancer pain.

Contra-indications: Hypersensitivity to **aspirin** or other NSAID (urticaria, rhinitis, asthma, angioedema), *hypersensitivity to sulfonamides*, active GI ulceration, established ischaemic heart disease, peripheral arterial disease, cerebrovascular disease, severe heart failure, severe hepatic impairment, severe renal impairment, deteriorating renal function, inflammatory bowel disease.

Pharmacology

No significant COX-1 inhibition was observed in healthy volunteers on 400mg b.d.[1] Thus, despite its modest selectivity when tested *in vitro*,[2,3] celecoxib is correctly classified as a selective COX-2 inhibitor.[4]

Celecoxib is metabolized mainly via CYP2C9. *Slow (poor) metabolizers are at increased risk of undesirable effects.* In the USA, the manufacturer suggests that the dose should be *halved* in known or suspected slow metabolizers.[5] In contrast, the UK SPC merely suggests that such individuals should be treated with caution.[6]

In people of European ancestry, the CYP2C9∗3 variant is particularly important, slowing methylhydroxylation *in vitro* by 90% and more than doubling the AUC in single dose studies.[7] The APC trial using celecoxib to prevent development of sporadic colorectal adenomas in high risk individuals showed that higher doses of celecoxib provided additional 3-year risk reduction for adenomas only in individuals with this phenotype.[8]

Celecoxib is less lipophilic and is less bio-available than other coxibs. A high volume of distribution suggests widespread tissue binding. Non-COX-2 inhibitory properties may account for some of its activity, e.g. inhibition of endoplasmic reticulum Ca^{2+} $ATPase^9$ and inhibition of phosphodiesterase-5 activity.[10] The capacity to interact with non-COX-2 targets may be enhanced by accumulation of celecoxib within cells.[11] There is also evidence that central endogenous opioid and cannabinoid systems are involved in celecoxib analgesia.[12]

Celecoxib is as effective as non-selective NSAIDs in treating pain in rheumatoid arthritis[13,14] and osteoarthritis.[15,16] It is effective in postoperative pain[17] and dysmenorrhoea,[18] but *not in* renal colic.[19] There is a lack of data relating to cancer pain. Unlike opioids, celecoxib failed to control pain in mice with bone tumours.[20,21]

A meta-analysis of several hundred RCTs indicates that, compared with placebo, the risk of upper GI complications with coxibs is relatively low (about double), comparable with **diclofenac**, and half that seen with **ibuprofen** and **naproxen**.[22]

Coxibs increase the risk of a major cardiovascular event by about a third. The excess risk relates mainly to an increased risk of a major coronary event.[22] Accordingly, celecoxib is contra-indicated in patients with cardiovascular disease of any kind (see above). On the other hand, there is a trend towards less risk with celecoxib 200mg daily (the most widely used coxib regimen).[22]

Celecoxib has no effect on platelet function in healthy volunteers and can be used with low-dose aspirin.[23,24] Celecoxib does *not* cause new onset hypertension.[25,26] The risk of renal failure is comparable with other NSAIDs.[27]

Coxibs have been shown to have an anti-cancer effect in several situations.[28,29] The adjuvant use of celecoxib in chemotherapy is being investigated.[30–32] In mice, chronic administration of morphine stimulates angiogenesis, tumour growth, and metastasis and leads to earlier mortality; these effects are neutralized by the co-administration of celecoxib without compromising analgesia.[33] The relevance of these findings to clinical practice remains to be elucidated.

Celecoxib is also of benefit in cancer-related cachexia (see Progestogens, p.536), although such use remains experimental.

Bio-availability Not known in humans; 22–40% in dogs.[34]

Onset of action 60min.[35]

Time to peak plasma concentration 3h; high fat meals may delay peak by 1–2 hours; aluminium- and magnesium-containing antacids reduce peak concentration.

Plasma halflife 11h, celecoxib is eliminated almost entirely by hepatic excretion.

Duration of action 5h in single-dose post-dental extraction pain;[35] but given that recommended frequency of administration is once daily–b.d., presumably longer when given regularly.

Cautions

Renal and hepatic impairment (see p.316 and p.317). Correct hyperkalaemia before use. To minimize the potential for serious undesirable effects, use the lowest effective dose for the shortest treatment duration possible. Risk of aseptic meningitis in patients with SLE (very rare).

As with all NSAIDs, concurrent administration with an SSRI is associated with an increased risk of GI bleeding.

Drug interactions

Because they cause sodium and fluid retention, all NSAIDs can decrease the effect of diuretics, ACE inhibitors and antihypertensives.

Because an increase in INR occasionally occurs when celecoxib is prescribed for a patient already taking **warfarin**, monitor the INR weekly for 3–4 weeks and adjust the dose of **warfarin** if necessary.[36]

For general interactions between NSAIDs and other drugs, see Tables 8 and 9 (p.319 and p.320). Of particular importance is the risk of toxic plasma levels of **clofarabine**, **digoxin**, **lithium**, and **methotrexate** caused by reduced renal function and/or reduced tubular excretion. If an NSAID is prescribed, monitor the plasma drug concentration or haematological effect of these drugs as appropriate and reduce doses as necessary (see p.318).

CYP2C9 inhibitors (see Chapter 25, Table 8, p.775) may increase plasma concentrations of celecoxib. The manufacturer recommends halving the celecoxib dose if **fluconazole** is taken concurrently.[36] In known CYP2C9 slow metabolizers, avoid concurrent administration of CYP2C9 inhibitors and celecoxib. Conversely, CYP2C9 inducers (e.g., **carbamazepine**, **phenobarbital**, **rifampicin**) may reduce plasma concentrations of celecoxib.

Celecoxib is an inhibitor of CYP2D6 and theoretically may increase the plasma concentrations of other drugs metabolised by this enzyme (see Chapter 25, Table 8, p.775) if given concurrently.

Undesirable effects

Also see NSAIDs, p.307.

Common (<10%, >1%): abdominal pain, diarrhoea, dyspepsia, flatulence (but all comparable with or less than other NSAIDs), pharyngitis, rhinitis, allergy, pruritus, insomnia, dizziness, hypertonia, rash, flu-like symptoms, peripheral oedema, fluid retention.

Dose and use

For patients with, or at *very* high risk of, NSAID-related GI ulceration, see Box D, p.314.

- start with 100mg b.d. or 200mg once daily
- if necessary, increase to 200mg b.d.

Supply

Celebrex® (Pharmacia)

Capsules 100mg, 200mg, 28 days @ 200mg daily = £21.

1 Fries S et al. (2006) Marked interindividual variability in the response to selective inhibitors of cyclooxygenase-2. *Gastroenterology.* **130**: 55–64.
2 Warner TD and Mitchell JA (2008) COX-2 selectivity alone does not define the cardiovascular risks associated with non-steroidal anti-inflammatory drugs. *Lancet.* **371**: 270–273.
3 Riendeau D et al. (2001) Etoricoxib (MK-0663): Preclinical profile and comparison with other agents that selectively inhibit cyclooxygenase-2. *Journal of Pharmacology and Experimental Therapeutics.* **296**: 558–566.
4 Schwartz JI et al. (2008) Comparative inhibitory activity of etoricoxib, celecoxib, and diclofenac on COX-2 versus COX-1 in healthy subjects. *Journal of Clinical Pharmacology.* **48**: 745–754.
5 Pfizer (2012) Celebrex 200mg capsules. *US Prescribing information* www.accessdata.fda.gov/scripts/cder/drugsatfda/index.cfm
6 Pfizer (2011) Celebrex 100mg & 200mg capsules. *SPC* www.medicines.org.uk
7 Gong L et al. (2012) Celecoxib pathways: pharmacokinetics and pharmacodynamics. *Pharmacogenetics and Genomics.* **22**: 310–318.
8 Chan AT et al. (2009) Cytochrome P450 2C9 variants influence response to celecoxib for prevention of colorectal adenoma. *Gastroenterology.* **136**: 2127–2136 e2121.
9 Alloza I et al. (2006) Celecoxib inhibits interleukin-12 alphabeta and beta2 folding and secretion by a novel COX2-independent mechanism involving chaperones of the endoplasmic reticulum. *Molecular Pharmacology.* **69**: 1579–1587.
10 Klein T et al. (2007) Celecoxib dilates guinea-pig coronaries and rat aortic rings and amplifies NO/cGMP signaling by PDE5 inhibition. *Cardiovascular Research.* **75**: 390–397.
11 Maier TJ et al. (2009) Cellular membranes function as a storage compartment for celecoxib. *Journal of Molecular Medicine.* **87**: 981–993.
12 Rezende RM et al. (2012) Endogenous opioid and cannabinoid mechanisms are involved in the analgesic effects of celecoxib in the central nervous system. *Pharmacology.* **89**: 127–136.
13 Emery P et al. (1999) Celecoxib versus diclofenac in long-term management of rheumatoid arthritis: randomised double-blind comparison. *Lancet.* **354**: 2106–2111.
14 Simon LS et al. (1999) Anti-inflammatory and upper gastrointestinal effects of celecoxib in rheumatoid arthritis: a randomized controlled trial. *Journal of the American Medical Association.* **282**: 1921–1928.
15 Bensen WG et al. (1999) Treatment of osteoarthritis with celecoxib, a cyclooxygenase-2 inhibitor: a randomized controlled trial. *Mayo Clinic Proceedings.* **74**: 1095–1105.
16 Chen YF et al. (2008) Cyclooxygenase-2 selective non-steroidal anti-inflammatory drugs (etodolac, meloxicam, celecoxib, rofecoxib, etoricoxib, valdecoxib and lumiracoxib) for osteoarthritis and rheumatoid arthritis: a systematic review and economic evaluation. *Health Technology Assessment.* **12**: 1–278, iii.
17 Derry S (2008) Single dose oral celecoxib for acute postoperative pain in adults. *Cochrane Database of Systematic Reviews.* **4**: CD004233.
18 Daniels S et al. (2009) Celecoxib in the treatment of primary dysmenorrhea: results from two randomized, double-blind, active- and placebo-controlled, crossover studies. *Clinical Therapeutics.* **31**: 1192–1208.
19 Phillips E et al. (2009) Celecoxib in the management of acute renal colic: a randomized controlled clinical trial. *Urology.* **74**: 994–999.

20 Saito O et al. (2005) Analgesic effects of nonsteroidal antiinflammatory drugs, acetaminophen, and morphine in a mouse model of bone cancer pain. Journal of Anesthesia. 19: 218–224.

21 Mouedden ME and Meert TF (2007) Pharmacological evaluation of opioid and non-opioid analgesics in a murine bone cancer model of pain. Pharmacology, Biochemistry, and Behavior. 86: 458–467.

22 CNT Collaboration (2013) Vascular and upper gastrointestinal effects of non-steroidal anti-inflammatory drugs: meta-analyses of individual participant data from randomised trials. Lancet. 382: 769–779.

23 Leese PT et al. (2000) Effects of celecoxib, a novel cyclooxygenase-2 inhibitor, on platelet function in healthy adults: a randomized, controlled trial. Journal of Clinical Pharmacology. 40: 124–132.

24 Graff J et al. (2007) Effects of selective COX-2 inhibition on prostanoids and platelet physiology in young healthy volunteers. Journal of Thrombosis and Haemostasis. 5: 2376–2385.

25 Chan CC et al. (2009) Do COX-2 inhibitors raise blood pressure more than nonselective NSAIDs and placebo? An updated meta-analysis. Journal of Hypertension. 27: 2332–2341.

26 Solomon DH et al. (2004) Relationship between COX-2 specific inhibitors and hypertension. Hypertension. 44: 140–145.

27 Schneider V et al. (2006) Association of selective and conventional nonsteroidal antiinflammatory drugs with acute renal failure: A population-based, nested case-control analysis. American Journal of Epidemiology. 164: 881–889.

28 Zhou R et al. (2010) Effect of celecoxib on proliferation, apoptosis, and survivin expression in human glioma cell line U251. Chinese Journal of Cancer. 29: 294–299.

29 Fujimura T et al. (2007) Cyclooxygenase-2 (COX-2) in carcinogenesis and selective COX-2 inhibitors for chemoprevention in gastrointestinal cancers. Journal of Gastrointestinal Cancer. 38: 78–82.

30 Lipton A et al. (2010) Phase II trial of gemcitabine, irinotecan, and celecoxib in patients with advanced pancreatic cancer. Journal of Clinical Gastroenterology. 44: 286–288.

31 Debucquoy A et al. (2009) Double blind randomized phase II study with radiation+5-fluorouracil+/-celecoxib for resectable rectal cancer. Radiotherapy and Oncology. 93: 273–278.

32 Schonthal AH et al. (2008) Celecoxib analogs that lack COX-2 inhibitory function: preclinical development of novel anticancer drugs. Expert Opinion on Investigational Drugs. 17: 197–208.

33 Farooqui M et al. (2007) COX-2 inhibitor celecoxib prevents chronic morphine-induced promotion of angiogenesis, tumour growth, metastasis and mortality, without compromising analgesia. British Journal of Cancer. 97: 1523–1531.

34 Paulson S et al. (2001) Pharmacokinetics of celecoxib after oral administration in dogs and humans: effects of food and site absorption. Journal of Pharmacology and Experimental Therapeutics. 297: 638–645.

35 Malmstrom K et al. (1999) Comparison of rofecoxib and celecoxib, two cyclooxygenase-2 inhibitors, in postoperative dental pain: a randomised, placebo- and active-comparator-controlled clinical trial. Clinical Therapeutics. 21: 1653–1663.

36 Baxter K and Preston CL Stockley's Drug Interactions. London: Pharmaceutical Press www.medicinescomplete.com (accessed December 2012).

Updated (minor change) May 2014

DICLOFENAC SODIUM   BNF 10.1.1

Class: Non-opioid analgesic, NSAID, preferential COX-2 inhibitor.

Indications: Pain and inflammation in arthritic conditions and other musculoskeletal disorders, postoperative pain, †dysmenorrhoea, acute gout, †cancer pain, †neoplastic fever.

Contra-indications: Hypersensitivity to **aspirin** or other NSAID (urticaria, rhinitis, asthma, angioedema), active GI ulceration, history of two or more distinct episodes of proven ulceration or bleeding, cerebrovascular bleeding or other bleeding disorders, ischaemic heart disease, peripheral arterial disease cerebrovascular disease, congestive heart failure (New York Heart Association [NYHA] classification II–IV), active liver disease or severe hepatic impairment, severe renal impairment, deteriorating renal function. (BNF advises *not* using IV diclofenac if plasma creatinine > 160micromol/L.)

Pharmacology

Diclofenac is a preferential COX-2 inhibitor (see Tables 1 and 2, p.309).[1–3] The analgesic effect of diclofenac has been shown in animals to be both peripheral and central.[4–6] In addition to inhibiting COX, diclofenac:

* activates the nitric oxide-cGMP nociceptive pathway[7]
* impacts on central nociception by increasing brain concentrations of kynurenic acid, an endogenous antagonist on the glycine recognition site of the NMDA-receptor-channel complex[8]
* facilitates inhibitory M-currents by opening potassium channels KCNQ2/3.[9,10]

It is possible that diclofenac is intrinsically more broad-spectrum in its central effects than other NSAIDs.[11]

It is a potent reversible inhibitor of platelet aggregation *in vitro*, but typical PO doses have no effect on bleeding time.[12] In contrast, IV diclofenac has a measurable effect on bleeding time, but most subjects remain within normal limits. However, with invasive procedures, bleeding time is a poor predictor of blood loss.[13] Using indicators which best correlate with peri-operative blood loss, diclofenac causes platelet dysfunction in about two thirds of healthy volunteers.[14]

In terms of effectiveness for osteoarthritis, diclofenac is non-inferior to other NSAIDs.[15] About 10–15% of patients experience undesirable effects (mainly gastric intolerance).[16] These are generally mild and transient; diclofenac needs to be withdrawn in only 2%.[12] Age[17] and renal or hepatic impairment do not have any significant effect on plasma concentrations of diclofenac, although metabolite concentrations increase in severe renal impairment. The principal metabolite, hydroxydiclofenac, possesses little anti-inflammatory effect.

A meta-analysis of several hundred RCTs indicates that, compared with placebo, the risk of upper GI complications with **diclofenac** is relatively low (about double), comparable with coxibs, and half that seen with **ibuprofen** and **naproxen**.[18]

Diclofenac carries a higher cardiovascular risk than non-selective NSAIDs,[18] and is now contra-indicated in individuals with vascular disease (see above).[19] The meta-analysis does not allow conclusions about how soon diclofenac increases the risk. The risk of renal failure with diclofenac is comparable with other NSAIDs.[20]

Severe local necrosis has been described anecdotally after IM and SC use.[21] Diclofenac is available as the *sodium* and *potassium* salts; diclofenac *potassium* is absorbed more quickly and peak plasma concentration is reached sooner. It is theoretically a better alternative in patients already troubled by Na^+ and water retention. However, it is much more expensive. Low dose (12.5mg tablets) are available OTC.

Bio-availability 50% PO (both immediate-release and m/r products); suppositories about 33%.
Onset of action 20–30min.
Time to peak plasma concentration diclofenac *sodium*: 2.5h e/c (fasting), 6h e/c (taken with food), ≥4h m/r, 1h suppositories; diclofenac *potassium* PO 20–60min (not significantly affected by food).
Plasma halflife 1–2h.
Duration of action 8h.

Cautions

Renal and hepatic impairment (see p.316 and p.317). Diclofenac treatment should be initiated only after careful consideration in patients with significant risk factors for cardiovascular events (e.g. hypertension, hyperlipidaemia, diabetes mellitus, smoking). Correct hyperkalaemia before use. To minimize the potential for serious undesirable effects, use the lowest effective dose for the shortest treatment duration possible. Risk of aseptic meningitis in patients with SLE (very rare).

Because of the increased risk of bleeding (from decreased platelet aggregation) try to avoid concurrent prescription of diclofenac and **warfarin**. As with all NSAIDs, concurrent administration with an SSRI is associated with an increased risk of GI bleeding.

The thromboprotective effect of **aspirin** for stroke is compromised in people taking a diclofenac concurrently.[22] Thus, people on **aspirin** for thromboprotection should *not* take diclofenac. If an NSAID is considered essential, stop the **aspirin** and prescribe **naproxen** b.d. (see p.315).

Drug interactions

Avoid taking antacids at the same time of day as e/c and m/r formulations.

Because they cause sodium and fluid retention, all NSAIDs can decrease the effect of diuretics, ACE inhibitors and antihypertensives.

In addition to the effect on platelet function (see Cautions), an increase in INR may occur when diclofenac is prescribed for a patient already taking **warfarin**; monitor the INR weekly for 3–4 weeks and adjust the dose of **warfarin** if necessary.[23]

For general interactions between NSAIDs and other drugs, see Tables 8 and 9 (p.319 and p.320). Of particular importance is the risk of toxic plasma levels of **clofarabine**, **digoxin**, **lithium**, and **methotrexate** caused by reduced renal function and/or reduced tubular excretion. If diclofenac is prescribed, monitor the plasma drug concentration or haematological effect of these drugs as appropriate and reduce doses as necessary (see p.318).

Concurrent use of diclofenac with **ciclosporin** may increase the plasma concentration of diclofenac (up to double), and decrease the plasma concentration of **ciclosporin**. If given concurrently, the manufacturer advises halving the dose of diclofenac.

Diclofenac plasma concentration may be *increased* by **voriconazole**. This may be due to inhibition by CYP2C9 hepatic enzyme; lower doses of diclofenac may be necessary. Conversely, **rifampicin** may *decrease* diclofenac plasma concentration due to CYP3A4 enzyme induction; consider an alternative NSAID if pain returns. Caution should be taken with concurrent use of other drugs which inhibit or induce these enzymes, particularly in those who are poor CYP2C9 metabolizers (see Chapter 25, p.775).

Undesirable effects

Also see NSAIDs, p.307.

Common (<10%, >1%): headache, dizziness, oedema, indigestion, abdominal discomfort, nausea, constipation or diarrhoea, pruritus, rash, ecchymosis.

Dose and use

For patients with, or at very high risk of, NSAID-related GI ulceration, see Box D, p.314.

The SPC recommends that diclofenac is taken with or after food, but this advice seems unnecessary; there is no evidence that this reduces upper GI complications (see p.321).

Typical regimens of diclofenac sodium are:
• 50mg PO b.d.–t.d.s.
• m/r 75mg PO b.d. or 100mg once daily
• 50mg PR b.d.–t.d.s.
Some patients obtain greater benefit from 200mg/24h with no immediately apparent increase in undesirable effects, e.g. m/r 100mg b.d. However, doses > 150mg/24h are unauthorized and are associated with an increased cardiovascular risk (see Pharmacology).

Diclofenac is available as an injection and is used primarily to relieve biliary and renal colic (75mg IM p.r.n., maximum 150mg/24h).[24,25] If given by CSCI, it must be given via a separate syringe driver (or other delivery device) because it is an alkaline solution and thus incompatible with other drugs (see p.701). A typical regimen is 75mg SC/IM stat and 150mg/24h CSCI.

For topical use, see p.584.

Supply

Diclofenac *sodium* (generic)
Tablets *e/c* 25mg, 50mg, 28 days @ 50mg t.d.s. = £1.
Suppositories 100mg, 10 = £3.50.

Voltarol® (Novartis)
Tablets *e/c* 25mg, 50mg, 28 days @ 50mg t.d.s. = £4.50
Tablets dispersible 50mg, 28 days @ 50mg t.d.s. = £25.
Injection 25mg/mL, 3mL amp = £1
Suppositories 12.5mg, 25mg, 50mg, 100mg; 50mg, 10 = £2; 100mg, 10 = £3.

Modified-release
Diclomax SR® (Galen)
Capsules *m/r* 75mg, 28 days @ 75mg b.d. = £11.

Diclomax Retard® (Galen)
Capsules *m/r* 100mg, 28 days @ 100mg once daily = £9.

Motifen® 75mg (Daiichi Sankyo)
Capsules (containing *e/c* **pellets 25mg and** *m/r* **pellets 50mg)** 75mg, 28 days @ 75mg b.d. = £8.

Voltarol® 75mg SR (Novartis)
Tablets *m/r* 75mg, 28 days @ 75mg b.d. = £13.

Voltarol® Retard (Novartis)
Tablets *m/r* 100mg, 28 days @ 100mg once daily = £10.

With **misoprostol**

Arthrotec® 50 (Pharmacia)

Tablets diclofenac sodium 50mg e/c + **misoprostol** 200microgram, 28 days @ 1 t.d.s. = £12. Note the cost of this product is approximately the same as prescribing the two drugs separately.

Arthrotec® 75 (Pfizer)

Tablets diclofenac sodium 75mg e/c + **misoprostol** 200microgram, 28 days @ 1 b.d. = £16. Note the cost of this product is cheaper than prescribing diclofenac 75mg capsules and misoprostol tablets separately (or equivalent in price to using the diclofenac 25mg tablets); however, it contains only half the **misoprostol** dose needed for optimal protection.

1 John V (1979) The pharmacokinetics and metabolism of diclofenac sodium (Voltarol) in animals and man. Rheumatology and Rehabilitation. (suppl 2): 22–37.

2 Patrignani P et al. (1997) Differential inhibition of human prostaglandin endoperoxide synthase-1 and -2 by nonsteroidal anti-inflammatory drugs. Journal of Physiology and Pharmacology. 48: 623–631.

3 Schwartz JI et al. (2008) Comparative inhibitory activity of etoricoxib, celecoxib, and diclofenac on COX-2 versus COX-1 in healthy subjects. Journal of Clinical Pharmacology. 48: 745–754.

4 McCormack K (1994) Nonsteroidal anti-inflammatory drugs and spinal nociceptive processing. Pain. 59: 9–43.

5 Svensson CI and Yaksh TL (2002) The spinal phospholipase-cyclooxygenase-prostanoid cascade in nociceptive processing. Annual Review of Pharmacology and Toxicology. 42: 553–583.

6 Ortiz MI et al. (2008) Additive interaction between peripheral and central mechanisms involved in the antinociceptive effect of diclofenac in the formalin test in rats. Pharmacology, Biochemistry and Behavior. 91: 32–37.

7 Ortiz MI et al. (2003) The NO-cGMP-K+ channel pathway participates in the antinociceptive effect of diclofenac, but not of indomethacin. Pharmacology, Biochemistry and Behavior. 76: 187–195.

8 Schwieler L et al. (2005) Prostaglandin-mediated control of rat brain kynurenic acid synthesis - opposite actions by COX-1 and COX-2 isoforms. Journal of Neural Transmission. 112: 863–872.

9 Peretz A et al. (2005) Meclofenamic acid and diclofenac, novel templates of KCNQ2/Q3 potassium channel openers, depress cortical neuron activity and exhibit anticonvulsant properties. Molecular Pharmacology. 67: 1053–1066.

10 Gan TJ (2010) Diclofenac: an update on its mechanism of action and safety profile. Current Medical Research Opinion. 26: 1715–1731.

11 McCormack K and Twycross RG (2001) Are COX-2 selective inhibitors effective analgesics. Pain Review. 8: 13–26.

12 Todd P and Sorkin E (1988) Diclofenac sodium: a reappraisal of its pharmacodynamic and pharmacokinetic properties, and therapeutic efficacy. Drugs. 35: 244–285.

13 Peterson P et al. (1998) The preoperative bleeding time test lacks clinical benefit: College of American Pathologists' and American Society of Clinical Pathologists' position article. Archives of Surgery. 133: 134–139.

14 Ng KF et al. (2008) Comprehensive preoperative evaluation of platelet function in total knee arthroplasty patients taking diclofenac. Journal of Arthroplasty. 23: 424–430.

15 Pavelka K (2012) A comparison of the therapeutic efficacy of diclofenac in osteoarthritis: a systematic review of randomised controlled trials. Current Medical Research Opinion. 28: 163–178.

16 Medsafe (2010) New Zealand Medicines and Medical Devices Safety Authority. Available from: http://www.medsafe.govt.nz/profs/datasheet/d/diclaxtab.htm

17 Willis JV and Kendall MJ (1978) Pharmacokinetic studies on diclofenac sodium in young and old volunteers. Scandinavian Journal of Rheumatology. Suppl: 36–41.

18 CNT Collaboration (2013) Vascular and upper gastrointestinal effects of non-steroidal anti-inflammatory drugs: meta-analyses of individual participant data from randomised trials. Lancet. 382: 769–779.

19 MHRA (2013) Diclofenac: new contraindications and warnings after a Europe-wide review of cardiovascular safety. Drug Safety Update. (6) 11: www.mhra.gov.uk/safetyinformation

20 Schneider V et al. (2006) Association of selective and conventional nonsteroidal antiinflammatory drugs with acute renal failure: A population-based, nested case-control analysis. American Journal of Epidemiology. 164: 881–889.

21 Kirkpatrick G (2003) SC diclofenac. In: Bulletin board discussion. Palliativedrugs.com. Available from: http://www.palliative-drugs.com/bulletin-board.html

22 Gladding PA et al. (2008) The antiplatelet effect of six non-steroidal anti-inflammatory drugs and their pharmacodynamic interaction with aspirin in healthy volunteers. American Journal of Cardiology. 101: 1060–1063.

23 Baxter K and Preston CL Stockley's Drug Interactions London: Pharmaceutical Press www.medicinescomplete.com (accessed December 2012).

24 Lundstam SOA et al. (1982) Prostaglandin-synthetase inhibition with diclofenac sodium in treatment of renal colic: comparison with use of a narcotic analgesic. Lancet. 1: 1096–1097.

25 Thompson JF et al. (1989) Rectal diclofenac compared with pethidine injection in acute renal colic. British Medical Journal. 299: 1140–1141.

Updated August 2013

FLURBIPROFEN   BNF 10.1.1

Class: Non-opioid analgesic, NSAID, preferential COX-1 inhibitor.

Indications: Pain and inflammation in arthritic conditions, musculoskeletal disorders and trauma, dental pain, dysmenorrhoea, migraine, postoperative analgesia, sore throat (lozenges, see p.604), †cancer pain, †neoplastic fever, †detrusor instability.[1]

Contra-indications: Hypersensitivity to **aspirin** or other NSAID (urticaria, rhinitis, asthma, angioedema), active GI ulceration, history of two or more distinct episodes of proven ulceration or bleeding, cerebrovascular bleeding or other bleeding disorders, severe heart failure, active liver disease or severe hepatic impairment, severe renal impairment, deteriorating renal function.

Pharmacology

Flurbiprofen is a propionic acid derivative and a highly potent COX inhibitor. It inhibits both COX-1 and COX-2 but, along with **indometacin**, **ketoprofen** and **ketorolac**, has higher COX-1 selectivity than many NSAIDs.[2] The molar potency for 50% inhibition of PGE_2 synthesis in vitro is >5,000 times that of **aspirin**, 250 times that of **ibuprofen**, and 125 times that of **naproxen**.[3] In animals, mg for mg, it is 8–20 times more potent than **aspirin**. Flurbiprofen is excreted in the urine both as unchanged drug and several hydroxylated metabolites.

Flurbiprofen has been used for many years by some palliative care services as the NSAID of choice (without routine gastroprotection). It is convenient to use and apparently very effective. Flurbiprofen does not feature in any of the recent surveys and meta-analyses, and it is in danger of becoming a forgotten drug even though there are no specific adverse GI data to justify its exclusion. However, a recent case-crossover study ranked the risk of myocardial infarction for oral flurbiprofen second only to ketorolac.[4]

In addition to its analgesic use, flurbiprofen has been used to relieve frequency caused by instability of the detrusor muscle of the bladder. Animal studies show that PGs are produced by the detrusor (bladder muscle) and that they increase tone and bladder contractile activity. In humans, frequency, urgency, and urge incontinence are all significantly decreased by flurbiprofen 50mg t.d.s.[1]

Bio-availability >85% PO.
Onset of action 30–60min.
Time to peak plasma concentration 1–2h PO; 4–6h m/r.
Plasma halflife 3–6h.
Duration of action 8–16h.[5]

Cautions

Renal, hepatic and cardiovascular impairment (see p.315–317). Correct hyperkalaemia before use. To minimize the potential for serious undesirable effects, use the lowest effective dose for the shortest treatment duration possible. Risk of aseptic meningitis in patients with SLE (very rare).

Because of the increased risk of bleeding (from decreased platelet aggregation) try to avoid concurrent prescription of flurbiprofen and **warfarin**. As with all NSAIDs, concurrent administration with an SSRI is associated with an increased risk of GI bleeding.

The thromboprotective effect of **aspirin** for stroke is compromised in people taking certain NSAIDs concurrently.[6] However, the preferential and intense COX-1 inhibition achieved with flurbiprofen is likely to produce prolonged platelet inhibition (as with **naproxen**). Thus, it is reasonable to stop **aspirin** when flurbiprofen is prescribed.

Drug interactions

Because they cause sodium and fluid retention, all NSAIDs can decrease the effect of diuretics, ACE inhibitors and antihypertensives.

In addition to the effect on platelet function (see Cautions), an increase in INR occasionally occurs when flurbiprofen is prescribed for a patient already taking **warfarin**; monitor the INR weekly for 3–4 weeks and adjust the dose of **warfarin** if necessary.[7]

For general interactions between NSAIDs and other drugs, see Tables 8 and 9 (p.319 and p.320). Of particular importance is the risk of toxic plasma levels of **clofarabine**, **digoxin**,

lithium, and **methotrexate** caused by reduced renal function and/or reduced tubular excretion. If flurbiprofen is prescribed, monitor the plasma drug concentration or haematological effect of these drugs and reduce doses as necessary (see p.318).

Flurbiprofen is metabolized by CYP2C9. Caution should be taken with concurrent use of drugs which inhibit or induce this enzyme, particularly in those who are poor CYP2C9 metabolizers (see Chapter 25, p.775). **Fluconazole** and possibly **voriconazole** (strong CYP2C9 inhibitors) increase flurbiprofen plasma concentration, and lower doses may be necessary.

Undesirable effects

Also see NSAIDs, p.307.

Common (<10%, >1%): headache, dizziness, oedema, indigestion, abdominal discomfort, nausea, constipation or diarrhoea, pruritus, rash, ecchymosis.

Dose and use

For patients with, or at *very* high risk of, NSAID-related GI ulceration, see Box D, p.314.

The SPC recommends that flurbiprofen is taken with or after food, but this advice seems unnecessary; there is no evidence that this reduces upper GI complications (see p.321).

Typical regimens for cancer pain:
*   start with 100mg b.d.
*   if necessary, increase to 100mg t.d.s.
*   in very elderly or debilitated:
    ▷ start with 50mg b.d.
    ▷ if necessary, increase to 100mg b.d.

For sore throat, see p.604.

Supply

Flurbiprofen (generic)
Tablets 50mg, 100mg, 28 days @ 100mg b.d. = £16.

Froben® (Abbott)
Tablets 50mg, 100mg, 28 days @ 100mg b.d. = £10.

1 Cardozo L et al. (1980) Evaluation of flurbiprofen in detrusor instability. British Medical Journal. **280**: 281–282.
2 Uzan A (2005) The unexpected side effects of new nonsteroidal anti-inflammatory drugs. Expert Opinion on Emerging Drugs. **10**: 687–688.
3 Crook D et al. (1976) Effect of aspirin-like drug therapy. Prostaglandin synthetase activity from human rheumatoid synovial microsomes. Annals of the Rheumatic Diseases. **35**: 327–332.
4 Shau WY et al. (2012) Risk of new acute myocardial infarction hospitalization associated with use of oral and parenteral non-steroidal anti-inflammation drugs (NSAIDS): a case crossover study of Taiwan's National health Insurance claims database and review of current evidence. Available from: www.biomedcentral.com/1471-2261/12/4
5 Kowanko I et al. (1981) Circadian variations in the signs and symptoms of rheumatoid arthritis and in the therapeutic effectiveness of flurbiprofen at different times of day. British Journal of Clinical Pharmacology. **11**: 477–484.
6 Gladding PA et al. (2008) The antiplatelet effect of six non-steroidal anti-inflammatory drugs and their pharmacodynamic interaction with aspirin in healthy volunteers. American Journal of Cardiology. **101**: 1060–1063.
7 Baxter K and Preston CL Stockley's Drug Interactions. London: Pharmaceutical Press www.medicinescomplete.com (accessed December 2012).

Updated August 2013

IBUPROFEN   BNF 10.1.1

Class: Non-opioid analgesic, NSAID, non-selective COX inhibitor.

Indications: Pain and inflammation in arthritic conditions and other musculoskeletal disorders, postoperative pain, dental pain, dysmenorrhoea, headache, migraine, fever, †cancer pain.

Contra-indications: Hypersensitivity to **aspirin** or other NSAID (urticaria, rhinitis, asthma, angioedema), active GI ulceration, history of two or more distinct episodes of proven ulceration or bleeding, cerebrovascular bleeding or other bleeding disorders, severe heart failure, active liver disease or severe hepatic impairment, severe renal impairment, deteriorating renal function.

Pharmacology

Ibuprofen is a non-selective COX inhibitor (see Tables 1 and 2, p.309). Like **flurbiprofen** and **naproxen**, it is a propionic acid derivative. The analgesic effect of ibuprofen is mediated by several non-COX mechanisms in addition to COX inhibition (see p.310).[1] Doses of 2,400mg/day are well tolerated by most patients. Ibuprofen is three times more potent than **aspirin**, i.e. 200mg is equivalent to 600mg of **aspirin**. Higher doses of ibuprofen have a greater analgesic effect than standard doses of **aspirin**. The antipyretic action of ibuprofen is mediated both by inhibition of prostaglandin synthesis and by COX-independent mechanisms.[2]

Ibuprofen is a chiral NSAID, i.e. it is a mixture of roughly equal amounts of S– and R– enantiomers, mirror-image molecules which rotate polarized light in opposite directions.[3,4] The anti-inflammatory activity resides mostly in the S–enantiomer, but about half the R–enantiomer is converted to the S– form in the GI tract and liver.[1] Thus, the clinical effects of the racemic mixture depend on absorption rate.[5]

Ibuprofen shares this property of enantiomeric inversion with similar NSAIDs, e.g. **ketoprofen**. This has led to the production of **dexibuprofen** and **dexketoprofen** (both authorized in the UK) which are pure S–enantiomers and thus theoretically more potent mg for mg. The enantiomers are metabolized via CYP450. Age also affects the S–enantiomer free drug concentrations and clearance; the S–enantiomer reaches higher levels and persists for longer in the elderly.[6]

Inversion takes time, and the time frame for single doses in acute situations is too short for inversion to play an important part.[7] Even so, a single dose of ibuprofen for acute postoperative pain is highly effective, with an NNT of around 2.5 for 200–400mg PO.[8] In arthritis, ibuprofen is concentrated at sites of inflammation, e.g. the joint synovium.[9] At low doses (200–400mg) it is as effective as **paracetamol** 1g, and efficacy increases as the dose increases.[10]

Low-dose ibuprofen (≤1,200mg/24h) has a low propensity for causing upper GI complications (ulceration, bleeding, perforation)[11,12] and, in consequence, is available OTC. However, with high dose ibuprofen (2,400mg/24h), the risk is quadrupled (as with high-dose **naproxen**).[13] This compares unfavourably with the doubled risk seen with **diclofenac** and the coxibs. Even at low doses ibuprofen causes significantly more ulcers than **celecoxib**.[14] On the other hand, a small RCT found that ibuprofen 2,400mg/24h + **misoprostol** 800mg/24h carries the same risk of endoscopic ulcers as **nabumetone** alone.[15] Concern has been expressed about the possibility that OTC ibuprofen may occasionally cause small bowel damage.[16]

A meta-analysis of several hundred RCTs showed that high-dose ibuprofen (2,400mg/24h) significantly increases major cardiovascular events, with a risk comparable with **diclofenac** and the coxibs.[13] However, there were many fewer events in RCTs of ibuprofen vs. coxib compared with placebo-controlled ones. Further, a meta-analysis of >50 epidemiological studies suggests that low-dose ibuprofen (<1200–1800mg/24h) carries no cardiovascular risk, even in patients with previous cardiovascular problems.[17]

The risk of renal failure with ibuprofen is comparable with other NSAIDs.[18] It is safe in overdose; only 14 deaths attributable to ibuprofen alone have been reported, involving overdoses of 36–200g.[19–23] It is definitely safer than two other commonly used antipyretic analgesics, **paracetamol** and **aspirin**.[1]

Ibuprofen is of benefit in cancer-related cachexia (see Progestogens, p.536), although such use is experimental.

Ibuprofen can be used topically (as a locally prepared preparation), particularly for sprains, strains and arthritis.[24] Although application to the skin produces plasma concentrations which are only 5% of those obtained with oral administration, the underlying muscle and fascial concentrations are 25 times greater.[25,26] An RCT showed that patients with sprains and bruises treated with TD ibuprofen did significantly better in relation to speed of resolution, relief of pain, reduction in swelling and return of function.[27]

A Health Technology Assessment found that topical and PO ibuprofen were equally effective for chronic knee pain in patients aged ≥50 years, although those with more severe or widespread pain preferred PO treatment.[28] The incidence of major undesirable effects were similar, but topical treatment led to fewer minor undesirable effects and less treatment discontinuation. Based on the cost per quality-adjusted life-year, topical ibuprofen was more cost-effective over the first year, whereas PO treatment was more cost-effective over 2 years.[28] Systemic undesirable effects with topical ibuprofen for acute pain are uncommon, and even local effects were not significantly different from placebo.[29]

Because it has a more rapid onset of action, IV ibuprofen (not UK) has a potential role in the management of acute pain.[30]

Bio-availability 90% PO.
Onset of action 20–30min.
Time to peak plasma concentration 1–2h.
Plasma halflife 2–3h.[1]
Duration of action 4–6h.

Cautions

Renal, hepatic and cardiovascular impairment (see p.315–317). Correct hyperkalaemia before use. To minimize the potential for serious undesirable effects, use the lowest effective dose for the shortest treatment duration possible. Risk of aseptic meningitis in patients with SLE (very rare).

Because of the increased risk of bleeding (from decreased platelet aggregation) try to avoid concurrent prescription of ibuprofen and **warfarin**. As with all NSAIDs, concurrent administration with an SSRI is associated with an increased risk of GI bleeding.

The thromboprotective effect of **aspirin** for stroke is compromised in people taking ibuprofen concurrently.[31–33] Thus, people on **aspirin** for thromboprotection should not take ibuprofen. If an NSAID is considered essential, stop the **aspirin** and prescribe **naproxen** b.d. (see p.315).

Drug interactions

Avoid taking antacids at the same time of day as m/r formulations.

Because they cause sodium and fluid retention, all NSAIDs can decrease the effect of diuretics, ACE inhibitors and antihypertensives.

In addition to the effect on platelet function (see Cautions), an increase in INR occasionally occurs when ibuprofen is prescribed for a patient already taking **warfarin**; monitor the INR weekly for 3–4 weeks and adjust the dose of **warfarin** if necessary.[34]

For general interactions between NSAIDs and other drugs, see Tables 8 and 9 (p.319 and p.320). Of particular importance is the risk of toxic plasma levels of **clofarabine**, **digoxin**, **lithium**, and **methotrexate** caused by reduced renal function and/or reduced tubular excretion. If ibuprofen is prescribed, monitor the plasma drug concentration or haematological effect of these drugs as appropriate and reduce doses as necessary (see p.318).

Ibuprofen is metabolized by CYP2C9. Caution should be taken with concurrent use of drugs which inhibit or induce this enzyme, particularly in those who are poor CYP2C9 metabolizers (see Chapter 25, p.775). **Fluconazole** and **voriconazole** (strong CYP2C9 inhibitors) increase ibuprofen plasma concentration, and lower doses may be necessary.

Undesirable effects

Also see NSAIDs, p.307.
Common (<10%, >1%): headache, dizziness, oedema, indigestion, abdominal discomfort, nausea, constipation or diarrhoea, pruritus, rash, ecchymosis.

Dose and use

For patients with, or at *very* high risk of, NSAID-related GI ulceration, see Box D, p.314.
The SPC recommends that ibuprofen is taken with or after food, but this advice seems unnecessary; there is no evidence that this reduces upper GI complications (see p.321).

- start with 400mg t.d.s.
- if necessary, increase to 600–800mg t.d.s.

For topical use, see p.584.

Supply

Ibuprofen tablets and capsules 200mg and 400mg, and ibuprofen suspension and gel are available OTC.

Ibuprofen (generic)
Tablets 200mg, 400mg, 600mg, 28 days @ 400mg t.d.s. = £2.
Oral suspension 100mg/5mL, 28 days @ 400mg t.d.s. = £30; *sugar free suspenstion also available.*

Brufen® (Abbott)
Tablets 200mg, 400mg, 600mg, 28 days @ 400mg t.d.s. = £7.
Oral syrup 100mg/5mL, 28 days @ 400mg t.d.s. = £30.
Granules 600mg/sachet, 28 days @ 600mg b.d. = £18 *(contains 6.5mmol Na^+/sachet).*

Modified-release
Brufen Retard® (Abbott)
Tablets *m/r* 800mg, 28 days @1,600mg once daily. = £7.

Fenbid® (Goldshield)
Capsules enclosing *m/r* pellets 300mg, 28 days @ 600mg b.d. = £9.

1   Rainsford KD (2009) Ibuprofen: pharmacology, efficacy and safety. *Inflammopharmacology.* **17**: 275–342.
2   Soares DM et al. (2011) Cyclooxygenase-independent mechanism of ibuprofen-induced antipyresis: the role of central vasopressin V(1) receptors. *Fundamental and Clinical Pharmacology.* **25**: 670–681.
3   Rudy AC et al. (1991) Stereoselective metabolism of ibuprofen in humans: administration of R-, S- and racemic ibuprofen. *Journal of Pharmacology and Experimental Therapeutics.* **259**: 1133–1139.
4   Jamali F et al. (1992) Human pharmacokinetics of ibuprofen enantiomers following different doses and formulations: intestinal chiral inversion. *Journal of Pharmaceutical Sciences.* **81**: 221–225.
5   Ding G et al. (2007) Effect of absorption rate on pharmacokinetics of ibuprofen in relation to chiral inversion in humans. *Journal of Pharmacy and Pharmacology.* **59**: 1509–1513
6   Tan SC et al. (2003) Influence of age on the enantiomeric disposition of ibuprofen in healthy volunteers. *British Journal of Clinical Pharmacology.* **55**: 579–587.
7   Evans AM (2001) Comparative pharmacology of S(+)-ibuprofen and (RS)-ibuprofen. *Clinical Rheumatology.* **20 Suppl 1**: S9–14.
8   Derry C et al. (2009) Single dose oral ibuprofen for acute postoperative pain in adults. *Cochrane Database of Systematic Reviews.* **3**: CD001548.
9   Glass RC and Swannell AJ (1978) Concentrations of ibuprofen in serum and synovial fluid from patients with arthritis [proceedings]. *British Journal of Clinical Pharmacology.* **6**: 453P–454P.
10 McQuay HJ and Moore RA (2007) Dose-response in direct comparisons of different doses of aspirin, ibuprofen and paracetamol (acetaminophen) in analgesic studies. *British Journal of Clinical Pharmacology.* **63**: 271–278.
11 Masso Gonzalez EL et al. (2010) Variability among nonsteroidal antiinflammatory drugs in risk of upper gastrointestinal bleeding. *Arthritis and Rheumatism.* **62**: 1592–1601.
12 Michels SL et al. (2012) Over-the-counter ibuprofen and risk of gastrointestinal bleeding complications: a systematic literature review. *Current Medical Research Opinion.* **28**: 89–99.
13 CNT Collaboration (2013) Vascular and upper gastrointestinal effects of non-steroidal anti-inflammatory drugs: meta-analyses of individual participant data from randomised trials. *Lancet.* **382**: 769–779.
14 Scheiman JM et al. (2004) A randomized, controlled comparison of ibuprofen at the maximal over-the-counter dose compared with prescription-dose celecoxib on upper gastrointestinal mucosal injury. *Clinical Gastroenterology and Hepatology.* **2**: 290–295.
15 Roth SH et al. (1993) A controlled study comparing the effects of nabumetone, ibuprofen, and ibuprofen plus misoprostol on the upper gastrointestinal tract mucosa. *Archives of Internal Medicine.* **153**: 2565–2571.
16 Sidhu M et al. (2010) Undisclosed use of nonsteroidal anti-inflammatory drugs may underlie small-bowel injury observed in capsule endoscopy. *Clinical Gastroenterology and Hepatology.* **8**: 992–995.
17 McGettigan P and Henry D (2011) Cardiovascular risk with non-steroidal anti-inflammatory drugs: systematic review of population-based controlled observational studies. *PLoS Med.* **8**: e1001098.

18 Schneider V et al. (2006) Association of selective and conventional nonsteroidal antiinflammatory drugs with acute renal failure: A population-based, nested case-control analysis. American Journal of Epidemiology. **164**: 881–889.

19 Wood DM et al. (2006) Fatality after deliberate ingestion of sustained-release ibuprofen: a case report. Critical Care. **10**: R44.

20 Krenova M and Pelclova D (2005) Fatal poisoning with ibuprofen. Clinical Toxicology. **43**: 537.

21 Volans G et al. (2003) Ibuprofen overdose. International Journal of Clinical Practice Supplement. 54–60.

22 Holubek W et al. (2007) A report of two deaths from massive ibuprofen ingestion. Journal of Medical Toxicology. **3**: 52–55.

23 Lodise M et al. (2012) Acute Ibuprofen intoxication: report on a case and review of the literature. American Journal of Forensic Medicine and Pathology. **33**: 242–246.

24 Chlud K and Wagener H (1987) Percutaneous nonsteroidal anti-inflammatory drug (NSAID) therapy with particular reference to pharmacokinetic factors. EULAR Bulletin. **2**: 40–43.

25 Mondino A et al. (1983) Kinetic studies of ibuprofen on humans. Comparative study for the determination of blood concentrations and metabolites following local and oral administration. Medizinische Welt. **34**: 1052–1054.

26 Kageyama T (1987) A double blind placebo controlled multicenter study of piroxicam 0.5% gel in osteoarthritis of the knee. European Journal of Rheumatology and Inflammation. **8**: 114–115.

27 Peters H et al. (1987) Percutaneous kinetics of ibuprofen (German). Aktuelle Rheumatologie. **12**: 208–211.

28 Underwood M et al. (2008) Topical or oral ibuprofen for chronic knee pain in older people. The TOIB study. Available from: www.hta.ac.uk/project/1302.asp

29 Massey T et al. (2010) Topical NSAIDS for acute pain in adults. Cochrane Database of Systematic Reviews. **6**: CD007402.

30 Smith HS and Voss B (2012) Pharmacokinetics of intravenous ibuprofen: implications of time of infusion in the treatment of pain and fever. Drugs. **72**: 327–337.

31 Gengo FM et al. (2008) Effects of ibuprofen on the magnitude and duration of aspirin's inhibition of platelet aggregation: clinical consequences in stroke prophylaxis. Journal of Clinical Pharmacology. **48**: 117–122.

32 Gladding PA et al. (2008) The antiplatelet effect of six non-steroidal anti-inflammatory drugs and their pharmacodynamic interaction with aspirin in healthy volunteers. American Journal of Cardiology. **101**: 1060–1063.

33 Awa K et al. (2012) Prediction of time-dependent interaction of aspirin with ibuprofen using a pharmacokinetic/ pharmacodynamic model. Journal of Clinical Pharmacy and Therapeutics. **37**: 469–474.

34 Baxter K and Preston CL Stockley's Drug Interactions. London: Pharmaceutical Press www.medicinescomplete.com (accessed December 2012).

Updated (minor change) May 2014

*KETOROLAC TROMETAMOL   BNF 15.1.4.2

Class: Non-opioid analgesic, NSAID, preferential COX-1 inhibitor.

Indications: Short-term management of moderate–severe acute postoperative pain, †intractable nociceptive cancer pain.

Contra-indications: Hypersensitivity to **aspirin** or other NSAID (urticaria, rhinitis, asthma, angioedema), syndrome of nasal polyps, angioedema and bronchospasm, history of asthma, history of or active GI ulceration, cerebrovascular bleeding or other bleeding disorders, severe heart failure, severe hepatic impairment, moderate or severe renal impairment (eGFR < 60mL/ min/1.73m^2), deteriorating renal function.

Concurrent prescription with **warfarin**, **heparin**, **aspirin**, other NSAID, **pentoxifylline** (increased risk of bleeding), **lithium** (increased plasma concentration and toxicity), and **probenecid** (increased ketorolac plasma concentration and halflife).

Pharmacology

Ketorolac is a cyclic propionate structurally related to the acetate NSAIDs, **tolmetin** and **indometacin**.[1,2] It inhibits both COX-1 and COX-2 but, along with **flurbiprofen**, **indometacin** and **ketoprofen**, has higher COX-1 selectivity than many NSAIDs.[3]

Ketorolac trometamol is more water-soluble than the parent substance. Over 99% of the oral dose is absorbed and about 75% of a dose is excreted in the urine within 7h, and over 90% within 2 days, over half as unmodified ketorolac.[4] The rest is excreted in the faeces. The analgesic and anti-inflammatory activity of ketorolac resides mainly in the S-enantiomer, which is cleared more rapidly than the less active R-enantiomer. The analgesic effect is far greater than the antipyretic and anti-inflammatory properties. In animal studies, ketorolac is about 350 times more potent than **aspirin** as an analgesic but only 20 times more potent as an antipyretic.[5] As an anti-inflammatory ketorolac is about half as potent as **indometacin** and twice as potent as **naproxen**. Like most inhibitors of COX-1, ketorolac inhibits platelet aggregation.

Of all the NSAIDs, ketorolac (PO or parenteral) appears to carry the highest risk for gastritis and duodenitis, and upper GI complications (ulceration, bleeding, perforation).[6] A meta-analysis calculated a 15 times increase in risk with ketorolac, which is three times the risk of non-selective NSAIDs generally.[7]

Likewise, ketorolac (PO or parenteral) possibly carries the highest risk of acute myocardial infarction of any NSAID.[8] A retrospective case-crossover study of 38,000 people with strokes found PO ketorolac to be associated with only a moderate increase in the risk of stroke (odds ratio 1.9) but parenterally the risk of ischaemic or haemorrhagic stroke was increased 4–6 times.[9]

However, other postoperative studies indicate that, compared with opioids, the short-term use of ketorolac is associated with only a small increased risk of GI and operative site bleeding.[10,11] The risk is largely related to old age, and increases significantly if treatment is continued for > 1 week.[10,12] Thus, authorization for ketorolac is restricted to short-term postoperative use.[13,14] In some countries, authorization has been withdrawn, e.g. France and Germany. Ketorolac has been used in emergency departments for post-traumatic pain.[11] However, high-dose ketorolac after spinal surgery is associated with an increased rate of bony non-union.[15]

Studies submitted to the FDA to obtain marketing authorization in the USA were on acute pain.[16] Data on management of chronic pain are scanty and of low quality. In palliative care, ketorolac has been used for extended periods but always with a gastroprotective drug.[5,17–19]

In a week-long RCT in cancer pain, PO ketorolac 10mg q.d.s. was no better than **paracetamol** 600mg + **codeine** 60mg q.d.s.[20] It was also found to be no better than PO **diclofenac**.[21] However, anecdotal clinical experience suggests that parenteral ketorolac may be effective in some patients, notably with bone pain, who fail to obtain relief with NSAIDs PO.[5,17–19]

Bio-availability 100% PO.
Onset of action 30min PO, 10–30min IM/IV.
Time to peak plasma concentration 44 min PO, 35min IM, 1.1min IV.
Plasma halflife 5h; 7h in the elderly;[22] 6–19h with renal impairment.[12]
Duration of action 6h PO, 4–6h IM.

Cautions

Renal, hepatic and cardiovascular impairment (see p.315–317). Correct hyperkalaemia before use. To minimize the potential for serious undesirable effects, use the lowest effective dose for the shortest treatment duration possible. Risk of aseptic meningitis in patients with SLE (very rare).

As with all NSAIDs, concurrent administration with an SSRI is associated with an increased risk of GI bleeding.

Drug interactions

Because they cause sodium and fluid retention, all NSAIDs can decrease the effect of diuretics, ACE inhibitors and antihypertensives.

See above for drugs contra-indicated with ketorolac. For general interactions between NSAIDs and other drugs, see Tables 8 and 9 (p.319 and p.320). Of particular importance is the risk of toxic plasma levels of **clofarabine**, **digoxin**, **lithium**, and **methotrexate** caused by reduced renal function and/or reduced tubular excretion (see p.318).

Undesirable effects

Also see NSAIDs, see p.307.
Very common (>10%): headache, dyspepsia, nausea, abdominal pain.
Common (<10%, >1%): dizziness, drowsiness, tinnitus, oedema, hypertension, anaemia, stomatitis, vomiting, bloating, flatulence, GI ulceration, diarrhoea, constipation, abnormal renal function, pruritus, purpura, rash, bleeding and pain at injection site (less with CSCI).

Dose and use

For patients with, or at very high risk of, NSAID-related GI ulceration, see Box D, p.314

Moderate–severe acute pain
Authorized in the UK for a maximum of 2 days IM/IV
For adults < 65 years, with normal renal function and weighing > 50kg:

- 10–30mg IM/IV q6h–q4h (or q2h in the initial post-operative period)
- maximum recommended daily dose 90mg IM/IV.

For those aged >65 years, those with renal impairment, and those weighing <50kg:
- 10mg IM/IV q8h–q6h
- maximum recommended daily dose 60mg IM/IV.

Cancer pain

Ketorolac is used at some centres when a parenteral NSAID is needed for a few weeks to help relieve metastatic bone pain while arranging and awaiting benefit from more definitive therapy, e.g. radiotherapy. However, ketorolac has been used for up to 6 months without causing serious GI events.[19]

Ketorolac can be given by intermittent injections 15–30mg SC t.d.s. but these are uncomfortable; it is better given by CSCI:
- *always prescribe a gastroprotective drug concurrently*, e.g. a PPI once daily or **misoprostol** 200microgram t.d.s.–q.d.s.[17]
- start with ketorolac 60mg/24h by CSCI; this is also the recommended maximum dose in people over 65 and those <50kg
- if necessary, increase by 15mg/24h to 90mg/24h.

CSCI: because ketorolac is irritant, dilute to the largest volume possible, and consider the use of 0.9% saline as the diluent (see p.697).

CSCI compatibility with other drugs: Ketorolac is alkaline in solution and there is a high risk of *incompatibility* when mixed with acidic drugs. There are 2-drug compatibility data for ketorolac in 0.9% saline with **diamorphine** and **oxycodone**.[23]

Incompatibility has been reported with **cyclizine, glycopyrronium, haloperidol, hydromorphone, hydroxyzine, levomepromazine, midazolam, morphine, pethidine**, and **promethazine** (see Chapter 20, p.701).

For more details, 2-drug and 3-drug compatibility charts can be found on the extended appendix section of the on-line PCF on www.palliativedrugs.com

For compatiblity charts for mixing drugs in WFI see Appendix 3 charts, p.817

Supply

There is no PO ketorolac product available in the UK.

Ketorolac trometamol (generic)
Injection 30mg/mL, 1mL amp = £1, *vehicle contains alcohol.*

1 Buckley MM-T and Brogden R (1990) Ketorolac: a review of its pharmacodynamic and pharmacokinetic properties, and therapeutic potential. *Drugs.* **39**: 86–109.
2 Gillis J and Brogden R (1997) Ketorolac: A reappraisal of its pharmacodynamic and pharmacokinetic properties and therapeutic use in pain management. *Drugs.* **53**: 139–188.
3 Uzan A (2005) The unexpected side effects of new nonsteroidal anti-inflammatory drugs. *Expert Opinion on Emerging Drugs.* **10**: 687–688.
4 Litvak K and McEvoy G (1990) Ketorolac: an injectable nonnarcotic analgesic. *Clinical Pharmacy.* **9**: 921–935.
5 Blackwell N et al. (1993) Subcutaneous ketorolac - a new development in pain control. *Palliative Medicine.* **7**: 63–65.
6 Chang CH et al. (2011) Risk of hospitalization for upper gastrointestinal adverse events associated with nonsteroidal anti-inflammatory drugs: a nationwide case-crossover study in Taiwan. *Pharmacoepidemiology and Drug Safety.* **20**: 763–771.
7 Masso Gonzalez EL et al. (2010) Variability among nonsteroidal antiinflammatory drugs in risk of upper gastrointestinal bleeding. *Arthritis and Rheumatism.* **62**: 1592–1601.
8 Shau WY et al. (2012) Risk of new acute myocardial infarction hospitalization associated with use of oral and parenteral non-steroidal anti-inflammation drugs (NSAIDS): a case crossover study of Taiwan's National health Insurance claims database and review of current evidence. Available from: www.biomedcentral.com/1471-2261/12/4
9 Chang CH et al. (2010) Increased risk of stroke associated with nonsteroidal anti-inflammatory drugs: a nationwide case-crossover study. *Stroke.* **41**: 1884–1890.
10 Strom B et al. (1996) Parenteral ketorolac and risk of gastrointestinal and operative site bleeding. A postmarketing surveillance study. *Journal of the American Medical Assocation.* **275**: 376–382.
11 Rainer T et al. (2000) Cost effectiveness analysis of intravenous ketorolac and morphine for treating pain after limb injury: double blind randomised controlled trial. *British Medical Journal.* **321**: 1247–1251.
12 Reinhart D (2000) Minimising the adverse effects of ketorolac. *Drug Safety.* **22**: 487–497.
13 Choo V and Lewis S (1993) Ketorolac doses reduced. *Lancet.* **342**: 109.
14 Lewis S (1994) Ketorolac in Europe. *Lancet.* **343**: 784.

15 Li Q *et al.* (2010) High-Dose Ketorolac Affects Adult Spinal Fusion: A Meta-Analysis of the Effect of Perioperative Nonsteroidal Anti-Inflammatory Drugs on Spinal Fusion. *Spine (Phila Pa 1976).* **36**: E461–E468.

16 Ridgway D (2004) Analgesics for acute pain: Meeting the United States Food and Drug Administration's requirements for proof of efficacy. *Clinical Journal of Pain.* **20**: 123–132.

17 Myers K and Trotman I (1994) Use of ketorolac by continuous subcutaneous infusion for the control of cancer-related pain. *Postgraduate Medical Journal.* **70**: 359–362.

18 Middleton RK *et al.* (1996) Ketorolac continuous infusion: a case report and review of the literature. *Journal of Pain and Symptom Management.* **12**: 190–194.

19 Hughes A *et al.* (1997) Ketorolac: continuous subcutaneous infusion for cancer pain. *Journal of Pain and Symptom Management.* **13**: 315–317.

20 Carlson RW *et al.* (1990) A multiinstitutional evaluation of the analgesic efficacy and safety of ketorolac tromethamine, acetaminophen plus codeine, and placebo in cancer pain. *Pharmacotherapy.* **10**: 211–216.

21 Pannuti F *et al.* (1999) A double-blind evaluation of the analgesic efficacy and toxicity of oral ketorolac and diclofenac in cancer pain. The TD/10 recordati Protocol Study Group. *Tumori.* **85**: 96–100.

22 Greenwald R (1992) Ketorolac: an innovative nonsteroidal analgesic. *Drugs of Today.* **28**: 41–61.

23 Dickman A *et al.* (2011) *The Syringe Driver: Continuous Subcutaneous Infusions in Palliative Care* (3e). Oxford University Press, Oxford.

Updated August 2013

NAPROXEN   BNF 10.1.1

Class: Non-opioid analgesic, NSAID, non-selective COX inhibitor.

Indications: Pain and inflammation in arthritic conditions and other musculoskeletal disorders, dysmenorrhoea, acute gout †cancer pain, †fever.

Contra-indications: Hypersensitivity to **aspirin** or other NSAID (urticaria, rhinitis, asthma, angioedema), active GI ulceration, history of two or more distinct episodes of proven ulceration or bleeding, cerebrovascular bleeding or other bleeding disorders, severe heart failure, active liver disease or severe hepatic impairment, severe renal impairment, deteriorating renal function.

Pharmacology

Naproxen is a non-selective COX inhibitor. Like **flurbiprofen** and **ibuprofen**, it is a propionic acid derivative. Absorption is not affected by food or antacids. A steady-state is achieved after 4–5 days of b.d. administration. Excretion is almost entirely urinary, mainly as conjugated naproxen, with some unchanged drug. Plasma concentrations do not increase with doses >500mg b.d. because of rapid urinary excretion.[1]

A meta-analysis of several hundred RCTs indicates that, compared with placebo, the risk the risk of upper GI complications is quadrupled with high-dose naproxen (500mg b.d.), comparable with high-dose **ibuprofen** (2,400mg/24h).[2] Although attempts have been made to improve naproxen's GI safety by linking it with an NO-donating moiety to produce naproxicinod, or by combining it with phosphatidylcholine (see p.312) to produce naproxen-PC,[3] in an RCT in nearly 1,000 volunteers naproxicinod was no better than naproxen.[4]

High-dose naproxen (500mg b.d.) appears *not* to increase the risk of a major cardiovascular event,[2] and is thus the safest NSAID to use in patients with cardiovascular disease or with cardiovascular risk factors. This is consistent with experimental studies showing that this dose of naproxen can produce sufficient COX-1 inhibition to achieve intense and prolonged platelet inhibition in some individuals, which could attenuate any adverse vascular effects of COX-2 inhibition.[5] Thus, in patients taking **aspirin** for thromboprotection, if prescribed naproxen 500mg b.d. regularly, consider stopping the **aspirin**.

As with all NSAIDs, naproxen should be avoided in severe heart failure.[6] Naproxen carries a similar risk of inducing acute renal failure as other NSAIDs.[7]

Although generally given b.d., a single dose of naproxen 500mg at bedtime was equal in efficacy to 250mg b.d. in patients with osteo-arthritis[8,9] and with rheumatoid arthritis.[10]

Naproxen *sodium* 275mg (discontinued in the UK) is equivalent to 250mg naproxen. Naproxen *sodium* is more rapidly absorbed, resulting in plasma concentrations about 1.5–2 times higher than those of naproxen over the first hour, and better analgesia from 4h onwards.[11]

Bio-availability 95% PO.
Onset of action 20–30min.
Time to peak plasma concentration 1.5–5h depending on dose and formulation.[12,13]
Plasma halflife 12–15h.
Duration of action 6–8h single dose; >12h multiple doses.

Cautions

Renal, hepatic and cardiovascular impairment (see p.315–317). Correct hyperkalaemia before use. To minimize the potential for serious undesirable effects, use the lowest effective dose for the shortest treatment duration possible. Risk of aseptic meningitis in patients with SLE (very rare).

Because of the increased risk of bleeding (from decreased platelet aggregation) try to avoid concurrent prescription of naproxen and **warfarin**. As with all NSAIDs, concurrent administration with an SSRI is associated with an increased risk of GI bleeding.

Naproxen *sodium* products (not UK) should be used with caution in patients on a salt-restricted diet.

Drug interactions

Avoid taking antacids at the same time of day as e/c and m/r formulations. Naproxen plasma concentrations are increased by **probenecid**.

Because they cause sodium and fluid retention, all NSAIDs can decrease the effect of diuretics, ACE inhibitors and antihypertensives.

In addition to the effect on platelet function (see Cautions), an increase in INR occasionally occurs when naproxen is prescribed for a patient already taking **warfarin**; monitor the INR weekly for 3–4 weeks and adjust the dose of **warfarin** if necessary.[14]

For general interactions between NSAIDs and other drugs, see Tables 8 and 9 (p.319 and p.320). Of particular importance is the risk of toxic plasma levels of **clofarabine**, **digoxin**, **lithium**, and **methotrexate** caused by reduced renal function and/or reduced tubular excretion. If naproxen is prescribed, monitor the plasma drug concentration or haematological effect of these drugs as appropriate and reduce doses as necessary (see p.318).

Undesirable effects

Also see NSAIDs, p.307.
Very common (>10%): headache.
Common (<10%, >1%): headache, dizziness, oedema, indigestion, abdominal discomfort, nausea, constipation or diarrhoea, pruritus, rash, ecchymosis.

Dose and use

For patients with, or at very high risk of, NSAID-related GI ulceration, see Box D, p.314.

The SPC recommends that naproxen is taken with or after food, but this advice seems unnecessary; there is no evidence that this reduces upper GI complications (see p.321).

Naproxen is the NSAID of choice at some centres:
• typically 250–500mg b.d.
• can be taken as a single daily dose, either each morning or each evening
• occasionally, with careful monitoring, it may be worth titrating up to a total daily dose of 1.5g (e.g. 500mg t.d.s.); this is higher than the manufacturer's recommended maximum daily doses of 1–1.25g (depending on indication) and should normally be done for only a limited period. This is comparable to doses used for severe rheumatoid arthritis.

Supply

Naproxen 250mg tablets are available OTC for dysmenorrhoea.

Naproxen (generic)
Tablets 250mg, 500mg, 28 days @ 500mg b.d. = £3.50.
Tablets e/c 250mg, 375mg, 500mg, 28 days @ 500mg b.d. = £5.

Oral solution 125mg/5mL (available as a special order from Martindale products, 500mL = £147, see Appendix 1, p.817).

Naprosyn® (Roche)
Tablets 250mg, 500mg, 28 days @ 500mg b.d. = £9.
Tablets e/c 250mg, 375mg, 500mg, 28 days @ 500mg b.d. = £9.

With **esomeprazole**
Vimovo® (Astra Zeneca)
Tablets m/r naproxen 500mg e/c + **esomeprazole** 20mg, 28 days @ 1 tablet b.d. = £15. *Note this product is cheaper than prescribing both drugs separately.*

With **misoprostol**
Napratec® (Pharmacia)
Tablets (combination pack) naproxen 500mg and **misoprostol** 200microgram as separate tablets, 28 days @ 1 tablet of each drug b.d. = £24. *Note: the combination pack is more expensive than prescribing both drugs separately and contains only half the **misoprostol** dose needed for optimal protection.*

1 Simon L and Mills J (1980) Nonsteroidal anti-inflammatory drugs. Part 2. *New England Journal of Medicine.* **302**: 1237–1243.
2 CNT Collaboration (2013) Vascular and upper gastrointestinal effects of non-steroidal anti-inflammatory drugs: meta-analyses of individual participant data from randomised trials. *Lancet.* **382**: 769–779.
3 Lichtenberger LM *et al.* (2009) Naproxen-PC: a GI safe and highly effective anti-inflammatory. *Inflammopharmacology.* **17**: 1–5.
4 Lohmander LS *et al.* (2005) A randomised, placebo controlled, comparative trial of the gastrointestinal safety and efficacy of AZD3582 versus naproxen in osteoarthritis. *Annals of the Rheumatic Diseases.* **64**: 449–456.
5 Capone ML *et al.* (2004) Clinical pharmacology of platelet, monocyte, and vascular cyclooxygenase inhibition by naproxen and low-dose aspirin in healthy subjects. *Circulation.* **109**: 1468–1471.
6 Gislason GH *et al.* (2009) Increased mortality and cardiovascular morbidity associated with use of nonsteroidal anti-inflammatory drugs in chronic heart failure. *Archives of Internal Medicine.* **169**: 141–149.
7 Schneider V *et al.* (2006) Association of selective and conventional nonsteroidal antiinflammatory drugs with acute renal failure: A population-based, nested case-control analysis. *American Journal of Epidemiology.* **164**: 881–889.
8 Brooks P *et al.* (1982) Evaluation of a single daily dose of naproxen in osteoarthritis. *Rheumatology and Rehabilitation.* **21**: 242–246.
9 Mendelsohn s (1991) Clinical efficacy and tolerability of naproxen in osteoarthritis patients using twice-daily and once-daily regimens. *Clinical Therapy.* **13 (suppl A)**: 8–15.
10 Graziano F (1991) Once-daily or twice-daily administration of naproxen in patients with rheumatoid arthritis. *Clinical Therapy.* **13 (suppl A)**: 20–25.
11 Sevelius H *et al.* (1980) Bioavailability of naproxen sodium and its relationship to clinical analgesic effects. *British Journal of Clinical Pharmacology.* **10**: 259–263.
12 Kelly J *et al.* (1989) Pharmacokinetic properties and clinical efficacy of once-daily sustained-release naproxen. *European Journal of Clinical Pharmacology.* **36**: 383–388.
13 Davies N and Anderson K (1997) Clinical pharmacokinetics of naproxen. *Clinical Pharmacokinetics.* **32**: 268–293.
14 Baxter K and Preston CL *Stockley's Drug Interactions* London: Pharmaceutical Press www.medicinescomplete.com (accessed December 2012).

Updated August 2013

NABUMETONE   BNF 10.1.1

Class: Non-opioid analgesic, NSAID, non-selective COX inhibitor.

Indications: Pain in osteo-arthritis and rheumatoid arthritis, †cancer pain.

Contra-indications: Hypersensitivity to **aspirin** or other NSAID (urticaria, rhinitis, asthma, angioedema), active GI ulceration, history of two or more distinct episodes of proven ulceration or bleeding, cerebrovascular bleeding or other bleeding disorders, severe heart failure, active liver disease or severe hepatic impairment, severe renal impairment, deteriorating renal function.

Pharmacology

Worldwide, nabumetone is one of the most commonly prescribed NSAIDs.[1] It is a unique NSAID in that it is both a pro-drug and non-acidic; this may explain its low risk for GI toxicity (see below).

Absorption is mainly unaffected by food, and is increased if taken with milk.[1] It undergoes rapid and extensive first-pass metabolism in the liver to mainly 6-methoxy-2-naphthylacetic acid (6-MNA), which is further metabolized by O-methylation and conjugation to inactive compounds.[2] Less than 1% is excreted as 6-MNA. Steady-state plasma concentrations of 6-MNA are not altered in patients with renal impairment even though the renal excretion of 6-MNA is reduced.[1] This could relate to non-linear protein-binding, changes in apparent volume of distribution[3] or increased excretion by other routes.

Although early studies suggested that nabumetone is COX-2 selective, later studies using whole blood assay indicate that it is non-selective.[4–6] Nabumetone has no effect on platelet aggregation in clinical studies.[1,5,7–9] In most patients, once daily administration is satisfactory.

A systematic review of single-dose nabumetone in postoperative pain failed to find any study showing significant benefit.[10] However, when given in a regular dose of 1g/24h in rheumatoid and osteo-arthritis and after acute soft tissue injury, nabumetone is as effective as other NSAIDs.[11–13]

In patients with osteo-arthritis, nabumetone is significantly less gastrotoxic than **diclofenac** and **piroxicam**; the incidence of serious GI events (ulceration, bleeding, perforation) over 6 months is 1.1% vs. 4.3%, and no hospitalizations vs. 1.4%.[14] Nabumetone produced fewer endoscopic ulcers over 12 weeks than **ibuprofen**, and was comparable to **ibuprofen** 2,400mg/24h + **misoprostol** 800microgram/24h.[15] It is less gastrotoxic than **naproxen** (endoscopic monitoring for 5 years).[16] This persistent low level of ulcer formation is unique to nabumetone; most NSAIDs have a high level of risk when started, which then diminishes but continues significantly above the baseline even at 5 years.

Meta-analysis of 13 studies, incorporating some 50,000 patients, showed that serious GI events were 10–36 times less likely than with the comparator NSAIDs. However, it should be noted that the confidence intervals for this were extremely wide, approximately 5–760.[17] Hospitalization for NSAID-related events was also less frequent (odds ratio 3.7, 95% CI 1–11).[17] A more recent review of the GI tolerability of nabumetone is also available.[18]

Over some 30 years on the ARAMIS database (for patients with rheumatoid arthritis; www.aramis.stanford.edu), nabumetone has had the least hospitalizations for serious GI events of all the NSAIDs.[19] In practice this means that, except when there is very high risk of gastrotoxicity, a gastroprotective drug need *not* be prescribed with nabumetone. Nabumetone's decreased propensity for causing gastroduodenal toxicity is probably related to the following features:
- it is non-acidic and thus does not damage phosphatidylcholine in the mucous layer and is not subject to acid-trapping (see p.312)
- because it is non-acidic, it has only a weak uncoupling effect on oxidative phosphorylation, and thus causes little disruption of the tight junctions which control mucosal permeability to acid
- it is a pro-drug activated in the liver, and thus causes little direct damage to the stomach and duodenum[20]
- there is no enterohepatic recirculation of the active metabolite.

The relative risk of major cardiovascular events with nabumetone is unclear.[21,22] Unlike several other non-selective NSAIDs, it has not been scrutinized in this respect in a major recent RCT.[23] In patients with treated hypertension, compared with **ibuprofen**, fewer on nabumetone had a significant increase in blood pressure (17% vs. 6%).[24]

Nabumetone is the NSAID of choice at one major UK palliative care service. The higher cost (vs. **diclofenac**, **ibuprofen** and **naproxen**) is largely offset by generally *not* needing to prescribe concurrent gastroprotection (e.g. a PPI or **misoprostol**).

Bio-availability of 6-MNA 38% (increased by administration with milk).[1,25]
Onset of action 1–2h.
Time to peak plasma concentration for 6-MNA 3–6h.[2]
Plasma halflife of 6-MNA about 24h.
Duration of action >24h.

Cautions

Renal, hepatic and cardiovascular impairment (see p.315–317). Correct hyperkalaemia before use. To minimize the potential for serious undesirable effects, use the lowest effective dose for the shortest treatment duration possible. Risk of aseptic meningitis in patients with SLE (very rare).

As with all NSAIDs, concurrent administration with an SSRI is associated with an increased risk of GI bleeding.

Drug interactions

Because they cause sodium and fluid retention, all NSAIDs can decrease the effect of diuretics, ACE inhibitors and antihypertensives.

Although nabumetone does not generally alter platelet aggregation or affect the INR in anticoagulated patients, there is an isolated report of haemarthrosis and raised INR in a patient taking **warfarin** concurrently.[26] Thus, if nabumetone is prescribed for a patient already taking **warfarin**, monitor the INR weekly for 3–4 weeks and adjust the dose of **warfarin** if necessary.[27]

6-MNA is highly protein-bound and theoretically may displace other highly bound drugs from plasma proteins, e.g. **phenytoin**, sulfonylureas, the clinical relevance of this is unknown. The main enzyme involved in metabolism of 6-MNA is CYP2C9, which has implications for possible drug interactions (see Chapter 25, p.767).[28]

For general interactions between NSAIDs and other drugs, see Tables 8 and 9 (p.319 and p.320). Of particular importance is the risk of toxic plasma levels of **clofarabine**, **digoxin**, **lithium**, and **methotrexate** caused by reduced renal function and/or reduced tubular excretion. If an NSAID is prescribed, monitor the plasma drug concentration or haematological effect of these drugs and reduce doses as necessary (see p.318).

Undesirable effects

Also see NSAIDs, p.307.

Common (<10%, >1%): tinnitus, dyspepsia, nausea, abdominal pain, diarrhoea, constipation, rash, pruritus, oedema.[29]

Dose and use

Generally, there is no need for gastroprotection with nabumetone (see above). For patients with, or at *very* high risk of, NSAID-related GI ulceration, see Box D, p.314.

The SPC recommends that nabumetone is taken with or after food, but this advice seems unnecessary; there is no evidence that this reduces upper GI complications (see p.321).

- start with 1g each evening
- if necessary, increase to 500mg each morning and 1g each evening
- if necessary, increase further to 1g b.d.
- in very elderly (80+ years) frail patients, start with 500mg, and limit to 1g once daily.

Dose reduction is not necessary in patients with mild–moderate renal impairment.[1]

Supply

Nabumetone (generic)
Tablets 500mg, 28 days @ 1g daily = £5.

Relifex® (Meda)
Tablets 500mg, 28 days @ 1g daily = £6.
Oral suspension 500mg/5mL, 28 days @ 1g daily = £24.

1 Hedner T et al. (2004) Nabumetone: Therapeutic use and safety profile in the management of osteoarthritis and rheumatoid arthritis. *Drugs*. **64**: 2315–2343; discussion 2344–2345.
2 Davies NM (1997) Clinical pharmacokinetics of nabumetone. The dawn of selective cyclo-oxygenase-2 inhibition? *Clinical Pharmacokinetics*. **33**: 404–416.
3 Brier ME et al. (1995) Population pharmacokinetics of the active metabolite of nabumetone in renal dysfunction. *Clinical Pharmacology and Therapeutics*. **57**: 622–627.
4 Patrignani P et al. (1994) Biochemical and pharmacological characterization of the cyclooxygenase activity of human blood prostaglandin endoperoxide synthases. *Journal of Pharmacology and Experimental Therapeutics*. **271**: 1705–1712.
5 Cipollone F et al. (1995) Effects of nabumetone on prostanoid biosynthesis in humans. *Clinical Pharmacology and Therapeutics*. **58**: 335–341.
6 van Kraaij DJ et al. (2002) A comparison of the effects of nabumetone vs meloxicam on serum thromboxane B2 and platelet function in healthy volunteers. *British Journal of Clinical Pharmacology*. **53**: 644–647.
7 Hilleman DE et al. (1993) Nonsteroidal antiinflammatory drug use in patients receiving warfarin: emphasis on nabumetone. *American Journal of Medicine*. **95 (Suppl 2A)**: 30S–34S.
8 Knijff-Dutmer EA et al. (1999) Effects of nabumetone compared with naproxen on platelet aggregation in patients with rheumatoid arthritis. *Annals of Rheumatic Diseases*. **58**: 257–259.

9 Jennings MB et al. (2009) A double-blind study of the effect of hemostasis of nabumetone (Relafen) compared to placebo. Journal of Foot and Ankle Surgery. **39**: 168–173.

10 Moore RA et al. (2009) Single dose oral nabumetone for acute postoperative pain in adults. Cochrane Database of Systematic Reviews. **4**: CD007548.

11 Friedel HA et al. (1993) Nabumetone. A reappraisal of its pharmacology and therapeutic use in rheumatic diseases. Drugs. **45**: 131–156.

12 Lister BJ et al. (1993) Efficacy of nabumetone versus diclofenac, naproxen, ibuprofen, and piroxicam in osteoarthritis and rheumatoid arthritis. American Journal of Medicine. **95 (Suppl 2A)**: 2S–9S.

13 Morgan GJ et al. (1993) Efficacy and safety of nabumetone versus diclofenac, naproxen, ibuprofen, and piroxicam in the elderly. American Journal of Medicine. **95 (Suppl 2A)**: 19S–27S.

14 Scott DL and Palmer RH (2000) Safety and efficacy of nabumetone in osteoarthritis: emphasis on gastrointestinal safety. Alimentary Pharmacology and Therapeutics. **14**: 443–452.

15 Roth SH et al. (1993) A controlled study comparing the effects of nabumetone, ibuprofen, and ibuprofen plus misoprostol on the upper gastrointestinal tract mucosa. Archives of Internal Medicine. **153**: 2565–2571.

16 Roth SH et al. (1994) A longterm endoscopic evaluation of patients with arthritis treated with nabumetone vs naproxen. Journal of Rheumatology. **21**: 1118–1123.

17 Huang JQ et al. (1999) Gastrointestinal safety profile of nabumetone: a meta-analysis. American Journal of Medicine. **107 (Suppl 2A)**: 55S–61S; discussion 61S–64S

18 Bannwarth B (2008) Safety of the nonselective NSAID nabumetone : focus on gastrointestinal tolerability. Drug Safety. **31**: 485–503.

19 Ashworth NL et al. (2004) A population based historical cohort study of the mortality associated with nabumetone, Arthrotec, diclofenac, and naproxen. Journal of Rheumatology. **31**: 951–956.

20 Jeremy JY et al. (1990) The effect of nabumetone and its principal active metabolite on in vitro human gastric mucosal prostanoid synthesis and platelet function. British Journal of Rheumatology. **29**: 116–119.

21 Helin-Salmivaara A et al. (2006) NSAID use and the risk of hospitalization for first myocardial infarction in the general population: a nationwide case-control study from Finland. European Heart Journal. **27**: 1657–1663.

22 Huang WF et al. (2006) Cardiovascular events associated with the use of four nonselective NSAIDs (etodolac, nabumetone, ibuprofen, or naproxen) versus a cyclooxygenase-2 inhibitor (celecoxib): a population-based analysis in Taiwanese adults. Clinical Therapeutics. **28**: 1827–1836.

23 CNT Collaboration (2013) Vascular and upper gastrointestinal effects of non-steroidal anti-inflammatory drugs: meta-analyses of individual participant data from randomised trials. Lancet. **382**: 769–779.

24 Palmer R et al. (2003) Effects of nabumetone, celecoxib, and ibuprofen on blood pressure control in hypertensive patients on angiotensin converting enzyme inhibitors. American Journal of Hypertension. **16**: 135–139.

25 Dollery C (1999) Therapeutic Drugs. (2e). Churchill Livingstone, Edinburgh.

26 Dennis VC et al. (2000) Potentiation of oral anticoagulation and hemarthrosis associated with nabumetone. Pharmacotherapy. **20**: 234–239.

27 Baxter K and Preston CL Stockley's Drug Interactions London: Pharmaceutical Press www.medicinescomplete.com (accessed December 2012).

28 Matsumoto K et al. (2011) In vitro characterization of the cytochrome P450 isoforms involved in the metabolism of 6-methoxy-2-napthylacetic acid, an active metabolite of the prodrug nabumetone. Biological and Pharmaceutical Bulletin. **34**: 734–739.

29 Willkens RF (1990) An overview of the long-term safety experience of nabumetone. Drugs. **40 (Suppl 5)**: 34–37.

Updated (minor change) June 2014

WEAK OPIOIDS   BNF 4.7.1 & 4.7.2

There is no pharmacological need for Step 2 of the WHO Analgesic Ladder. Low doses of **morphine**, or an alternative strong opioid, can generally be used instead.[1] Moving directly from Step 1 to Step 3 is now the preferred option in children[2] and, at some centres, in adults. However, from an international perspective, Step 2 remains a practical necessity because of the restricted availability (or non-availability) in many countries of oral **morphine** and other strong opioids.

Codeine is the archetypical weak opioid (and **morphine** the archetypical strong opioid).[3] However, the division of opioids into 'weak' and 'strong' is to a certain extent arbitrary. In reality, opioids manifest a range of strengths which is not fully reflected in two discrete categories. Increasingly, it may be preferable to refer more broadly to 'Step 2 analgesics', and include any drug which is generally used as an alternative to **codeine**. This eases the problem of how to categorize an atypical opioid like **tramadol** (Table 1).

By IM injection, weak opioids can all provide analgesia equivalent, or almost equivalent, to **morphine** 10mg but most weak opioids are not marketed as injections. High-dose **codeine** (or alternative) is comparable to low-dose **morphine** (or alternative), and vice versa.

Weak opioids are said to have a 'ceiling' effect for analgesia. This is an oversimplification; although mixed agonist-antagonists (e.g. **pentazocine**) have a true ceiling effect, the maximum

Table 1 Weak opioids

Drug	Bio-availability (%)	Time to peak plasma concentration (h)	Plasma halflife (h)	Duration of analgesia (h)[a]	Approximate potency ratio with codeine
Codeine	40 (12–84)	1–2	2.5–3.5	4–6	1
Dihydrocodeine	20	1.6–1.8	3.5–4.5	3–4	4/3
Tramadol	75[b]	2	6[c]	4–6	1[d]

a. when used in typical doses for mild–moderate pain
b. multiple doses >90%
c. active metabolite (M1) 7.4h; both figures double in cirrhosis and severe renal failure
d. estimated on basis of potency ratio with morphine.

effective dose of weak opioid agonists is arbitrary. At higher doses, there are progressively more undesirable effects, e.g. nausea and vomiting, which outweigh any additional analgesic effect. Other dose-limiting factors are the number of tablets which patients will readily accept and, in some combination products, the dose of the non-opioid, e.g. **paracetamol**.

There is little to choose between **codeine** and its alternatives in terms of efficacy[4] but there is no consensus about which is the weak opioid of choice. The following should be noted:

- **codeine** has little or no analgesic effect until metabolized to **morphine** mainly via CYP2D6. Thus, in poor metabolizers, it is essentially ineffective. In contrast, in ultra-rapid metabolizers, it is potentially toxic; in children this has led to rare postoperative deaths, and its use is discouraged (see p.348)
- **dihydrocodeine**, like **codeine**, is a substrate for CYP2D6 and its partial metabolism is limited in poor metabolizers and is blocked by CYP2D6 inhibitors. However, unlike **codeine**, there is no evidence that such inhibition reduces its analgesic effect, i.e. **dihydrocodeine** is an active substance, not a pro-drug like **codeine** (see p.350)
- **tramadol** is less constipating than **codeine** and **dihydrocodeine**, but causes more vomiting, dizziness and anorexia. Further, if used with another drug which affects serotonin metabolism or availability, it can lead to serotonin toxicity, particularly in the elderly. It lowers seizure threshold. Unless metabolized to O-desmethyltramadol (M1) via CYP2D6, **tramadol** has a much reduced analgesic effect; it is thus practically ineffective in poor metabolizers (see p.352)
- **pentazocine** should *not* be used; it often causes psychotomimetic effects (dysphoria, depersonalization, frightening dreams, hallucinations).[5]

Whichever weak opioid is used, the following general rules should be observed:

- a weak opioid should be added to, not substituted for, a non-opioid analgesic
- it is generally inappropriate to switch from one weak opioid to another weak opioid
- if a weak opioid is inadequate when given regularly, change to **morphine** (or an alternative strong opioid).

As with all opioids, patients must be monitored for undesirable effects (see p.360), particularly nausea and vomiting, and constipation. Depending on individual circumstances, an anti-emetic should be prescribed for regular or p.r.n. use, (see p.241) and, routinely, a laxative prescribed (see p.44).

1 Caraceni A et al. (2012) Use of opioid analgesics in the treatment of cancer pain: evidence-based recommendations from the EAPC. Lancet Oncology. 13: e58–68.
2 WHO (2012) Persisting pain in children package: WHO guidelines on the pharmacological treatment of persisiting pain in children with medical illness. World Health Organisation, Geneva. Available from: www.who.int/publications
3 WHO (1986) Cancer Pain Relief. World Health Organization, Geneva.
4 Moore RA and McQuay HJ (1997) Single-patient data meta-analysis of 3453 postoperative patients: oral tramadol versus placebo, codeine and combination analgesics. Pain. 69: 287–294.
5 Woods A et al. (1974) Medicines evaluation and monitoring group: central nervous system effects of pentazocine. British Medical Journal. 1: 305–307.

Updated (minor change) June 2014

CODEINE PHOSPHATE BNF 1.4.2, 3.9.1, 4.7.1 & 4.7.2

Class: Opioid analgesic.

Indications: Mild–moderate pain, cough, diarrhoea.

Note: there is no pharmacological need for weak opioids (Step 2) in the WHO Analgesic Ladder. Moving directly from non-opioids (Step 1) to strong opioids (Step 3) is now the preferred option in children and, at some centres, in adults (see Weak opioids, p.346).

Contra-indications: None absolute if titrated carefully to effect. Avoid use in children (see below).[1,2]

Pharmacology

Codeine (methylmorphine) is an opium alkaloid, about one tenth as potent as **morphine**. An increasing analgesic response has been reported with IM doses up to 360mg.[3] However, in practice, codeine is generally used PO in doses of 15–60mg, often in combination with a non-opioid. Although widely prescribed, there is a lack of RCT data on the efficacy and tolerability of fixed-dose **paracetamol**-codeine combinations in cancer pain.

Codeine is metabolized mainly (80%) by conjugation to codeine-6-glucuronide which may contribute to its analgesic effect.[4,5] However, most of its analgesic effect results from the ≤10% of codeine which is converted to **morphine** by O-demethylation via CYP2D6.[6,7] If this pathway is blocked by CYP2D6 inhibitors (see Chapter 25, Table 8, p.775), codeine lacks significant analgesic activity. However, because of genetic polymorphism, there is wide interindividual variation in the production of **morphine** (see Chapter 25, Table 3, p.771), which results in a wide range of responses to codeine.[8–12]

Compared with the general population (extensive metabolizers), poor metabolizers produce little or no **morphine**, and obtain little or no pain relief from codeine. On the other hand, undesirable effects are comparable in both groups.[11,13] In contrast, ultra-rapid metabolizers produce more **morphine**; this can lead to opioid intoxication. Rarely, in children, this has been fatal.[1,14–17]

Like **morphine**, codeine is antitussive and also slows GI transit.[18] Given that opioids can cause pruritus, it is noteworthy that a patient with primary biliary cirrhosis obtained relief with regular oral codeine (also see Chapter 28, p.793).[19] Because of constipation, codeine was stopped and the pruritus returned. When codeine was restarted, together with a laxative, the patient again obtained relief.

Bio-availability 40% (12–84%) PO.[6]
Onset of action 30–60min for analgesia; 1–2h for antitussive effect.
Time to peak plasma concentration 1–2h.
Plasma halflife 2.5–3.5h.[6]
Duration of action 4–6h.

Cautions

Because of the risk of opioid intoxication, codeine should be used with caution in patients known or likely to be ultra-rapid metabolizers.

Driving ability may be impaired by a dose of 50mg.[20,21] Like **morphine** and **dihydrocodeine**, codeine is more toxic in renal failure. This is because of accumulation of **morphine** and of other active metabolites (see p.367).

Codeine is generally best not used in patients with moderate–severe hepatic impairment; reduced metabolism could result in less being transformed into **morphine**, thereby reducing its analgesic effect.[22]

Drug interactions

CYP2D6 inhibitors (e.g. **fluoxetine**, **paroxetine**, **quinidine**) block the biotransformation of codeine to morphine, and will render codeine ineffective as an analgesic; see Chapter 25, Table 8, p.775 for more details.

Undesirable effects

Codeine can produce the whole range of opioid undesirable effects (see Strong opioids, Box B, p.361)

Dose and use

As with all opioids, patients must be monitored for undesirable effects, particularly nausea and vomiting, and constipation (see p.360). Depending on individual circumstances, an anti-emetic should be prescribed for regular or p.r.n. use, (see p.241) and, routinely, a laxative prescribed (see p.44).

It is bad practice to prescribe codeine to patients already taking **morphine** or any other strong opioid; if a greater effect is needed, the dose of **morphine** (or other strong opioid) should be increased.

Pain relief

Codeine is often given in a combination product with a non-opioid. The codeine content of these products is generally 8mg, 15mg, or 30mg (lower strengths, e.g. 8–12.8mg, are present in some OTC combination products containing, e.g. **aspirin, ibuprofen** or **paracetamol**). Thus patients with inadequate relief may benefit by changing to a higher strength product. When given alone, the dose is generally 30–60mg q4h. Higher doses can be given but equivalent analgesic doses of **morphine** (one tenth of the dose of codeine) may be less constipating.

Cough

Codeine is effective as an antitussive by any route. The dose is tailored to the patient's need, e.g. 15–30mg p.r.n., up to q4h. Administration as an oral linctus or syrup is not necessary.

Diarrhoea

To control diarrhoea, a dose of 30–60mg is used both p.r.n. and regularly up to q4h. However, loperamide may be preferable (see p.37).

Supply

Codeine phosphate (generic)
Tablets 15mg, 30mg, 60mg, 28 days @ 30mg q.d.s. = £5.
Oral syrup 25mg/5mL, 28 days @ 25mg q.d.s. = £6.
Injections CD are available but are not recommended.

Codeine linctus BP
Oral solution 15mg/5mL, 28 days @ 30mg q.d.s. = £8; sugar-free formulations are available.

With **aspirin**
Co-codaprin (generic)
Tablets dispersible codeine phosphate 8mg, **aspirin** 400mg, 28 days @ 2 q.d.s. = £94.

With **paracetamol**
Co-codamol 8/500 (generic)
Capsules codeine phosphate 8mg, **paracetamol** 500mg, 28 days @ 2 q.d.s. = £19.
Tablets codeine phosphate 8mg, **paracetamol** 500mg, 28 days @ 2 q.d.s. = £3.50.
Tablets dispersible codeine phosphate 8mg, **paracetamol** 500mg, 28 days @ 2 q.d.s. = £10.

Co-codamol 15/500
Codipar® (Goldshield)
Caplets (capsule-shaped tablets) codeine phosphate 15mg, **paracetamol** 500mg, 28 days @ 2 q.d.s. = £18.
Tablets dispersible codeine phosphate 15mg, **paracetamol** 500mg, 28 days @ 2 q.d.s. = £18.

Co-codamol 30/500 (generic)
Capsules codeine phosphate 30mg, **paracetamol** 500mg, 28 days @ 2 q.d.s. = £12.
Tablets/caplets codeine phosphate 30mg, **paracetamol** 500mg, 28 days @ 2 q.d.s. = £8.
Tablets effervescent codeine phosphate 30mg, **paracetamol** 500mg, 28 days @ 2 q.d.s. = £17.

This is not a complete list; see BNF for more information.

Note: Dispersible or effervescent formulations may contain Na^+ up to 20mmol/tablet or sachet. Check individual brand SPC and avoid high Na^+ formulations in renal impairment.

1   Racoosin JA et al. (2013) New Evidence about an Old Drug - Risk with Codeine after Adenotonsillectomy. New England Journal of Medicine. doi: 10.1056/NEJMp1302454.

2   MHRA (2013) Codeine: restricted use as an analgesic in children and adolescents after European safety review. Drug Safety Update (6) 11www.mhra.gov.uk/safetyinformation

3   Beaver W (1966) Mild analgesics: a review of their clinical pharmacology (Part II). American Journal of Medical Science. 251: 576–599.

4   Lotsch J et al. (2006) Evidence for morphine-independent central nervous opioid effects after administration of codeine: contribution of other codeine metabolites. Clinical Pharmacology and Therapeutics. 79: 35–48.

5   Vree TB et al. (2000) Codeine analgesia is due to codeine-6-glucuronide, not morphine. International Journal of Clinical Practice. 54: 395–398.

6   Persson K et al. (1992) The postoperative pharmacokinetics of codeine. European Journal of Clinical Pharmacology. 42: 663–666.

7   Findlay JWA et al. (1978) Plasma codeine and morphine concentrations after therapeutic oral doses of codeine-containing analgesics. Clinical Pharmacology and Therapeutics. 24: 60–68.

8   Sindrup SH and Brosen K (1995) The pharmacogenetics of codeine hypoalgesia. Pharmacogenetics. 5: 335–346.

9   Caraco Y et al. (1996) Pharmacogenetic determination of the effects of codeine and prediction of drug interactions. Journal of Pharmacology and Experimental Therapeutics. 278: 1165–1174.

10 Lurcott G (1999) The effects of the genetic absence and inhibition of CYP2D6 on the metabolism of codeine and its derivatives, hydrocodone and oxycodone. Anesthesia Progress. 45: 154–156.

11 Eckhardt K et al. (1998) Same incidence of adverse drug events after codeine administration irrespective of the genetically determined differences in morphine formation. Pain. 76: 27–33.

12 Lotsch J et al. (2004) Genetic predictors of the clinical response to opioid analgesics: clinical utility and future perspectives. Clinical Pharmacokinetics. 43: 983–1013.

13 Susce MT et al. (2006) Response to hydrocodone, codeine and oxycodone in a CYP2D6 poor metabolizer. Progress in Neuropsychopharmacology and Biological Psychiatry. 30: 1356–1358.

14 Gasche Y et al. (2004) Codeine intoxication associated with ultrarapid CYP2D6 metabolism. New England Journal of Medicine. 351: 2827–2831.

15 Koren G et al. (2006) Pharmacogenetics of morphine poisoning in a breastfed neonate of a codeine-prescribed mother. Lancet. 368: 704.

16 Kirchheiner J et al. (2007) Pharmacokinetics of codeine and its metabolite morphine in ultra-rapid metabolizers due to CYP2D6 duplication. Pharmacogenomics Journal. 7: 257–265.

17 Williams DG et al. (2002) Pharmacogenetics of codeine metabolism in an urban population of children and its implications for analgesic reliability. British Journal of Anaesthesia. 89: 839–845.

18 Anonymous (1989) Drugs in the management of acute diarrhoea in infants and young children. Bulletin of the World Health Organization. 67: 94–96.

19 Zylicz Z and Krajnik M (1999) Codeine for pruritus in primary biliary cirrhosis. Lancet. 353: 813.

20 Linnoila M and Hakkinen S (1974) Effects of diazepam and codeine, alone and in combination with alcohol, on simulated driving. Clinical Pharmacology and Therapeutics. 15: 368–373.

21 Linnoila M and Mattila MJ (1973) Proceedings: Drug interaction on driving skills as evaluated by laboratory tests and by a driving simulator. Pharmakopsychiatric Neuropsychopharmakologie. 6: 127–132.

22 Tegeder I et al. (1999) Pharmacokinetics of opioids in liver disease. Clinical Pharmacokinetics. 37: 17–40.

Updated (minor change) June 2014

DIHYDROCODEINE TARTRATE BNF 4.7.1 & 4.7.2

Class: Opioid analgesic.

Indication: Moderate–severe pain.

Note: there is no pharmacological need for weak opioids (Step 2) in the WHO Analgesic Ladder. Moving directly from non-opioids (Step 1) to strong opioids (Step 3) is now the preferred option in children and, at some centres, in adults (see Weak opioids p.346).

Contra-indications: None absolute if titrated carefully to effect.

Pharmacology

Dihydrocodeine is a semisynthetic analogue of **codeine**. It relieves pain and cough,[1–3] and causes constipation.[4] Like **codeine**, dihydrocodeine is a substrate for CYP2D6 and its partial metabolism to dihydromorphine is limited in poor metabolizers and is blocked by CYP2D6 inhibitors (see Chapter 25, Table 1, p.769).[5] However, unlike **codeine**, there is no evidence that such inhibition reduces the analgesic effect of dihydrocodeine.[6] In other words, dihydrocodeine is an active substance, not a pro-drug like **codeine**.[7,8]

By injection 60mg provides significantly more analgesia than 30mg and is comparable to morphine 10mg.[9,10] Dihydrocodeine is about twice as potent as **codeine** by injection but, because its oral bio-availability is low, the two drugs are essentially equipotent by mouth.[11]
Bio-availability 20% PO.
Onset of action 30min.
Time to peak plasma concentration 1.7h.
Plasma halflife 3.5–4.5h.
Duration of action 4h.

Cautions

May impair the ability to perform skilled tasks, e.g. driving. Prolonged erections have occurred when **sildenafil** was taken concurrently with dihydrocodeine, possibly because abnormally high concentrations of cyclic guanosine monophosphate were produced in peripheral nerve endings.[12]

Like **morphine** and **codeine**, dihydrocodeine is more toxic in renal failure, probably because of accumulation of an active glucuronide (also see p.367).[13]

Undesirable effects

Common (<10%, >1%): sedation, dizziness, disturbed dreams, headache, vertigo, nausea and vomiting, constipation, pruritus, rash.
Uncommon (<1%): hallucinations, paralytic ileus, urinary retention.

Dose and use

As with all opioids, patients must be monitored for undesirable effects, particularly nausea and vomiting, and constipation (see p.360). Depending on individual circumstances, an anti-emetic should be prescribed for regular or p.r.n. use, (see p.241) and, routinely, a laxative prescribed (see p.44).

It is bad practice to prescribe dihydrocodeine to patients already taking **morphine** *or any other strong opioid; if a greater effect is needed, the regular and p.r.n. doses of* **morphine** *(or other strong opioid) should be increased.*

As a single agent analgesic:
• start with 30mg q6h–q4h
• if necessary, increase to 60mg q6h–q4h
The higher dose is associated with a significant increase in undesirable effects.[14]

Supply

Dihydrocodeine tartrate (generic)
Tablets 30mg, 28 days @ 30mg q.d.s. = £6.
Oral solution 10mg/5mL, 28 days @ 30mg q.d.s. = £39.
Injection CD 50mg/mL, 1mL amp = £3.

DF118 Forte® (Martindale)
Tablets 40mg, 28 days @ 40mg t.d.s. = £10.

Modified-release
DHC Continus® (Napp)
Tablets m/r 60mg, 90mg, 120mg, 28 days @ 60mg b.d. = £5.

With **paracetamol**
Co-dydramol 10/500 (generic)
Tablets dihydrocodeine tartrate 10mg, **paracetamol** 500mg, 28 days @ 2 q.d.s. = £8.

Remedeine® (Napp)
Tablets dihydrocodeine tartrate 20mg, **paracetamol** 500mg, 28 days @ 2 q.d.s. = £21.
Tablets Forte dihydrocodeine tartrate 30mg, **paracetamol** 500mg, 28 days @ 2 q.d.s. = £26.

1 Keats AS et al. (1957) Studies of analgesic drugs: dihydrocodeine. *Journal of Pharmacology and Experimental Therapeutics.* 120: 354–360.
2 Weiss B (1959) Dihydrocodeine. A pharmacologic review. *American Journal of Pharmacy.* **August:** 286–301.
3 Luporini G et al. (1998) Efficacy and safety of levodropropizine and dihydrocodeine on nonproductive cough in primary and metastatic lung cancer. *European Respiratory Journal.* 12: 97–101.

4 Freye E *et al.* (2001) Dose-related effects of controlled release dihydrocodeine on oro-cecal transit and pupillary light reflex. A study in human volunteers. *Arzneimittelforschung.* 51: 60–66.
5 Fromm M *et al.* (1995) Dihydrocodeine: A new opioid substrate for the polymorphic CYP2D6 in humans. *Clinical Pharmacology and Therapeutics.* 58: 374–382.
6 Wilder-Smith CH *et al.* (1998) The visceral and somatic antinociceptive effects of dihydrocodeine and its metabolite, dihydromorphine. A cross-over study with extensive and quinidine-induced poor metabolizers. *British Journal of Clinical Pharmacology.* 45: 575–581.
7 Webb JA *et al.* (2001) Contribution of dihydrocodeine and dihydromorphine to analgesia following dihydrocodeine administration in man: a PK-PD modelling analysis. *British Journal of Clinical Pharmacology.* 52: 35–43.
8 Schmidt H *et al.* (2003) The role of active metabolites in dihydrocodeine effects. *International Journal of Clinical Pharmacology and Therapeutics.* 41: 95–106.
9 Seed JC *et al.* (1958) A comparison of the analgesic and respiratory effects of dihydrocodeine and morphine in main. *Archives Internationales de Pharmacodynamie et de Therapie.* 116: 293–339.
10 Palmer RN *et al.* (1966) Incidence of unwanted effects of dihydrocodeine bitartrate in healthy volunteers. *Lancet.* 2: 620–621.
11 Anonymous (1991) Dihydrocodeine (tartrate). In: C Dollery (ed) *Therapeutic Drugs.* Churchill Livingstone, Edinburgh, pp. 133–136.
12 Goldmeier D and Lamba H (2002) Prolonged erections produced by dihydrocodeine and sildenafil. *British Medical Journal.* 324: 1555.
13 Barnes J *et al.* (1985) Dihydrocodeine in renal failure: further evidence for an important role in the kidney in the handling of opioid drugs. *British Medical Journal.* 290: 740–742.
14 McQuay H *et al.* (1993) A multiple dose comparison of ibuprofen and dihydrocodeine after third molar surgery. *British Journal of Oral and Maxillofacial Surgery.* 31: 95–100.

Updated (minor change) June 2014

TRAMADOL   BNF 4.7.2

Class: Opioid analgesic (but see below).

Indications: Moderate–severe pain.

Note: there is no pharmacological need for weak opioids (Step 2) in the WHO Analgesic Ladder. Moving directly from non-opioids (Step 1) to strong opioids (Step 3) is now the preferred option in children and, at some centres, in adults (see Weak opioids p.346).

Contra-indications: Use of MAOIs concurrently or within 14 days, severe hepatic impairment, renal failure (creatinine clearance < 10mL/min), uncontrolled epilepsy.

Pharmacology

Tramadol, like **tapentadol** (p.448), is a synthetic centrally-acting analgesic with both non-opioid and opioid properties.[1,2] Efficacy appears comparable to **codeine** and other 'weak opioids' (see p.346) for moderate cancer and non-cancer pain, and thus it should be thought of as a Step 2 analgesic (despite sometimes being classified as a strong opioid).[3–6]

Tramadol is derived from **codeine** (p.348) and is structurally similar to **venlafaxine** (p.215). It exists as a racemic mixture which stimulates neuronal serotonin release and inhibits the presynaptic re-uptake of both serotonin (mainly mediated via (+) tramadol) and noradrenaline (norepinephrine; mainly mediated via (–) tramadol). The potentiation of noradrenaline appears the more relevant analgesic effect through activation of the descending pain inhibitory pathway. Conversely, serotonin acts as a neurotransmitter in both the descending inhibitory and excitatory pain pathways and, via the latter, could have a pro-nociceptive effect.[7]

Tramadol is also converted in the liver, mainly via CYP2D6, to the active metabolite O-desmethyltramadol (M1) which, in animals, is 6 times more potent than tramadol.[8] This is because the agonist effect at the μ-opioid receptor is mediated mainly via the (+) M1 enantiomer.[9,10] Thus, in regard to its opioid effects, tramadol can be considered a pro-drug. Further biotransformation of M1 results in many inactive metabolites which are excreted by the kidneys.

Changes in CYP2D6 activity, both acquired (e.g. drug-induced) and constitutional (≤10% of Caucasians are either CYP2D6 poor or ultra-rapid metabolizers)[11,12] can affect the response to tramadol. Decreased CYP2D6 activity will result in decreased response/higher dose requirements, and vice versa (see Drug interactions, below and Chapter 25, p.769).[13–17]

A comparison of μ-opioid receptor affinities and mono-amine re-uptake inhibition indicates that the analgesic effect of tramadol (and **tapentadol**) is the result of synergism between these two mechanisms (Tables 1 and 2).[2] In animal models, tramadol also has an anti-inflammatory effect which is independent of PG inhibition.[18]

Table I μ-opioid receptor affinities: K_i (micromol) values[9,7]

	Receptor affinity
Morphine	0.009
Tapentadol	0.16
Tramadol[b]	2.4

a. the lower the K_i value, the greater the receptor affinity
b. much lower for (+) MI, i.e. 0.003.

Table 2 Inhibition of mono-amine uptake: K_i (micromol) values[9,7]

	Norepinephrine	Serotonin
Morphine	>100	>100
Tapentadol	0.48	2.4
Tramadol	0.59[b]	0.87[c]

a. the lower the K_i value, the greater the functional uptake inhibition
b. (–) tramadol
c. (+) tramadol.

Although **naloxone** can only partially reverse the effects of tramadol,[9,19] in a series of 11 patients with a tramadol overdose, seven had a good response to **naloxone**, and only one had no response.[20]

In placebo-controlled trials, tramadol significantly relieves neuropathic pain (e.g. diabetic neuropathy, post-herpetic neuralgia, polyneuropathy), with an NNT of 3.8.[21] This is comparable with several anti-epileptics, but not as good as the TCAs (NNT = 2.3, see p.297). Further, **oxycodone** has an NNT of 2.5 in post-herpetic neuralgia[22] and, in an RCT of cancer and non-cancer patients with and without neuropathic pain, tramadol was indistinguishable from **morphine**.[23]

Tramadol is as effective as **codeine** as a cough suppressant.[24,25] Postoperatively, it causes less respiratory depression than equi-analgesic doses of **morphine**.[26] It also causes less constipation than **codeine, dihydrocodeine** and **morphine**;[27–29] but more vomiting, dizziness and anorexia than **codeine** and **dihydrocodeine**.[30] In contrast to **morphine**, tramadol reduces the basal pressure in the sphincter of Oddi (for <20min after IM administration) and does not increase the pressure in the common bile duct.[31]

Although the risk of dependence and misuse is considerably less compared with **morphine** and other opioids,[32] tramadol has been reclassified (in 2014) as a schedule 3 **CD**. As with other opioids, tramadol is associated with the development of physical dependence (see Dose and use below)[33] and, in overdose, CNS depression, respiratory depression and death.[34] There are also case reports of possible opioid-induced hyperalgesia (also see p.364).

By injection, tramadol is generally regarded as one tenth as potent as **morphine** (e.g. tramadol 100mg is equivalent to **morphine** 10mg).[35] In fact, various pre- and postoperative studies give a range of potency ratios, from 1:11–1:19,[36,37] suggesting that the figure of 1:10 is more of a 'convenient to remember' ratio than a scientifically precise one. Some of the postoperative studies also suggest that, to produce adequate analgesia, tramadol needs to be administered more frequently than **morphine** over the first few hours (by IV PCA), after which doses become less frequent. The need for the equivalent of a loading dose with tramadol may reflect its different mode of action from **morphine**. A delayed maximum effect has also been reported in an RCT of oral tramadol and **morphine**.[23]

By mouth compared with **morphine**, RCTs indicate a potency ratio of 1:5 and 1:4 respectively (i.e. tramadol 100mg PO = **morphine** 20–25mg PO).[38,39] However, extensive clinical experience

has led many physicians to regard the PO potency ratio for tramadol and **morphine** to be 1:10 (i.e. tramadol 100mg PO = **morphine** 10mg PO), i.e. the same as by injection.[40–42]
Bio-availability 65–75% PO; 90% with multiple doses;[43] 77% PR.[44,45]
Onset of action 30min–1h.
Time to peak plasma concentration 2h; 4–8h m/r.
Plasma halflife 6h; active metabolite 7.4h; these more than double in cirrhosis and severe renal failure.
Duration of action 4–9h.

Cautions

Epilepsy, head trauma or raised intracranial pressure. In hepatic impairment or severe renal impairment (creatinine clearance <30mL/min), because of impaired metabolism or elimination, halve the dose, e.g. by reducing frequency from q.d.s. to q12h. Despite renal failure being a contra-indication to the use of tramadol, some centres have successfully used it in this setting (see p.367).[46]

Tramadol has been associated with seizures, notably when the total daily dose exceeds 400mg or when tramadol is used concurrently with other medications which lower the seizure threshold, e.g. TCAs, SSRIs, antipsychotics, and other opioids.[20,47,48] Seizures have also been reported in patients after rapid IV injection of tramadol. Treat with standard measures, i.e. IV benzodiazepines (see p.148). Resolution generally occurs in <1 day.[20] Fatalities resulting from tramadol-induced seizures are rare.[8]

Serotonin toxicity has occasionally occurred when tramadol has been taken concurrently with a second drug which also interferes with presynaptic serotonin re-uptake (see p.195). Risk factors are those which increase the exposure to tramadol or the second drug, e.g. for tramadol, these include the use of higher doses, increasing age, the second drug being a CYP2D6 inhibitor, CYP2D6 poor metabolizer status and hepatic impairment.[49]

The FDA has warned of an increased risk of suicide in emotionally unstable patients taking tramadol, particularly if they are also taking antidepressants or tranquillizers.

Drug interactions

Because of the increased risk of seizures and serotonin toxicity, concurrent use of tramadol with an MAOI is contra-indicated, and its use with other antidepressants, particularly SSRIs or TCAs, requires caution (see Cautions and below).[49,50]

Carbamazepine and **rifampicin**[51] increase the metabolism of tramadol and M1, and thus may decrease analgesia (see Chapter 25, p.767). CYP2D6 inhibitors, e.g. **fluoxetine**, **paroxetine**, **quinidine**, and **ritonavir**, inhibit the conversion of tramadol to M1 and may decrease analgesia while increasing the risk of serotonin toxicity.[49,52,53]

Tramadol occasionally prolongs the INR of patients taking **warfarin**.[54,55] Monitor the INR closely for 3–4 weeks if tramadol is prescribed for a patient already taking **warfarin**.[53]

There are mixed reports of the analgesic effect of tramadol being reduced by **ondansetron** (possibly by blocking the action of serotonin at presynaptic 5HT$_3$-receptors on primary afferent nociceptive neurones in the spinal dorsal horn).[56] In one postoperative pain study, the dose of tramadol needed by IV PCA was 2–3 times greater in patients receiving **ondansetron**,[57] but was unaffected in another.[58]

Undesirable effects

Incidence and nature of undesirable effects (monoamine reuptake inhibition vs. opioid) may vary with activity of CYP2D6 (see Pharmacology). Urinary incontinence, recovering fully on cessation of tramadol, has been reported.[59]
Very common (>10%): dizziness, nausea, vomiting.
Common (<10%, >1%): headache, drowsiness, fatigue, sweating, dry mouth, constipation.
Rare (<0.1%): seizures (dose-dependent, see Cautions above).

Dose and use

As with all opioids, patients must be monitored for undesirable effects (see p.360), particularly nausea and vomiting, and constipation. Depending on individual circumstances, an anti-emetic should be prescribed for regular or p.r.n. use, (see p.241) and, routinely, a laxative prescribed (see p.44).

Most cancer patients prescribed tramadol will already be taking a non-opioid:
- start with 50mg q.d.s. or 200mg m/r once daily
- in severe renal impairment (creatinine clearance 10–30mL/min) or hepatic impairment, halve the starting dose to 50mg q12h or 100mg m/r once daily; likewise in very frail patients[1]
- if necessary, increase the dose in stages to a maximum recommended total daily dose of 400mg (less in those with severe renal or hepatic impairment and in very frail patients)
- higher doses have been given, e.g. 600mg/24h, and sometimes more[40,41,60]
- for break-through (episodic) pain when taking m/r tramadol, consider immediate-release tramadol or immediate-release **morphine** (p.372).

Stopping tramadol

Abruptly stopping tramadol, even after only a few days of use, can result in typical symptoms of opioid withdrawal (e.g. anxiety, restlessness, abdominal cramps, diarrhoea, goose flesh, sweating) and tapering the dose over several days is recommended.

However, opioid withdrawal should not occur when tramadol is being substituted by another μ-opioid agonist, e.g. **morphine**. Nonetheless, abruptly stopping tramadol has also sometimes resulted in symptoms not typical of opioid withdrawal (e.g. severe anxiety/panic attacks, delirium, paranoia, hallucinations, paraesthesia), particularly with doses >400mg/24h.[61,62] This suggests the potential for a discontinuation reaction similar to that seen with antidepressants (see p.201)[61] and is another reason why tapering the dose over several days is recommended.

Supply

All products are now schedule 3 **CD** (with storage exemption).

Immediate-release oral products
Tramadol (generic)
Capsules 50mg, 28 days @ 100mg q.d.s. = £8.
Orodispersible tablets 50mg, 28 days @ 100mg q.d.s. = £27.
Oral drops 100mg/mL (2.5mg/drop), 10mL, 28 days @100mg q.d.s. = £40.

Modified-release 12-hourly oral products
Tramadol (generic)
Tablets m/r 100mg, 150mg, 200mg, 28 days @ 200mg b.d. = £34.
Capsules m/r 50mg, 100mg, 150mg, 200mg, 28 days @ 200mg b.d. = £29.

Modified-release 24-hourly oral products
Tramadol (generic)
Tablets m/r 100mg, 150mg, 200mg, 300mg, 400mg, 28 days @ 400mg once daily = £29.

Parenteral products
Tramadol (generic)
Injection 50mg/mL, 2mL amp = £1.

With **paracetamol**
Tramacet® (Grünenthal)
Tablets tramadol hydrochloride 37.5mg, **paracetamol** 325mg, 28 days @ 2 q.d.s. = £36.
Tablets soluble tramadol hydrochloride 37.5mg, **paracetamol** 325mg, 28 days @ 2 q.d.s. = £36.

1 Grond S and Sablotzki A (2004) Clinical pharmacology of tramadol. Clinical Pharmacokinetics. 43: 879–923.
2 Dickman A (2007) Tramadol: a review of this atypical opioid. European Journal of Palliative Care. 14: 181–185.
3 Tassinari D et al. (2011) The second step of the analgesic ladder and oral tramadol in the treatment of mild to moderate cancer pain: a systematic review. Palliative Medicine. 25: 410–423.

4   Caraceni A et al. (2012) Use of opioid analgesics in the treatment of cancer pain: evidence-based recommendations from the EAPC. Lancet Oncology. 13: e58–68.
5   Cepeda MS et al. (2006) Tramadol for osteoarthritis. Cochrane Database of Systematic Reviews. 3: CD005522.
6   British National Formulary Section 4.7.2. Opioid analgesics. London: Pharmaceutical Press. www.bnf.org (accessed May 2014).
7   Tzschentke TM et al. (2014) The Mu-Opioid Receptor Agonist/Noradrenaline Reuptake Inhibition (MOR-NRI) concept in analgesia: The case of tapentadol. CNS Drugs. 28: 319–329.
8   Close BR (2005) Tramadol: does it have a role in emergency medicine? Emergency Medicine Australasia. 17: 73–83.
9   Raffa RB et al. (1992) Opioid and nonopioid components independently contribute to the mechanism of action of tramadol, an 'atypical' opioid analgesic. Journal of Pharmacology and Therapeutics. 260: 275–285.
10 Raffa RB et al. (1993) Complementary and synergistic antinociceptive interaction between enantiomers of tramadol. Journal of Pharmacology and Experimental Therapeutics. 267: 331–340.
11 Sachse C et al. (1997) Cytochrome P450 2D6 variants in a Caucasian population: allele frequencies and phenotypic consequences. American Journal of Human Genetics. 60: 284–295.
12 Zanger UM et al. (2004) Cytochrome P450 2D6: overview and update on pharmacology, genetics, biochemistry. Naunyn Schmiedebergs Archives of Pharmacology. 369: 23–37.
13 Stamer UM et al. (2003) Impact of CYP2D6 genotype on postoperative tramadol analgesia. Pain. 105: 231–238.
14 Poulsen L et al. (1996) The hypoalgesic effect of tramadol in relation to CYP2D6. Clinical Pharmacology and Therapeutics. 60: 636–644.
15 Collart L et al. (1993) [Duality of the analgesic effect of tramadol in humans]. Schweizerische Medizinische Wochenschrift. 123: 2241–2243.
16 Kim E et al. (2010) Adverse events in analgesic treatment with tramadol associated with CYP2D6 extensive-metaboliser and OPRM1 high-expression variants. Annals of the Rheumatic Diseases. 69: 1889–1890.
17 Elkalioubie A et al. (2011) Near-fatal tramadol cardiotoxicity in a CYP2D6 ultrarapid metabolizer. European Journal of Clinical Pharmacology. 67: 855–858.
18 Buccellati C et al. (2000) Tramadol anti-inflammatory activity is not related to a direct inhibitory action on prostaglandin endoperoxide synthases. European Journal of Pain. 4: 413–415.
19 Shipton EA (2000) Tramadol - present and future. Anaesthesia and Intensive Care. 28: 363–374.
20 Marquardt KA et al. (2005) Tramadol exposures reported to statewide poison control system. Annals of Pharmacotherapy. 39: 1039–1044.
21 Duehmke RM (2006) tramadol for neuropathic pain. Cochrane Database of Systematic Reviews. 3: CD003726.
22 Watson C and Babul N (1998) Efficacy of oxycodone in neuropathic pain: a randomized trial in postherpetic neuralgia. Neurology. 50: 1837–1841.
23 Leppert W (2001) Analgesic efficacy and side effects of oral tramadol and morphine administered orally in the treatment of cancer pain. Nowotwory. 51: 257–266.
24 Szekely SM and Vickers MD (1992) A comparison of the effects of codeine and tramadol on laryngeal reactivity. European Journal of Anaesthesiology. 9: 111–120.
25 Louly PG et al. (2009) N-of-1 double-blind, randomized controlled trial of tramadol to treat chronic cough. Clinical Therapeutics. 31: 1007–1013.
26 Houmes R et al. (1992) Efficacy and safety of tramadol versus morphine for moderate and severe postoperative pain with special regard to respiratory depression. Anesthesia and Analgesia. 74: 510–514.
27 Wilder-Smith C and Bettiga A (1997) The analgesic tramadol has minimal effect on gastrointestinal motor function. British Journal of Clinical Pharmacology. 43: 71–75.
28 Wilder-Smith CH et al. (1999) Effect of tramadol and morphine on pain and gastrointestinal motor function in patients with chronic pancreatitis. Digestive Diseases and Sciences. 44: 1107–1116.
29 Wilder-Smith C et al. (2001) Treatment of severe pain from osteoarthritis with slow-release tramadol or dihydrocodeine in combination with NSAID's: a randomised study comparing analgesia, antinociception and gastrointestinal effects. Pain. 91: 23–31.
30 Rodriguez RF et al. (2007) Incidence of weak opioids adverse events in the management of cancer pain: a double-blind comparative trial. Journal of Palliative Medicine. 10: 56–60.
31 Wu SD et al. (2004) Effects of narcotic analgesic drugs on human Oddi's sphincter motility. World Journal of Gastroenterology. 10: 2901–2904.
32 Preston K et al. (1991) Abuse potential and pharmacological comparison of tramadol and morphine. Drug and Alcohol Dependency. 27: 7–18.
33 Soyka M et al. (2004) Tramadol use and dependence in chronic noncancer pain patients. Pharmacopsychiatry. 37: 191–192.
34 FDA (2010) Ultram (tramadol hydrochloride), Ultracet (tramadol hydrochloride/acetaminophen): Label change. Safety Alerts for Human Medical Products www.fda.gov/Safety/MedWatch/SafetyInformation
35 Vickers M et al. (1992) Tramadol: pain relief by an opioid without depression of respiration. Anaesthesia. 47: 291–296.
36 Naguib M et al. (1998) Perioperative antinociceptive effects of tramadol. A prospective, randomized, double-blind comparison with morphine. Canadian Journal of Anaesthesia. 45: 1168–1175.
37 Pang WW et al. (1999) Comparison of patient-controlled analgesia (PCA) with tramadol or morphine. Canadian Journal of Anaesthesia. 46: 1030–1035.
38 Wilder-Smith CH et al. (1994) Oral tramadol, a mu-opioid agonist and monoamine reuptake-blocker, and morphine for strong cancer-related pain. Annals of Oncology. 5: 141–146.
39 Tawfik MO et al. (1990) Tramadol hydrochloride in the relief of cancer pain: a double blind comparison against sustained release morphine. Pain. 41(Suppl 1): S377.
40 Leppert W and Luczak J (2005) The role of tramadol in cancer pain treatment–a review. Supportive Care in Cancer. 13: 5–17.
41 Grond S et al. (1999) High-dose tramadol in comparison to low-dose morphine for cancer pain relief. Journal of Pain and Symptom Management. 18: 174–179.
42 Palliativedrugs.com (2008) Tramadol - What is your experience? March/April Survey. www.palliativedrugs.com
43 Gibson T (1996) Pharmacokinetics, efficacy, and safety of analgesia with a focus on tramadol HCl. American Journal of Medicine. 101 (Suppl 1A): 47s–53s.
44 Mercadante S et al. (2005) Randomized double-blind, double-dummy crossover clinical trial of oral tramadol versus rectal tramadol administration in opioid-naive cancer patients with pain. Supportive Care in Cancer. 13: 702–707.
45 Lintz W et al. (1998) Pharmacokinetics of tramadol and bioavailability of enteral tramadol formulations. 3rd Communication: suppositories. Arzneimittelforschung. 48: 889–899.

46 King S et al. (2011) A systematic review of the use of opioid medication for those with moderate to severe cancer pain and renal impairment. Palliative Medicine. 25: 454–470.
47 Boyd IW (2005) Tramadol and seizures. Medical Journal of Australia. 182: 595–596.
48 Spiller HA et al. (1997) Prospective multicenter evaluation of tramadol exposure. Journal of Toxicology and Clinical Toxicology. 35: 361–364.
49 Park SH et al. (2014) Serotonin syndrome: is it a reason to avoid the use of tramadol with antidepressants? Journal of Pharmacy Practice. 27: 71–78.
50 Pilgrim JL et al. (2011) Deaths involving contraindicated and inappropriate combinations of serotonergic drugs. International Journal of Legal Medicine. 125: 803–815.
51 Saarikoski T et al. (2013) Rifampicin markedly decreases the exposure to oral and intravenous tramadol. European Journal of Clinical Pharmacology. 69: 1293–1301.
52 Laugesen S et al. (2005) Paroxetine inhibits a cytochrome P450 2D6 inhibitor, diminishes the stereoselective O-demethylation and reduces the hypoalgesic effect of tramadol. Clin Pharmacol Ther. 77: 312–323.
53 Baxter K and Preston CL. Stockley's Drug Interactions. London: Pharmaceutical Press www.medicinescomplete.com (accessed January 2014).
54 Sabbe JR et al. (1998) Tramadol-warfarin interaction. Pharmacotherapy. 18: 871–873.
55 Juel J et al. (2013) Administration of tramadol or ibuprofen increases the INR level in patients on warfarin. European Journal of Clinical Pharmacology. 69: 291–292.
56 De Witte JL et al. (2001) The analgesic efficacy of tramadol is impaired by concurrent administration of ondansetron. Anesthesia and Analgesia. 92: 1319–1321.
57 Arcioni R et al. (2002) Ondansetron inhibits the analgesic effects of tramadol: a possible 5-HT(3) spinal receptor involvement in acute pain in humans. Anesthesia and Analgesia. 94: 1553–1557.
58 Rauers NI et al. (2010) Antagonistic effects of ondansetron and tramadol? A randomized placebo and active drug controlled study. Journal of Pain. 11: 1274–1281.
59 Gautam SK et al. (2013) Urinary incontinence induced by tramadol. Indian Journal of Palliative Care. 19: 76–77.
60 Osipova N et al. (1991) Analgesic effect of tramadol in cancer patients with chronic pain: A comparison with prolonged-action morphine sulfate. Current Therapeutic Research. 50: 812–815.
61 Senay EC et al. (2003) Physical dependence on Ultram (tramadol hydrochloride): both opioid-like and atypical withdrawal symptoms occur. Drug Alcohol Dependence. 69: 233–241.
62 Rajabizadeh G et al. (2009) Psychosis following Tramadol Withdrawal. Addiction and Health. 1: 58–61.

Updated June 2014

STRONG OPIOIDS   BNF 4.7.2

Strong opioids are essential drugs in palliative care; their use should be dictated by therapeutic need and response, not by brevity of prognosis.[1,2]

Contra-indications: Provided the dose of an opioid is carefully titrated against the patient's pain, there are generally no absolute contra-indications to the use of strong opioids in palliative care. However, there are circumstances, e.g. renal impairment, when it may be better to avoid the use of certain opioids and/or positively choose certain other ones (see p.367; also see Chapter 14, p.639).

Chemical classes

Opioids can be divided into four chemical classes (Table 1). Knowledge of the different chemical classes is of value when dealing with cases of intolerance (i.e. unacceptable undesirable effects) to a particular opioid, e.g. cutaneous histamine release causing a rash and pruritus. However, in many situations switching from one phenanthrene to another phenanthrene is satisfactory, e.g. neurotoxicity (see p.364).

Opioid receptors

There are four opioid receptors (μ, κ, δ, and ORL-1) distributed in varying densities throughout the body, particularly in nervous tissue. Their naturally-occurring ligands are peptides, and together they contribute to various physiological functions including the modulation of pain, hormones and the immune system (Table 2).[3,4]

In nervous tissue, the peptides function as neural transmitters. Like other peptides, they are synthesized as large inactive precursors in the neuronal cell body, and are then cleaved while being transported to the nerve terminals. The active fragment is released into the synapse and binds to one or more receptors.

Opioid receptors are found both pre- and post-synaptically, with the former predominating. Generally, opioid receptor agonists lead to an inhibitory effect. Pre-synaptic receptor activation controls the release of several neurotransmitters. Endogenous peptides are rapidly degraded, and

Table 1   Chemical classification of opioids

Phenanthrenes	Benzomorphans	Phenylpiperidines	Diphenylheptanes
Codeine	Diphenoxylate	Fentanils	Dextropropoxyphene
Dextromethorphan	Loperamide	Pethidine[a]	Methadone
Dihydrocodeine	Pentazocine[a]		
Hydrocodone			
Tramadol			
Morphine			
Diamorphine			
Buprenorphine			
Hydromorphone			
Oxycodone			
Oxymorphone			
Tapentadol			

a. *not* recommended for use in palliative care.

have a relatively short duration of action. In contrast, exogenous opioids such as **morphine** have a prolonged effect. They produce analgesia primarily by interacting with μ-opioid receptors in the CNS.

In the presence of local inflammation, opioids also have a peripheral analgesic action because inflammation activates otherwise dormant opioid receptors in the peripheral nerve terminals.

Undesirable effects relate to both central and peripheral receptors, mainly in the CNS and GI tract.

All clinically important opioid analgesics act as agonists at the μ-opioid receptor (Table 2), and some may also have significant effects on δ-opioid receptors (e.g. **methadone**, see p.433) and k-opioid receptors (e.g. **oxycodone**, see p.442). Some opioids are mixed agonist-antagonists (e.g. **buprenorphine** is a partial μ *agonist*, an opioid-receptor-like (ORL-1) *agonist*, and a κ and δ *antagonist*.)[5–8]

Some opioids also possess non-opioid activity. Thus, **methadone** blocks the pre-synaptic re-uptake of serotonin and the NMDA-receptor-channel (see p.433), **tapentadol** blocks re-uptake of noradrenaline (norepinephrine; see p.448), and **tramadol** (a Step 2 analgesic) blocks re-uptake of both serotonin and noradrenaline (see p.352).

Clinical use

The focus of this section of *PCF* is on the use of strong opioids for cancer pain. Although similar considerations exist regarding the use of strong opioids for chronic non-cancer pain, because generally benefits are lower and risks higher,[11] specialist advice should be followed (e.g. British Pain Society guidelines)[12] and/or sought from chronic pain teams.

Based on familiarity, availability and cost, **morphine** is the strong opioid of choice for cancer pain management (see p.372).[13–16] Other strong opioids are used mainly when:
• **morphine** is not readily available (e.g. **oxycodone**)
• the TD route is preferable (**buprenorphine, fentanyl**)
• the patient has unacceptable undesirable effects with **morphine**.[13]

Differences in receptor affinity (Table 2) may partly explain why some patients report better pain relief after switching opioids (see p.365). Similarly, the pattern and severity of undesirable effects may be altered, e.g. when switching from **morphine** to **oxycodone** (p.442) or TD **fentanyl** (p.403).

Both **methadone** (p.433) and **tapentadol** (p.448) have opioid and non-opioid effects which, in the case of **tapentadol**, are analgesically synergistic.

Strong opioids are not the panacea for cancer pain; effective analgesia generally requires the use of both a strong opioid and a non-opioid. Further, even combined use does not guarantee success, particularly with neuropathic pain or if the psychosocial dimension of suffering is ignored. Other reasons for poor relief include:
• underdosing (failure to titrate the dose upwards or dose at the correct interval)

Table 2 Opioid receptors,[9,10] ligands, and effects[a]

Receptors	Mu (μ)	Delta (δ)	Kappa (κ)	ORL-1
Endogenous opioid	β-Endorphin Endormorphins	Enkephalins	Dynorphins	Nociceptin
Exogenous agonist	Morphine Buprenorphine[b] Codeine Dextropropoxphene Dihydrocodeine Fentanils Hydromorphone Methadone Oxycodone Pethidine Tapentadol Tramadol	DSTBULET Methadone (?)	U50488H Oxycodone (?)	Buprenorphine
Antagonists	Naloxone Naltrexone	Buprenorphine Naloxone	Buprenorphine Naloxone	
Effector mechanism	G protein opens K$^+$channel	G protein opens K$^+$channel	G protein closes Ca^{++}channel	G protein opens K$^+$ channel
Effects[c]	*Hyperpolarization of neurons, inhibition of neurotransmitter release* Analgesia Euphoria Nausea Constipation Cough suppression Dependence Respiratory depession Miosis	Similar to μ but less marked	Analgesia Aversion Diuresis	Mixed analgesia (spinal) and anti-opioid (brain)

a. also see individual drug monographs
b. partial agonist
c. not an exhaustive list; other roles include hormone and immune system regulation.

- poor patient adherence (patient not taking medication)
- poor alimentary absorption, e.g. because of vomiting.

Pentazocine should *not* be used; it is a weak opioid by mouth,[17,18] and often causes psychotomimetic effects (dysphoria, depersonalization, frightening dreams, hallucinations).[19] **Pethidine** also should *not* be used (Box A).

Although branded and generic versions of the same formulations are often bio-equivalent, names and appearance vary. Consequently, to avoid confusing patients and carers, prescribing by brand is recommended;[20] recent advice relating to TD formulations repeats this recommendation.[21]

Box A   Pethidine

The use of pethidine is actively discouraged in palliative care.

Pethidine is a synthetic μ agonist. In typical doses PO it is little more than a weak opioid (see Table 4, p.366). It has a relatively short duration of action (2–3h) and is thus a bad choice for round-the-clock analgesia.

Pethidine has a toxic metabolite, norpethidine, which accumulates when pethidine is given regularly. Particularly in renal impairment, norpethidine causes tremors, multifocal myoclonus, agitation, and occasionally seizures.[22]

Pethidine:
- is not antitussive
- is less constipating than morphine but causes more vomiting
- causes less smooth muscle spasm (e.g. sphincter of Oddi)
- is antimuscarinic (anticholinergic)
- does not cause constriction of the pupils.[23]

Drug-drug interaction with:
- phenobarbital ⎫
- chlorpromazine ⎬   increase production of norpethidine.
- MAOIs ⎭

Serotonin toxicity
Pethidine must not be given concurrently with an MAOI because of the risk of serotonin toxicity (see p.195).[24–26]

Overdose and effect of naloxone
Overdose is a mixed picture of CNS depression (pethidine) and excitation (norpethidine), with both stupor and seizures.

Naloxone will reverse the pethidine-induced stupor but not the stimulant effects of norpethidine. Seizures should be treated with a benzodiazepine (see p.148).

Undesirable effects

Strong opioids tend to cause the same undesirable effects (Box B), although to a varying degree. Strategies are necessary to deal with the undesirable effects of **morphine** and other strong opioids, particularly nausea and vomiting (see p.241), and constipation (see p.44).[27] For opioid-induced pruritus, see Chapter 28, p.795.

Respiratory depression
Pain is a physiological antagonist to the central depressant effects of opioids.
When appropriately titrated against the patient's pain, strong opioids do not cause clinically important respiratory depression in patients in pain.[28–30] Strong opioids also relieve moderate–severe breathlessness at rest at doses which do not cause respiratory depression (see p.379).

Naloxone, a specific opioid antagonist, is rarely needed in palliative care (see p.450). In contrast to postoperative patients, cancer patients with pain:
- have generally been receiving a weak opioid for some time, i.e. are not opioid-naïve
- take medication PO (slower absorption, lower peak concentration)
- titrate the dose upwards step by step (less likelihood of an excessive dose being given).

Box B   Undesirable effects of opioids when used for analgesia

Common initial
Nausea and vomiting[a]
Drowsiness
Lightheadedness/unsteadiness
Delirium (acute confusional state)

Common ongoing
Constipation
Nausea and vomiting[a]
Dry mouth

Possible ongoing
Suppression of hypothalamic-pituitary axis
Suppression of immune system

Less common
Neurotoxicity:
  hyperalgesia
  allodynia
  myoclonus
  cognitive failure/delirium
  hallucinations
Sweating
Urinary retention
Postural hypotension
Spasm of the sphincter of Oddi
Pruritus (see Chapter 28, p.795)

Rare
Respiratory depression
Psychological dependence

---

a. generally, opioid-related nausea and vomiting is transient and improves after 5–7 days; if persistent despite an anti-emetic (see p.241), consider other possible causes before switching to another opioid (see p.365).

The relationship of the therapeutic dose to the lethal dose of a strong opioid (the therapeutic ratio) is greater than commonly supposed. For example, patients who take a double dose of **morphine** at bedtime are no more likely to die during the night than those who do not.[31]

The *belief* that the lethal dose of **morphine** is the weight of the patient in kg given as mg of **morphine** is *false*, and, in any case, is irrelevant to palliative care practice. Patients receiving an individually titrated dose of PO **morphine** on a regular basis to relieve pain are not the same physiologically as people without pain who receive *de novo* **morphine** 40–80mg by injection.

Tolerance and dependence

Generally, tolerance to strong opioids is not a practical problem.[32,33] Psychological dependence (addiction) to **morphine** is rare in patients with cancer pain.[30,34,35] Caution in this respect should be reserved for patients with a present or past history of substance abuse (Box C); but even then strong opioids should be used when there is clinical need.[36,37] Physical dependence does not prevent a reduction in the dose if the patient's pain ameliorates, e.g. as a result of radio therapy or a nerve block.[38]

Box C   Example of a contract for controlled substance prescriptions with addicts[a]

Controlled substance medications (narcotics, tranquillizers and barbiturates) are very useful, but have high potential for misuse and are therefore closely controlled by the local, state, and federal government. They are intended to relieve pain, to improve function and/or ability to work, not simply to feel good. Because my physician is prescribing such medication for me to help manage my condition, I agree to the following conditions:

1 I am responsible for my controlled substance medications. If the prescription of medication is lost, misplaced, or stolen, or if I use it up sooner than prescribed, I understand that it will not be replaced.

2 I will not request or accept controlled substance medication from any other physicians or individual while I am receiving such medication from Dr._____. Besides being illegal to do so, it may endanger my health. The only exception is if it is prescribed while I am admitted in a hospital.

continued

Box C Continued

3 Refills of controlled substance medication:
- Will be made only during Dr._____ regular office hours, in person, once each month during a scheduled office visit. Refills will not be made at night, on holidays, or weekends.
- Will not be made if I 'run out early'. I am responsible for taking the medication in the dose prescribed and for keeping track of the amount remaining.
- Will not be made as an 'emergency', such as on Friday afternoon because I suddenly realize I will 'run out tomorrow'. I will call at least seventy-two hours ahead if I need assistance with a controlled substance medication prescription.

4 I will bring in the containers of all medications prescribed by Dr. _____ each time I see him even if there is no medication remaining. These will be in the original containers from the pharmacy for each medication.

5 I understand that if I violate any of the above conditions, my controlled substances prescription and/or treatment with Dr._____ may be ended immediately. If the violation involves obtaining controlled substances from another individual, as described above, I may also be reported to my physician, medical facilities, and other authorities.

6 I understand that the main treatment goal is to improve my ability to function and/or work. In consideration of that goal and the fact that I am being given potent medication to help me reach that goal, I agree to help myself by the following better health habits: exercise, weight control, and the non-use of tobacco and alcohol. I understand that only through following a healthier life-style can I hope to have the most successful outcome to my treatment.

I have been fully informed by Dr._____ and his staff regarding psychological dependence (addiction) of a controlled substance, which I understand is rare. I know that some persons may develop a tolerance, which is the need to increase the dose of the medication to achieve the same effect of pain control, and I do know that I will become physically dependent on the medication. This will occur if I am on the medication for several weeks, and, when I stop the medication, I must do so slowly and under medical supervision or I may have withdrawal symptoms.

I have read this contract and it has been explained to me by Dr._____ and/or his staff. In addition, I fully understand the consequences of violating said contract.

_____ _____ _____ _____
Patient's Signature   Date   Witness   Date

a. reproduced with permission from Hansen 1999.[39] © Southern Medical Association.

However, with the dramatic increase in the use of opioids for chronic non-cancer pain there have been corresponding increases in rates of addiction and fatal overdose. These concerns have led to a re-appraisal of the place of opioids in chronic non-cancer pain and to the introduction of opioid products which reduce abuse potential. For example, some m/r formulations form insoluble precipitates if an attempt is made to crush and dissolve them, preventing their injection.[40] Others contain a sequestered opioid antagonist which, if the tablet is crushed or dissolved, is released in sufficient amounts to antagonize the opioid and prevent a 'high'. (see p.450).

Opioid-related serotonin toxicity
Serotonin toxicity results from the ingestion of drug(s) which increase brain serotonin above a critical level (see p.195).[41] Toxicity manifests as a triad of neuro-excitatory features:

- *autonomic hyperactivity*; sweating, fever, mydriasis, tachycardia, hypertension, tachypnea, sialorrhoea, diarrhoea
- *neuromuscular hyperactivity*; tremor, clonus, myoclonus, hyperreflexia, and pyramidal rigidity (advanced stage)
- *altered mental status*; agitation, hypomania, and delirium (advanced stage).

Clonus (inducible, spontaneous or ocular), agitation, sweating, tremor and hyperreflexia are essential features. Spontaneous clonus, in the presence of a serotoninergic drug, is the most reliable indicator of serotonin toxicity.[42]

Opioids are relatively weak serotonin re-uptake inhibitors and only cause symptoms in higher doses or susceptible individuals, or when used concurrently with a second drug with serotoninergic potency, notably an MAOI but also with many other antidepressants and some psychostimulants (see Antidepressants, Box B, p.195).

Fatalities from serotonin toxicity have occurred with **dextromethorphan, pethidine** (see Box A), **tramadol**, and possibly **fentanyl**.[43] Non-fatal serotonin toxicity has also been observed with other fentanils, **dextropropoxyphene, methadone**, and **pentazocine**. It has *not* been observed with other opioids, and the 'blanket' warning against the concurrent use of an MAOI and other opioids is misplaced (Box D).

Box D A misleading report about morphine and MAOIs[44]

A patient who regularly took an MAOI and trifluoperazine 20mg/24h was given pre-operative promethazine 50mg IM and morphine 1mg IV followed by two doses of morphine 2.5mg IV. About 3min later she became unresponsive and hypotensive (systolic pressure 40mmHg); responding within 2min to IV naloxone.

Although repeatedly referenced as such, this was *not* MAOI-related serotonin toxicity; it was a hypotensive response to IV morphine in someone chronically taking trifluoperazine, an α antagonist.

The onset of toxicity is generally rapid and progressive, typically as the second drug reaches effective blood levels (one or two doses). Occasionally, recurrent mild symptoms may occur for weeks before the development of severe toxicity. The patient is often alert or agitated, with tremor (sometimes severe), myoclonus and hyperreflexia. Ankle clonus is generally demonstrable or, in severe toxicity, occurs spontaneously. Neuromuscular signs are initially greater in the lower limbs, then become more generalized as toxicity increases. Other symptoms include shaking, shivering (often including chattering of the teeth), and sometimes trismus. Pyramidal rigidity is a late development in severe cases, and can impair respiration. Rigidity, a fever of $> 38.5\,°C$ or deteriorating blood gases indicate life-threatening toxicity.

Opioids and hypothalamic–pituitary function

Chronic administration of opioids can interfere with hypothalamic-pituitary function:[45]
- inhibition of hypothalamic gonadotrophin-releasing hormone from the hypothalamus:
  ▷ ↓ luteinizing hormone (LH) release from the pituitary → ↓ production of testosterone (testes) or oestrogen (ovaries)
  ▷ ↓ follicle-stimulating hormone (FSH) release from the pituitary → ↓ production of sperm or ovarian follicles
  ▷ associated with loss of libido, impotence, irregular menses or amenorrhoea, subfertility and other consequences of hypogonadism, e.g. reduced muscle mass, osteoporosis
- inhibition of adrenocorticotrophic hormone (ACTH) from the pituitary:[46]
  ▷ ↓ cortisol production and release (adrenals)
  ▷ associated with symptoms such as fatigue, weight loss, anorexia, vomiting, diarrhoea, abdominal pain, hypoglycaemia, hypotension
- inhibition of growth hormone from the pituitary:
  ▷ associated with decreased exercise tolerance, decreased mood and general wellbeing, reduced bone remodelling activity, altered body fat distribution (increased central adiposity), hyperlipidaemia and increased predisposition to atherogenesis.[47]

In patients with chronic non-cancer pain, hormone suppression is evident after 1 week of opioid administration and appears dose-related; in one study, abnormally low levels of sex hormones were found in three quarters of men receiving opioids by mouth equivalent to < 150mg morphine/24h, and in all receiving > 150mg/24h.[48]

IT **morphine** (mean doses 5–12mg/24h) produced hypogonadism in most subjects, both men and women.[49–51] In one study, one third of patients also developed hypocortisolism ± growth hormone deficiency, leading to an Addisonian crisis in one patient.[49] Thus, in patients due to receive long-term IT opioids, it is recommended to measure sex hormone levels at baseline, and annually thereafter (see Spinal analgesia, Table 5, p.718).

However, when any patient receiving long-term opioids for non-cancer pain has symptoms suggestive of hypothalamic dysfunction, it may be necessary to refer to an endocrinologist for investigation and possible replacement hormone therapy.[49]

Compared with **morphine** and other opioids, **buprenorphine** appears less likely to suppress the gonadal axis or testosterone levels (see p.392).

Opioids and immune function

Opioids modulate immune cell function directly and indirectly via activation of the hypothalamic-pituitary-adrenal axis (HPA) and the autonomic nervous system. Lymphocytes and mononuclear phagocytes express μ-, k- and δ-opioid receptors, which when activated trigger cellular apoptosis. Immune function is suppressed by the opioid-induced release of glucocorticoids and catecholamines (e.g. adrenaline (epinephrine), noradrenaline (norepinephrine) and dopamine) from the adrenal medulla and the release of catecholamines from sympathetic nerve fibres which innervate lymphoid tissue (e.g. lymph nodes, spleen).[52] Thus, **morphine** depresses natural killer cell activity, T-lymphocyte proliferation, monocyte/macrophage function and cytokine function (e.g. interleukin (IL)-2, interferon (IFN)-γ), potentially reducing host resistance to bacterial, fungal and viral infections.[53–55] Further, partly through its effects on the immune system, **morphine** can influence cancer cell growth and metastasis. However, it is unclear if the overall effect is beneficial or deleterious.[56]

Compared with **morphine** (and **diamorphine**), other opioids are less immunosuppressive and **buprenorphine**, **hydromorphone**, **methadone**, **oxycodone**, **oxymorphone** and **tramadol** have little or no effect.[57–60] Neither **buprenorphine** nor **fentanyl** affect CD4+/CD8+ counts in patients with AIDS.[61] In one small retrospective study in patients with cancer pain, the incidence of infections was less in those receiving **oxycodone** compared to **morphine**.[62]

The clinical implications of these effects are uncertain.[56,60,63] However, they may help to explain the increased susceptibility to infection seen in opioid abusers.[64] On the other hand, because pain is immunosuppressive, opioid analgesia may improve immune function in patients with pain.[65]

Opioid-induced hyperalgesia

Opioid-induced hyperalgesia (OIH) appears important in both acute and chronic pain. Although poorly understood, it appears to result from sustained sensitization of the nervous system in which the excitatory amino acid neurotransmitter system and the NMDA-receptor-channel complex play important roles.[66,67] Possible causes include:

- opioid-induced activation of glial cells, which play a role in inflammation, pain signal transmission, pain hypersensitivity and opioid tolerance[68–70]
- alteration in the G protein coupling of opioid receptors, i.e. Gs rather than Gi/o; the Gs variant has an excitatory rather than an inhibitory effect[71]
- in the case of **morphine**, accumulation of M3G.[72]

Genetic make-up probably plays an important part in its development.

Clinical features

In surgical pain, OIH may contribute to exaggerated levels of pain in the immediate postoperative period and the development of a chronic pain state. In patients with cancer, OIH may manifest in various ways:

- rapidly developing tolerance to opioids
- short-lived benefit from increased doses
- a change of pain pattern (Table 3).

The extreme upper end of the spectrum may be those patients who manifest evidence of severe neural hyperexcitability (myoclonus, allodynia, and/or hyperalgesia), particularly when taking high doses of **morphine** or an alternative strong opioid. This may be accompanied by sedation and delirium (when it is often described as opioid neurotoxicity). However, OIH:

- is *not* limited to very high doses, or to any one opioid
- is probably under-diagnosed
- is more common than generally thought.

Severe pain which does not respond to increasing doses of opioids, or is complicated by severe undesirable effects, should raise the *possibility* of OIH.[73]

Table 3 Opioid-induced hyperalgesia[73]

What the patient says	What the doctor finds
Increased sensitivity to pain stimulus (hyperalgesia)	Any dose of any opioid, but particularly with high-dose morphine or hydromorphone, and in renal failure
Worsening pain despite increasing doses of opioids	Pain elicited from ordinary non-painful stimuli, e.g. stroking skin with cotton (allodynia)
Pain which becomes more diffuse, extending beyond the distribution of the pre-existing pain	Presence of other manifestations of opioid-induced neural hyperexcitability: myoclonus, seizures, delirium

Evaluation

A diagnosis of OIH is generally made on the basis of a high level of clinical suspicion, probability, and pattern recognition. OIH must be differentiated from increased pain caused by disease progression or the development of opioid tolerance, both of which may be managed by increasing the opioid dose.

Management

Management is based largely on theoretical grounds and clinical observation.

Prophylaxis

Use a multimodal approach to analgesia, e.g.:

- an NSAID may help to reduce the production of excitatory amino acid neurotransmitters which activate the pronociceptive and anti-opioid systems
- **gabapentin** may block calcium channels which may contribute to hyperalgesia in nerve pain.

Treatment

- progressively and rapidly reduce the dose of the causal opioid to about 25% of the peak dose
- switch to an opioid with less risk of OIH, i.e. **fentanyl** (highest) → **morphine** → **methadone** → **buprenorphine** (lowest)[74]
- (rarely) if occurring at very low doses (< 10mg/24h), discontinue the opioid completely
- use a multimodal approach to analgesia, i.e. use non-opioids, e.g. **paracetamol** or an NSAID, and adjuvant analgesics, e.g. **gabapentin**
- start oral or parenteral **ketamine** (an NMDA-receptor-channel blocker).[75]

Note that when switching from **morphine** because of severe neural hyperexcitability, a lower than expected dose of the alternative opioid is likely to be needed unless the dose of **morphine** has been much reduced (as suggested above).[76,79] If these steps do not lead to a resolution of the OIH:

- consider spinal, regional or local analgesia (with local anaesthetics), and tail off systemic opioids completely
- check for hypomagnesaemia because this can aggravate OIH.[78,79]
- consider treatment with ultralow doses of an opioid antagonist.[80–82]

Opioid switching ('rotation')

It is crucial to appreciate that conversion ratios are *never* more than an approximate guide. Thus, careful monitoring during conversion is necessary to avoid both underdosing and excessive dosing.

Generally, switching from **morphine** (or other strong opioid) to an alternative is undertaken in an attempt to improve analgesia and/or reduce undesirable effects. Before switching, it is worth considering if other options may be more appropriate, e.g. the use of adjuvant analgesics or modifying the management of the undesirable effects.

Switching is necessary in about 20% of patients according to one prospective survey.[83] Changes from **morphine** to TD **fentanyl** (or vice versa) are included in this figure. Higher figures have been published elsewhere, e.g. 44%.[84] The lower figure better reflects clinical experience in the UK.[85] Examples of when switching may be appropriate include:

- poor adherence (→ TD **fentanyl**)
- poor response to **morphine** plus an NSAID (→ **methadone**)[86]
- intolerable undesirable effects, e.g. *intractable* constipation (→ TD **fentanyl**)
- significant decline in the patient's renal function (**morphine** → **methadone**, TD **fentanyl** or **hydromorphone**)
- opioid-induced hyperalgesia or other manifestations of neurotoxicity, e.g. cognitive failure/delirium, hallucinations, myoclonus, allodynia.

In cases of neurotoxicity, **hydromorphone**, **oxycodone** and **methadone** have all been substituted successfully for **morphine**.[87–89] Similarly, in the presence of inadequate pain relief and intolerable undesirable effects, TD **buprenorphine** has been substituted successfully for TD **fentanyl**, and vice versa.[90]

When converting from **morphine** to an alternative strong opioid, or vice versa, the initial dose depends on the relative potency of the two drugs (Table 4). (See also Chapter 15, p.661).

Table 4 Approximate PO opioid potency ratios (morphine = 1)[a]

Analgesic	Potency ratio with morphine	Duration of action (h)[b]
Codeine ⎫ Dihydrocodeine ⎬ Dextropropoxyphene ⎭	1/10	3–6
Tramadol	1/10	4–6
Pethidine	1/8	2–4
Hydrocodone (not UK)	2/3	4–8
Papaveretum	2/3[c]	3–5
Oxycodone	1.5 (2)[d]	3–4
Methadone	5–10[e]	8–12
Hydromorphone	4–5 (5–7.5)[d]	4–5
Buprenorphine (SL)	80	6–8
Buprenorphine (TD)	100 (75–115)[d]	Formulation dependent
Fentanyl (TD)	100 (150)[d]	72

a. multiply dose of opioid by its potency ratio to determine the equivalent dose of morphine sulfate/hydrochloride; conversely, divide morphine dose by the appropriate potency ratio to determine the equivalent dose of another opioid
b. dependent in part on severity of pain and on dose; often longer lasting in very elderly and those with renal impairment
c. papaveretum (strong opium) is standardized to contain 50% morphine base; potency expressed in relation to morphine sulfate
d. the numbers in parenthesis are the manufacturers' preferred ratios; for explanation of divergence, see individual drug monographs
e. a single 5mg dose of methadone is equivalent to morphine 7.5mg, but a variable long plasma halflife and broad-spectrum receptor affinity result in a much higher than expected potency ratio when administered regularly, sometimes much higher than the range given above (see p.433).[76,91]

However, potency and thus conversion ratios are *never* more than an approximate guide because of:[92–95]

- wide interindividual variation in opioid pharmacokinetics; influencing factors include age, ethnicity, renal or hepatic impairment
- other variables including dose and duration of opioid treatment, direction of switch in opioid, nutritional status and concurrent medications
- their method of derivation, e.g. single dose rather than chronic dose studies, using typical doses.

Thus, careful monitoring during conversion is necessary to avoid both underdosing and excessive dosing.

Providing explicit guidance on switching opioids is difficult because the reasons for switching are varied, as are the patient's circumstances. One guideline, based on expert consensus, recommends routinely reducing the calculated equivalent dose of the new opioid by 25–50%.[96] Various patient factors are then taken into account to modify the reduction, which potentially could see it removed (e.g. young patient, no undesirable effects, in severe pain, switching at low dose) or increased further (e.g. older patient, delirious, in moderate pain, switching at high dose).

Certainly, a dose reduction of at least 50% would seem prudent when switching at high doses (e.g. **morphine** or equivalent doses of $\geqslant 1g/24h$), in elderly or frail patients, because of intolerable undesirable effects (e.g. delirium), or when there has been a recent rapid escalation of the first opioid (possibly due to opioid-induced hyperalgesia). In such circumstances, p.r.n. doses can be relied on to make up any deficit while re-titrating to a satisfactory dose of the new opioid.

A separate strategy is necessary for **methadone** (see p.433).

Combining opioids

It is generally considered to be bad practice to prescribe two or more opioids for simultaneous use. Thus, for example, regular **morphine** is best backed up by p.r.n **morphine** for breakthrough (episodic) pain. However, there are circumstances when the p.r.n. opioid differs from the regular opioid, for example TD **fentanyl** backed up by p.r.n. **morphine** (see p.411). Also, someone with good pain relief from a regular weak opioid may have a supply of **morphine** for back-up use in case of severe break-through (episodic) pain.

However, there are reports of two strong opioids being used successfully in combination, i.e. providing better pain relief at relatively lower doses and reduced undesirable effects.[97–99] For example, in one, regular **oxycodone** plus p.r.n. **morphine** was more beneficial than regular **morphine** plus p.r.n. **morphine**.[97] In another, patients on regular morphine benefited from the addition of a second regular opioid in low dose (either **methadone** or TD **fentanyl**).[98] However, the quality of this evidence is low or very low.[100] Better evidence exists for a synergistic effect between **morphine** and **oxycodone**, with a combination product in development (see p.442). Nonetheless, despite such reports, patients should *not* normally have two opioids prescribed concurrently on a regular basis.[101,102]

Opioids in renal impairment and end-stage renal failure

In renal impairment and end-stage renal failure, regardless of the opioid used, extra caution is *always* required whether or not the patient is on dialysis. This is particularly necessary in patients with rapidly deteriorating renal function or when acutely unwell, e.g. because of sepsis.

Clear written instructions regarding analgesic drug regimens should routinely be provided together with close monitoring. Patients and their carers should be educated about the early symptoms of opioid toxicity and the actions required should they occur.

Opioids differ in their potential to cause toxicity when renal function is impaired. However, the evidence base from clinical studies is limited,[103] and stratification of risk is based on the presence of active metabolites, risk of accumulation, and expert opinion.

The pharmacokinetics and pharmacodynamics of opioids are altered by renal impairment (see p.654). Accumulation of an opioid or active metabolite will lead to a prolonged duration of action and increased toxicity. Changes in plasma protein concentrations or alterations in the blood–brain barrier also increase the potential for toxicity with any opioid. Thus in renal impairment, when possible optimize the use of adjuvant analgesics before introducing an opioid, e.g. in neuropathic pain (see p.295). If an opioid is necessary, it is important to:

- start at lower than usual doses
- consider increasing the intervals between doses
- monitor closely for toxicity, both immediate and delayed (also see p.654).

Weak and strong opioids with active metabolites (e.g. **codeine, hydromorphone, morphine, oxycodone, tramadol**) can be used with caution in patients with *mild–moderate* renal impairment. However, in *severe* renal impairment (and in renal *failure*), it is generally preferable to use a strong opioid which has no active metabolite and is not removed by dialysis (Table 5). On the other hand, expert opinion (with a limited objective evidence base) suggests that **tramadol** and **hydromorphone** can still be used with caution in this setting, e.g. by reducing the upper dose limit (Figure 1).[103–106]

Table 5 Opioid analgesia and severe renal impairment or renal failure [13,103,107–109]

Opioid[a]	Main metabolite(s)	Active metabolite(s)[b]	Effect of renal impairment	Removed by dialysis[c]	Comment
Recommended for chronic use					
Alfentanil	Noralfentanil	No	No accumulation. Possible increase in unbound fraction but clinical significance unknown	No	When used as a rescue analgesic, its short duration of action may necessitate frequent p.r.n. use
Buprenorphine	Norbuprenorphine	Yes[d]	Possible accumulation of metabolites but clinical significance unknown	No	Less experience of its use in this setting compared with fentanyl
Fentanyl	Norfentanyl	No	Possible accumulation of parent drug but clinical significance unknown	No[e]	
Methadone	Methadol, EDDP, EMDP[f]	No	No accumulation	No	Use requires caution; unpredictable accumulation and toxicity even in the absence of renal impairment (see p.433)
Use cautiously					
Hydromorphone	Hydromorphone-3-glucuronide (H3G)	Yes	Accumulation of H3G can occur to a clinically significant degree	Yes	H3G has no analgesic effect but may cause neurotoxicity. Generally, no additional dose required with dialysis
Tramadol	O-desmethyltramadol (M1)	Yes	Accumulation of parent drug and metabolites can occur to a clinically significant degree	Yes	Generally, no additional dose required with dialysis
Not recommended for chronic use					
Codeine	Codeine-6-glucuronide, morphine-3-glucuronide (M3G), morphine-6-glucuronide (M6G)	Yes	Accumulation of M3G and M6G can occur to a clinically significant degree	Yes	
Morphine	M3G, M6G	Yes	Accumulation of M3G and M6G can occur to a clinically significant degree	Yes	M6G more active than morphine. Human studies suggest M3G has no analgesic effect but may cause neurotoxicity
Oxycodone	Noroxycodone, oxymorphone	Yes	Accumulation of oxycodone and metabolites can occur to a clinically significant degree	Yes	

a. close monitoring of the patient is required whichever opioid is used
b. in sufficient quantities with the potential to produce a clinical effect
c. the removal of the parent drug or metabolites when patients are undergoing regular dialysis depends on several factors, and evidence is limited and contradictory. If loss of analgesia occurs either prior to or soon after dialysis, consider giving an additional dose of the opioid
d. norbuprenorphine has similar receptor binding to buprenorphine but does not readily cross the blood-brain barrier
e. certain dialysis membranes may remove fentanyl, e.g. cellulose triacetate 190

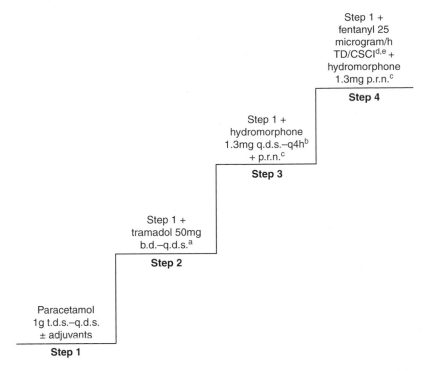

Figure 1 Example of an analgesic ladder for patients with severe renal impairment or failure; doses PO unless stated otherwise.

a. equivalent to about morphine 10–20mg/24h PO; the maximum dose of tramadol is limited to 100mg/24h in patients not on dialysis and 200mg/24h in those on dialysis
b. equivalent to about morphine 20–30mg/24h PO; start with q.d.s and increase if necessary and if tolerated to q4h. Fentanyl TD/CSCI 12microgram/h is an alternative to q4h hydromorphone and is preferred in patients *not* on dialysis
c. equivalent to about morphine 5mg PO
d. equivalent to about morphine 60mg/24h PO; use when unacceptable pain relief in step 3 despite frequent p.r.n. use, i.e. 4–6/24h
e. CSCI alfentanil can be substituted for CSCI fentanyl: it is about one quarter as potent as fentanyl (see p.385).

Fentanyl (see p.403) can be administered continuously TD or CSCI.[103,106,110] There is also an increasing range of SL, buccal and nasal fentanyl products suitable for p.r.n. use, although these are authorized only for break-through (episodic) cancer pain (see p.413).

Buprenorphine, like **fentanyl**, is not removed by haemodialysis and it could become a popular choice in patients with renal impairment.[13,109,111,112] It does have an active metabolite (norbuprenorphine) with similar opioid receptor-binding affinities to **buprenorphine**, but this does not generally cross the blood-brain barrier and thus has little, if any, central effect (see p.392).[113,114] However, renal impairment increases the permeability of the blood-brain barrier and more experience is required with **buprenorphine** in this setting.[103]

At the end of life, consensus guidelines[110] favour **fentanyl** for analgesia in patients with severe renal impairment or failure (GFR <30mL/min). Consequently, experience with this approach has increased (also see fentanyl, p.403). However, in some centres or settings, the cautious use of a familiar opioid may be preferred to switching to an unfamiliar (albeit 'renally safer') one.

Ketamine may also have a role to play in some patients with renal impairment (see p.625).[115]

1 Portenoy RK *et al.* (2006) Opioid use and survival at the end of life: a survey of a hospice population. *Journal of Pain and Symptom Management.* **32**: 532–540.
2 Ballantyne JC (2007) Regulation of opioid prescribing. *British Medical Journal.* **334**: 811–812.
3 Mika J (2008) The opioid systems and the role of glial cells in the effects of opioids. *Advances in Palliative Medicine.* **7**: 185–196.
4 Sauriyal DS *et al.* (2011) Extending pharmacological spectrum of opioids beyond analgesia: Multifunctional aspects in different pathophysiological states. *Neuropeptides.* **45**: 175–188.
5 Rothman R (1995) Buprenorphine: a review of the binding literature. In: A Cowan and J Lewis (eds) *Buprenorphine: combatting drug abuse with a unique opioid.* Wiley-Liss, New York, pp. 19–29.
6 Zaki P *et al.* (2000) Ligand-induced changes in surface mu-opioid receptor number: relationship to G protein activation? *Journal of Pharmacology and Experimental Therapeutics.* **292**: 1127–1134.
7 Lutfy K *et al.* (2003) Buprenorphine-induced antinociception is mediated by mu-opioid receptors and compromised by concomitant activation of opioid receptor-like receptors. *Journal of Neuroscience.* **23**: 10331–10337.
8 Lewis JW and Husbands SM (2004) The orvinols and related opioids–high affinity ligands with diverse efficacy profiles. *Current Pharmaceutical Design.* **10**: 717–732.
9 Hill RG (1992) Multiple opioid receptors and their ligands. *Frontiers of Pain.* **4**: 1–4.
10 Corbett AD *et al.* (1993) Selectivity of ligands for opioid receptors. In: A Herz (ed) *Opioids.* Springer-Verlag, London, pp. 657–672.
11 Manchikanti L *et al.* (2012) American Society of Interventional Pain Physicians (ASIPP) guidelines for responsible opioid prescribing in chronic non-cancer pain: Part I–evidence assessment. *Pain Physician.* **15**: S1–65.
12 British Pain Society (2010) Opioids for persistent pain: Good practice. London. Available from: www.britishpainsociety.org
13 Caraceni A *et al.* (2012) Use of opioid analgesics in the treatment of cancer pain: evidence-based recommendations from the EAPC. *Lancet Oncology.* **13**: e58–68.
14 WHO (1986) *Cancer Pain Relief.* World Health Organization, Geneva.
15 Quigley C (2005) The role of opioids in cancer pain. *British Medical Journal.* **331**: 825–829.
16 NICE (2012) Opioids in palliative care: safe and effective prescribing of strong opioids for pain in palliative care adults. *Clinical Guideline.* CG104. www.nice.org.uk
17 Hoskin P and Hanks G (1991) Opioid agonist-antagonist drugs in acute and chronic pain states. *Drugs.* **41**: 326–344.
18 Twycross RG (1994) Pentazocine. In: *Pain Relief in Advanced Cancer.* Churchill Livingstone, Edinburgh, pp. 247–248.
19 Woods S *et al.* (1974) Medicines evaluation and monitoring group: central nervous system effects of pentazocine. *British Medical Journal.* **1**: 305–307.
20 Smith J (2004) Building a safer NHS for patients - Improving medication safety. A Report by the Chief Pharmacuetical Officer. Gateway ref 1459. 105–111 Department of Health, London.
21 Care Quality Commission and NHS England (2013) Safer use of controlled drugs - preventing harms from fentanyl and buprenorphine transdermal patches. *Use of controlled drugs supporting information.* www.cqc.org.uk
22 Plummer JL *et al.* (2001) Norpethidine toxicity. *Pain Reviews.* **8**: 159–170.
23 Sweetman SC (ed) (2005) Martindale: The Complete Drug Reference. (34e). Pharmaceutical Press, London, pp. 80–82.
24 Shee JC (1960) Dangerous potentiation of pethidine by iproniazid, and its treatment. *British Medical Journal.* **ii**: 507–509.
25 Taylor D (1962) Alarming reaction to pethidine in patients on phenelzine. *Lancet.* **2**: 401–402.
26 Rogers KJ and Thornton JA (1969) The interaction between monoamine oxidase inhibitors and narcotic analgesics in mice. *British Journal of Pharmacology.* **36**: 470–480.
27 Cherny N *et al.* (2001) Strategies to manage the adverse effects of oral morphine: an evidence-based report. *Journal of Clinical Oncology.* **19**: 2542–2554.
28 Borgbjerg FM *et al.* (1996) Experimental pain stimulates respiration and attenuates morphine-induced respiratory depression: a controlled study in human volunteers. *Pain.* **64**: 123–128.
29 Estfan B *et al.* (2007) Respiratory function during parenteral opioid titration for cancer pain. *Palliative Medicine.* **21**: 81–86.
30 Sykes NP (2007) Morphine kills the pain, not the patient. *Lancet.* **369**: 1325–1326.
31 Regnard CFB and Badger C (1987) Opioids, sleep and the time of death. *Palliative Medicine.* **1**: 107–110.
32 Collin E *et al.* (1993) Is disease progression the major factor in morphine 'tolerance' in cancer pain treatment? *Pain.* **55**: 319–326.
33 Portenoy RK (1994) Tolerance to opioid analgesics: clinical aspects. *Cancer Surveys.* **21**: 49–65.
34 Passik S and Portenoy R (1998) Substance abuse issues in palliative care. In: A Berger (ed) *Principles and Practice of Supportive Oncology.* Lippincott-Raven, Philadelphia, pp. 513–529.
35 Joranson D *et al.* (2000) Trends in medical use and abuse of opioid analgesics. *Journal of the American Medical Association.* **283**: 1710–1714.
36 Passik S *et al.* (1998) Substance abuse issues in cancer patients. Part 1: prevalence and diagnosis. *Oncology.* **12**: 517–521.
37 Passik S *et al.* (1998) Substance abuse issues in cancer patients. Part 2: evaluation and treatment. *Oncology.* **12**: 729–734.
38 Twycross RG and Wald SJ (1976) Longterm use of diamorphine in advanced cancer. In: JJ Bonica and D Albe-Fessard (eds) *Advances in Pain Research and Therapy* Vol 1. Raven Press, New York, pp. 653–661.
39 Hansen H (1999) Treatment of chronic pain with antiepileptic drugs. *Southern Medical Journal.* **92**: 642–649.
40 Cicero TJ *et al.* (2012) Effect of abuse-deterrent formulation of OxyContin. *New England Journal of Medicine.* **367**: 187–189.
41 Gillman K (2006) Serotonin toxicity, serotonin syndrome. *Psycho Tropical Research.* www.psychotropical.com (accessed April 2013).
42 Dunkley EJ *et al.* (2003) The Hunter Serotonin Toxicity Criteria: simple and accurate diagnostic decision rules for serotonin toxicity. *Quarterly Journal of Medicine.* **96**: 635–642.
43 Gillman PK (2005) Monoamine oxidase inhibitors, opioid analgesics and serotonin toxicity. *British Journal of Anaesthesia.* **95**: 434–441.
44 Barry B (1979) Adverse effects of MAO inhibitors with narcotics reversed with naloxone. *Anaesthesia and Intensive Care.* **7**: 194.
45 McWilliams K *et al.* (2014) A systematic review of opioid effects on the hypogonadal axis of cancer patients. *Supportive Care in Cancer.* **22**: 1699–1704.
46 Debono M *et al.* (2011) Tramadol-induced adrenal insufficiency. *European Journal of Clinical Pharmacology.* **67**: 865–867.
47 NICE (2003) Human Growth hormone (somatropin) in adults with growth hormone deficiency. *Technology appraisal guidance.* **TA64.** www.nice.org.uk
48 Daniell HW (2002) Hypogonadism in men consuming sustained-action oral opioids. *The Journal of Pain.* **3**: 377–384.
49 Abs R *et al.* (2000) Endocrine consequences of long-term intrathecal administration of opioids. *Journal of Clinical Endocrinology and Metabolism.* **85**: 2215–2222.
50 Finch PM *et al.* (2000) Hypogonadism in patients treated with intrathecal morphine. *Clinical Journal of Pain.* **16**: 251–254.

51 Roberts LJ et al. (2002) Sex hormone suppression by intrathecal opioids: a prospective study. Clinical Journal of Pain. 18: 144–148.

52 Vallejo R et al. (2004) Opioid therapy and immunosuppression: a review. American Journal of Therapeutics. 11: 354–365.

53 Sacerdote P et al. (1997) Antinociceptive and immunosuppressive effects of opiate drugs: a structure-related activity study. British Journal of Pharmacology. 121: 834–840.

54 Risdahl JM et al. (1998) Opiates and infection. Journal of Neuroimmunology. 83: 4–18.

55 McCarthy L et al. (2001) Opioids, opioid receptors, and the immune response. Drug and Alcohol Dependence. 62: 111–123.

56 Afsharimani B et al. (2011) Morphine and tumor growth and metastasis. Cancer Metastasis Reviews. 30: 225–238.

57 Sacerdote P et al. (2000) The effects of tramadol and morphine on immune responses and pain after surgery in cancer patients. Anesthesia and Analgesia. 90: 1411–1414.

58 Budd K and Shipton E (2004) Acute pain and the immune system and opioimmunosuppression. Acute Pain. 6: 123–135.

59 Budd K and Raffa R (eds) (2005) Buprenorphine - the unique opioid analgesic. Georg Thieme Verlag, Stuttgart, Germany, p. 134.

60 Sacerdote P et al. (2008) Buprenorphine and methadone maintenance treatment of heroin addicts preserves immune function. Brain, Behavior, and Immunity. 22: 606–613.

61 Canneti A et al. (2013) Safety and efficacy of transdermal buprenorphine and transdermal fentanyl in the treatment of neuropathic pain in AIDS patients. Minerva Anestesiologica. 79: 871–883.

62 Suzuki M et al. (2013) Correlation between the administration of morphine or oxycodone and the development of infections in patients with cancer pain. American Journal of Hospice and Palliative Care. 30: 712–716.

63 Rittner HL et al. (2010) The clinical (ir)relevance of opioid-induced immune suppression. Current Opinion in Anaesthesiology. 23: 588–592.

64 Alonzo NC and Bayer BM (2002) Opioids, immunology, and host defenses of intravenous drug abusers. Infectious Disease Clinics of North America. 16: 553–569.

65 Page GG (2005) Immunologic effects of opioids in the presence or absence of pain. Journal of Pain and Symptom Management. 29: S25–31.

66 Simonnet G (2008) Preemptive antihyperalgesia to improve preemptive analgesia. Anesthesiology. 108: 352–354.

67 Bekhit MH (2010) Opioid-induced hyperalgesia and tolerance. American Journal of Therapeutics. 17: 498–510.

68 Ren K and Dubner R (2008) Neuron-glia crosstalk gets serious: role in pain hypersensitivity. Current Opinion in Anaesthesiology. 21: 570–579.

69 Romero-Sandoval EA et al. (2008) Neuroimmune interactions and pain: focus on glial-modulating targets. Current Opinion in Investigational Drugs. 9: 726–734.

70 Milligan ED and Watkins LR (2009) Pathological and protective roles of glia in chronic pain. Nature Reviews Neuroscience. 10: 23–36.

71 Crain S and Shen K (2000) Antagonists of excitatory opioid receptor functions enhance morphine's analgesic potency and attenuate opioid tolerance/dependence liability. Pain. 84: 121–131.

72 Bartlett S et al. (1994) Pharmacology of morphine and morphine-3-glucuronide at opioid, excitatory amino acid, GABA and glycine binding sites. Pharmacology and Toxicology. 75: 73–81.

73 Zylicz Z and Twycross R (2008) Opioid-induced hyperalgesia may be more frequent than previously thought. Journal of Clinical Oncology. 26: 1564; author reply 1565.

74 Filitz J et al. (2008) Supra-additive effects of tramadol and acetaminophen in a human pain model. Pain. 136: 262–270.

75 Walker SM and Cousins MJ (1997) Reduction in hyperalgesia and intrathecal morphine requirements by low-dose ketamine infusion. Journal of Pain and Symptom Management. 14: 129–133.

76 Bruera E et al. (1996) Opioid rotation in patients with cancer pain. Cancer. 78: 852–857.

77 Lawlor P et al. (1998) Dose ratio between morphine and methadone in patients with cancer pain. Cancer. 82: 1167–1173.

78 Dubray C et al. (1997) Magnesium deficiency induces an hyperalgesia reversed by the NMDA receptor antagonist MK801. Neuroreport. 8: 1383–1386.

79 Begon S et al. (2002) Magnesium increases morphine analgesic effect in different experimental models of pain. Anesthesiology. 96: 627–632.

80 Gan T et al. (1997) Opioid-sparing effects of a low-dose infusion of naloxone in patient-administered morphine sulfate. Anesthesiology. 87: 1075–1081.

81 Chindalore VL et al. (2005) Adding ultralow-dose naltrexone to oxycodone enhances and prolongs analgesia: a randomized, controlled trial of Oxytrex. Journal of Pain. 6: 392–399.

82 Rauck RL et al. (2006) A randomized, double-blind, placebo-controlled study of intrathecal ziconotide in adults with severe chronic pain. Journal of Pain and Symptom Management. 31: 393–406.

83 Sarhill N et al. (2001) Parenteral opioid rotation in advanced cancer: A prospective study. Abstracts of the MASCC/ISOO 13th International Symposium Supportive Care in Cancer, Copenhagen, Denmark, June 14–16. Supportive Care Cancer. 9: 307.

84 Cherny NJ et al. (1995) Opioid pharmacotherapy in the management of cancer pain: a survey of strategies used by pain physicians for the selection of analgesic drugs and routes of administration. Cancer. 76: 1283–1293.

85 Twycross RG Unpublished work.

86 Morley J and Makin M (1998) The use of methadone in cancer pain poorly responsive to other opioids. Pain Reviews. 5: 51–58.

87 Sjogren P et al. (1994) Disappearance of morphine-induced hyperalgesia after discontinuing or substituting morphine with other opioid agonists. Pain. 59: 313–316.

88 Hagen N and Swanson R (1997) Strychnine-like multifocal myoclonus and seizures in extremely high-dose opioid administration: treatment strategies. Journal of Pain and Symptom Management. 14: 51–58.

89 Ashby M et al. (1999) Opioid substitution to reduce adverse effects in cancer pain management. Medical Journal of Australia. 170: 68–71.

90 Aurilio C et al. (2009) Opioids switching with transdermal systems in chronic cancer pain. Journal of Experimental and Clinical Cancer Research. 28: 61.

91 Nixon AJ (2005) Methadone for cancer pain: a case report. American Journal of Hospice and Palliative Care. 22: 337.

92 Anderson R et al. (2001) Accuracy in equianalgesic dosing: conversion dilemmas. Journal of Pain and Symptom Management. 21: 397–406.

93 Pasternak G (2001) Incomplete cross tolerance and multiple mu opioid peptide receptors. Trends in Pharmacological Sciences. 22: 67–70.

94 Pereira J et al. (2001) Equianalgesic dose ratios for opioids: a critical review and proposals for long-term dosing. Journal of Pain and Symptom Management. 22: 672–687.

95 Knotkova H et al. (2009) Opioid rotation: the science and the limitations of the equianalgesic dose table. Journal of Pain and Symptom Management. **38**: 426–439.
96 Fine PG and Portenoy RK (2009) Establishing "best practices" for opioid rotation: conclusions of an expert panel. Journal of Pain and Symptom Management. **38**: 418–425.
97 Lauretti GR et al. (2003) Comparison of sustained-release morphine with sustained-release oxycodone in advanced cancer patients. British Journal of Cancer. **89**: 2027–2030.
98 Mercadante S et al. (2004) Addition of a second opioid may improve opioid response in cancer pain: preliminary data. Supportive Care Cancer. **12**: 762–766.
99 Kotlinska-Lemieszek A (2010) Rotation, partial rotation (semi-switch), combining opioids, and titration. Does "opioid plus opioid" strategy make a step forward on our way to improving the outcome of pain treatment? Journal of Pain and Symptom Management. **40**: e10–12.
100 Fallon MT and Laird BJA (2011) A systematic review of comination strong opioid therapy in cancer pain. Palliative Medicine. **25**: 597–603.
101 Davis MP et al. (2005) Look before leaping: combined opioids may not be the rave. Supportive Care in Cancer. **13**: 769–774.
102 Strasser F (2005) Promoting science in a pragmatic world: not (yet) time for partial opioid rotation. Supportive Care in Cancer. **13**: 765–768.
103 King S et al. (2011) A systematic review of the use of opioid medication for those with moderate to severe cancer pain and renal impairment. Palliative Medicine. **25**: 454–470.
104 Clemens KE and Klaschik E (2009) Morphine and hydromorphone in palliative care patients with renal impairment. Anasthesiologie and Intensivmedizin. **50**: 70–76.
105 Lee MA et al. (2001) Retrospective study of the use of hydromorphone in palliative care patients with normal and abnormal urea and creatinine. Palliative Medicine. **15**: 26–34.
106 Ferro CJ et al. (2004) Management of pain in renal failure. In: EJ Chambers et al. (eds) Supportive Care for the Renal Patient. Oxford University Press, Oxford, UK, pp. 105–153.
107 Dean M (2004) Opioids in renal failure and dialysis patients. Journal of Pain and Symptom Management. **28**: 497–504.
108 Davison SN et al. (2010) Management of pain in renal failure. In: EJ Chambers et al. (eds) Supportive Care for the Renal Patient (2e). Oxford University Press, Oxford, pp. 139–188.
109 Niscola P et al. (2010) The use of major analgesics in patients with renal dysfunction. Current Drug Targets. **11**: 752–758.
110 Douglas C et al. (2009) Symptom management for the adult patient dying with advanced chronic kidney disease: a review of the literature and development of evidence-based guidelines by a United Kingdom Expert Consensus Group. Palliative Medicine. **23**: 103–110.
111 Murtagh FE et al. (2007) The use of opioid analgesia in end-stage renal disease patients managed without dialysis: recommendations for practice. Journal of Pain and Palliative Care Pharmacotherapy. **21**: 5–16.
112 Boger RH (2006) Renal impairment: a challenge for opioid treatment? The role of buprenorphine. Palliative Medicine. **20 Suppl 1**: s17–23.
113 Hand CW et al. (1990) Buprenorphine disposition in patients with renal impairment: single and continuous dosing, with special reference to metabolites. British Journal of Anaesthesia. **64**: 276–282.
114 Elkader A and Sproule B (2005) Buprenorphine: clinical pharmacokinetics in the treatment of opioid dependence. Clinical Pharmacokinetics. **44**: 661–680.
115 Murphy EJ (2005) Acute pain management pharmacology for the patient with concurrent renal or hepatic disease. Anaesthesia and Intensive Care. **33**: 311–322.

Updated June 2014

MORPHINE   BNF 4.7.2

Class: Opioid analgesic.

Indications: Severe or †moderate pain, diarrhoea, †cough, †dyspnoea.

Contra-indications: None absolute if titrated carefully against a patient's pain (also see Strong opioids, p.357).

Pharmacology

Morphine is the main pharmacologically active constituent of opium. Its effects are mediated by specific opioid receptors both within the CNS and peripherally. Under normal circumstances, its main peripheral action is on smooth muscle. However, in the presence of inflammation, normally silent peripheral receptors become activated.[1,2] The liver is the principal site of morphine metabolism.[3] Metabolism also occurs in other organs,[4] including the CNS.[5] Glucuronidation is rarely impaired except in severe hepatic impairment, and morphine is well tolerated in patients with mild–moderate hepatic impairment.[6] However, with impairment severe enough to prolong the prothrombin time, the plasma halflife of morphine may be increased[4] and the dose of morphine may need to be reduced or given less often, e.g. q6h or even q8h (see p.651).

The major metabolites of morphine are morphine-3-glucuronide (M3G; 55–80%) and morphine-6-glucuronide (M6G; 10–15%) which are excreted by the kidneys.[7] M6G binds to opioid receptors and contributes substantially to the effects of morphine, both desirable (e.g. analgesia) and undesirable (e.g. nausea and vomiting, sedation and respiratory depression).[8–10] In renal failure, the plasma halflife of M6G increases from 2.5h up to 7.5h, and is likely to lead to accumulation and enhanced toxicity unless the frequency of administration and/or the dose of morphine is reduced (see p.367). M3G will also accumulate, but the significance of this is unclear; it binds poorly to opioid receptors and is considered devoid of an analgesic effect. Although animal studies suggest a neuro-excitatory effect, this has not been clearly demonstrated in humans.[11]

Morphine is administered by a range of routes. Systemic absorption from topical application to ulcers or inflamed surfaces varies with the amount and concentration of the gel used; bio-availability ranges from negligible (with 0.06–0.125% gel) to almost the same as SC (0.125–0.5% gel applied to large ulcers).[12–15]

Bio-availability 35% PO, ranging from 15–64%; 25% PR.

Peak effect ≤60min PO (immediate-release tablets); 20min IV; 30–60min IM; 50–90min SC.

Time to peak plasma concentration 15–60min PO (immediate-release tablets), 1–6h m/r (product dependent); 10–20min IM; 15min SC; 45–60min PR.

Plasma halflife 1.5–4.5h PO; 1.5h IV.

Duration of action 3–6h; 12–24h m/r (product dependent).

Cautions

Renal impairment; avoid in renal failure (see p.367)

Undesirable effects

See Table 1 and Strong opioids, Box B, p.361.

Dose and use

As with all opioids, patients must be monitored for undesirable effects, particularly nausea and vomiting, and constipation (see p.360). Depending on individual circumstances, an anti-emetic should be prescribed for regular or p.r.n. use (see p.241) and, routinely, a laxative prescribed (see p.44).

Based on familiarity, availability and cost, morphine is the strong opioid of choice for cancer pain.[17] However, in terms of efficacy and undesirable effects, morphine, **hydromorphone** and **oxycodone** are essentially similar.[18] Morphine is generally prescribed with a non-opioid when the non-opioid + a weak opioid does not provide adequate relief (see p.291).

Note: the WHO recommends that weak opioids are not used in children, and that morphine is used whenever non-opioids are insufficient.[19] Some adult palliative care services also omit weak opioids (see below).

PO

Morphine is available as immediate-release tablets and solutions, and m/r tablets, capsules and suspensions. Most m/r products are administered b.d., some once daily. Because the pharmacokinetic profiles of m/r products differ,[20–22] it is best to keep individual patients on the same brand. M/r tablets should be swallowed whole; crushing or chewing them will lead to a rapid release of an overdose of morphine. For administration of immediate-release and m/r morphine to patients with swallowing difficulties or enteral feeding tubes, see p.725.

Patients can be started on either an ordinary (immediate-release) or an m/r formulation (Box A).[23,24] An observational study supports a starting dose of 5mg q4h as generally safe for opioid-naïve patients, and 10mg q4h for those being switched from a regular weak opioid.[25] However, slight variation exists between guidelines, e.g. in the recommended starting dose.[26] It is important to recognize that guidelines are just guidelines; and for each patient, when deciding the starting dose, it is necessary to consider the individual circumstances, e.g. severity of the pain, current analgesia, presence of renal impairment, increasing age or frailty. In every case, the patient must be monitored closely, and the dose titrated as necessary.

Table I Potential intolerable effects of morphine

Type	Effects	Initial action	Comment
For general undesirable effects of opioid analgesics, see Strong opioids, Box B, p.361.			
Gastric stasis	Epigastric fullness, flatulence, anorexia, hiccup, persistent nausea	Prescribe a prokinetic, e.g. metoclopramide 10–20mg t.d.s.–q.d.s. (see p.242)	If the problem persists, change to an alternative opioid, with less impact on the GI tract
Sedation	Intolerable persistent sedation	Reduce dose of morphine; consider a psychostimulant, e.g. methylphenidate 5mg b.d. (see p.224)	Sedation may be caused by other factors; stimulant rarely appropriate
Cognitive failure	Agitated delirium with hallucinations	Prescribe an antipsychotic, e.g. haloperidol 1mg stat & q2h p.r.n. (see p.177); reduce dose of morphine and, if no improvement, switch to an alternative opioid	Some patients develop intractable delirium with one opioid but not with an alternative opioid
Myoclonus	Multifocal twitching ± jerking of limbs	Prescribe a benzodiazepine, e.g. diazepam/ midazolam 5mg or lorazepam 500microgram stat & q1h p.r.n.; reduce dose of morphine but increase again if pain recurs	Uncommon with typical oral doses; more common with high dose IV and spinal morphine
Neurotoxicity	Abdominal muscle spasms, symmetrical jerking of legs; whole-body allodynia, hyperalgesia (manifests as excruciating pain)	Prescribe a benzodiazepine, e.g. diazepam/ midazolam 5mg or lorazepam 500microgram stat & q1h p.r.n.; reduce dose of morphine; consider changing to an alternative opioid	A rare syndrome in patients receiving intrathecal or high dose IV morphine; occasionally seen with typical oral and SC doses
Vestibular stimulation	Movement-induced nausea and vomiting	Prescribe an antihistaminic antimuscarinic anti-emetic, e.g. cyclizine or promethazine 25–50mg q8h–q6h (see p.249)	If intractable, try levomepromazine or switch to an alternative opioid
Pruritus	Whole-body itch with systemic morphine; localized to upper body or face/nose with spinal morphine	With systemic opioids, prescribe PO H₁-antihistamine (e.g. chlorphenamine 4–8mg stat; if beneficial continue with 4mg t.d.s. or p.r.n. for 2–3 days). Possibly switch opioids, e.g. morphine → oxycodone. For spinal opioids, see p.720.	Pruritus after systemic opioids is uncommon. It can sometimes be caused by cutaneous histamine release and self-limiting but the most distressing cases are chronic and antihistamine-resistant. Centrally-acting opioid antagonists relieve the pruritus but also antagonize analgesia[16]
Histamine release	Bronchoconstriction → breathlessness	Treat as for anaphylaxis (see p.787); change to a chemically distinct opioid immediately;	Rare

---

Box A   Starting a patient on PO morphine

The starting dose of morphine is calculated to give a greater analgesic effect than the medication already in use:
- if the patient was previously receiving a weak opioid regularly (e.g. codeine 240mg/24h or equivalent), give 10mg q4h or m/r 20–30mg q12h, but less if suspected to be a poor codeine metabolizer (see p.348)
- if changing from an alternative strong opioid (e.g. fentanyl, methadone) a much higher dose of morphine may be needed
- if the patient is frail and elderly, or opioid-naïve, a lower dose helps to reduce initial drowsiness, confusion and unsteadiness, e.g. 5mg q4h
- because of accumulation of an active metabolite, a lower and/or less frequent regular dose may suffice in mild–moderate renal impairment, e.g. 5–10mg q8h–q6h (but the use of a 'renally safer' opioid is generally advisable with moderate–severe renal impairment, see p.367).

When adjusting the dose of morphine, p.r.n. use should be taken into account; increments should not exceed 33–50% every 24h.

As with all opioids, patients must be monitored for undesirable effects, particularly nausea and vomiting, and constipation (see Strong-opioids, Box B, p.361). Depending on individual circumstances, an anti-emetic should be prescribed for regular or p.r.n. use (see p.241) and, routinely, a laxative prescribed (see p.44).

Upward titration of the dose of morphine stops when either the pain is relieved or unacceptable undesirable effects occur. In the latter case, it is generally necessary to consider alternative measures. The aim is to have the patient free of pain and mentally alert after the initial drowsiness has cleared.

Because of poor absorption, m/r morphine may not be satisfactory in patients troubled by frequent vomiting or those with diarrhoea or an ileostomy.

Scheme 1: immediate-release morphine solution or tablets
- morphine given q4h 'by the clock' with p.r.n. doses 1/10–1/6 of the 24h dose
- after 1–2 days, recalculate q4h dose by dividing the total used in previous 24h (regular + p.r.n. use) by 6
- continue q4h and p.r.n. doses
- increase the regular dose until there is adequate relief throughout each 4h period, taking p.r.n. use into account
- a double dose at bedtime obviates the need to wake the patient for a dose during the night
- >90% of patients achieve satisfactory pain relief within 5 days.

Scheme 2: immediate-release morphine and modified-release (m/r) morphine
- begin as for Scheme 1
- when the q4h dose is stable, replace with m/r morphine q12h, or once daily if a 24h product is prescribed
- the q12h dose will be three times the previous q4h dose; a q24h dose will be six times the previous q4h dose, rounded to a convenient number of tablets or capsules
- continue to provide immediate-morphine solution or tablets for p.r.n. use; give 1/10–1/6 of the 24h dose.

Scheme 3: m/r morphine and immediate-release morphine
- generally start with m/r morphine 20–30mg q12h, or 10mg q12h in frail elderly patients
- use immediate-release morphine solution or tablets for p.r.n. medication; give 1/10–1/6 of the 24h dose
- if necessary, increase the dose of m/r morphine every 2–3 days until there is adequate relief throughout each 12h period, guided by p.r.n. use.

Traditionally, to make things easier for patients, morphine q4h has been given on waking, 1000h, 1400h, 1800h with a double dose at bedtime. Despite contrary results in a non-blinded study,[27] RCT evidence has shown that this approach results in less pain through the night, better sleep, and no increase in early morning pain.[28]

When adjusting the dose of morphine, p.r.n. use should be taken into account; increments should not exceed 33–50% every 24h.[29] Two-thirds of patients never need > 30mg q4h (or m/r morphine 100mg q12h); the rest need up to 200mg q4h (or m/r morphine 600mg q12h), and occasionally more.[30] Instructions must be clear: extra p.r.n. morphine does not mean that the next regular dose is omitted.

P.r.n. doses of morphine for break-through pain are typically 1/10-1/6 of the regular 24h dose but, as with the regular dose, there is need to consider individual variation. In practice, satisfactory p.r.n. doses vary from 1/20 (5%) to 1/5 (20%) of the 24h dose.[31]

As a general rule, the p.r.n. dose should be increased when the regular dose is increased. A p.r.n. dose is generally permitted every q2–4h as required (up to q1h when pain severe, or in the last days of life). However, frequent use of p.r.n. doses, i.e. ≥2 a day, should prompt a review of pain management. The time to peak plasma concentration is significantly shorter with a solution of morphine compared with an immediate-release tablet (median 1h vs. 2h),[32] suggesting that morphine solution is the better option for p.r.n. use (also see p.413).

An anti-emetic, e.g. **haloperidol** 1.5mg stat and at bedtime, should be supplied for p.r.n. use during the first week or prescribed regularly if the patient has had nausea with a weak opioid. Warn patients about the possibility of initial drowsiness. A laxative should be prescribed routinely unless there is a definite reason for not doing so, e.g. the patient has an ileostomy (see p.44). *Constipation may be more difficult to manage than the pain.* Laxative suppositories and enemas continue to be necessary in about one third of patients.[33]

SC/CSCI

In the UK, if the PO route becomes an unreliable means of administering regular morphine, e.g. because of difficulty swallowing or vomiting, generally the CSCI route is used (see Chapter 20, p.697).

The oral to SC potency ratio of morphine is between 1:2 and 1:3 (i.e. the SC dose is 2–3 times more potent than a PO dose) and, correspondingly, the SC dose is 1/2–1/3 of the oral dose. The same ratio holds true for IM and IV injections.[34,35] In practice, most centres divide the PO dose by 2, and re-titrate as necessary, e.g.:
- patient taking m/r morphine 30mg b.d. PO = 60mg/24h PO
- 60mg/24h divided by 2 = 30mg/24h CSCI
- the p.r.n. dose is 1/10–1/6 of the 24h dose, i.e. 3–5mg SC.

For CSCI dilute with WFI, 0.9% saline or 5% glucose.

> **CSCI compatibility with other drugs:** There are 2-drug compatibility data for morphine sulfate in WFI with **clonazepam, cyclizine, glycopyrronium, hyoscine *butylbromide*, hyoscine *hydrobromide*, ketamine, levomepromazine, metoclopramide,** and **octreotide.**
>
> Morphine sulfate is *incompatible* with **ketorolac** and may be *incompatible* with higher concentrations of **haloperidol** or **midazolam.**
>
> For more details and 3-drug compatibility data, see Appendix 3, Chart 1 (p.824) and Chart 5 (p.832).
>
> Compatibility charts for mixing drugs in 0.9% saline can be found in the extended appendix of the on-line PCF on www.palliativedrugs.com

IV/CIVI

IV morphine is widely used for the rapid relief of severe pain caused by acute trauma or medical emergencies. In opioid-naïve patients:
- give a prophylactic anti-emetic IV, e.g. **metoclopramide** 10mg
- give morphine 5–10mg (2.5–5mg in the elderly) IV over 5–10min
- when insufficient, give additional morphine at a rate not exceeding 1–2mg/min until satisfactory relief obtained; monitor for undesirable effects, e.g. excessive sedation, respiratory depression
- the dose can be repeated q2–4h as required.

Although uncommon in UK, CIVI morphine and/or p.r.n. IV morphine are used in palliative care units in Europe and North America.[36,37] Generally, this is in the context of the first few days of an inpatient admission for pain control.

When subsequently switching from IV to PO, a potency ratio of between 2:1 and 3:1 appears to hold true (i.e. the PO dose should be 2–3 greater than the IV dose). In a recent observational study, about 80% of patients achieved a satisfactory 24h PO dose at 3 times the previous 24h IV dose, rounded down to convenient strength m/r tablets.[38]

Rapid IV/SC titration of morphine dose for severe cancer pain

Although rapid IV/SC titration of morphine is generally *not* necessary, it can be useful in patients with severe acute pain, whether already taking opioids ('opioid-tolerant') or 'opioid-naïve'.[39,40] Further, because of difficulties in relation to follow-up, rapid IV titration is the norm at some centres in India for new patients presenting with pain of ≥5/10.

Two IV methods are included here; the first with 10min and the second with 1min intervals between each IV bolus (Box B and Box C).[40–44] In India, a single cumulative IV dose is given, followed immediately by PO medication (Box B). About 80% of patients obtain relief with 10mg or less.[41,42] At the Cleveland Clinic (USA), patients are maintained on CIVI for several days before conversion to PO medication (Box C). Although these methods have been used safely in many patients, **naloxone** should be readily available (see p.455).

Box B Rapid titration of morphine dose in 'opioid-naïve' patients (Institute of Palliative Medicine, India)[41,42]

Prerequisites
Pain ≥5/10 on a numerical scale.
Probability of a partial or complete response to morphine.[a]

Method
Obtain venous access with a butterfly cannula.
Give metoclopramide 10mg IV routinely.
Dilute the contents of 15mg morphine ampoule in a 10mL syringe.[b]
Inject 1.5mg (1mL) every 10min until the patient is pain-free or complains of undue sedation.[c]
If patients experience nausea, give additional metoclopramide 5mg IV.

Results
Dose required (with approximate percentages):
• 1.5–4.5mg (40%)
• 6–9mg (40%)
• 10.5–15mg (15%)
• >15mg (5%).
Complete relief in 80%; none in 1%.
Drop outs 2%.
Undesirable effects: sedation 32%; other 3%.

Ongoing treatment
Prescribe a dose of oral morphine q4h similar to the IV dose, rounded to nearest 5mg, e.g. needed morphine 3–6mg IV → 5mg PO; the minimum dose is 5mg. Advise about p.r.n. doses and, if >2/24h needed, to increase the dose the next day. In practice, 20% of patients need a dose increase within 3 days.

---

a. most patients will already be taking an NSAID
b. ampoule strengths varies from country to country; use local standard
c. if ampoule = 10mg/mL (diluted to 10mg in 10mL), a bolus dose of 2mg would be reasonable.

IV patient-controlled analgesia (PCA) can also be used but is more costly, requires inpatient admission and may take >10h to achieve relief.[45,46] Some centres use a more rapidly acting strong opioid, e.g. IV **fentanyl**, with subsequent doses given after pauses of only 5–10min.[47]

Note: patients who have required a rapid escalation in opioid requirements must be monitored closely. The underlying cause may be transient, e.g. haemorrhage into a liver metastasis, and a subsequent reduction in dose will be necessary.

Box C Rapid titration of morphine dose in both 'opioid-tolerant' and 'opioid-naïve' patients (based on practice at Cleveland Clinic, Ohio, USA)[39,43,44]

Sequence	IV	SC
Dose	1mg/min up to 10mg	2mg q5min up to 10mg
Pause	5min	10min
Dose	1mg/min up to 10mg	2mg q5min up to 10mg
Pause	5min	10min
Dose	1mg/min up to 10mg[a]	2mg q5min up to 10mg[a]

Maintenance IV/SC dose
Regard cumulative effective dose as the equivalent of a q4h dose, and prescribe accordingly.

Example
Cumulative effective IV dose = 9mg.
If giving intermittent injections, dose = 9mg q4h, rounded to 10mg.
If CIVI, total daily IV dose = 9mg x 6 = 54mg/24h.
Round this up or down to convenient number of ampoules, i.e. 50mg or 60mg.
P.r.n. dose = 5–10mg q1h.

a. review cause if relief inadequate after a total of 30mg.

Alternative routes
Buccal morphine
Morphine is slowly absorbed through the buccal mucosa.[48] However, most of a morphine solution given sublingually or into the gingival gutter will be swallowed and absorbed from the GI tract. Nonetheless, in the past, this route was successfully used in moribund patients.

Rectal morphine
Morphine is absorbed from suppositories.[49] From the lower and middle rectum, it will enter the systemic circulation bypassing the liver. From the upper rectum, it will undergo hepatic first-pass metabolism after it enters the portal circulation. However, there are extensive anastomoses between the rectal veins which make it impossible to predict how much will enter the portal circulation.[50,51] Despite the uncertainty, in practice the same dose is given PR as PO and titrated as necessary.

Although not authorized for this route and not generaly recommended, m/r morphine tablets have been used PR to provide analgesia in moribund patients, generally while organizing a more reliable delivery method.[52]

Spinal morphine
In the UK, <5% of cancer patients needing morphine receive it spinally, i.e. ED or IT. This route of administration (see p.713) is normally undertaken by an anaesthetist. Particularly with neuropathic pain, morphine is generally combined with a local anaesthetic (e.g. **bupivacaine**), and sometimes with **clonidine**.

Topical morphine
Nociceptive afferent nerve fibres contain peripheral opioid receptors which are silent except in the presence of local inflammation.[1,2,13,53] This property is exploited in joint surgery where morphine is given intra-articularly at the end of the operation.[54] Topical morphine has also been used successfully to relieve otherwise intractable pain associated with cutaneous ulceration, often decubitus ulcers.[55–58] It is often given as a 0.1% (1mg/mL) gel, using IntraSite®. If prepared under sterile conditions, morphine sulfate is stable for at least 28 days when mixed with IntraSite® gel at a concentration of 0.125% (1.25mg/mL). This preparation can be made by thoroughly mixing 1mL of morphine sulfate 10mg/mL injection with an 8g sachet of IntraSite® gel.[59]

Higher concentrations, namely 0.3–0.5%, have been used when managing pain associated with:
• vaginal inflammation associated with a fistula
• rectal ulceration.[56]

The amount of gel applied varies according to the size and the site of the ulcer, but is typically 5–10mL applied b.d.–t.d.s. The topical morphine is kept in place with either a non-absorbable pad or dressing, e.g. Opsite® or Tegaderm®, or gauze coated with petroleum jelly. Other opioids, e.g. **diamorphine, methadone**, and other carriers, e.g. Stomahesive® paste, **medronidazole** gel have also been used.[60]

A 0.2% (2mg/mL) morphine solution without alcohol, (15mL used to rinse the mouth for 2min and then spat out, q2–3h) has also been used for cancer treatment-related mucositis (see p.604). It provides better pain relief than a placebo mouthwash, or one containing **co-magaldrox + lidocaine + diphenhydramine.**[61,62] Significant relief occurs after about 30min, and lasts about 3.5h.[63]

Morphine for breathlessness

Generally, opioids are more beneficial in patients who are breathless at rest than in those who are breathless only on exertion. Even with maximal exertion, breathlessness generally recovers within a few minutes, much quicker than the time it takes to locate, administer and obtain benefit from an opioid. Thus, non-drug measures are of primary importance in this circumstance.[64]

A systematic review supports the use of opioids by the oral and parenteral but *not* the nebulized route, and the latter should not be used outside of a clinical trial.[65–71]

Morphine and other opioids reduce the ventilatory response to hypercapnia, hypoxia and exercise, decreasing respiratory effort and breathlessness.[64] Improvements are seen at doses that *do not* cause respiratory depression.[72–77] In opioid-naïve patients:
• start with small doses of morphine, e.g. 2.5–5mg PO p.r.n.; larger doses can be poorly tolerated
• if ≥2 doses/24h are needed, prescribe morphine regularly and titrate the dose according to response, duration of effect and undesirable effects
• relatively small doses may suffice, e.g. 20–60mg/24h.[68,69,72–76,78–81]
In patients already taking morphine for pain and with:
• severe breathlessness (i.e. ≥7/10), a dose that is 100% or more of the q4h analgesic dose may be needed
• moderate breathlessness (i.e. 4–6/10), a dose equivalent to 50–100% of the q4h analgesic dose may suffice
• mild breathlessness (i.e. ≤3/10), a dose equivalent to 25–50% of the q4h analgesic dose may suffice.
However, as with pain, individual titration is required for optimal benefit. In some patients, morphine by CSCI is better tolerated and provides greater relief, possibly by avoiding the peaks (with undesirable effects) and troughs (with loss of effect) of oral medication. If using an alternative opioid to morphine, adopt the same approach as above.

Opioids are also used in patients with severe COPD who have distressing breathlessness despite usual treatments. A low-dose and slow titration is generally advocated, e.g.:
• start with morphine 1mg PO b.d., increasing to 1–2.5mg q4h over one week
• thereafter, increase dose by 25% each week until satisfactory relief obtained
• when a stable dose is found, consider switching to a m/r formulation.[82]
For severe breathlessness in the last days of life:
• patients often fear suffocating to death and a positive approach to the patient, their family and colleagues about the relief of terminal breathlessness is important
• no patient should die with distressing breathlessness
• failure to relieve terminal breathlessness is a failure to utilize drug treatment correctly.
Because of the distress, inability to sleep and exhaustion, patients and their carers generally accept that drug-related drowsiness may need to be the price paid for greater comfort. However, unless there is overwhelming distress, sedation is not the primary aim of treatment and some patients become mentally brighter when their breathlessness is reduced.

Even so, because increasing drowsiness also generally reflects the deteriorating clinical condition, it is important to stress the gravity of the situation and the aim of treatment to the relatives. Drug treatment typically comprises:[83]
• parenteral administration of an opioid and a sedative-anxiolytic, e.g. morphine and **midazolam** by CSCI and p.r.n.
• **haloperidol** or **levomepromazine** if the patient develops an agitated delirium (may be aggravated by a benzodiazepine).

Supply
Unless indicated otherwise, all products are **CD**.

Immediate-release oral products

> Morphine solution is available in two strengths, 2mg/mL and a high potency concentrate of 20mg/mL supplied with a calibrated syringe. *Deaths have occurred from accidental overdose with the concentrated solution*, mostly when doses prescribed in *mg* were administered as *mL*, resulting in *20 times* the prescribed dose being given.[84]

Sevredol® (Napp)
Tablets 10mg, 20mg, 50mg; 10mg and 100mg dose = £0.10 and £1 respectively.

Morphine sulfate (Martindale)
Oral solution 2mg/mL (**PoM**, not **CD**); 10mg dose = £0.10; *contains alcohol.*
Oral solution 2mg/mL (**PoM** not **CD**), 10mg dose = £12; *alcohol-free* (Unauthorized, available as a special order; see Appendix 1, p.817).

Oramorph® (Boehringer Ingelheim)
Oral solution 2mg/mL (**PoM**, not **CD**); 10mg dose = £0.10; *contains alcohol.*
Concentrated oral solution 20mg/mL, 100mg dose = £1.

Modified-release 12-hourly oral products

> Because the pharmacokinetic profiles of m/r products differ, and to minimize the risk of mistakes (e.g. mixing up immediate-release and m/r products), it is best to keep individual patients on the same m/r brand, and to label with both the generic and proprietary names.

Filnarine® SR (Teva)
Tablets m/r 10mg, 30mg, 60mg, 100mg, 200mg, 28 days @ 30mg q12h = £8.

Morphgesic® SR (Amdipharm)
Tablets m/r 10mg, 30mg, 60mg, 100mg, 28 days @ 30mg q12h = £9.

MST Continus® (Napp)
Tablets m/r 5mg, 10mg, 15mg, 30mg, 60mg, 100mg, 200mg, 28 days @ 30mg q12h = £12.
Oral suspension (sachet of m/r granules) 20mg, 30mg, 60mg, 100mg, 200mg/sachet, 28 days @ 30mg q12h = £51. *May be mixed with 10mL water, or the granules sprinkled on cold soft food and swallowed whole.*

Zomorph® (Archimedes)
Capsules containing m/r granules 10mg, 30mg, 60mg, 100mg, 200mg, 28 days @ 30mg q12h = £8. *May be swallowed whole or opened and the granules sprinkled on cold soft food and swallowed whole.*

Modified-release 24-hourly oral products
MXL® (Napp)
Capsules containing m/r granules 30mg, 60mg, 90mg, 120mg, 150mg, 200mg, 28 days @ 60mg once daily = £15. *May be swallowed whole or opened and the granules sprinkled on cold soft food and swallowed whole.*

Immediate-release rectal products
Morphine *sulfate* (generic)
Suppositories 10mg, 15mg, 20mg, 30mg; 10mg dose = £1; *the salt should be specified on the prescription.*

Parenteral products
Morphine *sulfate* (generic)
Injection 10, 15, 20 and 30mg/mL, 1mL and 2mL amp = £1.
Infusion 1mg/mL 50mL vial = £5, 2mg/mL 50mL vial = £6.

Other injectable morphine formulations are available including morphine sulfate 1mg/mL (10mL disposable syringe, Minijet®), combination products with anti-emetics, e.g. cyclimorph® and an epidural modified-release formulation, Depodur®.

1 Krajnik M et al. (1998) Opioids affect inflammation and the immune system. Pain Reviews. 5: 147–154.
2 Smith HS (2008) Peripherally-acting opioids. Pain Physician. 11: S121–132.
3 Hasselstrom J et al. (1986) The metabolism and bioavailability of morphine in patients with severe liver cirrhosis. British Journal of Clinical Pharmacology. 29: 289–297.
4 Mazoit J-X et al. (1987) Pharmacokinetics of unchanged morphine in normal and cirrhotic subjects. Anesthesia and Analgesia. 66: 293–298.
5 Sandouk P et al. (1991) Presence of morphine metabolites in human cerebrospinal fluid after intracerebroventricular administration of morphine. European Journal of Drug Metabolism and Pharmacology. 16: 166–171.
6 Regnard CFB and Twycross RG (1984) Metabolism of narcotics (letter). British Medical Journal. 288: 860.
7 McQuay HJ et al. (1990) Oral morphine in cancer pain: influences on morphine and metabolite concentration. Clinical Pharmacology and Therapeutics. 48: 236–244
8 Osborne RJ et al. (1986) Morphine intoxication in renal failure: the role of morphine-6-glucuronide. British Medical Journal. 292: 1548–1549.
9 Thompson P et al. (1992) Mophine-6-glucuronide: a metabolite of morphine with greater emetic potency than morphine in the ferret. British Journal of Pharmacology. 106: 3–8.
10 Buetler TM et al. (2000) Analgesic action of i.v. morphine-6-glucuronide in healthy volunteers. British Journal of Anaesthesia. 84: 97–99.
11 Gretton S and Riley J (2008) Morphine metabolites: a review of their clinical effects. European Journal of Palliative Care. 15: 110–114.
12 Westerling D et al. (1994) Transdermal administration of morphine to healthy subjects. British Journal of Clinical Pharmacology. 37: 571–576.
13 Ribeiro MD et al. (2004) The bioavailability of morphine applied topically to cutaneous ulcers. Journal of Pain and Symptom Management. 27: 434–439.
14 Watterson G et al. (2004) Peripheral opioids in inflammatory pain. Archives of Disease in Childhood. 89: 679–681.
15 Jansen M (2006) Morphine gel. Palliativedrugs.com bulletin board message. Available from:www.palliativedrugs.com/forum51/read.php?1,9189,9271#msg-9271
16 Twycross RG et al. (2003) Itch: scratching more than the surface. Quarterly Journal of Medicine. 96: 7–26.
17 Caraceni A et al. (2012) Use of opioid analgesics in the treatment of cancer pain: evidence-based recommendations from the EAPC. Lancet Oncology. 13: e58–68
18 Caraceni A et al. (2011) Is oral morphine still the first choice opioid for moderate to severe cancer pain? A systematic review within the European Palliative Care Research Collaborative guidelines project. Palliative Medicine. 25: 402–409.
19 WHO (2012) WHO guidelines on the pharmacological treatment of persistent pain in children with medical illness. Available from: http://www.palliativedrugs.com/news/march/who-guidelines-for-treating-persistent-pain-in-children.html
20 Bloomfield S et al. (1993) Analgesic efficacy and potency of two oral controlled-release morphine preparations. Clinical Pharmacology and Therapeutics. 53: 469–478.
21 Gourlay G et al. (1993) A comparison of Kapanol (a new sustained-release morphine formulation), MST Continus and morphine solution in cancer patients: pharmacokinetic aspects. In: The Seventh World Congress on Pain; Seattle. IASP Press.
22 West R and Maccarrone C (1993) Single dose pharmacokinetics of a new oral sustained-release morphine formulation, Kapanol capsules. In: The Seventh World Congress on Pain; Seattle. IASP Press.
23 Mercadante S (2007) Opioid titration in cancer pain: a critical review. European Journal of Pain. 11: 823–830.
24 De Conno F et al. (2008) The MERITO Study: a multicentre trial of the analgesic effect and tolerability of normal-release oral morphine during 'titration phase' in patients with cancer pain. Palliative Medicine. 22: 214–221.
25 Ripamonti CI et al. (2009) Normal-release oral morphine starting dose in cancer patients with pain. Clinical Journal of Pain. 25: 386–390
26 Taubert M et al. (2010) Re: Update on cancer pain guidelines. Journal of Pain and Symptom Management. 24: 1–5
27 Todd J et al. (2002) An assessment of the efficacy and tolerability of a 'double dose' of normal-release morphine sulphate at bedtime. Palliative Medicine. 16: 507–512.
28 Dale O et al. (2009) A double-blind, randomized, crossover comparison between single-dose and double-dose immediate-release oral morphine at bedtime in cancer patients. Journal of Pain and Symptom Management. 37: 68–76.
29 Carver AC and Foley KM (2001) Symptom assessment and management. Neurologic Clinics. 19: 921–947.
30 Schug SA et al. (1992) A long-term survey of morphine in cancer pain patients. Journal of Pain and Symptom Management. 7: 259–266.
31 Donnelly S et al. (2002) Morphine in cancer pain management: a practical guide. Supportive Care in Cancer. 10: 13–35.
32 Sawe J et al. (1983) Steady-state kinetics and analgesic effect of oral morphine in cancer patients. European Journal of Clinical Pharmacology. 24: 537–542.
33 Twycross RG and Harcourt JMV (1991) The use of laxatives at a palliative care centre. Palliative Medicine. 5: 27–33
34 Hanks G et al. (2001) Morphine and alternative opioids in cancer pain: the EAPC recommendations. British Journal of Cancer. 84: 587–593.
35 Takahashi M et al. (2003) The oral-to-intravenous equianalgesic ratio of morphine based on plasma concentrations of morphine and metabolites in advanced cancer patients receiving chronic morphine treatment. Palliative Medicine. 17: 673–678.
36 Mercadante S et al. (2008) Intravenous morphine for breakthrough (episodic-) pain in an acute palliative care unit: a confirmatory study. Journal of Pain and Symptom Management. 35: 307–313.
37 Mercadante S (2010) Intravenous morphine for management of cancer pain. Lancet Oncology. 11: 484–489.
38 Lasheen W et al. (2010) The intravenous to oral relative milligram potency ratio of morphine during chronic dosing in cancer pain. Palliative Medicine. 24: 9–16.
39 Hagen N et al. (1997) Cancer pain emergencies: a protocol for management. Journal of Pain and Symptom Management. 14: 45–50.
40 Davis MP et al. (2004) Opioid dose titration for severe cancer pain: a systematic evidence-based review. Journal of Palliative Medicine. 7: 462–468.
41 Kumar K et al. (2000) Intravenous morphine for emergency treatment of cancer pain. Palliative Medicine. 14: 183–188.
42 Harris JT et al. (2003) Intravenous morphine for rapid control of severe cancer pain. Palliative Medicine. 17: 248–256.
43 Davis MP (2004) Acute pain in advanced cancer: an opioid dosing strategy and illustration. American Journal of Hospice and Palliative Care. 21: 47–50.
44 Davis MP (2005) Rapid opioid titration in severe cancer pain. European Journal of Palliative Care. 12: 11–14.

45 Radbruch L et al. (1999) Intravenous titration with morphine for severe cancer pain: report of 28 cases. Clinical Journal of Pain. 15: 173–178.

46 Schiessl C et al. (2010) Rhythmic pattern of PCA opioid demand in adults with cancer pain. European Journal of Pain. 14: 372–379

47 Soares LG et al. (2003) Intravenous fentanyl for cancer pain: a "fast titration" protocol for the emergency room. Journal of Pain and Symptom Management. 26: 876–881.

48 Coluzzi P (1998) Sublingual morphine: efficacy reviewed. Journal of Pain and Symptom Management. 16: 184–192

49 deBoer AG et al. (1982) Rectal drug administration: clinical pharmacokinetic considerations. Clinical Pharmacokinetics. 7: 285–311.

50 Johnson AG and Lux G (1988) Progress in the Treatment of Gastrointestinal Motility Disorder. The role of cisapride. Excerpta Medica, Amsterdam.

51 Ripamonti C and Bruera E (1991) Rectal, buccal and sublingual narcotics for the management of cancer pain. Journal of Palliative Care. 7: 30–35.

52 Wilkinson T et al. (1992) Pharmacokinetics and efficacy of rectal versus oral sustained-release morphine in cancer patients. Cancer Chemotherapy and Pharmacology. 31: 251–254.

53 Krajnik M and Zylicz Z (1997) Topical opioids - fact or fiction? Progress in Palliative Care. 5: 101–106.

54 Likar R et al. (1999) Dose-dependency of intra-articular morphine analgesia. British Journal of Anaesthesia. 83: 241–244.

55 Back NI and Finlay I (1995) Analgesic effect of topical opioids on painful skin ulcers. Journal of Pain and Symptom Management. 10: 493.

56 Krajnik M et al. (1999) Potential uses of topical opioids in palliative care - report of 6 cases. Pain. 80: 121–125.

57 Twillman R et al. (1999) Treatment of painful skin ulcers with topical opioids. Journal of Pain and Symptom Management. 17: 288–292.

58 Zeppetella G et al. (2003) Analgesic efficacy of morphine applied topically to painful ulcers. Journal of Pain and Symptom Management. 25: 555–558.

59 Zeppetella G and Ribeiro MD (2005) Morphine in intrasite gel applied topically to painful ulcers. Journal of Pain and Symptom Management. 29: 118–119.

60 Le Bon B et al. (2009) Effectiveness of topical administration of opiods inpalliative care a systematic review. Journal of Pain and Symptom Management. 37: 913–917.

61 Cerchietti LC et al. (2002) Effect of topical morphine for mucositis-associated pain following concomitant chemoradiotherapy for head and neck carcinoma. Cancer. 95: 2230–2236.

62 Vayne-Bossert P et al. (2010) Effect of topical morphine (mouthwash) on oral pain due to chemotherapy- and/or radiotherapy-induced mucositis: a randomized double-blinded study. Journal of Palliative Medicine.13: 125–128.

63 Cerchietti LC et al. (2003) Potential utility of the peripheral analgesic properties of morphine in stomatitis-related pain: a pilot study. Pain. 105: 265–273.

64 Twycross R et al. (2009) Symptom Management in Advanced Cancer (4e). palliativedrugs.com, pp. 145–158.

65 Davis C (1999) Nebulized opioids should not be prescribed outside a clinical trial. American Journal of Hospice and Palliative Care. 16: 543.

66 Jennings A et al. (2002) A systematic review of the use of opioids in the management of dyspnoea. Thorax. 57: 939–944.

67 Foral PA et al. (2004) Nebulized opioids use in COPD. Chest. 125: 691–694.

68 Brown SJ et al. (2005) Nebulized morphine for relief of dyspnea due to chronic lung disease. Annals of Pharmacotherapy. 39: 1088–1092.

69 Bruera E et al. (2005) Nebulized versus subcutaneous morphine for patients with cancer dyspnea: a preliminary study. Journal of Pain and Symptom Management. 29: 613–618.

70 Bruera E et al. (2006) Can we really say that nebulized morphine works? (authors response). Journal of Pain and Symptom Management. 32: 102–103.

71 Lasheen W et al. (2006) Can we really say that nebulized morphine works? Journal of Pain and Symptom Management. 32: 101–102; author reply 102–103.

72 Bruera E et al. (1990) Effects of morphine on the dyspnea of terminal cancer patients. Journal of Pain and Symptom Management. 5: 341–344.

73 Bruera E et al. (1993) Subcutaneous morphine for dyspnoea in cancer patients. Annals of internal medicine. 119: 906–907.

74 Mazzocato C et al. (1999) The effects of morphine on dyspnoea and ventilatory function in elderly patients with advanced cancer: A randomized double-blind controlled trial. Annals of Oncology. 10: 1511–1514.

75 Abernethy AP et al. (2003) Randomised, double blind, placebo controlled crossover trial of sustained release morphine for the management of refractory dyspnoea. British Medical Journal. 327: 523–528.

76 Allen S et al. (2005) Low dose diamorphine reduces breathlessness without causing a fall in oxygen saturation in elderly patients with end-stage idiopathic pulmonary fibrosis. Palliative Medicine. 19: 128–130.

77 Clemens KE et al. (2008) Is there a higher risk of respiratory depression in opioid-naive palliative care patients during symptomatic therapy of dyspnea with strong opioids? Journal of Palliative Medicine. 11: 204–216.

78 Cohen M et al. (1991) Continuous intravenous infusion of morphine for severe dyspnoea. Southern Medical Journal. 84: 229–234.

79 Boyd K and Kelly M (1997) Oral morphine as symptomatic treatment of dyspnoea in patients with advanced cancer. Palliative Medicine. 11: 277–281.

80 Poole PJ et al. (1998) The effect of sustained-release morphine on breathlessness and quality of life in severe chronic obstructive pulmonary disease. American Journal of Respiratory and Critical Care Medicine. 157: 1877–1880.

81 Allard P et al. (1999) How effective are supplementary doses of opioids for dyspnea in terminally ill cancer patients? A randomized continuous sequential clinical trial. Journal of Pain and Symptom Management. 17: 256–265.

82 Rocker G et al. (2009) Palliation of dyspnoea in advanced COPD: revisiting a role for opioids. Thorax. 64: 910–915.

83 Navigante AH et al. (2006) Midazolam as adjunct therapy to morphine in the alleviation of severe dyspnea perception in patients with advanced cancer. Journal of Pain and Symptom Management. 31: 38–47.

84 FDA (2011) Medwatch safety alert. Morphine sulfate oral solution 100mg per 5mL (20mg/mL): medication use error - reports of accidental overdose. Available from: www.fda.gov/Safety/MedWatch/SafetyInformation/SafetyAlertsforHumanMedical Products/ucm239559.htm?sms_ss = email&at_xt = 4d372d1d29c3a5e2%2C0

Updated October 2013

DIAMORPHINE   BNF 4.7.2

Class: Strong opioid analgesic (available only in the UK).

Indications: As for **morphine**; used in the UK instead of parenteral **morphine** because of its greater solubility, particularly when large doses are necessary.

Contra-indications: None absolute if titrated carefully against a patient's pain (also see Strong opioids, p.357 and p.362).

Pharmacology

Diamorphine (di-acetylmorphine, heroin) is available for medicinal analgesic use only in the UK. It is generally considered to be a pro-drug without intrinsic activity.[1] *In vivo*, it is rapidly de-acetylated (plasma halflife 3min) to an active metabolite, 6-mono-acetylmorphine (6-MAM) (plasma halflife 20min), and then to **morphine** itself.[2] Thus, similar considerations as for **morphine** apply regarding the use of diamorphine in patients with renal or hepatic impairment/failure (see p.372).[3]

IM diamorphine is more than twice as potent as IM **morphine**.[4–6] The greater potency of parenteral diamorphine could be because 6-MAM is more potent than **morphine**[7] or because diamorphine and 6-MAM cross the blood-brain barrier more readily than **morphine**. However, by mouth the two opioids are almost equipotent.[8]

Diamorphine IM acts more quickly than **morphine**,[6,9] but **morphine** acts more quickly IV.[10] This paradox is not easily explained, but it could relate to differences in plasma protein-binding (diamorphine 40%, **morphine** 20%).

In terms of analgesic efficacy and effect on mood, diamorphine has no clinical advantage over **morphine** by oral or SC/IM routes.[4,5,8] Diamorphine hydrochloride is much more water-soluble than **morphine** sulfate/hydrochloride and, in the UK, is the strong opioid of choice when high-dose injections are needed (Table 1). In some countries, **hydromorphone** is used instead (see p.430).

Table 1   Solubility of selected opioids[11]

Preparation	Amount of water needed to dissolve 1g at 25°C (mL)
Morphine	5,000
Morphine hydrochloride	24
Morphine sulfate	21
Diamorphine hydrochloride	1.6[a]
Hydromorphone	3

a. 1g of diamorphine hydrochloride dissolved in 1.6mL has a volume of 2.4mL.

Like **morphine**, diamorphine can be given by many different routes, including spinally. Diamorphine can also be given intranasally using a nasal dosing device, a route used mainly in children.[12] It can be used for the same range of indications as **morphine**, including bladder spasms (intravesical administration)[13,14] and painful decubitus ulcers (topically in Intrasite® gel).[15,16]

Bio-availability (as 6-MAM) no data.
Onset of action 5–10min SC.
Time to peak plasma concentration 1.5–2h PO as 6-MAM and **morphine**.
Plasma halflife 3min IV; metabolized to active metabolites.
Duration of action 4h.

Stability

Diamorphine hydrochloride is stable indefinitely when stored as a powder[17] but de-acetylates when in solution, first to 6-mono-acetylmorphine (6-MAM) and then to **morphine**. The rate of de-acetylation is situation dependent. Thus, *in vivo*, diamorphine is converted to 6-MAM in minutes, whereas the stability of diamorphine hydrochloride in simple solution is much longer. Further, because 6-MAM is the primary active agent, there is no loss of potency until 6-MAM is degraded to **morphine**.[7]

In one study, after 3 months in simple solution, 30% of the diamorphine had degraded to 6-MAM, but it was only at 12 months that a trace of **morphine** became detectable.[18] A second study looked at the effect of ambient temperature.[19,20] The loss of 10% of diamorphine to 6-MAM took 8 weeks when kept at 22°C, but only 2 weeks at 37°C. Other studies have produced comparable results.[21,22]

Undesirable effects

See Strong opioids, Box B, p.361.

Dose and use

As with all opioids, patients must be monitored for undesirable effects, particularly nausea and vomiting, and constipation (see p.360). Depending on individual circumstances, an anti-emetic should be prescribed for regular or p.r.n. use (see p.241) and a laxative prescribed routinely (see p.44).

In the UK, diamorphine has been used for all the same indications as **morphine**, and by the same range of routes, including topically and spinally (see p.372). Although in the past it was widely used PO, diamorphine is now generally reserved for parenteral use (see p.697). The following are practical clinical conversion ratios:

• PO **morphine** to SC diamorphine, give one third of the PO dose
• PO diamorphine to SC diamorphine, give one half of the PO dose.

For CSCI dilute with WFI, concentration-dependent *incompatibility* occurs with 0.9% saline at higher doses (see CSCI).

CSCI compatibility with other drugs: There are 2-drug compatibility data for diamorphine in WFI with **clonazepam, dexamethasone, glycopyrronium, hyoscine *butylbromide*, hyoscine *hydrobromide*, ketorolac, levomepromazine, metoclopramide, midazolam, octreotide,** and **ondansetron**.

Concentration-dependent *incompatibility* occurs with **cyclizine** or **haloperidol** at higher concentrations. For more details and 3-drug compatibility data, see Appendix 3 Chart 1 (p.824) and Chart 3 (p.828).

Compatibility charts for mixing drugs in 0.9% saline can be found in the extended appendix section of the on-line PCF on www.palliativedrugs.com

An intranasal spray is now commercially available, authorized for the relief of acute severe pain in children 2–15 years of age in a hospital setting, originating from off-label use in Emergency Departments in England and Wales.[12,23,24]

Supply

Because diamorphine ampoules cost about 3 times more than **morphine** ampoules, many palliative care units in the UK now use **morphine** as their standard parenteral strong opioid, unless the need for high doses makes diamorphine more convenient because of its greater solubility.[25] All preparations are Schedule 2 **CD**.

Diamorphine (generic)
Tablets 10mg, 10mg dose = £0.23.
Injection (powder for reconstitution) 5mg amp = £2.50; 10mg amp = £3; 30mg amp = £3; 100mg amp = £9; 500mg amp = £39.

Ayendi (Wockhardt)
Nasal Spray (powder for reconstitution with 0.5% saline and 9 disposable nasal tips provided for multiple patient use) 720microgram/metered dose spray, 1600microgram/metered dose spray, 160 metered dose spray bottle = £113 and £124 respectively; *stable for 14 days after reconstitution*.

1 Inturrisi CE *et al.* (1984) The pharmacokinetics of heroin in patients with chronic pain. *New England Journal of Medicine.* **310**: 1213–1217.
2 Barrett DA *et al.* (1992) The effect of temperature and pH on the deacetylation of diamorphine in aqueous solution and in human plasma. *Journal of Pharmacy and Pharmacology.* **44**: 606–608.

3   King S et al. (2011) A systematic review of the use of opioid medication for those with moderate to severe cancer pain and renal impairment. *Palliative Medicine.* **25**: 525–552.

4   Kaiko RF et al. (1981) Analgesic and mood effects of heroin and morphine in cancer patients with postoperative pain. *New England Journal of Medicine.* **304**: 1501–1505.

5   Beaver WT et al. (1981) Comparison of the analgesic effect of intramuscular heroin and morphine in patients with cancer pain. *Clinical Pharmacology and Therapeutics.* **29**: 232.

6   Reichle CW et al. (1962) Comparative analgesic potency of heroin and morphine in postoperative patients. *Journal of Pharmacology and Experimental Therapeutics.* **136**: 43–46.

7   Wright CI and Barbour FA (1935) The respiratory effects of morphine, codeine and related substances. *Journal of Pharmacology and Experimental Therapeutics.* **54**: 25–33.

8   Twycross RG (1977) Choice of strong analgesic in terminal cancer: diamorphine or morphine? *Pain* **3**: 93–104.

9   Dundee JW et al. (1966) Studies of drugs given before anaesthesia XI: diamorphine (heroin) and morphine. *British Journal of Anaesthesia.* **38**: 610–619.

10 Morrison L et al. (1991) Comparison of speed of onset of analgesic effect of diamorphine and morphine. *British Journal of Anaesthesia.* **66**: 656–659.

11 Hanks GW and Hoskin PJ (1987) Opioid analgesics in the management of pain in patients with cancer: a review. *Palliative Medicine.* **1**: 1–25.

12 Kendall J et al. (2014) A novel multipatient intranasal diamorphine spray for use in acute pain in children: pharmacovigilance data from an observational study. *Emergency Medical Journal.* Epub ahead of print.

13 McCoubrie R and Jeffrey D (2003) Intravesical diamorphine for bladder spasm. *Journal of Pain and Symptom Management.* **25**: 1–3.

14 Duckett J (1997) Intravesical morphine analgesia after bladder surgery. *Journal of Urology.* **157**: 1407–1409.

15 Abbas SQ (2004) Diamorphine-Intrasite dressings for painful pressure ulcers. *Journal of Pain and Symptom Management.* **28**: 532–534.

16 Flock P (2003) Pilot study to determine the effectiveness of diamorphine gel to control pressure ulcer pain. *Journal of Pain and Symptom Management.* **25**: 547–554.

17 Lerner M and Mills A (1963) Some modern aspects of heroin analysis. *Bulletin on Narcotics.* **15**: 37–42.

18 Rizzotti G (1935) Contributo allo studio delle alterazioni delle soluzioni acquose di eroina. *Archives Internationales de Pharmacodynamie et de Therapie.* **52**: 87–96.

19 Twycross RG and Gilhooley RA (1973) Euporiant elixirs. *British Medical Journal.* **4**: 552.

20 Twycross RG (1974) Diamorphine and cocaine elixir BPC. *Pharmaceutical Journal.* **212**: 153 & 159.

21 Omar OA et al. (1989) Diamorphine stability in aqueous solution for subcutaneous infusion. *Journal of Pharmcy and Pharmacology.* **41**: 275–277.

22 Kleinberg ML et al. (1990) Stability of heroin hydrochloride in infusion devices and containers for intravenous administration. *American Journal of Hospital Pharmacy.* **47**: 377–381.

23 Shelley K and Paech MJ (2008) The clinical applications of intranasal opioids. *Current Drug Delivery.* **5**: 55–58.

24 Hadley G et al. (2010) A survey of intranasal medication use in the paediatric emergency setting in England and Wales. *Emergency Medical Journal.* **27**: 553–554.

25 Palliativedrugs.com (2010) Diamorphine essential opioid or time to say goodbye? Available from: www.palliativedrugs.com/ download/100223_diamorphine_essential_opioid.pdf

Updated May 2014

*ALFENTANIL   BNF 4.7.2

Class: Strong opioid analgesic.

Indications: Intra-operative analgesia, analgesia and procedure-related pain in mechanically ventilated patients on intensive care units, †an alternative in cases of intolerance to other strong opioids, particularly in renal failure,[1] †procedure-related pain in non-ventilated patients,[2–4] †break-through (episodic) pain.[5,6]

Contra-indications: Do not administer concurrently with MAOIs or within two weeks of their discontinuation. Generally no absolute if titrated carefully against a patient's pain (also see Strong opioids, p.357).

Pharmacology

Alfentanil is a synthetic lipophilic opioid in the same class as **fentanyl** and **sufentanil** (not UK). Compared with these, it has a more rapid onset of action and time to peak effect, and a shorter duration of action (Table 1). Its potency is approximately one quarter that of **fentanyl**[7] (and 10–20 times more than parenteral **morphine**).

Alfentanil is less lipophilic than **fentanyl** and is 90% bound to mainly α_1-acid glycoprotein.[8] However, because most of the unbound alfentanil is unionized, it rapidly enters the CNS. It is metabolized in the liver by CYP3A4 to inactive metabolites that are excreted in the urine. Alfentanil can accumulate with chronic administration, particularly when clearance is reduced, e.g. in the elderly and the obese, and when there is hepatic impairment.[9] In consequence, if switching from an alfentanil infusion to another opioid, it is safer to use conservative dose estimates. It has been suggested that analgesic tolerance occurs rapidly with alfentanil,[10] but this has been refuted.[11] Certainly, tolerance does not seem to be a problem in palliative care.[1]

Although dose reductions may be necessary in patients with even relatively mild hepatic impairment,[12] this is not necessary in renal failure. Consequently, alfentanil is used at some centres when a parenteral opioid is required in end-stage renal failure (see p.367).[1] Because alfentanil is available in a more concentrated form (500microgram/mL) than **fentanyl** (50microgram/mL), a smaller equivalent dose volume is needed, and this facilitates administration by CSCI or SL. For similar reasons, in countries where alfentanil is not available, **sufentanil** is used instead (Table 1 and Box A).[13] However, unless the volume is prohibitive, **fentanyl** is generally recommended first-line in these circumstances.[1] Other guidelines recommend **buprenorphine** (SC/IV) as an alternative first-line parenteral opioid in renal failure (see p.367).[14]

Alfentanil has been used successfully by short-term PCA or CSCI for dressing changes in burns or trauma patients.[2,3] It can be used SL and nasally for episodic pain, including severe intractable angina in inoperable coronary artery disease.[5,15,16] In the UK, a spray bottle containing alfentanil 5mg in 5mL is manufactured from alfentanil powder, delivering 140microgram/0.14mL spray. Details and instructions for use can be downloaded from palliativedrugs.com.[6] In an audit of patients already on regular strong opioids, about three quarters benefited from SL alfentanil in doses of 560–1,680microgram (4–12 sprays; titrated as necessary). Pain relief was seen within 10min.

Spinal administration of lipophilic opioids remains controversial because of the rapid clearance into the systemic circulation (see Chapter 21, p.713).[17]

Opioid withdrawal symptoms can occur when switching from **morphine** (or other less lipophilic/less potent opioid) to CSCI alfentanil.[18] These manifest with symptoms like gastric flu and last for a few days; p.r.n. doses of the original opioid will relieve troublesome symptoms.

Table 1 Pharmacokinetics of single IV doses of fentanils[19–21]

	Alfentanil	Sufentanil	Fentanyl
Onset of action (min)	0.75[a]	1	1.5[b]
Time to peak effect (min)	1.5	2.5	4.5
Plasma halflife (min)	95	165	220
Duration of action (min)	30[a]	60	60

a. onset slower if given IM (<5min), and duration of action longer (60min)
b. onset slower if given IM (7–15min), and duration of action longer (1–2h).

Box A Sufentanil (not UK)

A lipophilic opioid with a strong affinity for the μ-opioid receptor. Time to onset of action and to peak effect is mid-way between that of alfentanil and fentanyl (see Table 1).[20]

Sufentanil is about 7.5–10 times more potent than fentanyl,[22,23] and this allows a smaller volume to be given. Divide the dose of fentanyl by 10 to obtain an easy-to-calculate starting dose.

Example
Fentanyl 1,000microgram/24h CSCI (i.e. 20mL of 50microgram/mL)
→ sufentanil 100microgram/24h CSCI (i.e. 2mL of 50microgram/mL).

Sufentanil can be administered SC, IV or spinally.[24] By CSCI, it is compatible with other commonly prescribed drugs.[25]

Also given by intranasal or SL routes as pre-operative sedation, analgesia for moderare–severe acute trauma pain[26] and for rescue analgesia for episodic cancer pain.[27]

Accumulates in fat tissue when given continuously;[28] monitor carefully when switching to another opioid.

Is not dependent on renal function for elimination, and is thus useful in renal impairment.

Cautions

Hepatic impairment. Elderly or debilitated.

Drug interactions

Alfentanil is metabolized by CYP3A4. Caution is required with concurrent use of drugs which inhibit or induce these enzymes, (see Chapter 25, p.770). Reports of interactions where closer monitoring ± dose adjustment are required are listed in Table 2.[29]

Table 2   Interactions between alfentanil and other drugs involving CYP450

Alfentanil plasma concentration	
Increased by	Decreased by
Aprepitant[a]	Aprepitant[a]
Azoles, e.g. fluconazole, voriconazole	Efavirenz
Cimetidine	Rifampicin
Diltiazem	
Macrolide antibiotics, e.g. clarithromycin, erythromycin	
Protease inhibitors, e.g. indinavir, nelfinavir, ritonavir	

a. aprepitant can increase the exposure to CYP3A4 substrates in the short-term, then reduce their exposure within 2 weeks.

Undesirable effects

See Strong opioids, Box B, p.361.

Dose and use

As with all opioids, patients must be monitored for undesirable effects, particularly nausea and vomiting, and constipation (see p.360). Depending on individual circumstances, an anti-emetic should be prescribed for regular or p.r.n. use (see p.241) and a laxative prescribed routinely (see p.44).

Procedure-related pain (see Quick Prescribing Guide, p.390)
• 250–500microgram SL (using the 500microgram/mL injection formulation) or SC/IV.

As an alternative to morphine
Used mostly for patients in renal failure in whom there is evidence of **morphine** neurotoxicity (see p.364). Given the shorter duration of action of alfentanil, it is difficult to give a single precise dose conversion ratio. However, the following are safe practical conversion ratios:
• PO **morphine** to CSCI alfentanil, give one thirtieth of the 24h dose, e.g.
  morphine 60mg/24h PO = alfentanil 2mg/24h CSCI
• CSCI **morphine** to CSCI alfentanil, give one fifteenth of the 24h dose, e.g.
  morphine 30mg/24h = alfentanil 2mg/24h
• CSCI **diamorphine** to CSCI alfentanil, give one tenth of the 24h dose, e.g.
  diamorphine 30mg/24h = alfentanil 3mg/24h.
Conventionally, SC p.r.n. doses of alfentanil are 1/6–1/10 of the total 24h CSCI dose. Because of the short duration of action of alfentanil (≤30min), even with an optimally titrated p.r.n. dose, frequent dosing may be required; this is one reason why **fentanyl** and **buprenorphine** are recommended first-line in these circumstances (see Pharmacology). The CSCI dose of alfentanil should be reviewed at least daily, and titrated accordingly. For CSCI dilute with WFI, 0.9% saline or 5% glucose.

An alternative dosing schedule
The recommendations above may well be too conservative for some patients. It is important to review sooner rather than later, and increase the dose if necessary. At one centre, a conversion ratio for **diamorphine** to alfentanil of one sixth has been used for many years without clinical evidence of respiratory depression.[30]

At this centre, p.r.n. **diamorphine/morphine** is given to supplement CSCI alfentanil, giving the same p.r.n. dose as used before the switch to alfentanil. When the switch has been prompted by opioid neurotoxicity, a recurrence has not been observed with 1–2 p.r.n. doses/24h of **diamorphine/morphine.**

Break-through (episodic) cancer pain, SL administration
Given the variability in the intensity of break-through pains, p.r.n. recommendations are best expressed as a range of doses rather than a single fixed dose. There is a poor relationship between the effective SL p.r.n. dose and regular CSCI dose. Individual dose titration is necessary, e.g. starting with 1/10–1/6 of the daily alfentanil dose, and titrating upwards if necessary. Retaining even 2mL in the mouth (sublingually or buccally) for 5–10min is difficult. Thus, the smaller the volume, the easier it is for the patient (see Table 3).

Table 3 Equivalent volumes of parenteral formulations of alfentanil, sufentanil and fentanyl for SL use[a]

Alfentanil (500microgram/mL)		Sufentanil (50microgram/mL)		Fentanyl (50microgram/mL)	
Dose (microgram)	Volume (mL)	Dose (microgram)	Volume (mL)	Dose (microgram)	Volume (mL)
100	0.2	2.5	N/A	25	0.5
200	0.4	5	0.1	50	1
300	0.6	7.5	0.15	75	1.5
400	0.8	10	0.2	100	2
500	1	12.5	0.25	125	N/O[b]
600	1.2	15	0.3	150	N/O
800	1.6	20	0.4	200	N/O
1,000	2	25	0.5	250	N/O
2,000	N/O[b]	50	1	500	N/O
3,000	N/O	75	1.5	750	N/O
4,000	N/O	100	2	1,000	N/O

a. this is *not* a true dose conversion chart. Alfentanil, sufentanil and fentanyl have differing properties and, although bio-availability and onset of effect are broadly similar, duration of effect differs (fentanyl > sufentanil > alfentanil). As always with analgesics, individual patient dose titration is required
b. N/O = not optimal, because > 2mL.

Supply
All preparations are Schedule 2 **CD**.

The high-strength 5mg/mL injection is used at some centres when the CSCI/CIVI dose is > 5mg/24h. However, to avoid the risk of the high-strength injection being administered by mistake, in many hospitals its availability is restricted to the Intensive Care Unit.

Alfentanil (generic)
Nasal spray (with attachment for buccal/SL use) 5mg/5mL, 5mL bottle = £14; minimum order value = £50. (Unauthorized, available as a special order from the pharmacy manufacturing unit, Torbay hospital, see Appendix 1, p.817). *Telephone number for enquiries: 01803 664707; orders must be faxed to the manufacturing unit on 01803 664354. The solution is stable for 1 year unopened and for 28 days after opening.*
Injection 500microgram/mL, 2mL amp = £1, 10mL amp = £3.50.
Injection (for dilution and use as a continuous infusion) 5mg/mL, 1mL amp = £2.50.

1 King S et al. (2011) A systematic review of the use of opioid medication for those with moderate to severe cancer pain and renal impairment. *Palliative Medicine.* **25**: 525–552.
2 Sim KM et al. (1996) Use of patient-controlled analgesia with alfentanil for burns dressing procedures: a preliminary report of five patients. *Burns.* **22**: 238–241.
3 Gallagher G et al. (2001) Target-controlled alfentanil analgesia for dressing change following extensive reconstructive surgery for trauma. *Journal of Pain and Symptom Management.* **21**: 1–2.
4 Miner JR et al. (2011) Alfentanil for procedural sedation in the emergency department. *Annals of Emergency Medicine.* **57**: 117–121.
5 Duncan A (2002) The use of fentanyl and alfentanil sprays for episodic pain. *Palliative Medicine.* **16**: 550.
6 Palliativedrugs.com (2003) Hot Topics: alternatives to sublingual fentanyl. In: *August Newsletter.* Available from: www.palliativedrugs.com
7 Larijani G and Goldberg M (1987) Alfentanil hydrochloride: a new short acting narcotic analgesic for surgical procedures. *Clinical Pharmacy.* **6**: 275–282.
8 Bernards C (1999) Clinical implications of physicochemical properties of opioids. In: C Stein (ed) *Opioids in Pain Control: basic and clinical aspects.* Cambridge University Press, Cambridge, pp. 166–187.
9 Bodenham A and Park GR (1988) Alfentanil infusions in patients requiring intensive care. *Clinical Pharmacokinetics.* **15**: 216–226.
10 Kissin I et al (2000) Acute tolerance to continuously infused alfentanil: the role of cholecystokinin and N-methyl-D-aspartate-nitric oxide systems. *Anesthesia and Analgesia.* **91**: 110–116.
11 Schraag S et al. (1999) Lack of rapid development of opioid tolerance during alfentanil and remifentanil infusions for postoperative pain. *Anesthesia and Analgesia.* **89**: 753–757.
12 Bosilkovska M et al. (2012) Analgesics in patients with hepatic impairment: pharmacology and clinical implications. *Drugs.* **72**: 1645–1669.
13 Gardner-Nix J (2001) Oral transmucosal fentanyl and sufentanil for incident pain. *Journal of Pain and Symptom Management.* **22**: 627–630.
14 Caraceni A et al. (2012) Use of opioid analgesics in the treatment of cancer pain: evidence-based recommendations from the EAPC. *Lancet Oncology.* **13**: e58–68.
15 Osborn H and Jefferson M (2010) Intranasal alfentanil for severe intractable angina in inoperable coronary artery disease. *Palliative Medicine.* **24**: 94–95.
16 Brenchley J and Ramlakhan S (2006) Intranasal alfentanil for acute pain in children. *Emergency Medical Journal.* **23**: 488.
17 Bujedo BM (2013) Spinal opioid bioavailability in postoperative pain. *Pain Practice.* **14**: 350–364
18 Carmichael JP and Lee MA (2010) Symptoms of opioid withdrawal syndrome after switch from oxycodone to alfentanil. *Journal of Pain and Symptom Management.* **40**: e4–6.
19 Willens JS and Myslinski NR (1993) Pharmacodynamics, pharmacokinetics, and clinical uses of fentanyl, sufentanil, and alfentanil. *Heart Lung.* **22**: 239–251.
20 Scholz J et al. (1996) Clinical pharmacokinetics of alfentanil, fentanyl and sufentanil. An update. *Clinical Pharmacokinetics.* **31**: 275–292.
21 Hall T and Hardy J (2005) The lipophilic opioids: fentanyl, alfentanil, sufentanil and remifentanil. In: M Davis et al. (eds) *Opioids in Cancer Pain.* Oxford University Press, Oxford.
22 Reynolds L et al. (2004) Relative analgesic potency of fentanyl and sufentanil during intermediate-term infusions in patients after long-term opioid treatment for chronic pain. *Pain.* **110**: 182–188.
23 Scott JC et al. (1991) Electroencephalographic quantitation of opioid effect: comparative pharmacodynamics of fentanyl and sufentanil. *Anesthesiology.* **74**: 34–42.
24 Waara-Wolleat KL et al. (2006) A review of intrathecal fentanyl and sufentanil for the treatment of chronic pain. *Pain Medicine.* **7**: 251–259.
25 White C et al. (2008) Subcutaneous sufentanil for palliative care patients in a hospital setting. *Palliative Medicine.* **22**: 89–90.
26 Steenblik J et al. (2012) Intranasal sufentanil for the treatment of acute pain in a winter resort clinic. *American Journal of Emergency Medicine.* **30**: 1817–1821.
27 Good P et al. (2009) Intranasal sufentanil for cancer-associated breakthrough pain. *Palliative Medicine.* **23**: 54–58.
28 Alazia M et al. (1992) Pharmacokinetics of long term sufentanil infusion (72 hours) used for sedation in ICU patients. *Anesthesiology.* **77**: A364 (abstract).
29 Baxter K and Preston CL. *Stockley's Drug Interactions.* London: Pharmaceutical Press www.medicinescomplete.com (accessed March 2014).
30 Dorman S (2014). *Personal communication.*

Updated May 2014

Quick Prescribing Guide: Management of procedure-related pain

I Palliative care patients may experience pain while undergoing procedures, e.g.:

- position change
- investigation, e.g. MRI
- wound dressing change
- venous cannulation
- urethral catheterization
- removing impacted faeces

- insertion of nasogastric tube
- insertion/removal of central line
- insertion/removal of spinal line
- drainage of chest/abdomen
- treatment, e.g. radiation therapy.

2 The goal is adequate pain relief without undesirable effects. What is appropriate depends on the anticipated pain severity, procedure duration, current opioid use, and the patient's past personal experience. Thus, severe procedure-related pain may necessitate parenteral analgesia and sedation as first-line therapy.

3 Always include non-drug approaches:

- discuss past experiences of procedure-related pain, identify what was helpful or unhelpful, and clarify present concerns
- explain the procedure thoroughly before starting
- assure that you will stop immediately if requested
- as far as possible, choose the most comfortable position for the patient
- distract and relax, e.g. through talking, music, hypnosis and other relaxation techniques.

4 Use a local anaesthetic for:

- venous cannulation; use EMLA® cream if needle phobic or if requested (wait 60min)
- urethral catheterization; use lidocaine gel (wait 5min)
- chest aspiration; use lidocaine for tissue infiltration (wait 5min).

5 If available, consider nitrous oxide-oxygen (Entonox®) inhalation if the procedure is short and the patient is able to use the mask or mouthpiece effectively.

6 Give analgesia from the appropriate step of the ladder. (General anaesthetic approaches are beyond the scope of these guidelines.)

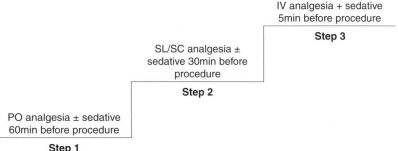

7 If pain relief inadequate, give a repeat dose and wait again; if still inadequate, move to the next step.

8 When a sedative or sedative analgesic is used, practitioners must be competent in airway management. Monitor the patient to ensure that the airway remains patent, and intervene if the patient becomes cyanosed because of severely depressed respiration.

Examples of analgesia for procedure-related pain

Step 1: If anticipating mild-moderate pain
Give 60min before the procedure:
PO morphine, give the patient's usual rescue dose for break-through (episodic) pain. If necessary, combine with:
- PO diazepam 5mg *or*
- SL lorazepam 500microgram–1mg *or*
- an alternative sedative.

Step 2: If anticipating moderate-severe pain
Give 30min before procedure:
SC morphine, give 50% of the patient's usual PO morphine rescue dose. If necessary, combine with:
- SL/SC midazolam 2.5–5mg *or*
- SL lorazepam 500microgram–1mg *or*
- an alternative sedative.

Step 3: If anticipating severe-excruciating pain
Give 5min before procedure:
IV morphine, give 50% of the patient's usual PO morphine rescue dose *or*
IV ketamine 0.5–1mg/kg (typically 25–50mg). Combine with:
- IV midazolam 2.5–5mg *or*
- an alternative sedative.

Note: there is a risk of marked sedation when ketamine and a sedative such as midazolam are combined in this way; use only if competent in airway management.

Alternatives to SC/IV morphine
- fentanyl 50–100microgram or more transmucosally using an authorized product (see p.413)
- alfentanil 250–500microgram SL (*from ampoule for injection or spray*) or SC/IV
- fentanyl 50–100microgram SL (*from ampoule for injection*) or SC/IV
- sufentanil 12.5–25microgram SL (*from ampoule for injection*) or SC/IV.

---

9 An opioid antagonist (naloxone) and a benzodiazepine antagonist (flumazenil) should be available in case of need. To prevent the complete reversal of any background regular opioid analgesic therapy, use naloxone 20–100microgram IV, repeated every 2min until the respiratory rate and cyanosis have improved. The initial dose of flumazenil is 200microgram IV over 15 seconds. If the desired level of consciousness is not obtained after 1 minute, further 100microgram doses can be given at 1 minute intervals p.r.n. up to a maximum total dose of 1mg.

10 If the procedure is to be repeated, give analgesia based on previous experience, e.g. drugs used and the patient's comments.

BUPRENORPHINE   BNF 4.7.2

Buprenorphine is experiencing a renaissance in the management of chronic cancer and non-cancer pain, and opioid dependence (high-dose SL formulation ± **naloxone**).[1-7] Preliminary data suggests that compared to **morphine** and other opioids, buprenorphine appears to cause less hyperalgesia (see p.364) and tolerance, and has less effect on the immune and endocrine systems. However, clinical trials are needed to find out whether such differences represent real clinical advantages.

Class: Strong opioid analgesic.

Indications: *SL tablet (200 and 400microgram) and injection* moderate–severe pain, premedication and peri-operative analgesia, †intolerance to other strong opioids.
SL higher-dose tablet (400microgram, 2mg, 8mg) withthdrawal and maintenance therapy for opioid addicts (also available as a combined formulation with naloxone, to prevent parenteral misuse).
TD moderate (BuTrans®) or severe (Transtec®, Hapoctasin®) non-cancer pain; moderate–severe cancer pain (Transtec®, Hapoctasin®), †intolerance to other strong opioids.

Contra-indications: None absolute if titrated carefully against a patient's pain (also see Strong opioids, p.357). TD buprenorphine should not be used for acute (transient, intermittent or short-term) pain, e.g. postoperative, or when there is need for rapid dose titration for severe uncontrolled pain.

Pharmacology

Buprenorphine is a partial μ-opioid receptor and opioid-receptor-like (ORL-1) *agonist* and a k- and δ-opioid receptor *antagonist*.[8-10] It has high affinity at the μ-, k- and δ-opioid receptors, but affinity at the ORL-1 receptor is 500-fold less. It associates and dissociates slowly from receptors.[11] Subjective and physiological effects are generally similar to **morphine** (μ agonist).

Studies in volunteers suggest that compared with **morphine** and other opioids, buprenorphine exerts a more prominent antihyperalgesic than analgesic effect;[12,13] however, this is not a consistent finding.[14] Animal studies and case reports also suggest that buprenorphine may be of particular benefit in neuropathic pain,[2,15] but controlled studies are needed to confirm this.[6,16-18] The co-administration of an ultra-low dose of an opioid antagonist potentiated the analgesic effect of buprenorphine (as with other opioids) in healthy volunteers but not patients (also see p.450).[19,20]

Antagonist effects at the k-opioid receptor may limit spinal analgesia, sedation and psychotomimetic effects.[21] In animal studies, buprenorphine shows a ceiling effect or a bell-shaped dose-response curve for analgesic (> 1mg/kg) and respiratory effects (0.1mg/kg). This is thought to be due to its partial agonist effect at the μ-opioid receptor. An agonist effect at the pronociceptive supraspinal ORL-1 receptor may also contribute.[22] In humans, a ceiling effect has been shown for respiratory depression (~200microgram/70kg IV)[23,24] and other effects, e.g. euphoria (4–8mg SL),[25,26] but not for analgesia.[24] Total daily doses up to 24mg SL are reported to provide effective analgesia;[27-29] anecdotally, even higher doses have been used, with no upper dose limit clearly established.[30] Thus, the ceiling dose for analgesia in humans is much higher than the 'maximum' TD dose recommended by the UK manufacturers, namely 3.36mg/day (70microgram/h patches x 2).

Studies of buprenorphine TD or SL up to 1.6mg/day have confirmed that it is possible to use **morphine** (or other μ agonist) for break-through (episodic) pain,[31] and to switch either way between buprenorphine and **morphine** (or other μ agonist) without loss of analgesia.[32,33]

However, greater difficulties are experienced when switching patients on higher doses of opioids, using larger doses of buprenorphine.[29] When patients on various opioids (oral morphine equivalent 15–450mg/24h) were switched using doses of buprenorphine 2mg SL (resulting in maximum post-switch doses of 6–24mg/24h), over half experienced intolerable undesirable effects and abandoned the switch. Generally, undesirable effects related to opioid excess in patients receiving low doses of oral morphine equivalent (≤20mg/24h) and opioid withdrawal in those receiving high doses (> 300mg/24h). This experience guided the development of a clinical protocol, although the dosing algorithm has not yet been tested formally.[29]

The use of other μ agonists for break-through (episodic) pain in patients on higher doses of buprenorphine may also be less straightforward (see SL opioid-maintenance therapy in addicts). Nonetheless, various μ agonists have been used in patients on SL buprenorphine 2–32mg/24h, although higher doses than usual may be required.[28,34]

Buprenorphine has either no effect or a smaller effect than **morphine** on pressure within the biliary and pancreatic ducts.[35,36] Buprenorphine does slow intestinal transit, but possibly less so than **morphine**.[37,38] Constipation may be less severe.[39]

Compared with **morphine** and other opioids, buprenorphine appears less likely to suppress the gonadal axis or testosterone levels (see p.372).[40] This may relate to its k *antagonist* effect.[41] Because hypogonadism is associated with reduced sexual desire and function, mood disturbance, fatigue and other physiological effects, e.g. muscle wasting, osteoporosis, this may become an important consideration in patients requiring long-term opioid therapy.[42–44]

Compared with **morphine** and other opioids, buprenorphine has little or no immunosuppressive effect (see p.372).[2,45–48]

Compared with **methadone**, buprenorphine has less effect on the QT interval (see p.433).[49,50]

In an anecdotal report, 2 out of 5 patients with cholestatic pruritus responded to treatment with buprenorphine.[51,52] However, there are insufficient data at present to recommend its use in this circumstance.

TD buprenorphine

Buprenorphine is highly lipid-soluble making it suitable for TD delivery. It is available in the UK in formulations delivering lower and higher doses, i.e. 5, 10 or 20microgram/h as 7-day patches (BuTrans[®])[53–55] and 35, 52.5 or 70microgram/h as 3-day (Hapoctasin[®]) or 4-day patches (Transtec[®]).[56] Like other strong opioids, buprenorphine is an alternative to both weak opioids and **morphine**.[57] Buprenorphine is evenly distributed in a drug-in-adhesive matrix. Its release is controlled by the physical characteristics of the matrix and is proportional to the surface area of the patch. Absorption of the buprenorphine through the skin and into the systemic circulation is influenced by the stratum corneum and blood flow. Thus, if the skin is warm and vasodilated, the rate of absorption increases.

There are few practical differences in the use of the buprenorphine or **fentanyl** matrix patches, and similar safety considerations apply, e.g. not to expose the patch to external sources of heat. Compared with **fentanyl**, TD buprenorphine (as Transtec[®]) adheres better. However, after patch removal, it is associated with more persistent erythema (± localized pruritus), and sometimes a more definite dermatitis.[58] This is generally caused by the adhesive, but occasionally buprenorphine itself causes a contact dermatitis ± more widespread skin rash.[59]

Retrospective analysis suggests that, compared with TD **fentanyl**, patients receiving TD buprenorphine (as Transtec[®]) have a slower rate of dose increase and longer periods of dose stability.[60] This requires confirmation in an RCT. Indeed, systematic reviews have highlighted a lack of high quality studies of TD buprenorphine.[61,62]

SL opioid-maintenance therapy in addicts

Buprenorphine binds to the μ-opioid receptor with a higher affinity than other μ-opioid agonists. Studies in addicts indicate that buprenorphine ≥16mg SL is required to suppress illicit opioid use;[63] at this dose level, ≥80% of the μ-opioid receptors in the brain are occupied by buprenorphine which is sufficient to antagonize the subjective and respiratory depressant effects of **hydromorphone**, a μ agonist.[11,64] This has implications for the management of acute pain in these patients, e.g. postoperative or traumatic pain (see Chapter 18, p.687) and potentially for patients on higher-dose buprenorphine for chronic pain (see above).

Respiratory depression

Significant respiratory depression is rarely seen with clinically recommended doses. A lower risk of respiratory depression may also explain why buprenorphine (mainly SL ± **naloxone**) appears to have a better safety profile than **methadone**.[65] However, serious or fatal respiratory depression has occurred in addicts misusing buprenorphine, generally in high-dose IV and in combination with benzodiazepines or other CNS depressants, e.g. alcohol.[66,67] Because buprenorphine has very strong receptor affinity (reflected in its high relative potency with **morphine**), **naloxone** in standard doses does not reverse the effects of buprenorphine and higher doses must be used (Box A).[2,68] The non-specific respiratory stimulant **doxapram** can also be used, 1–1.5mg/kg IV over 30sec, repeated if necessary at hourly intervals or 1.5–4mg/min CIVI.[68–70]

> **Box A**   Reversal of buprenorphine-induced respiratory depression
>
> 1 Discontinue buprenorphine (stop CSCI/CIVI, remove TD patch).
>
> 2 Give oxygen by mask.
>
> 3 Give IV naloxone 2mg stat over 90sec.
>
> 4 Commence naloxone 4mg/h by CIVI.
>
> 5 Continue CIVI until the patient's condition is satisfactory (probably <90min).
>
> 6 Monitor the patient frequently for the next 24h, and restart CIVI if respiratory depression recurs.
>
> 7 If the patient's condition remains satisfactory, restart buprenorphine at a reduced dose, e.g. half the previous dose.

Potency

Buprenorphine has a longer duration of action than **morphine**. In postoperative single-dose studies, buprenorphine provided analgesia for 6–7h compared with 4–5h with **morphine**.[71] This is reflected in the recommended dose frequency (q8h–q6h vs. q4h for **morphine**). However, the longer duration of action of buprenorphine almost certainly means that potency ratios based on *single-dose* studies will *underestimate* the potency of buprenorphine. Thus, the following ratios should be *not* be regarded as 'cast iron'. They merely provide a rough guide for use when switching route or opioids (see Chapter 15, p.661):

- SL buprenorphine is about half as potent as IV/IM/SC buprenorphine; thus, in round figures, 200microgram SL is equivalent to 100microgram by injection[72,73]
- SL buprenorphine is about 80 times more potent than PO **morphine**;[32] thus, in round figures, 200microgram SL buprenorphine is equivalent to 15mg PO **morphine**
- IV/IM/SC buprenorphine is 30–40 times more potent than IV/IM/SC **morphine**;[74] thus, in round figures, 300microgram IV buprenorphine is equivalent to 10mg IV **morphine**
- TD buprenorphine is 70–115 times more potent than PO **morphine**.[75–77]

The lower limit of the last ratio is based on a small prospective study and the upper limit on a large retrospective chart review. Thus, *PCF* considers TD buprenorphine being 100 times more potent than PO **morphine** a convenient compromise. A PO **morphine**: TD buprenorphine conversion ratio of 100:1 makes a 5microgram/h TD buprenorphine patch equivalent to about 12mg/24h PO **morphine**. (Note: a lack of definitive data explains the wide variation seen in recommendations and clinical practice.[78–80]

A conversion ratio of PO **morphine**:TD buprenorphine of 100:1 also means that TD buprenorphine and TD **fentanyl** can be considered essentially equipotent (see Chapter 15, Table 2, p.664). However, others suggest that TD **fentanyl** is 1.4 times more potent than TD buprenorphine,[33,77] making TD **fentanyl** 25 and 50microgram/h patches equivalent to buprenorphine 35 and 70microgram/h patches respectively. Even so, when switching opioids because of possible opioid-induced hyperalgesia, it is prudent to reduce the calculated equivalent dose of the new opioid by 25–50% (see Opioid switching, p.365).

Switching opioids

As with any opioid switch, patients changing from another opioid to buprenorphine may experience worsening pain and/or opioid-withdrawal symptoms. Careful monitoring and titration of buprenorphine is required to ensure any worsening pain is dealt with promptly.

Opioid-withdrawal manifests with GI and flu-like symptoms, e.g. abdominal pain, diarrhoea, arthralgia, myalgia, and last for a few days. With TD and lower doses of SL buprenorphine, p.r.n. doses of the previous opioid will relieve troublesome symptoms.

However, in addiction medicine, when switching generally involves high-dose SL buprenorphine, the practice is to discontinue the first opioid, await the development of withdrawal symptoms and only then commence buprenorphine. In this way, opioid withdrawal will not be precipitated by buprenorphine (because of its greater affinity for the μ-opioid receptor) but, rather, once withdrawal symptoms are present, they should be relieved by it.

Pharmacokinetics

The bio-availability of PO buprenorphine is low (15%); it undergoes extensive first-pass metabolism in the GI mucosa and liver, where it is almost completely converted by CYP3A4 to norbuprenorphine. Norbuprenorphine has similar opioid receptor-binding affinities to buprenorphine but does not readily cross the blood-brain barrier and has little, if any, central effect.[81] Both buprenorphine and norbuprenorphine undergo glucuronidation to what have traditionally been considered inactive metabolites, although recent animal work has questioned this.[82,83]

The bio-availability of SL buprenorphine is about 50%; it is rapidly absorbed into the oral mucosa (2–3min), followed by a slower absorption into the systemic circulation (t_{max} 30min–3.5h after a single dose; 1–2h with repeat dosing).[81] This, together with a duration of action of 6–8h, suggests that SL buprenorphine is not ideal for the treatment of breakthrough (episodic) pain. Nonetheless, onset of analgesia in 10–20min is reported for SL buprenorphine,[37] and it has been successfully used as a rescue analgesic in patients receiving higher dose TD buprenorphine (i.e. Transtec®).[84] After parenteral and SL administration, 70% of buprenorphine is excreted unchanged in the faeces and some enterohepatic recirculation is likely; whereas norbuprenorphine is mainly excreted in the urine.[85] Vomiting is more common with SL administration than IM or TD.

Buprenorphine has a large volume of distribution and is highly protein-bound (96%; α- and β-globulins).[81] It does not accumulate in renal impairment nor is it removed by haemodialysis, and thus analgesia is unaffected.[86,87] Although accumulation of norbuprenorphine can occur, this may be of little clinical relevance given its lack of central effect.[81,86] Thus, buprenorphine is potentially a reasonable option for patients with renal impairment (see p.367). However, clinical experience is more limited compared to other opioids, e.g. **fentanyl** (p.403).[88]

Data are limited,[89] but smaller starting doses and careful titration are advisable in patients with severe (but not mild–moderate) hepatic impairment. Buprenorphine crosses the placenta and enters breast milk. The incidence, severity and duration of the neonatal abstinence syndrome appears to be less than with **methadone**.[90,91]

The bio-availability of IV buprenorphine is by definition 100%, and that of SC essentially the same. Bio-availability is irrelevant in relation to TD patches; the stated delivery rates reflect the mean amount of drug delivered to patients throughout the patch's recommended duration of use. Inevitably, there will be interindividual variation in the amount delivered. Extrapolating from data relating to TD fentanyl, the absorption of TD buprenorphine could also be impaired in patients with cachexia, possibly because of a loss of skin hydration.[92] Pharmacokinetic data are summarized in Table 1.

Table 1   Pharmacokinetic details for buprenorphine

	IV	TD (Hapoctasin®)	TD (Transtec®)	TD (BuTrans®)	SL
Onset of action	5–15min[71]	4–12h	21h for 35microgram/h patch; 11h for 70microgram/h patch	18–24h	10–20min[37]
Time to peak plasma concentration	5min	34h for 35microgram/h patch; 29h for 70microgram/h patch	60h	3 days	30min–3.5h single dose; 1–2h multiple doses[21,81]
Plasma halflife	3–16h[81]	24–27h[a]	25–36h[a]	13–35h[a]	24–69h[81]
Duration of action	6–8h	3 days	4 days	7 days	6–8h

a. the halflife after a patch has been removed and not replaced.

Cautions

Hepatic impairment. The combination of high-dose buprenorphine SL with antiretrovirals, particularly **delavirdine** and **ritonavir** increases the QT interval, but the clinical significance of this is uncertain.[93] Although the SPC contra-indicates the use of buprenorphine within 14 days of MAOI use, this appears a blanket precaution, see Strong opioids, p.362.

Drug interactions

A single case report describes respiratory depression when IM **ketorolac** was added to ED buprenorphine.[94]

Buprenorphine is mainly a substrate of CYP3A4, and the manufacturers and others advise caution if prescribed concurrently with CYP3A4 inhibitors (e.g. **clarithromycin, erythromycin, itraconazole**, protease inhibitors), or avoiding concurrent use, because of the potential to increase buprenorphine levels. Although for most CYP3A4 inhibitors this is a theoretical concern, **atazanavir, ritonavir** and **delavirdine** (not UK) have been shown to significantly increase buprenorphine levels in patients receiving high-doses SL (8–16mg/day).[95] Accordingly, it is recommended that the dose of buprenorphine is halved in patients receiving high-dose buprenorphine SL if used concurrently with a CYP3A4 inhibitor (see Chapter 25, Table 7, p.774).[95]

Conversely, CYP3A4 inducers (e.g. **carbamazepine, phenobarbital, phenytoin, rifampicin**) could reduce buprenorphine levels.

Undesirable effects

Also see Strong opioids, Box B, p.361.

Very common (>10%): nausea; erythema and pruritus at the patch application site.

Common (<10%, >1%): asthenia, drowsiness, dizziness, headache, oedema, vomiting, constipation, sweating.

Dose and use

In 2013, in response to large numbers of safety incident reports about buprenorphine and **fentanyl** TD patches, the Care Quality Commission highlighted the need to ensure that:
- use is appropriate, e.g. chronic *not* acute pain
- dose is appropriate, i.e. in line with published conversion charts
- dose is titrated appropriately, i.e. no more than 50% of the previous daily dose
- date and site of application are recorded to avoid inadvertent dose omission or duplication.

Further, to avoid confusing patients and carers, prescribing by brand was recommended.[96]

As with all opioids, patients must be monitored for undesirable effects (see p.360), particularly nausea and vomiting, and constipation. Depending on individual circumstances, an anti-emetic should be prescribed for regular or p.r.n. use, (see p.241) and, routinely, a laxative prescribed (see p.44).

In Europe, the TD patches are the commonest formulation of buprenorphine used in chronic cancer and non-cancer pain. Particularly for patients unable to swallow or take PO/SL products reliably, TD buprenorphine provide an alternative non-invasive route for opioid administration.[78]

Compared to the SL and parenteral routes, the TD patches permit smaller initial doses of buprenorphine to be delivered more consistently (without large peaks and troughs) and are thus better tolerated.[97]

TD

See Quick Prescribing Guide, p.401.

In the UK, TD buprenorphine patches are available as:
- 5, 10 and 20microgram/h 7-day patches (BuTrans®)
- 35, 52.5, 70microgram/h 3-day (Hapoctasin®) or 4-day patches (Transtec®).

For patients who have not already been taking an opioid, the lowest patch strength should be prescribed, i.e. 5microgram/h (equivalent to **morphine** 12mg/24h PO). General advice and recommended starting doses are detailed in the manufacturer's SPC. With inpatients, the use of a monitoring chart is recommended (see Document Library, www.palliativedrugs.com).[98]

SL

The tablet should not be chewed or swallowed as this will reduce efficacy:
- manufacturer's recommended starting dose 200microgram (equivalent to approximately **morphine** 15mg PO) q8h; this may be too much for some patients
- use with a sip of water if mouth is dry
- use an appropriate dose of a strong opioid as a rescue analgesic. Note. SL buprenorphine is *not* an ideal rescue analgesic but, if used, allow one tenth of the total daily dose, rounded to a convenient tablet size, q3h p.r.n.; some limit this to a maximum of four doses per 24h
- titrate the dose every 4–5 days, based on p.r.n. use
- typical dose 800–1,200microgram/day, given as 200–400microgram q8h–q6h
- doses of 2–24mg/day have been reported in chronic pain patients switched from other opioids.[27,29]

SC/IM/IV

- manufacturer's recommended starting dose 300microgram (equivalent to approximately **morphine** 10mg SC/IM/IV) q8h; this may be too much for some patients
- give IV over ⩾2min
- if necessary, titrate to 600microgram q8h–q6h (the recommended maximum in acute pain; in chronic pain higher doses may be required).

CSCI/CIVI

- buprenorphine has been given CIVI diluted in 0.9% saline or 5% glucose at a concentration of 15microgram/mL; there are no compatibility data for mixing with other drugs used in palliative care
- for patients receiving CSCI/CIVI buprenorphine, p.r.n. injections about one tenth of the total daily dose can be used for break-through (episodic) pain.

Supply

All preparations are Schedule 3 **CD**.

Temgesic® (RB Pharmaceuticals)
Tablets SL 200microgram, 400microgram, 28 days @ 200microgram t.d.s. = £9.
Injection 300microgram/mL, 1mL amp = £0.50.

Tephine® (Sandoz)
Tablets SL 200microgram, 400microgram, 28 days @ 200microgram t.d.s. = £9.
Note: SL buprenorphine tablets 400microgram, 2mg and 8mg for substitution treatment for opioid dependence are available in 7 tablet packs as a generic, and also as proprietary products (Prefibin®, Sandoz; Subutex®, Reckitt Benckiser). A combined formulation with **naloxone** is also available (Suboxone®, Reckitt Benckiser).

Transdermal products
BuTrans® (Napp)
Patches (for 7 days) 5microgram/h, 10microgram/h, 20microgram/h, 1 = £4.50, £8 and £14 respectively.

Hapoctasin® (Actavis)
Patches (for 3 days) 35microgram/h, 52.5microgram/h, 70microgram/h, 1 = £2.50, £3 and £5 respectively.

Transtec® (Napp)
Patches (for 4 days) 35microgram/h, 52.5microgram/h, 70microgram/h, 1 = £4, £6 and £8 respectively.

1 Resnick RB (2003) Food and Drug Administration approval of buprenorphine-naloxone for office treatment of addiction. *Annals of Internal Medicine*. **138**: 360.
2 Budd K and Raffa R (eds) (2005) Buprenorphine - the unique opioid analgesic. Georg Thieme Verlag, Stuttgart, Germany, p. 134.
3 Griessinger N et al. (2005) Transdermal buprenorphine in clinical practice–a post-marketing surveillance study in 13,179 patients. *Current Medical Research and Opinion*. **21**: 1147–1156.
4 Gowing L et al. (2006) Buprenorphine for the management of opioid withdrawal. *Cochrane Database Systematic Reviews*. CD002025.

5 Landau CJ et al. (2007) Buprenorphine transdermal delivery system in adults with persistent noncancer-related pain syndromes who require opioid therapy: a multicenter, 5-week run-in and randomized, double-blind maintenance-of-analgesia study. Clinical Therapeutics. 29: 2179–2193.

6 Kress HG (2009) Clinical update on the pharmacology, efficacy and safety of transdermal buprenorphine. European Journal of Pain. 13: 219–230.

7 Przeklasa-Muszynska A and Dobrogowski J (2011) Transdermal buprenorphine for the treatment of moderate to severe chronic pain: results from a large multicenter, non-interventional post-marketing study in Poland. Current Medical Research Opinion. 27: 1109–1117.

8 Rothman R (1995) Buprenorphine: a review of the binding literature. In: A Cowan and J Lewis (eds) Buprenorphine: combatting drug abuse with a unique opioid. Wiley-Liss, New York, pp. 19–29.

9 Zaki P et al. (2000) Ligand-induced changes in surface mu-opioid receptor number: relationship to G protein activation? Journal of Pharmacology and Experimental Therapeutics. 292: 1127–1134.

10 Lewis JW and Husbands SM (2004) The orvinols and related opioids–high affinity ligands with diverse efficacy profiles. Current Pharmaceutical Design. 10: 717–732.

11 Greenwald M et al. (2007) Buprenorphine duration of action: mu-opioid receptor availability and pharmacokinetic and behavioral indices. Biological Psychiatry. 61: 101–110.

12 Koppert W et al. (2005) Different profiles of buprenorphine-induced analgesia and antihyperalgesia in a human pain model. Pain. 118: 15–22.

13 Simonnet G (2005) Opioids: from analgesia to anti-hyperalgesia? Pain. 118: 8–9.

14 Ravn P et al. (2013) Morphine- and buprenorphine-induced analgesia and antihyperalgesia in a human inflammatory pain model: a double-blind, randomized, placebo-controlled, five-arm crossover study. Journal of Pain Research. 6: 23–38.

15 Hans G (2007) Buprenorphine–a review of its role in neuropathic pain. Journal of Opioid Management. 3: 195–206.

16 Sanchez-Blazquez P and Garzon J (1988) Pertussis toxin differentially reduces the efficacy of opioids to produce supraspinal analgesia in the mouse. European Journal of Pharmacology. 152: 357–361.

17 Likar R and Sittl R (2005) Transdermal buprenorphine for treating nociceptive and neuropathic pain: four case studies. Anesthesia and Analgesia. 100: 781–785.

18 Penza P et al. (2008) Short- and intermediate-term efficacy of buprenorphine TDS in chronic painful neuropathies. Journal of the Peripheral Nervous System. 13: 283–288.

19 Hay JL et al. (2011) Potentiation of buprenorphine antinociception with ultra-low dose naltrexone in healthy subjects. European Journal of Pain. 15: 293–298.

20 Ling W et al. (2012) Comparisons of analgesic potency and side effects of buprenorphine and buprenorphine with ultra-low-dose naloxone. Journal of Addiction Medicine. 6: 118–123.

21 Johnson RE et al. (2005) Buprenorphine: considerations for pain management. Journal of Pain and Symptom Management. 29: 297–326.

22 Lutfy K et al. (2003) Buprenorphine-induced antinociception is mediated by mu-opioid receptors and compromised by concomitant activation of opioid receptor-like receptors. Journal of Neuroscience. 23: 10331–10337.

23 Dahan A et al. (2005) Comparison of the respiratory effects of intravenous buprenorphine and fentanyl in humans and rats. British Journal Anaesthesia. 94: 825–834.

24 Dahan A et al. (2006) Buprenorphine induces ceiling in respiratory depression but not in analgesia. British Journal of Anaesthesia. 96: 627–632.

25 Budd K (2002) Buprenorphine: a review. Evidence Based Medicine in Practice. Hayward Medical Communications, Newmarket.

26 Walsh S et al. (1994) Clinical pharmacology of buprenorphine: ceiling effects at high doses. Clinical Pharmacology and Therapeutics. 55: 569–580.

27 Malinoff HL et al. (2005) Sublingual buprenorphine is effective in the treatment of chronic pain syndrome. American Journal of Therapeutics. 12: 379–384.

28 Heit HA and Gourlay DL (2008) Buprenorphine: new tricks with an old molecule for pain management. Clinical Journal of Pain. 24: 93–97.

29 Rosenblum A et al. (2012) Sublingual buprenorphine/naloxone for chronic pain in at-risk patients: development and pilot test of a clinical protocol. Journal of Opioid Management. 8: 369–382.

30 Portenoy R (2013) Personal communication.

31 Mercadante S et al. (2006) Safety and effectiveness of intravenous morphine for episodic breakthrough pain in patients receiving transdermal buprenorphine. Journal of Pain and Symptom Management. 32: 175–179.

32 Atkinson R et al. (1990) The efficacy in sequential use of buprenorphine and morphine in advanced cancer pain. In: D Doyle (ed) Opioids in the treatment of cancer pain. Royal Society of Medicine Services, London, pp. 81–87.

33 Mercadante S et al. (2007) Switching from transdermal drugs: an observational "N of 1" study of fentanyl and buprenorphine. Journal of Pain and Symptom Management. 34: 532–538.

34 Kornfeld H and Manfredi L (2010) Effectiveness of full agonist opioids in patients stabilized on buprenorphine undergoing major surgery: a case series. American Journal of Therapeutics. 17: 523–528.

35 Pausawasdi S et al. (1984) The effect of buprenorphine and morphine on intraluminal pressure of the common bile duct. Journal of the Medical Association of Thailand. 67: 329–333.

36 Staritz M et al. (1986) Effect of modern analgesic drugs (tramadol, pentazocine, and buprenorphine) on the bile duct sphincter in man. Gut. 27: 567–569.

37 Robbie DS (1979) A trial of sublingual buprenorphine in cancer pain. British Journal of Clinical Pharmacology. 7 (Suppl 3): S315–S317.

38 Bach V et al. (1991) Buprenorphine and sustained release morphine - effect and side-effects in chronic use. The Pain Clinic. 4: 87–93.

39 Pace MC et al. (2007) Buprenorphine in long-term control of chronic pain in cancer patients. Frontiers in Bioscience. 12: 1291–1299.

40 Hallinan R et al. (2009) Hypogonadism in men receiving methadone and buprenorphine maintenance treatment. International Journal of Andrology. 32: 131–139.

41 Bliesener N et al. (2005) Plasma testosterone and sexual function in men receiving buprenorphine maintenance for opioid dependence. Journal of Clinical Endocrinology and Metabolism. 90: 203–206.

42 Daniell HW (2002) Hypogonadism in men consuming sustained-action oral opioids. The Journal of Pain. 3: 377–384.

43 Rajagopal A et al. (2004) Symptomatic hypogonadism in male survivors of cancer with chronic exposure to opioids. Cancer. 100: 851–858.

44 Hallinan R et al. (2008) Erectile dysfunction in men receiving methadone and buprenorphine maintenance treatment. Journal of Sexual Medicine. **5**: 684–692.

45 Sacerdote P et al. (2000) The effects of tramadol and morphine on immune responses and pain after surgery in cancer patients. Anesthesia and Analgesia. **90**: 1411–1414.

46 Budd K and Shipton E (2004) Acute pain and the immune system and opioimmunosuppression. Acute Pain. **6**: 123–135.

47 Sacerdote P et al. (2008) Buprenorphine and methadone maintenance treatment of heroin addicts preserves immune function. Brain, Behavior, and Immunity. **22**: 606–613.

48 Canneti A et al. (2013) Safety and efficacy of transdermal buprenorphine and transdermal fentanyl in the treatment of neuropathic pain in AIDS patients. Minerva Anestesiologica. **79**: 871 883.

49 Wedam EF et al. (2007) QT-interval effects of methadone, levomethadyl, and buprenorphine in a randomized trial. Archives of Internal Medicine. **167**: 2469–2475.

50 Esses JL et al. (2008) Successful transition to buprenorphine in a patient with methadone-induced torsades de pointes. Journal of Interventional Cardiac Electrophysiology. **23**: 117–119.

51 Juby L et al. (1994) Buprenorphine and hepatic pruritus. British Journal of Clinical Practice. **48**: 331.

52 Reddy L et al. (2007) Transdermal buprenorphine may be effective in the treatment of pruritus in primary biliary cirrhosis. Journal of Pain and Symptom Management. **34**: 455–456.

53 Steiner DJ et al. (2011) Efficacy and safety of the seven-day buprenorphine transdermal system in opioid-naive patients with moderate to severe chronic low back pain: an enriched, randomized, double-blind, placebo-controlled study. Journal of Pain and Symptom Management. **42**: 903–917.

54 Conaghan PG et al. (2011) Transdermal buprenorphine plus oral paracetamol vs an oral codeine-paracetamol combination for osteoarthritis of hip and/or knee: a randomised trial. Osteoarthritis and Cartilage. **19**: 930–938.

55 Steiner D et al. (2011) Efficacy and safety of buprenorphine transdermal system (BTDS) for chronic moderate to severe low back pain: a randomized, double-blind study. Journal of Pain and Symptom Management. **12**: 1163–1173.

56 Likar R et al. (2007) Transdermal buprenorphine patches applied in a 4-day regimen versus a 3-day regimen: a single-site, Phase III, randomized, open-label, crossover comparison. Clinical Therapeutics. **29**: 1591–1606.

57 Davis MP (2005) Buprenorphine in cancer pain. Supportive Care in Cancer. **13**: 878–887.

58 Schmid-Grendelmeier P et al. (2006) A comparison of the skin irritation potential of transdermal fentanyl versus transdermal buprenorphine in middle-aged to elderly healthy volunteers. Current Medical Research Opinion. **22**: 501–509.

59 Vander Hulst K et al. (2008) Allergic contact dermatitis from transdermal buprenorphine. Contact Dermatitis. **59**: 366–369.

60 Sittl R et al. (2006) Patterns of dosage changes with transdermal buprenorphine and transdermal fentanyl for the treatment of noncancer and cancer pain: a retrospective data analysis in Germany. Clinical Therapeutics. **28**: 1144–1154.

61 Deandrea S et al. (2009) Managing severe cancer pain: the role of transdermal buprenorphine: a systematic review. Therapeutics and Clinical Risk Management. **5**: 707–718.

62 Tassinari D et al. (2011) Transdermal opioids as front line treatment of moderate to severe cancer pain: a systemic review. Palliative Medicine. **25**: 478–487.

63 Mattick RP et al. (2014) Buprenorphine maintenance versus placebo or methadone maintenance for opioid dependence. Cochrane Database of Systematic Reviews. **2**: CD002207.

64 Greenwald MK. et al. (2003) Effects of buprenorphine maintenance dose on mu-opioid receptor availability, plasma concentrations, and antagonist blockade in heroin-dependent volunteers. Neuropsychopharmacology. **28**: 2000–2009.

65 Dasgupta N et al. (2010) Post-marketing surveillance of methadone and buprenorphine in the United States. Pain Medicine. **11**: 1078–1091.

66 Kintz P (2001) Deaths involving buprenorphine: a compendium of French cases. Forensic Science International. **121**: 65–69.

67 Hakkinen M et al. (2012) Benzodiazepines and alcohol are associated with cases of fatal buprenorphine poisoning. European Journal of Clinical Pharmacology. **68**: 301–309.

68 Dahan A et al. (2010) Incidence, Reversal, and Prevention of Opioid-induced Respiratory Depression. Anesthesiology. **112**: 226–238.

69 British National Formulary Section 3.5.1 Respiratory stimulants London: BMJ Group and Pharmaceutical Press www.bnf.org (accessed December 2012).

70 Orwin JM (1977) The effect of doxapram on buprenorphine induced respiratory depression. Acta anaesthesiologica Belgica. **28**: 93–106.

71 Heel RC et al. (1979) Buprenorphine: a review of its pharmacological properties and therapeutic efficiency. Drugs. **17**: 81–110.

72 Ellis R et al. (1982) Pain relief after abdominal surgery-a comparison of i.m. morphine, sublingual buprenorphine and self-administered i.v. pethidine. British Journal of Anaesthesia. **54**: 421–428.

73 Bullingham RE et al. (1984) Mandatory sublingual buprenorphine for postoperative pain. Anaesthesia. **39**: 329–334.

74 Cuschieri RJ et al. (1984) Comparison of morphine and sublingual buprenorphine following abdominal surgery. British Journal of Anaesthesia. **56**: 855–859.

75 Sittl R et al. (2005) Equipotent doses of transdermal fentanyl and transdermal buprenorphine in patients with cancer and noncancer pain: results of a retrospective cohort study. Clinical Therapeutics. **27**: 225–237.

76 Likar R et al. (2008) Challenging the equipotency calculation for transdermal buprenorphine: four case studies. International Journal of Clinical Practice. **62**: 152–156.

77 Mercadante S et al. (2009) Equipotent doses to switch from high doses of opioids to transdermal buprenorphine. Supportive Care in Cancer. **17**: 715–718.

78 Caraceni A et al. (2012) Use of opioid analgesics in the treatment of cancer pain: evidence-based recommendations from the EAPC. Lancet Oncology. **13**: e58–68.

79 NICE (2012) Opioids in palliative care: safe and effective prescribing of strong opioids for pain in palliative care adults. Clinical Guideline. CG140. www.nice.org.uk

80 Palliativedrugs.com (2013) The oral morphine equivalent of buprenorphine TD patches - What conversion do you use? Survey Results. Additions Archive. **March**: www.palliativedrugs.com

81 Elkader A and Sproule B (2005) Buprenorphine: clinical pharmacokinetics in the treatment of opioid dependence. Clinical Pharmacokinetics. **44**: 661–680.

82 McQuay H and Moore R (1995) Buprenorphine kinetics in humans. In: A Cowan and J Lewis (eds) Buprenorphine: combatting drug abuse with a unique opioid. Wiley-Liss, New York, pp. 137–147.

83 Brown SM et al. (2011) Buprenorphine metabolites, buprenorphine-3-glucuronide and norbuprenorphine-3-glucuronide, are biologically active. Anesthesiology. **115**: 1251–1260.

84 Poulain P et al. (2008) Efficacy and safety of transdermal buprenorphine: a randomized, placebo-controlled trial in 289 patients with severe cancer pain. *Journal of Pain and Symptom Management*. **36**: 117–125.

85 Cone EJ et al. (1984) The metabolism and excretion of buprenorphine in humans. *Drug Metabolism and Disposition*. **12**: 577–581.

86 Hand CW et al. (1990) Buprenorphine disposition in patients with renal impairment: single and continuous dosing, with special reference to metabolites. *British Journal of Anaesthesia*. **64**: 276–282.

87 Filitz J et al. (2006) Effect of intermittent hemodialysis on buprenorphine and norbuprenorphine plasma concentrations in chronic pain patients treated with transdermal buprenorphine. *European Journal of Pain*. **10**: 743–748.

88 King S et al. (2011) A systematic review of the use of opioid medication for those with moderate to severe cancer pain and renal impairment. *Palliative Medicine*. **25**: 525–552.

89 Bosilkovska M et al. (2012) Analgesics in patients with hepatic impairment: pharmacology and clinical implications. *Drugs*. **72**: 1645–1669.

90 Fischer G (2000) Treatment of opioid dependence in pregnant women. *Addiction*. **95**: 1141–1144.

91 Lacroix I et al. (2004) Buprenorphine in pregnant opioid-dependent women: first results of a prospective study. *Addiction*. **99**: 209–214.

92 Heiskanen T et al. (2009) Transdermal fentanyl in cachectic cancer patients. *Pain*. **144**: 218–222.

93 Baker JR et al. (2006) Effect of buprenorphine and antiretroviral agents on the QT interval in opioid-dependent patients. *Annals of Pharmacotherpy*. **40**: 392–396.

94 Jain PN and Shah SC (1993) Respiratory depression following combination of epidural buprenorphine and intramuscular ketorolac. *Anaesthesia*. **48**: 898–899.

95 Baxter K and Preston CL (2012). *Stockley's Drug Interactions*. London: Pharmaceutical Press www.medicinescomplete.com (accessed December 2012).

96 Care Quality Commission and NHS England (2013) Safer use of controlled drugs - preventing harms from fentanyl and buprenorphine transdermal patches. *Use of controlled drugs supporting information*. www.cqc.org.uk

97 James IG et al. (2010) A randomized, double-blind, double-dummy comparison of the efficacy and tolerability of low-dose transdermal buprenorphine (BuTrans seven-day patches) with buprenorphine sublingual tablets (Temgesic) in patients with osteoarthritis pain. *Journal of Pain and Symptom Management*. **40**: 266–278.

98 Palliativedrugs.com (2014) Strong opioid transdermal patch monitoring chart. *Document Library*. **Pain (strong opioids)**: www.palliativedrugs.com

Updated June 2014

Quick Prescribing Guide: Use of transdermal buprenorphine

1 Indications for using transdermal (TD) buprenorphine instead of morphine include:
  • intolerable undesirable effects with morphine, e.g. nausea and vomiting, constipation, hallucinations, dysphagia
  • renal failure (no centrally active metabolites)
  • 'tablet phobia' or poor compliance with oral medication
  • high risk of tablet misuse/diversion (although the patch can still be abused).

2 TD buprenorphine is contra-indicated in patients with acute (short-term) pain and in those who need rapid dose titration for severe uncontrolled pain.

3 TD buprenorphine patches are available in two formulations:
  • 5, 10 and 20microgram/h 7-day patches (BuTrans®)
  • 35, 52.5, 70microgram/h 3-day (Hapoctasin®) or 4-day patches (Transtec®).
The maximum *authorized* dose is two 70microgram/h patches.

Use the Table below to decide a safe starting dose for TD buprenorphine and an appropriate rescue dose of morphine. These recommendations are based on a PO morphine:TD buprenorphine dose conversion ratio of 100:1 derived from published data, which is in keeping with the manufacturer's dose ratio range of 75–115:1 (see SPC). It is an approximation, and inevitably there will be individual variation. If switching to buprenorphine because of possible opioid-induced hyperalgesia, reduce the calculated equivalent dose by 25–50%.

4 Patients not previously receiving opioids should start on 5 or 10microgram/h patches; patients with unrelieved pain despite maximum dose of a Step 2 analgesic should commence on 20 or 35microgram/h patches, according to circumstances.

5 For patients taking a dose of morphine that is not the exact equivalent of a buprenorphine patch, it will be necessary to opt for a patch which is either slightly more or slightly less than the morphine dose. Thus, if the patient still has pain, round up to a higher patch strength; if pain-free and frail, round down.

Comparative doses based on dose conversion ratio 100:1

PO Morphine[a]		SC/IV Morphine[a]		TD Buprenorphine	
mg/24h	p.r.n. mg[b]	mg/24h[c]	p.r.n. mg[b]	microgram/h	microgram/24h
				BuTrans®	
12	2[d]	6	1	5	120
24	5[d]	12	2.5	10	240
48	10	24	5	20	480
				Transtec®, Hapoctasin®	
84	15	42	7.5	35	840
126	20	63	10	52.5	1,260
168	30	84	15	70[e]	1,680

a. an alternative strong opioid can be used, calculated using the appropriate conversion factor. Note. SL buprenorphine is *not* an ideal rescue medication but some centres use an initial dose of 200microgram SL q3h, up to 4 doses per 24h, for patients receiving any strength of Transtec® or Hapoctasin®
b. using traditional one sixth of total daily dose as p.r.n. dose and rounded to a convenient dose; give up to q1h; some centres opt for one tenth of total daily dose
c. assuming potency ratio of morphine SC/IV to PO of 2:1
d. at these doses, p.r.n. codeine/dihydrocodeine (30–60mg) or tramadol (50mg) may suffice
e. for combinations of patches, add the p.r.n. doses together, e.g. 70 + 52.5microgram/h patches = 15 + 10mg morphine SC/IV = 25mg morphine SC/IV, but can round up to 30mg or down to 20mg for convenience.

6 The date of application and/or the date for renewal should be written in a consistent manner on the patch. Apply to dry, non-inflamed, non-irradiated, hairless skin on the upper trunk or arm. Body hair may be clipped with scissors but not shaved. If the skin is washed beforehand, use only water; do not use soap and do not apply oils, cream or ointment to the area. Press patch firmly in place for at least 30 seconds. Micropore® or Tegaderm® can be used to ensure adherence. Careful removal of the patch helps to minimize local skin irritation.

7 Systemic analgesic concentrations are generally reached within 12–24h but levels continue to rise for 32–54h. If converting from:
   • 4-hourly PO morphine, give regular doses for the first 12h after applying the patch
   • 12-hourly m/r morphine, apply the patch and the final m/r dose at the same time
   • 24-hourly m/r morphine, apply the patch 12h after the final m/r dose
   • CSCI/CIVI opioids, continue the infusion for about 12h after applying the patch.

8 Steady-state plasma concentrations of buprenorphine are reached after 9 days (1–2 days with patch strength of ≤20microgram/h); the patient should use p.r.n. doses liberally, particularly during the first 24h, either the previously used weak opioid, or morphine/other strong opioid, or buprenorphine (see Table above).

9 After 72h, if a patient continues to need 2 or more rescue doses of analgesic/day, the next strength patch should be used.

10 Patients could experience opioid-withdrawal symptoms when changed from another opioid (particularly large doses) to TD buprenorphine. These manifest with symptoms like gastric flu and last for a few days; p.r.n. doses of the previous opioid will relieve troublesome symptoms.

11 Buprenorphine is less constipating than morphine; halve the dose of laxatives when starting buprenorphine and re-titrate.

12 Buprenorphine may cause nausea and vomiting; if necessary, prescribe an anti-emetic, e.g. haloperidol 1.5mg PO stat & at bedtime.

13 In febrile patients, the rate of absorption of buprenorphine increases, and may cause toxicity, e.g. drowsiness. Absorption is also enhanced by an external heat source over the patch, e.g. electric blanket or hot-water bottle; patients should be warned about this. Patients may swim or shower with a patch but should not soak in a hot bath.

14 Remove and replace patches once (7-day patch) or twice (3- and 4-day patches) a week. The 4-day patch (Transtec®) can be replaced on fixed days in the week, i.e. after 3 and 4 days alternatively. Change the position of the new patches so as to rest the underlying skin for at least 9 days.

15 A reservoir of buprenorphine cumulates in the body, particularly in adipose tissue, and significant plasma levels persist for at least 24h after discontinuing TD buprenorphine.

16 TD buprenorphine is unsatisfactory in <5% of patients.

17 In moribund patients, continue TD buprenorphine and give additional SC morphine p.r.n. (see Table above). If >2 p.r.n. doses are required/24h, give morphine by CSCI, starting with a dose equal to the sum of the p.r.n. doses over the preceding 24h. If necessary, adjust the p.r.n. dose taking into account the total opioid dose (i.e. TD buprenorphine + CSCI morphine).

18 Used patches still contain buprenorphine; after removal, fold the patch with the adhesive side inwards, and then discard in a sharps container (hospital) or dustbin (home), and wash hands. Ultimately, any unused patches should be returned to a pharmacy.

FENTANYL   BNF 4.7.2 & 15.1.4.3

For transmucosal fentanyl for cancer-related breakthrough (episodic) pain or procedure-related pain, see p.413.

Class: Strong opioid analgesic.

Indications: *TD* severe chronic (persistent, long-term) pain, including cancer, †AIDS,[1,2] †intolerance to other strong opioids.[3] *Injection* severe pain, premedication and peri-operative analgesia, analgesic/respiratory depressant in patients requiring assisted ventilation, neuroleptanalgesia (i.e. in combination with an antipsychotic/neuroleptic), †intolerance to other strong opioids.

Contra-indications: TD fentanyl should not be used for acute (transient, intermittent or short-term) pain, e.g. postoperative, or when there is need for rapid dose titration for severe uncontrolled pain.

In the UK, most manufacturers and the Care Quality Commission/NHS England recommend against its use in opioid-naïve patients (see Dose and use).[4]

In the USA and Canada, TD fentanyl is contra-indicated in opioid-naïve patients because of reports of unintentional overdoses, with serious (sometimes fatal) consequences.[5]

Pharmacology

Fentanyl (*like* **morphine**) is a strong μ-opioid receptor agonist. It has a relatively low molecular weight and (*unlike* **morphine**) is lipophilic. This makes it suitable for TD and transmucosal administration (see p.413). Generally, TD fentanyl is used only when PO opioids, e.g. **morphine**, **oxycodone**, are not tolerated.[3] In some patients, it may be the preferred strong opioid, e.g. those unable to swallow.[6]

Fentanyl is sequestrated in body fats, including epidural fat and the white matter of the CNS.[7,8] Thus, by any route (including spinally), after systemic redistribution, fentanyl acts supraspinally mainly in the thalamus (white matter). Any effect in the dorsal horn (grey matter) is probably minimal.[7]

The lipophilic nature of fentanyl also provides one explanation for the difference in undesirable effects compared with **morphine** (Figure 1).[9] Thus, when converting from PO or parenteral **morphine** to TD or parenteral fentanyl, there is a massive decrease in opioid molecules outside the CNS with, in consequence, less constipation. This also explains why peripherally-mediated withdrawal symptoms are also sometimes seen.

TD fentanyl is used in the management of chronic severe pain,[10–12] particularly in cancer.[13–18] Steady-state plasma concentrations of fentanyl are generally achieved after 36–48h[1] but, according to manufacturer data[19] this is sometimes achieved only after 9–12 days.

Elimination of fentanyl mainly involves biotransformation in the liver by CYP3A4 to inactive norfentanyl which is excreted in the urine. Less than 7% is excreted unchanged. The SPCs generally advise caution in patients with moderate–severe liver or renal impairment, but this is based on limited data which suggest reduced clearance of fentanyl because of, for example, alterations in metabolic clearance and plasma protein-binding. Given the risk of accumulation, close monitoring is indicated. Nonetheless, fentanyl is a reasonable option for patients with renal impairment or failure (see below and also p.367),[20] including those with hepatorenal syndrome.[21]

If pain relief does not last for 3 days, the correct response is to increase the patch strength. Even so, a small percentage of patients do best if the patch is changed every 2 days.[17,22]

Matrix and reservoir patches are now available from several manufacturers. All the SPCs contain dose conversion recommendations from PO morphine which, although broadly similar, do vary. The original manufacturer in the UK initially recommended a dose conversion ratio for **morphine** and fentanyl of 150:1. However, several RCTs support a smaller ratio, ranging 70–125:1. Indeed, at the same time in Germany, the original manufacturer promoted 100:1. Consequently, *PCF* has opted for a ratio of 100:1, as have others.[6,23,24]

The original manufacturer's SPC in the UK and in Germany now contain conversion tables based on both 150:1 and 100:1, with the former recommended for patients who have only been on morphine or other strong opioid for 'several weeks' and the latter for 'highly opioid-tolerant patients on a stable and well-tolerated opioid regimen for long periods' (see Chapter 15, Box B, p.666). It is unclear on what evidence this distinction is made.

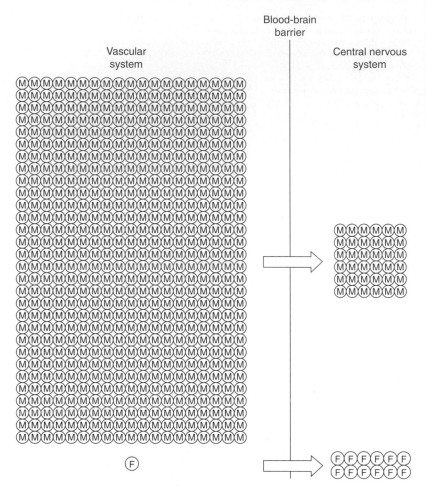

Figure 1 Distribution of equipotent doses of morphine and fentanyl in the vascular and central nervous systems based on animal data.[9]

PCF also favours a PO **morphine**:TD **buprenorphine** conversion ratio of 100:1 and this means that TD **buprenorphine** and TD fentanyl can be considered essentially equipotent (see Chapter 15, Table 2, p.664). However, others suggest that fentanyl is 1.4 times more potent than TD **buprenorphine**,[25,26] which would make TD fentanyl 25 and 50microgram/h patches equivalent to **buprenorphine** 35 and 70microgram/h patches respectively. Even so, when switching opioids because of possible opioid-induced hyperalgesia, it is prudent to reduce the calculated equivalent dose of the new opioid by 25–50% (see p.365).

Because fentanyl is less constipating than **morphine**,[18,22,27,28] when converting from **morphine** to fentanyl, the dose of laxative should be halved and subsequently adjusted according to need. Some patients experience withdrawal symptoms (e.g. diarrhoea, colic, nausea, sweating, restlessness) when changed from PO **morphine** to TD fentanyl despite satisfactory pain relief. This is probably related to differences between the two opioids in relation to their relative impact on peripheral and central μ-opioid receptors (see Figure 1). Such symptoms are easily treatable by using rescue doses of **morphine** until they resolve after a few days. Like **buprenorphine**, fentanyl appears to have little effect on the sphincter of Oddi.[29]

At one PCU, it was noted that patients admitted on fentanyl TD were receiving relatively higher equivalent opioid doses than other patients.[30] The reasons for this are not clear but may include a failure to appreciate the potency of fentanyl, and the induction of opioid-induced hyperalgesia by inappropriately high doses. It is noteworthy that fentanyl TD was successfully reduced or discontinued in 60% of patients.[30]

Pharmacokinetic data are summarized in Table 1. Bio-availability is irrelevant in relation to TD patches; the stated delivery rates reflect the mean amount of drug delivered to patients throughout the patch's recommended duration of use. Inevitably, there will be interindividual variation in the amount delivered, e.g. for the 100microgram/h patch, the mean ($\pm$SD) delivery is 97 ($\pm$15) microgram/h,[31] and the amount of unused fentanyl in the patch after 3 days can vary from 30–85% of the original contents.[32]

In cachectic patients, plasma concentrations of fentanyl are reduced by 1/3–1/2.[33] The reason for this is unclear; it appears not to relate to loss of subcutaneous adipose tissue,[34] but loss of skin hydration is a possibility.[33]

Table 1 Pharmacokinetic data for fentanyl

	TD	SC/IM	IV
Onset of action	3–23h[35]	7–15min IM	1.5min
Time to peak plasma concentration	24–72h	Median 15min, range 10–30min [36]	<5min
Plasma halflife	13–22h[a,37]	Median 10h, range 6–16h[36]	4h
Duration of action	72h; for some patients, 48h[38]	1–2h IM	60min

a. the halflife after a patch has been removed and not replaced.

Cautions

The reservoir patches should not be cut because damage to the rate-controlling membrane can lead to a rapid release of fentanyl and overdose. Although cutting matrix patches is theoretically safer, some strongly discourage it because of similar concerns.[39] However, cutting has become unnecessary with the introduction of a 12microgram/h patch.

After reports of serious adverse events (overdoses and deaths), regulatory authorities in the UK, USA and Canada have issued safety warnings about the use of TD fentanyl.[4,5,40,41] Factors contributing to adverse drug events include:
- lack of appreciation that fentanyl is a strong opioid analgesic
- inappropriate use for short-term, intermittent or postoperative pain in patients who had not previously been receiving a strong opioid
- lack of patient education regarding directions for safe use, storage and disposal
- lack of awareness of the signs of an overdose and when to seek attention
- lack of awareness that the rate of absorption of fentanyl may be increased if the skin under the patch becomes vasodilated, e.g. in febrile patients, high ambient temperatures,[42] or by an external heat source, e.g. electric blanket, heat lamps, saunas, hot tubs
- lack of awareness of drug interactions which can increase fentanyl levels.

Deaths continue to occur from incorrect use.[43] Additional errors include the failure to remove old patches, the dispensing and application of higher strength patches than prescribed and incorrect disposal. The latter is associated with accidental exposure and deaths in others, particularly children.

Patients with COPD or other medical conditions which predispose to respiratory depression (e.g. myasthenia gravis) or who are susceptible to the intracranial effects of hypercapnia (e.g. those with raised intracranial pressure). Caution is also needed if bradyarrhythmic (symptomatic bradycardia can occur),[44] elderly, cachectic, debilitated, moderate–severe hepatic or renal impairment, hypovolaemic, hypotensive, and if a history or high risk of abuse or diversion. Muscle rigidity can occur (generally transiently following IV injection).

Although fentanyl analgesia is generally unaffected by haemodialysis,[45] there are rare reports of pain recurring in patients on TD fentanyl during and after haemodialysis.[46] This probably relates only to certain dialysis membranes (see p.367) and may reflect loss of fentanyl through membrane adsorption rather than loss into the dialysate solution.[45]

Addicts misuse TD fentanyl in various ways, e.g. heating the patch, applying buccally, chewing, ingesting, inhaling, IV injection of patch contents, sometimes with fatal consequences.[47,48]

Drug interactions

Fentanyl is metabolized by CYP3A4. Caution is required with concurrent use of drugs which inhibit or induce these enzymes, (see Chapter 25, p.775). Reports of interactions where closer monitoring ± dose adjustment are required are listed in Table 2.[49–53]

Table 2   Interactions between fentanyl and other drugs involving CYP450

Fentanyl plasma concentration	
Increased by	*Decreased by*
Aprepitant[a]	Aprepitant[a]
Azoles, e.g. fluconazole[b], voriconazole	Carbamazepine
Cimetidine	Phenytoin
Macrolide antibiotics, e.g. clarithromycin, erythromycin	Phenobarbital
Protease inhibitors, e.g. indinavir, nelfinavir, ritonavir	Rifampicin

a. aprepitant can increase the exposure to CYP3A4 substrates in the short-term, then reduce their exposure within 2 weeks
b. a case report of a fatality with oral fluconazole and TD fentanyl has been attributed to this interaction.

Fentanyl has been reported to reduce the metabolism of midazolam, reducing the clearance by 30% and extending the half-life by 50%.[49]

Fentanyl is best avoided in patients who have used a MAOI within the past 2 weeks. Although they have been used safely together, serotonin toxicity (sometimes fatal) has occurred (also see p.195), manufacturers' SPCs warn of a risk of serotonin toxicity when fentanyl is *used in combination* with other serotoninergic drugs.[49]

Undesirable effects

Also see Strong opioids. Box B, p.361.
Very common (>10%): drowsiness, dizziness, headache, insomnia, nausea, vomiting, constipation; muscle rigidity (including thoracic muscles) when given IV.
Common (<10%, >1%): anxiety, visual disturbance, palpitations, dry mouth, anorexia, dyspepsia, abdominal pain, diarrhoea, sweating, vasodilation.
Topical effects: Occasional skin irritation, hypersensitivity.

Dose and use

As with all opioids, patients must be monitored for undesirable effects, particularly nausea and vomiting, and constipation (see p.360). Depending on individual circumstances, an anti-emetic should be prescribed for regular or p.r.n. use, (see p.241) and, routinely, a laxative prescribed (see p.44).

TD fentanyl

The use of TD fentanyl patches is summarized in the Quick Prescribing Guide (see p.411). These and the comments in this section are based on a dose conversion ratio of PO **morphine** to TD fentanyl of 100:1. Prescribers using the manufacturer's ratio of 150:1 should follow the dose conversion guidelines in the SPC (Chapter 15, Box B, p.666).

Prescribers considering the use of TD fentanyl as a first-line strong opioid, particularly in opioid-naïve patients, should be sufficiently experienced and able to closely monitor the patient; otherwise seek specialist advice.

In 2013, in response to large numbers of safety incident reports about **buprenorphine** and fentanyl TD patches, the Care Quality Commission highlighted the need to ensure that:
• use is appropriate, e.g. chronic *not* acute pain
• dose is appropriate, i.e. in line with published conversion charts
• dose is titrated appropriately, i.e. no more than 50% of the previous daily dose
• date and site of application are recorded to avoid inadvertent dose omission or duplication.
Further, to avoid confusing patients and carers, prescribing by brand was recommended.[4]
   Under no circumstances should a *reservoir* patch be cut in an attempt to reduce the dose. Leakage from the cut reservoir could result in either the patient receiving minimal or no fentanyl or, alternatively, an overdose from the rapid absorption of fentanyl through the surrounding skin.

Two different TD formulations are currently available:
• *reservoir* patch (e.g. Fentalis®, Tilofyl®) the fentanyl is contained within a reservoir, and the release of fentanyl is controlled by a rate-limiting membrane
• *matrix* patch (e.g. Durogesic DTrans®, Matrifen®) the fentanyl is evenly distributed throughout a drug-in-adhesive matrix, and the release of fentanyl is controlled by the physical characteristics of the matrix.
Absorption of the fentanyl through the skin and into the systemic circulation is influenced by both the condition of the skin and cutaneous blood flow. Thus, if the skin is warm and vasodilated, the rate of absorption will be increased.
   Bio-equivalence has been demonstrated between two different makes of *matrix* patches, and between the *matrix* and *reservoir* patches.[19,54–56] However, the matrix patch is thinner (because there is no reservoir) and, for equal strengths, more than one-third smaller. Consequently, to avoid confusing patients and carers, prescribing by brand is recommended.[4]
   In North America, the manufacturer stresses that TD fentanyl should be commenced *only* in patients who have been receiving strong opioids in a dose at least equivalent to a 25microgram/h patch for ⩾1 week, such as:
• **morphine** 60mg/day PO
• **oxycodone** 30mg/day PO
• **hydromorphone** 8mg/day PO.
In the UK, most manufacturers and the Care Quality Commission/NHS England recommend against use in opioid-naïve patients, advising initial titration with immediate-release **morphine**.[4] Nonetheless, there are reports where TD fentanyl has been used satisfactorily as a first-line strong opioid in, for example, patients with severe dysphagia, renal failure or who are living in social circumstances where there is a high risk of diversion and tablet misuse. (Note: misuse of TD fentanyl can also occur; see Cautions). TD fentanyl is also used in totally opioid-naïve patients at centres which skip Step 2 of the WHO analgesic ladder.[57–59] However, prescribers considering the use of TD fentanyl as a first-line strong opioid, particularly in opioid-naïve patients, should be sufficiently experienced and able to closely monitor the patient; otherwise specialist advice should be sought. Authorized starting doses for TD fentanyl as a first-line strong opioid in the UK are 12–25microgram/h, depending on the individual product, equivalent to **morphine** 30–60mg/24h PO. Thus, the 12microgram/h dose will be a safer starting dose for *totally opioid-naïve* patients and for some *strong* (but not weak) *opioid-naïve* patients, e.g. frail patients using low doses of weak opioid with moderate pain. Undesirable effects, e.g. nausea and vomiting, are more frequent in strong opioid-naïve patients and, in separate studies, resulted in one-sixth and one-third of patients discontinuing TD fentanyl 12microgram/h and 25microgram/h respectively.[60,61]
   It is important to give adequate rescue doses of **morphine** (see Quick Prescribing Guide, p.411) or other strong opioid. Adjusting the patch strength on a daily basis is not recommended.[62] With inpatients, the use of a monitoring chart is recommended (for an example, see www.palliativedrugs.com).[63]

SC/IM/IV

• start with a stat dose of 50–200microgram, and subsequently 50microgram p.r.n.
• reduce the dose in the elderly and debilitated, e.g. 12.5–25microgram SC p.r.n.
• traditionally p.r.n. dosing intervals are q1h, but more frequent dosing with close monitoring may be required in severe acute pain
• give IV by slow injection; this reduces the risk of muscular rigidity.

CSCI

In the UK, this route is recommended mostly in the setting of severe and end-stage renal impairment (eGFR < 30mL/min) when pain is uncontrolled:[20]
opioid-naïve
- initial dose 100–300microgram/24h CSCI
- allow 12.5–25microgram SC p.r.n q1h
converting from another opioid
- calculate equivalent dose (see Chapter 15, p.661)
- reduce by 20% and use as initial dose
- allow a suitable p.r.n. dose (traditionally 1/6–1/10 of the total daily regular dose).

If the patient is not in the last days of life, a switch to TD fentanyl may be possible once stable pain control is achieved. Select a patch which delivers a similar rate of fentanyl in microgram/h as the CSCI, discontinuing the CSCI at the same time as the first patch is applied.

For CSCI, dilute with WFI, 0.9% saline or 5% glucose. There are limited compatibility data for mixing fentanyl with other drugs for CSCI. Health professionals are encouraged to add details of any successful or unsuccessful combinations to the existing list of fentanyl combinations on the www.palliativedrugs.com Syringe Driver Survey Database (SDSD).

If the required dose of CSCI fentanyl causes volume issues, consider using **alfentanil** instead (see p.385). However, because **alfentanil** has a shorter half-life, continue to use fentanyl SC p.r.n. for break-through pain.

Transmucosal fentanyl formulations could be used as an alternative p.r.n. analgesic, but only when the patient has sufficient time and ability to co-operate with the necessary titration (see p.413). Because bio-availability of transmucosal fentanyl is less than SC and varies widely, apply an appropriate reduction when adjusting the background CSCI dose based on the p.r.n. dose and frequency of use. Monitor the patient closely for signs of toxicity.

CIVI

Fentanyl CIVI is used in some centres (generally *not* UK) for initial control of cancer pain. When an effective stable dose is found, the route is switched to TD over 6h:
- start by applying patch(es) which deliver the same dose/h as the CIVI, rounded for convenience
- after 6h, discontinue the CIVI.[64]

This appears satisfactory for most patients; other methods exist, but are more complex.[64]

Supply

All preparations are schedule 2 **CD**.

Fentanyl

Reservoir patches (for 3 days) 12microgram/h, 1 = £2.50, 25microgram/h, 1 = £3.50; 50microgram/h, 1 = £7; 75microgram/h, 1 = £10; 100microgram/h, 1 = £12. Products include *Tilofyl®, Fentalis®*.

Matrix patches (for 3 days)
12microgram/h, 1 = £2.50; 25microgram/h, 1 = £3.50; 37.5microgram/h (Mezolar® only), 1 = £3; 50microgram/h, 1 = £7; 75microgram/h, 1 = £10; 100microgram/h, 1 = £12.
Products include *Durogesic Dtrans®, Fencino®, Matrifen®, Mezolar®, Opiodur®, Osmanil®, Victanyl®*.

Fentanyl citrate (generic)

Injection 50microgram/mL, 2mL amp = £0.50, 10mL amp = £1.

1 Newshan G and Lefkowitz M (2001) Transdermal fentanyl for chronic pain in AIDS: a pilot study. *Journal of Pain and Symptom Management.* 21: 69–77.
2 Canneti A *et al.* (2013) Safety and efficacy of transdermal buprenorphine and transdermal fentanyl in the treatment of neuropathic pain in AIDS patients. *Minerva Anestesiologica.* 79: 871–883.
3 Tassinari D *et al.* (2011) Transdermal opioids as front line treatment of moderate to severe cancer pain: a systemic review. *Palliative Medicine.* 25: 478–487.
4 Care Quality Commission and NHS England (2013) Safer use of controlled drugs - preventing harms from fentanyl and buprenorphine transdermal patches. *Use of controlled drugs supporting information.* www.cqc.org.uk
5 Health Canada (2008) Fentanyl transdermal patch and fatal adverse reactions. *Canadian Adverse Reaction Newsletter.* 18(3): 1–2.
6 Caraceni A *et al.* (2012) Use of opioid analgesics in the treatment of cancer pain: evidence-based recommendations from the EAPC. *Lancet Oncology.* 13: e58–68.

7 Bernards C (1999) Clinical implications of physicochemical properties of opioids. In: C Stein (ed) *Opioids in Pain Control: basic and clinical aspects*. Cambridge University Press, Cambridge, pp. 166–187.

8 Ummenhofer W et al. (2000) Comparative spinal distribution and clearance kinetics of intrathecally administered morphine, fentanyl, alfentanil, and sufentanil. *Anesthesiology*. **92**: 739–953.

9 Herz A and Teschemacher H-J (1971) Activities and sites of antinociceptive action of morphine-like analgesics and kinetics of distribution following intravenous, intracerebral and intraventricular application. *Advances in Drug Research*. **6**: 79–119.

10 Simpson R et al. (1997) Transdermal fentanyl as treatment for chronic low back pain. *Journal of Pain and Symptom Management*. **14**: 218–224.

11 Milligan K and Campbell C (1999) Transdermal fentanyl in patients with chronic, nonmalignant pain: a case study series. *Advances in Therapy*. **16**: 73–77.

12 Allan L et al. (2001) Randomised crossover trial of transdermal fentanyl and sustained release oral morphine for treating chronic non-cancer pain. *British Medical Journal*. **322**: 1154–1158.

13 Yeo W et al. (1997) Transdermal fentanyl for severe cancer-related pain. *Palliative Medicine*. **11**: 233–239.

14 Payne R et al. (1998) Quality of life and cancer pain: satisfaction and side effects with transdermal fentanyl versus oral morphine. *Journal of Clinical Oncology*. **16**: 1588–1593.

15 Sloan P et al. (1998) A clinical evaluation of transdermal therapeutic system fentanyl for the treatment of cancer pain. *Journal of Pain and Symptom Management*. **16**: 102–111.

16 Nugent M et al. (2001) Long-term observations of patients receiving transdermal fentanyl after a randomized trial. *Journal of Pain and Symptom Management*. **21**: 385–391.

17 Radbruch L et al. (2001) Transdermal fentanyl for the management of cancer pain: a survey of 1005 patients. *Palliative Medicine*. **15**: 309–321.

18 Hadley G et al. (2013) Transdermal fentanyl for cancer pain. *Cochrane Database of Systematic Reviews*. **10**: CD010270.

19 Janssen-Cilag Ltd Data on file.

20 King S et al. (2011) A systematic review of the use of opioid medication for those with moderate to severe cancer pain and renal impairment. *Palliative Medicine*. **25**: 525–552.

21 Bosilkovska M et al. (2012) Analgesics in patients with hepatic impairment: pharmacology and clinical implications. *Drugs*. **72**: 1645–1669.

22 Donner B et al. (1998) Long-term treatment of cancer pain with transdermal fentanyl. *Journal of Pain and Symptom Management*. **15**: 168–175.

23 Donner B et al. (1996) Direct conversion from oral morphine to transdermal fentanyl: a multicenter study in patients with cancer pain. *Pain*. **64**: 527–534.

24 Mercadante S and Caraceni A (2011) Conversion ratios for opioid switching in the treatment of cancer pain: a systematic review. *Palliative Medicine*. **25**: 504–515.

25 Mercadante S et al. (2007) Switching from transdermal drugs: an observational "N of 1" study of fentanyl and buprenorphine. *Journal of Pain and Symptom Management*. **34**: 532–538.

26 Mercadante S et al. (2009) Equipotent doses to switch from high doses of opioids to transdermal buprenorphine. *Supportive Care in Cancer*. **17**: 715–718.

27 Tassinari D et al. (2008) Adverse effects of transdermal opiates treating moderate-severe cancer pain in comparison to long-acting morphine: a meta-analysis and systematic review of the literature. *Journal of Palliative Medicine*. **11**: 492–501.

28 Hannon B et al. (2013) The role of fentanyl in refractory opioid-related acute colonic pseudo-obstruction. *Journal of Pain and Symptom Management*. **45**: e1–3.

29 Koo HC et al. (2010) Effect of transdermal fentanyl patches on the motility of the sphincter of oddi. *Gut and Liver*. **4**: 368–372.

30 Botterman J and Criel N (2011) Inappropriate use of high doses of transdermal fentanyl at admission to a palliative care unit. *Palliative Medicine*. **25**: 111–116.

31 Van Nimmen NF et al. (2010) Fentanyl transdermal absorption linked to pharmacokinetic characteristics in patients undergoing palliative care. *Journal of Clinical Pharmacology*. **50**: 667–678.

32 Marquardt KA et al. (1995) Fentanyl remaining in a transdermal system following three days of continuous use. *Annals of Pharmacotherpy*. **29**: 969–971.

33 Heiskanen T et al. (2009) Transdermal fentanyl in cachectic cancer patients. *Pain*. **144**: 218–222.

34 Hadgraft J and Lane ME (2005) Skin permeation: the years of enlightenment.[see comment]. *International Journal of Pharmaceutics*. **305**: 2–12.

35 Gourlay GK et al. (1989) The transdermal administration of fentanyl in the treatment of post-operative pain: pharmacokinetics and pharmacodynamic effects. *Pain*. **37**: 193–202.

36 Capper SJ et al. (2010) Pharmacokinetics of fentanyl after subcutaneous administration in volunteers. *European Journal of Anaesthesiology*. **27**: 241–246.

37 Portenoy RK et al. (1993) Transdermal fentanyl for cancer pain. *Anesthesiology*. **78**: 36–43.

38 Smith J and Ellershaw J (1999) Improvement in pain control by change of fentanyl patch after 48 hours compared with 72 hours. *Poster EAPC Congress, Geneva*. POI/1376.

39 Anonymous (2007) Safe use of fentanyl (Duragesic) patches. *Pharmacist's Letter/Prescriber's Letter*. **23**: 1–5.

40 FDA (2007) Fentanyl transdermal system (marketed as Duragesic) Information. *Post market drug safety information for patients and providers*. www.fda.gov/Drugs/DrugSafety.

41 MHRA (2008) Fentanyl patches: serious and fatal overdose from dosing errors, accidental exposure, and inappropriate use. *Drug Safety Update*. **2**. www.mhra.gov.uk/safetyinformation

42 Sindali K et al. (2012) Life-threatening coma and full-thickness sunburn in a patient treated with transdermal fentanyl patches: a case report. *Journal of Medical Case Reports*. **6**: 220.

43 Jumbelic MI (2010) Deaths with transdermal fentanyl patches. *American Journal of Forensic Medicine and Pathology*. **31**: 18–21.

44 Hawley P (2013) Case report of severe bradycardia due to transdermal fentanyl. *Palliative Medicine*. **27**: 793–795.

45 Dean M (2004) Opioids in renal failure and dialysis patients. *Journal of Pain and Symptom Management*. **28**: 497–504.

46 Hardy JR et al. (2007) Opioids in patients on renal dialysis. *Journal of Pain and Symptom Management*. **33**: 1–2.

47 Prosser JM et al. (2010) Complications of oral exposure to fentanyl transdermal delivery system patches. *Journal of Medical Toxicology*. **6**: 443–447.

48 Carson HJ et al. (2010) A fatality involving an unusual route of fentanyl delivery: Chewing and aspirating the transdermal patch. *Legal Medicine (Tokyo)*. **12**: 157–159.

49 Baxter K and Preston CL. *Stockley's Drug Interactions*. London: Pharmaceutical Press www.medicinescomplete.com (accessed April 2014).

50 Kharasch ED *et al.* (2004) Influence of hepatic and intestinal cytochrome P4503A activity on the acute disposition and effects of oral transmucosal fentanyl citrate. *Anesthesiology.* **101**: 729–737.

51 Takane H *et al.* (2005) Rifampin reduces the analgesic effect of transdermal fentanyl. *Annals of Pharmacotherpy.* **39**: 2139–2140.

52 Sasson M and Shvartzman P (2006) Fentanyl patch sufficient analgesia for only one day. *Journal of Pain and Symptom Management.* **31**: 389–391.

53 Morii H et al. (2007) Failure of pain control using transdermal fentanyl during rifampicin treatment. *Journal of Pain and Symptom Management.* **33**: 5–6.

54 Freynhagen R *et al.* (2005) Switching from reservoir to matrix systems for the transdermal delivery of fentanyl: a prospective, multicenter pilot study in outpatients with chronic pain. *Journal of Pain and Symptom Management.* **30**: 289–297.

55 Marier JF *et al.* (2006) Pharmacokinetics, tolerability, and performance of a novel matrix transdermal delivery system of fentanyl relative to the commercially available reservoir formulation in healthy subjects. *Journal of Clinical Pharmacology.* **46**: 642–653.

56 Kress HG *et al.* (2010) Transdermal fentanyl matrix patches Matrifen and Durogesic DTrans are bioequivalent. *European Journal of Pharmceutics and Biopharmaceutics.* **75**: 225–231.

57 Vielvoye-Kerkmeer A *et al.* (2000) Transdermal fentanyl in opioid-naive cancer pain patients: an open trial using transdermal fentanyl for the treatment of chronic cancer pain in opioid-naive patients and a group using codeine. *Journal of Pain and Symptom Management.* **19**: 185–192.

58 van Seventer R *et al.* (2003) Comparison of TTS-fentanyl with sustained-release oral morphine in the treatment of patients not using opioids for mild-to-moderate pain. *Current Medical Research Opinion.* **19**: 457–469.

59 Tawfik MO *et al.* (2004) Use of transdermal fentanyl without prior opioid stabilization in patients with cancer pain. *Current Medical Research Opinion.* **20**: 259–267.

60 Mercadante S *et al.* (2010) Low doses of transdermal fentanyl in opioid-naive patients with cancer pain. *Current Medical Research Opinion.* **26**: 2765–2768.

61 Chang JT *et al.* (2010) Transdermal fentanyl for pain caused by radiotherapy in head and neck cancer patients treated in an outpatient setting: a multicenter trial in Taiwan. *Japanese Journal of Clinical Oncology.* **40**: 307–312.

62 Korte W *et al.* (1996) Day-to-day titration to initiate transdermal fentanyl in patients with cancer pain: short and long term experiences in a prospective study of 39 patients. *Journal of Pain and Symptom Management.* **11**: 139–146.

63 Palliativedrugs.com (2014) Strong opioid transdermal patch monitoring chart. *Document Library.* Pain (strong opioids) www.palliativedrugs.com

64 Samal R *et al.* Efficacy and safety of a six hour continuous overlap method for converting intravenous to transdermal fentanyl in cancer pain. *Journal of Pain and Symptom Management.* **48**: 132–136.

Updated June 2014

Quick Prescribing Guide: Use of transdermal fentanyl patches

These recommendations use a dose conversion ratio for PO morphine to TD fentanyl of 100:1 and, as such, differ from those in UK SPCs. It is an approximation, and inevitably there will be individual variation.
Note: pain not relieved by morphine will generally not be relieved by fentanyl. If in doubt, seek specialist advice before prescribing TD fentanyl.

1 **Indications for using TD fentanyl instead of morphine include:**
   • intolerable undesirable effects with morphine, e.g. nausea and vomiting, constipation, hallucinations, dysphagia
   • renal failure (fentanyl has no active metabolite)
   • 'tablet phobia' or poor compliance with oral medication
   • high risk of tablet misuse/diversion.

2 TD fentanyl is contra-indicated in patients with acute (short-term) pain and in those who need rapid dose titration for severe uncontrolled pain. Generally, it is *not* recommended as a first-line strong opioid (seek specialist advice). Thus, TD fentanyl is most appropriate for patients already on a stable dose of morphine (or other strong opioid) for ⩾1 week.

3 TD fentanyl patches are available in six strengths: 12, 25, 37.5, 50, 75 and 100microgram/h for 3 days.

4 Use the table below to decide a safe starting dose for TD fentanyl, and an appropriate rescue dose. The starting dose for patients taking a weak opioid should be 12microgram/h.

5 For patients taking a dose of morphine that is not the exact equivalent of a fentanyl patch, it will be necessary to opt for a patch which is either slightly more or slightly less than the morphine dose. Thus, if the patient still has pain, round up to a higher patch strength; if pain-free and frail, round down. However, if switching because of possible opioid-induced hyperalgesia, reduce the calculated equivalent dose by 25–50%.

Comparative doses of PO morphine and TD fentanyl (based on dose ratio 100:1)

PO Morphine		SC/IV Morphine		TD Fentanyl	
mg/24h	p.r.n mg[a]	mg/24h[b]	p.r.n mg[a]	microgram/h	mg/24h
30	5	15	2.5	12	0.3
60	10	30	5	25	0.6
90	15	45	7.5	37.5	0.9
120	20	60	10	50	1.2
180	30	90	15	75	1.8
240	40	120	20	100[c]	2.4

a. using traditional 1/6 of total daily dose as p.r.n. dose
b. assuming morphine SC/IV is twice as potent as PO
c. for combinations of patches, add the p.r.n. doses together, e.g. 100 + 75microgram/h patches = 20 + 15mg morphine SC/IV = 35mg morphine SC/IV, but can round up to 40mg or down to 30mg for convenience.

6 The date of application and/or the date for renewal should be written on the patch. Apply to dry, non-inflamed, non-irradiated, hairless skin on the upper trunk or arm. Body hair may be clipped with scissors but not shaved. If the skin is washed beforehand, use only water; do not use soap and do not apply oils, cream or ointment to the area. Press patch firmly in place for at least 30 seconds. Micropore® or Tegaderm® can be used to ensure adherence. Careful removal of the patch helps to minimize local skin irritation.

7 Effective systemic analgesic concentrations are generally reached in < 12h. When converting from:

- 4-hourly PO morphine, give regular doses for the first 12h after applying the patch
- 12-hourly m/r morphine, apply the patch and the final m/r dose at the same time
- 24-hourly m/r morphine, apply the patch 12h after the final m/r dose
- CSCI/CIVI morphine, continue the infusion unchanged for 8–12h after applying the patch, then discontinue
- CSCI/CIVI fentanyl, continue the infusion unchanged for 6h after applying the patch, then discontinue.

8 Steady-state plasma concentrations of fentanyl are generally achieved in 36–48h; the patient should use p.r.n. doses liberally during the first 3 days, particularly the first 24h. Safe rescue doses of PO morphine are given in the table above.

9 After 48h, if a patient still needs 2 or more rescue doses of morphine/day, the strength of the next patch to be applied should be increased by 12–25microgram/h. (Note: with the manufacturer's recommended starting doses, about 50% of patients need to increase the patch strength after the first 3 days).

10 About 10% of patients experience opioid withdrawal symptoms when changed from morphine to TD fentanyl. These manifest with symptoms like gastric flu and last for a few days; p.r.n. doses of morphine will relieve troublesome symptoms.

11 Fentanyl is less constipating than morphine; halve the dose of laxatives when starting fentanyl and re-titrate.

12 Fentanyl may cause nausea and vomiting; if necessary, prescribe an anti-emetic, e.g. haloperidol 1.5mg stat & at bedtime.

13 In febrile patients, the rate of absorption of fentanyl increases, and may cause toxicity, e.g. drowsiness. Absorption is also enhanced by high ambient temperatures or external heat sources over the patch, e.g. electric blanket or hot-water bottle; patients should be warned about this. Patients may shower with a patch but should not soak in a hot bath.

14 Remove patches after 72h; change the position of the new patches so as to rest the underlying skin for 3–6 days.

15 A reservoir of fentanyl accumulates in the body, and significant blood concentrations persist for at least 24h after discontinuing TD fentanyl.

16 TD fentanyl is unsatisfactory in < 5% of patients. However, discontinuation is more common when TD fentanyl is used in strong opioid-naïve patients.

17 Additional or alternative analgesic approaches should be considered when the dose exceeds 300microgram/h.

18 In moribund patients, continue TD fentanyl and give additional SC morphine p.r.n. (see Table). If > 2 p.r.n. doses are required/24h, give morphine by CSCI, starting with a dose equal to the sum of the p.r.n. doses over the preceding 24h. If necessary, adjust the p.r.n. dose taking into account the total opioid dose (i.e. TD fentanyl + CSCI morphine).

19 Used patches still contain fentanyl; after removal, fold the patch with the adhesive side inwards and discard in a sharps container (hospital) or dustbin (home), and wash hands. Ultimately, any unused patches should be returned to a pharmacy.

FENTANYL (TRANSMUCOSAL) BNF 4.7.2

Relative to PO opioids, transmucosal fentanyl products are expensive (about £5–12/episode). They are more effective than placebo, but direct comparison with PO morphine, or each other, is limited. Careful patient selection, training, titration and monitoring are required to ensure optimum use. They are *not* interchangeable.

Medicine advisory boards (Scottish Medicines Consortium, All Wales Medicines Strategy Group) have recommended restricting their use to patients unsuitable for other short-acting opioids, e.g. PO morphine.

Class: Strong opioid analgesic.

Indications: Break-through (episodic) pain in patients on regular strong opioids. The use of fentanyl injection SL or nasally is off-label.

Contra-indications: Use in strong opioid-naïve patients, acute non-cancer pain (e.g. postoperative pain, migraine), severe obstructive airways disease. *Instanyl®:* previous facial radiotherapy, recurrent epistaxis.

Pharmacology

Fentanyl (*like* **morphine**) is a strong μ-opioid receptor agonist. It has a relatively low molecular weight and (*unlike* **morphine**) is lipophilic, which makes it suitable for TD (see p.403) and transmucosal administration. Multiple formulations are now authorized for the treatment of break-through (episodic) cancer pain, including a SL tablet (Abstral®), a lozenge (Actiq®), a buccal/SL tablet (Effentora®), a buccal film (Breakyl®) and nasal sprays (Instanyl®, Pecfent®). Others are in development, e.g. SL spray.[1]

Break-through cancer pain generally has a relatively rapid onset (median 5–10min) and short duration (45–60min), but ranges from < 1min to 4–6h (see p.291).[2] By comparison, PO opioids such as **morphine**, on average, take about 30–40min to achieve meaningful pain relief and have a longer duration of effect (3–6h).[3] Thus, transmucosal fentanyl products aim to provide rapid onset pain relief which better matches the time course of a typical break-through pain.

Pharmacokinetics

The transmucosal formulations range from an aqueous solution of fentanyl (Instanyl®) to combinations with bio-adhesive substances, e.g. croscarmellose (Abstral®), pectin (Pecfent®) or cellulose-based polymers (Breakyl®). The pharmacokinetic characteristics of the products vary and they are *not* interchangeable (Tables 1 and 2). Fentanyl is readily absorbed transmucosally and the bio-adhesive substances tend to *slow* its rate of absorption. Various justifications are given (e.g. to aid mucosal adherence, to attenuate the peak plasma concentration) but the fact that a novel delivery system can be patented (although not fentanyl itself) is also relevant.

With the buccal/SL products, the amount of fentanyl absorbed directly across the mucosa or swallowed varies with formulation and route of administration. About two thirds of any swallowed fentanyl will be eliminated by intestinal or hepatic first-pass metabolism. Nonetheless, significant amounts of swallowed fentanyl are absorbed, e.g. about 25%, 20% and 15% of the systemically available Actiq®, Breakyl® and Effentora® respectively is via GI absorption.[6,8,15] The effects of the GI absorption on the plasma concentration of fentanyl include producing a 'double peak', maintaining high levels for longer (e.g. > 2h) and contributing to the wide range in T_{max}.[7]

The rate and degree of absorption of fentanyl from the nasal cavity is dependent on mucosal perfusion. Vasoconstrictive nasal decongestants, e.g. **oxymetazoline**, double the time to maximum plasma concentration and halve the maximum plasma concentration of a dose of nasal fentanyl. Thus, the concurrent use of vasoconstrictive nasal decongestants with Instanyl® or Pecfent® should be avoided.

Once absorbed, fentanyl is rapidly distributed to the best perfused tissues, i.e. brain, heart, lungs, and then to fat, muscle and other tissues. Subsequently, fentanyl is redistributed between the deep tissue compartment and plasma. This pattern of rapid distribution, followed by a slower redistribution explains why fentanyl has a relatively short duration of action despite a long halflife (Tables 1 and 2). However, with repeat administration, saturation of the deep tissue compartment can occur, resulting in higher peak plasma concentrations of fentanyl and a more prolonged effect.

Table I Selected characteristics and pharmacokinetic data for oromucosal fentanyl products[a,b]

	Abstral®	Actiq®	Breakyl®	Effentora® [c]
Formulation	SL tablet	Buccal lozenge	Buccal film	Buccal/SL tablet
Dose range and presentation	100, 200, 300, 400, 600, 800microgram. Different shapes; packs of 10 or 30	200, 400, 600, 800, 1,200, 1,600microgram. On a stick, marked with dose and different colours; packs of 3 or 30	200, 400, 800microgram. Size increases with dose; marked with 2, 4, etc., packs of 10 or 28 (800microgram)	100, 200, 400, 600, 800microgram. 100 smaller in size; embossed 1, 2, etc.; packs of 4 or 28
Maximum dose/episode	800microgram	1,600microgram	1,200microgram	800microgram
Maximum frequency of use	Maximum 4 episodes/24h, ideally ≥4h apart (see Dose and use)	Maximum 4 episodes/24h, ideally ≥4h apart (see Dose and use)	Maximum 4 episodes/24h, ≥4h apart	Maximum 4 episodes/24h, ≥4h apart
Approximate cost per tablet	£5	£7	£5	£5
Time to dissolution	<2min	Applied over 15min	15–30min	Buccal 14–25min; SL quicker
Onset of action[d]	10min	15min	15min	10min
Time to peak plasma concentration, median (range)	30–60min (15–240). Longer with highest dose	Across dose range 90min (30–480)[4,5]. Longer with highest dose	60–180min (45–240). Longer with highest dose, and when 800microgram administered as 4 × 200microgram films rather than single film (150 vs. 90min)[6]	Pooled data 53min (20–240)[7]. Longer with highest dose

Table 1 Continued

	Abstral®	Actiq®	Breakyl®	Effentora® c
Plasma halflife	Mean 5–14h	Median 18h (7–49) 800microgram[4]	Mean 8–14h, longer with higher doses	Median 12h (2–44), pooled data[7]
Duration of action	≥1h	≥1h (≤3.5h reported with higher doses)[8]	≥1h	≥2h
Bio-availability	55%	50% (25% transmucosal, 25% PO)[8]	70% (50% transmucosal, 20% PO)[6]	65% (50% transmucosal, 15% PO)
Comments		Requires continual movement around the mouth; less effective if finished <15min as more is swallowed	Absorption not affected by mild (grade 1) mucositis or by heat (e.g. a hot drink)[9,10]	Absorption not affected by mild (grade 1) mucositis[11]

a. the source (i.e. healthy volunteers vs. patients) and quality (e.g. small number of subjects, whole dose range not studied, use of massage over buccal tablet) of the data varies widely
b. data based on venous blood sampling; with arterial sampling, a higher maximum concentration is achieved about 15min quicker[12]
c. pharmacokinetics are similar for either buccal or SL placement
d. earliest *statistically significant* difference between fentanyl product and placebo in mean pain intensity difference; a *clinically meaningful* difference has been variably defined and generally takes longer (see text).

Table 2 Selected characteristics and pharmacokinetic data for intranasal fentanyl products[a]

	Instanyl®	Pecfent®
Formulation	Nasal spray	Nasal spray
Dose range and presentation	50, 100, 200microgram/spray (100microL) 1 dose repeated once after 10min p.r.n.; colour coded and in single, 10 and 20 dose bottles	100, 200, 400 and 800microgram; given as 1 or 2 doses of 100 or 400microgram/spray (100microL); colour coded and in 8 and 32 dose bottles
Maximum dose/episode	400microgram	800microgram
Maximum frequency of use	Maximum 4 episodes/24h, ≥4h apart	Maximum 4 episodes/24h, ≥4h apart
Approximate cost per spray	£6; up to 1/2 require 2 doses, thus average cost up to £9	£4; about 1/2 require 200 or 800microgram dose, thus average cost = £7
Onset of action[b]	5min	10min
Time to peak plasma concentration, median (range)	Across dose range 12–15min (6–90min)[13]	Across dose range 15–21min (5–180min)[5]
Plasma halflife	Median 19h (8–30); 200microgram, 2 doses 10min apart[14]	Mean 15–25h
Duration of action	≥1h	≥1h
Bio-availability	90%	No data
Comments	Non-preserved solution, pH 6.6, osmolality ~0.9% saline	Preserved solution containing pectin, adjusted for pH and osmolality. Cmax is about 1/3 of that of Instanyl. Audible click denotes dose administered; visual priming guide and dose counter, end-of-use lock

a. the source (i.e. healthy volunteers vs. patients) and quality (e.g. small number of subjects, whole dose range not studied) of the data varies widely
b. earliest *statistically significant* difference between fentanyl product and placebo in mean pain intensity difference; a *clinically meaningful* difference has been variably defined and can take longer (see text).

Up to 85% of fentanyl is protein bound, mainly to α_1-acid glycoprotein, but also to albumin and lipoproteins. Elimination mainly involves biotransformation in the liver by CYP3A4 to inactive norfentanyl, which is excreted in the urine. Less than 7% is excreted unchanged. The SPCs of all of the transmucosal fentanyl products advise caution in their use in patients with moderate–severe hepatic or renal impairment, but this is based on limited data which suggests a reduced clearance of fentanyl, e.g. via alterations in metabolic clearance and plasma protein binding. Nonetheless, fentanyl is a reasonable option for patients with renal impairment or failure (also see p.403 and p.367),[16] including those with hepatorenal syndrome.[17]

Pharmacokinetic studies of repeat/chronic dosing of the transmucosal products are limited. Repeating three single doses of Breakyl® at 1h intervals results in a maximum plasma concentration three times higher than after a single dose.[18] Similarly, repeating a dose of Pecfent® after an interval of 1 or 2h significantly increases the maximum plasma concentration, but not when given 4h apart.[5] Accumulation of fentanyl can occur with regular use; when Abstral® (whole of dose range) or Effentora[®] (400microgram) are given q6h, steady state is reached after about 3–5 days, and the maximum plasma concentration becomes double that of the initial dose.[19,20] Thus, even when an effective and tolerable dose is identified through titration, with subsequent regular use, accumulation, and undesirable effects could occur.

Pharmacodynamics

Generally, patients recruited to the development studies for the fentanyl transmucosal products were relatively young (mean age 50–60 years), had a good performance status (ECOG PS 0–2), no clinically relevant renal or hepatic impairment and were taking regular scheduled doses of an opioid equivalent to 160–280mg morphine PO/24h. Thus, additional caution is required when giving these products to patients with characteristics which differ from this group, particularly those who are elderly. A sober critique of the published papers is also required for various reasons, including:

- many studies are sponsored by the manufacturer and thus lack impartiality
- although similar methods of evaluation are used across studies, the criteria used to define a response vary, making direct comparison difficult (see below)
- some approaches undertaken in the studies do not reflect recommended clinical practice, e.g.:
  ▷ only single doses of Abstral[®] were used for titration and maintenance in the study on which its safety data is based, with the effective dose confirmed over several consecutive episodes; by comparison, in the SPC, a second dose is permitted during titration, with no mention of confirmation of the effective dose[21]
  ▷ Effentora[®] tablet remnants were 'massaged' after 10–15min in the pharmacokinetic and some efficacy studies, potentially artificially enhancing absorption and efficacy data[22]
  ▷ patients who had already used Instanyl[®] were enrolled into an efficacy study, artificially enhancing the proportion achieving successful titration (>90% vs. more usual 60–70%)[14]
  ▷ in some instances the regulatory authorities expressed concerns about the amount and/or the quality of the data, e.g. Abstral[®] pharmacokinetic data, Instanyl[®] safety reporting.[14,23]

For speed of onset of analgesia, generally what is promoted is the earliest *statistically significant* difference in pain intensity between the fentanyl product and placebo (generally 5–15min). Although some patients report a reduction in pain intensity which is considered *clinically meaningful* by this time, this generally takes longer for most products. Reliable comparison of the different products is difficult because the definition and calculation of a clinically meaningful change varies, e.g. reduction in pain intensity score from baseline of ⩾2/10 or 30–33%, by episode (at least one or all) or by patient. Further, applying different criteria to the same data can produce different times, e.g. for Pecfent[®], half of the patients experience a reduction in pain intensity score of ⩾2 by 15min, but a ⩾33% reduction takes 30min.[5,24] (Note: it has been suggested that a ⩾50% improvement in pain intensity is required to be of *substantial* clinical importance.[25]) However, data suggest that for half of the episodes, an improvement in pain intensity of at least moderate clinical importance appears by about 10min (Instanyl[®,26]), 15min (Pecfent[®,24]) or 30min (Abstral[®,27] Actiq[®,28] Breakyl[®,29] Effentora[®,30]). Even so, in up to a quarter of episodes, an alternative rescue analgesic is needed because of an inadequate response to the fentanyl product. Clinicians must provide careful explanation to ensure the patient uses both rescue analgesics correctly.

High-quality comparative data, either between products or with PO analgesics, are limited.[31] Generally, the transmucosal products perform statistically significantly better than the immediate-release PO formulations tested, but the absolute differences in outcomes are relatively small, making their clinical relevance uncertain (Box A).

Given the mismatch between the time-action relationship of PO **morphine** and the typical time course of a break-through pain, it is interesting how well PO **morphine** performs in these studies. Unlike the fentanyl product, the PO **morphine** was not optimized in a titration phase and was given as *tablets* rather than as a *solution*, which is absorbed and acts more quickly. Studies have reported a median (range) T_{max} of 60min (20–90) vs. 125min (40–240) and mean time to meaningful pain relief of about 15min vs. 30min for morphine solution vs. tablets respectively.[37,38] Only an inadequate comparison of Abstral[®] with PO **morphine** *solution* is currently available.[39]

The lack of high quality comparative data among the transmucosal products prevents conclusions about the best to use. However, the practical aspects of using some of the products have been compared in a patient satisfaction survey.[40] Following instruction, 30 patients were asked to use a single *placebo* version of Abstral[®], Effentora[®] and Instanyl[®] and to rate factors such as ease of access from packaging, ease of administration and palatability; they also rated their current rescue analgesic (generally PO **morphine** or **oxycodone**) similarly. They were asked to

---

Box A   Higher quality active comparator studies of transmucosal fentanyl products

Actiq® vs. PO morphine tablets[28]

Actiq®, titrated to an effective dose, has been compared with morphine *tablets* (previously identified effective dose, encapsulated to maintain blinding) in a double-blind, double-dummy, multiple cross-over study. For the primary and secondary outcomes, Actiq® was statistically superior to PO morphine tablets. However, the differences were small and their clinical relevance uncertain.

For example, for Actiq® vs. PO morphine tablets, the proportion of episodes after 15min with clinical meaningful pain relief (defined as a ⩾33% reduction in pain intensity) was 42 vs. 32%. Nonetheless, >90% of patients chose to continue with Actiq®.

Effentora® vs. PO oxycodone tablets[32,33]

Effentora® titrated to an effective dose, has been compared with oxycodone *tablets* (titrated to an effective dose and encapsulated to maintain blinding) in double-blind, double-dummy, cross-over studies in opioid-tolerant patients mostly with non-cancer break-through pain (only two had cancer pain). Findings were similar in both studies; for primary and most secondary outcomes, Effentora® was statistically superior to PO oxycodone tablets. However, the differences were small and their clinical relevance uncertain.

For example, in the larger of the two studies,[32] for Effentora® vs. PO oxycodone tablets:
- mean (SD) pain intensity difference at 15min (primary outcome) was 0.8 (1.1) vs. 0.6 (0.9)
- % of episodes with a reduction in pain intensity of ⩾33% was 13 vs. 9% (15min) and 41 vs. 32% (30min); for a reduction ⩾50%, it was 6 vs. 4% (15min) and 21 vs. 16% (30min)
- patients rated the overall medication performance as 'good' to 'excellent' in 41 vs. 26% of episodes at 30min and 79 vs. 71% at 60min.

Pecfent® vs. PO morphine tablets[34,35]

Pecfent®, titrated to an effective dose, has been compared with encapsulated morphine *tablets* (one sixth of the total daily dose, or previously identified effective dose) in a double-blind, double-dummy, multiple cross-over study. For the primary and most secondary outcomes, Pecfent® was statistically superior to PO morphine tablets. However, the differences were small and their clinical relevance uncertain.

For example, for Pecfent® vs. PO morphine tablets:
- mean (SD) pain intensity difference at 15min (primary outcome) was 3.0 (0.2) vs. 2.7 (0.2)
- % of episodes with clinical meaningful pain relief (defined as a ⩾2 reduction in pain intensity) was 25 vs. 23% (5min); 52 vs. 45% (10min) and 76 vs. 69% (15min).

Instanyl® vs. Actiq® [14,36]

Instanyl® and Actiq® (both titrated to an effective dose) have been compared in an open label RCT. The primary outcome was time to meaningful pain relief, measured by stopwatch. The fastest time to meaningful pain relief was significantly more likely with Instanyl® than Actiq®, with a median difference of 5min (11 vs. 16min respectively). A second dose of Instanyl® or Actiq® was required in about 60% and 30% of episodes respectively. For Instanyl® this was permitted 10min after the first dose, and for Actiq® 15min after fully consuming the first dose, i.e. at least 30min after starting the first dose. Usual rescue analgesia was required in 5–8% of episodes. Patients found the administration of Instanyl® easier and overall preferred Instanyl® (75%) to Actiq® (25%).

---

indicate if they would be prepared to use the transmucosal product and, if so, which they felt was the best and why. Several themes emerged:
- *ease of access:* the fentanyl products were generally more difficult to access than usual rescue analgesia, particularly the child-proof container for Instanyl®
- *ease of use:* Abstral® and the usual rescue analgesia were equal best
- *palatability:* Abstral® was rated best
- *patients willing to use:* Abstral® (90%) vs. Effentora® and Instanyl® (about 60% each); three patients would not use any (did not like the product or could not open the packaging)
- *which is best and why?:*

▷ Abstral® (~70%); easy to access and use, dissolved quickly
▷ Instanyl® (~20%); quick to use (once you get into package), route familiar
▷ Effentora® (~10%); liked sensation in the mouth
▷ one could not choose between Abstral® and Effentora®.

The use of placebos means that overall satisfaction with the products could not be compared. Nonetheless, taking these practical issues and other factors into account, the PCF suggests the following in patients with cancer taking regular strong opioids and experiencing cancer-related break-through pain:

• use immediate-release PO strong opioids first-line and titrate accordingly (include a trial of a PO solution if tablets not adequate); only when inadequate with regards to speed of onset of action or prolonged undesirable effects should the transmucosal products be considered (echoed in recent NICE guidance)[41]
• a patient's circumstances should be considered carefully to ensure they fulfil the necessary requirements for use of a transmucosal product, e.g. current opioid dose, ability to access, use, store and dispose of the product reliably etc. (see Dose and use)
• decide which route and product is the most appropriate, i.e.:
  ▷ nasal: generally works quicker and shorter lasting (less PO absorption) than the SL/buccal route; Pecfent® works slightly slower than Instanyl®, but has a safer, accountable delivery system, and is cheaper
  ▷ SL/buccal: there is little to choose from in terms of efficacy; Abstral® dissolves the quickest, making it the most convenient to use. Breakyl® is less likely to cause dental caries and mucosal irritation compared with Actiq® and Effentora® respectively.

There may be other more specific reasons which guide choice of route, e.g. patient preference, presence of severe dry mouth or mucositis (use nasal), or frequent nose bleeds (use SL/buccal).

In contrast to PCF and NICE guidance,[41] European guidelines recommend that either PO or transmucosal fentanyl products can be used for break-through pain without clearly distinguishing a first-line preference.[42]

Unauthorized alternatives

As a cheaper alternative to authorized transmucosal fentanyl products, some palliative care services use the parenteral formulation of various fentanils for SL administration, e.g. fentanyl (50microgram/mL), sufentanil (50microgram/mL, not UK) and alfentanil (500microgram/mL and 5mg/mL).[43–45] Onset of analgesic effect may be broadly similar (5–10min) but duration of effect is likely to differ (fentanyl > sufentanil > alfentanil) (see Alfentanil, p.385). Several small doses can be given until pain relief is obtained. Using a 1mL graduated oral syringe:

• start with fentanyl 25–50microgram (0.5–1mL of 50microgram/mL)
• if necessary, increase to 50–100microgram; many patients do not need more than this
• doses > 100microgram are impractical because 2mL is the maximum volume that can be reliably kept in the mouth for transmucosal absorption.[44]

Drawing up the correct amount of the parenteral formulation into a syringe is inconvenient, but this can be overcome by the use of a spray bottle.[45,46]

The 50microgram/mL fentanyl injection solution has also been administered as a nasal spray. In adults this approach is limited by the large dose volume. However, it has provided effective analgesia in children 1–18 years old presenting pre-hospital or to the emergency department with acute moderate–severe pain.[47,48] A 1mL syringe attached to a mucosal atomizer device permits the appropriate amount of fentanyl to be converted into a spray. The initial dose is generally 1–2microgram/kg, administered in divided doses to a maximum of 1mL in each nostril, with some centres permitting a second dose of 0.5microgram/kg after 10min if required.[49]

To overcome the dose/volume issues, higher concentration fentanyl solutions up to 300microgram/mL have also been used. However, compared with the standard solution, they are less readily available, more expensive and, at least in children < 50kg, no more effective.[48,50] Obviously, the authorized products avoid the dose/volume issue, and the use of Instanyl® 50–100microgram by paramedics for acute severe pain has been reported.[51]

Further dilution of the 50microgram/mL fentanyl injection solution to produce 10 and 25microgram/mL solutions, has permitted 1 and 2.5microgram/0.1mL doses to be administered intranasally to dying neonates and infants with respiratory distress.[52] However, evidence supporting the use of transmucosal fentanyl to relieve breathlessness in other circumstances is limited.[53,54]

Cautions

All companies provide additional information for prescribers, pharmacists and patients; these include check-lists to ensure proper patient selection and education around use, signs of opioid overdose, safe storage and disposal. Store out of reach of children (accidental deaths have occurred).

In 2007, after reports of serious overdoses and deaths in the USA, the FDA issued a safety warning about the use of Fentora® (Effentora®). Factors which contributed to the adverse drug events included improper:
• patient selection, e.g. non-opioid tolerant, acute (non-cancer) pain
• dosing, e.g. wrong dose prescribed, exceeding recommended maximum use
• product substitution, e.g. like for like swap from Actiq® to Fentora®.
Thus, these products need to be used correctly, specifically:
• do *not* use in opioid naïve (non-tolerant) patients, including those who only take strong opioids p.r.n.
• they are contra-indicated in the management of acute or postoperative pain, including headache/migraine
• they are not interchangeable; do *not* convert patients on a microgram per microgram basis from one to another; it is necessary to titrate the new formulation
• when dispensing, do *not* substitute one product for another.

Use with caution in patients with COPD or other medical conditions predisposing them to respiratory depression (e.g. myasthenia gravis) or susceptible to the intracranial effects of hypercapnia (e.g. those with raised intracranial pressure). Also if bradyarrhythmia, elderly, cachectic, debilitated, moderate–severe hepatic or renal impairment, hypovolaemia, hypotension; and if a history or high risk of abuse or diversion.

Mouth wounds, mucositis (may enhance absorption); nasal vasoconstrictive decongestants (reduce the effect), other nasal medications (the SPC for Instanyl® recommends avoiding because of lack of data, whereas that for Pecfent® advises avoiding within 15min of a dose), epistaxis.

Actiq® contains 2g of sugars; inform diabetic patients, also risk of tooth decay (uncommon).

Drug interactions

Fentanyl is metabolized by CYP3A4. Caution is required with concurrent use of drugs which inhibit or induce these enzymes, (see Chapter 25, p.775). Reports of interactions where closer monitoring ± dose adjustment are required are listed in Table 3.[55–59]

Table 3 Interactions between fentanyl and other drugs involving CYP450

Fentanyl plasma concentration	
Increased by	*Decreased by*
Aprepitant[a]	Aprepitant[a]
Azoles, e.g. fluconazole[b], voriconazole	Carbamazepine
Cimetidine	Phenytoin
Macrolide antibiotics, e.g. clarithromycin, erythromycin	Phenobarbital
Protease inhibitors, e.g. indinavir, nelfinavir, ritonavir	Rifampicin

a. more pronounced with PO midazolam
b. monitor for excessive sedation and titrate midazolam dose accordingly (any route).

Fentanyl has been reported to reduce the metabolism of **midazolam**, reducing the clearance by 30% and extending the halflife by 50%.[59]

Fentanyl is best avoided in patients who have used a MAOI within the past 2 weeks. Although they have been used safely together, serotonin toxicity (sometimes fatal) has occurred (also see p.195), manufacturers' SPCs warn of a risk of serotonin toxicity when fentanyl is *used in combination* with other serotoninergic drugs.[59]

Undesirable effects

Also see Strong opioids, Box B, p.361.

Very common (>1/10): drowsiness, dizziness, headache, confusion, nausea, vomiting, sweating.

Topical effects: less common and formulation-dependent, but include: oral and nasal discomfort, inflammation or ulceration, rhinorrhoea, epistaxis, sore throat, dysguesia, dental caries with Actiq® (uncommon).

Dose and use

As with all opioids, patients must be monitored for undesirable effects, particularly nausea and vomiting, and constipation (see p.360). Depending on individual circumstances, an anti-emetic should be prescribed for regular or p.r.n. use, (see p.241) and, routinely, a laxative prescribed (see p.44)

For TD and SC routes of administration, see p.403.

Prescribers of transmucosal fentanyl products should:
- be experienced in the management of opioid-therapy in cancer patients
- limit use to opioid-tolerant patients who can adhere to the instructions regarding indication, administration, storage and returns
- provide ongoing supervision
- keep in mind the potential for fentanyl to be misused[60–63]
- understand that the formulations are *not* bio-equivalent and thus *not* interchangeable; when switching products, de novo titration from the lowest available dose is required.

Transmucosal fentanyl products should be used only in adults on a regular strong opioid for chronic cancer pain for ≥1 week:
- **morphine** 60mg/24h PO
- fentanyl 25microgram/h TD (50microgram/h required in some studies)
- **hydromorphone** 8mg/24h PO
- **oxycodone** 30mg/24h PO
- an equivalent dose of another opioid.

Individual titration is required because the effective dose cannot be reliably predicted from the maintenance dose of opioid[22,32,36,64–66] Despite this, the use of doses proportional to the maintenance dose has been suggested.[67]

Careful monitoring is required during initial or subsequent titration; the complexity of the titration schedules varies between products (Box B–G). Even so, transmucosal fentanyl products are unsatisfactory in about 1/4–1/3 of patients, either because they fail to provide relief at the highest practical dose or cause unacceptable undesirable effects.

The optimal dose found during successful titration (Box B–G) can be used to treat up to 4 break-through pain episodes/24h. The recommended minimum interval between treatments is generally ≥4h apart. This varies between products (e.g. Abstral® specifies ≥2h and Actiq® does not specify a minimum) and even for the same product between countries (e.g. Breakyl® and Pecfent® in the UK and USA). However, applying the ≥4h apart rule across all products would be reasonable because it was used by most studies and more frequent dosing than q4h appears to increase the maximum plasma concentration achieved with the subsequent dose of fentanyl.[5] Thus, an alternative p.r.n. analgesic, e.g. **morphine** PO, will be required to treat any additional, more frequent episodes. Further, in about 5–25% of episodes, the transmucosal products fail to provide adequate relief and an alternate analgesic is required.[66,68]

Box B   Abstral® dose and use

Follow the manufacturer's guidance on administration, titration, storage and disposal in the SPC, Prescribers guide, Dose titration guide, and Patient Information Leaflet. A hospital/ hospice referral pad for GPs is also available.

Abstral® is a SL tablet, placed in the deepest part under the tongue. The tablets must not be chewed or sucked and patients should not eat or drink until they have dissolved. Those with a dry mouth may moisten it with water beforehand. The tablet generally dissolves quickly (<5min), with the particles produced adhering to the oral mucosa from which the fentanyl is subsequently absorbed.

Evaluate each dose after 15–30min and if effective, i.e. a *single* dose provides adequate analgesia with little or no undesirable effects, this is the maintenance dose. If unsuccessful, during titration, a further dose can be given and subsequently a higher dose used for the next episode:
- start with 100microgram, if unsuccessful, give an additional 100microgram dose
- for the next episode give 200microgram, if unsuccessful, give an additional 100microgram tablet
- for the next episode give 300microgram, if unsuccessful, give an additional 100microgram tablet
- for the next episode give 400microgram, if unsuccessful, give an additional 200microgram tablet
- for the next episode give 600microgram, if unsuccessful, give an additional 200microgram tablet
- for the next episode give 800microgram, the maximum dose.

The SPC suggests that intermediate doses of 500 and 700microgram can be considered if there is adequate analgesia but undesirable effects at either the 600 or 800microgam doses. However, in practice, such doses are rarely used. It requires the use of a 100microgram tablet plus a 400 or 600microgram tablet, and doubles the cost of treating an episode (£10).

Note: in the efficacy and safety study, only single doses of Abstral® were used for titration and maintenance, with the effective dose confirmed over several consecutive episodes.[21]

More than two-thirds of patients find an effective and tolerable dose; about one quarter require 800microgram.[69] However, because of inadequate relief after 30min, an alternative rescue analgesic is needed in about 10% of episodes.[21]

A maximum of 4 break-through pain episodes/24h can be treated. In studies, this had to be ≥2h apart (each pain episode was limited to treatment with a single dose)[21,70] and is the recommended interval in the SPC; nonetheless, ≥4h apart is the ideal (see text). Regular daily use of break-through medication (traditionally ≥2/24h) should prompt a review and possible increase in the dose of the regular strong opioid. Subsequently, if a single dose of Abstral® fails to provide consistent relief, the dose should be further titrated as above.

Abstral® is generally well tolerated and remains effective. Use of a median dose of 600microgram treating a mean of 3 episodes/day for 5–6 months showed that:
- opioid-related undesirable effects (e.g. nausea) are common but not a major cause of discontinuation
- application site irritation rarely occurred
- about 75% of patients were satisfied or very satisfied with its use.[21,70]

Although only authorized for break-through cancer pain, some data exists for the use of Abstral® in non-cancer pain.[71]

Box C Actiq® dose and use

Follow the manufacturer's guidance on administration, titration, storage and disposal in the SPC, Patients and caregivers guide and Patient Information Leaflet.

Actiq® is a 'lozenge on a stick' containing fentanyl in a hard sweet matrix. In order to achieve maximum mucosal exposure to the fentanyl, the lozenge should be placed between the cheek and the gum and moved constantly up and down, and changed at intervals from one cheek to the other. It should not be chewed. The lozenge should be consumed completely over 15min; quicker than this and more fentanyl is swallowed. Patients with xerostomia (dry mouth) may find it hard to consume it in this time period.[72] If necessary, moisten the mouth with water beforehand. Initially, prescribe 6 doses of one strength at a time:

- start with fentanyl 200microgram and consume over 15min; drinking or eating is not permitted during administration
- wait 15min; if there is inadequate analgesia, use a second 200microgram lozenge
- not more than two lozenges should be used for any one episode of pain
- continue with 200microgram for a further 2 episodes of pain, allowing a second lozenge when necessary
- if on review, the break-through (episodic) pain is not controlled satisfactorily with a single 200microgram dose, increase to 400microgram
- wait 15min; use a second 400microgram lozenge if necessary
- continue this upwards titration through the available dose strengths until a *single* dose provides adequate analgesia with little or no undesirable effects; this is the maintenance dose
- the maximum dose is 1,600microgram.

The lozenge should be removed from the mouth once the pain is relieved; partly consumed lozenges should be dissolved under hot running water and the handle discarded in a waste container out of reach of children.

About three quarters of patients find an effective and tolerable dose. An alternative rescue analgesic is required in 5–15% of episodes (permitted if inadequate response 15min after Actiq® dose fully completed).

A maximum of 4 break-through pain episodes/24h can be treated. In studies, this generally had to be ≥2h apart (each pain episode was limited to treatment with a single dose);[28] ≥4h apart is the ideal (see text). Regular daily use of break-through medication (traditionally ≥2/24h) should prompt a review and possible increase in the dose of the regular strong opioid. Subsequently, if a single dose of Actiq® fails to provide consistent relief, the dose should be further titrated as detailed above.

Actiq® is generally well tolerated and remains effective. Follow up over a mean of about 3 months showed that:

- opioid-related undesirable effects are common (e.g. nausea) but not a major cause of discontinuation
- a single dose is effective in 85–90% of episodes
- about 1/2–3/4 of patients require a dose adjustment; mostly upwards, but sometimes downwards
- patient ratings of global medication performance remain the same (generally 'very good').[73,74]

Box D   Breakyl® dose and use

Follow the manufacturer's guidance on administration, titration, storage and disposal in the SPC and Patient Information Leaflet.

Breakyl® is a soluble film which is placed on the inside of the cheek. After removal from its package, Breakyl® should be used immediately to prevent it drying out. Before application, the inside of the cheek is wetted either with the tongue or by rinsing with water. Using a dry finger, the pink side of the film is held against the inside of the cheek for 5 seconds to ensure adherence to the mucosa. Subsequently, the film should not be touched or moved. Drinking is permitted after 5min, but food should be avoided until the film has dissolved completely (generally 15–30min). Most patients notice a taste, which is considered pleasant/acceptable by >90%.

Breakyl® must not be cut, torn, rubbed with the tongue, chewed or swallowed. Mild mucositis (grade 1) does not affect absorption,[9] but avoid use in more severe grades because the impact on absorption has not been examined.

Evaluate each dose after 30min and, if effective, this is the maintenance dose. If ineffective, an alternative rescue analgesic can be given. Up to four 200microgram films may be applied, two on either side of the mouth, placed so as not to overlap:

- start with 200microgram
- if unsuccessful, for the next episode, give 400microgram (2 × 200microgram films)
- if unsuccessful, for the next episode, give 600microgram (3 × 200microgram films)
- if unsuccessful, for the next episode, give 800microgram (4 × 200microgram films)
- if unsuccessful, for the next episode, increase to the maximum dose of 1,200microgram (1 × 800microgram and 1 × 400microgram).

About two thirds of patients find an effective and tolerable dose. Subsequently only a *single* film of the appropriate strength is used per episode. An alternative rescue analgesic is required in about 10–30% of episodes.

A maximum of 4 break-through pain episodes/24h can be treated. The SPC recommends ≥4h between doses. Regular daily use of break-through medication (traditionally ≥2/24h) should prompt a review and possible increase in the dose of the regular strong opioid. Subsequently, if a single dose of Breakyl® fails to provide consistent relief, the dose may require further titration as above.

Breakyl® is generally well tolerated and remains effective. Follow up over a mean of 4 months (in a study which permitted doses up to 2,400microgram) showed that:

- opioid-related undesirable effects are common (e.g. nausea) but not a major cause of discontinuation
- application site problems (e.g. pain, irritation, ulceration) are seen in <3% but are generally mild and do not necessitate discontinuation
- about three quarters of patients continue on the same dose
- patient ratings of global medication performance were 'good' to 'excellent' in 85% of episodes.[75]

Box E Effentora® dose and use

Follow the manufacturer's guidance on administration, titration, storage and disposal in the SPC, Patients and caregivers guide and Patient Information Leaflet.

Effentora® is a tablet which can be placed either buccally (between the cheek and gum near a molar tooth) or SL. Absorption is similar from both sites, but it dissolves quicker SL.[76] A dry mouth should be moistened with water beforehand. Mild mucositis (grade 1) does not affect absorption,[11] but avoid use in more severe grades because the impact on absorption has not been examined.

The tablets must not be chewed or sucked and patients should not eat or drink until they have dissolved. The time to dissolution is generally 15–25min but can be longer. However, any tablet remnants should be swallowed after 30min with a glass of water.

Evaluate each dose after 30min and, if effective, this is the maintenance dose. If unsuccessful, during the titration phase, a further dose can be given and subsequently a higher dose used for the next episode. Titration packs, each containing 4 tablets, are available; prescribing 1 pack of 100microgram and 3 packs of 200microgram is sufficient to escalate through the dose range over 5 break-through episodes:

- start with 100microgram, if unsuccessful, give an additional 100microgram dose
- for the next episode give 200microgram (2 x 100microgram tablets), if unsuccessful, give an additional 200microgram tablet
- for the next episode give 400microgram (2 x 200microgram tablets), if unsuccessful, give an additional 200microgram tablet
- for the next episode give 600microgram (3 x 200microgram tablets), if unsuccessful, give an additional 200microgram tablet
- for the next episode give the maximum dose of 800microgram (4 x 200microgram tablets).

About two thirds of patients find an effective and tolerable dose. Subsequently only a *single* dose of the appropriate strength tablet is used per episode, which can be prescribed in 28 tablet packs. An alternative rescue analgesic is required in about 10–25% of episodes.

A maximum of 4 break-through pain episodes/24h can be treated, with at least 4h between doses (including any other rescue analgesic used). Regular daily use of break-through medication (traditionally ≥2/24h) should prompt a review and possible increase in the dose of the regular strong opioid. Subsequently, if a single dose of Effentora® fails to provide consistent relief, the dose may require further titration as above.

Effentora® is generally well tolerated and remains effective. Follow up over a mean of 6 months showed that:

- opioid-related undesirable effects are common (e.g. nausea) but not a major cause of discontinuation
- application site problems (e.g. pain, irritation, ulceration) are seen in 6% and lead to discontinuation in <2%
- 70% of patients continue on the same dose
- patient ratings of global medication performance remain the same (generally 'good').[77]

Although only authorized for up to ≤800microgram in break-through cancer pain, data exist for the use of Effentora® in:

- highly opioid-tolerant cancer patients (>700mg oral morphine equivalent/24h) in doses of 1,200–3,200microgram[78]
- opioid-tolerant patients with non-cancer break-through pain, e.g. degenerative back pain, complex regional pain syndrome[32,60,79–81]
- opioid-naïve patients with severe pain attending emergency departments with possible or definite fractures or dislocations (single dose of 100microgram).[82]

The use of Effentora® in non-cancer patients is controversial, and concerns exist around safety and the potential for misuse.[60–62]

Box F   Instanyl® dose and use

Follow the guidance on priming, administration, storage and disposal in the manufacturer's SPC, Physician and Pharmacist guides, Patient brochure/Information Leaflet.

Instanyl® is a nasal spray. Not all patients feel the spray and they should be warned not to repeat the dose because of this. There is no dose counter.

Evaluate each dose after 10min and if effective, this is the maintenance dose; if unsuccessful, a maximum of one further dose can be given.

Evaluate each dose strength over 3–4 episodes; increase to the next higher strength if there is frequent need for a second dose:
- start with 50microgram in one nostril, if unsuccessful give an additional 50microgram in the other nostril
- if unsuccessful over several episodes, give 100microgram in one nostril, if necessary give an additional 100microgram in the other nostril
- if unsuccessful over several episodes, give 200microgram in one nostril, if necessary give an additional 200microgram in the other nostril; this is the *maximum* dose.

About 2/3–3/4 of patients find an effective and tolerable dose. Although the aim is to use only one dose per episode, 30–50% require a second dose. An alternative rescue analgesic is required in about 15% of episodes; this is given after waiting ⩾10min after a dose of Instanyl®.

A maximum of 4 break-through pain episodes/24h can be treated, with at least 4h between doses (including any other rescue analgesic used). Regular daily use of break-through medication (traditionally ⩾2/24h) should prompt a review and possible increase in the dose of the regular strong opioid. The dose of Instanyl® may subsequently need to be re-titrated.

Instanyl® is generally well tolerated; opioid-related undesirable effects are common (e.g. nausea) but not a major cause of discontinuation.

Instanyl® is generally well tolerated and remains effective. Follow up for ⩽3 months showed that:
- 65% of patients continue on the same dose
- <3% of patients dropped out because of drug-related undesirable effects
- 15% of patients dropped out because of a lack of efficacy.[83]

The multi-dose bottles should be stored upright in the child-resistant container for safety; if not used for >1 week, they need to be primed again by spraying a single dose in the air.

Supply

All preparations are fentanyl citrate and schedule 2 **CD**. All costs per dose for each transmucosal product are independent of strength or pack size.

Oromucosal products
Abstral® (ProStrakan)
Tablets sublingual 100microgram, 200microgram, 300microgram, 400microgram, 600microgram, 800microgram, pack sizes 10 and 30, 1 tablet = £5.

Actiq® (Flynn)
Lozenge buccal with oromucosal applicator 200microgram, 400microgram, 600microgram, 800microgram, 1,200microgram and 1,600microgram, pack sizes 3 and 30, 1 lozenge = £7.

Breakyl® (Meda)
Soluble film buccal 200microgram, 400microgram, 800microgram, pack sizes 10 and 28 (800microgram), 1 film = £5.

Box G   Pecfent® dose and use

Follow the guidance on priming, administration, storage and disposal in the manufacturer's SPC, Physician and Pharmacist guides, Patient brochure/Information Leaflet.

Pecfent® is a nasal spray. Not all patients feel the spray, but there is an audible click when the dose is administered, and the dose counter advances by one. Advise patients not to blow their nose for 1h after administration:
- start with 100microgram in one nostril
- if unsuccessful, for the next episode, give 200microgram (100microgram in each nostril)
- if uneffective, for the next episode, prescribe higher concentration formulation and give 400microgram in one nostril
- if uneffective, for the next episode, increase to the maximum dose of 800microgram (400microgram in each nostril).

Evaluate each dose after 30min and, if ineffective, an alternative rescue analgesic can be given.

If any of the above doses are effective, this should be confirmed in the next episode. About three quarters of patients find an effective and tolerable dose; an alternative rescue analgesic is needed in about 5–10% of episodes. Subsequently, if a previously effective dose fails to provide relief over several episodes, consider titration to a higher dose.

A maximum of 4 break-through pain episodes/24h can be treated, with at least 4h between doses (including any other rescue analgesic used). Regular daily use of break-through medication (traditionally ≥2/24h) should prompt a review and a possible increase in the dose of the regular strong opioid. The dose of Pecfent® may subsequently need to be re-titrated.

Pecfent® is generally well tolerated and remains effective.[24,68] Follow up over a mean of about 10 months showed that:
- 70% continued on the same dose
- <7% of patients dropped out because of drug-related undesirable effects
- <3% of patients dropped out because of a lack of efficacy.[84]

The bottles should be kept in the child-resistant container for safety; if not used for >5 days, they need to be primed again by spraying a single dose in the air. Discard 60 days after first opening.

Effentora® (Teva UK)
Tablets buccal 100microgram, 200microgram, 400microgram, 600microgram, 800microgram, pack sizes 4 and 28, 1 tablet = £5.

Intranasal products
Instanyl® (Takeda)
Nasal spray 50micrograms/metered dose spray, 100microgram/metered dose spray and 200microgram/metered dose spray, single-dose, 10 and 20 dose, 1 spray = £6.

Pecfent® (Archimedes)
Nasal spray 100microgram/metered dose spray, 400microgram/metered dose spray, 8 or 32 dose, 1 spray = £4.50; the dose required may consist of 1 or 2 sprays.

Injection
Fentanyl citrate (generic)
Injection 50microgram/mL, 2mL amp = £0.50, 10mL amp = £1.

1 Parikh N et al. (2013) Single-dose pharmacokinetics of fentanyl sublingual spray and oral transmucosal fentanyl citrate in healthy volunteers: a randomized crossover study. Clinical Therapeutics. 35: 236–243.
2 Davies A et al. (2013) Breakthrough cancer pain: an observational study of 1000 European oncology patients. Journal of Pain and Symptom Management. 46: 619–628.

3   Zeppetella G (2008) Opioids for cancer breakthrough pain: a pilot study reporting patient assessment of time to meaningful pain relief. *Journal of Pain and Symptom Management*. **35**: 563–567.

4   Darwish M et al. (2007) Absolute and relative bioavailability of fentanyl buccal tablet and oral transmucosal fentanyl citrate. *Journal of Clinical Pharmacology*. **47**: 343–350.

5   European Medicines Agency (2010) Assessment report for Pecfent. Procedure No. EMA/H/C/001164.

6   Vasisht N et al. (2010) Single-dose pharmacokinetics of fentanyl buccal soluble film. *Pain Medicine*. **11**: 1017–1023.

7   European Medicines Agency (2008) Effentora: EPAR - Scientific discussion.

8   Lichtor J et al. (1999) The relative potency of oral transmucosal fentanyl citrate compared with intravenous morphine in the treatment of moderate to severe postoperative pain. *Anesthesia and Analgesia*. **89**: 732–738.

9   Finn AL et al. (2011) Absorption and tolerability of fentanyl buccal soluble film (FBSF) in patients with cancer in the presence of oral mucositis. *Journal of Pain Research*. **4**: 245–251.

10 FDA (2009) Center for drug evaluation and research. Summary Review. Application number 22–266.

11 Darwish M et al. (2007) Absorption of fentanyl from fentanyl buccal tablet in cancer patients with or without oral mucositis: a pilot study. *Clinical Drug Investigation*. **27**: 605–611.

12 Darwish M et al. (2006) Comparison of equivalent doses of fentanyl buccal tablets and arteriovenous differences in fentanyl pharmacokinetics. *Clinical Pharmacokinetics*. **45**: 843–850.

13 Kaasa S et al. (2010) Pharmacokinetics of intranasal fentanyl spray in patients with cancer and breakthrough pain. *Journal of Opioid Management*. **6**: 17–26.

14 European Medicines Agency (2009) Assessment report for Instanyl. Procedure No. EMEA/H/C/959. London.

15 Darwish M et al. (2006) Pharmacokinetic properties of fentanyl effervescent buccal tablets: a phase I, open-label, crossover study of single-dose 100, 200, 400, and 800 microgram in healthy adult volunteers. *Clinical Therapeutics*. **28**: 707–714.

16 King S et al. (2011) A systematic review of the use of opioid medication for those with moderate to severe cancer pain and renal impairment. *Palliative Medicine*. **25**: 525–552.

17 Bosilkovska M et al. (2012) Analgesics in patients with hepatic impairment: pharmacology and clinical implications. *Drugs*. **72**: 1645–1669.

18 Vasisht N et al. (2010) Evaluation of the single- and multiple-dose fentanyl buccal soluble film in normal healthy volunteers. *Journal of Clinical Pharmacology*. **50**: 785–791.

19 Darwish M et al. (2007) Single-dose and steady-state pharmacokinetics of fentanyl buccal tablet in healthy volunteers. *Journal of Clinical Pharmacology*. **47**: 56–63.

20 Lister N et al. (2011) Pharmacokinetics, safety, and tolerability of ascending doses of sublingual fentanyl, with and without naltrexone, in Japanese subjects. *Journal of Clinical Pharmacology*. **51**: 1195–1204.

21 Rauck RL et al. (2009) Efficacy and long-term tolerability of sublingual fentanyl orally disintegrating tablet in the treatment of breakthrough cancer pain. *Current Medical Research Opinion*. **25**: 2877–2885.

22 Slatkin NE et al. (2007) Fentanyl buccal tablet for relief of breakthrough pain in opioid-tolerant patients with cancer-related chronic pain. *Journal of Supportive Oncology*. **5**: 327–334.

23 European Medicines Agency (2008) Committee for medicinal products for human use (CHMP). Opinion following article 29(4) referral for Rapinyl.

24 Portenoy RK et al. (2010) A multicenter, placebo-controlled, double-blind, multiple-crossover study of Fentanyl Pectin Nasal Spray (FPNS) in the treatment of breakthrough cancer pain. *Pain*. **151**: 617–624.

25 Dworkin RH et al. (2008) Interpreting the clinical importance of treatment outcomes in chronic pain clinical trials: IMMPACT recommendations. *Journal of Pain*. **9**: 105–121.

26 Kress HG et al. (2009) Efficacy and tolerability of intranasal fentanyl spray 50 to 200 microg for breakthrough pain in patients with cancer: a phase III, multinational, randomized, double-blind, placebo-controlled, crossover trial with a 10-month, open-label treatment period. *Clinical Therapeutics*. **31**: 1177–1191.

27 Prostraken (2010) *Personal communication*.

28 Coluzzi P et al. (2001) Breakthrough cancer pain: a randomized trial comparing oral transmucosal fentanyl citrate (OTFC) and morphine sulfate immediate release (MSIR). *Pain*. **91**: 123–130.

29 Rauck R et al. (2010) Fentanyl buccal soluble film (FBSF) for breakthrough pain in patients with cancer: a randomized, double-blind, placebo-controlled study. *Annals of Oncology*. **21**: 1308–1314.

30 Zeppetella G et al. (2010) Consistent and clinically relevant effects with fentanyl buccal tablet in the treatment of patients receiving maintenance opioid therapy and experiencing cancer-related breakthrough pain. *Pain Practice*. **10**: 287–293.

31 Zeppetella G and Davies AN (2013) Opioids for the management of breakthrough pain in cancer patients. *Cochrane Database of Systematic Reviews*. **10**: CD004311.

32 Ashburn MA et al. (2011) The efficacy and safety of fentanyl buccal tablet compared with immediate-release oxycodone for the management of breakthrough pain in opioid-tolerant patients with chronic pain. *Anesthesia and Analgesia*. **112**: 693–702.

33 Webster LR et al. (2013) Fentanyl buccal tablet compared with immediate-release oxycodone for the management of breakthrough pain in opioid-tolerant patients with chronic cancer and noncancer pain: a randomized, double-blind, crossover study followed by a 12-week open-label phase to evaluate patient outcomes. *Pain Medicine*. **14**: 1332–1345.

34 Fallon M et al. (2011) Efficacy and safety of fentanyl pectin nasal spray compared with immediate-release morphine sulfate tablets in the treatment of breakthrough cancer pain: a multicenter, randomized, controlled, double-blind, double-dummy multiple-crossover study. *Journal of Supportive Oncology*. **9**: 224–231.

35 Davies A et al. (2011) Consistency of efficacy, patient acceptability, and nasal tolerability of fentanyl pectin nasal spray compared with immediate-release morphine sulfate in breakthrough cancer pain. *Journal of Pain and Symptom Management*. **41**: 358–366.

36 Mercadante S et al. (2009) A comparison of intranasal fentanyl spray with oral transmucosal fentanyl citrate for the treatment of breakthrough cancer pain: an open label, randomised, crossover trial. *Current Medical Research Opinion*. **25**: 2805–2815.

37 Sawe J et al. (1983) Steady-state kinetics and analgesic effect of oral morphine in cancer patients. *European Journal of Clinical Pharmacology*. **24**: 537–542.

38 Freye E et al. (2007) Effervescent morphine results in faster relief of breakthrough pain in patients compared to immediate release morphine sulfate tablet. *Pain Practice*. **7**: 324–331.

39 Velazquez Rivera I et al. (2014) Efficacy of sublingual fentanyl vs. oral morphine for cancer-related breakthrough pain. *Advances in Therapy*. **31**: 107–117.

40 England R et al. (2011) How practical are transmuscosal fentanyl products for breakthrough cancer pain? Novel use of placebo formulations to survey user opinion. BMJ Supportive and Palliative Care. 1: 349–351.

41 NICE (2012) Opioids in palliative care: safe and effective prescribing of strong opioids for pain in palliative care adults. Clinical Guideline. CG104. www.nice.org.uk

42 Caraceni A et al. (2012) Use of opioid analgesics in the treatment of cancer pain: evidence-based recommendations from the EAPC. Lancet Oncology. 13: e58–68.

43 Gardner-Nix J (2001) Oral transmucosal fentanyl and sufentanil for incident pain. Journal of Pain and Symptom Management. 22: 627–630.

44 Zeppetella G (2001) Sublingual fentanyl citrate for cancer-related breakthrough pain: a pilot study. Palliative Medicine. 15: 323–328.

45 Palliativedrugs.com (2003) Hot Topics: alternatives to sublingual fentanyl. Newsletter. August: www.palliativedrugs.com

46 Duncan A (2002) The use of fentanyl and alfentanil sprays for episodic pain. Palliative Medicine. 16: 550.

47 Hansen MS and Dahl JB (2013) Limited evidence for intranasal fentanyl in the emergency department and the prehospital setting–a systematic review. Danish Medical Journal. 60: A4563.

48 Mudd S (2011) Intranasal fentanyl for pain management in children: a systematic review of the literature. Journal of Pediatric Health Care. 25: 316–322.

49 Cole J et al. (2009) Intranasal fentanyl in 1-3-year-olds: a prospective study of the effectiveness of intranasal fentanyl as acute analgesia. Emergency Medicine Australasia. 21: 395–400.

50 Borland M et al. (2011) Equivalency of two concentrations of fentanyl administered by the intranasal route for acute analgesia in children in a paediatric emergency department: a randomized controlled trial. Emergency Medicine Australasia. 23: 202–208.

51 Karlsen AP et al. (2013) Safety of Intranasal Fentanyl in the Out-of-Hospital Setting: A Prospective Observational Study. Annals of Emergency Medicine.

52 Harlos MS et al. (2013) Intranasal fentanyl in the palliative care of newborns and infants. Journal of Pain amd Symptom Management. 46: 265–274.

53 Simon ST et al. (2013) Fentanyl for the relief of refractory breathlessness: a systematic review. Journal of Pain and Symptom Management. 46: 874–886.

54 Pinna MA et al. (2013) A Randomized Crossover Clinical Trial to Evaluate the Efficacy of Oral Transmucosal Fentanyl Citrate in the Treatment of Dyspnea on Exertion in Patients With Advanced Cancer. American Journal of Hospice and Palliative Care.

55 Kharasch ED et al. (2004) Influence of hepatic and intestinal cytochrome P4503A activity on the acute disposition and effects of oral transmucosal fentanyl citrate. Anesthesiology. 101: 729–737.

56 Takane H et al. (2005) Rifampin reduces the analgesic effect of transdermal fentanyl. Annals of Pharmacotherpy. 39: 2139–2140.

57 Sasson M and Shvartzman P (2006) Fentanyl patch sufficient analgesia for only one day. Journal of Pain and Symptom Management. 31: 389–391.

58 Morii H et al. (2007) Failure of pain control using transdermal fentanyl during rifampicin treatment. Journal of Pain and Symptom Management. 33: 5–6.

59 Baxter K and Preston CL. Stockley's Drug Interactions. London: Pharmaceutical Press www.medicinescomplete.com (accessed April 2014).

60 Fine PG et al. (2010) Long-term safety and tolerability of fentanyl buccal tablet for the treatment of breakthrough pain in opioid-tolerant patients with chronic pain: an 18-month study. Journal of Pain and Symptom Management. 40: 747–760.

61 Markman JD (2008) Not so fast: the reformulation of fentanyl and breakthrough chronic non-cancer pain. Pain. 136: 227–229.

62 Passik SD et al. (2011) Aberrant Drug-Related Behavior Observed During Clinical Studies Involving Patients Taking Chronic Opioid Therapy for Persistent Pain and Fentanyl Buccal Tablet for Breakthrough Pain. Journal of Pain and Symptom Management. 41: 116–125.

63 Nunez-Olarte JM and Alvarez-Jimenez P (2011) Emerging opioid abuse in terminal cancer patients taking oral transmucosal fentanyl citrate for breakthrough pain. Journal of Pain and Symptom Management. 42: e6–8.

64 Christie J et al. (1998) Dose-titration, multicenter study of oral transmucosal fentanyl citrate for the treatment of breakthrough pain in cancer patients using transdermal fentanyl for persistent pain. Journal of Clinical Oncology. 16: 3238–3248.

65 Portenoy R et al. (1999) Oral transmucosal fentanyl citrate (OTFC) for the treatment of breakthrough pain in cancer patients: a controlled use titration study. Pain. 79: 303–312.

66 Portenoy RK et al. (2006) A randomized, placebo-controlled study of fentanyl buccal tablet for breakthrough pain in opioid-treated patients with cancer. Clinical Journal of Pain. 22: 805–811.

67 Mercadante S et al. (2013) The use of fentanyl buccal tablets for breakthrough pain by using doses proportional to opioid basal regimen in a home care setting. Supportive Care Cancer in Cancer. 21: 2335–2339.

68 Portenoy RK et al. (2010) Long-term safety, tolerability, and consistency of effect of fentanyl pectin nasal spray for breakthrough cancer pain in opioid-tolerant patients. Journal of Opioid Management. 6: 319–328.

69 Nalamachu SR et al. (2012) Successful dose finding with sublingual fentanyl tablet: combined results from 2 open-label titration studies. Pain Practice 12: 449–456.

70 Nalamachu S et al. (2011) Long-term effectiveness and tolerability of sublingual fentanyl orally disintegrating tablet for the treatment of breakthrough cancer pain. Current Medical Research Opinion. 27: 519–530.

71 Guitart J et al. (2013) Efficacy and safety of sublingual fentanyl orally disintegrating tablets in patients with breakthrough pain: multicentre prospective study. Clinical Drug Investigation. 33: 675–683.

72 Davies AN and Vriens J (2005) Oral transmucosal fentanyl citrate and xerostomia. Journal of Pain and Symptom Management. 30: 496–497.

73 Payne R et al. (2001) Long-term safety of oral transmucosal fentanyl citrate for breakthrough cancer pain. Journal of Pain and Symptom Management. 22: 575–583.

74 Hanks GW et al. (2004) Oral transmucosal fentanyl citrate in the management of breakthrough pain in cancer: an open, multicentre, dose-titration and long-term use study. Palliative Medicine. 18: 698–704.

75 Meda Pharmaceuticals Ltd (2012) Personal communication.

76 Darwish M et al. (2008) Bioequivalence following buccal and sublingual placement of fentanyl buccal tablet 400 microg in healthy subjects. Clinical Drug Investigation. 28: 1–7.

77 Weinstein SM et al. (2009) Fentanyl buccal tablet for the treatment of breakthrough pain in opioid-tolerant patients with chronic cancer pain: A long-term, open-label safety study. Cancer. 115: 2571–2579.

78 Mercadante S et al. (2011) Fentanyl buccal tablets for breakthrough pain in highly tolerant cancer patients: preliminary data on the proportionality between breakthrough pain dose and background dose. Journal of Pain and Symptom Management. 42: 464–469.

79 Simpson DM et al. (2007) Fentanyl buccal tablet for the relief of breakthrough pain in opioid-tolerant adult patients with chronic neuropathic pain: a multicenter, randomized, double-blind, placebo-controlled study. Clinical Therapy. 29: 588–601.

80 Portenoy RK et al. (2007) Fentanyl buccal tablet (FBT) for relief of breakthrough pain in opioid-treated patients with chronic low back pain: a randomized, placebo-controlled study. Current Medical Research Opinion. 23: 223–233.

81 Farrar JT et al. (2010) A novel 12-week study, with three randomized, double-blind placebo-controlled periods to evaluate fentanyl buccal tablets for the relief of breakthrough pain in opioid-tolerant patients with noncancer-related chronic pain. Pain Medicine. 11: 1313–1327.

82 Shear ML et al. (2010) Transbuccal fentanyl for rapid relief of orthopedic pain in the ED. American Journal of Emergency Medicine. 28: 847–852.

83 Kongsgaard UE et al. (2014) The use of Instanyl(R) in the treatment of breakthrough pain in cancer patients: a 3-month observational, prospective, cohort study. Supportive Care in Cancer 22: 1655–1662.

84 Taylor D et al. (2014) A report on the long-term use of fentanyl pectin nasal spray in patients with recurrent breakthrough pain. Journal of Pain Symptom Management 47: 1001–1007.

Updated June 2014

HYDROMORPHONE   BNF 4.7.2

Class: Opioid analgesic.

Indications: Severe pain in cancer; †an alternative in cases of intolerance to other strong opioids.[1,2]

Contra-indications: None absolute if titrated carefully against a patient's pain. (Also see Cautions below, and Strong opioids, p.357).

Pharmacology

Hydromorphone is an analogue of **morphine** with similar pharmacokinetic and pharmacodynamic properties.[3] Thus, it is both analgesic and antitussive. Hydromorphone, **morphine** and **oxycodone** are comparable in terms of analgesic efficacy, although differ in potency.[1,2] Undesirable effects are similar but, as with all opioids, these can vary in severity between individuals. Hydromorphone can be used as an alternative in cases of intolerance to **morphine** or another opioid.[1]

PO hydromorphone is absorbed mainly in the small intestine. As with **morphine**, bio-availability is subject to wide inter-individual variation.[4] Hydromorphone is metabolized in the liver by 6-ketoreduction with subsequent glucuronidation. The main metabolite is hydromorphone-3-glucuronide (H3G). All the metabolites are renally excreted and can accumulate in renal impairment.[5]

H3G has no analgesic activity but is estimated to be about 2.5 times more potent than morphine-3-glucuronide as a neuro-excitant.[6] In animal studies, dose-dependent allodynia, myoclonus, and seizures are seen.[7] Neurotoxicity (e.g. tremor, myoclonus, delirium) has been reported with hydromorphone, generally with higher doses and/or renal impairment.[8]

Hydromorphone is available in PO (immediate-release, modified-release) and injectable formulations (not UK). Compared with **morphine**, hydromorphone costs more. However, hydromorphone is more soluble than **morphine**, and is available as a high concentration injection (50mg/mL). Because hydromorphone is more potent (see below), this permits a high dose to be delivered in a small volume. Thus, in countries where **diamorphine** (p.383) is not available, hydromorphone is used CSCI, particularly when higher doses are required.

An osmotic-release oral delivery system (OROS®) for once daily administration has been developed, but as yet is unauthorized in the UK and Ireland. This 'extended-release' hydromorphone displays dose-dependent linear pharmacokinetics which are not significantly affected by food or alcohol.[9,10]

According to the UK manufacturer, hydromorphone PO and SC/IM is about 7.5 times more potent than **morphine**,[11,12] and this accounts for the choice of capsule content (1.3mg and 2.6mg; stated to be equivalent to **morphine** 10mg and 20mg PO respectively). However, independent reviews and guidelines recommend that when switching from **morphine** to hydromorphone, a conversion ratio of 5:1 is used, i.e. the hydromorphone dose should be one fifth of the **morphine** dose.[2,13] (Also see Opioid switching, p.365 and Chapter 15, Table 1, p.663).

Bio-availability 37–62% PO.[4]

Onset of action <5min IV;[14] 15min SC/IM; 30min PO.[15]

Time to peak plasma concentration 45min PO.[16]

Plasma halflife 2.5h early phase, with a prolonged late phase.

Duration of action 4–5h immediate-release; 12–24h m/r (product-dependent).[17–19]

Cautions

In 2005, the FDA warned that the concurrent ingestion of alcohol could hasten the release of hydromorphone from one m/r product resulting in 'dose dumping', i.e. a rapid rise in plasma concentrations. In 2011, the EMEA reported the results of a review of the interaction between alcohol and opioid m/r mechanisms, and concluded that the risk is minor for most m/r products except those using polymethylmethacrylate-triethylcitrate (none in the UK).[20]

The SPC for hydromorphone lists hepatic impairment as a contra-indication. In moderate hepatic impairment, because of increased bio-availability, both C_{max} and overall exposure to hydromorphone (i.e. the AUC) are quadrupled, but halflife is unchanged. Thus, lower than usual starting doses given at standard time intervals are advised.[21,22] With severe liver impairment, the halflife could increase, and the dosing interval may need to be increased. Hydromorphone is advised against in hepatorenal syndrome because of the additional impact of the renal impairment.[22]

In patients with moderate renal impairment, the AUC is about doubled; in severe impairment AUC is quadrupled and the halflife more than doubled.[23] Thus, lower than usual starting doses are advised in moderate or severe renal impairment, along with increased dosing intervals in the latter.

Despite the risk of accumulation of H3G and other glucuronide metabolites, hydromorphone is successfully used in some centres as a preferred strong opioid in severe renal impairment (see p.367).[5]

Haemodialysis reduces plasma concentrations of hydromorphone by about one-half, which could result in worsening pain or symptoms of opioid withdrawal.[24] Treat with a dose of an immediate-release formulation; if recurrent, consider giving a prophylactic dose at the start of each session of dialysis.

Undesirable effects
Also see Strong opioids, Box B, p.361.

Dose and use

As with all opioids, patients must be monitored for undesirable effects, particularly nausea and vomiting, and constipation (see p.360). Depending on individual circumstances, an anti-emetic should be prescribed for regular or p.r.n. use, (see p.241) and, routinely, a laxative prescribed (see p.44).

PO hydromorphone is used in the same way as PO **morphine**, generally q4h as immediate-release capsules or q12h as m/r capsules; both formulations can be swallowed whole or, if necessary, opened and the contents sprinkled on a small amount of soft food, e.g. yoghurt. Note:
- the m/r granules should not be crushed or chewed because this could lead to a rapid release of an overdose (see Chapter 22, Box B, p.728)
- when converting hydromorphone from PO to SC, use half the PO dose
- if given byCSCI, high potency ampoules can be used (unauthorized in the UK)
- for CSCI dilute with WFI, 0.9% saline or 5% glucose.

CSCI compatibility with other drugs: Although most data are for dilution in 0.9% saline, there are 2-drug compatibility data for hydromorphone in WFI with **glycopyrronium, hyoscine butylbromide, hyoscine hydrobromide, ketamine, levomepromazine metoclopramide** and **midazolam**.

Concentration-dependent *incompatibility* may occur with **cyclizine, dexamethasone, haloperidol** and **ketorolac**. For more details and 3-drug compatibility data, see Appendix 3 Chart 1, p.824 and Chart 4, p.830.

Compatibility charts for mixing drugs in 0.9% saline can be found in the extended appendix of the on-line PCF on www.palliativedrugs.com.

In the UK, hydromorphone is unlikely to be used primarily as an antitussive but theoretically could be (see Antitussives, p.142).

Supply

Unless indicated otherwise, all products are **CD**.

Immediate-release oral formulation
Palladone® (Napp)
Capsules 1.3mg, 2.6mg, 1.3mg dose = £0.16.

Modified-release oral formulation
Palladone® SR (Napp)
Capsules enclosing m/r granules 2mg, 4mg, 8mg, 16mg, 24mg, 28 days @ 2mg, 8mg or 24mg every 12h = £21, £56 and £160 respectively.

Parenteral formulation
Hydromorphone hydrochloride
Injection 10mg/mL, 1mL amp = £9; 20mg/mL, 1mL amp = £11; high-potency 50mg/mL, 1mL amp = £13. (Unauthorized, available as a special order from Martindale; See Appendix 1).

1 Pigni A et al. (2011) The role of hydromorphone in cancer pain treatment: a systematic review. Palliative Medicine. **25**: 471–477.
2 Caraceni A et al. (2012) Use of opioid analgesics in the treatment of cancer pain: evidence-based recommendations from the EAPC. Lancet Oncology. **13**: e58–68.
3 Quigley C and Glare P (2009) Hydromorphone. In: M Davis et al. (eds) Opioids in Cancer Pain (2e). Oxford University Press, Oxford, pp. 245–252.
4 Vallner J et al. (1981) Pharmacokinetics and bioavailability of hydromorphone following intravenous and oral administration to human subjects. Journal of Clinical Pharmacology. **21**: 152–156.
5 King S et al. (2011) A systematic review of the use of opioid medication for those with moderate to severe cancer pain and renal impairment. Palliative Medicine. **25**: 525–552.
6 Wright AW et al. (2001) Hydromorphone-3-glucuronide: a more potent neuro-excitant than its structural analogue, morphine-3-glucuronide. Life Sciences. **69**: 409–420.
7 Babul N and Darke AC (1992) Putative role of hydromorphone metabolites in myoclonus. Pain. **51**: 260–261.
8 Paramanandam G et al. (2011) Adverse effects in hospice patients with chronic kidney disease receiving hydromorphone. Journal of Palliative Medicine. **14**: 1029–1033.
9 Hale ME et al. (2012) Safety and tolerability of OROS(R) hydromorphone ER in adults with chronic noncancer and cancer pain: pooled analysis of 13 studies. Journal of Opioid Management. **8**: 299–314.
10 Vandenbossche J et al. (2012) Repeat-dose steady-state pharmacokinetic evaluation of once-daily hydromorphone extended-release (OROS((R)) hydromorphone ER) in patients with chronic pain. Journal of Pain Research. **5**: 523–533.
11 McDonald C and Miller A (1997) A comparative potency study of a controlled release tablet formulation of hydromorphone with controlled release morphine in patients with cancer pain. European Journal of Palliative Care Abstracts of the Fifth Congress.
12 Moriarty M et al. (1999) A randomised crossover comparison of controlled release hydromorphone tablets with controlled release morphine tablets in patients with cancer pain. Journal of Clinical Research. **2**: 1–8.
13 Mercadante S and Caraceni A (2011) Conversion ratios for opioid switching in the treatment of cancer pain: a systematic review. Palliative Medicine. **25**: 504–515.
14 Coda B et al. (1997) Hydromorphone analgesia after intravenous bolus administration. Pain. **71**: 41–48.
15 Benedetti CB and Butler SH (1990) Systemic analgesics. In: Bonica J.J (ed) The Management of Pain. Lea and Febiger, Philedelphia.
16 Durnin C et al. (2001) Pharmacokinetics of oral immediate-release hydromorphone (Dilaudid IR) in young and elderly subjects. Proceedings of the Western Pharmacology Society. **44**: 79–80.
17 Hagen N et al. (1995) Steady-state pharmacokinetics of hydromorphone and hydromorphone-3-glucuronide in cancer patients after immediate and controlled-release hydromorphone. Journal of Clinical Pharmacology. **35**: 37–44.
18 Bruera E et al. (1996) A randomized, double-blind, double-dummy, crossover trial comparing the safety and efficacy of oral sustained-release hydromorphone with immediate-release hydromorphone in patients with cancer pain. Canadian Palliative Care Clinical Trials Group. Journal of Clinical Oncology. **14**: 1713–1717.
19 Hays H et al. (1994) Comparative clinical efficacy and safety of immediate release and controlled release hydromorphone for chronic severe cancer pain. Cancer. **74**: 1808–1816.
20 European Medicines Agency (2010) Concludes review of modified-release oral opioids of the WHO level III. Available from: www.ema.europa.eu/ema/index.jsp?curl = pages/medicines/human/public_health_alerts/2010/09/human_pha_detail_000008.jsp&murl = menus/medicines/medicines.jsp&mid = WC0b01ac058001d126
21 Durnin C et al. (2001) Pharmacokinetics of oral immediate-release hydromorphone (Dilaudid IR) in subjects with moderate hepatic impairment. Proceedings of the Western Pharmacology Society. **44**: 83–84.

22 Bosilkovska M et al. (2012) Analgesics in patients with hepatic impairment: pharmacology and clinical implications. *Drugs.* **72**: 1645–1669.

23 Durnin C et al. (2001) Pharmacokinetics of oral immediate-release hydromorphone (Dilaudid IR) in subjects with renal impairment. *Proceedings of the Western Pharmacology Society.* **44**: 81–82.

24 Perlman R et al. (2013) Intradialytic clearance of opioids: methadone versus hydromorphone. *Pain.* **154**: 2794–2800.

Updated June 2014

*METHADONE   BNF 4.7.2

Class: Strong opioid analgesic.

Methadone should be used as a strong opioid analgesic only by those fully conversant with its pharmacology.[1] It is generally best reserved for patients who fail to respond well to **morphine** or another μ-opioid receptor agonist. Important facts about methadone include:

- a widely variable plasma halflife
- dosing which is more complicated than for other strong opioids
- metabolism which is modified to a clinically important extent by other drugs which may be used in palliative care
- an association with a potentially fatal cardiac arrhythmia (see Cautions below and Chapter 24, p.759).

In addition, because methadone is used to treat opioid addiction, there is a social stigma attached to its use.

Indications: Moderate–severe pain, cough, †an alternative in cases of intolerance to other strong opioids, †**morphine** poorly-responsive pain, †pain relief in severe renal impairment.[2,3] Also treatment of opioid addiction.

Contra-indications: None absolute if titrated carefully against a patient's pain (also see Strong opioids, p.357).

Pharmacology

Methadone is a synthetic strong opioid with mixed properties.[4,5] Thus, it is a μ-opioid receptor agonist, possibly a δ-opioid receptor agonist,[6] an NMDA-receptor-channel blocker,[7,8] and a pre-synaptic blocker of serotonin re-uptake.[9] It also has immunomodulatory and anti-inflammatory effects.[10] Methadone is a racemic mixture (R- and S-enantiomers); R-methadone is responsible for most of the analgesic and undesirable effects, whereas S-methadone is antitussive and has a more potent effect on cardiac conduction. Methadone is a non-acidic and lipophilic drug which is generally well absorbed from all routes of administration. However, PO bio-availability shows wide variation, in part explained by methadone being a substrate for p-glycoprotein (see Chapter 25 p.767).

Partly because of its lipid-solubility methadone has a high volume of distribution with only about 1% of the drug in the blood.[11] Methadone accumulates in tissues when given repeatedly, creating an extensive reservoir.[12] Protein-binding (principally to a glycoprotein) is 60–90%;[13] this is double that of **morphine**. Both volume of distribution and protein-binding contribute to the long plasma halflife (it takes 4–7 days to achieve steady state), and accumulation is a potential problem. Methadone is metabolized mainly in the liver by cytochrome P450 to several inactive metabolites.[14] About half of the drug and its metabolites are excreted by the intestines and half by the kidneys, most of the latter unchanged.[15] Renal and hepatic impairment do not affect methadone clearance.[16,17] Even so, in renal and hepatic failure (see Chapter 14, p.639), it is generally best to reduce the starting dose, e.g. by at least 50%, and titrate according to response.

In single doses, methadone PO is about one half as potent as IM,[18] and IM a single dose of methadone is marginally more potent than **morphine**. With repeated doses, methadone is several times more potent and longer-acting; analgesia lasts 8–12h and sometimes more.[19,20] There is no single potency ratio between methadone and **morphine**. When patients with inadequate pain relief or undesirable effects with **morphine** are switched, the eventual 24h dose of methadone is typically 5–10 times smaller than the previous dose of **morphine**, but sometimes 20–30 times smaller, and occasionally even smaller.[21–25] The potency ratio tends to increase as the dose of **morphine** increases, i.e. proportionately less methadone is required as the **morphine** dose increases.[22–25]

When considering the use of methadone, the difficulty of a subsequent switch from methadone to another opioid should also be borne in mind. For such switches, typically the PO **morphine** equivalent dose will be 5–10 times greater than the PO methadone dose with a wide range again reported, e.g. from 1–75 times.[22,26] Thus, it is prudent to use conservative dose calculations and monitor the patient closely.

Methadone is used in several different settings. RCT evidence is limited for both cancer and non-cancer pain, and insufficient for meta-analysis.[27–29] Nonetheless, when used first-line in cancer pain, methadone appears to provide similar analgesia to **morphine** but, in some studies, more undesirable effects.[1] For example, in one RCT, 20% of patients allocated to PO methadone 7.5mg b.d. discontinued treatment compared with 5% of those who received **morphine** 15mg b.d. Half of the withdrawals occurred in the first week, and most were because of sedation or nausea. For patients remaining in the study, there was no difference in efficacy or undesirable effects.[20] This suggests that a smaller starting dose of PO methadone (e.g. 2.5–5mg b.d., or even 1–2mg b.d.) would have been more appropriate.[30,31] Indeed, in one large case series of patients with cancer and non-cancer pain receiving methadone first-line, the median effective PO dose was 2.5mg b.d., with only 20% requiring ≥10mg/24h.[32]

Second-line, patients who experience inadequate analgesia with **morphine**, with or without unacceptable undesirable effects such as nausea, vomiting, hallucinations or sedation, when switched to relatively low-dose methadone can obtain good relief with few undesirable effects.[33–35] Patients who experience more specific neurotoxicity with **morphine**, e.g. hyperalgesia, allodynia and/or myoclonus ± sedation and delirium, generally also benefit by switching to methadone. However, switching to other opioids also helps.[36–39] Thus, when switching from **morphine**, it would seem sensible to choose an opioid which is easier and safer to use than methadone, e.g. **oxycodone**, **hydromorphone**, **fentanyl**.

Methadone is an alternative strong opioid for patients with severe renal impairment at risk of excessive drowsiness ± delirium with **morphine** because of accumulation of morphine-6-glucuronide.[3] Methadone is poorly removed by haemodialysis.[40] However, for moribund patients, **alfentanil** or **fentanyl** are probably better choices (see p.367). Methadone can also be used as a strong opioid analgesic in former opioid addicts who are being maintained on methadone.[41,42] The once daily maintenance dose (typically 60–120mg) is halved and given q12h and subsequently titrated as necessary. Successful use of a locally prepared TD gel has been described in patients unable to tolerate administration by other routes.[43]

Methadone has been successfully used for cancer break-through (episodic) pain, either PO or SL (1mL of extemporaneously produced solutions ranging 1–40mg/mL held for 2min); the average time to meaningful pain relief is 30min and 10min respectively.[44,45] However, given that the time to peak plasma concentration takes ≤4h, together with a long halflife and duration of action, this approach is unsuitable for patients with frequent short-lasting episodes of break-through pain.

Bio-availability 80% (range 40–100%) PO.

Onset of action <30min PO, 15min IM.

Time to peak plasma concentration 4h PO; 1h IM.

Plasma halflife highly variable, mean 20–35h (range 5–130h);[46] longer in older patients; acidifying the urine results in a shorter halflife (20h) and raising the pH with sodium bicarbonate a longer halflife (>40h).[47]

Duration of action 4–5h PO and 3–5h IM single dose; 8–12h repeated doses.

Cautions

In 2006, after a review of deaths and life-threatening adverse events (e.g. respiratory depression, cardiac arrhythmia) associated with unintentional overdose, drug interactions, and prolongation of the QT interval, the FDA in the USA issued a safety warning about the use of methadone. This highlighted the need for:
- physicians to be fully aware of the pharmacology of methadone

- close monitoring of the patient when starting methadone, particularly when switching from a high dose of another opioid
- slow dose titration, and close monitoring of the patient when changing the dose of methadone
- warning the patient not to exceed the prescribed dose.

Because methadone generally has a long plasma halflife, accumulation to a variable extent should be anticipated, particularly in the elderly. Drowsiness and respiratory depression may develop after several days/weeks on a steady dose. PCF recommends p.r.n. dose titration to minimize the risk of this occurring (see below).[48]

QT interval prolongation and, rarely, a serious ventricular arrhythmia (torsade de pointes) have been observed during treatment with methadone. Generally, the latter is associated with, but not limited to, higher dose treatment (> 120mg/24h) (see Chapter 24, p.759).[49] The SPC recommends that methadone is administered with caution to patients at risk of developing QT prolongation, e.g. those with:

- a history of cardiac conduction abnormalities
- a family history of sudden death
- advanced heart disease or ischaemic heart disease
- liver disease
- electrolyte abnormalities
- concurrent treatment with drugs which:
  ▷ may cause electrolyte abnormalities
  ▷ have a potential to prolong QT
  ▷ inhibit CYP3A4.

Note: the IV formulation of methadone in the USA (but not the UK), contains a preservative chlorobutanol, which has an additive QT prolonging effect.[50]

The risk this rare but potentially fatal cardiac complication poses must be considered in the context of the patient's circumstances. A commonsense approach should prevail, and ECG monitoring will be largely irrelevant in the last days of life. On the other hand, for a patient with a prognosis of several months or longer, it may be appropriate to identify any risk factors for QT prolongation and consider ECG ± electrolyte monitoring (see Chapter 24, p.759).

Even so, research is needed to establish the magnitude of the risk of torsade de pointes with methadone, and the overall value of monitoring in the palliative care setting.[49]

Plasma levels of methadone are increased in CYP2D6 poor metabolizers resulting in a greater risk of undesirable effects, including fatal overdose.[51] Similarly, plasma levels of S-methadone are increased in CYP2B6 poor metabolizers which, because it is a more potent blocker of the potassium channels in the cardiac myocytes than R-methadone, may increase their risk of prolonged QTc and arrhythmia (also see Chapter 25, p.767).[52]

Drug interactions

Methadone is metabolized by several cytochrome P450 iso-enzymes, mainly CYP3A4 and CYP2B6, with CYP2D6, CYP2C9, CYP2C19, and CYP1A2 also involved to varying degrees; this differs between the enantiomers with CYP3A4 and CYP2B6 preferentially metabolizing R-methadone and S-methadone respectively. Clinically relevant and well-established CYP-related drug-drug interactions are listed in Table 1. Note particularly that **carbamazepine, phenobarbital, phenytoin, rifampicin** and **St John's wort** increase the metabolism of methadone, and may reverse previously satisfactory pain relief, or even precipitate withdrawal symptoms.[53,54] Conversely, methadone overdose has occurred when such inducers have been stopped, including after cessation of smoking (polycyclic aromatic hydrocarbons in tobacco smoke are CYP1A2 inducers).[55]

Symptomatic bradycardia has been reported in a patient on **thalidomide** given methadone.[56] Avoid concurrent use with other drugs that prolong the QT interval.

Risk of serotonin toxicity when used in combination with other serotoninergic drugs, e.g. **selegiline**, SSRIs, see Antidepressants, Box B, p.195.

The concurrent use of MAOIs and methadone is contra-indicated in the SPC, however see Strong opioids, p.362.

Table I Cytochrome P450 interactions with methadone resulting in changed drug plasma concentrations[53]

Methadone increased by	Methadone decreased by	Increased by methadone	Decreased by methadone
SSRIs	Carbamazepine	Desipramine	Amprenavir
Cimetidine	Phenobarbital	Zidovudine (AZT)	
Ciprofloxacin	Phenytoin		
Diazepam (high-dose)	Rifampicin		
Itraconazole	St John's wort		
Fluconazole	Antiretroviral, e.g. abacavir,		
Voriconazole	amprenavir, efavirenz,		
	lopinavir, nelfinavir,		
	nevirapine, ritonavir,		
	saquinavir,		
	telaprevir, tipranavir		
	Tobacco smoking		

Undesirable effects

See Strong opioids, Box B, p.361. Methadone may occasionally cause neurotoxicity, e.g. myoclonus,[57] or more florid opioid-induced hyperalgesia.[58,59] Local erythema and induration when given by CSCI.[60]

Rarely, hypoglycaemia (in a patient receiving IV methadone; animal work confirms a dose-related effect)[61,62] and sensorineural hearing loss (generally following overdose; can be permanent).[63,64]

Dose and use

As with all opioids, monitor for undesirable effects, particularly nausea and vomiting, and constipation (see p.360). Depending on individual circumstances, an anti-emetic should be prescribed for regular or p.r.n. use (see p.241) and a laxative prescribed routinely (see p.44).

Because of the wide interindividual variation in the pharmacokinetics of methadone, dose titration is different from **morphine**. Several methods exist for switching from **morphine** to methadone, but none has been shown to be definitely superior.[22] However, all require practitioners to be experienced in the use of methadone and close observation of the patient, generally as an inpatient.[3,21,33–35,65–69] Some have reported carefully controlled outpatient regimens, but pain relief can take weeks rather than days to achieve.[66,69]

With methadone, the implication of its large volume of distribution must be considered. During the first few days, while the body tissues become saturated, a greater daily dose of methadone will be required for satisfactory analgesia than subsequently; once saturation is complete, a smaller daily dose of methadone will then be sufficient. Continuing on the initial daily dose is likely to result in sedation after a few days, and possibly respiratory depression and even death.[70,71]

PCF favours a 'stop and go' approach, i.e. the abrupt cessation of the **morphine** and introduction of methadone p.r.n. (see, p.440). These guidelines are an evolution from earlier ones, incorporating feedback to www.palliativedrugs.com from clinicians.[3,21,72] A single loading dose aids tissue saturation and helps to reduce the number of p.r.n. doses required in the first 48h.[21] The recommendations may be overcautious but are safer, particularly in the elderly and for those switching from large doses of **morphine**.

Several other methods for switching from **morphine** or from another strong opioid have been published, some with supporting pharmacokinetic data.[34,68,73–81] Regardless of the method used, the importance of close supervision cannot be overemphasized. Caution is also required when there has been rapid dose escalation of the pre-switch opioid; in these circumstances it is probably safer to calculate the initial dose of methadone using the pre-escalation dose.[82] Maintenance doses vary considerably, but most are <80mg/24h.[67] Subsequent switching from methadone to other opioids can be difficult. In one series 12/13 patients experienced increased pain ± dysphoria.[83]

Because of the difficulties associated with a complete swap from **morphine** to methadone, some clinicians add a small dose of methadone (as per first-line use) alongside **morphine** (or other strong opioid).[84,85] The dose of **morphine** is progressively reduced if opioid toxicity occurs. Although simpler, this approach does *not* avoid the need for close supervision. Only low-level evidence (grade D) exists to support this approach.[86]

Methadone SC (generally doses >25mg) or CSCI can cause marked local inflammation necessitating site rotation, and possibly other measures (see, p.440).[87,88] When switching from methadone PO to SC, a safe conversion is to halve the methadone PO dose. However, for some patients, particularly those receiving a small dose of methadone (<80mg/24h), a 1:1 conversion ratio may be more appropriate and subsequent upwards dose titration may be required.[88] Methadone can also be given SL, PR, IV, CIVI ± PCA.[73,89–91] It has also been used as a topical analgesic for mouth ulcers (as a mouthwash),[92] and for open wounds and ulcers (in powder form mixed with Stomahesive®).[93]

For CSCI, dilute with WFI, 0.9% saline or 5% glucose. There are limited compatibility data for mixing methadone with other drugs for CSCI. Health professionals are encouraged to add details of any successful or unsuccessful combinations to the existing list of methadone combinations on the www.palliativedrugs.com Syringe Driver Survey Database (SDSD).

Supply

All preparations are schedule 2 **CD**.

Methadone (generic)
Tablets 5mg, 28 days @ 5mg b.d. = £3.50.
Oral solution 1mg/mL, 28 days @ 5mg b.d. = £4.
Injection 10mg/mL, 1mL amp = £1, 2mL amp = £2, 3.5mL amp = £1.50, 5mL amp = £2; 25mg/mL, 2mL amp = £2; 50mg/mL, 1mL amp = £2.

Do not confuse methadone oral solution 1mg/mL with methadone linctus 2mg/5mL (authorized for cough) or with methadone oral concentrates 10mg/mL and 20mg/mL (authorized for opioid dependence) which require further dilution with Methadose® diluent to the required strength.

1 Caraceni A et al. (2012) Use of opioid analgesics in the treatment of cancer pain: evidence-based recommendations from the EAPC. Lancet Oncology. 13: e58–68.
2 Gannon C (1997) The use of methadone in the care of the dying. European Journal of Palliative Care. 4: 152–158.
3 Morley J and Makin M (1998) The use of methadone in cancer pain poorly responsive to other opioids. Pain Reviews. 5: 51–58.
4 Watanabe S (2001) Methadone the renaissance. Journal of Palliative Care. 17 (2): 117–120.
5 Davis MP and Walsh D (2001) Methadone for relief of cancer pain: a review of pharmacokinetics, pharmacodynamics, drug interactions and protocols of administration. Supportive Care in Cancer. 9: 73–83.
6 Raynor K et al. (1994) Pharmacological characterization of the cloned kappa-, delta-, and mu-opioid receptors. Molecular Pharmacology. 45: 330–334.
7 Ebert B et al. (1995) Ketobemidone, methadone and pethidine are non-competitive N-methyl-D-aspartate (NMDA) antagonists in the rat cortex and spinal cord. Neuroscience Letter. 187: 165–168.
8 Gorman A et al. (1997) The d- and l- isomers of methadone bind to the non-competitive site on the N-methyl-D-aspartate (NMDA) receptor in rat forebrain and spinal cord. Neuroscience Letters. 223: 5–8.
9 Codd E et al. (1995) Serotonin and norepinephrine uptake inhibiting activity of centrally acting analgesics: structural determinants and role in antinociception. Journal of Pharmacology and Experimental Therapeutics. 274: 1263–1270.
10 Kafami L et al. (2013) Methadone diminishes neuroinflammation and disease severity in EAE through modulating T cell function. Journal of Neuroimmunology. 255: 39–44.
11 Ferrari A et al. (2004) Methadone-metabolism, pharmacokinetics and interactions. Pharmacological Research. 50: 551–559.
12 Robinson AE and Williams FM (1971) The distribution of methadone in man. Journal of Pharmacy and Pharmacology. 23: 353–358.
13 Eap CB et al. (1990) Binding of D-methadone, L-methadone and DL-methadone to proteins in plasma of healthy volunteers: role of variants of X1-acid glycoprotein. Clinical Pharmacology and Therapeutics. 47: 338–346.
14 Fainsinger R et al. (1993) Methadone in the management of cancer pain: clinical review. Pain. 52: 137–147.
15 Inturrisi CE and Verebely K (1972) The levels of methadone in the plasma in methadone maintenance. Clinical Pharmacology and Therapeutics. 13: 633–637.
16 King S et al. (2011) A systematic review of the use of opioid medication for those with moderate to severe cancer pain and renal impairment. Palliative Medicine. 25: 525–552.
17 Bosilkovska M et al. (2012) Analgesics in patients with hepatic impairment: pharmacology and clinical implications. Drugs. 72: 1645–1669.
18 Beaver WT et al. (1967) A clinical comparison of the analgesic effects of methadone and morphine administered intramuscularly, and of orally and parenterally administered methadone. Clinical Pharmacology and Therapeutics. 8: 415–426.
19 Sawe J et al. (1981) Patient-controlled dose regimen of methadone for chronic cancer pain. British Medical Journal. 282: 771–773.

20 Bruera E et al. (2004) Methadone versus morphine as a first-line strong opioid for cancer pain: a randomized, double-blind study. Journal of Clinical Oncology. 22: 185–192.

21 Cornish CJ and Keen JC (2003) An alternative low-dose ad libitum schedule for conversion of other opioids to methadone. Palliative Medicine. 17: 643–644.

22 Weschules DJ and Bain KT (2008) A systematic review of opioid conversion ratios used with methadone for the treatment of pain. Pain Medicine. 9: 595-612.

23 Benitez-Rosario MA et al. (2009) Morphine-methadone opioid rotation in cancer patients: analysis of dose ratio predicting factors. Journal of Pain and Symptom Management. 37: 1061–1068.

24 Mercadante S and Caraceni A (2011) Conversion ratios for opioid switching in the treatment of cancer pain: a systematic review. Palliative Medicine. 25: 504–515.

25 Chatham MS et al. (2013) Dose ratios between high dose oral morphine or equivalents and oral methadone. Journal of Palliative Medicine. 16: 947–950.

26 Walker PW et al. (2008) Switching from methadone to a different opioid: what is the equianalgesic dose ratio? Journal of Palliative Medicine. 11: 1103–1108.

27 Nicholson AB (2007) Methadone for cancer pain. Cochrane Database of Systematic Reviews. 4: CD003971.

28 Cherny N (2011) Is oral methadone better than placebo or other oral/transdermal opioids in the management of pain? Palliative Medicine. 25: 488–493.

29 Haroutiunian S et al. (2012) Methadone for chronic non-cancer pain in adults. Cochrane Database of Systemic Reviews. 11: CD008025.

30 Mercadante S et al. (2008) Sustained-release oral morphine versus transdermal fentanyl and oral methadone in cancer pain management. European Journal of Pain. 12: 1040–1046.

31 Gallagher R (2009) Methadone: an effective, safe drug of first choice for pain management in frail older adults. Pain Medicine. 10: 319–326.

32 Salpeter SR et al. (2013) The use of very-low-dose methadone for palliative pain control and the prevention of opioid hyperalgesia. Journal of Palliative Medicine. 16: 616–622.

33 Tse DM et al. (2003) An ad libitum schedule for conversion of morphine to methadone in advanced cancer patients: an open uncontrolled prospective study in a Chinese population. Palliative Medicine. 17: 206–211.

34 Mercadante S et al. (2001) Switching from morphine to methadone to improve analgesia and tolerability in cancer patients: a prospective study. Journal of Clinical Oncology. 19: 2898–2904.

35 Mercadante S et al. (1999) Rapid switching from morphine to methadone in cancer patients with poor response to morphine. Journal of Clinical Oncology. 17: 3307–3312.

36 Sjogren P et al. (1994) Disappearance of morphine-induced hyperalgesia after discontinuing or substituting morphine with other opioid agonists. Pain. 59: 313–316.

37 Hagen N and Swanson R (1997) Strychnine-like multifocal myoclonus and seizures in extremely high-dose opioid administration: treatment strategies. Journal of Pain and Symptom Management. 14: 51–58.

38 Ashby M et al. (1999) Opioid substitution to reduce adverse effects in cancer pain management. Medical Journal of Australia. 170: 68–71.

39 Morita T et al. (2005) Opioid rotation from morphine to fentanyl in delirious cancer patients: an open-label trial. Journal of Pain and Symptom Management. 30: 96–103.

40 Furlan V et al. (1999) Methadone is poorly removed by haemodialysis. Nephrology, Dialysis, Transplantation. 14: 254–255.

41 Manfredi P et al. (2001) Methadone analgesia in cancer pain patients on chronic methadone maintenance therapy. Journal of Pain and Symptom Management. 21: 169–174.

42 Rowley D et al. (2011) Review of cancer pain management in patients receiving maintenance methadone therapy. American Journal of Hospice and Palliative Care. 28: 183–187.

43 Love R and Bourgeois K (2014) Topical methadone: an alternative for pain control in end-of-life management. Journal of Palliative Medicine. 17: 128.

44 Fisher K et al. (2004) Characterization of the early pharmacodynamic profile of oral methadone for cancer-related breakthrough pain: a pilot study. Journal of Pain and Symptom Management. 28: 619–625.

45 Hagen NA et al. (2010) A formal feasibility study of sublingual methadone for breakthrough cancer pain. Palliative Medicine. 24: 696–706.

46 Lugo RA et al. (2005) Pharmacokinetics of methadone. Journal of Pain and Palliative Care Pharmacotherapy. 19: 13–24.

47 Nilsson MI et al. (1982) Pharmacokinetics of methadone during maintenance treatment: adaptive changes during the induction phase. European Journal of Clinical Pharmarcology. 22: 343–349.

48 Hendra T et al. (1996) Fatal methadone overdose. British Medical Journal. 313: 481–482.

49 Wilcock A and Beattie JM (2009) Prolonged QT interval and methadone: implications for palliative care. Current Opinion in Supportive and Palliative Care. 3: 252–257.

50 Kornick CA et al. (2003) QTc interval prolongation associated with intravenous methadone. Pain. 105: 499–506.

51 Bunten H et al. (2011) CYP2B6 and OPRM1 gene variations predict methadone-related deaths. Addiction Biology. 16: 142–144.

52 Eap CB et al. (2007) Stereoselective block of hERG channel by (S)-methadone and QT interval prolongation in CYP2B6 slow metabolizers. Clinical Pharmacology and Therapeutics. 81: 719–728.

53 Baxter K and Preston CL. Stockley's Drug Interactions. London: Pharmaceutical Press www.medicinescomplete.com (accessed May 2014).

54 Kreek MJ et al. (1976) Rifampin-induced methadone withdrawal. New England Journal of Medicine. 294: 1104–1106.

55 Wahawisan J et al. (2011) Methadone toxicity due to smoking cessation–a case report on the drug-drug interaction involving cytochrome P450 isoenzyme 1A2. Annals of Pharmacotherapy. 45: e34.

56 Buchanan D (2010) Sinus bradycardia related to methadone in a patient with myeloma receiving thalidomide therapy. Palliative Medicine. 24: 742–743.

57 Sarhill N et al. (2001) Methadone-induced myoclonus in advanced cancer. American Journal of Hospice and Palliative Care. 18: 51–53.

58 Davis MP et al. (2007) When opioids cause pain. Journal of Clinical Oncology. 25: 4497–4498.

59 El Osta B et al. (2007) Intractable pain: intoxication or undermedication? Journal of Palliative Medicine. 10: 811–814.

60 Bruera E et al. (1991) Local toxicity with subcutaneous methadone. Experience of two centers. Pain. 45: 141–143.

61 Maingi S et al. (2008) Symptomatic hypoglycaemia due to escalating doses of intravenous methadone. Journal of Pain. 9 (Suppl 2): 37.

62 Faskowitz AJ et al. (2013) Methadone-induced hypoglycemia. Cell and Molecular Neurobiology. 33: 537–542.

63 Saifan C et al. (2013) Methadone induced sensorineural hearing loss. Case Reports in Medicine. **2013**: Article ID 242730.
64 Vorasubin N et al. (2013) Methadone-induced bilateral severe sensorineural hearing loss. American Journal of Otolaryngology. **34**: 735–738.
65 Ripamonti C et al. (1997) An update on the clinical use of methadone cancer pain. Pain. **70**: 109–115.
66 Hagen N and Wasylenko E (1999) Methadone: outpatient titration and monitoring strategies in cancer patients. Journal of Pain and Symptom Management. **18**: 369–375.
67 Scholes C et al. (1999) Methadone titration in opioid-resistant cancer pain. European Journal of Cancer Care. **8**: 26–29.
68 Nauck F et al. (2001) A German model for methadone conversion. American Journal of Hospice and Palliative Care. **18**. 200–202.
69 Soares LG (2005) Methadone for cancer pain: what have we learned from clinical studies? American Journal of Hospice and Palliative Care. **22**: 223–227.
70 Twycross RG (1977) A comparison of diamorphine with cocaine and methadone. British Journal of Clinical Pharmacology **4**: 691–692.
71 Lipman AG (2005) Methadone: effective analgesia, confusion, and risk. Journal of Pain and Palliative Care Pharmacotherapy. **19**. 3–5.
72 Palliativedrugs.com (2005) Hot Topics: new draft methadone monograph. September Newsletter. www.palliativedrugs.com
73 Santiago-Palma J et al. (2001) Intravenous methadone in the management of chronic cancer pain: safe and effective starting doses when substituting methadone for fentanyl. Cancer. **92**: 1919–1925.
74 Blackburn D et al. (2002) Methadone: an alternative conversion regime. European Journal of Palliative Care. **9**: 93–96.
75 Benitez-Rosario MA et al. (2004) Opioid switching from transdermal fentanyl to oral methadone in patients with cancer pain. Cancer. **101**: 2866–2873.
76 Blackburn D (2005) Methadone: the analgesic. European Journal of Palliative Care. **12**: 188–191.
77 Bruera E et al. (1996) Opioid rotation in patients with cancer pain. Cancer. **78**: 852–857.
78 Walmsley R et al. (2010) Use of methadone for uncontrolled pain: an alternative dosing regimen. Journal of Pain and Symptom Management. **40**: e3–4.
79 Auret K et al. (2006) Pharmacokinetics and pharmacodynamics of methadone enantiomers in hospice patients with cancer pain. Therapeutic Drug Monitoring. **28**: 359–366.
80 Moksnes K (2011) How to switch from morphine or oxycodone to methadone in cancer patients? a randomised clinical phase II trial. European Journal of Cancer. **47**: 2463–2470.
81 Moksnes K et al. (2012) Serum concentrations of opioids when comparing two switching strategies to methadone for cancer pain. European Journal of Clinical Pharmacology. **68**: 1147–1156.
82 Zimmermann C et al. (2005) Rotation to methadone after opioid dose escalation: How should individualization of dosing occur? Journal of Pain and Palliative Care Pharmacotherapy. **19 (2)**: 25–31.
83 Moryl N et al. (2002) Pitfalls of opioid rotation: substituting another opioid for methadone in patients with cancer pain. Pain. **96**: 325–328.
84 McKenna M and Nicholson AB (2011) Use of methadone as a coanalgesic. Journal of Pain and Symptom Management. **42**: e4–6.
85 Haughey C et al. (2012) Use of methadone as a coanalgesic: response to McKenna and Nicholson. Journal of Pain and Symptom Management. **43**: e5–6.
86 Fallon MT and Laird BJ (2011) A systematic review of combination step III opioid therapy in cancer pain: an EPCRC opioid guideline project. Palliative Medicine. **25**: 597–603.
87 Mathew P and Storey P (1999) Subcutaneous methadone in terminally ill patients: manageable local toxicity. Journal of Pain and Symptom Management. **18**: 49–52.
88 Centeno C and Vara F (2005) Intermittent subcutaneous methadone administration in the management of cancer pain. Journal of Pain and Palliative Care Pharmacotherapy. **19**: 7–12.
89 Fitzgibbon D and Ready L (1997) Intravenous high-dose methadone administered by patient controlled analgesia and continuous infusion for the treatment of cancer pain refractory to high-dose morphine. Pain. **73**: 259–261.
90 Davis M and Walsh D (2001) Methadone for relief of cancer pain: a review of pharmacokinetics, pharmacodynamics, drug interactions and protocols of administration. Supportive Care in Cancer. **9**: 73–83.
91 Manfredi PL and Houde RW (2003) Prescribing methadone, a unique analgesic. Journal of Supportive Oncology. **1**: 216–220.
92 Gallagher R (2004) Methadone mouthwash for the management of oral ulcer pain. Journal of Pain and Symptom Management. **27**: 390–391.
93 Gallagher RE et al. (2005) Analgesic effects of topical methadone: a report of four cases. Clinical Journal of Pain. **21**: 190–192.

Updated June 2014

Quick Prescribing Guide: Use of methadone for cancer pain

Methadone has both opioid and non-opioid properties, and a long variable halflife (range 5–130h vs. 2.5h for morphine). Thus there is no single potency ratio for methadone and other opioids. When switching from morphine, the eventual 24h dose of methadone is typically 5–10 times smaller than the dose of morphine, sometimes 20–30 times smaller, and occasionally even smaller. Inevitable accumulation is the reason for the week-long intervals between dose adjustments. *Switching must be closely supervised by specialists*, generally as an inpatient.

Indications for use

- neuropathic or mixed nociceptive-neuropathic pain not responding to an NSAID + morphine + adjuvant analgesics, e.g. an antidepressant ± an anti-epileptic
- neurotoxicity with morphine at any dose (e.g. myoclonus, allodynia, hyperalgesia) which does not respond to a reduction in morphine dose and switching to another easier-to-use opioid (e.g. fentanyl, hydromorphone, oxycodone) is not possible
- the strong opioid of choice, instead of morphine
- end-stage renal failure.

Dose titration

1 When prescribing PO methadone as first-line strong opioid:
- start with methadone 5mg (1–2.5mg in the elderly) q12h regularly and q3h p.r.n.
- if necessary, titrate the regular dose upwards once a week, guided by p.r.n. use
- continue with 5mg p.r.n., or 1–2.5mg in the elderly
- with doses ⩾30mg q12h, increase the p.r.n. dose to 1/6–1/10 of the q24h dose, rounded to a convenient tablet size or volume.

2 If the patient is already receiving morphine, use the following method.

PO morphine to PO methadone

Morphine is stopped abruptly when methadone is started.
If switching from:
- immediate-release morphine, give the first dose of methadone ⩾2h (pain present) or 4h (pain-free) after last dose of morphine
- m/r morphine, give the first dose of methadone ⩾6h (pain present) or 12h (pain-free) after the last dose of a 12h preparation, or ⩾12h (pain present) or 24h (pain-free) after the last dose of a 24h preparation.

Give a single loading dose of PO methadone one tenth of the previous total 24h PO morphine dose, up to a maximum of 30mg.

Give q3h p.r.n. doses of methadone one third of the loading dose (i.e. 1/30 of the previous total 24h PO morphine dose), rounded to a convenient tablet size or volume, up to a maximum of 30mg per dose.

> *Example 1:* Morphine 300mg/24h PO = loading dose of methadone 30mg PO, and 10mg q3h p.r.n.
>
> *Example 2:* Morphine 1,200mg/24h PO = loading dose of methadone 120mg PO, and 40mg q3h p.r.n.; however, both are limited to the maximum of 30mg.

For patients in severe pain who need more analgesia in <3h, see point 6 below.

On Day 6, the amount of methadone taken over the previous 2 days is noted and divided by 4 to give a regular q12h dose, with 1/6–1/10 of the 24h dose q3h p.r.n., e.g. *methadone 80mg PO in previous 48h → 20mg q12h and 5mg PO q3h p.r.n.*

If ⩾2 doses/day of p.r.n. methadone continue to be needed, the dose of regular methadone should be increased once a week, guided by p.r.n. use.

---

3 If using another strong opioid, calculate the morphine equivalent daily dose and then follow the guidelines for morphine.

4 If converting from PO methadone to SC/IV methadone, or from another CSCI/CIVI opioid, see the respective boxes below.

5 If there has been recent rapid escalation of the pre-switch opioid dose, calculate the initial dose of methadone using the pre-escalation dose of the opioid.

6 For patients in severe pain and who need more analgesia in <3h, options include:
- taking the previously used opioid q1h p.r.n. (50–100% of the p.r.n. dose used before switching)
- if neurotoxicity with the pre-switch opioid, use an appropriate dose of an alternative strong opioid
- ketamine.

7 The switch to methadone is successful (i.e. improved pain relief and/or reduced toxicity) in about 75% of patients.

8 If a patient:
- becomes oversedated, reduce the dose generally by 33–50% (some centres monitor the level of consciousness and respirations q4h for 24h)
- develops opioid abstinence symptoms, give p.r.n. doses of the previous opioid to control these.

PO methadone to SC/IV or CSCI/CIVI methadone

To convert PO methadone to SC/IV methadone, halve the PO dose, e.g. methadone 10mg/24h PO = 5mg/24h SC/IV. This is a safe conversion ratio; for some patients the SC/IV dose = PO dose.

Because of its long halflife, methadone (10mg/mL) can be given SC q12h–q8h. If SC injection is painful or causes local inflammation, give by CSCI/CIVI instead.

If CSCI methadone causes a skin reaction:
- administer as a more dilute solution in a 20–30mL syringe
- change the site daily
- consider applying hydrocortisone cream 1% topically around the needle entry site (under an occlusive dressing)
- consider adding dexamethasone 1mg to the diluted combination of drugs (compatibility data permitting).

For additional rescue doses of methadone SC/IV, give 1/6–1/10 of the 24h SC/IV dose q3h p.r.n., e.g. methadone 20mg CIVI/24h = 2mg q3h p.r.n. SC/IV.

If ≥2 p.r.n. doses/day continue to be needed, the 24h SC/IV dose should be increased once a week, guided by p.r.n. use.

For patients in severe pain who need more analgesia in <3h, see point 6 above.

Other CSCI/CIVI opioids to CSCI/CIVI methadone

The safest approach is to follow the method for PO switching, using bolus injections of SC/IV methadone instead of PO doses.

Convert the opioid 24h CSCI/CIVI dose to its PO equivalent and determine the PO methadone dose (Dose titration, point 2).

The SC/IV dose of methadone is half the PO dose; the maximum initial dose of SC/IV methadone will be 15mg. This is a safe conversion ratio; for some patients the SC/IV dose = PO dose.

OXYCODONE BNF 4.7.2

Class: Opioid analgesic.

Indications: Moderate–severe cancer and non-cancer pain, †an alternative in cases of intolerance to other strong opioids.[1,2]

Contra-indications: Renal failure (creatinine clearance < 10mL/min). Otherwise none absolute if titrated carefully against a patient's pain (also see Strong opioids, p.357).

Pharmacology

Oxycodone is a strong opioid with similar properties to **morphine**.[3–7] However, its opioid receptor site affinities remain a matter of controversy.[8] Studies with selective opioid antagonists suggest that oxycodone and **morphine** produce analgesia through different populations of opioid receptors.[9] Thus, in rats, naloxonazine (a selective μ-opioid receptor antagonist) completely blocks **morphine**-induced antinociception but does not attenuate the effect of oxycodone.[10] In contrast, norbinaltorphimine (a selective κ-opioid receptor antagonist) completely blocks oxycodone-induced antinociception but does not attenuate the effect of **morphine**. On the other hand, in other studies (rats, mice, and humans), oxycodone showed definite μ-opioid receptor activity.[11–13] However, some of this activity could have been mediated by active metabolites, e.g. **oxymorphone**.[13]

Synergy between **morphine** and oxycodone has been shown in animal and human studies, and a formulation which combines fixed doses of oxycodone and **morphine** in a ratio of 1:1.5 is in development.[14,15–17] At **morphine** equivalent doses, the combination is 1.5 times more potent than **morphine** alone.[17] In post-operative pain, compared to equivalent doses of either opioid given alone, the combination formulation provides similar analgesia but causes less undesirable effects, e.g. nausea and vomiting.[15,16] However, this difference was less apparent in patients with chronic non-cancer pain, possibly because they are already opioid-tolerant (also see p.357).[17]

Oxycodone is less immunosuppressive than **morphine** (see p.364). Although the clinical implications of this are uncertain, a small retrospective study in patients with cancer pain found that the incidence of infections was less in those receiving oxycodone compared to **morphine**.[18]

Oxycodone is metabolized principally to noroxycodone via CYP3A4, and 10% to **oxymorphone** via CYP2D6.[19,20] Parenteral **oxymorphone** is 10 times more potent than parenteral **morphine**.[21] However, after blocking CYP2D6 with **quinidine**, the non-analgesic effects of oxycodone in volunteers are unchanged.[19] Further, postoperatively, no differences are found between CYP2D6 rapid or slow metabolizers in the dose requirements or analgesic efficacy of oxycodone.[22] Thus it is unlikely that in most people **oxymorphone** contributes significantly to the analgesic effect of oxycodone. However, CYP2D6 ultra-rapid metabolizers may be at risk of undesirable CNS effects even with low-dose oxycodone.[23] This may relate to an enhanced production of **oxymorphone** (also see Chapter 25, p.767).

By mouth, oxycodone has a mean bio-availability of 75%, whereas **morphine**'s is about half this. This partly explains why PO oxycodone is more potent than PO **morphine** (i.e. fewer mg of oxycodone are needed than **morphine** to have a comparable analgesic effect).[24–29] The PO potency ratio for oxycodone to **morphine** is about 1.5:1, and thus the dose of oxycodone by mouth is about two thirds that of **morphine** (i.e. oxycodone 10mg is equivalent to **morphine** 15mg). Hence, the recommendation by the manufacturers to halve the dose of PO **morphine** when converting to PO oxycodone, although reasonable in terms of caution and safety, almost certainly exaggerates the actual potency of oxycodone.

Parenterally, when bio-availability is comparable, the situation is different. Despite a short-term (2h) postoperative PCA study which suggested that **morphine** is less potent parenterally than oxycodone (i.e. *more* mg of **morphine** will be needed, as with PO administration),[30] earlier single-dose studies and two more recent longer PCA studies (1–2 days) suggest that by injection **morphine** is more potent than oxycodone, in the region of 4:3. Thus, *fewer* mg of **morphine** will be needed (**morphine** 10mg being approximately equivalent to oxycodone 13mg).[21,24,31] However, given the modest difference in potency, together with the constraints of ampoule size, it is reasonable in clinical practice to use a parenteral potency ratio of 1:1 when converting from oxycodone injections to **morphine** injections (or vice versa), i.e. regard IV/SC oxycodone 10mg as equivalent to IV/SC **morphine** 10mg.

About 20% of oxycodone is excreted unchanged in the urine. In mild–moderate hepatic impairment, oxycodone and noroxycodone concentrations increase (but the **oxymorphone** concentration decreases) and the elimination halflife increases by about 2h. In renal impairment the clearance of oxycodone, noroxycodone and conjugated **oxymorphone** are reduced. Oxycodone plasma concentration increases by 50% and the halflife lengthens by 1h.[25,32] Oxycodone is contra-indicated in renal failure and is not recommended in severe renal impairment[1] (see p.367); nonetheless, it is used as an alternative to **morphine** in mild–moderate renal impairment.

Although reports are not consistent, most suggest that the clearance of oxycodone is unaffected by increasing age *per se*; any reduction most likely relating to associated renal impairment.[33,34]

Bio-availability 75% PO, ranging from 60–87%.[36,36]
Onset of action 20–30min PO.
Time to peak plasma concentration 1–1.5h; 3h m/r.
Plasma halflife 3.5h; 4.5h in renal failure.
Duration of action 4–6h; 12h m/r.

Cautions

Hepatic and renal impairment (see p.367).

Drug interactions

Inhibitors of CYP3A4 (e.g. **voriconazole**, **erythromycin**, **telithromycin** and **ritonavir**) can inhibit oxycodone metabolism, and may enhance its effects.[37–40] However, inhibition of CYP2D6 (e.g. with **quinidine**) appears to have no detectable clinical impact.[41]

The enzyme inducers **rifampicin** and **St John's Wort** decrease plasma concentrations of oxycodone.[37,42,43]

Undesirable effects

See Strong opioids, Box B, p.361. Various studies have suggested possible differences in the undesirable effect profiles of oxycodone and **morphine**.[44] However, a systematic review comparing efficacy and tolerability of oxycodone versus other opioids found no difference in the undesirable effect profile between oxycodone and either **morphine** or **hydromorphone**.[45]

Dose and use

As with all opioids, patients must be monitored for undesirable effects (see p.360), particularly nausea and vomiting, and constipation. Depending on individual circumstances, an anti-emetic should be prescribed for regular or p.r.n. use, (see p.241) and, routinely, a laxative prescribed (see p.44).

Although oxycodone is similar to **morphine** (and **hydromorphone**) in terms of efficacy and undesirable effects,[2] because it is more expensive it should generally be reserved for patients who cannot tolerate **morphine**. In Scotland, oxycodone injections are restricted to cancer patients who cannot tolerate **diamorphine** or **morphine** injections.

A combination product of oxycodone with **naloxone** is available (Targinact® Box A).

Note: remains of m/r tablets (Oxycontin®, Longtec® and Targinact®) may appear in the patient's faeces ('ghost tablets'), but these are inert residues, and do not affect the efficacy of the products.

Oral

Immediate-release oxycodone is generally given q4h but, in some patients, q6h is satisfactory.[58] Oxycodone m/r tablets are biphasic in their release of oxycodone, i.e. there is an initial fast release which leads to the early onset of analgesia and a slow release which provides a prolonged duration of action. M/r tablets should be swallowed whole; crushing or chewing them will lead to a rapid release of an overdose of oxycodone. For strong opioid-naïve patients:
• start with 5mg q6h–q4h for immediate-release capsules and oral solutions

---

Box A   Oxycodone combined with naloxone (Targinact®)

Targinact® is marketed as a range of tablets containing m/r formulations of oxycodone and naloxone in a fixed-dose ratio of 2:1, i.e. oxycodone 5mg/naloxone 2.5mg; 10mg/5mg; 20mg/10mg and 40mg/20mg. The addition of naloxone is to antagonize the constipating effect of oxycodone. The desire to develop a formulation which deters misuse (e.g. by crushing and injecting IV) is also relevant.

Targinact® is authorized for severe pain. Evidence to support claims of improved pain control, better GI tolerability, and improved quality of life are based mainly on uncontrolled, observational studies.[46–49]

RCTs have mostly involved relatively young non-cancer (mid-50s) and cancer patients (early 60s) with either moderate or severe pain, and with no significant hepatic or renal impairment. Reported use in older cancer patients (mean age 70) is limited to open-label studies.[47]

In the non-cancer studies, those unable to tolerate a 'restricted laxative regimen' were excluded, i.e. the most severely constipated. Although Targinact® improved bowel function and reduced the number of patients requiring laxatives, laxatives were taken only p.r.n.[50,51]

In a RCT in cancer patients, Targinact® improved bowel function and there was a trend towards a reduction in mean total laxative use. However, laxatives were again taken only p.r.n.[52]

Targinact® is 40% more expensive than the equivalent dose of m/r oxycodone alone, and 2–3 times more expensive than an equivalent dose of morphine + regular laxatives. Because the benefit of Targinact® in patients taking laxatives *regularly* is uncertain, the Scottish Medicines Consortium, the Drugs and Therapeutics Bulletin and *PCF* do *not* recommend its use.[53]

If clinicians choose to prescribe Targinact®, its use should be restricted to occasions when the upward titration of regularly administered laxatives is ineffective (see p.48). Because constipation is generally multifactorial in origin,[54] Targinact® is likely to augment rather than replace laxatives.[50,51]

The m/r formulation of naloxone avoids a 'bolus dose', and >97% is removed by first-pass metabolism in the liver. Thus, the main effect of naloxone is on the GI tract, with insufficient amounts reaching the systemic circulation to adversely affect analgesia.[55,56] However, plasma concentrations of naloxone can increase significantly in:
- *hepatic impairment:* use of Targinact® requires caution in mild impairment and is contra-indicated in moderate–severe impairment
- *renal impairment:* use Targinact® with caution.

Dose recommendations:
- in opioid-naïve patients, generally start with oxycodone/naloxone 10mg/5mg b.d.
- in elderly/frail patients, 5mg/2.5mg b.d. may be more appropriate
- in those already taking strong opioids, switch to the equivalent dose of oxycodone
- maximum dose 40mg/20mg b.d.

When higher analgesic doses are required, the manufacturer recommends supplemental oxycodone m/r tablets, taken at the same time as the m/r combination tablets. However, this reduces the impact of the naloxone, and oxycodone:naloxone ratios >4:1 have no significant effect on bowel function[51,57]

Common undesirable effects include nausea, vomiting, abdominal pain and diarrhoea. The manufacturer warns that patients on long-term opioids may develop opioid withdrawal symptoms when switched to Targinact®.

- start with 10mg b.d. for m/r tablets
- titrate the dose to optimize analgesia.

For patients transferring from PO **morphine**:
- start with a dose conversion ratio of 1.5:1 (e.g. replace **morphine** 15mg by oxycodone 10mg)
- titrate the dose to optimize analgesia.

Note: this recommendation differs from the manufacturer's dose conversion ratio of 2:1 (see Pharmacology above; also see Chapter 15, Table 1, p.663).

The manufacturer recommends that the initial dose is reduced in patients with mild hepatic impairment or mild–moderate renal impairment, i.e. start with 2.5mg q6h for oral solution or 5mg b.d. for m/r tablets. This will generally include most elderly/frail patients.

Injection
Oxycodone injection may be given IV or SC as a bolus or by infusion. For CSCI, dilute with WFI, 0.9% saline or 5% glucose.

For opioid-naïve patients:
- start with 7.5mg/day
- if necessary, titrate the dose upwards, guided by p.r.n. use.

When converting from PO oxycodone to SC/IV oxycodone:
- the manufacturer recommends giving half the PO dose by injection; however, because mean oral bio-availability is 75% (range 60–87%), some centres use a conversion ratio of 1.5:1, e.g. oxycodone 30mg/24h PO g oxycodone 20mg/24h SC/IV
- if necessary, titrate the dose upwards, guided by p.r.n. use.

For patients transferring from **morphine** injections, use a 1:1 dose ratio (e.g. replace SC **morphine** 10mg by SC oxycodone 10mg), and titrate to optimize analgesia.

Two strengths of injection are available, 10mg/mL and high-strength 50mg/mL. The latter may be useful in situations where high doses cause volume difficulties for CSCI. However, there is an increased risk of serious mistakes being made when more than one strength is readily available.[59,60] There are also differences in compatibility with other drugs (see below) and, on a mg for mg basis, the high-strength injection costs about twice as much.

CSCI with oxycodone 10mg/mL
There are 2-drug compatibility data for mixtures in WFI with **clonazepam, dexamethasone, glycopyrronium, haloperidol, hyoscine** *butylbromide***, hyoscine** *hydrobromide***, levomepromazine, metoclopramide, midazolam,** and **octreotide.**
Concentration-dependent incompatibility may occur when oxycodone (hydrochloride) is mixed with **cyclizine** (lactate); for more details see Appendix 3, Chart 1, p.824.
CSCI with oxycodone 50mg/mL
Differences in compatibility with other drugs for the 10mg/mL and 50mg/mL formulations of oxycodone have been reported.[61,62] This may be due to the different ratios of excipients in each formulation (see Appendix 3, Table 1, p.838). It is important *not* to extrapolate compatibility information from one formulation to the other.
More details
For 2-drug and 3-drug compatibility data for oxycodone 10mg/mL in WFI, and for currently available data for oxycodone 50mg/mL, see Appendix 3, Chart 1 (p.824), 6 (p.834) and Table 1 (p.838).
For compatibility charts for mixing drugs in 0.9% saline, see the extended appendix section of the on-line PCF on www.palliativedrugs.com

Supply
Unless indicated otherwise, all preparations are **CD**.

Immediate-release oral products

Oxycodone oral solution is available in two strengths, 1mg/mL and a high potency concentrate of 10mg/mL prescribing should be in *mg* not mL to minimise the risk of 10 times the intended dose being given.

Oxycodone (generic)
Capsules (Shortec®) 5mg, 10mg, 20mg, 5mg dose = £0.20.
Oral solution 5mg/5mL, 5mg dose = £0.20.
Concentrated oral solution 10mg/mL, 5mg dose = £0.20.
Injection 10mg/mL, 1mL amp = £1.50, 2mL amp = £3.

OxyNorm® (Napp)
Capsules 5mg, 10mg, 20mg, 5mg dose = £0.20.
Oral solution (sugar-free) 5mg/5mL, 5mg dose = £0.20.
Concentrated oral solution (sugar-free) 10mg/mL, 5mg dose = £0.20.
Injection 10mg/mL, 1mL amp = £1.50, 2mL amp = £3.
Injection 50mg/mL, 1mL amp = £14.

Modified-release 12-hourly oral products
Longtec® (Qdem)
Tablets m/r 5mg, 10mg, 20mg, 40mg, 80mg 28 days @ 10mg, 20mg, 40mg and 80mg b.d. = £21, £42, £85, and £170 respectively.

OxyContin® (Napp)
Tablets m/r 5mg, 10mg, 15mg, 20mg, 30mg, 40mg, 60mg, 80mg, 120mg 28 days @ 10mg, 15mg, 20mg, 30mg, 80mg and 120mg b.d. = £25, £37, £50, £75, £200 and £299 respectively.

Oxycodone/naloxone combined
Targinact® (Napp)
Tablets m/r containing oxycodone/naloxone in a fixed ratio of 2:1, 5mg/2.5mg, 10mg/5mg, 20mg/10mg, 40mg/20mg, 28 days @10mg/5mg b.d. = £35.

Note: Other products are anticipated in 2014, see on-line PCF for latest details.

1 King S et al. (2011) A systematic review of the use of opioid medication for those with moderate to severe cancer pain and renal impairment. Palliative Medicine. 25: 454–470.
2 Caraceni A et al. (2012) Use of opioid analgesics in the treatment of cancer pain: evidence-based recommendations from the EAPC. Lancet Oncology. 13: e58–68.
3 Glare PA and Walsh TD (1993) Dose-ranging study of oxycodone for chronic pain in advanced cancer. Journal of Clinical Oncology. 11: 973–978.
4 Poyhia R et al. (1993) Oxycodone: an alternative to morphine for cancer pain. A review. Journal of Pain and Symptom Management. 8: 63–67.
5 Shah S and Hardy J (2001) Oxycodone: a review of the literature. European Journal of Palliative Care. 8: 93–96.
6 Davis MP et al. (2003) Normal-release and controlled-release oxycodone: pharmacokinetics, pharmacodynamics, and controversy. Supportive Care in Cancer. 11: 84–92.
7 Kalso E (2005) Oxycodone. Journal of Pain and Symptom Management. 29 (Suppl 5): s47–s56.
8 Poyhia R and Kalso EA (1992) Antinociceptive effects and central nervous system depression caused by oxycodone and morphine in rats. Pharmacology and Toxicology. 70: 125–130.
9 Smith M et al. (2001) Oxycodone has a distinctly different pharmacology from morphine. European Journal of Pain. 15 (Suppl A): 135–136.
10 Ross F and Smith M (1997) The intrinsic antinociceptive effects of oxycodone appear to be kappa-opioid receptor mediated. Pain. 73: 151–157.
11 Yoburn B et al. (1995) Supersensitivity to opioid analgesics following chronic opioid antagonist treatment: relationship to receptor selectivity. Pharmacology, Biochemistry and Behavior. 51: 535–539.
12 Chen Z et al. (1991) Mu receptor binding of some commonly used opioids and their metabolites. Life Sciences. 48: 2165–2171.
13 Kalso E et al. (1990) Morphine and oxycodone in the management of cancer pain: plasma levels determined by chemical and radioreceptor assays. Pharmacology and Toxicology. 67: 322–328.
14 Ross FB et al. (2000) Co-administration of sub-antinociceptive doses of oxycodone and morphine produces marked antinociceptive synergy with reduced CNS side-effects in rats. Pain. 84: 421–428.
15 Webster L (2012) Efficacy and safety of dual-opioid therapy in acute pain. Pain Medicine. 13 (Suppl 1): S12–20.
16 Richards P et al. (2011) Analgesic and adverse effects of a fixed-ratio morphine-oxycodone combination (MoxDuo) in the treatment of postoperative pain. Journal of Opioid Management. 7: 217–228.
17 de la Iglesia FA et al. (2012) Tolerability and efficacy of two synergistic ratios of oral morphine and oxycodone combinations versus morphine in patients with chronic noncancer pain. Journal of Opioid Management. 8: 89–98.
18 Suzuki M et al. (2013) Correlation between the administration of morphine or oxycodone and the development of infections in patients with cancer pain. American Journal of Hospice and Palliative Care. 30: 712–716.
19 Heiskanen T et al. (1998) Effects of blocking CYP2D6 on oxycodone. Clinical Pharmacology and Therapeutics. 64: 603–611.
20 Lalovic B et al. (2006) Pharmacokinetics and pharmacodynamics of oral oxycodone in healthy human subjects: role of circulating active metabolites. Clin Pharmacol Ther. 79: 461–479.
21 Beaver WT et al. (1978) Analgesic studies of codeine and oxycodone in patients with cancer. II. Comparisons of intramuscular oxycodone with intramuscular morphine and codeine. Journal Pharmacology and Experiemental Therapeutics. 207: 101–108.
22 Zwisler ST et al. (2010) Impact of the CYP2D6 genotype on post-operative intravenous oxycodone analgesia. Acta Anaesthesiologica Scandinavica. 54: 232–240.

23 de Leon J et al. (2003) Adverse drug reactions to oxycodone and hydrocodone in CYP2D6 ultrarapid metabolizers. Journal of Clinical Psychopharmacology. 23: 420–421.

24 Kalso E and Vainio A (1990) Morphine and oxycodone in the management of cancer pain. Clinical Pharmacology and Therapeutics. 47: 639–646.

25 Heiskanen T and Kalso E (1997) Controlled-release oxycodone and morphine in cancer related pain. Pain. 73: 37–45.

26 Bruera E et al. (1998) Randomized, double-blind, cross-over trial comparing safety and efficacy of oral controlled-release oxycodone with controlled-release morphine in patients with cancer pain. Journal of Clinical Oncology. 16: 3222–3229.

27 Mucci-LoRusso P et al. (1998) Controlled-release oxycodone compared with controlled-release morphine in the treatment of cancer pain: a randomized, double-blind, parallel-group study. European Journal of Pain. 2: 239–249.

28 Curtis GB et al. (1999) Relative potency of controlled-release oxycodone and controlled-release morphine in a postoperative pain model. European Journal of Clinical Pharmacology. 55: 425–429.

29 Lauretti GR et al. (2003) Comparison of sustained-release morphine with sustained-release oxycodone in advanced cancer patients. British Journal of Cancer. 89: 2027–2030.

30 Kalso E et al. (1991) Intravenous morphine and oxycodone for pain after abdominal surgery. Acta anaesthesiologica Scandinavica. 35: 642–646.

31 Silvasti M et al. (1998) Comparison of analgesic efficacy of oxycodone and morphine in postoperative intravenous patient-controlled analgesia. Acta anaesthesiologica Scandinavica. 42: 576–580.

32 Glare P and Davis MP (2009) Oxycodone. In: MP Davis et al. (eds) Opioids in Cancer Pain (2e). Oxford University Press, Oxford, pp. 155–173.

33 Liukas A et al. (2011) Elimination of intravenous oxycodone in the elderly: a pharmacokinetic study in postoperative orthopaedic patients of different age groups. Drugs Aging. 28: 41–50.

34 Charles B et al. (2014) Should the dosage of controlled-release oxycodone in advanced cancer be modified on the basis of patient characteristics? Supportive Care in Cancer. 22: 325–330.

35 Leow K et al. (1992) Single-dose and steady-state pharmacokinetics and pharmacodynamics of oxycodone in patients with cancer. Clinical Pharmacology and Therapeutics. 52: 487–495.

36 Poyhia R et al. (1992) The pharmacokinetics and metabolism of oxycodone after intramuscular and oral administration to healthy subjects. British Journal of Clinical Pharmacology. 33: 617–621.

37 Baxter K, Preston CL Stockley's Drug Interactions. London: Pharmaceutical Press www.medicinescomplete.com (accessed October 2013).

38 Hagelberg NM et al. (2009) Voriconazole drastically increases exposure to oral oxycodone. European Journal of Clinical Pharmacology. 65: 263–271.

39 Nieminen TH et al. (2010) Oxycodone concentrations are greatly increased by the concomitant use of ritonavir or lopinavir/ritonavir. European Journal of Clinical Pharmacology. 66: 977–985.

40 Hagelberg NM et al. (2011) Interaction of oxycodone and voriconazole-a case series of patients with cancer pain supports the findings of randomised controlled studies with healthy subjects. European Journal of Clinical Pharmacology. 67: 863–864.

41 Kleine-Bruggeney (2010) Pharmacogenetics in palliative care. Forensic Science International. epub doi:10.1016/j.forsciint.2010.1007.1003.

42 Nieminen TH et al. (2009) Rifampin greatly reduces the plasma concentrations of intravenous and oral oxycodone. Anesthesiology. 110: 1371–1378.

43 Nieminen TH et al. (2010) St John's wort greatly reduces the concentrations of oral oxycodone. European Journal of Pain. 14: 854–859.

44 Leppert W (2010) Role of oxycodone and oxycodone/naloxone in cancer pain management. Pharmacological Reports. 62: 578–591.

45 Reid CM et al. (2006) Oxycodone for cancer-related pain: meta-analysis of randomized controlled trials. Archives of Internal Medicine. 166: 837–843.

46 Schutter U et al. (2010) Innovative pain therapy with a fixed combination of prolonged-release oxycodone/naloxone: a large observational study under conditions of daily practice. Current Medical Research Opinion. 26: 1377–1387.

47 Clemens KE et al. (2011) Bowel function during pain therapy with oxycodone/naloxone prolonged-release tablets in patients with advanced cancer. International Journal of Clinical Practice. 65: 472–478.

48 Hermanns K et al. (2012) Prolonged-release oxycodone/naloxone in the treatment of neuropathic pain - results from a large observational study. Expert Opinion on Pharmacotherapy. 13: 299–311.

49 Gatti A et al. (2013) Prolonged-release oxycodone/naloxone in nonmalignant pain: single-center study in patients with constipation. Advances in Therapy. 30: 41–59.

50 Simpson K et al. (2008) Fixed-ratio combination oxycodone/naloxone compared with oxycodone alone for the relief of opioid-induced constipation in moderate-to-severe noncancer pain. Current Medical Research Opinion. 24: 3503–3512.

51 Lowenstein O et al. (2009) Combined prolonged-release oxycodone and naloxone improves bowel function in patients receiving opioids for moderate-to-severe non-malignant chronic pain: a randomised controlled trial. Expert Opinion in Pharmacotherapy. 10: 531–543.

52 Ahmedzai SH et al. (2012) A randomized, double-blind, active-controlled, double-dummy, parallel-group study to determine the safety and efficacy of oxycodone/naloxone prolonged-release tablets in patients with moderate/severe, chronic cancer pain. Palliative Medicine. 26: 50–60.

53 Anonymous (2010) Targinact - opioid relief without constipation? Drugs and Therapeutics Bulletin. 48: 138–141.

54 Larkin PJ et al. (2008) The management of constipation in palliative care: clinical practice recommendations. Palliative Medicine. 22: 796–807.

55 Vondrackova D et al. (2008) Analgesic efficacy and safety of oxycodone in combination with naloxone as prolonged release tablets in patients with moderate to severe chronic pain. Journal of Pain. 9: 1144–1154.

56 Sandner-Kiesling A et al. (2010) Long-term efficacy and safety of combined prolonged-release oxycodone and naloxone in the management of non-cancer chronic pain. International Journal of Clinical Practice. 64: 763–774.

57 Meissner W et al. (2009) A randomised controlled trial with prolonged-release oral oxycodone and naloxone to prevent and reverse opioid-induced constipation. European Journal of Pain. 13: 56–64.

58 Lugo RA and Kern SE (2004) The pharmacokinetics of oxycodone. Journal of Pain and Palliative Care Pharmacotherapy. 18: 17–30.

59 National Patient Safety Agency (2008) Reducing risk of overdose with midazolam injection in adults. Rapid response report. NPSA/2008/RRR011. www.nrls.npsa.uk

60 National Patient Safety Agency (2006) Ensuring safer practice with high dose ampoules of diamorphine and morphine. Safer Practice Notice. NPSA/2006/12. www.nrls.npsa.nhs.uk

61 Gardiner P (2003) Compatibility of an injectable oxycodone formulation with typical diluents, syringes, tubings, infusion bags and drugs for potential co-administration. *Hospital Pharmacist* **10**: 354–361.

62 Hines S and Pleasance S (2009) Compatibility of an injectable high strength oxycodone formulation with typical diluents, syrings, tubings and infusion bags and drugs for potential co-administration. *European Journal of Hospital Pharmacy Practice.* **15**: 32–38.

Updated (minor change) August 2014

TAPENTADOL   BNF 4.7.2

Class: Strong opioid analgesic (but see below).

Indications: Moderate-severe acute pain (immediate-release formulation); severe chronic pain (m/r formulation).

Contra-indications: None absolute if titrated carefully against a patient's pain. (Also see Cautions below, and Strong opioids, p.357).

Pharmacology

Tapentadol is a centrally-acting analgesic which is both a μ agonist and an inhibitor of synaptic re-uptake of noradrenaline (norepinephrine); the latter enhances the action of the descending pain inhibitory pathway, contributing to a synergistic analgesic effect.[1–3] This possibly explains why tapentadol is only about ≤3 times less potent than **morphine**, despite an affinity for the μ-opioid receptor some ⩾18 times lower (see Tramadol, Table 1, p.353).[1–3] Tapentadol also has some serotoninergic activity, but this is not considered relevant to its analgesic effect.

Tramadol, like tapentadol, is also a synthetic centrally-acting analgesic with both non-opioid and opioid properties. However, at recommended maximum doses, tapentadol is equivalent to a much higher dose of PO **morphine** than **tramadol**, namely 150–200mg/24h vs. 40mg/24h (see p.352). Thus, for practical purposes, **tramadol** is best considered a Step 2 weak opioid (alongside **codeine**) and tapentadol a Step 3 strong opioid (alongside **morphine**; see p.291).

RCTs of tapentadol, using mainly **oxycodone** as the comparator, have been conducted in both acute (e.g. postoperative orthopaedic, low back pain)[4–6] and chronic pain (e.g. osteo-arthritis, low back pain, diabetic neuropathy, cancer-related).[7,8] These have shown tapentadol to be superior to placebo and/or non-inferior to **oxycodone** *at the lower end of its dose range*, i.e. in the chronic pain studies, the maximum comparative dose was **oxycodone** m/r ≤50mg b.d.

Tapentadol is comparable in cost to m/r **oxycodone**. However, a lack of comparative studies with other cheaper strong opioid products has resulted in recommendations *against* its use in acute pain,[9] and its restriction in chronic pain to patients who fail to get satisfactory analgesia from **morphine**.[10]

Undesirable effects include those typical of an opioid agonist. However, GI effects are significantly less than with **oxycodone** (less nausea, vomiting, constipation).[11] In non-cancer chronic pain studies, drug-related treatment withdrawals were about 20% for tapentadol vs. 40% for **oxycodone**.[7] In the cancer pain study, compared with **oxycodone**, rates of constipation and nausea were about 7% lower with tapentadol, with a similar rate of treatment withdrawal for both (≤8%).[8]

Food does not alter absorption to a clinically relevant degree. Tapentadol is extensively metabolized in the liver to inactive metabolites by glucuronidation, with ≤15% of a dose metabolized via CYP450 (mostly 2C9 and 2C19), thus reducing the likelihood of pharmacokinetic drug-drug interactions; only 3% is excreted unchanged in the urine. Systemic exposure to tapentadol is increased by hepatic but not renal impairment, although in the latter, levels of tapentadol-O-glucuronide (considered inactive) are increased. It has no effect on the QT interval (see Chapter 24, p.759).

By mouth, it is about 5 times *less* potent than **oxycodone** (i.e. tapentadol 50mg is approximately equivalent to **oxycodone** 10mg). By extrapolation, this suggests that it is about 3 times *less* potent than **morphine** (i.e. tapentadol 50mg is approximately equivalent to **morphine** 15–20mg) and recent study data supports this.[12] Thus, the maximum recommended m/r dose of

tapentadol 250mg b.d. is approximately equivalent to **oxycodone** 50mg b.d. or **morphine** 75–100mg b.d.
Bio-availability 32% PO.
Onset of action
Time to peak plasma concentration 75min immediate-release; 3–6h m/r.
Plasma halflife 4h immediate-release; 5–6h m/r.
Duration of action 4–6h immediate-release; 12h m/r.

Cautions

In moderate hepatic impairment, systemic exposure to tapentadol is increased >4 times, and the maximum recommended starting dose is 50mg q8h (immediate-release formulation) or once daily (m/r formulation).

Because of a lack of clinical trial data, the SPC recommends against the use of tapentadol in patients with severe hepatic or renal impairment, and those with, or at risk of, epilepsy.

Switching from another μ agonist (e.g. **morphine**, **oxycodone**) to tapentadol may cause low-grade opioid withdrawal, and p.r.n. doses of the original opioid should be used to counter this (e.g. give an immediate-release formulation at 1/4–1/2 of the original dose).

Abrupt discontinuation of tapentadol may result in symptoms of opioid withdrawal and the SPC advises tapering gradually. On the other hand, the SPC also notes that even with ≤12 months of use, withdrawal symptoms were either absent or mild.

Tapentadol has the potential for abuse and addiction.[13]

Drug interactions

Avoid concurrent administration with an MAOI, or within 2 weeks of the cessation of one, due to potential additive effects on synaptic noradrenaline concentrations.

Tapentadol is not completely devoid of serotoninergic activity.[1] There have been isolated reports of serotonin toxicity involving the use of tapentadol in conjunction with serotoninergic drugs (e.g. SSRIs); also see p.195.

Undesirable effects

See Strong opioids, Box B, p.361.

Dose and use

As with all opioids, patients must be monitored for undesirable effects (see p.360), particularly nausea and vomiting, and constipation. Depending on individual circumstances, an anti-emetic should be prescribed for regular or p.r.n. use (see p.241) and, routinely, a laxative prescribed (see p.44).

Immediate-release; moderate–severe acute pain:
* start with 50mg PO q4–6h if moderate pain/strong opioid naïve
* a higher starting dose may be necessary for severe pain/previous strong opioid use
* if the first dose is inadequate, a second dose can be taken after 1h (once only)
* if required, increase progressively to 100mg q4h or 150mg q6h
* maximum dose 600mg/24h (700mg in first 24h of use).

M/r; severe chronic pain:
* start with 50mg PO q12h if strong opioid naïve
* a higher starting dose may be necessary when switching from another strong opioid; non-cancer chronic pain trials have used the following starting doses based on existing oral morphine equivalent (OME) use:[12,14]
  ▷ OME ≤100mg/24h → tapentadol 50mg b.d.
  ▷ 101–160mg/24h → 100mg b.d.
  ▷ >160mg/24h → 150mg b.d.
  ▷ Note: all represent a reduction in opioid dose (see Pharmacology)
* if necessary, increase by 50mg b.d. every 3 days
* maximum dose 250mg b.d.

Supply
All products are **CD**.

Immediate-release oral formulation
Palexia® (Grünenthal)
Tablets 50mg, 75mg, 50mg dose = £0.45.
Oral solution 20mg/mL, 50mg dose = £0.45; *can be diluted in water or a non-alcoholic cold drink and is suitable for administration via EFT.*

Modified-release oral formulation
Palexia® SR (Grünenthal)
Tablets m/r 50mg, 100mg, 150mg, 200mg, 250mg 28 days @ 100mg q12h = £50.

---

1   Hoy SM (2012) Tapentadol extended release: in adults with chronic pain. *Drugs.* **72**: 375–393.
2   Schroder W et al. (2011) Synergistic interaction between the two mechanisms of action of tapentadol in analgesia. *Journal of Pharmacology and Experimental Therapeutics.* **337**: 312–320.
3   Tzschentke TM et al. (2014) The Mu-Opioid Receptor Agonist/Noradrenaline Reuptake Inhibition (MOR-NRI) concept in analgesia: The case of tapentadol. *CNS Drugs.* **28**: 319–329.
4   Frampton JE (2010) Tapentadol immediate release: a review of its use in the treatment of moderate to severe acute pain. *Drugs.* **70**: 1719–1743.
5   Biondi D et al. (2013) Tapentadol immediate release versus oxycodone immediate release for treatment of acute low back pain. *Pain Physician.* **16**: E237–246.
6   Vorsanger GJ et al. (2013) Immediate-release tapentadol or oxycodone for treatment of acute postoperative pain after elective arthroscopic shoulder surgery: a randomized, phase IIIb study. *Journal of Opioid Management.* **9**: 281–290.
7   Afilalo M and Morlion B (2013) Efficacy of tapentadol ER for managing moderate to severe chronic pain. *Pain Physician.* **16**: 27–40.
8   Imanaka K et al. (2013) Efficacy and safety of oral tapentadol extended release in Japanese and Korean patients with moderate to severe, chronic malignant tumor-related pain. *Current Medical Research Opinion.* **29**: 1399–1409.
9   Anonymous (2012) Tapentadol (Palexia) for moderate to severe acute pain. *Drug and Therapeutics Bulletin.* **50**: 30–33.
10 Scottish Medicines Consortium (2011) Tapentadol prolonged-release tablets (Palexia SR). www.scottishmedicines.org
11 Etropolski M et al. (2011) Comparable efficacy and superior gastrointestinal tolerability (nausea, vomiting, constipation) of tapentadol compared with oxycodone hydrochloride. *Advances in Therapy.* **28**: 401–417.
12 Galvez R et al. (2013) Tapentadol prolonged release versus strong opioids for severe, chronic low back pain: results of an open-label, phase 3b study. *Advances in Therapy.* **30**: 229–259.
13 Cepeda MS et al. (2013) Comparison of opioid doctor shopping for tapentadol and oxycodone: a cohort study. *Journal of Pain.* **14**: 158–164.
14 Steigerwald I et al. (2013) Effectiveness and tolerability of tapentadol prolonged release compared with prior opioid therapy for the management of severe, chronic osteoarthritis pain. *Clinical Drug Investigation.* **33**: 607–619.

Updated (minor change) August 2014

OPIOID ANTAGONISTS   BNF 1.6.6, 4.10.3 & 15.1.7

Indications: Reversal of opioid-induced respiratory depression (**naloxone**), acute opioid overdose (**naloxone**), prevention of relapse in opioid and †alcohol addiction (**naloxone, naltrexone**), opioid-induced constipation or post-operative ileus (**methylnaltrexone**), †pruritus caused by cholestasis[1] or spinal opioids (**naloxone, naltrexone**), and possibly, chronic renal failure (**naltrexone**).[2,3]

Contra-indications: Vary between products; consult SPC for details, e.g.:
Naloxone: none when used to reverse opioid-induced respiratory depression or acute opioid overdose
Naltrexone: patients physically dependent on opioids (i.e. after 2 weeks of regular PO use); acute hepatitis or hepatic failure; severe renal impairment (creatinine clearance < 30mL/min)
Methylnaltrexone: known or suspected bowel obstruction.

Pharmacology
Naloxone, naltrexone and **nalmefene** (not UK) are generally thought of as pure antagonists; they have a high affinity for opioid receptors but no intrinsic activity. They reversibly block access to the opioid receptors and, if given after an opioid agonist, they displace the latter because of their higher receptor affinity.[4]

However, the discovery that ultra-low doses of **naloxone** and **nalmefene** given post-operatively potentiate the analgesic effect of **morphine** and/or reduce undesirable effects (nausea and vomiting, and pruritus) means that the situation is more complex.[5–9]

In fact, it is over 30 years since it was shown in post-dental extraction pain that **naloxone** could produce either analgesia (low-dose) or hyperalgesia (high-dose).[10] Further, in the same circumstances, **naloxone** 400microgram neutralizes the analgesic effect of **morphine** 8mg IV (as expected) but more than doubles the analgesic effect of **pentazocine** 60mg IV.[11] (Pentazocine is a partial μ and κ agonist and δ antagonist.)[12] **Naltrexone** appears to demonstrate similar effects.[13–15] In patients, *ultra-low* dose **naltrexone** potentiates the analgesic effect of **methadone, oxycodone** and IT **morphine**.[13,16,17]

These phenomena are best explained by opioid antagonists having other effects in addition to classical opioid receptor antagonism. For example, a ligand binding to an opioid receptor can trigger either an inhibitory or excitatory response, dependent on the type of G protein coupled to the receptor, either G_I/G_O (inhibitory) or G_s (excitatory). Typically, with an opioid agonist, the G_I/G_O (inhibitory) activity predominates resulting in analgesia and other opioid effects. In such circumstances, a typical clinical dose of an opioid antagonist like **naloxone** will displace the opioid agonist from the receptor and thereby reverse its effects. However, the G_s excitatory response can increase in various circumstances, e.g. chronic opioid use, nerve damage.[18] This may contribute to opioid tolerance and, when predominant, to opioid-induced hyperalgesia.[19] Ultra-low levels of **naloxone** interfere with the scaffolding protein (filamin A), which couples G_s to the opioid receptor and thereby inhibits the excitatory response.[20]

Naloxone also binds to the non-opioid toll-like receptor 4 on glial cells; this interaction inhibits glial cell activation, which appears important in CNS sensitization.[21,22] Glial cell activation is associated with a reduction in glutamate transporters, which impedes the synaptic clearance of this excitatory neurotransmitter. In an animal model of neuropathic pain, ultra-low dose **naloxone** prevented the loss of glutamate transporters and enhanced the analgesic effect of **morphine**.[23]

These effects of ultra-low dose **naloxone** at non-opioid receptor binding sites, which can improve analgesia, are lost with higher doses because of classical opioid receptor antagonism. Thus, despite the potential benefits of ultra-low dose **naloxone**, the inherent risk of reversal of analgesia limits the widespread clinical application of this approach and it should only be undertaken by specialists in pain or palliative medicine. In practice, if opioid-induced hyperalgesia is suspected, the first and most important step is to reduce the dose of the offending opioid (also see p.364).

Opioid antagonists are used in various clinical settings:

Reversal of opioid-induced respiratory depression: The most important clinical property of naloxone is reversal of opioid-induced respiratory depression (and other opioid effects) caused by either an overdose of an opioid or an exaggerated response to conventional doses. Compared with other opioids, antagonism of buprenorphine requires higher doses of **naloxone** because **buprenorphine** also has high receptor affinity (see p.393).

Naloxone has been reported to be only partially effective in reversing the effects of **tramadol**.[24,25] However, in a series of 11 patients with a **tramadol** overdose, seven had a good response to **naloxone**, and only one had no response.[26]

Patients with opioid overdose may develop pulmonary oedema. The exact mechanism is unclear. Because pulmonary oedema has been seen both in older patients with typical doses of **naloxone**, e.g. 200–400microgram, and in healthy teenagers with doses as low as 40–80microgram, it has been suggested that **naloxone** can trigger a central neurogenic response which leads to vasoconstriction of the pulmonary vasculature followed by pulmonary oedema.[27] Alternatively, because pulmonary oedema is almost universal in fatal opioid overdose,[28,29] **naloxone**, by increasing respiratory rate and tidal volume, may simply unmask pulmonary oedema which has developed secondary to severe hypoxaemia and acidaemia.[30]

Delayed-onset pulmonary oedema (48h after overdose treated with **naloxone**) due to acute cardiomyopathy has also been reported, possibly the result of cardiac muscle damage caused by hypoxaemia.[31]

Prevention of relapse in opioid addiction: **Naltrexone** 100mg blocks the effect of a challenge of IV **diamorphine** 25mg by 96% at 24h, and 46% at 72h.[32] Thus, **naltrexone** is primarily used to prevent relapse in opioid addiction by blocking opioid 'highs'. It is also used PO off-label to reduce the relapse rate in alcohol addiction. **Naltrexone** is given PO either once daily or three times per week. It is also available as a long-acting depot IM injection (duration of action > 1 month; authorized for use in alcohol and opioid addiction) and a SC pellet implant (duration of action weeks–months).[33–35] Both injectable products are unauthorized in the UK, but are available through private addiction clinics.

Opioid combination products to deter opioid abuse: In an attempt to reduce the risk of opioid abuse, PO formulations containing both a strong opioid and an opioid antagonist have been developed, e.g.:
- Suboxone® (**buprenorphine + naloxone**) given SL for opioid dependency
- Targinact® (**oxycodone + naloxone**, see p.444)

When administered PO, the opioid antagonist either remains sequestered or the amount released is insufficient to antagonize the analgesic effect of the opioid. However, if abused (e.g. the tablets crushed and administered by insufflation or IV), the opioid antagonist is then released in sufficient amounts to antagonize the opioid.

Opioid-induced GI disorders: **Methylnaltrexone** and **alvimopan** (not UK) are quaternary compounds which do not readily cross the blood-brain barrier and thus act as peripheral opioid antagonists. SC **methylnaltrexone** is authorized for use in 'advanced illness' to treat opioid-induced constipation despite treatment with laxatives (see Dose and use). In this situation, **methylnaltrexone** has an NNT of 3 (95% CI 2–10) and an NNH of 14 (95% CI 9–33).[36] PO **alvimopan** is indicated in postoperative ileus.[37,38]

In the past, PO **naloxone** and **naltrexone** have been used to correct delayed gastric emptying and constipation.[37] However, because both are centrally acting, there is a risk of reversal of analgesia and systemic withdrawal and **methylnaltrexone** is now preferable.

Because constipation in advanced disease is generally multifactorial in origin,[39] **methylnaltrexone** augments rather than replaces laxatives. Off-label uses include opioid-induced constipation in post-operative[40,41] or non-surgical critical care patients[42] and opioid-related acute colonic pseudo-obstruction.[43] **Methylnaltrexone** may also improve other peripheral effects of opioids, e.g. urinary retention.[40]

Targinact® (m/r **oxycodone** + m/r **naloxone**) is also marketed as a product which helps reduce opioid-induced constipation. Although primarily added to deter abuse (see above), the naloxone appears to reduce the impact of the opioid on the GI tract (see p.442). The m/r formulation helps ensure that most of the naloxone is removed by first-pass metabolism, minimizing the amount reaching the systemic circulation and the risk of reversal of analgesia.

Pruritus: In cholestasis, pruritus is a consequence of increased opioidergic tone caused by a raised plasma enkephalin concentration.[44–47] Opioid antagonists counteract the increased tone, and thus relieve the pruritus.

Naloxone by CIVI/CSCI decreases scratching activity by patients with cholestatic pruritus[48–50] and has a place in the emergency treatment of acute exacerbations of cholestatic pruritus. PO **naltrexone**[1,51] (or **nalmefene**;[52] not UK) can then be used long-term.

However, opioid antagonists can precipitate an opioid withdrawal-like reaction in patients with cholestasis, including hallucinations and dysphoria.[46,53] To avoid or minimize such a reaction, treatment must be started cautiously with a low-dose (see Dose and use).

The use of **naltrexone** to relieve cholestatic jaundice may sometimes unmask or exacerbate underlying pain, necessitating discontinuation of **naltrexone**.[54] Thus, patients with cholestatic jaundice and pruritus and severe pain should *not* be treated with an opioid antagonist.[55] Instead, an alternative treatment for pruritus should be used (see Chapter 28, Table 1, p.796) and the pain treated appropriately with both non-opioid and opioid analgesics.

There are reports of patients with cholestatic pruritus who have responded to **buprenorphine** alone or in combination with ultra-low doses of **naloxone**.[56–59] Sometimes ultra-low doses of **naloxone** or **naltrexone** improved both the pruritus and the pain.[60] However, there are insufficient data at present to recommend this approach.

In uremic pruritus, the situation is more complex because there are several causal mechanisms, both peripheral (cutaneous) and central (neural).[61] The opioid system is involved, but in uraemia there is no increase in opioidergic tone (and thus no danger of a withdrawal syndrome if an opioid antagonist is given). Instead, the ratio between μ-opioid (pruritus-inducible) and κ-opioid (pruritus-suppressive) receptors alters in favour of the former.[62,63] This predisposes to the onset or exacerbation of pruritus. It also suggests that both κ *agonists* and μ *antagonists* could bring relief. Thus, in an RCT lasting 2–4 weeks of **nalfurafine** (not UK), a novel κ agonist, 36% of subjects responded (at least 50% reduction in worst itching) compared with 15% in the placebo group.[64]

Naltrexone has also been tried in this setting.[65] However, RCTs have given conflicting results, e.g. benefit was seen in uraemic patients with very severe pruritus[2] but not in those with moderately severe pruritus.[3] One explanation is that, in uraemia, an opioid mechanism is important only in severe pruritus. The fact that **naltrexone** is non-selective and antagonizes both μ- and κ-opioid receptors may also be relevant.

In an open study of patients with various skin and systemic disorders associated with pruritus, good relief was obtained with **naltrexone** in 70% of patients.[45] However, in the absence of controlled data, the results should be interpreted with caution. Pruritus associated with chronic disease generally requires alternative specific measures (see Chapter 28, p.797).

Ultra-low dose **naloxone** is also used to relieve pruritus caused by spinal opioids, when other treatments have failed (see Spinal analgesia, p.720).

Miscellaneous: **Naloxone** is reported to benefit patients with septic shock,[66] **morphine**-induced peripheral vasodilation,[67] ischaemic central neurological deficits[68,69] and post-stroke central pain.[70]

Endogenous opioids inhibit cell proliferation, an effect which intermittent low-dose **naltrexone** appears to augment by provoking a compensatory elevation in opioid growth factor (OGF, an enkephalin) and OGF receptor, (a non-classical opioid receptor). This interaction impacts upon the cell cycle, inhibiting proliferation. The potential roles of low-dose **naltrexone** and OGF in cancer and auto-immune diseases (e.g. multiple sclerosis, Crohn's disease) are being explored.[71–73]

Pharmacokinetics: Table 1 contains selected pharmacokinetic data. Compared with **naloxone**, **naltrexone** has a higher PO bio-availability and a longer duration of action; it undergoes extensive first-pass metabolism.[74,75] The major metabolite, 6-β-naltrexol, is a *neutral* antagonist, i.e. it inhibits activation of opioid receptors but, unlike **naloxone** and **naltrexone**, it does not suppress basal receptor signalling, thereby reducing the risk of severe withdrawal. The antagonist effect of 6-β-naltrexol also shows peripheral selectivity. Accordingly, it may be developed commercially as a treatment for opioid-induced GI disorders.[76]

Table 1 Pharmacokinetic profiles of selected opioid antagonists

	Naloxone	Naltrexone
Bio-availability (%)	6 PO	5–40 PO
Onset of action	1–2min IV; 2–5min SC/IM	May precipitate withdrawal symptoms in <5min in opioid-dependent patients
Time to peak plasma concentration		1–2h PO
Plasma halflife	about 1h	4h; 13h for 6-β-naltrexol[77]
Duration of action	IV 15–90min	1–3 days

Cautions

In patients receiving opioids for pain relief, **naloxone** should *not* be used for drowsiness and/or delirium which is not life-threatening because of the danger of reversing the opioid analgesia and precipitating a major physical withdrawal syndrome. Instead, omit or reduce the next regular dose, and subsequently continue at a reduced dose.

The use of **naltrexone** will also impede opioid analgesia (see below),[78] and can precipitate an opioid withdrawal-like syndrome in patients with cholestatic pruritus. **Naltrexone** may cause occasional hepatotoxicity;[79] the manufacturer advises checking LFTs before and at intervals during treatment.

The dose of **methylnaltrexone** should be reduced in severe renal impairment.

Undesirable effects

Naloxone: nausea and vomiting; occasionally severe hypertension, pulmonary oedema (see above), rarely tachycardia, arrhythmias, and even cardiac arrest.[80]

Naltrexone: very common (> 10% in detoxifying opioid addicts) insomnia, headaches, anxiety, nausea and vomiting, intestinal colic, lack of energy, joint and muscle pain.

The long-term use of **naltrexone** increases the concentration of opioid receptors in the CNS and results in a temporary enhanced response to the subsequent administration of opioid analgesics.[81] The management of severe acute and postoperative pain in patients receiving long-term **naltrexone** requires careful consideration (Box A).[78]

Box A   Management of acute pain in patients receiving naltrexone

Elective surgery

The use of naltrexone must be identified well before the operation.

Ensure effective liaison between the substance misuse and acute pain teams.

Consider switching patients on IM depot injections to PO tablets before surgery.

For minor surgery, when non-opioids are considered sufficient to manage the postoperative pain, leave SC pellet *in situ*; if severe postoperative pain anticipated, remove SC pellet.

Discontinue PO naltrexone 72h before the operation.

Maximize the use of non-opioid analgesics, e.g. IV paracetamol, NSAID.

Note: if an opioid analgesic is required, a bigger than usual dose may be needed but, conversely, there may be an increased response to opioids (see Pharmacology above).

Unexpected severe acute pain, e.g. trauma, emergency surgery

If possible use non-opioid analgesics, e.g.:
• IV paracetamol and/or NSAID
• ketamine 100microgram/kg IV every 5min until satisfactory analgesia obtained, plus a single dose of midazolam 20–40microgram/kg IV to minimize dysphoria; may be repeated after 30min; give further midazolam only if dysphoria present.

Note: there is a risk of marked sedation when ketamine and midazolam are combined in this way; to be used only by those competent in airway management.

If venous access is difficult, ketamine can be given SC; use the same doses as for IV but allow 15min between doses.

The above are generally used to achieve rapid pain relief until other measures can be instituted, e.g.:
• local anaesthetic blocks
• epidural analgesia (local anaesthetic ± clonidine).

Methylnaltrexone: *common* abdominal pain/colic (generally mild–moderate),[82] diarrhoea, flatulence, nausea (these generally resolve after a bowel movement), dizziness (postural hypotension can occur). *Rare* syncope, severe diarrhoea and cardiovascular collapse, and GI perforation (stomach, small and large bowel).[83]

Dose and use
Naloxone is best given IV but, if not practical, may be given IM or SC.

Opioid overdose (naloxone)
Dose recommendations vary, and the following is offered as a guide. Assess each dose after 1min and if no response, move to the next dose:
• start with 400microgram → 800microgram → 800microgram → 2–4mg
• if no response to 2–4mg consider an alternate diagnosis
• if necessary, set up an IVI set to deliver an hourly dose which is 50–100% of the stat dose which had previously maintained satisfactory ventilation for ⩾15min
• the recommended IVI concentration is 200microgram/mL, diluted in 0.9% saline or 5% glucose
• titrate the IVI as necessary.[84]

Because **buprenorphine** has very strong receptor affinity (reflected in its high relative potency with **morphine**), **naloxone** in standard doses does *not* reverse the effects of **buprenorphine** and higher doses must be used (see Buprenorphine, Box A, p.394).

After the administration of **naloxone**, if there is unexpected breathlessness and persistent hypoxaemia despite **oxygen**, the possibility of pulmonary oedema should be considered. Delayed-onset pulmonary oedema (48h after overdose) may also occur, associated with acute cardiomyopathy, and possibly the result of hypoxaemic cardiac muscle damage.[31] Treat as necessary with **oxygen**, IV **furosemide**, IVI nitrates, and ventilation. The pulmonary oedema generally responds to these measures and resolves within 24–48h.

Reversal of respiratory depression caused by the medicinal use of opioids (naloxone)

Small doses must be used: total antagonism with **naloxone** 400microgram (a standard ampoule) will lead to severe pain and, if physically opioid-dependent, hyperalgesia and marked agitation, together with an acute withdrawal syndrome.[85] Thus, it is important to titrate the dose against respiratory function and *not* the level of consciousness.

If respiratory rate ≥8 breaths/min, and the patient easily rousable and not cyanosed, adopt a policy of 'wait and see'; consider omitting or reducing the next regular dose, and subsequently continuing at a reduced dose.

If respiratory rate <8 breaths/min, and the patient comatose/unconscious and/or cyanosed:
• give **naloxone** 100–200microgram IV stat
• then give 100microgram IV every 2min until respiratory function is satisfactory.

If the overdose is associated with a long-acting opioid, e.g. m/r formulation or **methadone**, the duration of action of the opioid will exceed that of **naloxone**. Thus, even if there is an initial response to **naloxone**, further IV doses are likely to be needed, and it may be necessary to continue treatment with a closely monitored IVI of **naloxone** for up to 24h, and sometimes longer. Lower doses have been recommended by the American Pain Society (Box B).[86]

Box B Naloxone for iatrogenic opioid overdose (American Pain Society)[86]

If respiratory rate ≥8 breaths/min, and the patient easily rousable and not cyanosed, adopt a policy of 'wait and see'; consider reducing or omitting the next regular dose of opioid.

If respiratory rate <8 breaths/min, and the patient comatose/unconscious and/or cyanosed:
• dilute a 1mL ampoule containing naloxone 400microgram to 10mL with 0.9% saline for injection
• administer 0.5mL (20microgram) IV every 2min until the patient's respiratory status is satisfactory
• further boluses may be necessary because naloxone is shorter-acting than morphine (and other opioids)
• wait until there has been a sustained improvement in consciousness before restarting a lower dose of opioid.

In addition, consider possible cause(s) for the opioid overdose, e.g. excessive use in an opioid poorly-responsive pain, accumulation because of a long halflife (**methadone**) or reduced elimination because of renal impairment (**morphine, hydromorphone**). Wait until there has been a sustained improvement in consciousness before restarting a lower dose of opioid. It may be preferable to switch the type of opioid; seek specialist advice.

Rarely, following an opioid overdose, pulmonary oedema can occur but the signs may be absent until **naloxone** administration improves the respiratory rate and tidal volume. Consider also when there is unexpected breathlessness and persistent hypoxaemia despite **oxygen**. Delayed onset pulmonary oedema (48h after overdose) has also been reported due to acute cardiomyopathy, possibly as a result of cardiac muscle damage caused by hypoxaemia.[29] Treat the pulmonary oedema with **oxygen**, IV **furosemide**, IVI nitrates, and ventilation as necessary. Generally the pulmonary oedema responds to these approaches and resolves within 24–48h.

Treatment of opioid-induced constipation (methylnaltrexone)

Methylnaltexone is relatively expensive and should be considered only as a supplement to a stimulant laxative (e.g. **senna**, see p.40) when an optimized dose of the latter is insufficient. A survey in the USA found that about one quarter of prescriptions for **methylnaltrexone** (mainly by generalists) were inappropriate with regard to indication or dose.[87]

Methylnaltrexone is contra-indicated in cases of known or suspected bowel obstruction; it should be used with caution in patients with conditions which may predispose to perforation (e.g. GI cancer, peptic ulcer, colonic pseudo-obstruction).

Between 1/3–1/2 of patients given **methylnaltrexone** defaecate within 30min–4h without loss of analgesia or the development of opioid withdrawal symptoms.[88–92] Dose recommendations:
- for patients weighing 38–61kg, start with 8mg on alternate days
- for patients weighing 62–114kg, start with 12mg on alternate days
- outside this range, give 150microgram/kg on alternate days
- the interval between administrations can be varied, either extended or reduced, but not more than once daily.

In severe renal impairment (creatinine clearance <30mL/min) reduce the dose:
- for patients weighing 62–114kg, reduce to 8mg
- outside this range, reduce to 75*microgram/kg*, rounding up the dose volume to the nearest 0.1mL.

Cholestatic pruritus (naloxone, nalmefene, naltrexone)

To try and avoid or minimize an opioid withdrawal-like syndrome, start with a low dose. Although some recommend the initial use of **naloxone**, others have successfully used **naltrexone** *de novo* 12.5–25mg PO b.d. and subsequently titrated as below:
- start with a low dose of **naloxone** by CIVI, e.g. 0.002microgram/kg/min (about 160–200 microgram/24h)[46]; long-term administration by CSCI has also been reported[50]
- if no withdrawal-like symptoms occur, the rate can be doubled every 3–4h; but if symptoms occur, continue with the current dose until resolved
- after 18–24h, when a rate known to be associated with opioid antagonistic effects is reached (0.2microgram/kg/min), the infusion is stopped and **naltrexone** 12.5–25mg PO b.d. is started)[46,51,53]
- the dose is increased every few days until a satisfactory clinical response is obtained; at this stage the effective dose should be consolidated into a single daily maintenance dose
- the effective dose range for PO **naltrexone** is 25–250mg once daily[46]
- for **nalmefene** (not UK) start with 2mg PO b.d.; double the dose every 2 days until pruritus is relieved or no further improvement; individual maximum doses 30–120mg b.d.[93]

Uraemic pruritus (naltrexone)
- start with **naltrexone** 50mg PO once daily[2,3]
- if ineffective after 1 week, consider increasing dose to 100mg once daily.

Supply

Naloxone

Naloxone hydrochloride (generic)
Injection 20microgram/mL, 2mL amp = £6; 400microgram/mL, 1mL amp = £4; 1mg/mL, 2mL prefilled syringe = £17.

Minijet® Naloxone (UCB Pharma)
Injection (prefilled syringe) 400microgram/mL, 1mL = £20, 2mL = £13, 5mL = £21.

Naltrexone

Naltrexone hydrochloride (generic)
Tablets (scored) 50mg, 28 days @ 50mg once daily = £22.
Capsules 0.5mg, 1mg, 1.5mg, 3mg, 4mg, 4.5mg; 100 x all strengths = £180 (unauthorized, available as a special order from Martindale, see Appendix 1, p.817).
Oral suspension 5mg/mL, 28 days @ 50mg once daily = £674 (unauthorized, available as a special order, see Appendix 1, p.817); *price based on specials tariff in community.*

Methylnaltrexone

Relistor® (Wyeth)
Injection methylnaltrexone bromide 20mg/mL, 0.6mL = £21.

1 Wolfhagen F et al. (1997) Oral naltrexone treatment for cholestatic pruritus: A double-blind, placebo-controlled study. Gastroenterology. 113: 1264–1269.
2 Peer G et al. (1996) Randomised crossover trial of naltrexone in uraemic pruritus. Lancet. 348: 1552–1554.
3 Pauli-Magnus C et al. (2000) Naltrexone does not relieve uremic pruritus. Journal of the American Society of Nephrology. 11: 514–519.
4 Choi YS and Billings JA (2002) Opioid antagonists: a review of their role in palliative care, focusing on use in opioid-related constipation. Journal of Pain and Symptom Management. 24: 71–90.
5 Gan T et al. (1997) Opioid-sparing effects of a low-dose infusion of naloxone in patient-administered morphine sulfate. Anesthesiology. 87: 1075–1081.
6 Joshi G et al. (1999) Effects of prophylactic nalmefene on the incidence of morphine-related side effects in patients receiving intravenous patient-controlled analgesia. Anesthesiology. 90: 1007–1011.
7 Cepeda MS et al. (2004) Addition of ultralow dose naloxone to postoperative morphine PCA: unchanged analgesia and opioid requirement but decreased incidence of opioid side effects. Pain. 107: 41–46.
8 Maxwell LG et al. (2005) The effects of a small-dose naloxone infusion on opioid-induced side effects and analgesia in children and adolescents treated with intravenous patient-controlled analgesia: a double-blind, prospective, randomized, controlled study. Anesthesia and Analgesia. 100: 953–958.
9 Murphy JD et al. (2011) Analgesic efficacy of intravenous naloxone for the treatment of postoperative pruritus: a meta-analysis. Journal of Opioid Management. 7: 321–327.
10 Levine JD et al. (1979) Naloxone dose dependently produces analgesia and hyperalgesia in postoperative pain. Nature. 278: 740–741.
11 Levine J and Gordon N (1988) Synergism between the analgesic actions of morphine and pentazocine. Pain. 33: 369–372.
12 Hill RG (1992) Multiple opioid receptors and their ligands. Frontiers of Pain. 4: 1–4.
13 Chindalore VL et al. (2005) Adding ultralow-dose naltrexone to oxycodone enhances and prolongs analgesia: a randomized, controlled trial of Oxytrex. Journal of Pain. 6: 392–399.
14 Largent-Milnes TM et al. (2008) Oxycodone plus ultra-low-dose naltrexone attenuates neuropathic pain and associated mu-opioid receptor-Gs coupling. Journal of Pain. 9: 700–713.
15 Hay JL et al. (2011) Potentiation of buprenorphine antinociception with ultra-low dose naltrexone in healthy subjects. European Journal of Pain. 15: 293–298.
16 Cruciani RA et al. (2003) Ultra-low dose oral naltrexone decreases side effects and potentiates the effect of methadone. Journal of Pain and Symptom Management. 25: 491–494.
17 Hamann S and Sloan P (2007) Oral naltrexone to enhance analgesia in patients receiving continuous intrathecal morphine for chronic pain: a randomized, double-blind, prospective pilot study. Journal of Opioid Management. 3: 137–144.
18 Crain S and Shen K (2000) Antagonists of excitatory opioid receptor functions enhance morphine's analgesic potency and attenuate opioid tolerance/dependence liability. Pain. 84: 121–131.
19 Sjogren P et al. (1994) Disappearance of morphine-induced hyperalgesia after discontinuing or substituting morphine with other opioid antagonists. Pain. 59: 313–316.
20 Wang HY and Burns LH (2009) Naloxone's pentapeptide binding site on filamin A blocks Mu opioid receptor-Gs coupling and CREB activation of acute morphine. PLoS One. 4: e4282.
21 Milligan ED and Watkins LR (2009) Pathological and protective roles of glia in chronic pain. Nature Reviews Neuroscience. 10: 23–36.
22 Ren K and Dubner R (2008) Neuron-glia crosstalk gets serious: role in pain hypersensitivity. Current Opinion in Anaesthesiology. 21: 570–579.
23 Yang CP et al. (2011) Intrathecal ultra-low dose naloxone enhances the antinociceptive effect of morphine by enhancing the reuptake of excitatory amino acids from the synaptic cleft in the spinal cord of partial sciatic nerve-transected rats. Anesthesia and Analgesia. 113: 1490–1500.
24 Raffa RB et al. (1992) Opioid and nonopioid components independently contribute to the mechanism of action of tramadol, an 'atypical' opioid analgesic. Journal of Pharmacology and Therapeutics. 260: 275–285.
25 Shipton EA (2000) Tramadol - present and future. Anaesthesia and Intensive Care. 28: 363–374.
26 Marquardt KA et al. (2005) Tramadol exposures reported to statewide poison control system. Annals of Pharmacotherapy. 39: 1039–1044.
27 Horng HC et al. (2010) Negative pressure pulmonary edema following naloxone administration in a patient with fentanyl-induced respiratory depression. Acta Anaesthesiology Taiwan. 48: 155–157.
28 Ridgway ZA and Pountney AJ (2007) Acute respiratory distress syndrome induced by oral methadone managed with non-invasive ventilation. Emergency Medicine Journal. 24: 681.
29 Feeney C et al. (2011) Morphine-induced cardiogenic shock. Annals of Pharmacotherpy. 45: e30.
30 Clarke SF et al. (2005) Naloxone in opioid poisoning: walking the tightrope. Emergency Medicine Journal. 22: 612–616.
31 Paranthaman SK and Khan F (1976) Acute cardiomyopathy with recurrent pulmonary edema and hypotension following heroin overdosage. Chest. 69: 117–119.
32 Verebey K (1981) The clinical pharmacology of naltrexone: pharmacology and pharmacodynamics. NIDA Research Monograph. 28: 147–158.
33 Volpicelli JR et al. (1992) Naltrexone in the treatment of alcohol dependence. Archives of General Psychiatry. 49: 876–880.
34 Swift RM et al. (1994) Naltrexone-induced alterations in human ethanol intoxication. American Journal of Psychiatry. 151: 1463–1467.
35 Krupitsky E et al. (2011) Injectable extended-release naltrexone for opioid dependence: a double-blind, placebo-controlled, multicentre randomised trial. Lancet. 377: 1506–1513.
36 Ford AC et al. (2013) Efficacy of pharmacological therapies for the treatment of opioid-induced constipation: systematic review and meta-analysis. American Journal of Gastroenterology. 108: 1566–1574.
37 McNicol ED (2008) Mu-opioid antagonists for opioid-induced bowel dysfunction. Cochrane Database of Systematic Reviews. 2: CD006332.
38 Becker G and Blum HE (2009) Novel opioid antagonists for opioid-induced bowel dysfunction and postoperative ileus. Lancet. 373: 1198–1206.
39 Larkin PJ et al. (2008) The management of constipation in palliative care: clinical practice recommendations. Palliative Medicine. 22: 796–807.

40 Deibert P et al. (2010) Methylnaltrexone: the evidence for its use in the management of opioid-induced constipation. *Core Evidence*. **4**: 247–258.

41 Anissian L et al. (2012) Subcutaneous methylnaltrexone for treatment of acute opioid-induced constipation: phase 2 study in rehabilitation after orthopedic surgery. *Journal of Hospital Medicine*. **7**: 67–72.

42 Sawh SB et al. (2012) Use of methylnaltrexone for the treatment of opioid-induced constipation in critical care patients. *Mayo Clinic Proceedings*. **87**: 255–259.

43 Weinstock LB and Chang AC (2011) Methylnaltrexone for treatment of acute colonic pseudo-obstruction. *Journal of Clinical Gastroenterology*. **45**: 883–884.

44 Davis M (2007) Cholestasis and endogenous opioids: liver disease and exogenous opioid pharmacokinetics. *Clinical Pharmacokinetics*. **46**: 825–850.

45 Metze D et al. (1999) Efficacy and safety of naltrexone, an oral opiate receptor antagonist, in the treatment of pruritus in internal and dermatological diseases. *Journal of the American Academy of Dermatology*. **41**: 533–539.

46 Jones E et al. (2002) Opiate antagonist therapy for the pruritus of cholestasis: the avoidance of opioid withdrawal-like reactions. *Quarterly Journal of Medicine*. **95**: 547–552.

47 Tandon P et al. (2007) The efficacy and safety of bile acid binding agents, opioid antagonists, or rifampin in the treatment of cholestasis-associated pruritus. *American Journal of Gastroenterology*. **102**: 1528–1536.

48 Bergasa N et al. (1992) A controlled trial of naloxone infusions for the pruritus of chronic cholestasis. *Gastroenterology*. **102**: 544–549.

49 Bergasa N et al. (1995) Effects of naloxone infusions in patients with the pruritus of cholestasis. *Annals of Internal Medicine*. **123**: 161–167.

50 Kumar N et al. (2013) Opiate receptor antagonists for treatment of severe pruritus associated with advanced cholestatic liver disease. *Journal of Palliative Medicine*. **16**: 122–123.

51 Terg R et al. (2002) Efficacy and safety of oral naltrexone treatment for pruritus of cholestasis, a crossover, double blind, placebo-controlled study. *Journal of Hepatology*. **37**: 717–722.

52 Bergasa N et al. (1999) Oral nalmefene therapy reduces scratching activity due to the pruritus of cholestasis: a controlled study. *Journal of the American Academy of Dermatology*. **41**: 431–434.

53 Jones E and Dekker L (2000) Florid opioid withdrawal-like reaction precipitated by naltrexone in a patient with chronic cholestasis. *Gastroenterology*. **118**: 431–432.

54 McRae CA et al. (2003) Pain as a complication of use of opiate antagonists for symptom control in cholestasis. *Gastroenterology*. **125**: 591–596.

55 Lonsdale-Eccles AA and Carmichael AJ (2009) Opioid antagonist for pruritus of cholestasis unmasking bony metastases. *Acta Dermato Venereologica*. **89**: 90.

56 Juby L et al. (1994) Buprenorphine and hepatic pruritus. *British Journal of Clinical Practice*. **48**: 331.

57 Reddy L et al. (2007) Transdermal buprenorphine may be effective in the treatment of pruritus in primary biliary cirrhosis. *Journal of Pain and Symptom Management*. **34**: 455–456.

58 Marinangeli F et al. (2009) Intravenous naloxone plus transdermal buprenorphine in cancer pain associated with intractable cholestatic pruritus. *Journal of Pain and Symptom Management*. **38**: e5–8.

59 Zylicz Z et al. (2005) Severe pruritus of cholestasis in disseminated cancer: developing a rational treatment strategy. A case report. *Journal of Pain and Symptom Management*. **29**: 100–103.

60 Jones EA and Zylicz Z (2005) Treatment of pruritus caused by cholestasis with opioid antagonists. *Journal of Palliative Medicine*. **8**: 1290–1294.

61 Manenti L et al. (2009) Uraemic pruritus: clinical characteristics, pathophysiology and treatment. *Drugs*. **69**: 251–263.

62 Kumagai H et al. (2000) Endogenous opioid system in uraemic patients. In: *Joint Meeting of the Seventh World Conference on Clinical Pharmacology and IUPHAR - Division of Clinical Pharmacology and the Fourth Congress of the European Association for Clinical Pharmacology and Therapeutics*.

63 Odou P et al. (2001) A hypothesis for endogenous opioid peptides in uraemic pruritus: role of enkephalin. *Nephrology, Dialysis, Transplantation*. **16**: 1953–1954.

64 Wikstrom B et al. (2005) Kappa-opioid system in uremic pruritus: multicenter, randomized, double-blind, placebo-controlled clinical studies. *Journal of the American Society of Nephrology*. **16**: 3742–3747.

65 Quan Phan N (2010) Antipruritic treatment with systemic u-opioid receptor antagonists; a review. *Journal of the American Academy of Dermatology*. **63**: 680–688.

66 Peters WP et al. (1981) Pressor effect of naloxone in septic shock. *Lancet*. **i**: 529–532.

67 Cohen RA and Coffman JD (1980) Naloxone reversal of morphine-induced peripheral vasodilatation. *Clinical Pharmacology and Therapeutics*. **28**: 541–544.

68 Baskin DS and Hosobuchi Y (1981) Naloxone reversal of ischaemic neurological deficits in man. *Lancet*. **ii**: 272–275.

69 Bousigue J-Y et al. (1982) Naloxone reversal of neurological deficit. *Lancet*. **ii**: 618–619.

70 Ray D and Tai Y (1988) Infusions of naloxone in thalamic pain. *British Medical Journal*. **296**: 969–970.

71 Smith JP et al. (2010) Opioid growth factor improves clinical benefit and survival in patients with advanced pancreatic cancer. *Open Access Journal of Clinical Trials*. **2010**: 37–48.

72 Donahue RN et al. (2011) Low-dose naltrexone targets the opioid growth factor-opioid growth factor receptor pathway to inhibit cell proliferation: mechanistic evidence from a tissue culture model. *Experimental Biology and Medicine*. **236**: 1036–1050.

73 McLaughlin PJ and Zagon IS (2012) The opioid growth factor-opioid growth factor receptor axis: homeostatic regulator of cell proliferation and its implications for health and disease. *Biochemical Pharmacology*. **84**: 746–755.

74 Gonzalez J and Brogden R (1988) Naltrexone: a review of its pharmacodynamic and pharmacokinetic properties and therapeutic efficacy in the management of opioid dependence. *Drugs*. **35**: 192–213.

75 Crabtree B (1984) Review of naltrexone: a long-acting opiate antagonist. *Clinical Pharmacy*. **3**: 273–280.

76 Yancey-Wrona J et al. (2011) 6beta-naltrexol, a peripherally selective opioid antagonist that inhibits morphine-induced slowing of gastrointestinal transit: an exploratory study. *Pain Medicine*. **12**: 1727–1737.

77 Gutstein H and Akil H (2001) Opioid analgesics. In: J Hardman et al. (eds) *Goodman & Gilman's The Pharmacological Basis of Therapeutics* (10e). McGraw-Hill, New York ; London.

78 Vickers AP and Jolly A (2006) Naltrexone and problems in pain management. *British Medical Journal*. **332 (7534)**: 132–133.

79 Mitchell J (1986) Naltrexone and hepatotoxicity. *Lancet*. **1**: 1215.

80 Partridge BL and Ward CF (1986) Pulmonary oedema following low-dose naloxone administration. *Anesthesiology*. **65**: 709–710.

81 Yoburn BC et al. (1988) Upregulation of opioid receptor subtypes correlates with potency changes of morphine and DADLE. Life Sci. **43**: 1319–1324.

82 Slatkin NE et al. (2011) Characterization of abdominal pain during methylnaltrexone treatment of opioid-induced constipation in advanced illness: a post hoc analysis of two clinical trials. Journal of Pain and Symptom Management. **42**: 754–760.

83 Mackey AC et al. (2010) Methylnaltrexone and gastrointestinal perforation. Journal of Pain and Symptom Management. **40**: e1–3.

84 Sweetman SC Martindale: The Complete Drug Reference. London: Pharmaceutical Press. www.medicinescomplete.com (accessed May 2014).

85 Cleary J (2000) Incidence and characteristics of naloxone administration in medical oncology patients with cancer pain. Journal of Pharmaceutical Care in Pain and Symptom Control. **8**: 65–73.

86 Miaskowski C et al. (2008) Principles of analgesic use in the treatment of acute pain and cancer pain (6e). American Pain Society, Skokie, Illinois, p. 31.

87 Watkins JL et al. (2011) Utilization of methylnaltrexone (relistor) for opioid-induced constipation in an oncology hospital. Pharmacy and Therapeutics. **36**: 33–36.

88 Portenoy RK et al. (2008) Subcutaneous methylnaltrexone for the treatment of opioid-induced constipation in patients with advanced illness: a double-blind, randomized, parallel group, dose-ranging study. Journal of Pain and Symptom Management. **35**: 458–468.

89 Thomas J et al. (2008) Methylnaltrexone for opioid-induced constipation in advanced illness. N Engl J Med. **358**: 2332–2343.

90 Slatkin N et al. (2009) Methylnaltrexone for treatment of opioid-induced constipation in advanced illness patients. Journal of Supportive Oncology. **7**: 39–46.

91 Michna E et al. (2011) Subcutaneous methylnaltrexone for treatment of opioid-induced constipation in patients with chronic, nonmalignant pain: a randomized controlled Study. Journal of Pain. **12**: 554–562.

92 andy B et al. (2011) Laxatives or methylnaltrexone for the management of constipation in palliative care patients. Cochrane Database of Systematic Reviews. **19**: CD003448.

93 Bergasa N et al. (1998) Open-label trial of oral nalmefene therapy for the pruritus of cholestasis. Hepatology. **27**: 679–684.

Updated June 2014

6: INFECTIONS

ANTIBACTERIALS IN PALLIATIVE CARE   BNF 5

Remember: always ask about drug allergies before prescribing an antibacterial.
The dose and frequency of many antibacterials are reduced in renal impairment.

BNF Section 5 contains a comprehensive account of antibacterial use,[1] and many hospitals have antibacterial policies which govern local infection control and treatment, e.g. the prevention of methicillin-resistant Staphylococcus aureus (MRSA) infection and the prevention of Clostridium difficile infection. Thus, any specific recommendations about antibacterials in PCF should be considered in conjunction with local policy. When in doubt, seek advice from a local medical microbiologist.

Be aware that rigorously applied screening and infection control protocols will impose significant burdens at the end of life.[2]

Penicillin allergy
Allergic reactions to penicillins occur in 1–10% of exposed individuals, and anaphylaxis in <0.05%. Those with a history of urticaria, rash or anaphylaxis immediately after starting a course of a penicillin should not be prescribed a penicillin, a cephalosporin, or other beta-lactam antibacterial.
    Those with a history of a minor rash (e.g. non-confluent, non-pruritic rash restricted to a small area of the body) or a rash which occurs >72h after a penicillin is started are probably not allergic to penicillin, and a penicillin need not be withheld if indicated. However, the possibility of an allergic reaction should be kept in mind. Other beta-lactam antibacterials (including cephalosporins) can be used in these patients.[1]

Stop and think!
In a moribund patient with progressive incurable disease, are you justified in giving antibacterials for an intercurrent infection which may be the natural endpoint of the dying process?
Antibacterials in end-stage disease should have the primary purpose of ameliorating distressing symptoms (including fever and malaise), and not simply delaying inevitable death. It is important to *stop and think*: if antibacterials are automatically prescribed when infection is diagnosed, they may simply serve to prolong suffering.[3–5]
    The potential for antibacterials to impact on the survival of patients with advanced cancer varies with the type of infection and setting of the patient. For example, in hospital inpatients referred to a palliative care service, a prolonged survival was associated with the recent use of antibacterials for septicaemia but not focal infection.[6] Overall, compared to patients with infections who did not receive antibacterials, this amounted to a difference in median survival of

about 2–3 weeks. However, median survival differed by about 5 months (septicaemia) and 2 months (focal infection) between patients deemed to have had a good vs. a poor initial response to the antibacterials, with the latter only surviving about 1 and 3 weeks respectively.[6] On the other hand, in a community-based hospice programme, the presence of infection or the use of antibacterials made no difference to the median survival of patients of about 30 days.[7]

Nonetheless, whatever the setting, in addition to symptom relief, clinicians should balance the potential for any benefit from extra time gained by the use of antibacterials with the burden of irreversible progressive physical deterioration. Thus, antibacterials are generally appropriate for a patient with advanced cancer who develops a chest infection while still relatively active and independent. However, in someone who has become bedbound as a result of general progressive deterioration and who seems close to death, pneumonia should still be allowed to be 'the old person's friend'. In such circumstances it is generally appropriate *not* to prescribe antibacterials and to 'give death a chance'.

Although some terminally ill patients recover from a chest infection without an antibacterial, others progress to a 'grumbling pneumonia'. A continuing wet cough may cause much distress, and possibly loss of sleep. If this is the case, an antibacterial may well be indicated for symptom relief.

When it is difficult to make a decision, a '2-day rule' could be invoked: if after 2 days of general symptom management the patient is clinically stable, prescribe an antibacterial but, if the patient is clearly much worse, do not. Conversely, given the poor survival of those who fail to have a good initial response to antibacterials,[6] there is need also for a reverse '2-day rule', namely discontinue antibacterials after a few days if there is no apparent response, particularly if the patient is now moribund.

General considerations

Evidence for symptom improvement with antibacterials at the end of life remains patchy. Only 8 of 11 studies in a recent systematic review of antibacterial use in hospice patients considered symptom response as an outcome following antibacterial therapy.[8]

Several surveys give similar prevalence rates for *symptomatic* infection in palliative care patients, namely about 40%,[7] and show that the response to antibacterials varies according to the site of infection (Table 1). Provided a patient does not have an indwelling urinary catheter, UTIs should generally be treated routinely unless there is an overriding reason for not doing so (see p.471).[6,9] Cough caused by infection is also significantly reduced by antibacterials.[9] On the other hand, in patients with end-stage progressive disease being cared for at home, the use of antibacterials to treat septicaemia in a patient is generally futile (Table 1).

Table 1 Response to antimicrobials[a] in >600 home care patients[7]

Type of infection	Number	Response (%)[b]
UTI	265	79
RTI	221	43
Oral cavity[a]	63	46
Skin or SC	59	41
Septicaemia	25	0

a. includes the use of antibacterials for infections at all sites, and of antifungals for oropharyngeal candidosis
b. reduction of fever ± amelioration of site-specific symptoms within 3 days.

Specific recommendations

The specific information given in this chapter is limited to selected situations which may occur in palliative care:
- local infection causing severe pain
- ascending cholangitis associated with a biliary stent
- infection associated with an airway stent
- respiratory tract infection in the dying patient
- cellulitis in patients with lymphoedema (see p.476).

Antibacterials to relieve infection-related pain

Antibacterials are essential in some patients for the relief of severe pain associated with infection around a malignant tumour in, for example, the neck, the gluteal muscles underlying an ulcerated cancer, or the perineum.[6] Sometimes there is a history of a rapid increase in pain intensity over several days which is poorly responsive to escalating doses of a strong opioid. The pain is often associated with fever and malaise, and may be complicated by delirium. Commonly, there will be a mixture of more superficial aerobic infection with deeper anaerobic infection. Treatment is similar to that recommended for ascending cholangitis (see below).

Ascending cholangitis

Ascending cholangitis may occur in patients with a partially obstructed or stented common bile duct. It often causes severe systemic disturbance and should be treated promptly:

- **co-amoxiclav** 1.2g IV t.d.s.
- if a minor rash with a penicillin in the past (see p.461), **cefuroxime** 1.5g IV t.d.s. plus **metronidazole** 500mg IV t.d.s.
- if the patient is in septic shock, also give a single dose of **gentamicin** 5mg/kg (maximum dose 500mg) IV over 20–30min
- if a risk of multiresistant Gram-negative bacilli, serious penicillin allergy or in any doubt, consult a medical microbiologist.

When IV administration is difficult, alternatives include:

- **ceftazidime** 1g IM t.d.s., reconstituted with 3mL of WFI or 0.5–1% **lidocaine hydrochloride** solution (total injection volume ~3.8mL)
- in countries where it is available (not UK) **cefepime** 1g SC t.d.s. reconstituted with 2.4mL of either 0.9% saline, 5% glucose (dextrose), WFI or 0.5–1% **lidocaine hydrochloride** solution (total injection volume ~3.6mL).

The doses and/or frequency of **co-amoxiclav, cefuroxime, ceftazidime, cefepime,** and **gentamicin** should be reduced in renal impairment.

Infection associated with an airway stent

The presence of an airway stent, whether for cancer or other obstruction, increases the risk of serious respiratory tract infection.[11] In a systematic review of 500 patients, mortality rate was almost 70%.[12] Commonest pathogens are *Staphylococcus aureus* and *Pseudomonas aeruginosa*. Treatment should be commenced promptly and guided by the advice of a medical microbiologist.

Respiratory tract infection in the imminently dying patient

Occasionally, death rattle (noisy respiratory secretions) is caused by profuse purulent sputum from a chest infection, and an antibacterial is prescribed in the hope that it will reduce the copious purulent malodorous discharge from the mouth.[13] In this circumstance, the IV route is generally the best. However, if not practical, the IM or SC routes can be used instead.[14,15]

Some centres use single doses of **ceftriaxone**; either 1–2g IV, or 1g IM reconstituted with 3.5mL **lidocaine** 1% (total injection volume ~4.1mL).[13] **Ceftriaxone** is a broad-spectrum antibacterial and has a long duration of action. Patients who responded did so within hours (marked reduction in purulent sputum and resolution of associated halitosis). Non-responders appeared not to benefit from a second dose after 24h.

Other centres give **ceftriaxone** by SC injection[16,17] and administer multiple doses if a patient survives > 1 day, e.g. **ceftriaxone** 1g vial reconstituted with 2.2mL **lidocaine** 1% (total injection volume ~2.8mL) 250mg–1g SC once daily. If a larger volume of **lidocaine** is added, e.g. 3.3mL (total injection volume ~3.9mL), the mixture can be administered as a divided dose, given at the same time but using two or more separate SC/IM sites[18] (see manufacturer's SPC for additional information and guidance).

The results of a survey suggest that the above are reasonably well tolerated, and have been used for up to 10 days when patients have not been imminently dying.[14]

The bio-availability (in volunteers) of **cefepime** SC is comparable with IM.[19] Further, when 1g is infused over 30min, pain at the injection site is absent or minimal. Thus, **cefepime** (not UK) could be a better option. Concern about the safety of **cefepime**[20] has been shown to be groundless.[21]

Supply

Co-amoxiclav (generic)
Injection (powder for reconstitution) co-amoxiclav 500/100 (amoxicillin 500mg as sodium salt, clavulanic acid 100mg as potassium salt), co-amoxiclav 1000/200 (amoxicillin 1g as sodium salt, clavulanic acid 200mg as potassium salt), 2 days @ 1.2g t.d.s = £16.

Cefuroxime
Zinacef® (GSK)
Injection (powder for reconstitution) 250mg, 750mg, 1.5g (IV only), 2 days @ 1.5g t.d.s. = £28.

Ceftazidime (generic)
Injection (powder for reconstitution) 1g, 2g, 2 days @ 1g t.d.s. = £51.

Ceftriaxone (generic)
Injection (powder for reconstitution) 1g vial = £10, 2g vial = £20.

Gentamicin sulphate (generic)
Injection 40mg/mL, 1mL amp, 2mL vial = £1.50; 2mL amp = £1.

Also see **metronidazole**, p.468.

1 British National Formulary Section 5 Infections. London: BMJ Group and Pharmaceutical Press. www.bnf.org (accessed April 2014).
2 Bukki J et al. (2013) Methicillin-resistant Staphylococcus aureus (MRSA) management in palliative care units and hospices in Germany: a nationwide survey on patient isolation policies and quality of life. Palliative Medicine. 27: 84–90.
3 Lam PT et al. (2005) Retrospective analysis of antibiotic use and survival in advanced cancer patients with infections. Journal of Pain and Symptom Management. 30: 536–543.
4 Thompson AJ et al. (2012) Antimicrobial use at the end of life among hospitalized patients with advanced cancer. American Journal of Hospice and Palliative Care. 29: 599–603.
5 Albrecht JS et al. (2013) A nationwide analysis of antibiotic use in hospice care in the final week of life. Journal of Pain and Symptom Management. 46: 483–490.
6 Thai V et al. (2012) Impact of infections on the survival of hospitalized advanced cancer patients. Journal of Pain and Symptom Management. 43: 549–557.
7 Reinbolt RE et al. (2005) Symptomatic treatment of infections in patients with advanced cancer receiving hospice care. Journal of Pain and Symptom Management. 30: 175–182.
8 Rosenberg JH et al. (2013) Antimicrobial use for symptom management in patients receiving hospice and palliative care: a systematic review. Journal of Palliative Medicine. 16: 1568–1574.
9 Mirhosseini M et al. (2006) The role of antibiotics in the management of infection-related symptoms in advanced cancer patients. Journal of Palliative Care. 22: 69–74.
10 Bruera E and MacDonald N (1986) Intractable pain in patients with advanced head and neck tumors: a possible role of local infection. Cancer Treatment Reports. 70: 691–692.
11 Grosu HB et al. (2013) Stents are associated with increased risk of respiratory infections in patients undergoing airway interventions for malignant airways disease. Chest. 144: 441–449.
12 Agrafiotis M et al. (2009) Infections related to airway stenting: a systematic review. Respiration. 78: 69–74.
13 Spruyt O and Kausae A (1998) Antibiotic use for infective terminal respiratory secretions. Journal of Pain and Symptom Management. 15: 263–264.
14 palliativedrugs.com. (2010) Survey: SC/IM antibiotics - Do you use this route? Available from: www.palliativedrugs.com
15 Azevedo EF (2012) Administration of antibiotics subcutaneously: an integrative literature review. Acta Paulista de Enfermagem. 25: 817–822.
16 Borner K et al. (1985) Comparative pharmacokinetics of ceftriaxone after subcutaneous and intravenous administration. Chemotherapy. 31: 237–245.
17 Bricaire F et al. (1988) [Pharmacokinetics and tolerance of ceftriaxone after subcutaneous administration]. Pathologie Biologie (Paris). 36: 702–705.
18 Tahmasebi M (2005) SC injection of antibiotics Bulletin board. www.palliativedrugs.com (posted 26-08-05).
19 Walker P et al. (2005) Subcutaneous administration of cefepime. Journal of Pain and Symptom Management. 30: 170–174.
20 Yahav D et al. (2007) Efficacy and safety of cefepime: a systematic review and meta-analysis. The Lancet Infectious Diseases. 7: 338–348.
21 FDA (2009) Cefepime (marketed as Maxipime) update of ongoing safety review. Available from: www.fda.gov/Safety/MedWatch/SafetyInformation/SafetyAlertsforHumanMedicalProducts/ucm167427.htm

Updated (minor change) April 2014

OROPHARYNGEAL CANDIDOSIS BNF 5.2 & 12.3.2

Oral yeast carriage is present in about 1/3 of the general population. The prevalence in patients with advanced cancer is significantly higher (about 50–90%).[1] Thus, it is not surprising that oropharyngeal candidosis is a common fungal infection in the palliative care population of patients (13–30%).[2,3]

Many patients with oropharyngeal candidosis have concurrent oesophageal infection,[4] and some patients develop systemic fungal infections. Oral candidosis is associated with:

- poor performance status
- dry mouth
- dentures
- topical antibacterials and/or corticosteroids
- in AIDS with CD4 cell count <200cells/mm^3.[1–3]

Oral candidosis is not associated with the use of oral/parenteral antibacterials, and most data suggest that it is not associated with the use of oral/parenteral corticosteroids.[5]

Non-Candida albicans species are increasingly being isolated from patients with oral candidosis.[2,3] The reason for this is thought to be related to increased use of antifungal drugs; the consequence of this change is an increased incidence of azole drug resistance (many non-Candida albicans species exhibit inherent azole drug resistance).[6]

Management strategy

Correct the correctable

Underlying causal factors must be considered and corrected if possible, particularly dry mouth and poor denture hygiene.

Dentures must be thoroughly cleaned at least once daily, brushing the denture with a nailbrush or denture brush, and using soap and water or an appropriate commercial product.[7] Dentures should also be soaked overnight in an appropriate antiseptic, e.g. **chlorhexidine** or dilute **sodium hypochlorite**. The latter should not be used for dentures with metal parts. Failure to sterilize the denture will lead to failure of antifungal treatment. The dentures should be thoroughly rinsed before re-insertion to prevent drug inactivation.

Drug treatment

A systematic review concluded that there was limited evidence about the efficacy of antifungal drugs in patients with cancer, but that there was some evidence that drugs absorbed from the GI tract are more effective than drugs not absorbed from the GI tract.[8]

Nystatin is a good choice for mild oral candidosis in non-immunocompromised patients, whereas **fluconazole** is the preferred choice for moderate–severe infections, and in patients who cannot use **nystatin**.[9]

Cross-resistance and cross-infection do occur and, if there is a high prevalence of azole resistance within the local patient population, then even azole-naïve patients may be infected with azole-resistant organisms.[10] Local treatment protocols must take this into account.

Azole antifungals have an inhibitory effect on human cytochrome P450 enzymes (see Chapter 25, p.767). This results in inhibition of adrenal steroid synthesis (cortisol, testosterone, oestrogens and progesterone) and of the metabolism of many drugs. Drug interactions are most likely with **itraconazole**. They are generally less likely and less pronounced with **fluconazole** (a weaker CYP inhibitor), although several clinically important interactions have been reported with all of these.[11]

Potential topical treatments in resistant cases (or other special circumstances) include **chlorhexidine**,[1] **gentian violet** (e.g. 0.5–1%, 1.5mL applied twice daily),[12] and tea tree oil.[13]

Cautions

Because of a teratogenic risk with **fluconazole** and **itraconazole**, the manufacturers advise that women of child-bearing potential should use contraceptive precautions until the next menstrual period after completing treatment. Because of similar toxicological findings in animal studies with other azoles, it would be wise to extend this precaution to **miconazole**.

Itraconazole may cause or worsen left ventricular dysfunction or CHF. In hypochlorhydria, whereas absorption from **itraconazole** *capsules* is variable, it is reliable from the *oral solution*, and bio-availability is higher (also see Chapter 14, Box A, p.643). The absorption of **fluconazole** is not affected by antacids, **sucralfate**, H$_2$-receptor antagonists, PPIs or food.

Renal impairment: reduce dose of **fluconazole** by 50% if creatinine clearance is <50mL/min; the bio-availability of oral **itraconazole** may be reduced in renal impairment.

Hepatic impairment: serious or fatal hepatotoxicity may occur with **fluconazole** and **itraconazole**. The manufacturers advise monitoring liver function in patients receiving large doses and/or prolonged courses, and in patients with known liver dysfunction. With both drugs, treatment should be discontinued if symptoms suggestive of hepatotoxicity develop, e.g. jaundice, dark urine.

MHRA has issued an alert for products or medical devices containing **chlorhexidine** following reports of anaphylaxis.[14]

Drug interactions

Through inhibition of various cytochrome P450 enzymes, particularly CYP3A4, azoles produce clinically important increases in the plasma concentration of many drugs (see Chapter 25, p.767). Avoid concurrent administration of **itraconazole** or **miconazole** with **astemizole, pimozide** or **quinidine** because of a risk of fatal cardiac arrhythmias.

Fluconazole, itraconazole and **miconazole** increase the plasma concentration of **alfentanil, carbamazepine, dexamethasone, digoxin, glibenclamide, glipizide, methylprednisolone, midazolam, nifedipine, phenytoin, theophylline,** TCAs, most statins, and **warfarin,** and thus increase their toxicity and/or undesirable effects.

Strong CYP3A4 inducers, e.g. **carbamazepine, phenytoin, phenobarbital, rifampicin, rifabutin** and possibly *Hypericum perforatum* (St. John's wort), reduce **fluconazole** and **itraconazole** plasma concentrations, which may result in antifungal treatment failure.

Undesirable effects

Common (<10%, >1%): headache (azole antifungals), dizziness (**fluconazole** and **itraconazole**), GI symptoms, i.e. dyspepsia, nausea and vomiting, abdominal pain, diarrhoea (**fluconazole** and **itraconazole**), rashes, pruritus, hypokalaemia (**fluconazole** and **itraconazole**).

Uncommon, rare or very rare (<1%): anaphylaxis, hepatitis, cholestasis, hepatic failure, adrenal suppression (**itraconazole**), reduced libido, gynaecomastia, impotence, menstrual disturbances.

Dose and use

See Table 1. For patients being treated with topical **nystatin** suspension, **miconazole** oral gel or **amphotericin** lozenges (not UK), dentures should be removed temporarily before each dose is given. With all topical preparations and **itraconazole** *oral solution*, food and drink should be avoided for 1h after each dose. Note:

- because **chlorhexidine** binds to **nystatin** and leads to inactivation of both drugs, **chlorhexidine** mouthwash should *not* be used at the same time as **nystatin** oral suspension.[15] The problem can be avoided if **chlorhexidine** is used ≥30min before **nystatin**
- the absorption of **itraconazole** capsules is improved if taken with an acidic drink, e.g. cola.

Supply

Nystatin
Nystan$^®$ (Squibb)
Oral suspension 100,000 units/mL, 7 days @ 5mL q.d.s. = £10. *Note: the generic nystatin oral suspension is 10 times more expensive.*

Miconazole
Daktarin$^®$ (Janssen-Cilag)
Oral gel 24mg/mL, 7 days @ 5mL q.d.s = £12.

Loramyc$^®$ (Therabel)
Buccal tablet (muco-adhesive) 50mg, 7 days @ 50mg once daily = £23.

Table 1 Antifungal treatment[16]

Class	Drug	Recommended regimen	Comments
Polyene group	Nystatin	Oral suspension 100,000 units/mL; 5mL q.d.s for 7 days (continue for 48h after lesions disappear); hold against lesions for at least 1min, and then swallow	Smaller volumes make it more difficult to hold against lesions
	Amphotericin (not UK)	Lozenges 10mg; 1 lozenge q.d.s for 10–14 days (continue for 48h after lesions disappear); place in the mouth and allow to dissolve	Up to 2 lozenges q.d.s. in severe infections
Azole group (imidazoles)	Miconazole	Oral gel 24mg/mL; 5–10mL oral gel q.d.s for 5–7 days (continue for 48h after lesions disappear); hold against lesions for as long as possible, and then swallow. Buccal tablet 50mg; attach 1 tablet to the upper gum once daily for 7–14 days	Useful in management of angular cheilitis (has anti-staphylococcal action)
Azole group (triazoles)	Fluconazole	Capsules 50mg, 150mg, 200mg. Oral suspension 50mg/5mL and 200mg/5mL; 50–100mg once daily for 7 days	May need higher doses/longer courses in immunosuppressed patients, and patients with more severe infections
	Itraconazole	Capsules 100mg; 100mg once daily for 2 weeks. Oral solution 10mg/mL; 10–20mL b.d. for 2 weeks, use as a mouthwash and swallow	Not generally used as first-line treatment. May need higher doses in immunosuppressed patients, and patients with more severe infections

Fluconazole (generic)
Capsules 50mg, 150mg, 200mg, 7 days @ 50mg once daily = £1.

Diflucan® (Pfizer)
Capsules 50mg, 150mg, 200mg, 7 days @ 50mg once daily = £17.
Oral solution (powder for reconstitution) 50mg/5mL, 200mg/5mL, 7 days @ 50mg once daily = £17.

Itraconazole (generic)
Capsules (containing coated beads) 100mg, 14 days @100mg = £5.

Sporanox® (Janssen-Cilag)
Capsules (containing coated beads) 100mg, 14 days @ 100mg once daily = £14.
Oral solution 10mg/mL, 14 days @ 100mg b.d. = £110.

1 Finlay I and Davies A (2005) Fungal Infections. In: A Davies and I Finlay (eds) *Oral Care in Advanced Disease*. Oxford University Press, Oxford, pp. 55–71.
2 Davies AN *et al.* (2006) Oral candidosis in patients with advanced cancer. *Oral Oncology*. **42**: 698-702.
3 Davies AN *et al.* (2008) Oral candidosis in community-based patients with advanced cancer. *Journal of Pain and Symptom Management*. **35**: 508–514.
4 Samonis G *et al.* (1998) Oropharyngeal candidiasis as a marker for esophageal candidiasis in patients with cancer. *Clinical Infectious Diseases*. **27**: 283–286.
5 Samaranayake L (1990) Host factors and oral candidosis. In: L Samaranayake and T MacFarlane (eds) *Oral Candidosis*. Wright, London, pp. 66–103.
6 Bagg J *et al.* (2003) High prevalence of non-albicans yeasts and detection of anti-fungal resistance in the oral flora of patients with advanced cancer. *Palliative Medicine*. **17**: 477-481.
7 Sweeney P and Davies A (2010) Oral hygiene. In: A Davies and J Epstein (eds) *Oral Complications of Cancer and its Management*. Oxford University Press, Oxford, pp. 43-51.
8 Worthington HV *et al.* (2010) Interventions for treating oral candidiasis for patients with cancer receiving treatment. *Cochrane Database Systematic Reviews*. **7**: CD001972.
9 Pappas PG *et al.* (2009) Clinical practice guidelines for the management of candidiasis: 2009 update by the Infectious Diseases Society of America. *Clinical Infectious Diseases*. **48**: 503-535.
10 Davies A *et al.* (2006) Antifungal drug resistance amongst yeasts isolated from patients with advanced cancer. *Supportive Care in Cancer*. **14**: 645.
11 Baxter K and Preston CL. *Stockley's Drug Interactions*. London: Pharmaceutical Press www.medicinescomplete.com (accessed April 2014).
12 Nyst MJ *et al.* (1992) Gentian violet, ketoconazole and nystatin in oropharyngeal and esophageal candidiasis in Zairian AIDS patients. *Annales de la Societe Belge de Medecine Tropicale*. **72**: 45–52.
13 Vazquez J (1999) Options for the management of mucosal candidiasis in patients with AIDS and HIV infection. *Pharmacotherapy*. **19**: 76–87.
14 MHRA (2012) All medical devices and medicinal products containing chlorhexidine. *Medical Devices Alert*. MDA/2012/075 www.mhra.gov.uk/Safetyinformation
15 Barkvoll P and Attramadal A (1989) Effect of nystatin and chlorhexidine digluconate on Candida albicans. *Oral Surgery Oral Medicine and Oral Pathology*. **67**: 279–281.
16 Samaranayake K and Sitheeque M (2010) Oral fungal infections. In: A Davies and J Epstein (eds) *Oral Complications of Cancer and its Management*. Oxford University Press, Oxford, pp. 171–183.

Updated June 2014

METRONIDAZOLE BNF 5.1.11 & 13.10.1.2

Class: Antibacterial and antiprotozoal.

Indications: Anaerobic and protozoal infections, *Helicobacter pylori* gastritis (see p.486), malodour caused by fungating cancers (topical gel), †pseudomembranous colitis (see *Clostridium difficile* infection p.482), bacterial vaginosis.

Pharmacology

Metronidazole is highly active against anaerobic bacteria and protozoa. Although it has no activity against aerobic organisms *in vitro*, in mixed infections *in vivo* both aerobes and anaerobes appear susceptible. Unlike most other antibacterials, resistance to metronidazole among anaerobes is uncommon.

Metronidazole, either systemically (PO or IV) or topically, is used to reduce malodour from fungating cancers and decubitus ulcers.[1-4] The malodour is caused by volatile fatty acids produced by anaerobic bacteria colonizing moist necrotic tissue.

Metronidazole is hepatically metabolized; accumulation may occur in severe hepatic impairment, and the resulting high plasma concentrations may exacerbate hepatic encephalopathy.

Tinidazole is similar to metronidazole with a longer duration of action (is given either b.d. or once daily).[5] It is available only as a proprietary tablet, causes less GI disturbance but costs several times more than metronidazole.

Bio-availability 80–100% PO; 60–80% PR; 60% gel PV, 25% pessary PV.
Onset of action 20–60min PO; 5–12h PR.
Time to peak plasma concentration 1–2h PO; 3h PR.
Plasma halflife 6–11h.
Duration of action 8–12h.

Cautions

Concurrent use of alcohol (see Drug interactions). Monitoring of FBC and LFTs advised with systemic use > 10 days (see Undesirable effects). May exacerbate existing neurological disease. Photosensitivity (topical gel).

Drug interactions

Metronidazole impairs the metabolism or excretion of several drugs, e.g. **ciclosporin, fluorouracil, lithium, phenytoin, warfarin** and coumarins thus potentially increasing their toxicity. On the other hand, plasma concentrations of metronidazole are decreased by **phenobarbital** and **phenytoin**; consider a 2–3 fold increase in dose of metronidazole if not achieving the desired clinical effect.

Metronidazole precipitates a **disulfiram**-like reaction with alcohol in about 25% of patients.[6,7] Like **disulfiram**, metabolites of metronidazole inhibit alcohol dehydrogenase, xanthine oxidase and aldehyde dehydrogenase. Inhibition of alcohol dehydrogenase leads to activation of microsomal enzyme oxidative pathways, generating ketones and lactate which may cause acidosis.[8] Xanthine oxidase inhibition can lead to noradrenaline (norepinephrine) excess.[8] Accumulation of acetaldehyde is probably responsible for most of the symptoms, e.g. flushing of the face and neck, headaches, epigastric discomfort, nausea and vomiting, and a fall in blood pressure.

Patients should be warned that if they drink alcohol when taking metronidazole they may have an unpleasant reaction, although generally this is little more than mild anorexia. Very rarely, a patient may vomit profusely. The risk of a reaction with topical or PV metronidazole is small because of lower doses ± absorption.[9] In the USA, but not the UK, patients are also advised to avoid liquid medicines containing alcohol during metronidazole treatment. This is probably overcautious; indeed, metronidazole oral suspension (Flagyl S®) contains alcohol 32mg/5mL.

Undesirable effects

Very common (>10%): abdominal pain, nausea and vomiting, diarrhoea.
Common (<10%, >1%): skin irritation (topical use).
Very rare (<0.01%): epilepsy, encephalopathy, aseptic meningitis, optic and peripheral neuropathy (sometimes irreversible), blood dyscrasias (neutropenia, thrombocytopenia, pancytopenia), cholestatic hepatitis, pancreatitis (generally reversible on discontinuation), darkening of urine (due to metabolite).

Dose and use

Limit dose to a maximum of 400mg PO b.d. in elderly debilitated patients and 400mg PO once daily if significant hepatic impairment, i.e. patients with incipient or actual hepatic encephalopathy.

PO tablets (with or after food) is generally preferable because of the much lower cost than other routes of administration. Oral suspensions are available but are more expensive and best taken on an empty stomach (also see Chapter 22, Table 2, p.733).

If PO is not possible, metronidazole can be given IV or PR. Standard practice is 500mg IV or 1g PR, both q8h. Because prolonged rectal use causes proctitis, try to limit PR administration to 2–3 days or reduce to 1g PR q12h if PO medication cannot be restarted.

Topical application to a malodorous fungating cancer can be considered when:
- the cancer is relatively small (and thus easily accessible for topical application)
- the cancer is very sloughy and poorly vascularized (which will reduce systemic access by metronidazole)
- systemic therapy is impractical, e.g. because of dysphagia
- systemic therapy causes unacceptable undesirable effects.

High quality RCT evidence of topical use is limited,[10,11] but most patients benefit. About half report complete control of the odour; improvement generally occurs within 2 days but can take up to one month.[1,12]

Anaerobic infections
Metronidazole 400mg PO t.d.s. for 7 days.

Malodour caused by fungating cancers
- **systemic:**
  - ▷ metronidazole 200–400mg PO t.d.s. for 2 weeks[3]
  - ▷ if malodour recurs, re-treat for 2 weeks, then continue indefinitely with 200mg b.d.
- **topical:**
  - ▷ metronidazole 0.75% gel is commercially available[1-3,13]
  - ▷ after cleansing the wound, apply the gel liberally, about 1g/cm^2
  - ▷ pack large cavities with paraffin gauze smeared in the gel
  - ▷ cover with a non-adherent and then an absorbent dressing
  - ▷ repeat once daily–b.d. as long as beneficial.

As a cheaper alternative to commercial gels, some centres use a crushed 200mg tablet in lubricating gel.[14]

Clostridium difficile infection (see p.482).
Helicobacter pylori gastritis (see p.486).

Supply
Metronidazole (generic)
Tablets 200mg, 400mg, 14 days @ 400mg t.d.s. = £3.
Tablets 500mg, 14 days @ 500mg t.d.s.= £62.
Oral suspension (as benzoate) 200mg/5mL, 14 days @ 400mg t.d.s. = £47.
IV infusion 5mg/mL, 20mL amp = £1.50, 100mL = £3.50 (note: based on BNF pricing, this is *more expensive* than proprietary Metrolyl® injection).

Flagyl® (Winthrop)
Tablets 200mg, 400mg, 14 days @ 400mg t.d.s. = £19.
Oral suspension (as benzoate; Flagyl S®) 200mg/5mL, 14 days @ 400mg t.d.s. = £47; *contains alcohol. Discontinued in the UK April 2013.*
Suppositories 500mg, 1g, 3 days @ 1g t.d.s. and 11 days @ 1g b.d. = £72.

Metrolyl® (Sandoz)
Suppositories 500mg, 1g, 3 days @ 1g t.d.s. and 11 days @ 1g b.d. = £57.
IV infusion 5mg/mL, 100mL = £1.50 (note: based on BNF pricing, this is *cheaper* than generic injection); *contains sodium 15mmol/100mL.*

Topical products
Anabact® (CHS)
Gel 0.75%, 15g = £4.50, 30g = £8.

Metrogel® (Galderma)
Gel 0.75%, 40g = £7.

Other topical metronidazole gels are available; they are authorized for exacerbation of rosacea and are generally more expensive.

Crushed tablets in lubricating gel cost about £0.70 per topical application compared with £4.50 for proprietary gel.

Zidoval® (Meda)

Vaginal gel 0.75%, 40g pack with 5 applicators = £4.50.

1 Newman V et al. (1989) The use of metronidazole gel to control the smell of malodorous lesions. *Palliative Medicine.* **3**: 303–305.
2 Editorial (1990) Management of smelly tumours. *Lancet.* **335**: 141–142.
3 Ashford R et al. (1984) Double-blind trial of metronidazole in malodorous ulcerating tumours. *Lancet.* **I**: 1232–1233.
4 Finlay IG et al. (1996) The effect of topical 0.75% metronidazole gel on malodorous cutaneous ulcers. *Journal of Pain and Symptom Management.* **I I**: 158–162.
5 Carmine AA et al. (1982) Tinidazole in anaerobic infections: a review of its antibacterial activity, pharmacological properties and therapeutic efficacy. *Drugs.* **24**: 85–117.
6 deMattos H (1968) Relations between alcoholism and the gastrointestinal system. Experience using metronidazole. [In Portuguese]. *Hospital (Rio J).* **74**: 1669–1676.
7 Penick S et al. (1969) Metronidazole in the treatment of alcoholism. *American Journal of Psychiatry.* **125**: 1063–1066.
8 Harries D et al. (1990) Metronidazole and alcohol: potential problems. *Scottish Medical Journal.* **35**: 179–180.
9 Plosker G (1987) Possible interaction between ethanol and vaginally administered metronidazole. *Clinical Pharmacy.* **6**: 189–193.
10 Adderley U and Smith R (2007) Topical agents and dressings for fungating wounds. *Cochrane Database of Systematic Reviews.* CD003948.
11 Bower M et al. (1992) A double-blind study of the efficacy of metronidazole gel in the treatment of malodorous fungating tumours. *European Journal of Cancer.* **28A**: 888–889.
12 Kalinski C et al. (2005) Effectiveness of a topical formulation containing metronidazole for wound odor and exudate control. *Wounds.* **17**: 84–90.
13 Thomas S and Hay N (1991) The antimicrobial properties of two metronidazole medicated dressings used to treat malodorous wounds. *Pharmaceutical Journal.* **246**: 264–266.
14 Twycross R et al. (2009) *Symptom Management in Advanced Cancer* (4e). palliativedrugs.com, Nottingham, p. 344.

Updated (minor change) June 2014

URINARY TRACT INFECTIONS   BNF 5.1.1, 5.1.8 & 5.1.13

Infections with strains of Escherichia coli and other Gram-negative bacilli which are resistant to several antibacterials, i.e. ESBL (Extended Spectrum Beta-Lactamase) positive enterobacteria, are increasing. Some are resistant to **gentamicin**, quinolones and cephalosporins as well as other antibacterials.[1]

This possibility should be considered in patients with recurrent urinary infection. Appropriate specimens (including blood cultures) should be taken and any previous microbiology reviewed.

If a multiresistant isolate has been identified previously, e.g. a **gentamicin**-resistant coliform in urine, treatment should be discussed with a medical microbiologist because the usual first-line treatment may not be appropriate.

Cystitis is the commonest form of urinary tract infection (UTI) in terminally ill patients and, as in general medicine, is often caused by *E. coli.*[2,3] UTIs are more common in women and, in the community, 60% of women with suggestive symptoms have a UTI confirmed by microscopy and culture.[4]

UTIs are generally classified as 'uncomplicated' if they occur in otherwise healthy, premenopausal women with normal urinary tracts. 'Complicated' UTIs occur in men, children, pregnant women, women with abnormal urinary tracts and the elderly particularly if they have co-morbidities, e.g. dementia, that make diagnosis challenging. Complicated UTIs are caused by a broader range of bacteria that are more likely to be resistant to antibacterials.[5]

Pyelonephritis should be suspected if the patient has a fever >38°C, loin pain and/or costovertebral angle tenderness, whether or not there are associated symptoms of cystitis. Pyelonephritis *without* evidence of urosepsis (i.e. septicaemia secondary to UTI) in a woman with a normal urinary tract may be classed as 'uncomplicated'. Pyelonephritis occurring in any other patient group or with evidence of urosepsis is classed as 'complicated'.[6]

Diagnosis
Uncomplicated UTI

If a woman has typical or severe symptoms and signs of a UTI, without vaginal irritation or discharge suggestive of an alternative diagnosis, prompt empirical antibacterial treatment is indicated; *dipstick testing (see below) and urine culture are irrelevant.*[4]

In the community in non-catheterized women, three symptoms independently predict UTI: cloudy urine, dysuria and recent-onset nocturia:
- presence of all three symptoms has a positive predictive value of 82%
- absence of all three symptoms had a negative predictive value of 67%.[4,7]

Thus, using a symptom score alone will lead to a missed diagnosis in about 1/3 of UTIs.

With dipsticks, nitrites are most predictive, followed by leucocytes (leucocyte esterase+ or greater) and blood (haemolysed trace or greater). For dipstick tests in combination:
- nitrite+ and *either* blood+ *or* leucocyte esterase+; positive predictive value 92%
- nitrite+ or leucocyte esterase and blood *both*+; positive predictive value about 80%
- nitrite, leucocyte esterase and blood *all*−; negative predictive value 76% (Box A).[4,7]

Thus, the use of a dipstick alone will lead to a missed diagnosis in about 1/4 of UTIs.

A negative culture may suggest an alternative diagnosis, e.g. urethritis caused by sexually transmitted infections (STIs, e.g. *Chlamydia*, *Neisseria*, *Trichomonas*) or interstitial cystitis. Although

---

Box A   Urine dipsticks and the diagnosis of UTIs in non-catheterized women with few or mild symptoms

Use a urine dipstick which measures urinary pH and specific gravity, and the presence and amount of:
- glucose
- ketone
- blood
- protein
- nitrite, a bacterial metabolite
- leucocyte esterase (produced by inflammation/infection).

When to do the test
- if patient has few or mild symptoms of UTI
- if typical or severe symptoms of UTI, prescribe an antibacterial in accord with local policy without using a dipstick.

How to do the test
- clean external genitalia with sterile 0.9% sodium chloride
- take a mid-stream specimen of urine (or in-and-out catheter sample under aseptic conditions)
- dip the whole strip into the urine container and remove immediately
- drag the edge of the strip against the container rim to remove excess urine and start timing
- compare each test pad on the strip to the corresponding row of colour blocks on the bottle label
- read each test pad at the time shown on the bottle, starting with the shortest time first. *Late readings are of no value.*

Significance of the results
Nitrite positive or leucocyte and blood positive or all three positive: make a working diagnosis of UTI; prescribe an antibacterial in accord with local policy. Urine specimen for culture *not* required unless risk factors present, e.g. recent hospital admission, recurrent UTIs.

Nitrite, leucocyte and blood all negative: tentatively exclude UTI; do *not* send urine specimen for culture unless definite urinary tract symptoms.

---

the traditional criterion for a positive urine culture is 10^5 colony-forming units (cfu)/mL, some studies have demonstrated that this is insensitive in 30–50% of women who have lower UTI confirmed by bladder aspirate but have only 10^2–10^4 cfu/mL in voided urine. Thus, in a woman with symptoms of uncomplicated UTI, a culture report of 'no growth' should be treated with caution and a colony count of $\geqslant 10^3$ cfu/mL is microbiologically diagnostic.[3,5,8]

Complicated UTI

To confirm the presence of bacteria and identify antibacterial sensitivity, mid-stream urine should be collected before starting antibacterial therapy in patients at risk of a complicated UTI, i.e. those associated with:

- recurrent UTI
- suspected pyelonephritis
- impaired immunity, e.g. from immunosuppressive treatment or poorly controlled diabetes mellitus
- moderate-severe renal impairment
- an abnormal urinary tract
- a recent hospital admission
- men.

In frail, elderly and hospitalized patients, diagnosis of a UTI is harder because a complicated UTI may present with atypical clinical symptoms (e.g. features of systemic infection but no localizing features such as dysuria, frequency, urgency or loin pain, or just suspected because of the onset of delirium). When there are *no* urinary symptoms and *no* signs of systemic infection, delay starting an antibacterial until the results of urine culture is available, even if urinalysis is positive.[4,9,10,11] *Dipsticks are less reliable in these circumstances.*

Management

Remember: always ask about drug allergies before prescribing an antibacterial.
The dose and frequency of many antibacterials are reduced in renal impairment.

Uncomplicated UTIs

If symptoms are moderate-severe, or urine dipstick test is positive (unless elderly, see above), start antibacterial treatment according to local guidelines. Alternatively, consider:

- **nitrofurantoin** 50mg PO q.d.s. or 100mg m/r PO b.d.; avoid when creatinine clearance <60mL/min, or
- **co-amoxiclav** 375mg PO t.d.s. and **amoxicillin** 250mg PO t.d.s. (or **co-amoxiclav** 625mg PO t.d.s. whichever is cheaper locally)
- **trimethoprim** 200mg PO b.d. (*now third-line because of increasing resistance*[5,12] unless history of penicillin allergy and/or renal impairment)[4,11]
- **ciprofloxacin** 500mg PO b.d. is sometimes recommended for uncomplicated pyelonephritis in the outpatient setting.[12]

Recommendations vary in relation to duration of antibacterial treatment:

- for an uncomplicated UTI in a woman, 3 days is generally sufficient[13,14]
- for complicated UTI, e.g. in diabetic patients, those who have undergone recent urinary surgery, children, men, and women with fever and/or loin pain (i.e. possible pyelonephritis), 7–14 days is recommended.

Note:

- fully sensitive bacteria respond to two 3g doses of **amoxicillin** given 12h apart[15]
- in some European countries **fosfomycin trometamol** (not UK) 3g single dose is recommended as first-line treatment for premenopausal women with uncomplicated UTI.[5,12]

Single dose treatment may be useful for frail patients. However, when compared in elderly patients, the *bacteriological* cure rate is higher in short (3–6 days) and long courses (7–14 days). On the other hand, *clinical* cure rates are similar and the acceptability of single-dose treatment is greater. The longer half-lives of fluoroquinolones, **co-trimoxazole** and **fosfomycin trometamol** (not UK) may make them more efficacious for single-dose therapy, compared with the short half-lives of several penicillins and cephalosporins.[16]

MRSA UTI

In confirmed MRSA UTI, treat according to local guidelines. Alternatively, consider:
- *lower UTI without systemic sepsis:* **nitrofurantoin** 50mg PO q.d.s. or 100mg m/r PO b.d. for 7 days; *avoid when creatinine clearance < 60mL/min*
- *if pyelonephritis or with systemic sepsis:* **vancomycin** 1–1.5g IVI q12h at a maximum rate of 10mg/min; reduce to 500mg IVI q12h in patients ≥65 years and in renal impairment (see SPC); each 500mg must be diluted in 100mL 0.9% saline or 5% glucose and given via a large peripheral vein; plasma concentration monitoring is required.

Systemically unwell patients

If the patient is systemically unwell, or has pyelonephritis, consider:
- IV **co-amoxiclav** 1.2g t.d.s.
- if history of penicillin allergy, give **ciprofloxacin** 500mg PO b.d. or 400mg IVI q12h over 60min via a large peripheral vein, according to local guidelines.

A single dose of IV **gentamicin** 5mg/kg should be given if there is severe sepsis or septic shock. Second-line antibacterials vary from region to region; if necessary, consult a medical microbiologist.[11]

Catheter-Associated UTI (CA-UTI)

In catheterized patients, bacterial colonization is common, occurring in up to 30% of patients catheterized for >7 days and almost universally in those catheterized for >28 days. It should not be investigated or treated unless symptomatic because generally bacteriuria does not progress to UTI.

Unfortunately, patients who develop CA-UTI are unlikely to present with fever or symptoms referable to the urinary tract. Non-specific symptoms such as rigors and new-onset delirium are more commonly associated with CA-UTI, so thorough evaluation for alternative sources of infection should also be conducted.[17]

If UTI is clinically suspected, do *not* perform a urine dipstick test because it is unreliable but send urine for culture, and then start empirical treatment with either **nitrofurantoin** or **co-amoxiclav** (as above) for 7 days.[11,18] Changing the catheter before starting antibacterials for UTI improves clinical and bacteriological cure rates,[4,19] and should be considered particularly if the catheter has been in place for >7 days.[20]

Prophylactic antibacterials for routine catheter changes are *not* recommended unless the patient has a history of UTI associated with catheter changes, is significantly immunosuppressed (e.g. neutropenic from recent chemotherapy) or experiences trauma during catheter change, i.e. frank haematuria following two or more attempts at catheterization. In such cases, single dose treatment according to local guidelines is sufficient.[4,21]

Because of the risk of increasing antibacterial resistance, continuous prophylaxis against UTI in catheterized patients is not recommended, even though there is some evidence to suggest it reduces the risk of symptomatic UTI.[22-24]

Elderly female patients may require treatment of persistent bacteriuria following catheter removal to reduce the risk of symptomatic UTI. Antibacterial treatment for 2 days before or at the time of catheter removal significantly reduces the risk of a subsequent UTI.[25-27] In patients with symptoms of a UTI after catheter removal, the cure rate for a single dose of **trimethoprim** was 79%, compared with a 10-day treatment cure rate of 81%, i.e. statistically identical.[25]

Alternative approaches

In catheterized patients, consider a urinary antiseptic to help prevent recurrent UTIs (but *not* for treatment), e.g. **methenamine hippurate** (see p.554) or **cranberry juice** (see p.555).

For women with recurrent uncomplicated UTI, prophylaxis with **cranberry juice** (see p.555), or PO/intravaginal probiotics containing *Lactobacillus rhamnosus GR-1* and *L. reuteri RC-14* may be considered.[5]

Supply

Amoxicillin (generic)
Capsules 250mg, 500mg, 7 days @ 250mg t.d.s. = £1; two doses of 3g = £2.50.
Oral suspension 125mg/5mL, 250mg/5mL, 7 days @ 250mg t.d.s. = £1.50.
Oral suspension (sachet of powder to mix with water) 3g, two doses = £9.

Co-amoxiclav (generic)
Tablets 250/125 (amoxicillin 250mg, clavulanic acid 125mg), 7 days @ 375mg t.d.s. = £2.50.
Tablets 500/125 (amoxicillin 500mg, clavulanic acid 125mg), 7 days @ 625mg t.d.s. = £3.50.
Oral suspension 250/62 (amoxicillin 250mg as trihydrate, clavulanic acid 62.5mg as potassium salt)/5mL 7 days @ 10mL t.d.s = £14.
Injection (powder for reconstitution) 1000/200 (amoxicillin 1,000mg as sodium salt, clavulanic acid 200mg as potassium salt) 1.2g = £2.50.

Ciprofloxacin (generic)
Tablets 100mg, 250mg, 500mg, 750mg, 7 days @ 500mg b.d. = £1.
Infusion 2mg/mL, 400mg (200mL) bottle = £22.

Gentamicin sulphate (generic)
Injection 40mg/mL, 1mL amp and 2mL vial = £1.50, 2mL amp = £1.

Nitrofurantoin (generic)
Tablets 50mg, 100mg, 7 days @ 50mg q.d.s. = £2.
Oral suspension 25mg/5mL, 7 days @ 50mg q.d.s. = £99.

Macrobid® (Goldshield)
Capsules m/r 100mg, 7 days @ 100mg b.d. = £5.

Trimethoprim (generic)
Tablets 100mg, 200mg, 7 days @ 200mg b.d. = £1.
Oral suspension 50mg/5mL, 7 days @ 200mg b.d. = £6.

Vancomycin (generic)
Injection (powder for reconstitution) for IVI 500mg = £7.50, 1g = £15.

1 Nicolle LE (2011) Update in adult urinary tract infection. *Current Infectious Disease Reports*. **13**: 552–560.
2 Vitetta L et al. (2000) Bacterial infections in terminally ill hospice patients. *Journal of Pain and Symptom Management*. **20**: 326–334.
3 Hooton TM (2012) Clinical practice. Uncomplicated urinary tract infection. *New England Journal of Medicine*. **366**: 1028–1037.
4 CKS (2009) UTI in women. Available from: www.cks.nhs.uk/urinary_tract_infection_lower_women (accessed May 2012)
5 Grabe M et al. (2012) Guidelines on Urological Infections. *European Association of Urology*. 1–110.
6 Johansen TE et al. (2011) Critical review of current definitions of urinary tract infections and proposal of an EAU/ESIU classification system. *International Journal of Antimicrobial Agents*. **38 Suppl**: 64–70.
7 Little P et al. (2009) Dipsticks and diagnostic algorithms in urinary tract infection: development and validation, randomised trial, economic analysis, observational cohort and qualitative study. *Health Technology Assessment*. **13**: iii-iv, ix-xi, 1–73.
8 Stamm WE et al. (1982) Diagnosis of coliform infection in acutely dysuric women. *New England Journal of Medicine*. **307**: 463–468.
9 Singh S et al. (2007) *Treatment of Urinary Tract Iinfections in the Older Person. Medicines Information Leaflet*. Vol 4 No.10. Oxford Radcliffe Hospital, Oxford.
10 CKS (2010) UTI in men. Available from: www.cks.nhs.uk/uringary_tract_infection_lower_men (accessed May 2012)
11 Oxford Hospitals Adult Inpatient Pocket Antimicrobial Guide (2011) *Urinary tract infection*.
12 Gupta K et al. (2011) International clinical practice guidelines for the treatment of acute uncomplicated cystitis and pyelonephritis in women: A 2010 update by the Infectious Diseases Society of America and the European Society for Microbiology and Infectious Diseases. *Clinical Infectious Diseases*. **52**: e103–120.
13 Guay DR (2008) Contemporary management of uncomplicated urinary tract infections. *Drugs*. **68**: 1169–1205.
14 Milo G et al. (2005) Duration of antibacterial treatment for uncomplicated urinary tract infection in women. *Cochrane Database of Systematic Reviews*. CD004682.
15 BNF (2012) 5.1.13 Urinrary-tract infections. In: *British National Formulary No 63*. British Medical Association and the Royal Pharmaceutical Society of Great Britain, London.
16 Lutters M and Vogt-Ferrier MB (2008) Antibiotic duration for treating uncomplicated, symptomatic lower urinary tract infections in elderly women. *Cochrane Database of Systematic Reviews*. CD001535.
17 Hooton TM et al. (2010) Diagnosis, prevention, and treatment of catheter-associated urinary tract infection in adults: 2009 International Clinical Practice Guidelines from the Infectious Diseases Society of America. *Clinical Infectious Diseases*. **50**: 625–663.
18 Schwartz DS and Barone JE (2006) Correlation of urinalysis and dipstick results with catheter-associated urinary tract infections in surgical ICU patients. *Intensive Care Medicine*. **32**: 1797–1801.
19 Raz R et al. (2000) Chronic indwelling catheter replacement before antimicrobial therapy for symptomatic urinary tract infection. *Journal of Urology*. **164**: 1254–1258.
20 Tenke P et al. (2008) European and Asian gudelines on management and prevention of catheter-associated urinary tract infections. *International Journal of Antimicrobial Agents*. **31 (suppl 1)**: 68–78.
21 National Clinical Guidelines Centre (2012) Infection: prevention and control of healthcare-associated infections in primary and community care RCP. National Clinical Gudeline Centre at The Royal College of Physicians. Available from: http://www.nice.org.uk/guidancew/CG139

22 Rutschmann O and Zwahlen A (1995) Use of norfloxacin for prevention of symptomatic urinary tract infection in chronically catheterized patients. *Journal of Clinical Microbiology and Infectious Diseases.* 14: 441–444.

23 Niel-Weise BS and van den Broek PJ (2005) Urinary catheter policies for long-term bladder drainage. *Cochrane Database of Systematic Reviews.* CD004201.

24 Niel-Weise BS and van den Broek PJ (2005) Antibiotic policies for short-term catheter bladder drainage in adults. *Cochrane Database of Systematic Reviews.* CD005428.

25 Harding GK et al. (1991) How long should catheter-acquired urinary tract infection in women be treated? A randomized controlled study. *Annals of Internal Medicine.* 114: 713–719.

26 Hustinx W et al. (1991) Impact of concurrent antimicrobial therapy on catheter-associated urinary tract infection. *Journal of Hospital Infection.* 18: 45–56.

27 Pfefferkorn U et al. (2009) Antibiotic prophylaxis at urinary catheter removal prevents urinary tract infections: a prospective randomized trial. *Annals of Surgery.* 249: 573–575.

Updated September 2013

CELLULITIS IN A LYMPHOEDEMATOUS LIMB

Cellulitis, also called an acute inflammatory episode (AIE), is common in lymphoedema:
- mild: pain, increased swelling, erythema (well-defined or blotchy)
- severe: extensive erythema with well-defined margins, increased swelling, blistering and weeping skin; often accompanied by fever, nausea and vomiting, pain and, when the leg is affected, difficulty in walking.[1]

Management strategy
Preventive measures
Patients should be educated about:
- why they are susceptible to cellulitis, i.e. skin crevices harbour bacteria, reduced immunity[2]
- the consequences of cellulitis, i.e. increased swelling, more fibrosis, decreased response to compression treatment
- the importance of daily skin care to improve and maintain skin integrity. Risk factors for cellulitis include cracked or macerated interdigital skin, dermatitis, limb wounds (including leg ulcers), and weeping lymphangiectasia (leaking lymph blisters on the skin surface)
- reducing risk by, for example, reducing the swelling, protecting hands when gardening, cleaning cuts, treating fungal infections (e.g. **clotrimazole** 1% or **terbinafine** 1% cream b.d. for 2 weeks) and ingrowing toenails[3]
- the importance of seeking prompt medical attention and treatment if they suspect they may be developing cellulitis.

Patients who have had cellulitis in the past and who are travelling away from home should be supplied with an emergency 2-week supply of **amoxicillin** 500mg t.d.s. (or **erythromycin** 500mg q.d.s. for those allergic to penicillin).

Non-drug treatment
- compression garments should not be worn until the limb is comfortable
- daily skin hygiene should be continued; washing and gentle drying
- emollients should not be used in the affected area if the skin is broken
- if severe, bed rest is essential with the affected limb elevated in a comfortable position and supported on pillows.[3,4]

Drug treatment

The dose and frequency of many antibacterials are reduced in renal impairment.

Cellulitis should be treated promptly with antibacterials to prevent increased morbidity from increased swelling and accelerated fibrosis (see Quick Prescribing Guide, p.480). However, it is often difficult to isolate the responsible pathogen. The traditional advice of the British Lymphology Society (BLS) and Lymphoedema Support Network (LSN) was based on the predominant view among lymphoedema specialists in the UK that, in lymphoedematous limbs, beta-haemolytic *Streptococci* are the most common causal pathogens[1,5,6] and not *Staphylococcus aureus*.[7]

Accordingly, in the past, BLS/LSN recommended **amoxicillin** as the first-line antibacterial, noting that:

- the minimum inhibitory concentration (MIC) for **amoxicillin** is lower than that for **flucloxacillin**
- of the two drugs, **amoxicillin** probably penetrates lymphoedematous tissues better
- patients seem to tolerate **amoxicillin** better, although it causes more skin rashes.[8]

However, clinicians unaware of the traditional BLS/LSN advice will probably prescribe **flucloxacillin** in line with CREST recommendations.[9] These are based on the premise that *Staph. aureus* and *Streptococci* are both common causes of cellulitis, and that antibacterial therapy should be targeted at both, thus **flucloxacillin** rather than **amoxicillin** (ineffective against *Staph. aureus*). The prevailing consensus is that IV **flucloxacillin** in typical large doses will exceed the MIC, will penetrate lymphoedematous tissues adequately, and provides antibacterial activity against both *Streptococci* and *Staph. aureus*.

Such reasoning makes **flucloxacillin** first choice rather than **amoxicillin**. To avoid confusion among clinicians, BLS/LSN have modified their advice, and they too are now recommending IV **flucloxacillin** as first choice for acute cellulitis with associated septicaemia (Table 1).[10]

The advice of a medical microbiologist should be obtained in unusual circumstances, e.g.:

- in anogenital cellulitis
- cellulitis developing shortly after an animal lick or bite
- when the inflammation fails to respond to the recommended antibacterials.

Remember: Cellulitis is painful: analgesics should be prescribed regularly and p.r.n. Because of a possible relationship between skin infections, NSAIDs and necrotizing fasciitis,[11] paracetamol and opioids are the preferred analgesics.[12]

Supply

Amoxicillin (generic)
Capsules 250mg, 500mg, 14 days @ 500mg t.d.s.=£2.50.
Oral suspension 125mg/5mL, 250mg/5mL, 14 days @ 500mg t.d.s.=£6.
Injection (powder for reconstitution) 250mg, 500mg, 1g vial, 2g dose = £2.

Clarithromycin (generic)
Tablets 250mg, 500mg, 14 days @ 500mg b.d. = £11.
Oral suspension 125mg/5mL, 250mg/5mL, 14 days @ 500mg b.d. = £44.

Clindamycin (generic)
Capsules 150mg, 14 days @ 300mg q.d.s. £32.
Injection 150mg/mL, 2mL, 4mL amp, 600mg dose = £12.

Erythromycin (generic)
Capsules (enclosing e/c granules) 250mg, 14 days @ 500mg q.d.s. = £60.
Tablets e/c 250mg, 14 days @ 500mg q.d.s. = £7.
Oral suspension (as ethyl succinate) 125mg/5mL, 250mg/5mL, 500mg/5mL, 14 days @ 500mg q.d.s. = £13.

Flucloxacillin (generic)
Capsules 250mg, 500mg, 14 days @ 500mg q.d.s. = £6.
Oral solution 125mg/5mL, 250mg/5mL, 14 days @ 500mg q.d.s. = £168.
Injection (powder for reconstitution) 250mg, 500mg, 1g vial, 2g dose = £10.

Gentamicin sulphate (generic)
Injection 40mg/mL, 1mL amp, 2mL amp, 2mL vial all = £1.50.

Phenoxymethylpenicillin potassium (generic)
Tablets 250mg, 14 days @ 250mg b.d. = £1.50.
Oral solution 125mg/5mL, 250mg/5mL, 14 days @ 250mg b.d. = £4.

Table 1 Antibacterials for cellulitis[a,b]

Situation	First-line antibacterials	If allergic to penicillin	Second-line antibacterials	Comments
Acute cellulitis + septicaemia (inpatient admission)	Flucloxacillin 1–2g IV q6h[c,6] or amoxicillin 2g IV q8h[c] (see main text)	Clindamycin 600mg IV q6h[13]	Clindamycin 600mg IV q6h (if poor or no response by 48h)	Switch to PO flucloxacillin 500mg q.d.s. or amoxicillin 500mg t.d.s. or clindamycin 300mg PO q.d.s. when: • no fever for 48h and • inflammation much resolved and • falling CRP. Then continue as below.
Acute cellulitis (home care) or emergency back-up supply of antibacterials	Flucloxacillin 500mg q.d.s or amoxicillin 500mg t.d.s.[d]	Erythromycin[e] 500mg b.d. q.d.s. or clarithromycin[e] 500mg b.d.	Clindamycin 300mg q.d.s. If fails to resolve, convert to first-line IV regimen above	Give for a minimum of 2 weeks. Continue antibacterials until the acute inflammation has completely resolved; in severe cases this may take 1–2 months. (Note: residual 'staining' may persist beyond this.)
Prophylaxis if 2+ episodes of cellulitis per year	Phenoxymethylpenicillin 250mg b.d. (500mg b.d. if BMI ≥33)[4]	Erythromycin[e] 250mg once daily or clarithromycin[e] 250mg once daily	Clindamycin 150mg once daily or cefalexin 250mg once daily or doxycycline 50mg once daily[f]	Continue for 2 years, after 1 year, halve the dose of phenoxymethylpenicillin; if an AIE develops after dose reduction/discontinuation, treat the acute episode and then commence life-long prophylaxis.

a. but follow local guidelines, particularly for IV antibacterials
b. PO unless stated otherwise
c. add gentamicin 5mg/kg IV daily for 1 week if anogenital region involved, adjust dose according to renal function and gentamicin plasma concentration
d. if Staph. aureus infection suspected (folliculitis, pus formation, crusted dermatitis), flucloxacillin 500mg q.d.s. should definitely be used
e. for patients taking astemizole, tolterodine or statins, do not prescribe macrolide antibacterials (clarithromycin, erythromycin); use cefalexin (but not in patients with a history of serious penicillin allergy, i.e. anaphylaxis) or doxycycline; see, p.480
f. in these circumstances, review by local specialist lymphoedema services and advice from a microbiologist is recommended. There is a need to balance the use of certain antibiotics (e.g. clindamycin, cefalexin) as prophylaxis against the risk of predisposing to C. difficile infection.

1 Mortimer P (2000) Acute inflammatory episodes. In: RG Twycross *et al.* (eds) *Lymphoedema*. Radcliffe Medical Press, Oxford, pp. 130–139.
2 Mallon E *et al.* (1997) Evidence for altered cell-mediated immunity in postmastectomy lymphoedema. *British Journal of Dermatology.* 137: 928–933.
3 Twycross R *et al.* (2000) *Lymphoedema*. Radcliffe Medical Press, Oxford.
4 Twycross RG *et al.* (2007) *Symptom Management in Advanced Cancer* (4e). Palliativedrugs.com Ltd, Nottingham.
5 Cox NH (2008) Streptococcal cellulitis/erysipelas of the lower leg. In: William H et al (ed) *Evidence-Based Dermatology 2nd edition*. Blackwell Publishing, Oxford, pp. 406–417.
6 Leman P and Mukherjee D (2005) Flucloxacillin alone or combined with benzylpenicillin to treat lower limb cellulitis: a randomised controlled trial. *Emergency Medical Journal.* 22: 342–346.
7 Chira S and Miller LG (2010) Staphylococcus aureus is the most common identified cause of cellulitis: a systematic review. *Epidemiology Infection.* 138: 313–317.
8 British Lymphology Society (2010) Revised consensus document on the management of cellulitis in lymphoedema: flucloxacillin versus amoxicillin. Available from: www.thebls.com
9 CREST (2005) Guidelines on the management of cellulitis in adults. Available from: http://www.gain-ni.org/images/Uploads/Guidelines/cellulitis-guide.pdf
10 British Lymphology Society (2013) Revised consensus document on the management of cellulitis in lymphodema. Available from: www.thebls.com
11 Sultan HY *et al.* (2012) Necrotising fasciitis. *British Medical Journal.* 345: e4274.
12 Anonymous (2007) Necrotising fasciitis, dermal infections and NSAIDs: caution. *Prescrire International.* 16: 17.
13 Bisno AL and Stevens DL (1996) Streptococcal infections of skin and soft tissues. *New England Journal of Medicine.* 334: 240–245.
14 Team UKDCTNsPT *et al.* (2012) Prophylactic antibiotics for the prevention of cellulitis (erysipelas) of the leg: results of the UK Dermatology Clinical Trials Network's PATCH II trial. *British Journal of Dermatology.* 166: 169–178.

Updated October 2013

Quick Prescribing Guide: Cellulitis in lymphoedema

Cellulitis is often associated with septicaemia (e.g. fever, flu-like symptoms, hypotension, tachycardia, delirium, nausea and vomiting). It may be difficult to identify the pathogen but, in lymphoedema, *Streptococcus* is the most common.

Evaluation

1 Clinical features
- mild: pain, increased swelling, erythema (well-defined or blotchy)
- severe: extensive erythema with well-defined margins, increased swelling, blistering and weeping skin; often accompanied by fever, nausea and vomiting, pain and, when the leg is affected, difficulty in walking.

2 Diagnosis is based on pattern recognition and clinical judgement. Solicit:
- present history: date of onset, precipitating factor (e.g. insect bite or trauma), treatment received to date
- past history: details of past cellulitis, precipitating factors, antibacterials taken
- examination: include sites of lymphatic drainage to and from inflamed area.

3 Establish a baseline
- extent and severity of rash: if well demarcated outline with pen and date
- level of systemic upset: temperature, pulse, BP, CRP, WBC
- swab cuts or breaks in skin for microbiology before starting antibacterials.

4 Arrange admission to hospital for patients with septicaemia or who deteriorate or fail to improve despite PO antibacterials.

Antibacterials

5 To prevent increased swelling and accelerated fibrosis, cellulitis should be treated promptly with antibacterials *for a minimum of 2 weeks*. Continue antibacterials until the acute inflammation has completely resolved; this may take 1–2 months.

6 The advice of a microbiologist should be obtained in unusual circumstances, e.g. cellulitis developing shortly after an animal bite, and when the inflammation fails to respond to the recommended antibacterials.

7 Standard treatment at home (PO)

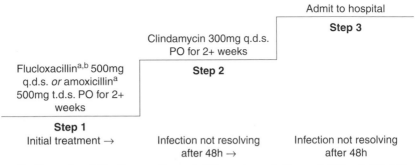

a. if a history of penicillin allergy, erythromycin 500mg q.d.s. or clarithromycin 500mg b.d. (but also see point 11 below).
b. if features suggest *Staph. aureus* infection (e.g. folliculitis, pus, crusted dermatitis), flucloxacillin should definitely be used.

8 Standard treatment in hospital (IV): follow local guidelines. The following reflect the recommendations of the British Lymphology Society and Lymphoedema Support Network. Switch to PO amoxicillin, flucloxacillin or clindamycin when no fever for 48h, inflammation settling and CRP falling (see 7 above).

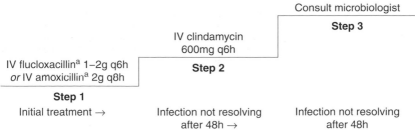

		Consult microbiologist
	IV clindamycin 600mg q6h	**Step 3**
IV flucloxacillin[a] 1–2g q6h *or* IV amoxicillin[a] 2g q8h	**Step 2**	
Step 1		
Initial treatment →	Infection not resolving after 48h →	Infection not resolving after 48h

a. if a history of penicillin allergy, start on Step 2.

9 For anogenital cellulitis, first line treatment is amoxicillin 2g IV q8h plus gentamicin 5mg/kg IV once daily; the dose of the latter to be adjusted according to renal function and gentamicin plasma concentration.

10 If ≥2 episodes of cellulitis/year, review skin condition and skin care regimen, and consider further steps to reduce limb swelling. Start antibacterial prophylaxis with:
- phenoxymethylpenicillin 250mg b.d. (500mg b.d. if BMI ≥33) for two years; halve the dose after one year if no recurrence
- if allergic to penicillins, prescribe erythromycin or clarithromycin 250mg once daily (but see 11 below)
- if cellulitis develops despite antibacterials, consider other once daily prophylactic antibacterials e.g. clindamycin 150mg, cefalexin 250mg or doxycycline 50mg; advice from a medical microbiologist and local specialist lymphoedema service is advised
- If cellulitis develops after discontinuation of antibacterials after 2 years, treat the acute episode, and then commence life-long prophylaxis
- if recurrent anogenital cellulitis, prescribe trimethoprim 100mg at bedtime.

11 Check for important drug interactions between macrolides (clarithromycin, erythromycin) and, in particular, statins, astemizole and tolterodine (avoid concurrent use). Alternative antibacterials: cefalexin 500mg t.d.s. (but not if a history of severe penicillin allergy) or doxycycline 200mg once daily stat, then 100mg once daily. For prophylaxis, prescribe cefalexin 250mg or doxycycline 50mg once daily.

General

12 Remember:
- if severe, bed rest and elevation of the affected limb on pillows are essential
- cellulitis is painful; analgesics should be prescribed regularly and p.r.n. Avoid NSAIDs because there may be an increased risk of necrotizing fasciitis
- compression garments should not be worn until limb is comfortable
- daily skin hygiene should be continued; washing and gentle drying
- emollients should not be used in the affected area if the skin is broken.

13 Patients should be educated about cellulitis:
- why susceptible (skin crevices harbour bacteria, reduced immunity)
- causes increased swelling, more fibrosis, decreased response to compression
- daily skin care to improve and maintain skin integrity
- reduce risk, e.g. protect hands when gardening, clean cuts, treat fungal infections (terbinafine cream once daily for two weeks) and ingrowing toenails
- obtaining prompt medical attention if cellulitis occurs
- if a history of cellulitis, take a 2-week supply of PO flucloxacillin 500mg q.d.s. or amoxicillin 500mg t.d.s. for emergency use when away from home. If allergic to penicillins, erythromycin 500mg q.d.s or clarithromycin 500mg b.d. (also see point 11 above).

Updated October 2013

CLOSTRIDIUM DIFFICILE INFECTION

BNF 1.5, 5.1.7 & 5.1.11

Clostridium difficile infection (CDI) is associated with hospital admission, the use of antibacterials, and the presence of other risk factors (Box A). However, community-acquired infection is increasing and now accounts for about one third of all cases, many of which lack 'traditional' risk factors, including antibacterial use.[1-3] Possible explanations include exposure to spores of *C. difficile* from infants (most are asymptomatic carriers), animals or foods.[2]

Box A   Clinical features and risk factors for *Clostridium difficile* infection

Clinical features
Watery diarrhoea + mucus ± blood
Abdominal pain and tenderness ± tenesmus
Fever and malaise
± Nausea, vomiting, and anorexia
± Dehydration and delirium
± Leukocytosis
Symptoms generally begin within 1 week of starting antibacterial treatment or shortly after stopping, but may occur up to 2 months later.[5]

Patient-related factors
Age > 65 years
Previous infection with *C. difficile*

Treatment-related factors
Prolonged hospital admission: 1% incidence if < 1 week but 50% if >4 weeks[6]
GI procedures (non-surgical or surgical)
Nasogastric tubes
PPIs
Radiation therapy

Antibacterial use[7]
Prolonged antibacterial treatment

Highest risk	*Low risk*
Cephalosporins (second/third generation)	Aminoglycosides
Clindamycin	Benzylpenicillin
Fluoroquinolones	Piptazobactam
	Tetracyclines
Medium risk	Trimethoprim
Amoxicillin/ampicillin	Vancomycin
Co-amoxiclav	
Macrolides	

Underlying disease states
Cancer
COPD
Renal failure
Immunosuppression

Toxins are produced which damage the intestinal mucosa, and in severe cases a pseudomembranous colitis develops, with sloughing of the inflamed colonic epithelium. This manifests as foul-smelling diarrhoea mingled with mucus and blood. CDI has a mortality of ≤40% in the frail elderly.[4]

In England, NHS Trusts are obliged to report all cases of CDI in anyone over 2 years old, and regular updates on infection rates and outcomes are published by the Health Protection Agency (available from: www.hpa.org.uk/Topics/InfectiousDiseases/InfectionsAZ/ClostridiumDifficile/).

C. difficile is spread indirectly by the faecal-oral route by spores left on surfaces:
- asymptomatic colonization in the general population is about 5%
- asymptomatic colonization in hospital and nursing home populations may be ≤30%[5]
- in about 33% of those colonized, *C. difficile* produces diarrhoea-producing toxins.[8]

A failure to mount an immune response is associated with colonization and toxin production. The presence of toxin correlates with mortality and is a better indicator of infection than the presence *per se* of toxigenic strains of *C. difficile* (see Diagnosis below). In the absence of toxin, outcomes are the same for patients with toxigenic *C. difficile* positive or negative samples. Nonetheless, identifying patients excreting toxigenic strains of *C. difficile* is important for infection control.[9]

Diagnosis

Based on current NHS advice:[9]
When to test for C. difficile
- a faecal sample should be sent as soon as possible for testing in patients with diarrhoea (ranging from soft 'blobs' to watery faeces) not clearly attributable to another cause, e.g. laxatives; this includes any hospital patient ≥2 years and all community patients ≥65 years (or those <65 years when clinically indicated)
- if *C. difficile* infection is suspected in the absence of diarrhoea, e.g. with ileus or toxic megacolon, alternative investigations may be required, e.g. colonoscopy, CT abdomen; *seek specialist advice.*

How to test for C. difficile
  C. difficile is difficult to culture. A two stage testing approach is recommended:
- initial screening test using either:
  ▷ a glutamate dehydrogenase test which detects an antigen produced by all *C. difficile* strains, including those which are not toxigenic *or*
  ▷ a toxin gene test, which detects the presence of toxin gene(s)
- when the screening test is positive, a second test is undertaken, either:
  ▷ a sensitive toxin test, which detects toxin(s) specific for *C. difficile* colitis *or*
  ▷ a cytotoxin assay, which detects toxins, but takes longer.

The screening test confirms the likely presence of *C. difficile* and the second test the presence or absence of toxins, which indicates if the patient has *C. difficile* infection or is merely colonized by *C. difficile*. For the latter, a toxin gene test (if not already done) can be used as an optional third test to identify toxigenic strains of *C. difficile*, which would make the patient a cross-infection risk to others. The presence of non-toxigenic strains of *C. difficile* can be regarded as normal bowel flora and are of no clinical or infection control relevance.

For those patients with a negative screening test, or who are toxin negative *C. difficile* excretors, other causes for their diarrhoea should be considered.

Management strategy
Prevention

Spread of *C. difficile* is by the ingestion of spores from the environment around symptomatic patients. Environmental controls ('universal precautions') will generally prevent the spread of outbreaks:
- patients should be isolated while they have diarrhoea, and have their own commode or separate en suite toilet
- carers should use gloves, gowns and disposable aprons when caring for infected patients and handling body fluids
- carers should thoroughly wash their hands before and after patient contact using antibacterial soap and water; *alcohol-based hand rubs are ineffective against C. difficile spores*[1]
  ▷ the WHO produces a downloadable chart illustrating correct hand-washing technique (available from: www.who.int/gpsc/tools/Pocket-Leaflet.pdf)
- areas where there are patients with *C. difficile* should be thoroughly cleaned using chlorine disinfectants.[10,11]

Antibacterial prescribing policies should aim to minimize the use of broad-spectrum antibacterials, and to regulate treatment duration.[1,7,10,11]

Acid-suppressing drugs, particularly PPIs, may be a risk factor for infection with *C. difficile*. Thus, it is important to review the need for PPIs in patients with or at high risk of CDI.[11]

General measures

Attention should be given to hydration, electrolytes and nutrition. Antiperistaltic drugs should be avoided because of the theoretical risk of precipitating toxic megacolon by slowing the clearance of *C. difficile* toxin from the intestine.[11]

Drug treatment

When there is high clinical suspicion of CDI, particularly when severe, consider starting treatment before test results are available. Ideally, discontinue all other antibacterial therapy.[7]

Metronidazole PO (see p.468) is the treatment of choice for mild–moderate infections; it is as effective as **vancomycin** and much cheaper.[1,11,12] IV **metronidazole** has been used in patients unable to take oral formulations but treatment failures have occurred.[5]

Current UK guidelines recommend **vancomycin** for severe infection, manifesting as any of the following:

* temperature $> 38.5°C$
* tachycardia > 100 beats/min
* WBC $> 15 \times 10^9/L$
* acutely rising plasma creatinine ($> 50\%$ above baseline)
* clinical or radiographic evidence of severe colitis, e.g. abdominal signs, hypotension, ileus.[11]

Vancomycin must be given PO or PR, because it is not secreted into the GI tract after IV administration.[13]

In severe cases not responding to **vancomycin**, PO **fidaxomicin** is an alternative or high-dose PO **vancomycin** ± IV **metronidazole**. The addition of oral **rifampicin** 300 mg b.d. or IV immunoglobulin 400 mg/kg should be considered.[11]

Fidaxomicin should also be considered for patients with severe CDI who are considered at high risk for recurrence. These include elderly patients with multiple comorbidities who are receiving antibacterials.

Most patients show some symptom improvement in < 2 days, e.g. reduction of fever. However, resolution of diarrhoea may take $\geqslant 6$ days.[1]

Relapse

About 20% of patients relapse, most in $\leqslant 3$ weeks.[11,14] This may be caused by germination of residual spores within the colon (more likely if recurrence within 14 days),[15] re-infection with *C. difficile* or further antibacterial treatment. Relapse because of antibacterial resistance in *C. difficile* is rare.[16]

* the same antibiotic may be used to treat the first relapse[11]
* for a second or third relapse, oral **fidaxomicin** is recommended; oral **vancomycin** is an alternative[11]
* for repeated relapses, *seek specialist microbiological/gastro-enterological advice.*

Options include more **fidaxomicin** or prolonged treatment with a slowly decreasing dose of **vancomycin**, e.g. over 6 weeks:[11,15]

* week 1, 125mg q.d.s.
* week 2, 125mg b.d.
* week 3, 125mg once daily
* week 4, 125mg every other day
* week 5 and 6, 125mg every 3 days.

Intermittent therapy in week 4 and 5 allows spores to germinate on 'no antibacterial' days with subsequent destruction on 'antibacterial' days. However, the use of such a regimen must be balanced against the risk of colonization with **vancomycin** resistant organisms such as enterococcus.

Probiotics may reduce the incidence of relapse,[17–19] but are not used routinely, and are not recommended by UK guidelines.[11] Various other approaches, including monoclonal antibodies against *C. difficile* toxins A and B, are being investigated for the prevention of recurrent CDI in patients already being treated with **metronidazole** or **vancomycin**.[20–22]

Dose and use
Metronidazole:

* 400–500mg PO t.d.s. for 10–14 days for initial treatment of mild–moderate cases[11,15,16]
* 500mg IV t.d.s. may be given in addition to high-dose PO or intracolonic **vancomycin** in severe cases which have not responded to low-dose **vancomycin** or in life-threatening infection[11]

Vancomycin:

- 125mg PO q.d.s. for 10–14 days[11]
- an oral solution can be prepared using the injection powder and is significantly cheaper than the capsules (see Supply)
- increase to 500mg PO (or by nasogastric tube) q.d.s. if infection is severe, life-threatening, or fails to respond to low-dose treatment[11] or
- if life-threatening, 500mg q.d.s. may be administered by the intracolonic (rectal) route.[11]

Fidaxomicin:

- 200mg b.d. for 10–14 days for treatment of severe infection where there is considered to be a high risk of recurrence[11]
- 200mg b.d. for 10–14 days for treatment of recurrent disease.[11]

Supply
See **metronidazole**, p.468.

Vancomycin (generic)
Capsules 125mg, 250mg, 10 days @ 125mg q.d.s. = £190.
Injection (powder for reconstitution) 500mg, 1g vial = £7 and £13 respectively.

Vancocin® (Flynn)
Matrigel capsules 125mg, 10 days @ 125mg q.d.s. = £126.
Injection (powder for reconstitution) 500mg, 1g vial = £7 and £13 respectively.

Vancomycin injection powder is authorized to prepare an oral solution; add 10mL WFI to a 500mg vial of powder and give 2.5mL (125mg) q.d.s. diluted with 30mL water or fruit juice (other than grapefruit), 10-day course = £70 (based on using 1 vial/day).

Fidaxomicin
Dificlir® (Astellas)
Tablets 200mg, 10 days @ 200mg b.d. = £1350.

1 Shannon-Lowe J et al. (2010) Prevention and medical management of Clostridium difficile infection. British Medical Journal. 340: c1296.
2 Leffler DA and Lamont JT (2012) Editorial: not so nosocomial anymore: the growing threat of community-acquired Clostridium difficile. American Journal of Gastroenterology. 107: 96–98.
3 Wilcox MH et al. (2008) A case-control study of community-associated Clostridium difficile infection. Journal of Antimicrobial Chemotherpy. 62: 388–396.
4 Mitchell BG and Gardner A (2012) Mortality and Clostridium difficile infection: a review. Antimicrobial Resistance and Infection Control. 1: 20.
5 Fekety R (1997) Guidelines for the diagnosis and management of Clostridium difficile-associated diarrhea and colitis. American College of Gastroenterology, Practice Parameters Committee. American Journal of Gastroenterology. 92: 739–750.
6 Johnson S et al. (1990) Nosocomial Clostridium difficile colonisation and disease. Lancet. 336: 97–100.
7 Monaghan T et al. (2008) Recent advances in Clostridium difficile-associated disease. Gut. 57: 850–860.
8 Starr J (2005) Clostridium difficile associated diarrhoea: diagnosis and treatment. British Medical Journal. 331: 498–501.
9 Department of Health (2012) Updated guidance on diagnosis and reporting of Clostridium Difficile. Available from: www.dh.gov.uk
10 Donaldson L and Beasley C (2005) Infection caused by Clostridium difficile. Letter from the Chief Medical Officer and Chief Nursing Officer. Department of Health. Available from: www.dh.gov.uk/en/Publicationsandstatistics/Lettersandcirculars/Professionalletters/Chiefmedicalofficerletters/DH_4125069
11 Department of Health (2013) Updated guidance on the management and treatment of Clostridum difficle infection. Available from: http://www.hpa.org.uk
12 British National Formulary Section 1.5 Chronic bowel disorders. London: BMJ Group and Pharmaceutical Press. www.bnf.org (accessed April 2014).
13 Durai R (2007) Epidemiology, pathogenesis, and management of Clostridium difficile infection. Digestive Diseases and Sciences. 52: 2958–2962.
14 Gilbert DN et al. (eds) (2008) The Sanford guide to antimicrobial therapy 2008. Antimicrobial Therapy Inc, Sperryville.
15 Figueroa I et al. (2012) Relapse versus reinfection: recurrent Clostridium difficile infection following treatment with fidaxomicin or vancomycin. Clinical and Infectious Diseases. 55 (Suppl 2): S104–109.
16 Freeman J et al. (2010) The changing epidemiology of Clostridium difficile infections. Clinical Microbiology Reviews. 23: 529–549.
17 Surawicz CM et al. (2000) The search for a better treatment for recurrent Clostridium difficile disease: use of high-dose vancomycin combined with Saccharomyces boulardii. Clinical Infectious Diseases. 31: 1012–1017.

18 Dendukuri N et al. (2005) Probiotic therapy for the prevention and treatment of Clostridium difficile-associated diarrhea: a systematic review. Canadian Medical Association Journal. 173: 167–170.
19 Venuto C et al. (2010) Alternative therapies for Clostridium difficile infections. Pharmacotherapy. 30: 1266–1278.
20 Lowy I et al. (2010) Treatment with monoclonal antibodies against Clostridium difficile toxins. New England Journal of Medicine. 362: 197–205.
21 Kyne L (2010) Clostridium difficile–beyond antibiotics. New England Journal of Medicine. 362: 264–265.
22 Lo Vecchio A and Zacur GM (2012) Clostridium difficile infection: an update on epidemiology, risk factors, and therapeutic options. Current Opinion in Gastroenterology. 28: 1–9.

Updated April 2014

HELICOBACTER PYLORI GASTRITIS   BNF 1.3

Helicobacter pylori infection of the stomach is ubiquitous, with a global prevalence of about 50% in the adult population. Overall, the prevalence is falling, but infection rates vary widely, being higher in developing countries and in low socio-economic groups. Infection is generally acquired in childhood, and long-term infection predisposes to chronic gastritis, GI ulceration and subsequent gastric cancer.[1,2] Eradication of H. pylori with antibacterials and PPIs is more cost-effective than acid suppression alone in relation to:

- relieving non-ulcer dyspepsia[3]
- healing peptic ulcers[3,4]
- preventing recurrent ulceration and bleeding.[4,5]

Evidence that eradication of H. pylori infection lowers the risk of gastric cancer is accumulating.[6–10] Current European guidelines recommend eradication after gastric cancer resection, and in first-degree relatives of gastric cancer patients.[3] In patients with early-stage mucosa-associated lymphoid tissue (MALT) lymphoma, eradication often leads to remission, and is recommended for this by European guidelines.[3]

H. pylori infection is associated with an increased risk of peptic ulcers in NSAID and low-dose aspirin users. Thus, eradication is beneficial before starting NSAID treatment,[11,12] and is mandatory in patients with a peptic ulcer history. However, H. pylori eradication alone does not prevent peptic ulceration in patients already receiving long-term NSAID treatment. For optimum prophylaxis, such patients require long-term treatment with a PPI as well.[3,13]

Management strategy
If possible, stop the NSAID
Patients on an NSAID who develop symptoms suggesting a GI ulcer should ideally stop taking the NSAID (or minimize the dose if this is not possible), start on a gastric acid suppressant, and be tested for H. pylori.[14,15]

Test for H. pylori
For patients starting on regular NSAID treatment or those with symptoms suggestive of an uncomplicated ulcer (e.g. gnawing or burning epigastric pain, worse at night or when the stomach is empty, and relieved by food or antacids), non-invasive tests are appropriate:

- faecal antigen tests detect H. pylori-associated antigens in faeces using specific antibodies. These tests have a specificity and sensitivity of >90% when performed accurately[16,17]
- urea breath tests involve ingesting ^{16}C-labelled urea, which is broken down by H. pylori to produce ammonia and labelled CO_2. This is then detected in expired air. These tests have excellent specificity, sensitivity and reliability.[16,18] However, to avoid false-positive results, PPIs or H_2-receptor antagonists must be stopped 1–2 weeks before the test, and patients must fast for 6h immediately before.[18]

Both types of test are better markers of active infection than a serological antibody test, which does not distinguish between present and past infection with H. pylori. ^{16}C-labelled urea breath tests are preferred in the UK, based on patient acceptability, convenience and overall laboratory costs.[16]

An endoscopic examination and biopsy is recommended for patients with symptoms suggesting a complicated ulcer or gastric cancer (i.e. otherwise unexplained GI bleeding, iron-deficiency anaemia, GI obstruction or mass, dysphagia, persistent vomiting, anorexia or weight loss, severe abdominal pain suggesting perforation, or suspicious barium meal). Endoscopy is also recommended for patients >55 years old who have unexplained persistent dyspepsia alone.[15]

Eradication

H. pylori infection is generally treated with a PPI and at least two antibacterials. Globally, *H. pylori* antibacterial resistance, mainly to **clarithromycin**, is increasing, and this causes a significant degree of treatment failure.[19,20] Recent data suggest that, in areas with a high level of resistance, conventional regimens may cure only a maximum of 70% of patients.[21]

At present, Northern Europe is an area of low **clarithromycin** resistance.[3] In the UK, 1-week triple therapy regimens (two antibacterials and a gastroprotective drug; Box A) are recommended because they are more or less as effective as quadruple therapy regimens.[14,22]

Box A   Examples of first-line eradication regimens for in the UK

Three drugs are taken b.d. for 1 week:
- a standard-dose PPI, e.g. lansoprazole 30mg, omeprazole 20mg or pantoprazole 40mg
- and *either*:
  ▷ clarithromycin 500mg with amoxicillin 1g, *or*
  ▷ clarithromycin 250mg with metronidazole 400mg (suitable for patients allergic to penicillin).

Resistance to amoxicillin is rare, whereas resistance to either clarithromycin or metronidazole is common and can arise during treatment. Thus, if the patient has recently been treated with clarithromycin or an alternative macrolide for a different infection, use amoxicillin + metronidazole. Similarly, if recent treatment with metronidazole, use clarithromycin + amoxicillin.

The cost of a 1-week course is £4–£10.

Note: clarithromycin predisposes to QT interval prolongation (see Chapter 24, p.759); it is metabolized by and inhibits CYP3A4/5 and thus potentially modifies the metabolism of several other drugs (see Chapter 25, p.767).

If a regimen including a PPI and **clarithromycin** fails to eradicate the infection, either a **bismuth**-containing quadruple therapy[14] or **levofloxacin**-containing triple therapy is recommended.[3] Alternatively, the patient can be referred for endoscopy and treatment based on culture and sensitivity testing.

Confirm eradication

Patients with or at high risk of ulcer complications (e.g. perforation or bleeding) and those with MALT lymphoma should be retested to confirm eradication. The urea breath test is the test of choice. However, because the results can be affected by antibacterials and PPIs, the test should only be carried out 4 weeks after finishing antibacterial-containing eradication regimens and 2 weeks after completing a course of PPIs.[14]

The faecal antigen test is an alternative but less accurate test. Serological testing does not help because antibodies persist long after *H. pylori* has been eradicated.[16]

Supply

For **lansoprazole** and **omeprazole**, see Proton pump inhibitors, p.31.
For **amoxicillin** and **clarithromycin**, see Cellulitis in a lymphoedematous limb, p.476.
For **metronidazole**, p.468.

[13]C-labelled urea breath tests

diabact UBT® (MDE)
Tablets 50mg, 1 kit (including 1 tablet, 4 breath-sample containers, straws) = £22 (analysis included).

Pylobactell® (Torbet) **Tablets soluble** 100mg, 1 kit (including 6 breath-sample containers, 30mL mixing and administration vial, straws) = £21 (analysis included).

Helicobacter Test INFAI® (Infai)
Oral powder 75mg, 1 kit (including 4 breath-sample containers, straws) = £20 (analysis included).
A 45mg kit for children age 3–11 is also available. However, the appropriateness of testing for H. pylori infection in children has not been established.

---

1 Czinn SJ (2005) Helicobacter pylori infection: detection, investigation, and management. *Journal of Pediatrics*. **146 (Suppl 3)**: s21–26.

2 Guarner J (2004) The spectrum of gastric disease associated with Helicobacter pylori and other infectious gastritides. *Current Gastroenterology Reports*. **6**: 441–446.

3 Malfertheiner P et al. (2012) Management of Helicobacter pylori infection–the Maastricht IV/ Florence Consensus Report. *Gut*. **61**: 646–664.

4 Ford A et al. (2009) Eradication therapy for peptic ulcer disease in Helicobacter pylori positive patients. *Cochrane Database of Systematic Reviews*. **4**: CD003840.

5 Gisbert JP et al. (2010) Helicobacter pylori eradication therapy vs. antisecretory non-eradication therapy (with or without long-term maintenance antisecretory therapy) for the prevention of recurrent bleeding from peptic ulcer. *Cochrane Database of Systematic Reviews*. **2**: CD004062.

6 McCormack K (1989) Mathematical model for assessing risk of gastrointestinal reactions to NSAIDs. In: K Rainsford (ed) *Azapropazone - over two decades of clinical use*. Kluwer Academic Publishers, Boston, pp. 81–93.

7 Di Leo V et al. (2005) Effect of Helicobacter pylori and eradication therapy on gastrointestinal permeability. Implications for patients with seronegative spondyloarthritis. *Journal of Rheumatology*. **32**: 295–300.

8 De Vries AC and Kuipers EJ (2007) Review article: Helicobacter pylori eradication for the prevention of gastric cancer. *Alimentary Pharmacology and Therapeutics*. **26 (Suppl 2)**: 25–35.

9 Fuccio L et al. (2009) Meta-analysis: can Helicobacter pylori eradication treatment reduce the risk for gastric cancer? *Annals of internal medicine*. **151**: 121–128.

10 Hartgrink HH et al. (2009) Gastric cancer. *Lancet*. **374**: 477–490.

11 Chan FK et al. (2002) Eradication of Helicobacter pylori and risk of peptic ulcers in patients starting long-term treatment with non-steroidal anti-inflammatory drugs: a randomised trial. *Lancet*. **359**: 9–13.

12 de Leest HT et al. (2007) Eradication of Helicobacter pylori does not reduce the incidence of gastroduodenal ulcers in patients on long-term NSAID treatment: double-blind, randomized, placebo-controlled trial. *Helicobacter*. **12**: 477–485.

13 Vergara M et al. (2005) Meta-analysis: role of Helicobacter pylori eradication in the prevention of peptic ulcer in NSAID users. *Alimentary Pharmacology and Therapeutics*. **21**: 1411–1418.

14 British National Formulary Section 1.3. Antisecretory drugs and mucosal protectants. London: BMJ Group and Pharmaceutical Press. ww.bnf.org (accessed April 2014).

15 NICE (2004) Dyspepsia. Management of dyspepsia in adults in primary care. *Clinical Guideline*. CG17. www.nice.org.uk

16 DTB (2005) H. pylori eradication in NSAID-associated ulcers. *Drug and Therapeutics Bulletin*. **43**: 37–40.

17 Schenk BE et al. (2000) Effect of Helicobacter pylori eradication on chronic gastritis during omeprazole therapy. *Gut*. **46**: 615–621.

18 Fallone CA et al. (2000) The urea breath test for Helicobacter pylori infection: taking the wind out of the sails of endoscopy. *Canadian Medical Association Journal*. **162**: 371–372.

19 Chuah SK et al. (2011) A new look at anti-Helicobacter pylori therapy. *World Journal of Gastroenterology*. **17**: 3971–3975.

20 Marin AC et al. (2013) A review of rescue regimens after clarithromycin-containing triple therapy failure (for Helicobacter pylori eradication). *Expert Opinion on Pharmacotherapy*. **14**: 843–861.

21 Graham DY and Fischbach L (2010) Helicobacter pylori treatment in the era of increasing antibiotic resistance. *Gut*. **59**: 1143–1153.

22 Luther J et al. (2010) Empiric quadruple vs. triple therapy for primary treatment of Helicobacter pylori infection: Systematic review and meta-analysis of efficacy and tolerability. *American Journal of Gastroenterology*. **105**: 65–73.

Updated May 2014

7: ENDOCRINE SYSTEM AND IMMUNOMODULATION

BISPHOSPHONATES   BNF 6.6.2 & 9.5.1.2

Indications: Authorized indications vary between products; consult SPC for details. They include hypercalcaemia; prophylaxis to reduce skeletal-related events (SRE) associated with osteolytic bone metastases, including pain; osteoporosis; Paget's disease.

Contra-indications: *Ibandronic acid PO*: Oesophageal abnormality (e.g. stricture or achalasia), inability to sit upright for 60min.

Pharmacology
The bisphosphonates are stable analogues of pyrophosphate, a naturally occurring regulator of bone metabolism. They have a high affinity for calcium ions, and bind rapidly to hydroxyapatite crystals in mineralized bone. Bisphosphonates are subsequently released and taken up by osteoclasts, interfering with their function and/or inducing their apoptosis (programmed cell death). Nitrogen-containing bisphosphonates (e.g. **alendronate, ibandronic acid, pamidronate disodium, zoledronic acid**) inhibit the mevalonate pathway vital for normal cellular function (e.g. vesicular trafficking, cell signalling, cytoskeleton function) and non-nitrogen-containing bisphosphonates (**sodium clodronate, disodium etidronate**) form cytotoxic adenosine triphosphate (ATP) analogues.[1,2] These cellular effects also extend to macrophages, reducing the production of cytokines, and this anti-inflammatory effect may contribute to the analgesic effect of bisphosphonates.[3,4] Bisphosphonates interfere with the cancer-related increase in the number and activity of osteoclasts which cause bone pain by:
- producing an increasingly acidic environment (stimulating acid-sensing receptors on sensory nerves)
- destroying sensory nerves (producing neuropathic pain)
- causing mechanical instability as a result of the loss of bone mineral (stimulating mechanoreceptors on sensory nerves in the periosteum).[5]

In vitro and in animals, bisphosphonates also have a direct anticancer effect via inhibition of matrix metalloproteinase, altered cell adhesion, anti-angiogenic activity, reduction in release of local growth factors from bone and induction of apoptosis.[6,7] However, a cancer-promoting effect has been seen in some animal studies.[8] Bisphosphonates have no impact on the effect of parathyroid hormone-related protein (PTHrP) or on renal tubular resorption of calcium.

Bisphosphonates are poorly absorbed PO and this is reduced further by food (see Chapter 14, Box A, p.643). They are rapidly taken up by the skeleton, particularly at sites of bone resorption and where the mineral is more exposed, and they remain there for weeks–months.[9] Most of the remainder is bound to plasma proteins. Bisphosphonates are not metabolized and are excreted unchanged via the kidneys. The plasma proportion of the drug is eliminated generally within 24h. Thereafter, elimination is much slower as the remainder gradually seeps out of bone.[10] Comparison of the halflives of different bisphosphonates is complicated by this multiphasic elimination.

Tumour-induced hypercalcaemia

Bisphosphonates given IV are the treatment of choice for hypercalcaemia of malignancy (Table 1).[11] With **zoledronic acid**, normocalcaemia is achieved after a median of 4 days (ranging up to 10), and pain relief ≤14 days.

Table 1 Bisphosphonates and the initial treatment of hypercalcaemia[12-14]

	Zoledronic acid	Pamidronate disodium	Ibandronic acid
IV dose	4mg	30–90mg	2–6mg
Onset of effect	<4 days	<3 days	<4 days
Maximum effect	4–7 days	5–7 days	7 days
Duration of effect	4 weeks	2.5 weeks	2.5 weeks (4mg)
			4 weeks (6mg)
Restores normocalcaemia	90%	70–75%	75%

Zoledronic acid 8mg has been given to patients who do not respond to 4mg or to **pamidronate disodium**, and those who relapse within a few days of treatment. Normocalcaemia is achieved in 50% but the median duration of response is only 2 weeks.[3] However, because the incidence of renal impairment doubles with the 8mg dose, its use was abandoned in clinical trials and it is unauthorized.[4]

Prevention of skeletal-related events (SRE) in patients with myeloma or bone metastases

Pamidronate disodium IV, **zoledronic acid** IV and **ibandronic acid** PO/IV are given long-term to patients with bone metastases to decrease the incidence of SREs (definition varies but includes pathological fracture, radiotherapy to bone, spinal cord compression or surgery to bone).[15-20] Various national guidelines recommend with provisos the routine use of bisphosphonates for the treatment and prevention of SRE in patients with:
- breast cancer with bone metastases[20-23]
- myeloma whether or not bone lesions are evident.[24,25]

They are also recommended for the relief of pain from bone metastases in patients with hormone-resistant prostate cancer when analgesia and radiotherapy have failed.[26-28] There is no consensus on the use of bisphosphonates in other cancers, although it has been suggested that in any patient with a prognosis of ≥4–6 months and multiple bone metastases, it is reasonable to consider their use.[29,30]

Only studies ≥6 months in duration have shown a reduction in fractures, hypercalcaemia, and the need for radiotherapy. Patients treated with **zoledronic acid** on a regular basis for more than 12 months had better outcomes in terms of reduced risk of SRE and possibly improved survival.[31-33] Studies ≥2 years in duration have also shown a reduced need for orthopaedic surgery. The incidence and severity of pain is reduced with an NNT of 11 at 1 month and 7 at 3 months. There is no impact on the occurrence of spinal cord compression. The optimal duration of treatment is unclear, but bisphosphonates are generally continued for as long as they are tolerated, or there is a substantial decline in the patient's performance status.

In patients with breast cancer, bisphosphonates delay time to developing first SRE, reduce the risk of developing an SRE and the rate at which SREs develop.[20] **Zoledronic acid** 4mg IV given monthly for 1 year reduces the risk of a SRE by about 40%, compared with placebo.[5] Treatment every 2 weeks provides no greater benefit.[6] After 1 year, a 12-weekly regimen has been shown to maintain beneficial effects.[34]

Zoledronic acid is at least as effective as **pamidronate disodium** in reducing SRE and pain scores in patients with multiple myeloma or breast cancer.[7-9] In one RCT, patients receiving **zoledronic acid** required less radiotherapy and less surgery than those receiving **pamidronate disodium**; NNTs were 4 and 20 respectively.[4] **Zoledronic acid** has reduced pain and markers of bone turnover in patients with breast cancer who have developed a SRE or progressive bone disease despite receiving **pamidronate disodium** or **disodium clodronate**.[9] The use of

zoledronic acid in early stage breast cancer as adjuvant therapy may improve overall survival.[29] In patients with multiple myeloma, **zoledronic acid** is a cost-effective alternative to **disodium clodronate** in the prevention of SRE.[24,26]

In prostate cancer, there is little benefit from bisphosphonates in relation to SRE, quality of life, or survival; this explains the more limited recommendation regarding their use in this setting (see above).[19,28]

Bisphosphonates as adjuvant analgesics

Bisphosphonates have been used for metastatic bone pain and several regimens have been recommended for use when more conventional methods have been exhausted.[3,35–38] An effect is generally seen within 2 weeks. The evidence suggests that benefit is more likely in patients with breast cancer or myeloma, and with an IV bisphosphonate.[20,38]

In patients with prostate cancer, a systematic review of ten studies showed a trend in favour of bisphosphonates compared to placebo for relief of bone pain. However, there was no consistent reduction in analgesic use between the groups.[19,28] In a further study, about one third of patients receiving **zoledronic acid** had a clinically relevant improvement in bone pain ($\geqslant 2$ point change in their pain score). However, baseline bone pain levels were low (mean composite Brief Pain Inventory score of 2/10) and over the course of the study, pain increased slightly in both groups.[12] Thus, bisphosphonate treatment is reserved for patients with bone pain unresponsive to analgesia or radiotherapy.

Primary prevention of bone loss in patients treated for breast or prostate cancer

Oestrogen deficiency is induced in women treated for breast cancer by chemotherapy $\pm$ aromatase inhibitors. This increases the rate of bone loss and risk of fracture.[39] Oral bisphosphonates, e.g. **risedronate** 35mg once a week, can prevent the loss following chemotherapy and ongoing studies are examining their use with aromatase inhibitors.[39,40]

The increased bone loss associated with androgen deprivation treatment in men with prostate cancer is also prevented by bisphosphonates, e.g. **zoledronic acid** 4mg every 3 months.[41] NICE guidelines recommend that bisphosphonate treatment is offered to men receiving androgen deprivation therapy who have osteoporosis.[28]

Cautions

Renal impairment (correct hypovolaemia before treatment and monitor renal function); vitamin D deficiency (increased risk of hypocalcaemia);[42] invasive dental procedures (risk of jaw osteonecrosis).

Drug interactions

Concurrent use increases the risk of:
- prolonged hypocalcaemia and hypomagnesaemia with an aminoglycoside[43]
- hypocalcaemia and dehydration with loop diuretics
- renal impairment with other nephrotoxic drugs
- renal impairment with **thalidomide** in multiple myeloma.

Undesirable effects

Very common (>10%): transient pyrexia and flu-like symptoms (more common with IV nitrogen-containing bisphosphonates see below), fatigue, headache, anxiety, hypertension, anaemia, thrombocytopenia, cough, arthralgia, myalgia, bone pain, *asymptomatic hypocalcaemia, hypomagne-saemia, hypophosphataemia.*

Oral products in particular may cause anorexia, dyspepsia, nausea, vomiting, abdominal pain, diarrhoea or constipation.

Common (<10%, >1%): sleep disturbance, psychosis, tachycardia, atrial fibrillation or flutter, syncope, breathlessness, leucopenia, infusion site reactions, deterioration in renal function (see below), hypokalaemia, jaw osteonecrosis (see below).

Rare (<0.1%, >0.01%): ocular inflammation (see below), angioedema, collapsing focal segmental glomerulosclerosis (**pamidronate disodium**), nephrotic syndrome (**pamidronate disodium**), symptomatic hypocalcaemia (e.g. tetany), atypical femoral fractures, usually in patients treated for >5 years for osteoporosis.[44]

Very rare (<0.01%): anaphylaxis, bronchospasm.

Systemic reactions after IV bisphosphonates

Acute systemic inflammatory reactions causing symptoms such as fever, myalgia, arthralgia, nausea and vomiting, occur in 25–50% of patients after IV bisphosphonates. They are possibly related to the release of cytokines from inflammatory cells. Generally, the onset is within 2 days of the infusion; the fever is mild, although rigors occasionally occur. There may be bone pain, generally <12h of the infusion. These effects can be treated with **paracetamol** or NSAIDs, and resolve completely within 1–2 days. They generally lessen with repeat doses or with prophylactic **paracetamol** or NSAID.[45]

Renal toxicity

Bisphosphonates can affect renal function. **Pamidronate disodium** rarely causes collapsing focal segmental glomerulosclerosis, particularly in high doses, e.g. 180mg every 2–4 weeks. The probable mechanism is a direct toxic effect on glomerular capillary podocytes and renal tubules.[46]

The more potent third-generation bisphosphonates are given in much smaller doses and reach lower concentrations in the renal tubules. Renal impairment has occurred with **zoledronic acid** but is uncommon with **ibandronic acid**.[47–51] In direct comparisons, the incidence of decreased renal function with **zoledronic acid** 4mg (about 10%) is similar to **pamidronate disodium** 90mg over 2h.[4,13]

With **zoledronic acid** 4mg, increases in plasma creatinine lead to treatment delay or discontinuation in about 1% and 3% of patients respectively. Increases in creatinine levels >3 times the upper limit of normal were seen in 0.4% of patients.[7,15] There have been reports of life-threatening renal failure caused by toxic acute tubular necrosis in patients treated with **zoledronic acid**, e.g. 72 cases among >430,000 patients (i.e. <0.02%).[16–18] Other risk factors were often present, including dehydration, pre-existing renal impairment, and concurrent use of other nephrotoxic drugs.

Onset of decreased renal function varies, but often manifests within 2 months of starting treatment. Mild impairment tends to recover a few days–several months after discontinuing **zoledronic acid**. In those with renal failure, the damage is generally permanent.[20]

The risk of renal toxicity is reduced by adhering to the recommended dose and infusion rate, ensuring adequate hydration, monitoring renal function and adjusting the dose of bisphosphonate as appropriate or discontinuing treatment if there is deterioration, and avoiding the concurrent use of other nephrotoxic drugs. **Ibandronic acid** (see Box B) and **denosumab** (see Box C) are authorized for use in severe renal failure.

Jaw osteonecrosis

All bisphosphonates (and **denosumab**) have been implicated as a risk factor for jaw osteonecrosis.[52–55] Most reports involve the long-term use of **zoledronic acid** or **pamidronate disodium** for metastatic bone disease.[56] Although osteonecrosis has been reported after as little as 4 months of bisphosphonate use, generally, patients have been receiving bisphosphonates for years (mean and median duration of use vary around 1 and 2–3 years respectively). The true incidence of osteonecrosis is difficult to identify, but some studies put it as high as 10% of patients receiving long-term **zoledronic acid** and 4% of those receiving **pamidronate disodium**.[56] Other risk factors for jaw osteonecrosis include dental procedures (reported in about 60% of patients), poor dental health, blood clotting disorders, anaemia, and possibly chemotherapy and corticosteroids.

The jaw bones may be particularly susceptible to osteonecrosis because of the combination of repeated low-level local trauma (e.g. from chewing, dentures) and ease of infection from microbes. Trauma and infection increase the demand for bone repair which the bisphosphonate-inhibited bone cannot meet, resulting in localized bone necrosis; the anti-angiogenic effect of bisphosphonates may also contribute.[56]

Osteonecrosis can present as an asymptomatic bony exposure in one or more sites in the mandible or maxilla, or with orofacial pain, trismus, offensive discharge from a cutaneous fistula, chronic sinusitis because of an oro-antral fistula and numbness in the mandible or maxilla.[45] If probed, the necrotic bone is usually non-tender and may not bleed. There may be osteomyelitis with oral-cavity flora or *Actinomyces* species. Osteonecrosis may show as mottled bone on a plain radiograph and be confused with bone metastases on a bone scan. Pathological fracture can occur. Management is based on clinical experience. Long-term outcomes are generally poor with relatively few patients experiencing improvement or resolution. Thus, prevention is an important part of the recommended approach:[45]

• *preventive dental treatment* before commencing long-term bisphosphonates, e.g. treat infection, teeth extractions
• *encourage good dental hygiene* including regular dental cleaning by a dentist or dental hygienist
• *avoid invasive dental procedures* during treatment
• *minimize trauma*, e.g. patients with dentures should wear soft liners.

If osteonecrosis occurs:

• *discontinue the bisphosphonate* but new lesions may continue to appear
• *treat infection*, e.g. antimicrobials, **chlorhexidine** mouthwash, periodic minor debridement and wound irrigation (major debridement is avoided as it may worsen the situation)
• *avoid major surgery* unless there is no alternative, e.g. due to sequestered bone, pathological fracture, or oro-antral fistula.

If urgent treatment precludes a prior dental examination, a dental referral and any treatment should be undertaken within 1–2 months for patients expected to receive long-term bisphosphonates.[56]

Ocular toxicity

A rare undesirable effect is ocular inflammation, causing eye pain, redness, swelling, abnormal vision or impaired eye movement (due to rectus muscle oedema).[57,58] Typically, the onset is within 2 days of the first or second infusion and affects both eyes. There may be other symptoms of an acute systemic inflammatory reaction (see above). An urgent ophthalmology assessment is required, followed by appropriate treatment. Patients with mild reactions, e.g. those which settle quickly without treatment, can generally continue to receive the same bisphosphonate. Those with more severe reactions, e.g. uveitis or scleritis, should not receive the same bisphosphonate again; some tolerate a switch to a non-nitrogen-containing bisphosphonate, but specialist advice should be sought from the ophthalmologist ± endocrinologist.[45]

Other emerging toxicities

Severe (sometimes incapacitating) musculoskeletal pain has been reported after days, months or years of bisphosphonate treatment. It has generally occurred with PO bisphosphonates used for osteoporosis and Paget's disease, but the FDA is also investigating a possible link with IV bisphosphonates. The pain is distinct from the arthralgia/myalgia associated with an acute systemic inflammatory reaction (see above), and may respond to temporary or permanent discontinuation of the bisphosphonate.[59]

Dose and use

Unless being treated for tumour-related hypercalcaemia, daily oral supplements of elemental **calcium** 500mg and **vitamin D** 400 units are recommended e.g. Calcichew® D3 Forte.

Because **zoledronic acid** is more effective and now available as a generic, it is replacing **pamidronate disodium** as bisphosphonate of first choice.

Tumour-induced hypercalcaemia

Stop and think! Are you justified in correcting a potentially fatal complication in a moribund patient?

For **zoledronic acid**:

• patients should be well hydrated
• give 4mg IVI in 100mL 0.9% saline or 5% glucose over 15min
• if plasma calcium does not normalize, repeat after 1 week[11]
• 8mg has been used in refractory hypercalcaemia[3] but is unauthorized because of concerns relating to renal impairment (see Pharmacology)
• measure plasma creatinine before each dose; no dose adjustment is needed in mild–moderate renal impairment for patients being treated for hypercalcaemia.

For **pamidronate disodium**: The SPC recommends a dose dependent on the initial albumin-corrected plasma calcium concentration (Box A and Table 2). However, it has been suggested that

the higher dose should be given irrespective of the initial calcium level to increase the probability of a response and prolong its duration.[11] Patients should be well hydrated, using 0.9% saline if necessary:
- standard and maximum recommended dose is 90mg IVI/treatment
- dilute the dose in 0.9% saline or 5% glucose; the concentration should not exceed 60mg/250mL
- the infusion rate should not exceed 1mg/min in patients with normal renal function; patients with mild–moderate renal impairment (creatinine clearance 30–90mL/min) do not require dose reduction but the infusion rate should not exceed 90mg/4h (about 20–22mg/h)
- for patients with severe renal impairment (creatinine clearance <30mL/min) see below
- repeat after 1 week if initial response inadequate
- repeat every 3–4 weeks according to plasma calcium concentration
- measure plasma creatinine before each dose, no dose adjustment is required in mild–moderate renal impairment.

Box A   Correcting plasma calcium concentrations[a]

If the mean normal albumin for the local laboratory is 40g/L
Corrected calcium (mmol/L) = measured calcium + (0.022 × (40 − albumin g/L))
  e.g. measured calcium = 2.45; albumin = 32
      corrected calcium = 2.45 + (0.022 × 8) = 2.63mmol/L
      (normal range = 2.12–2.65mmol/L)

---

a. most UK pathology laboratories will now automatically report an albumin-corrected plasma calcium concentration based on locally validated data.

Table 2   IV pamidronate disodium for hypercalcaemia[a]

Corrected plasma calcium concentration (mmol/L)	Dose (mg)
<3	15 or 30
3–3.5	30 or 60
3.5–4	60 or 90
>4	90

a. manufacturer's recommendations.

If the IV route is inaccessible, bisphosphonates can be administered by CSCI, together with SC hydration.[60,61]
- **pamidronate disodium** 90mg in 1L 0.9% saline over 12–24h
- **sodium clodronate** (not UK) 1,500mg in 50–250mL 0.9% saline or 5% glucose over 2–3h.
Denosumab is an alternative (see Box C).

In palliative care, treatment with a bisphosphonate is unlikely to be started in patients with hypercalcaemia and severe renal impairment (creatinine clearance <30mL/min). If appropriate, consider using **ibandronic acid** (see Box B) or **denosumab** (see Box C) and seek specialist renal/endocrinology advice.

Prophylactic use to reduce the incidence of skeletal-related events
For **zoledronic acid**:
- patients should be well hydrated
- give 4mg IVI in 100mL 0.9% saline or 5% glucose over 15min every 3–4 weeks; with appropriate support, these can be given in the home setting[21,22]
- for dose in patients with renal impairment, see Table 3.[25]

For **pamidronate disodium**:
- patients should be well hydrated, using 0.9% saline if necessary
- dilute 90mg in a minimum of 375mL of 0.9% saline or 5% glucose; the concentration should not exceed 60mg/250mL
- in *breast cancer with bone metastases* give 90mg IVI over 1.5h every 3–4 weeks
- in *multiple myeloma* a slower infusion rate is recommended because of the greater risk of renal impairment/renal toxicity; give 90mg IVI over 4h every 4 weeks.

Box B   Ibandronic acid

Ibandronic acid is a third-generation bisphosphonate which can be taken PO. It is smaller and more easily swallowed than sodium clodronate. It is the only bisphosphonate authorized for use in severe renal impairment (creatinine clearance <30mL/min).

Adverse events are similar to other bisphosphonates (see main text), but the incidence is low.[3,11,15] Renal impairment is no more frequent than with placebo.

Dose and use
For details, see SPC.

To maximize absorption and to minimize undesirable gastro-oesophageal effects, patients should take ibandronic acid tablets whole after an overnight fast with a glass of *plain tap water*, followed by no food for ⩾30min and remaining upright for 60min.

Tumour-induced hypercalcaemia
- if the corrected plasma calcium is >3mmol/L give 4mg IV
- if the corrected plasma calcium is <3mmol/L give 2mg IV
- for both, the dose is given IVI in 500mL 0.9% saline *or* 5% glucose over 2h.

Prevention of skeletal events in patients with bone metastases from breast cancer or metastatic bone pain
- 50mg PO once daily *or*
- 6mg IVI in 100mL 0.9% saline *or* 5% glucose over 15min every 3–4 weeks.

The dose should be reduced in moderate and severe renal impairment (creatinine clearance <50–30mL/min and <30mL/min respectively):
- PO:
  - ▷ in moderate renal impairment, give 50mg PO *alternate days*
  - ▷ in severe renal impairment, give 50mg PO *once a week*
- IV:
  - ▷ in moderate renal impairment, give 4mg over 1h in 500mL 0.9% saline or 5% glucose *every 3–4 weeks*
  - ▷ in severe renal impairment, give 2mg over 1h in 500mL *every 3–4 weeks*.

Box C   Denosumab

Indications: recommended by NICE for patients in whom bisphosphonates are contra-indicated or poorly tolerated in the following settings:
- prevention of osteoporotic fragility fractures in postmenopausal women[62]
- prevention of SRE in adults with bone metastases from breast cancer and other solid cancers (except prostate)[63]
- treatment of bone loss in men with prostate cancer receiving androgen deprivation therapy.[28]

Denosumab is also an option for treating refractory hypercalcaemia of malignancy (unauthorized indication).

Contra-indication: untreated severe hypocalcaemia.

Pharmacology
Denosumab is a human monoclonal antibody that binds with receptor activator of nuclear factor kappa β ligand (RANKL), preventing the RANKL-RANK interaction and resulting in reduced osteoclast number and function, thus decreasing bone resorption and cancer-induced bone destruction.

continued

Box C Continued

There is evidence that denosumab is superior to zoledronic acid in preventing SRE (including pain)[64,65] in patients with bone metastases from advanced cancer.[34,66–71] However, this benefit does not translate into improvement in survival. Although superior in preventing SRE, denosumab may not be a cost-effective alternative to zoledronic acid, particularly in prostate cancer.[52,72,73]

Denosumab can be used in patients with renal impairment; it does not need dose adjustment and can be given SC. However, its long-term efficacy and safety are unknown.

Undesirable effects
Very common (> 10%): dyspnoea, diarrhoea.
Common (< 10%, > 1%): hypocalcaemia, hypophosphataemia, hyperhidrosis, osteonecrosis of jaw, tooth extraction.
Uncommon (< 1%, > 0.1%): cellulitis, drug hypersensitivity.
The incidence of osteonecrosis of jaw is comparable with zoledronic acid; hypocalcaemia is more common with denosumab.

Dose and use
- *for prevention of SRE in patients with bone metastases form solid cancers*: 120mg administered as a single SC injection once every 4 weeks into the thigh, abdomen or upper arm (XGEVA®)
- *for treatment of postmenopausal osteoporosis in women at increased risk of fracture, and bone loss in men with prostate cancer receiving androgen deprivation therapy*: 60mg SC into thigh or upper arm once every 6 months (Prolia®).
The manufacturer recommends daily supplementation with ⩾500mg calcium and 400 IU Vitamin D unless the patient is hypercalcaemic.

Table 3 Dose reduction for zoledronic acid in patients with cancer involving the bones and mild–moderate renal impairment[a,b,c]

Baseline creatinine clearance (mL/min)	Recommended dose (mg)
> 60	4 (i.e. no reduction)
50–60	3.5
40–49	3.3
30–39	3

a. manufacturer's recommendations for patients with multiple myeloma or bone metastases
b. no data exist for severe renal impairment (creatinine clearance < 30mL/min) because these patients were excluded from the studies
c. reduced doses are diluted in 100mL 0.9% saline or 5% glucose and given IVI over 15min; see SPC for preparation details.

For **zoledronic acid** and **pamidronate disodium**:
- measure plasma creatinine before each dose; withhold treatment if creatinine increases by:
  ▷ ⩾44micromol/L in patients with a normal baseline creatinine concentration (i.e. < 124micromol/L), *or*
  ▷ ⩾88micromol/L in patients with a raised baseline creatinine concentration (i.e. > 124micromol/L)
- treatment may be resumed at the same dose as before when plasma creatinine returns to within 10% of the baseline value
- discontinue treatment permanently if plasma creatinine fails to improve after 4–8 weeks.

Metastatic bone pain

Several regimens have been recommended for when more conventional methods have been exhausted.

For **zoledronic acid**, see Prophylactic use to reduce the incidence of SRE (above).

For **pamidronate disodium**:
- **pamidronate disodium** 90mg IVI (50% of patients respond, generally within 1–2 weeks); if helpful repeat 60–90mg every 3–4 weeks for as long as benefit is maintained[3]
- **pamidronate disodium** 120mg IVI, repeated p.r.n. every 2–4 months[37]
- **pamidronate disodium** 90–120mg IVI or **sodium clodronate** 600–1,500mg IVI (not UK), repeated p.r.n. In patients not responding to a first treatment, a second can be tried but, if still no response, discontinue.[38]

Supply

Pamidronate disodium (generic)
Injection (concentrate for dilution and use as an infusion) 3mg/mL, 5mL and 10mL vial = £13 and £27 respectively; 6mg/mL, 10mL vial = £53; 9mg/mL, 10mL vial = £80; 15mg/mL, 1mL, 2mL, 4mL and 6mL vial = £30, £60, £119 and £170 respectively.

Aredia Dry Powder® (Novartis)
Injection (powder for reconstitution) 15mg vial = £30; 30mg vial = £60; 90mg vial = £170; *supplied with diluent for reconstitution.*

Zoledronic acid (generic)
Injection (concentrate for dilution and use as an infusion) 4mg/5mL, 5mL vial = £9.
Infusion 4mg/100mL, 100mL vial = £15.

Zometa® (Novartis)
Injection (concentrate for dilution and use as an infusion) 4mg/5mL, 5mL vial = £174.
Infusion 4mg/100mL, 100mL vial = £174.

Note: zoledronic acid 50microgram/mL, 100mL (Aclasta®) given IVI over 15min is authorized for the treatment of Paget's disease and as an annual dose for osteoporosis in women (postmenopausal) or men.

Ibandronic acid (generic)
Tablets 50mg, 28 days @ 50mg once daily = £12.

Bondronat® (Roche)
Tablets 50mg, 28 days @ 50mg once daily = £184.
Injection (concentrate for dilution and use as an infusion) 1mg/mL, 2mL vial = £89; 6mL vial = £184.

Note: ibandronic acid 150mg tablets and 1mg/mL, 3mL pre-filled syringe (Bonviva®) given once a month and every 3 months respectively are authorized for the treatment of postmenopausal osteoporosis.

Denosumab
Xgeva® (Amgen)
Injection 70mg/mL, 120mg vial = £310.

Note: denosumab 60mg/mL, 1mL pre-filled syringe (Prolia®) given SC every 6 months is authorized for the treatment of postmenopausal osteoporosis in women and treatment of bone loss in men with prostate cancer receiving androgen deprivation therapy.

1   Fleisch H (1998) Bisphosphonates: mechanisms of action. *Endocrine Reviews.* **19**: 80–100.
2   Russell R et al. (1999) Bisphosphonates: pharmacology, mechanisms of action and clinical uses. *Osteoporosis International.* **9** (Suppl 2): s66–s80.
3   Crosby V et al. (1998) A randomized controlled trial of intravenous clodronate. *Journal of Pain and Symptom Management.* **15**: 266–268.
4   Harada H et al. (2004) Effects of bisphosphonates on joint damage and bone loss in rat adjuvant-induced arthritis. *Inflammation Research.* **53**: 45–52.
5   Mantyh PW (2006) Cancer pain and its impact on diagnosis, survival and quality of life. *Nature Reviews Neuroscience.* **7**: 797–809.

6   Neville-Webbe H et al. (2002) The anti-tumour activity of bisphosphonates. Cancer Treatment Reviews. **28**: 305–319.
7   Green JR (2004) Bisphosphonates: preclinical review. Oncologist. **9 (Suppl 4)**: 3–13.
8   Sevcik MA et al. (2004) Bone cancer pain: the effects of the bisphosphonate alendronate on pain, skeletal remodeling, tumor growth and tumor necrosis. Pain. **111**: 169–180.
9   Rogers MJ et al. (2000) Cellular and molecular mechanisms of action of bisphosphonates. Cancer. **88 (Suppl 12)**: 2961–2978.
10 Barrett J et al. (2004) Ibandronate: a clinical pharmacological and pharmacokinetic update. Journal of Clinical Pharmacology. **44**: 951–965.
11 Saunders Y et al. (2004) Systematic review of bisphosphonates for hypercalcaemia of malignancy. Palliative Medicine. **18**: 418–431.
12 Purohit O et al. (1995) A randomised, double-blind comparison of intravenous pamidronate and clodronate in hypercalcaemia of malignancy. British Journal of Cancer. **72**: 1289–1293.
13 Major P et al. (2001) Zoledronic acid is superior to pamidronate in the treatment of hypercalcaemia of malignancy: a pooled analysis of two randomized, controlled clinical trials. Journal of Clinical Oncology. **19**: 558–567.
14 Ralston SH et al. (1997) Dose-response study of ibandronate in the treatment of cancer-associated hypercalcaemia. British Journal of Cancer. **75**: 295–300.
15 Wong R and Wiffen PJ (2002) Bisphosphonates for the relief of pain secondary to bone metastases. Cochrane Database Systematic Reviews. **2**: CD002068.
16 Ross JR et al. (2003) Systematic review of role of bisphosphonates on skeletal morbidity in metastatic cancer. British Medical Journal. **327**: 469.
17 Body JJ et al. (2004) Oral ibandronate improves bone pain and preserves quality of life in patients with skeletal metastases due to breast cancer. Pain. **111**: 306–312.
18 Body JJ et al. (2004) Oral ibandronate reduces the risk of skeletal complications in breast cancer patients with metastatic bone disease: results from two randomised, placebo-controlled phase III studies. British Journal of Cancer. **90**: 1133–1137.
19 Yuen KK et al. (2006) Bisphosphonates for advanced prostate cancer. Cochrane Database Systematic Reviews. CD006250.
20 Wong MH et al. (2012) Bisphosphonates and other bone agents for breast cancer. Cochrane Database of Systematic Reviews. **2**: CD003474.
21 Warr D et al. (2004) Use of biphosphonates in women with breast cancer. Practice guideline report #1-11. In: Cancer Care Ontario program in evidence-based care. Available from: www.cancercare.on.ca/common/pages/UserFile.aspx?fileId = 34182
22 SIGN (Scottish Intercollegiate Guidelines Network) (2005) Management of breast cancer in women. A national clinical guideline. (No. 84). SIGN publication, Edinburgh (Scotland).
23 NICE (2009) Advanced breast cancer: diagnosis and treatment. Clinical Guideline. CG81. www.nice.org.uk
24 Imrie K et al. (2007) The role of biphosphonates in the management of skeletal complications for patients with multiple myeloma: a clinical practice guideline. In: Cancer Care Ontario program in evidence-based care. Available from: www.cancercare.on.ca/common/pages/UserFile.aspx?fileId=14146
25 Bird JM et al. (2014) Guidelines for the Diagnosis and Management of Multiple Myeloma. British society for Standards in Haematology Guidelines. www.bcshguidelines.com
26 British Association of Urological Surgeons (2005) Systemic management of metastatic bone disease. In: Guidelines on the management and treatment of metastatic prostate cancer, UK.
27 Berry S et al. (2005) The use of biphosphonates in men with hormone-refractory prostate cancer. Practice guideline report #3-14. In: Cancer Care Ontario program in evidence-based care. Available from: www.cancercare.on.ca/common/pages/userFile.aspx?fileId=14032
28 NICE (2014) Prostate cancer: diagnosis and treatment. Clinical Guideline. CG157. www.nice.org.uk
29 Body JJ (2006) Bisphosphonates for malignancy-related bone disease: current status, future developments. Supportive Care in Cancer. **14**: 408–418.
30 Costa L et al. (2011) Anticancer evidence for zoledronic acid across the cancer continuum. Critical Reviews in Oncology Hematology. **77 (Suppl 1)**: S31–37.
31 Henk H et al. (2012) Evaluation of the clinical benefit of long-term (beyond 2 years) treatment of skeletal-related events in advanced cancers with zoledronic acid. Current Medical Research Opinion. **28**: 1119–1127.
32 Henk HJ et al. (2012) Retrospective evaluation of the clinical benefit of long-term continuous use of zoledronic acid in patients with lung cancer and bone metastases. Journal of Medical Economics. **15**: 195–204.
33 Henk HJ and Kaura S (2012) Retrospective database analysis of the effect of zoledronic acid on skeletal-related events and mortality in women with breast cancer and bone metastasis in a managed care plan. Journal of Medical Economics. **15**: 175–184.
34 Stopeck AT et al. (2010) Denosumab compared with zoledronic acid for the treatment of bone metastases in patients with advanced breast cancer: a randomized, double-blind study. Journal of Clinical Oncology. **28**: 5132–5139.
35 Vorreuther R (1993) Biphosphonates as an adjunct to palliative therapy of bone metastases from prostatic carcinoma. A pilot study on clodronate. British Journal of Urology. **72**: 792–795.
36 O'Rourke N et al. (1995) Double-blind, placebo-controlled, dose response trial of oral clodronate in patients with bone metastases. Journal of Clinical Oncology. **13**: 929–934.
37 Vinholes J et al. (1996) Metabolic effects of pamidronate in patients with metastatic bone disease. British Journal of Cancer. **73**: 1089–1095.
38 Mannix K et al. (2000) Using bisphosphonates to control the pain of bone metastases: evidence-based guidelines for palliative care. Palliative Medicine. **14**: 455–461.
39 Eastell R (2007) Breast cancer and the risk of osteoporotic fracture: a paradox. Journal of Clinical Endocrinology and Metaboloism. **92**: 42–43.
40 Greenspan SL et al. (2007) Prevention of bone loss in survivors of breast cancer: a randomized, double-blind, placebo-controlled clinical trial. Journal of Clinical Endocrinology and Metabolism. **92**: 131–136.
41 Smith MR (2003) Bisphosphonates to prevent osteoporosis in men receiving androgen deprivation therapy for prostate cancer. Drugs Aging. **20**: 175–183.
42 Broadbent A et al. (2005) Bisphosphonate-induced hypocalcemia associated with vitamin D deficiency in a patient with advanced cancer. American Journal of Hospice and Palliative Care. **22**: 382–384.
43 Johnson M and Fallon M (1998) Symptomatic hypocalcaemia with oral clodronate. Journal of Pain and Symptom Management. **15**: 140–142.
44 MHRA (2011) Bisphosphonates: atypical femoral fractures. Drug Safety Update. **(4)** 11: www.mhra.gov.uk/Safetyinformation

45 Tanvetyanon T and Stiff PJ (2006) Management of the adverse effects associated with intravenous bisphosphonates. *Annals of Oncology.* **17**: 897–907.

46 Markowitz GS et al. (2001) Collapsing focal segmental glomerulosclerosis following treatment with high-dose pamidronate. *Journal of the American Society of Nephrology.* **12**: 1164–1172.

47 Rosen LS et al. (2001) Zoledronic acid versus pamidronate in the treatment of skeletal metastases in patients with breast cancer or osteolytic lesions of multiple myeloma: a phase III, double-blind, comparative trial. *Cancer Journal.* **7**: 377–387.

48 Rosen LS et al. (2004) Zoledronic acid is superior to pamidronate for the treatment of bone metastases in breast carcinoma patients with at least one osteolytic lesion. *Cancer.* **100**: 36–43.

49 Markowitz GS et al. (2003) Toxic acute tubular necrosis following treatment with zoledronate (Zometa). *Kidney International.* **64**: 281–289.

50 Chang JT et al. (2003) Renal failure with the use of zoledronic acid. *New England Journal of Medicine.* **349**: 1676–1679.

51 Diel I et al. (2003) Renal safety of oral and intravenous ibandronate in metastatic bone disease: phase III clinical trial results. In: *15th Annual MASCC Meeting*; Berlin, 18–21 June.

52 West H (2011) Denosumab for prevention of skeletal-related events in patients with bone metastases from solid tumors: incremental benefit, debatable value. *Journal of Clinical Oncology.* **29**: 1095–1098.

53 FDA (2004) Drug Safety Revisions: Food and Drugs Administration Update. *P&T.* **29**: 733.

54 Ruggiero SL et al. (2004) Osteonecrosis of the jaws associated with the use of bisphosphonates: a review of 63 cases. *Journal of Oral and Maxillofacial Surgery.* **62**: 527–534.

55 MHRA (2006) Osteonecrosis of the jaw with bisphosphonates. In: *Current problems in pharmacovigilance*. Commission on Human Medicines. Available from: www.mhra.gov.uk/Publications/Safetyguidance/CurrentProblemsinPharmacovigilance/CON2023859

56 Woo SB et al. (2006) Narrative review: bisphosphonates and osteonecrosis of the jaws. *Annals of Internal Medicine.* **144**: 753–761.

57 Fraunfelder FW and Fraunfelder FT (2003) Bisphosphonates and ocular inflammation. *N Engl J Med.* **348**: 1187–1188.

58 Australian Adverse Drug Reactions Bulletin (2004) Bisphosphonates and ocular inflammation. www.tga.gov.au

59 FDA (2008) Bisphosphonates (marketed as Actonel, Actonel+Ca, Aredia, Boniva, Didronel, Fosamax, Fosamax+D, Reclast, Skelid, and Zometa). Information for healthcare professionals. *Postmarket drug safety information for patients and providers.* www.fda.gov/Drugs/DrugSafety (posted 1 July 2008).

60 Roemer-Becuwe C et al. (2003) Safety of subcutaneous clodronate and efficacy in hypercalcemia of malignancy: a novel route of administration. *Journal of Pain and Symptom Management.* **26**: 843–848.

61 Duncan AR (2003) The use of subcutaneous pamidronate. *Journal of Pain and Symptom Management.* **26**: 592–593.

62 NICE (2010) Denosumab for the prevention of osteoporotic fractures in postmenopausal women. *Technology appraisal guidance*: TA204. www.nice.org.uk

63 NICE (2012) Technology appraisal guidance 265. Denosumab for the prevention of skeletal-related events in adults with bone metastases from solid tumours.

64 Henry D et al. (2014) Delaying skeletal-related events in a randomized phase 3 study of denosumab versus zoledronic acid in patients with advanced cancer: an analysis of data from patients with solid tumors. *Supportive Care in Cancer.* **22**: 679–687.

65 Vadhan-Raj S et al. (2012) Clinical benefit in patients with metastatic bone disease: results of a phase 3 study of denosumab versus zoledronic acid. *Annals of Oncology.* **23**: 3045–3051.

66 Fizazi K et al. (2011) Denosumab versus zoledronic acid for treatment of bone metastases in men with castration-resistant prostate cancer: a randomised, double-blind study. *Lancet.* **377**: 813–822.

67 Henry DH et al. (2011) Randomized, double-blind study of denosumab versus zoledronic acid in the treatment of bone metastases in patients with advanced cancer (excluding breast and prostate cancer) or multiple myeloma. *Journal of Clinical Oncology.* **29**: 1125–1132.

68 Lipton A et al. (2012) Superiority of denosumab to zoledronic acid for prevention of skeletal-related events: a combined analysis of 3 pivotal, randomised, phase 3 trials. *European Journal of Cancer.* **48**: 3082–3092.

69 Sun L and Yu S (2013) Efficacy and safety of denosumab versus zoledronic acid in patients with bone metastases: a systematic review and meta-analysis. *American Journal of Clinical Oncology.* **36**: 399–403.

70 Peddi P et al. (2013) Denosumab in patients with cancer and skeletal metastases: a systematic review and meta-analysis. *Cancer Treatment Reviews.* **39**: 97–104.

71 Martin M et al. (2012) Bone-related complications and quality of life in advanced breast cancer: results from a randomized phase III trial of denosumab versus zoledronic acid. *Clinical Cancer Research.* **18**: 4841–4849.

72 Xie J et al. (2012) Cost-effectiveness of denosumab compared with zoledronic acid in patients with breast cancer and bone metastases. *Clinical Breast Cancer.* **12**: 247–258.

73 Snedecor SJ et al. (2013) Denosumab versus zoledronic acid for treatment of bone metastases in men with castration-resistant prostate cancer: a cost-effectiveness analysis. *Journal of Medical Economics.* **16**: 19–29.

Updated June 2014

SYSTEMIC CORTICOSTEROIDS   BNF 6.3.2

Indications: Suppression of inflammatory and allergic disorders, cerebral oedema, nausea and vomiting with chemotherapy; †see Box A.

Contra-indications: Systemic infection, unless considered to be life-saving and specific anti-infective therapy is employed.

Box A   Off-label indications for systemic corticosteroids in advanced cancer[1,2]

This list of off-label uses does not claim to be totally comprehensive. Further, inclusion does not mean that a systemic corticosteroid is necessarily the treatment of choice. Further, the evidence-base for some indications is only 'expert opinion'.

Specific
Spinal cord compression[3]
Nerve compression
Breathlessness
  pneumonitis (after radiotherapy)
  lymphangitic carcinomatosis
  tracheal compression/stridor
Superior vena caval obstruction[4]
Obstruction of hollow viscus
  bronchus[5]
  ureter
  GI[6,7]
Radiation-induced inflammation
Discharge from rectal tumour (can give either PO or PR)
Paraneoplastic fever
Nausea and vomiting in cancer resistant to standard measures (see p.241)
Hypercalcaemia associated with cancer (an adjunct to SC calcitonin)[8,9]

Pain relief
Pain caused by a tumour in a confined organ or body cavity, e.g. raised intracranial pressure, bone pain

Anticancer hormone therapy
Breast cancer[10]
Prostate cancer[11]
Haematological malignancies
Lymphoproliferative disorders

General ('tonic')
To improve appetite
To enhance sense of wellbeing

Pharmacology

The adrenal cortex secretes **hydrocortisone** (cortisol) which has glucocorticoid activity and weak mineralocorticoid activity.[12] It also secretes aldosterone which has mineralocorticoid activity. Thus, in deficiency states, physiological replacement is best achieved with a combination of **hydrocortisone** and **fludrocortisone**, a mineralocorticoid.

In many disease states, corticosteroids are used primarily as potent anti-inflammatory agents. The anti-inflammatory action is mediated via several interacting mechanisms,[12] in contrast to the more specific impact of NSAIDs on prostaglandin synthesis (see p.308). Thus, as anti-inflammatory agents, corticosteroids are potentially more effective than NSAIDs. However, certainly when used long-term, corticosteroids are likely to cause more numerous and more serious undesirable effects (see below).

When comparing the relative anti-inflammatory (glucocorticoid) potencies of corticosteroids, their water-retaining properties (mineralocorticoid effect) should also be borne in mind (Table 1). Thus, **hydrocortisone** is not used for long-term disease suppression because large doses would be required and these would cause troublesome fluid retention. On the other hand, the moderate anti-inflammatory effect of **hydrocortisone** makes it a useful corticosteroid for topical use in inflammatory skin conditions; both topical and systemic undesirable effects are minimal.

Prednisolone is the most frequently used corticosteroid for disease suppression. **Dexamethasone**, with high glucocorticoid activity but insignificant mineralocorticoid effect, is particularly suitable for high-dose anti-inflammatory therapy. It is 6–12 times more potent than **prednisolone**, i.e. 2mg of **dexamethasone** is approximately equivalent to 15–25mg of **prednisolone** (Box B) and it has a long duration of action (Table 1). Some corticosteroid esters, e.g. of **betamethasone** and of **beclometasone**, exert a marked topical effect; use is made of this property with skin applications and bronchial inhalations (see p.611 and p.125).

General 'tonic' use

The non-specific 'tonic' use of corticosteroids is based on the known general effects of this group of drugs. In patients with advanced cancer, treatment with corticosteroids may result in increased appetite, reduced nausea and improved well-being. In a recent qualitative study, patients initially

---

reported distressing symptoms, physical deterioration, decreased autonomy, and a feeling of apprehension and foreboding. After treatment for one week with **betamethasone** 4mg once daily, most patients had improved symptom relief, and reported enhanced physical abilities, increased autonomy, and renewed hope.[13]

RCTs of corticosteroids specifically as appetite stimulants have used daily doses of **prednisolone** 15–40mg (or equivalent).[14–16] All showed benefit compared with placebo. In one, benefit was comparable for daily doses of **dexamethasone** of either 3mg or 6mg (equivalent to **prednisolone** 20mg or 40mg). Overall, over 50% of the patients reported benefit, which was still apparent after 4 weeks.[14,15,17]

However, both corticosteroids and progestogens (see p.536) should not be regarded as 'anticachexia' agents. Any weight gain relates to fluid retention ± increased fat, rather than to increased skeletal muscle mass. This could make mobilizing more difficult in an already debilitated patient. In addition, the catabolic effect of corticosteroids on skeletal muscle, exacerbated by reduced levels of physical activity, may well further weaken the patient, rendering corticosteroids suitable for short-term use only.

Nausea and vomiting
Dexamethasone is an integral part of standard management of severe chemotherapeutic vomiting.[18] The anti-emetic effect is possibly mediated by a corticosteroid-induced reduction in the permeability of the chemoreceptor trigger zone and of the blood–brain barrier to emetogenic substances, and a reduction in the neuronal content of gamma-aminobutyric acid (GABA) in the brain stem.

In palliative care, **dexamethasone** is often used when all else fails as an 'add-on' anti-emetic (see p.241). However, there is some evidence that **dexamethasone** does not add to the anti-emetic efficacy of **metoclopramide** or phenothiazines in patients with advanced cancer.[19–21]

Obstructive syndromes
In obstructive syndromes (Box A), corticosteroids may help by reducing inflammation at the site of the obstruction, thereby increasing the lumen of the obstructed hollow viscus. Corticosteroids (**dexamethasone** equivalent 6–16mg/24h) may improve bowel obstruction but do not affect survival. The incidence of undesirable events is low.[6] High-dose corticosteroids (**dexamethasone** equivalent 20–40mg/24h) relieved stridor within 12h in 3 patients with upper airway obstruction from infiltrating tumour.[5]

Brain metastases
Dexamethasone is recommended for treatment of adults with symptomatic brain metastases; no benefit is seen in patients with asymptomatic brain metastases. **Dexamethasone** 4–8mg/24h provides temporary symptomatic relief for patients with mild symptoms related to raised intracranial pressure from cerebral oedema. If patients have severe symptoms or are at risk of herniation, doses of ≥16mg/24h are recommended. Symptom relief from **dexamethasone** reduces over time and undesirable effects increase. Thus, ideally, the dose of **dexamethasone** should be reduced after one week and discontinued after 2–4 weeks.[22] However, unless patients receive additional treatment (e.g. palliative radiotherapy), they will experience a recurrence of their symptoms at some point as the dose of **dexamethasone** is decreased. Thus, it may be necessary to taper more slowly or continue 'maintenance' **dexamethasone** indefinitely in some patients.

Whole brain radiotherapy may cause nausea, vomiting, headache, fever and a transient worsening of neurological symptoms. **Dexamethasone** should be continued for one week after treatment and then tapered over 2–4 weeks.[23,24]

Spinal cord compression
Spinal cord compression must be treated as an emergency; patients with paraparesis do better than those who are totally paraplegic.[3,25–27] Because corticosteroids inhibit inflammation, stabilize vascular membranes, and reduce spinal cord oedema, their use in spinal cord compression often results in a dramatic reduction in pain,[28] and an early improvement in the patient's physical status.

Traditionally, **dexamethasone** has been used as the corticosteroid of choice, sometimes initially given IV. However, given its high PO bio-availability (see Table 1), IV administration seems unnecessary. A typical PO regimen would be:
- a stat dose of 16mg PO
- continue with 16mg PO each morning for a further 3–4 days
- maintain on 8mg PO each morning until the completion of radiotherapy
- taper (and discontinue) over 2 weeks after the completion of radiotherapy.[29]

If there is neurological deterioration during the dose reduction, the dose should be increased again to the previous satisfactory dose, and maintained at that level for a further 2 weeks before attempting to taper the dose again. About 1/4 require maintenance **dexamethasone** in order to preserve neural function.

Very high initial doses of **dexamethasone** (96–100mg stat and once daily for 3 days, then tapering to zero over 2 weeks) are not justified. They provide little or no more benefit than 16mg,[30] but are associated with a definite risk of a major adverse event (> 10%), particularly acute GI perforation (3%, at any level from the stomach to the sigmoid colon), GI haemorrhage, and sepsis, and possibly even death.[31–33]

For pharmacokinetic details, see Table 1.

Box B   Approximate equivalent anti-inflammatory doses of corticosteroids[a]

Cortisone acetate	25mg
Hydrocortisone	20mg
Prednisone	5mg
Prednisolone	5mg
Methylprednisolone	4mg
Triamcinolone	4mg
Betamethasone	750microgram
Dexamethasone	750microgram

a. this list takes no account of either mineralocorticoid effects or variations in duration of action.

Cautions

Diabetes mellitus, psychotic illness. Although there is only a small increased risk of peptic ulceration with corticosteroids alone,[36] when given concurrently with NSAIDs, the risk is increased up to 15 times.[37,38]

Prolonged courses of corticosteroids increase susceptibility to infections and their severity. Clinical presentation may be atypical; the signs of infection (including peritonitis) may be masked. Serious infections (e.g. septicaemia and tuberculosis) may reach an advanced stage before diagnosis. Live vaccines should not be given; the antibody response to other vaccines may be diminished.

In patients who have taken >10mg **prednisolone** (or equivalent) daily for 3 weeks, the occurrence of any significant intercurrent illness, trauma or surgical procedure necessitates a temporary increase in corticosteroid dose (or, if stopped within the past 3 months, a temporary re-introduction) to compensate for a reduced adrenocortical response caused by the corticosteroid treatment.[39]

Drug interactions

Corticosteroids antagonize oral hypoglycaemics and **insulin** (glucocorticoid effect), antihypertensives and diuretics (mineralocorticoid effect). Increased risk of hypokalaemia if high doses of corticosteroids are prescribed with β_2 agonists (e.g. **salbutamol, terbutaline**).

The metabolism of corticosteroids is accelerated by anti-epileptics (**carbamazepine, phenobarbital, phenytoin, primidone**), and rifamycins (**rifabutin, rifampicin**). This is more pronounced with long-acting glucocorticoids; thus **phenytoin** may reduce the bioavailability of **dexamethasone** to 25–50%, and larger doses (double or more) will be needed when prescribed concurrently.[40] **Dexamethasone** itself can affect plasma **phenytoin** concentrations (may either rise or fall).

Concurrent prescription of a corticosteroid increases the INR in patients already taking **warfarin**, necessitating a dose reduction in about 50% of patients.[41] Thus, the INR should be checked weekly for 2–3 weeks when a corticosteroid is started or dose altered.

Table 1 Selected pharmacokinetic details of commonly used corticosteroids[34,35]

Drug	Anti-inflammatory potency	Approximate equivalent dose (mg)	Sodium-retaining potency	Oral bio-availability (%)	Onset of action	Peak plasma concentration	Plasma halflife (h)	Duration of action (h)	Relative affinity for lung tissue	Daily dose (mg) above which adrenal suppression possible	
										Male	Female
Hydrocortisone	1	20	1	96	No data	1h PO	1.5	8–12	1	20–30	15–25
Prednisone[a] / Prednisolone	4	5	0.25	75–85	No data	1h PO	3.5	12–36	1.6	7.5–10	7.5
Dexamethasone / Betamethasone	25–50[b]	0.5–1	<0.01	78 / 98	8–24h IM[c] / No data	1–2h PO / 10–36min IV	4.5 / 6.5	36–54 / 24–48	1	1–1.15	1

a. biologically inert prednisone is converted by the liver to prednisolone
b. thymic involution assay
c. acute allergic reactions.

Undesirable effects

See Box C–Box F.

Box C   Undesirable effects of corticosteroids[38]

Glucocorticoid effects

Avascular bone necrosis

Cataract (prednisolone 15mg/24h or
equivalent for several years = 75% risk;
also seen with long-term inhaled
steroids)[42]

Diabetes mellitus or deterioration of
glycaemic control in known diabetics
(see p.524)

Infection (increased susceptibility):
candidosis (debatable, see p.465)
septicaemia (may delay recognition)
tuberculosis (may delay recognition)
chickenpox[a] measles (increased severity)

Mental disturbances (Box D)

Muscle wasting and weakness (Box E)

Osteoporosis

Peptic ulceration (if given with an NSAID)[34]

Suppression of growth (in child)

Mineralocorticoid effects

Sodium and water retention
→ oedema

Potassium loss

Hypertension

Cushingoid features

Lipodystrophy after ⩾8 weeks of treatment
in 30–70% of patients (reversible on
stopping treatment):
moon face
buffalo hump
increased abdominal fat
reduced subcutaneous fat in limbs

Acne

Bruising

Hirsuitism

Striae

---

a. if exposed to infection, non-immune patients should be given varicella-zoster immunoglobulin (see BNF section 6.3.2).

Box D   Corticosteroid-induced psychiatric disturbances[44–47]

Incidence

Reports range from 13–62% of those prescribed a corticosteroid.
Prevalence is higher in women, and more likely with higher doses.

Clinical manifestations

Symptoms generally occur 4–6 days after starting a corticosteroid, but this is highly variable
and can occur even after cessation of treatment.

Manifestations are mostly mild or moderate, but can be severe, and include:
• depression (40%)
• mania (25%)
• paranoid ('steroid') psychosis (15%)
• delirium (10%)
• bipolar disorder (5%).[45]
Educating patients about the possible risk of undesirable psychiatric effects may improve the
reporting of symptoms.

Management

Reduce or discontinue the causal corticosteroid if possible.[44]
Environmental conditions should be optimized to minimize agitation.[48]
Symptoms may take 1–2 weeks to resolve.[46]
If the corticosteroid cannot be stopped, or symptoms are intolerable, atypical antipsychotics
should be prescribed for patients with psychosis, aggression or agitation.

continued

Box D   Continued

Although antidepressants may exacerbate agitation and psychosis, they are generally helpful in depressed patients who require long-term corticosteroids.

All patients with corticosteroid-induced psychiatric disturbance should be evaluated for suicidal ideation.

Prognosis
A history of:
- psychiatric disease does not make a corticosteroid-induced psychiatric disturbance more likely
- previous corticosteroid-induced disturbance does not necessarily mean that a second disturbance will occur if corticosteroids are represcribed.[47]

Box E   Systemic corticosteroid myopathy[49,50]

Glucocorticoids cause atrophy of limb and respiratory muscles. It is a dose-related effect which generally manifests only after $\geqslant 2$ months of treatment with dexamethasone > 4mg/24h or prednisolone > 40mg/24h. Can occur earlier and with lower doses.

If the chronological sequence fits with corticosteroid myopathy, a presumptive diagnosis should be made and the following steps taken:
- explanation to patient and family
- discuss need to compromise between maximizing therapeutic benefit and minimizing undesirable effects
- halve corticosteroid dose (generally possible as a single step)
- consider changing from dexamethasone to prednisolone (non-fluorinated corticosteroids cause less myopathy)
- attempt further reductions in dose at intervals of 1–2 weeks
- arrange for physiotherapy (disuse exacerbates myopathy)
- emphasize that weakness should improve after 3–4 weeks (provided cancer-induced weakness does not supervene).

Box F   Pseudorheumatism

Patients receiving corticosteroids for rheumatoid arthritis occasionally develop myalgia, arthralgia, malaise, rhinitis, conjunctivitis, painful itchy skin nodules, weight loss and pyrexia; so-called steroid pseudorheumatism.[51]

It is sometimes also seen in cancer patients receiving large doses of corticosteroids or when a very high dose is reduced rapidly to a lower dose. Most likely to be affected are those:
- receiving 100mg of prednisolone/24h for several days in association with chemotherapy
- with spinal cord compression given dexamethasone 96mg IV/24h for 3 days[52] (followed by a rapidly reducing oral dose)[a]
- on high doses of dexamethasone to reduce raised intracranial pressure associated with brain metastases
- reducing to an ordinary maintenance dose after a prolonged course.

a. such a high dose is unnecessary; 10mg IV is as effective as 96mg.[30,53]

Dose and use

Given the many and significant undesirable effects of corticosteroids, and the potentially deleterious effect of rapid withdrawal, corticosteroids should be prescribed cautiously:
- for defined symptoms potentially responsive to corticosteroid therapy
- always bearing in mind potential benefit vs. risk
- at a low–moderate dose, titrated to clinical effect
- for a time-limited trial
- discontinued if no clinical/symptomatic benefit seen *or*
- weaned to the lowest effective dose.[54]

If expected to take corticosteroids for ⩾3 weeks, patients should be given a *Steroid Treatment* card (Box G).

Box G Example of a *Steroid Treatment* card

I am a patient on STEROID treatment which must not be stopped suddenly.

- If you have been taking this medicine for more than 3 weeks, the dose should be reduced gradually when you stop taking steroids unless your doctor says otherwise.
- Read the patient information leaflet given with the medicine.
- Always carry this card with you and show it to anyone who treats you (for example a doctor, nurse, pharmacist, or dentist).
- For 1 year after you stop the treatment, you must mention that you have taken steroids.
- If you become ill, or if you come into contact with anyone who has an infectious disease, consult your doctor promptly.
- If you have never had chickenpox, you should avoid close contact with people who have chickenpox or shingles. If you do come into contact with chickenpox, see your doctor urgently.
- Make sure that the information on the card about your current dose is kept up to date.

Except for **hydrocortisone**, corticosteroids can be given in a single daily dose each morning. However, when 'tablet burden' is an issue, higher doses of **dexamethasone** (i.e. >8mg) can be halved and administered as a morning and a lunchtime dose. Giving doses later in the day should generally be avoided, as this increases the risk of corticosteroid-induced insomnia. Nonetheless, even with morning doses, **temazepam** or **diazepam** at bedtime is sometimes needed to counter insomnia or agitation.

The initial dose varies according to indication. The list below gives typical starting doses; all are PO unless otherwise stated. **Dexamethasone** has a PO bio-availability of about 80%; and, when necessary, many centres convert to SC/IV dexamethasone on a 1:1 basis (i.e. use the same dose for either route). For more information about dose adjustment and duration of treatment, see the relevant sections in Pharmacology above.

CSCI compatibility of dexamethasone with other drugs: Because it is an alkaline drug, therapeutic doses of **dexamethasone** often cause compatibility problems. To minimize the risk of precipitation, it should always be the last drug added to an already dilute combination of drugs. However, because **dexamethasone** has a long duration of action, it can generally be given as a bolus SC injection once daily (see Chapter 20, p.697).

Note: to reduce CSCI site reactions, **dexamethasone** 1mg is sometimes added to other drugs, when compatibility data permits (see Chapter 20, p.704).

Replacement therapy
- **hydrocortisone** 20mg each morning, 10mg each evening with **fludrocortisone** 100–300microgram each morning.

Anti-emetic
- e.g. **dexamethasone** 8–20mg each morning (see Pharmacology section above; also Quick Prescribing Guide: Management of nausea and vomiting, p.241).[55–57]

Anorexia
- **dexamethasone** 2–6mg or **prednisolone** 15–40mg each morning.[14–17]

Raised intracranial pressure
- **dexamethasone** 8–16mg each morning.[58,59]

Obstruction of hollow viscus
- **dexamethasone** 6–16mg each morning.[6]

Spinal cord compression:
- **dexamethasone** 16mg each morning.[30]

Discharge from rectal tumour or acute post-radiation proctitis
- retention enema of **hydrocortisoneacetate** 125mg PR or **prednisolone** 20mg PR every 1–2 days. If local application is impractical, PO corticosteroids can be used instead.

For use in management of anaphylaxis, see p.787.
For use CSCI, see p.697.
For inhaled corticosteroids, see p.125.
For depot corticosteroid injections, see p.583.
For topical corticosteroids, see p.611.

Stopping corticosteroids

If after 7–10 days the corticosteroid fails to achieve the desired effect, it should be stopped. It is often possible to stop corticosteroids abruptly (Box H).[60]

However, if there is uncertainty about disease or symptom resolution, withdrawal should be guided by monitoring disease activity or the symptom.

Particularly if it has been taken for >3 weeks, rapid withdrawal of a corticosteroid may result in a corticosteroid withdrawal syndrome. This may cause an array of symptoms and signs similar to those of pseudorheumatism (Box F) together with adrenal insufficiency. The syndrome is treated by restarting the corticosteroid or increasing the dose to that given before the onset of withdrawal symptoms.[61]

In patients who are moribund and no longer able to swallow tablets, it is generally acceptable to discontinue corticosteroids abruptly,[54] although sometimes a maintenance dose may be indicated to prevent distress from symptomatic hypo-adrenalism.

Occasionally, a patient with a brain tumour or multiple brain metastases requests that **dexamethasone** is stopped because, despite its continued use, there is progressive physical deterioration and/or cognitive impairment. In this circumstance, it is often best to reduce the **dexamethasone** step by step on a daily basis. This gives the patient time to reconsider. Extra analgesics should be prescribed in case headache develops as the intracranial pressure increases:
- if already taking **paracetamol**, prescribe a weak opioid or a weak opioid-**paracetamol** combination p.r.n.
- if already taking a weak opioid, prescribe **morphine** 10–20mg PO or **morphine** 5–10mg SC p.r.n.
- if >2 p.r.n. doses have been given in the last 24h, increase the regular analgesic dose
- if the patient becomes drowsy or swallowing becomes difficult, switch PO anti-epileptics to one which can be given parenterally, e.g. **midazolam** (see p.157) or **phenobarbital** (see p.286).
If the patient becomes semicomatose and cannot communicate clearly, the presence of headache may manifest as grimacing or general restlessness. However, as in all moribund patients, it is important to exclude other common reasons for agitation, e.g. a full bladder or rectum, and discomfort and stiffness secondary to immobility.

Box H	Recommendations for withdrawing systemic corticosteroids[60]

Abrupt withdrawal
Systemic corticosteroids may be stopped abruptly in those whose disease is unlikely to relapse *and* have received treatment for <3 weeks *and* are not in the groups below.

continued

Box H Continued

Gradual withdrawal

Gradual withdrawal of systemic corticosteroids is advisable in patients who:
- have received more than 3 weeks treatment
- have received prednisolone >40mg/24h or equivalent, e.g. dexamethasone 4–6mg
- have had a second dose in the evening
- have received repeated treatments
- are taking a short course within 1 year of stopping long-term treatment
- have other possible causes of adrenal suppression.

During corticosteroid withdrawal the dose may initially be reduced rapidly (e.g. halving the dose daily) to physiological doses (prednisolone 7.5mg/24h or equivalent) and then more slowly (e.g. 1–2mg per week) to allow the adrenals to recover and to prevent a hypo-adrenal crisis (malaise, profound weakness, hypotension, etc.). The patient should be monitored during withdrawal in case of deterioration.

Supply

Dexamethasone formulations in the UK[62]

PO tablets are formulated as dexamethasone *base,* the two parenteral preparations available are formulated as dexamethasone *sodium phosphate,* but are different strengths (Table 2). BNF, SPCs and product labels now all use dexamethasone *base* for labelling and dosing advice.

For simplicity, the Organon/MSD 4mg/mL ampoule is the preferable injectable brand when prescribing for patients who may need to switch between PO tablets and parenteral administration.

Table 2 Dexamethasone base and salt content in UK parenteral formulations

Manufacturer	Presentation	Dexamethasone base (as on the label)[a]	Dexamethasone sodium phosphate
Organon/MSD	1mL amp	4mg	5.2mg
Hospira/Hamelyn	1mL amp	3.3mg	4.3mg
Hospira/Hamelyn	2mL vial	6.6mg	8.6mg

a. dexamethasone base 1mg = dexamethasone sodium phosphate 1.3mg approximately.

Dexamethasone (generic)
Tablets 500microgram, 2mg, 28 days @ 2mg once daily = £4.
Oral solution (sugar-free) 2mg/5mL, 28 days @ 2mg once daily = £40. (In countries where an oral solution of dexamethasone is not available, the contents of an ampoule for injection can be used PO.)
Injection 4mg/mL, 1mL amp = £1.
Injection 3.3mg/mL, 1mL amp = £1, 2mL vial = £2.

Hydrocortisone (generic)
Tablets (scored) 10mg, 20mg 28 days @ 20mg each morning and 10mg each evening = £90.

Fludrocortisone
Florinef® (Squibb)
Tablets (scored) 100microgram, 28 days @ 100microgram each morning = £1.50.

Prednisolone (generic)
Tablets 1mg, 5mg, 25mg, 28 days @ 15mg once daily = £4.
Tablets e/c 2.5mg, 5mg, 28 days @ 15mg once daily = £30.
Tablets soluble 5mg, 28 days @ 15mg once daily = £29.

Rectal products
Hydrocortisone
Colifoam® (Meda)
Retention foam enema **hydrocortisone** *acetate* 10% (100mg/mL), 1 metered application = 125mg **hydrocortisone** *acetate*, 14-application cannister with applicator = £9.

Prednisolone (generic)
Retention foam enema **prednisolone** (as *metasulfobenzoate sodium*) 20mg/metered application, 14-application canister with applicators = £48.

Predsol® (UCB Pharma)
Retention enema **prednisolone** (as *sodium phosphate*) 20mg in 100mL, 7-single enemas = £7.50.
Suppositories **prednisolone** (as *sodium phosphate*) 5mg, 10 = £1.50.

Note: **budesonide** rectal products are also available, but are much more expensive.

1 Hanks GW et al. (1983) Corticosteroids in terminal cancer - a prospective analysis of current practice. *Postgraduate Medical Journal.* **59**: 702–706.
2 Hardy J et al. (2001) A prospective survey of the use of dexamethasone on a palliative care unit. *Palliative Medicine.* **15**: 3–8.
3 NICE (2008) Metastatic spinal cord compression: diagnosis and management of patients at risk of or with metastatic spinal cord compression. (Clinical guideline 75.). National Institute for Health and Clinical Excellence, London. Available from: www.nice.org.uk/CG75
4 Rowell NP and Gleeson FV (2001) Steroids, radiotherapy, chemotherapy and stents for superior vena caval obstruction in carcinoma of the bronchus. *Cochrane Database of Systematic Reviews.* CD001316.
5 Elsayem A and Bruera E (2007) High-dose corticosteroids for the management of dyspnea in patients with tumor obstruction of the upper airway. *Supportive Care in Cancer.* **15**: 1437–1439.
6 Feuer DJ and Broadley KE (2009) Corticosteroids for the resolution of malignant bowel obstruction in advanced gynaecological and gastrointestinal cancer 2000 (2). Update 2009. *Cochrane Database of Systematic Reviews.* CD001219.
7 Laval G et al. (2000) The use of steroids in the management of inoperable intestinal obstruction in terminal cancer patients: do they remove the obstruction? *Palliative Medicine.* **14**: 3–10.
8 Ralston S et al. (1985) Comparison of aminohydroxypropylidene diphosphonate, mithramycin, and corticosteroids/calcitonin in treatment of cancer-associated hypercalcaemia. *Lancet.* **ii**: 907–910.
9 Percival R et al. (1984) Role of glucocorticoids in management of malignant hypercalcaemia. *British Medical Journal.* **289**: 287.
10 Minton MJ et al. (1981) Corticosteroids for elderly patients with breast cancer. *Cancer.* **48**: 883–887.
11 Tannock IF et al. (1996) Chemotherapy with mitoxantrone plus prednisone or prednisone alone for symptomatic hormone-resistant prostate cancer: a Canadian randomized trial with palliative end points. *Journal of Clinical Oncology.* **14**: 1756–1764.
12 Rhen T and Cidlowski JA (2005) Antiinflammatory action of glucocorticoids–new mechanisms for old drugs. *New England Journal of Medicine.* **353**: 1711–1723.
13 Lundstrom S et al. (2009) The existential impact of starting corticosteroid treatment as symptom control in advanced metastatic cancer. *Palliative Medicine.* **23**: 165–170.
14 Bruera E et al. (1985) Action of oral methylprednisolone in terminal cancer patients: a prospective randomized double-blind study. *Cancer Treatment Reports.* **69**: 751–754.
15 Moertel C et al. (1974) Corticosteroid therapy for preterminal gastrointestinal cancer. *Cancer.* **33**: 1607–1609.
16 Twycross RG and Guppy D (1985) Prednisolone in terminal breast and bronchogenic cancer. *Practitioner.* **229**: 57–59.
17 Willox JC et al. (1984) Prednisolone as an appetite stimulant in patients with cancer. *British Medical Journal.* **288**: 27.
18 Ioannidis JP et al. (2000) Contribution of dexamethasone to control of chemotherapy-induced nausea and vomiting: a meta-analysis of randomized evidence. *Journal of Clinical Oncology.* **18**: 3409–3422.
19 Glare PA et al. (2008) Treatment of nausea and vomiting in terminally ill cancer patients. *Drugs.* **68**: 2575–2590.
20 Davis MP et al. (2010) A systematic review of the treatment of nausea and/or vomiting in cancer unrelated to chemotherapy or radiation. *Journal of Pain and Symptom Management.* **39**: 756–767.
21 Bruera E et al. (2004) Dexamethasone in addition to metoclopramide for chronic nausea in patients with advanced cancer: a randomized controlled trial. *Journal of Pain and Symptom Management.* **28**: 381–388.
22 Vecht C et al. (1994) Dose-effect relationship of dexamethasone on Karnofsky performance in metastatic brain tumors. A randomized study of doses of 4, 8 and 16 mg per day. *Neurology.* **44**: 675–680.
23 Soffetti et al. (2006) EFNS guidelines on diagnosis and treatment of brain metastases. *European Journal of Neurology.* **13**: 674–681.
24 Ryken TC et al. (2010) The role of steroids in the management of brain metastases: a systematic review and evidence-based clinical practice guideline. *Journal of Neuro-oncology.* **96**: 103–114.
25 Cowap J et al. (2000) Outcome of malignant spinal cord compression at a cancer center: implications for palliative care services. *Journal of Pain and Symptom Management.* **19**: 257–264.
26 Loblaw DA et al. (2005) Systematic review of the diagnosis and management of malignant extradural spinal cord compression: the Cancer Care Ontario Practice Guidelines Initiative's Neuro-Oncology Disease Site Group. *Journal of Clinical Oncology.* **23**: 2028–2037.
27 White BD et al. (2008) Diagnosis and management of patients at risk of or with metastatic spinal cord compression: summary of NICE guidance. *British Medical Journal.* **337**: a2538.
28 Greenberg HS et al. (1980) Epidural spinal cord compression from metastatic tumor: results with a new treatment protocol. *Annals of Neurology.* **8**: 361–366.
29 Klimo P, Jr. and Schmidt MH (2004) Surgical management of spinal metastases. *Oncologist.* **9**: 188–196.
30 Vecht C et al. (1989) Initial bolus of conventional versus high-dose dexamethasone in metastatic spinal cord compression. *Neurology.* **39**: 1255–1257.

31 Graham PH et al. (2006) A pilot randomised comparison of dexamethasone 96 mg vs 16 mg per day for malignant spinal-cord compression treated by radiotherapy: TROG 01.05 Superdex study. Clinical Oncology (R Coll Radiol). 18: 70–76.

32 Heimdal K et al. (1992) High incidence of serious side effects of high-dose dexamethasone treatment in patients with epidural spinal cord compression. Journal of Neuro-oncology. 12: 141–144.

33 Sorensen S et al. (1994) Effect of high-dose dexamethasone in carcinomatous metastatic spinal cord compression treated with radiotherapy: a randomised trial. European Journal of Cancer. 30A: 22–27.

34 Swartz S and Dluhy R (1978) Corticosteroids: clinical pharmacology and therapeutic use. Drugs. 16: 238–255.

35 Demoly P and Chung K (1998) Pharmacology of corticosteroids. Respiratory Medicine. 92: 385–394.

36 Ellershaw J and Kelly M (1994) Corticosteroids and peptic ulceration. Palliative Medicine. 8: 313–319.

37 Naesdal J and Brown K (2006) NSAID-associated adverse effects and acid control aids to prevent them: a review of current treatment options. Drug Safety. 29: 119–132.

38 Fardet L et al. (2007) Corticosteroid-induced adverse events in adults: frequency, screening and prevention. Drug Safety. 30: 861–881.

39 BNF (2012) Section 6.3.2. In: British National Formulary No 63. British Medical Association and the Royal Pharmaceutical Society of Great Britain, London.

40 Chalk J et al. (1984) Phenytoin impairs the bioavailability of dexamethasone in neurological and neurosurgical patients. Journal of Neurology, Neurosurgery, and Psychiatry. 47: 1087–1090.

41 Hazlewood KA et al. (2006) Effect of oral corticosteroids on chronic warfarin therapy. Annals of Pharmacotherapy. 40: 2101–2106.

42 Jick S et al. (2001) The risk of cataract among users of inhaled steroids. Epidemiology. 12: 229–234.

43 Piper JM et al. (1991) Corticosteroid use and peptic ulcer disease: role of nonsteroidal anti-inflammatory drugs. Annals of internal medicine. 114: 735–740.

44 Warrington TP and Bostwick JM (2006) Psychiatric adverse effects of corticosteroids. Mayo Clinic Proceedings. 81: 1361–1367.

45 Hall R Psychiatric adverse drug reactions: steroid psychosis. Available from: www.drrichardhall.com/steroid.htm

46 Brown ES and Suppes T (1998) Mood symptoms during corticosteroid therapy: a review. Harvard Review of Psychiatry. 5: 239–246.

47 Stiefel FC et al. (1989) Corticosteroids in cancer: neuropsychiatric complications. Cancer Investigation. 7: 479–491.

48 Twycross R et al. (2009) Symptom Management in Advanced Cancer (4e). palliativedrugs.com, Nottingham, pp. 209–210.

49 Eidelberg D (1991) Steroid myopathy. In: DA Rottenberg (ed) Neurological Complications of Cancer Treatment. Butterworth-Heineman, Boston, pp. 185–191.

50 Schakman O et al. (2008) Mechanisms of glucocorticoid-induced myopathy. Journal of Endocrinology. 197: 1–10.

51 Rotstein J and Good R (1957) Steroid pseudorheumatism. AMA Archives of Internal Medicine. 99: 545–555.

52 Greenberg H et al. (1979) Epidural spinal cord compression from metastatic tumour: results with a new treatment protocol. Annals of Neurology. 8: 361–366.

53 Delattre J-Y et al. (1988) High dose versus low dose dexamethasone in experimental epidural spinal cord compression. Neurosurgery. 22: 1005–1007.

54 Rousseau P (2004) Sudden withdrawal of corticosteroids: a commentary. American Journal of Hospice and Palliative Care. 21: 169–171.

55 Gralla R et al. (1999) Recommendations for the use of antiemetics: evidence-based, clinical practice guidelines. Journal of Clinical Oncology. 17: 2971–2994.

56 Sridhar K et al. (1992) Five-drug antiemetic combination for cisplatin chemotherapy. Cancer Investigation. 10: 191–199.

57 Editorial (1991) Ondansetron versus dexamethasone for chemotherapy-induced emesis. Lancet. 338: 478.

58 Galicich JH and French LA (1961) The use of dexamethasone in the treatment of cerebral oedema resulting from brain tumours and brain surgery. American Practitioner. 12: 169.

59 Kirkham S (1988) The palliation of cerebral tumours with high-dose dexamethasone: a review. Palliative Medicine. 2: 27–33.

60 CSM (Committee on Safety of Medicines and Medicines Control Agency) (1998) Withdrawal of systemic corticosteroids. Current Problems in Pharmacovigilance. 24: 5–7.

61 Margolin L et al. (2007) The steroid withdrawal syndrome: a review of the implications, etiology, and treatments. Journal of Pain and Symptom Management. 33: 224–228.

62 Palliativedrugs.com (2010) Clarifying label changes to parenteral formulations of dexamethasone. Available from: www.palliativedrugs.com/news/december/clarifying-dexamethasone-prescribing.html

Updated October 2013

DEMECLOCYCLINE   BNF 5.1.3 & 6.5.2

Class: Tetracycline antibacterial and vasopressin receptor antagonist.

Indications: Symptomatic hyponatraemia caused by paraneoplastic syndrome of inappropriate antidiuretic hormone (ADH) secretion (SIADH).

Contra-indications: Patients with hypovolaemic hyponatraemia, e.g. caused by severe diarrhoea, vomiting, or adrenal insufficiency.

Pharmacology

Demeclocycline is a tetracycline derivative. It induces nephrogenic diabetes insipidus, i.e. inhibits the action of ADH on renal tubules, probably by antagonism of arginine-vasopressin V_2-receptors.[1-3] There are at least three arginine-vasopressin receptor subtypes. V_2-receptors are concentrated in renal collecting tubules where antagonism leads to aquaresis, i.e. the excretion of water without significantly changing the total level of electrolyte excretion. V_2-receptors also occur in vascular endothelium where antagonism results in vasodilation.

The SPC states that, in paraneoplastic SIADH, demeclocycline should be used only if fluid restriction is ineffective. However, in palliative care, fluid restriction to 700–1,000mL/24h (or a daily urine output of <500mL) is burdensome and treatment with demeclocycline is generally preferable. The effect of demeclocycline is apparent after 3–5 days, and persists for several days after stopping treatment. There is no need to restrict fluid during treatment.

Tolvaptan is a recently introduced alternative arginine-vasopressin V_2-receptor antagonist (see Box C, p.513).
Bio-availability 60–80%.
Onset of action 3–5days.
Time to peak plasma concentration 3–4h.
Plasma halflife 12h.
Duration of action several days.

Pathogenesis and clinical features of SIADH

There are many causes of SIADH, including a range of drugs (Box A). In paraneoplastic SIADH there is ectopic secretion of arginine vasopressin (ADH) or vasopressin-like peptides by the cancer.[4,5] In SCLC an elevated arginine vasopressin can be detected in about 40% of patients, but in most it is asymptomatic.

Hyponatraemia (with consequential intracellular cerebral oedema), possibly caused by SIADH, should be considered in all patients who develop drowsiness, confusion or seizures while taking a TCA or SSRI. Risk factors for the development of SIADH with SSRIs include older age, female gender, low body weight and concurrent use of diuretics.[6]

Box A Causes of SIADH

Cancer
Small cell lung
Head and neck
Pancreas
Prostate
Carcinoid
Lymphoma
Acute myeloid leukaemia

Treatment
After neurosurgery
Chemotherapy, e.g.
   cyclophosphamide
   vincristine
Drugs
   barbiturates
   carbamazepine
   lorazepam
   phenothiazines
   SSRIs
   TCAs

Miscellaneous
Pulmonary
   pneumonia
   tuberculosis
   lung abscess
   positive pressure ventilation
Central nervous system
   meningitis
   encephalitis
   subarachnoid
   haemorrhage
   cerebral thrombosis
   head injury
Psychiatric
   schizophrenia
   psychosis
Recreational drugs
   ethanol
   nicotine

Clinical features of SIADH depend on both the level and the rate of decline of the plasma sodium concentration (Box B). Asymptomatic hyponatraemia indicates chronic rather than acute SIADH. Treatment is necessary only if the hyponatraemia is symptomatic.

If suspected, paired urine and serum samples should be obtained from the patient. The diagnosis of SIADH is based on the following criteria:
• hyponatraemia (<130mmol/L)
• low plasma osmolality (<270mosmol/L)
• urine osmolality >300mosmol/L (i.e. higher than plasma osmolality)
• urine sodium concentration always >20mmol/L, and generally >40mmol/L
• normal or moderately expanded plasma volume.[7]

> **Box B**   Clinical features of SIADH
>
> | **Plasma sodium 110–120mmol/L** | **Plasma sodium <110mmol/L** |
> |---|---|
> | Anorexia | Multifocal myoclonus |
> | Nausea and vomiting | Drowsiness |
> | Lassitude | Seizures |
> | Confusion | Coma |

Urine osmolality > 100mosm/L but < 300mosm/L may be consistent with a diagnosis of SIADH if there is co-existent renal tubular dysfunction, diuretic use or reset osmostat syndrome. In such cases, a raised urine sodium concentration (> 30mmol/L) is more diagnostically reliable.[8-10]

In practice, a plasma sodium concentration of ≤120mmol/L is sufficient to make a clinical diagnosis of SIADH in the absence of:
- severe vomiting
- diuretic therapy
- hypo-adrenalism
- hypothyroidism
- severe renal impairment.

Cautions

Renal and hepatic impairment; lower doses advised to avoid excessive systemic accumulation. Risk of photosensitivity; warn patients not to expose skin to direct sunlight or sunlamps.

Drug interactions

The absorption of demeclocycline is reduced by the concurrent administration of **iron**, **calcium**, **magnesium**, **aluminium** and **zinc**.

Demeclocycline depresses plasma prothrombin activity and, if used concurrently, the dose of **warfarin** may need to be reduced. Risk of oral contraceptive failure (as with all antibacterials). Avoid concurrent **penicillin** use (tetracyclines possibly antagonize the effect of penicillins).

Undesirable effects

Nausea, vomiting, diarrhoea, renal impairment (more likely with daily dose of 1,200mg),[11] photosensitivity (see Cautions), oesophagitis, discolouration of teeth during tooth development. Higher doses may lead to uraemia.

Dose and use

Treat the patient and not the biochemical results.
If feasible, stop the causal drug and/or treat the underlying cause.

If symptomatic and cause of SIADH irreversible:
- start with 300mg b.d. on an empty stomach, e.g. 1h a.c.; to reduce the risk of oesophagitis take with plenty of water and in an upright position; avoid milk, antacids, **iron** and **zinc** preparations at the same time
- if necessary, increase to 300mg q.d.s. after 1 week
- typical maintenance dose = 150mg b.d.–t.d.s.

In patients unable to take drugs PO, demeclocycline can be given PR dispersed in 5mL of a methylcellulose carrier.[12] However, the powder may cause local irritation and inflammation.

Supply

Demeclocycline hydrochloride (generic)
Capsules 150mg, 28 days @ 300mg b.d. = £50.

Tolvaptan (see Box C)
Samsca® (Otsuka)
Tablets 15mg, 30mg, 28 days @ 15mg or 30mg daily = £2,100.

Box C   Tolvaptan

Tolvaptan is an alternative arginine-vasopressin V_2-receptor antagonist (VRA).[13–15] In the EU, tolvaptan is approved for treatment of SIADH. In the USA, it is also licensed for hyponatraemia associated with heart failure or cirrhosis.

Tolvaptan decreases expression of aquaporin channels in the renal collecting ducts, resulting in increased free water clearance.[16]

In patients who are not fluid-restricted, the plasma sodium concentration generally increases by 2–3mmol/L in the first 24h of treatment. There is a mean increase of 7mmol/L after 1 month, with 60% of patients achieving a normal plasma sodium concentration.

Tolvaptan has *not* been compared with fluid restriction and/or demeclocyline. The impact of tolvaptan on long-term morbidity or mortality in SIADH of any cause is not known, although one study demonstrated acceptable safety in patients with various causes of hyponatraemia after 1 year.[17–19]

Like demeclocycline, tolvaptan is contra-indicated in patients with hypovolaemic hyponatraemia, e.g. caused by severe diarrhoea, vomiting, or adrenal insufficiency.[20,21] The effects of vasopressin analogues may be attenuated by tolvaptan, e.g. desmopressin used to control bleeding.[22]

A too rapid rise in plasma sodium risks irreversible osmotic demyelination (see below). Thus, when starting tolvaptan, plasma sodium levels should be checked at least every 6h for the first 48h. If the rise in plasma sodium exceeds 6mmol/L in the first 6h, 8mmol/L in the first 12h, 12mmol/L in 24h or 18mmol/L in 48h, discontinue tolvaptan and administer hypotonic fluid while continuing to monitor plasma sodium.

In RCTs, patients who were fluid restricted were at greater risk of a too rapid rise in plasma sodium. Patients receiving tolvaptan should *not* be fluid-restricted, and should *not* receive IV normal or hypertonic saline.[23]

Post-marketing pharmacovigilance monitoring for tolvaptan has revealed several cases of irreversible osmotic demyelination (both pontine and extrapontine) caused by too rapid correction in plasma sodium (> 12mmol/L in 24h).[24] Risk factors include a baseline plasma sodium < 120mmol/L, malnutrition, hypokalaemia, hypoxia, and excessive alcohol use.

Note:
- osmotic demyelination is a risk with any treatment which causes a too rapid rise in plasma sodium
- RCTs have generally excluded patients with a plasma sodium of < 120mmol/L, thus reducing the likelihood of causing osmotic demyelination[20]
- patients with paraneoplastic SIADH may be more sensitive to tolvaptan, necessitating a lower starting dose, e.g. 7.5mg once daily or alternate days.[25]

Undesirable effects include:
Very common (≥10%): dry mouth and thirst, weakness, hypernatraemia.
Common (<10%, >1%): nausea, constipation, urinary frequency, dizziness, hyperglycaemia.

The cost of tolvaptan (about £75/day) and the need to closely monitor plasma sodium will restrict the use of tolvaptan in palliative care. However, it may have a role in recurrent severe hyponatraemia unresponsive to fluid restriction and demeclocycline.[26]

---

1 deTroyer A (1977) Demeclocycline. Treatment for syndrome of inappropriate antidiuretic hormone secretion. *Journal of the American Medical Association.* **237**: 2723–2726.
2 Forrest J et al. (1978) Superiority of demeclocycline over lithium in the treatment of chronic syndrome of inappropriate secretion of antidiuretic hormone. *New England Journal of Medicine.* **298**: 173–177.

3 Miyagawa C (1986) The pharmacologic management of the syndrome of inapprorpiate secretion of antidiuretic hormone. *Drug Intelligence and Clinical Pharmacy.* **20**: 527–531.
4 Meinders A (1993) Hyponatraemia: SIADH or SIAD? *Netherlands Journal of Medicine.* **43**: 1–4.
5 Sorensen J et al. (1995) Syndrome of inappropriate secretion of antidiuretic hormone (SIADH) in malignant disease. *Journal of Internal Medicine.* **238**: 97–110.
6 Jacob S and Spinler SA (2006) Hyponatremia associated with selective serotonin-reuptake inhibitors in older adults. *Annals of Pharmacotherapy.* **40**: 1618–1622.
7 Burtis CA et al. (eds) (2008) *Pituitary disorders.* (6e). WB Saunders, Philadelphia, pp. 746–747.
8 Gross (2012) Clinical management of SIADH. *Therapeutic Advances in Endocrinology and Metabolism.* **3**: 61–73.
9 Smellie WS and Heald A (2007) Hyponatraemia and hypernatraemia: pitfalls in testing. *British Medical Journal.* **334**: 473–476.
10 Ellison DH and Berl T (2007) Clinical practice. The syndrome of inappropriate antidiuresis. *New England Journal of Medicine.* **356**: 2064–2072.
11 Trump D (1981) Serious hyponatremia in patients with cancer: management with demeclocycline. *Cancer.* **47**: 2908–2912.
12 Hussain I et al. (1998) Rectal administration of demeclocycline in a patient with syndrome of inappropriate ADH secretion. *International Journal of Clinical Practice.* **52**: 59.
13 Schrier RW et al. (2006) Tolvaptan, a selective oral vasopressin V_2-receptor antagonist, for hyponatremia. *New England Journal of Medicine.* **355**: 2099–2112.
14 Amin A and Meeran K (2011) New drugs for hyponatraemia. *British Medical Journal.* **342**: 559–560.
15 Plosker GL (2010) Tolvaptan: Adis drug profile. *Drugs.* **70**: 443–454.
16 Dubois EA et al. (2012) Tolvaptan. *British Journal of Clinical Pharmacology.* **73**: 9–11.
17 Berl T et al. (2010) Oral tolvaptan is safe and effective in chronic hyponatremia. *Journal of the American Society of Nephrology.* **21**: 705–712.
18 Amin A and Meeran K (2010) New drugs for hyponatraemia. *British Medical Journal.* **341**: c6219.
19 Verbalis JG et al. (2011) Efficacy and safety of oral tolvaptan therapy in patients with the syndrome of inappropriate antidiuretic hormone secretion. *European Journal of Endocrinology.* **164**: 725–732.
20 Decaux G et al. (2008) Non-peptide arginine-vasopressin antagonists: the vaptans. *Lancet.* **371**: 1624–1632.
21 Ali F et al. (2007) Therapeutic potential of vasopressin receptor antagonists. *Drugs.* **67**: 847–858.
22 MHRA (2012). Available from: www.mhra.gov.uk/Safetyinformation/DrugSafetyUpdate/CON149776
23 Peri A and Combe C (2012) Considerations regarding the management of hyponatraemia secondary to SIADH. *Best Practice and Research Clinical Endocrinology and Metabolism.* **26 (Suppl 1)**: S16–26.
24 Harb S et al. (2012) Dysarthria and ataxia in a middle aged women. *Journal of Hospital Medicine.* **7**: S194–S195.
25 Kenz S et al. (2011) High sensitivity to tolvaptan in paraneoplastic syndrome of inappropriate ADH secretion (SIADH). *Annals of Oncology.* **22**: 2696.
26 Mumby C and Adam S (2012) Tolvaptan use in a patient with metastatic small cell lung cancer. *Lung Cancer.* **75**: S59–S60.

Updated November 2012

DESMOPRESSIN   BNF 6.5.2

Class: Vasopressin analogue.

Indications: Authorized indications vary between products and formulations (Table 1); see SPCs for details. Pituitary diabetes insipidus, primary nocturnal enuresis and nocturia, mild–moderate haemophilia and von Willebrand's disease, headache from a lumbar puncture, testing renal concentration capacity, testing fibrinolytic response, †treatment of bleeding from anti-platelet therapy, †treatment of severe surface bleeding associated with acquired platelet dysfunction, e.g. renal or hepatic impairment, paraproteinaemia.[1]

Contra-indications: See SPCs for details. Age >65 years, current or previous hyponatraemia, coronary insufficiency, unstable angina, hypertension, concurrent use with diuretics, psychogenic and alcohol abuse-related polydipsia, moderate–severe renal impairment (creatinine clearance <50mL/min), type IIB or platelet-type (pseudo) von Willebrand's disease.

Pharmacology

Desmopressin is an analogue of the pituitary antidiuretic hormone, **vasopressin**. It stimulates arginine-vasopressin V_2-receptors in the medullary collecting tubules, increasing water resorption by the renal tubules, thereby reducing urine volume. The antidiuretic effect of desmopressin is 3–10 times greater than that of **vasopressin**, and it has a longer duration of action. Unlike **vasopressin**, it has no vasoconstrictor effect. Desmopressin is ineffective in nephrogenic diabetes insipidus.[2]

Desmopressin also stimulates V_2-receptors on endothelial cells, leading to the release of stored von Willebrand factor and factor VIII. This augments platelet function and enhances haemostasis; hence its use in certain bleeding states, including those associated with severe renal or hepatic impairment.[1,3–5]

Bio-availability 3–4% intranasal; 0.1–5% PO.
Onset of action 1h intranasal; 2h PO.
Plasma halflife 0.4–4h intranasal; 1.5–2.5h PO.
Duration of action 5–24h intranasal; 6–8h PO.

Cautions

CHF, raised intracranial pressure, cystic fibrosis. Take care to avoid fluid overload because with excessive water intake there is an increased risk of hyponatraemia. The effect of desmopressin may be potentiated by drugs which cause fluid retention, e.g. NSAIDs and corticosteroids. In renal impairment, the antidiuretic effect is less. Food may reduce the absorption of tablets.

Drug interactions

Loperamide triples the desmopressin plasma concentration after PO administration.[6] The concurrent use of drugs which increase the endogenous secretion of vasopressin increases the risk of symptomatic hyponatraemia, notably **carbamazepine, chlorpromazine, lamotrigine,** NSAIDs, opioids, SSRIs, TCAs.

Undesirable effects

Water retention and hyponatraemia is a risk particularly in patients treated with desmopressin for an indication other than pituitary diabetes insipidus. In extreme cases this may result in hyponatraemic seizures.
Common (<10%, >1%): tablets and high doses of nasal spray (≥40microgram/24h): headache, abdominal pain, nausea. Nasal spray: nosebleeds, nasal congestion or rhinitis, sore throat. IV: facial flushing, tachycardia, mild transient systemic arterial hypotension.[1]
Rare or very rare (<0.1%): IV: increase in thrombo-embolic events, e.g. myocardial infarction,[1] aggression in children.

Dose and use

Global post-marketing data indicate a higher incidence of hyponatraemia in patients treated intranasally compared with PO,[3] reflecting the more favourable intranasal pharmacokinetics.

To minimize the risk of symptomatic hyponatraemia, keep to the recommended starting doses and take precautions to avoid fluid overload:
• advise all patients to avoid drinking large amounts of fluid (including when swimming)
• restrict fluid to the minimum which satisfies thirst:
   ▷ from 1h before until 8h after the dose given for enuresis/nocturia
   ▷ continually with repeated doses for bleeding.
The degree of monitoring required for fluid retention (weight, blood pressure) ± hyponatraemia (plasma sodium) varies between indications; *see SPC and obtain advice from an endocrinologist.*
   Treatment should be stopped and fluid restricted if any of the following develop:
• unusually severe or prolonged headache, nausea or vomiting, confusion (symptoms associated with hyponatraemia); *advise patient to seek immediate medical help*
• progressive increase in blood pressure and/or body weight
• plasma sodium concentration < 130mmol/L
• plasma osmolality < 270mosmol/kg.
When a patient has fully recovered from an episode of fluid overload, desmopressin can be restarted at an appropriate dose, with strict fluid restriction enforced.
   When given for enuresis/nocturia, desmopressin should also be stopped during an acute intercurrent illness impacting on fluid/electrolyte balance, e.g. diarrhoea, vomiting.

Pituitary diabetes insipidus

Tablets should be used first-line. The nasal spray should be used only where PO or SL are not suitable.

- start with 100microgram PO t.d.s., 60microgram SL t.d.s. (or 10–20microgram intranasally at bedtime)
- if ineffective, increase dose progressively every few days
- effective dose is generally 100–400microgram PO t.d.s., 120–240microgram SL t.d.s. (or 10–20microgram intranasally at bedtime–b.d.).

Primary nocturnal enuresis (children >5 years, adults)

Exclude other causes of nocturia, e.g. diabetes mellitus. Treat only with PO or SL tablets:

- start with 200microgram PO or 120microgram SL at bedtime
- after 1–2 weeks, if ineffective, increase dose to 400microgram PO or 240microgram SL at bedtime.[2]

Note: women are more sensitive to the effects of desmopressin and more likely to develop hyponatraemia. A lower starting dose of desmopressin may thus be advisable in women, particularly those with other risk factors for hyponatraemia.[7]

Nocturia associated with multiple sclerosis

Give only when other treatments have failed in adults aged <65 years:

- 10–20microgram intranasally at bedtime to reduce nocturia or in the morning to reduce daytime frequency[8,9]
- occasionally, a trial of 40microgram may be justifiable; however, higher doses (e.g. 60microgram) are associated with a higher risk of hyponatraemia and generally do not provide additional symptomatic benefit[10]
- do *not* give >1 dose/24h.[2,10,11]

Severe surface bleeding and bleeding in renal impairment

The clinical benefit from using desmopressin to treat bleeding disorders associated with acquired defects of platelet functioning is small. Thus, use only when other interventions are insufficient:

- give a single dose of desmopressin 0.3–0.4microgram/kg IVI in 50mL 0.9% saline over 20min or by SC injection (using the Octim® formulation to minimize injection volume)[4]
- if necessary, give repeat injections once daily up to a total of 4 days[12]
- if inadequate, consider giving cryoprecipitate, e.g. 2 pooled packs.[13]

Because of the mechanism of action of desmopressin (releasing stored von Willebrand factor and factor VIII from the vascular endothelium), the second and subsequent injections provide only about two thirds of the benefit of the first injection.[14]

Severe non-variceal surface bleeding in hepatic impairment

If **phytomenadione** injection (Konakion® MM) 10mg IV is insufficient (see p.566), administer desmopressin as for bleeding in renal impairment.[14–16]

Supply

Desmopressin (generic)
Tablets 100microgram, 200microgram, 28 days @ 200microgram t.d.s. = £68.
Nasal spray 10microgram/metered spray, 60 dose bottle = £24.

DDAVP® (Ferring)
Tablets 100microgram, 200microgram, 28 days @ 200microgram t.d.s. = £88.
Tablets SL (DDAVP® Melt) 60microgram, 120microgram, 240microgram, 28 days @ 120microgram t.d.s. = £90.
Intranasal solution 100microgram/mL, 2.5mL dropper bottle and catheter = £10; *store in refrigerator at 2–8°C and protect from light.*
Injection 4microgram/mL, 1mL amp = £1; for SC/IM/IV injection or IVI.

Desmotabs® (Ferring)
Tablets 200microgram, 28 days @ 200microgram t.d.s. = £88.

Desmomelt® (Ferring)
Tablets SL 120microgram, 240microgram, 28 days @ 120microgram t.d.s. = £91.

Desmospray® (Ferring)
Nasal spray 10microgram/metered spray, 60 dose bottle = £25; *store at room temperature and protect from light.*

Octim® (Ferring)
Nasal spray 150microgram/metered spray, 25 dose bottle = £577.
Injection 15microgram/mL, 1mL amp = £20; for SC injection or IVI; *store at room temperature and protect from light.*

Table 1 Main authorized indications for UK desmopressin formulations

	Pituitary diabetes insipidus[b]	Primary nocturnal enuresis	Nocturia associated with MS	Haemophilia or Von Willebrands' disease
PO formulations				
Desmopressin generic	Yes	Yes		
DDAVP® tablets	Yes			
DDAVP® Melt SL tablets	Yes			
Desmotabs®		Yes		
Desmomelt®		Yes		
Nasal formulations				
Desmopressin generic	Yes		Yes	
DDAVP® intranasal solution	Yes		Yes	
Desmospray®	Yes		Yes	
Injection formulations				
DDAVP® injection	Yes			Yes
Octim® injection				Yes

a. for full authorized indications see manufacturer's SPC
b. tablets should be used first-line following post-marketing data recommendations.

1 Ozier Y and Bellamy L (2010) Pharmacological agents: antifibrinolytics and desmopressin. *Best Practice and Research Clinical Anaesthesiology.* **24**: 107–119.
2 Cvetkovic RS and Plosker GL (2005) Desmopressin: in adults with nocturia. *Drugs.* **65**: 99–107; discussion 108–109.
3 Van de Walle et al. (2007) Desmopressin 30 years in clinical use: A safety review. *Current Drug Safety.* **2**: 232–238.
4 Hedges SJ et al. (2006) Evidence-based treatment recommendations for uremic bleeding. *Nature Clinical Practice Oncology.* **3**: 138–153.
5 Mannucci P (1997) Desmopressin (DDAVP) in the treatment of bleeding disorders: the first 20 years. *Blood.* **90**: 2515–2521.
6 Callreus T et al. (1999) Changes in gastrointestinal motility influence the absorption of desmopressin. *European Journal of Clinical Pharmacology.* **55**: 305–309.
7 Juul KV et al. (2011) Gender difference in antidiuretic response to desmopressin. *American Journal of Renal Physiology.* **300**: F1116–1122.
8 Bosma R et al. (2005) Efficacy of desmopressin in patients with multiple sclerosis suffering from bladder dysfunction: a meta-analysis. *Acta Neurologica Scandinavica.* **112**: 1–5.
9 Eckford SD et al. (2003) An open, inpatient incremental safety and efficacy study of desmopression in women with multiple sclerosis and nocturia. *British Journal of Urology.* **74**: 459–463.
10 Fowler CJ et al. (2009) A UK consensus on the management of the bladder in multiple sclerosis. *Postgraduate Medical Journal.* **85**: 552–559.
11 Zahariou A et al. (2008) Maximal bladder capacity is a positive predictor of response to desmopressin treatment in patients with MS and nocturia. *International Urology and Nephrology.* **40**: 65–69.
12 Mannucci PM et al. (1992) Patterns of development of tachyphylaxis in patients with haemophilia and von Willebrand disease after repeated doses of desmopressin (DDAVP). *British Journal of Haematology.* **82**: 87–93.
13 Mannucci PM and Levi M (2007) Prevention and treatment of major blood loss. *New England Journal of Medicine.* **356**: 2301–2311.
14 Manucci (1992) Patterns of development of tachyphylaxis in patient with haernophilia and von Willebrand disease after repeated doses of desmopression (DDAVP). *British Journal of Haematology.* **82**: 87–93.
15 Blonski W et al. (2007) Coagulopathy in liver disease. *Current Treatment Options in Gastroenterology.* **10**: 464–473.
16 Lisman T et al. (2010) Hemostasis and thrombosis in patients with liver disease: the ups and downs. *Journal of Hepatology.* **53**: 362–371.

Updated December 2012

DRUGS FOR DIABETES MELLITUS   BNF 6.1

Diabetes UK have commissioned and published recommendations on the management of patients with diabetes at the end of life.[1] These should be read in conjunction with this monograph.

Indications: Diabetes mellitus not controlled by diet.

Contra-indications: Oral hypoglycaemics should not be used during severe infection, after major trauma, or peri-operatively.

Glibenclamide, Glimepiride and **chlorpropamide** (not UK) should not be used in the elderly and those with severe renal (eGFR < 30mL/min/1.73m^2, see Chapter 14, p.656) or hepatic impairment because of their long plasma halflives and risk of hypoglycaemia. They should be avoided or used at reduced dose in those with mild to moderate renal impairment.[2]

Metformin should not be used in patients with severe renal impairment, and should be withheld during and for 48h after testing with IV iodinated contrast agents or until renal function is normal. Because of the risk of developing lactic acidosis, it should be withheld in patients with acute conditions which may cause tissue hypoxia or sudden deterioration in renal function, e.g. dehydration, severe infection, sepsis, shock, acute heart failure, respiratory failure, hepatic impairment, excessive alcohol intake.

Thiazolidinediones, e.g. **pioglitazone**, should not be used in patients with CHF, severe hepatic impairment, at higher risk of fracture, with bladder cancer or at risk of developing of bladder cancer.[3]

Background

Diabetes mellitus comprises a group of metabolic diseases characterized by hyperglycaemia resulting from defects in insulin secretion, insulin action or both. There are two main types of diabetes mellitus (Box A). Some patients can exhibit features of both type 1 and type 2 diabetes, making a definite classification difficult.

Box A   Classification of diabetes mellitus

Type 1 (the minority, < 10%)
Typically develops in children, young people, and adults < 30 years old, but can occur at any age. There is a lack of insulin because of immune-mediated destruction of the β-cells in the pancreas. Symptoms develop rapidly and the diagnosis is based on the presence of characteristic symptoms plus a high blood glucose concentration.

Type 2 (the majority)
Typically develops in adults > 40 years old, although it is increasingly manifesting in younger people because of obesity. The pancreas does not produce sufficient insulin for the body's needs and generally there is also marked insulin resistance, i.e. cells are not able to respond to the insulin that is produced. Symptoms tend to develop gradually, with a long delay (possibly years) before diagnosis. Treatment is based on modification of diet and weight loss, together with various glucose-lowering drugs. *Some patients with Type 2 diabetes need insulin.*

In the UK, 7% of the general population have diabetes mellitus,[4,5] and nearly 40% of cancer patients have impaired glucose tolerance demonstrated by an oral or IV glucose tolerance test.[6,7] In cancer, corticosteroids are the most common cause of drug-induced hyperglycaemia[8] (see Box B, p.525), but thiazides, **levothyroxine**, **furosemide**, **octreotide** and atypical antipsychotics (e.g. **risperidone, olanzapine**) are also potential precipitants.[9]

In patients with symptoms suggestive of diabetes mellitus (e.g. thirst, polydipsia and/or polyuria), a diagnosis can be made on the basis of the following criteria:
- fasting blood glucose concentrations of ≥7mmol/L (normal <5.6mmol/L) *or*
- random blood glucose concentrations of ≥11.1mmol/L *or*
- 2h post-load blood glucose ≥11.1mmol/L (normal = <7.8mmol/L) during oral glucose tolerance test *or*
- glycated haemoglobin (HbA$_{1c}$) ≥48mmol/mol (≥6.5%).

In *asymptomatic* patients, ≥2 of the above must be present. Measurement of HbA$_{1c}$ is the recommended diagnostic test for diabetes mellitus and is convenient because it does not require the patient to fast. However, HbA$_{1c}$ reflects glycaemia in the preceding 2–3 months. Thus, it is not suitable as the sole diagnostic test in palliative care patients with recent onset hyperglycaemia, e.g. in those:
- at high risk of diabetes and acutely ill
- taking medications which may cause a rapid rise in blood glucose, e.g. corticosteroids, atypical antipsychotics (see list above)
- with short duration of symptoms suggestive of diabetes mellitus
- with symptoms suggestive of type 1 diabetes at any age
- with acute pancreatitis or recent pancreatic surgery
- all symptomatic children and young people.[10–12]

Pharmacology
Drug treatment in type 1 diabetes mellitus
Insulin is an essential life-long treatment in type 1 diabetes and is sometimes needed in type 2 diabetes. Human sequence insulin can be produced by bacteria using recombinant DNA technology, or semi-synthetically by enzymatic modification of animal insulin (mainly porcine, sometimes beef). Care must be taken when prescribing animal insulin for patients of particular faith groups.

Insulin preparations can be divided into three types: short-acting (including the rapid-acting insulin analogues), intermediate, and long-acting (Table 1). Because the plasma halflife for insulin is a few minutes, its time-activity profile is determined by its absorption characteristics, e.g. insulin dose, injection route, injection site, thickness of SC fat. Thus, there is significant intra- and inter-individual variation in the pharmacokinetics of a given dose of insulin. Further, sensitivity to insulin varies with body weight and renal function. Individual dose titration is required to identify the appropriate dose.

Table 1 Pharmacokinetics of different types of insulin given by SC administration

Duration of action	Short		Intermediate	Long
	Rapid	Short		
Example	Aspart	Soluble	Isophane	Glargine
Onset of action	10–20min	30min	2h	2h
Time to peak plasma concentration	40min	1.5–2.5h	5–8h	Plateau <4h[a]
Duration of action	3–5h	7–8h	13–22h	>30h

a. SC insulin glargine once daily takes 2–4 days to reach steady state.[13]

Most patients with type 1 diabetes will be on a multiple injection **insulin** regimen, e.g. short-acting insulin or a rapid-acting insulin analogue before meals and intermediate or long-acting insulin once or twice daily. Some may be using mixtures of insulin preparations, e.g. **biphasic insulin aspart** or **biphasic insulin lispro**, or omitting pre-meal insulin, particularly if they have difficulty with or prefer not to use multiple injection therapy. The ability of the patient to use the necessary equipment for insulin delivery also influences the type of insulin used and the regimen, e.g. those with poor eyesight may not be able to safely use a insulin pen injector. Insulin pump therapy is used increasingly to manage patients with type 1 diabetes mellitus (see below).

Patients starting treatment with **insulin** must inform the Driver and Vehicle Licensing Agency (DVLA) if they intend to drive. Patients with impaired awareness of the onset of hypoglycaemia or who have had two hypoglycaemic episodes requiring assistance in the last 12 months are not allowed to drive. This includes some patients who are only taking oral hypoglycaemic drugs. Detailed guidance on eligibility to drive is available from the DVLA www.gov.uk/diabetes-driving

Drug treatment in type 2 diabetes mellitus

There are several different classes of antidiabetic drugs, with differing modes of action (Table 2). **Insulin** is sometimes needed in patients with type 2 diabetes, and may be given in addition or as an alternative to other hypoglycaemic therapy. The risk of hypoglycaemia is greatest with **insulin** and sulfonylureas.

Metformin

Metformin is generally recommended as first-line therapy for patients with diabetes who are overweight or obese.[15,21] However, it is unlikely to be appropriate in patients with advanced cancer because it promotes weight loss, and initially may cause nausea and diarrhoea, or other undesirable effects, in ≤20% of patients.

Metformin is best *not* used in elderly debilitated patients, particularly those with hepatic impairment or COPD. The dose of **metformin** should be reduced in patients with an eGFR <45mL/min/1.73m^2 and avoided or withdrawn in those with an eGFR of <30mL/min/1.73m^2 (severe renal impairment) or creatinine > 150micromol/L.[1] It is contra-indicated in patients with acute heart failure, but not those with CHF controlled on treatment.

Although **metformin** has been linked to lactic acidosis in patients with deteriorating renal function, CHF or tissue hypoxia, recent evidence suggests that the risk of this has been overestimated.[4,22] Hypoglycaemia is rare with **metformin**.

Sulfonylureas

In debilitated or elderly patients, a short-acting sulfonylurea, i.e. **tolbutamide**, is generally the best choice, or intermediate-acting **gliclazide** (Table 3). These are also good choices in mild–moderate renal impairment. Initially monitor blood glucose closely e.g. by checking capillary (fingerstick) blood glucose twice daily before a meal.[2]

Dose adjustment may be necessary if liver function deteriorates. After discontinuation, **glibenclamide** and **chlorpropamide** (not UK) can produce hypoglycaemia for 2–3 days, and up to 4 days if there is renal or hepatic impairment.

The plasma concentration of sulfonylureas may be increased (effect enhanced) by **fluconazole** and **miconazole**, and decreased (effect reduced) by **rifampicin** and **rifabutin**.

Meglitinides

Meglitinides, e.g. **repaglinide**, are insulin secretagogues. They provide similar glucose control to sulfonylureas but act more rapidly and for a shorter time (see Table 3). This permits flexible 'pulse dosing' before meals, which may be useful in patients with a variable appetite and oral intake. Meglitinides are significantly more expensive than sulfonylureas. **Nateglinide** is authorized only for use with **metformin**.

Gemfibrozil (generally used as a second-line plasma lipid-lowering agent) increases plasma concentrations of **repaglinide** (and **pioglitazone**). Because this may result in severe hypoglycaemia, avoid concurrent use. However, in palliative care, the continued use of **gemfibrozil** will generally be unnecessary.

Pioglitazone

Pioglitazone is used as second- or third-line therapy with **metformin** and/or a sulfonylurea, or **insulin**. **Pioglitazone** is contra-indicated in patients with a high risk of fracture because it increases the risk of distal fracture, particularly in women,[23,24] or with CHF because it causes fluid retention. All patients taking **pioglitazone** should be monitored for symptoms and signs of CHF, e.g. excessive/rapid weight gain, cough, increasing breathlessness, and/or oedema.[15,25]

Gemfibrozil (generally used as a second-line lipid-lowering agent) increases plasma concentrations of **pioglitazone** (and **repaglinide**). Because this may result in severe hypoglycaemia, avoid concurrent use. However, in palliative care, the continued use of **gemfibrozil** will generally be unnecessary.

Table 2 Antidiabetic drugs

Class	Examples	Mechanism of action	Risk of hypoglycaemia	Comment
Biguanides	Metformin	Decrease hepatic gluconeogenesis, increase uptake of glucose by muscle	–	Tend to cause weight loss; may cause nausea and diarrhoea; low risk of lactic acidosis
Sulfonylureas	Gliclazide, tolbutamide, glibenclamide, chlorpropamide (not UK)	Increase insulin secretion	++ with longer-acting drugs, glibenclamide, chlorpropamide	Original class of oral antidiabetic drugs; relatively inexpensive
Meglitinides	Repaglinide, nateglinide	Increase insulin secretion	±	Relatively fast onset and short duration of action; permits a more flexible regimen
Glitazones (thiazolidinediones)	Pioglitazone	Reduce peripheral insulin resistance	±	2nd or 3rd line drug; causes fluid retention, exacerbates CHF. Contra-indicated in patients with macular oedema; increases risk of myocardial infarction;[14] fracture[15] and bladder cancer[3]
Gliptins (DPP-4/dipeptidyl peptidase-4 inhibitors)	Saxagliptin, sitagliptin, vildagliptin, linagliptin	Increase insulin secretion and lower glucagon secretion	±	Newly introduced; 2nd or 3rd line drugs, for use particularly if patient at high risk of hypoglycaemia.[15] Suitable for use in renal impairment/failure (seek advice). Linagliptin, sitagliptin and vildagliptin authorized as monotherapy if metformin inappropriate. Can use with insulin. Stop if symptoms of pancreatitis develop[a]
GLP-1 (glucagon-like peptide-1) receptor agonist	Exenatide SC b.d., liraglutide SC once daily	Increase insulin secretion and lower glucagon secretion: slow gastric emptying and increase satiety	±	Newly introduced; 2nd or 3rd line drugs, for use particularly in patients with a BMI ≥35kg/m²[15]. Stop if weight loss > 1.5kg weekly or if symptoms of pancreatitis develop.[16,a] Initial nausea and vomiting common

a. recent studies suggest that the risk of pancreatitis is about one extra case per 10,000 patients.[17,18] Concern has been expressed that incretin mimetics (gliptins and GLP-1 receptor agonists) may predispose to pancreatic cancer,[19] but evidence is inconclusive.[20]

Table 3 Pharmacokinetics of selected oral hypoglycaemic drugs

	Repaglinide	Tolbutamide	Gliclazide
Bio-availability	56%	>95%	78%
Onset of action	15–60min	1–3h	3–4h
Time to peak plasma concentration	1h	3–5h	2–4h
Plasma halflife	1h	4.5–6.5h	10–12h
Duration of action	4–6h	≤12h	12–24h

Insulin in type 2 diabetes

Insulin is sometimes needed in patients with type 2 diabetes. If the patient is already taking **metformin** or a sulfonylurea, usual practice is to start **insulin** in addition.[15] When adding **insulin** to oral hypoglycaemics to improve blood glucose control, 6–12 units of **isophane insulin** or long-acting **insulin** at bedtime may suffice. However, it may be easier for patients with advanced cancer to switch to an insulin-only regimen rather than combining insulin with existing oral therapy.[1] All patients started on insulin should be provided with an Insulin Passport and information booklet.[26]

Management

Patients with **insulin pumps** are likely to be able to adjust pump settings to manage moderate variations in oral intake. However, specialist advice from an diabetologist is essential when it is necessary to adjust pump settings in complex situations, e.g. marked reductions in oral intake, enteral feeding, commencement of corticosteroids.[27]

This section provides advice about the management of common clinical scenarios in *the last few weeks of life*. Guidance from a diabetologist should be sought if in doubt. For corticosteroid-induced diabetes mellitus see Box B, see p.525.

Because the patient's prognosis is short (days, weeks, a few months), it is *not* necessary to maintain rigid dietary control or target theoretically ideal blood glucose levels to avoid long-term complications.[28,29] Measuring HbA_{1c} to determine the overall level of glycaemic control over 6–8 weeks is also irrelevant for most palliative care patients.

The goal is to preserve quality of life. Thus, the aim of treatment is the prevention of symptoms from hyper- or hypoglycaemia, keto-acidosis and hyperosmolar non-ketotic states. Set a realistic safe target, e.g. a pre-meal capillary (fingerstick) blood glucose of 6–15mmol/L. However, because the threshold for symptomatic hyperglycaemia varies, the upper limit may need to be reduced in some patients.[1] When stable, monitor with a fasting fingerstick blood glucose test twice a week.

Although not as accurate, urine tests for glucose may well suffice; aim for < 1+ glycosuria before evening meal.

Management of existing type 1 diabetes mellitus

Injections of **insulin** are an essential life-long treatment, including the last days of life. However, in most patients, the **insulin** requirement decreases because of weight loss, anorexia, nausea and vomiting, renal and/or hepatic impairment.

Generally, short-acting **insulins** (given to cover mealtimes) which produce a more rapid peak and have a greater risk of hypoglycaemia, are reduced or discontinued first. Intermediate- or long-acting **insulins** (given once daily or b.d. to provide background control) may subsequently need to be reduced as well.

Likewise, patients receiving mixed **insulins** may need to reduce or discontinue the short-acting **insulin** component. However, if a patient has months or weeks to live, it would be prudent to liaise with a diabetologist before making major changes to an established insulin regimen.

Sick Day Management in type 1 diabetes mellitus

To avoid serious metabolic complications, e.g. diabetic keto-acidosis, apply sick day rules when the patient is feeling particularly unwell and unable to manage normal oral intake or levels of activity:[1]

- *do not stop the long-acting insulin*
- encourage the patient to sip sugar-free fluids, aiming for 100mL/h
- offer frequent small meals, e.g. soup, ice cream, milky drinks
- if the patient has symptoms of hyperglycaemia and dehydration, check fingerstick blood glucose and test urine or blood for ketones
- if ketones are present, test blood glucose and ketones every 2h:
  - ▷ if ketones ++ in urine or >1.5mmol in blood, give additional 10% of current daily average insulin as short-acting **insulin**, e.g. Actrapid®, NovoRapid®
  - ▷ if ketone levels do not improve, and the patient is vomiting, seek urgent advice from a diabetologist; consider transfer to hospital for IV **insulin** and rehydration.

Note: sick-day rules are generally *not* relevant for patients entering the last days or hours of life.

Withdrawing treatment in type 1 diabetes mellitus

A decision to stop **insulin** completely should generally be taken only after discussion with the patient (if still has capacity) and the family. It is generally appropriate to stop **insulin** injections completely when the patient has become irreversibly unconscious as part of the dying process, and not because of hypoglycaemia or diabetic keto-acidosis, and when all other life-prolonging treatments have been stopped.[8]

If it is felt strongly that the **insulin** should be continued, a simple regimen can be used, e.g. once daily long-acting, or b.d. intermediate-acting **insulin**, with the minimum of routine monitoring, e.g. fingerstick blood glucose test once daily at teatime:

- if blood glucose is <8mmol/L, reduce insulin by 10–20%
- if blood glucose >20mmol/L, increase insulin dose by 10–20%.[1,30]

Management of patients with advanced cancer and newly diagnosed type 2 diabetes mellitus

The relative advantages and disadvantages of **insulin** and oral hypoglycaemic drugs need to be taken into account together with factors such as the patient's prognosis, oral nutritional intake and presence of other co-morbidities. **Insulin** provides rapid, effective and more predictable control, is easier to titrate, and has less risk of prolonged hypoglycaemia compared with some oral hypoglycaemics. It is a better choice in patients with:

- a short prognosis (<3 months)
- co-morbidity contributing to hyperglycaemia, e.g. infection
- poor or erratic oral nutritional intake
- contra-indications to the use of oral hypoglycaemics
- severe symptoms from hyperglycaemia.

With oral hypoglycaemics, control may take several weeks, and be less effective, less predictable and harder to titrate than **insulin**.[9] If oral hypoglycaemics are preferred, start **tolbutamide** or **gliclazide**.

When deciding the starting dose of **insulin**, the patient's build, oral intake and the blood glucose levels must be taken into account. The dose is monitored to achieve a fasting blood glucose of 6–15mmol/L. Doses of 0.25 units/kg/day of a *long-acting* **insulin analogue**, e.g. **insulin glargine**, **insulin detemir** (both given once daily) or **isophane insulin** (given once daily or b.d.) will provide only a basal insulin supply, and thus it does not matter if a patient on this amount is not eating.

However, in patients who are still eating and require larger doses than this, **insulin glargine** or **insulin detemir** are a better choice than **isophane insulin** because there is less likelihood of interprandial hypoglycaemia, they still generally need be given only once daily, and need not be given at the same time each day, thus easing the burden of injections on the patient/carer.[4,15,31] Given these advantages, it may be beneficial for patients on oral hypoglycaemics troubled by hypoglycaemic episodes or a burdensome tablet load to be switched to once daily injections of **insulin glargine** or **insulin detemir**. Blood glucose should be monitored before each dose until the **insulin** dose is stable. The frequency can then be reduced and the time of testing varied to monitor control during different parts of the day.

A variable dose SC scale (previously called 'sliding scale') of a *rapid-acting* **insulin analogue** (e.g. **insulin aspart**, **insulin lispro**, available as pen devices) is occasionally necessary. Treatment with a variable rate, continuous IV infusion of rapid-acting regular **soluble insulin** is generally reserved for patients with diabetic keto-acidosis or peri-operatively.[2]

Isolated spikes of hyperglycaemia should *not* be treated with stat doses of short/rapid-acting **insulin**. Instead, monitor with regular fingerstick tests and adjust hypoglycaemic regimen if a particular pattern emerges.[32]

Rationalizing therapy in existing type 2 diabetes mellitus

If patients have a prognosis of weeks–months and are becoming increasingly dependent on carers to administer treatment, consider simplifying existing therapy:
- stop **pioglitazone**, GLP-1 agonists and DPP-4 inhibitors if part of dual or triple therapy
- switch from combination of oral hypoglycaemic and **insulin** to **insulin** alone
- switch from b.d. to once daily **insulin** (start with 75% of total b.d. dose).

If in doubt, consult a diabetologist.

Sick Day Management in type 2 diabetes mellitus

To avoid serious metabolic complications, apply sick day rules when the patient is feeling particularly unwell and unable to manage normal oral intake or levels of activity:
- encourage the patient to sip sugar-free fluids, aiming for 100mL/h
- offer frequent small meals, e.g. soup, ice cream, milky drinks
- check blood glucose only if symptoms of hyperglycaemia and dehydration develop.

For patients on diet alone, **metformin**, **pioglitazone** or **DPP4 inhibitor**:
- aim to maintain blood glucose ≤15mmol/L
- stop **metformin** if the patient develops vomiting or diarrhoea.

For patients on a **sulfonylurea**, **meglitinide**, **insulin** or **GLP1 agonist**:
- if blood glucose <6mmol/L, consider reducing dose of sulfonylurea or **insulin**
- if blood glucose >15mmol/L, consider increasing dose of sulfonylurea or **insulin**
- stop medicines for diabetes if the patient is not eating, has no symptoms of hyperglycaemia and blood glucose <15mmol/l.[1]

Note: sick-day rules are generally *not* relevant for patients entering the last days or hours of life.

Withdrawing treatment in patients with type 2 diabetes

In advanced cancer, patients with insulin-treated type 2 diabetes may be able to stop **insulin**, and those with tablet-treated type 2 diabetes may be able to stop tablets because of weight loss, anorexia, nausea and vomiting, renal and/or hepatic impairment.

As the patient approaches the last few days of life, they are unlikely to be able to swallow any remaining oral hypoglycaemic agents. These should be stopped, as should GLP-1 injections and blood glucose monitoring. Consider stopping low-dose **insulin** (e.g. intermediate or long-acting **insulin** <15 units total daily dose).

In most cases it will be appropriate to stop blood glucose monitoring too. However, if it is felt necessary to continue monitoring, conduct daily urinalysis:
- if urine glucose >2+, check fingerstick glucose
- if finger stick glucose >20mmol/L give 6 units SC rapid-acting **insulin**, e.g. Novorapid
- recheck finger stick glucose after 2h
- if rapid-acting **insulin** required more than b.d., consider starting daily **isophane insulin** or **insulin glargine**.

If a patient requires a total daily dose of >15 units of **insulin**, or a decision is made to continue **insulin** therapy, manage as for type 1 diabetes (see above).[1,33,34]

Corticosteroid-induced diabetes mellitus

Diabetes mellitus occurs in about 10% of patients treated with corticosteroids.[35] It can occur with any corticosteroid and any formulation (including inhaled and topical),[36] and is dose-related.[37] The greatest rise in blood glucose is likely to occur 2–3h after taking a corticosteroid, returning to normal <12h later.[33] Thus, treatment with a longer acting product, either a sulfonylurea (see Table 3) or **insulin**, may cause nocturnal hypoglycaemia. This should be taken into account when planning treatment.

If corticosteroids are given b.d., consider switching to a once daily morning dose (Box B). If tablet load is a concern, soluble **prednisolone** tablets are available and **dexamethasone** can be given as an oral solution (see p.499).

If not possible to switch to a corticosteroid once daily, consider prescribing **gliclazide** or **isophane insulin** b.d. However, there is a risk of early morning hypoglycaemia. If early morning hypoglycaemia occurs on several occasions or the patient is struggling to manage insulin b.d., give **glargine** once daily in the morning. Obtain early advice from a diabetologist.

Hypoglycaemia

Hypoglycaemia is a lower than physiologically normal blood glucose concentration. It can be described as 'mild' if self-treated and 'severe' if assistance by another person is needed.[38] Any blood glucose less than 4mmol/L should be treated (Box C). For patients at risk, it is helpful to have a 'hypo box' containing everything necessary for treating hypoglycaemia, and keep it in a prominent place.[32,38]

Box B Corticosteroids and diabetes: management of patients taking corticosteroids once daily in the morning[33,37]

Target glucose levels when antidiabetic treatment is indicated: fingerstick blood glucose 6–15mmol/L or <1+ glycosuria before evening meal.

Before starting corticosteroids

Check random *fingerstick* blood glucose, if >8mmol/L take random *venous* blood glucose:
- if >7.8mmol/L, the patient is at risk of developing diabetes with corticosteroid therapy; check blood glucose every 1–2 weeks
- if ≥11.1mmol/L, check fasting venous blood glucose; ≥7mmol/L indicates pre-existing undiagnosed diabetes mellitus; manage accordingly (see text above).

Corticosteroid-induced diabetes

Start antidiabetic drugs only if the patient has symptomatic hyperglycaemia and a prolonged course of corticosteroid treatment is planned, say >2 weeks.

If drug treatment is necessary, give corticosteroid + a once daily morning dose of:
- a sulfonylurea, e.g. gliclazide (see Dose and use below) *or*
- isophane insulin (e.g. 10 units). If blood glucose remains >15mmol/L before evening meal, increase insulin dose by 4 units.[1]

Corticosteroid-exacerbated pre-existing non-insulin dependent diabetes

If glycaemic control deteriorates when corticosteroids are started for a course of >3 days, antidiabetic treatment will need to be modified.

Diet controlled diabetes or patient taking metformin alone or metformin and DPP4 inhibitor

Check fingerstick blood glucose or urine glucose before evening meal.
If two consecutive readings of blood glucose >15mmol/L or >2+ urine glucose:
- start gliclazide 40mg each morning
- if necessary, increase gliclazide 40mg each morning until blood glucose 6–15mmol/L or <1+ urine glucose before evening meal
- if no hypoglycaemia and blood glucose >15mmol/L or >2+ urine glucose despite gliclazide 240mg each morning, add in evening meal dose of gliclazide 80mg
- if glucose remains above target levels, switch to a once daily morning dose of insulin, e.g. isophane insulin (see below).

Gliclazide controlled diabetes

Check fingerstick blood glucose or urine glucose before evening meal.
If two consecutive readings of blood glucose >15mmol/L or >2+ urine glucose:
- in patients taking <320mg gliclazide daily, adjust dose up to a maximum of 240mg each morning and 80mg with evening meal
- in patients taking gliclazide 320mg daily, switch to morning isophane insulin 10 units SC
- if blood glucose remains >15mmol/L before evening meal, increase morning insulin dose by 4 units.

Corticosteroid-exacerbated pre-existing insulin controlled diabetes mellitus

As above, target blood glucose is generally 6–15mmol/L. However, if a patient has episodes of hypoglycaemia despite between meals ('mid-meal') snacks or has long gaps between meals, aim for blood glucose of 8–15mmol/L.

continued

Box B Continued

Twice daily insulin
Check fingerstick blood glucose before evening meal.
If pre-evening meal blood glucose > 15mmol/L, increase morning insulin dose.
If pre-evening meal blood glucose 10–15mmol/L, consider increasing morning insulin dose if low risk of hypoglycaemia:
• if insulin dose <20 units, increase dose by 2–5 units
• if insulin dose 20–50 units, increase insulin dose by 5–10 units
• if insulin dose 50–100 units, increase dose by 10–20 units.

Basal bolus insulin
Check fingerstick blood glucose before lunch and evening meals:
• if blood glucose > 15mmol/L, increase breakfast or lunchtime insulin doses
• if blood glucose 10–15mmol/L, consider increasing breakfast or lunchtime insulin doses if low risk of hypoglycaemia.

Reducing the corticosteroid dose
Insulin requirements decline in parallel.
Review hypoglycaemic therapy following each change in corticosteroid dose, and consider reverting to pre-corticosteroid regimen.

Box C Treatment of hypoglycaemia[32,39]

1 If conscious, give quick-acting carbohydrate 15–20g PO of the patient's choice e.g:
  • 200mL of pure fruit juice
  • 100mL of Lucozade® (*not* diet version); this is preferable in renal patients
  • 150mL of Coca-Cola® (*not* diet version) or other non-diet fizzy drink
  • 5–7 Dextrosol® glucose tablets (or 4–5 Glucotabs®)
  • 3–4 heaped teaspoons or 4–5 lumps of sugar dissolved in water.

2 If the patient is not able to take tablets or drink but can still swallow, give 2 tubes of GlucoGel® or Dextrogel® squeezed into the mouth between the teeth and gums.

3 Repeat fingerstick test after 10–15min; if blood glucose <4mmol/L, repeat step 1 up to 3 times.

4 If blood glucose remains <4mmol/L after 45min or 3 cycles, give glucagon 1mg IM (can be given SC, but will act more slowly) *or* glucose 10% 100mL IV (if patient malnourished or cachectic).

5 When the blood glucose is >4mmol/L and the patient has recovered, give a long-acting carbohydrate of the patient's choice e.g.
  • two biscuits
  • one slice of bread/toast
  • 200–300mL glass of milk (not soya)
  • normal meal if due (must contain carbohydrate).
  Note: patients given glucagon require a larger portion of long-acting carbohydrate to replenish glycogen stores.

6 Review diabetes management, e.g. consider reducing the dose of insulin; in patients with type 2 diabetes consider need for oral hypoglycaemic therapy.

Drivers need to be particularly careful to avoid hypoglycaemia. Drivers treated with **insulin** should be advised to check their blood glucose before driving and, on long journeys, at 2-hour intervals as specified by the DVLA (www.gov.uk/diabetes-driving). These precautions may also be necessary for drivers taking oral antidiabetic drugs which carry a risk of hypoglycaemia (e.g. long-acting sulfonylureas, meglitinides). Drivers treated with **insulin** should ensure that a supply of sugar is always available in the vehicle, and they should avoid driving if a meal is delayed. If the warning signs hypoglycaemia develop, the driver should:
- stop the vehicle in a safe place
- switch off the ignition and move out of the driver's seat
- eat or drink a suitable source of sugar (see Box C)
- not drive again until 45 minutes after the blood glucose has returned to normal.

In patients with long-standing diabetes, autonomic neuropathy may remove both the warning symptoms (sweating, tremor, pounding heart beat) and the counter-regulatory mechanism of an adrenaline (epinephrine)-induced increase in blood glucose. Such patients tend to present with pallor, mental detachment ± drowsiness ± clumsiness. Some become irritable and aggressive, and others slip rapidly into hypoglycaemic coma. Malnourished patients with reduced hepatic glycogen stores also have a reduced capacity to counteract hypoglycaemia. **Glucagon** treatment in these patients is likely to be less effective.[40]

If the patient is unconscious or having seizures or is very aggressive, check the airway and give high-flow oxygen via a mask, check breathing and circulation and obtain IV access. If the patient has an **insulin** infusion in situ, stop immediately. Give **glucagon** 1mg IM. This will be less appropriate in malnourished patients, so instead give 20% glucose 75mL IV (over 10–15min) *or* 10% glucose 150mL IV (over 10–15min). Repeat fingerstick test 10min later and repeat if blood glucose <4mmol/L.[32]

If the patient is 'nil by mouth', give glucose IV as above until blood sugar >4mmol/L. Consider 10% glucose 100mL/h IV until the hypoglycaemic agent has been metabolized and blood glucose levels are stable.

If the patient is receiving enteral nutrition (PEG/NG feeding) and develops hypoglycaemia, give 15–20g quick-acting carbohydrate of the patient's choice, e.g. 25mL undiluted Ribena® (*not* diet version), 50–70mL of Ensure® Plus Juice or Fortijuice®, 3–4 heaped teaspoons of sugar dissolved in water. If necessary, proceed as above with IV glucose (**glucagon** is not recommended). When blood glucose is >4mmol/L and the patient has recovered, give a long acting carbohydrate, e.g. restart feed; if bolus feeding, give additional bolus feed (read nutritional information and calculate amount required to give 20g of carbohydrate).

Do *not* omit next **insulin** injection or start variable rate IV **insulin** infusion to 'stabilize' blood glucose. Instead, reduce the dose of hypoglycaemic to prevent further episodes of hypoglycaemia. If unsure of subsequent treatment, discuss with the diabetes team.

Dose and use

To maximize safety, all regular and single **insulin** (bolus) doses must be measured and administered using an **insulin** syringe or commercial **insulin** pen device. IV syringes must never be used because they are calibrated in mL and not in **insulin** units. *'Units' must always be written in full.* Abbreviations, e.g. 'U' or 'IU', should not be used; e.g. 10U could be mistakenly read as 100.[41,42]

Gliclazide
- start with 40–80mg each morning with breakfast
- if necessary, increase every 3 days to a maximum of 160mg b.d.

Tolbutamide
- start with 500mg b.d. with meals
- if necessary, increase every 3 days to a maximum of 1g b.d.

Metformin
- start with 500mg each morning with breakfast
- if necessary, increase by 500mg at weekly intervals
- maximum dose = 1g t.d.s.

Repaglinide
- start with 500microgram within 30min of main meals (or 1mg in patients previously treated with an alternative oral hypoglycaemic agent)
- if necessary, increase the dose at 1–2 week intervals to a maximum of 4mg q.d.s.

Insulin
- if the patient is already taking the maximum dose of an oral hypoglycaemic, and the fasting blood glucose is > 12mmol/L, prescribe **insulin glargine** 6–12 units once daily or **isophane insulin** 6–12 units once daily:
- adjust the dose according to the response
- a preprandial variable dose scale of SC short-acting **soluble insulin** is occasionally necessary (Table 4).

Table 4 Preprandial variable dose scale of SC soluble insulin[a]

Preprandial blood glucose (mmol/L)	Insulin dose (units)
10–15	6
15–18	8
18–22	10
>22[b]	12

a. responses to insulin vary widely and variable dose scales need to be individualized
b. patients with marked hyperglycaemia should have monitoring 2h after meals as well until the blood glucose is better controlled.

Supply
This is not a complete list; see BNF for additional details.
Gliclazide (generic)
Tablets 40mg, 80mg (scored), 28 days @ 80mg each morning = £1.
Oral suspension 80mg/5mL, 150mL ≈ £141, unauthorized; available as a special order (see Appendix 1, p.817).

Tolbutamide (generic)
Tablets 500mg, 28 days @ 500mg b.d. = £4.50

Metformin (generic)
Tablets 500mg, 850mg, 28 days @ 500mg each morning = £1.
Oral solution (sugar-free) 500mg/5mL, 28 days @ 500mg each morning = £78.

Glucophage® (Merck Serono)
Oral powder 500mg or 1g/sachet, 28 days @ 500mg each morning = £3.50; *mix with 150mL water.*

Repaglinide (generic)
Tablets 500microgram, 1mg, 2mg, 28 days @ 500microgram t.d.s. = £3.50.

Insulin
Most insulin products are also available as cartridges for use with dedicated re-usable injection pen devices or as prefilled disposable pen devices.

Note all insulin products are 100 units/mL with the exception of insulin degludec which is available in strengths of 100 units/mL and 200 units/mL.

Short-acting insulin
Actrapid® (Novo Nordisk)
Injection human sequence insulin 100 units/mL, 10mL multidose vial = £7.50.

Rapid-acting insulin analogues (e.g. aspart, glulisine, lispro) are double the price.

Intermediate-acting insulin
Isophane insulin

Insulatard® (Novo Nordisk)
Injection human sequence insulin 100 units/mL, 10mL multidose vial = £7.50.

Mixed preparations of short-acting with intermediate-acting insulins are available (biphasic isophane insulin, biphasic insulin aspart, biphasic insulin lispro).

Long-acting insulin (e.g. detemir, degludec, glargine, zinc suspension)
Insulin glargine Lantus® (Sanofi-Aventis)
Injection recombinant human insulin analogue 100 units/mL, 10mL multidose vial = £31; *once daily dosing.*

1 Diabetes UK (2012) End of Life Diabetes Care: A Strategy Document Commissed by Diabetes UK. *Clinical care recommendations.* Available from: www.diabetes.org.uk
2 British National Formulary. London: BMJ Group and Pharmaceutical Press www.bnf.org (accessed November 2013).
3 MHRA (2011) Pioglitazone: risk of bladder cancer. *Drug Safety Update.* **5**. www.mhra.gov.uk/Safetyinformation
4 National Collaborating Centre for Chronic Conditions (2008) *Type 2 diabetes: national clinical guideline for management in primary and secondary care (update).* London: Royal College of Physicians and NICE 2009.
5 Holman N et al. (2011) The Association of Public Health Observatories (APHO) Diabetes Prevalence Model: estimates of total diabetes prevalence for England, 2010–2030. *Diabetic Medicine.* **28**: 575–582.
6 McCoubrie R et al. (2005) Managing diabetes mellitus in patients with advanced cancer: a case note audit and guidelines. *European Journal of Cancer Care (Engl).* **14**: 244–248.
7 Glicksman A and Rawson R (1956) Diabetes and altered carbohydrate metabolism in patients with cancer. *Cancer.* **9**: 1127–1134.
8 Poulson J (1997) The management of diabetes in patients with advanced cancer. *Journal of Pain and Symptom Management.* **13**: 339–346.
9 Twycross R et al. (2009) *Symptom Management in Advanced Cancer* (4e). palliativedrugs.com Nottingham, pp. 221–225.
10 NHS Diabetes (2011) Use of Haemoglobin A1c (HbA$_{1c}$) in the diagnosis of diabetes mellitus: the implementation of World Health Organisation (WHO) guidance 2011. Available from: www.diabetes.nhs.uk
11 ADA (2012) Standards of medical care in diabetes. *Diabetes Care.* **35 (Suppl 1)**: 11–63.
12 International Expert Committee (2009) International Expert Committee report on the role of the A1C assay in the diagnosis of diabetes. *Diabetes Care.* **32**: 1327–1334.
13 Heinemann L et al. (2000) Time-action profile of the long-acting insulin analog insulin glargine (HOE901) in comparison with those of NPH insulin and placebo. *Diabetes Care.* **23**: 644–649.
14 Loke YK et al. (2011) Comparative cardiovascular effects of thiazolidinediones: systematic review and meta analysis of observational studies. *British Medical Journal.* **342**: d1309.
15 NICE (2010) The management of type 2 diabetes. *Clinical guideline.* CG87: Issued May 2009 updated September 2010 www.nice.org.uk
16 NICE (2010) Liraglutide for the treatment of type 2 diabetes mellitus. *Technology appraisal.* TA203. www.nice.org.uk
17 Li L et al. (2014) Incretin treatment and risk of pancreatitis in patients with type 2 diabetes mellitus: systematic review and meta-analysis of randomised and non-randomised studies. *British Medical Journal.* **348**: 2366.
18 Faillie JL et al. (2014) Incretin based drugs and risk of acute pancreatitis in patients with type 2 diabetes: cohort study. *British Medical Journal.* **348**: 2780.
19 Cohen D (2013) Has pancreatic damage from GLP-1diabetic drugs been underplayed? *British Medical Journal.* **346**: 16–21.
20 EMA (2013) Assessment report for GLP-1 based therapies. EMA/474117/2013. www.ema.europa.eu
21 ADA (American Diabetes Association) (2008) Diagnosis and classification of diabetes mellitus. *Diabetes Care.* **31 (Suppl 1)**: S55–60.
22 Salpeter S et al. (2003) Risk of fatal and nonfatal lactic acidosis with metformin use in type 2 diabetes mellitus. *Cochrane Database of Systematic Reviews.* CD002967.
23 Loke YK et al. (2009) Long-term use of thiazolidinediones and fractures in type 2 diabetes: a meta-analysis. *Canadian Medical Association Journal.* **180**: 32–39.
24 Habib ZA et al. (2010) Thiazolidinedione use and the longitudinal risk of fractures in patients with type 2 diabetes mellitus. *Journal of Clinical Endocrinology and Metabolism.* **95**: 592–600.
25 Yki-Jarvinen H et al. (1992) Comparison of insulin regimens in patients with non-insulin-dependent diabetes mellitus. *N Engl J Med.* **327**: 1426–1433.
26 National Patient Safety Agency (2011) The adult patient's passport for safer use of insulin. *Patient safety Alert.* NPSA/2011/PSA003. www.nrls.npsa.nhs.uk
27 Anonymous (2012) Insulin pump therapy. *Drug and Therapeutics Bulletin.* **50**: 105–108.
28 Angelo M et al. (2011) An approach to diabetes mellitus in hospice and palliative medicine. *Journal of Palliative Medicine.* **14**: 83–87.
29 Vandenhaute V (2010) Palliative Care and Type II Diabetes: A Need for New Guidelines? . *American Journal of Hospice and Palliative Care.* **27**: 444–445.
30 McCann M-A et al. (2006) Practical management of diabetes mellitus. *European Journal of Palliative Care.* **13**: 226–229.
31 Ciardullo AV et al. (2006) Effectiveness and safety of insulin glargine in the therapy of complicated or secondary diabetes: clinical audit. *Acta Diabetol.* **43**: 57–60.
32 NHS Diabetes (2010) Diabetes. The hospital management of hypoglycaemia in adults with diabetes mellitus. Available from: www.diabetes.nhs.uk/
33 Kilvert A et al. (2010) Diabetes and end of life care. Association of British Clinical Diabetologists. *ABCD Position Statement.* Available from: www.diabetologists-abcd.org.uk/
34 King EJ et al. (2012) The management of diabetes in terminal illness related to cancer. *Quarterly Journal of Medicine.* **105**: 3–9.
35 Pilkey J et al. (2012) Corticosteroid-induced diabetes in palliative care. *Journal of Palliative Medicine.* **15**: 681–689.
36 van der Linden MW et al. (2009) Topical corticosteroids and the risk of diabetes mellitus: a nested case-control study in the Netherlands. *Drug Safety.* **32**: 527–537.
37 Oyer DS et al. (2006) How to manage steroid diabetes in the patient with cancer. *Journal of Supportive Oncology.* **4**: 479–483.

38 DCCT (1993) The effect of intensive treatment of diabetes on the development and progression of long-term complications in insulin-dependent diabetes mellitus. The Diabetes Control and Complications Trial Research Group. *New England Journal of Medicine.* **329**: 977–986.
39 NHS Diabetes (2011) Recognition, treatment and prevention of hypoglycaemia in the community. Available from: http://www.diabetes.nhs.uk/
40 Holroyde C *et al.* (1975) Altered glucose metabolism in metastatic carcinoma. *Cancer Research.* **35**: 3710–3714.
41 National Patient Safety Agency (2010) Safer administration of insulin. *Patient Safety Alert.* NPSA/2010/RRR13. www.nrls.npsa.nhs.uk
42 NHS Diabetes (2010) Safe and Effective Use of Insulin in Hospitalised Patients. Available from: www.diabetes.nhs.uk

Updated (minor change) June 2014

*OCTREOTIDE   BNF 8.3.4.3

Class: Synthetic hormone.

Indications: Symptoms associated with unresectable hormone-secreting tumours, e.g. carcinoid, VIPomas, glucagonomas and acromegaly; prevention of complications after elective pancreatic surgery;[1] †salivary and enterocutaneous fistulas;[2,3] †intractable diarrhoea related to high output ileostomies,[4,5] AIDS, radiation therapy, chemotherapy or bone marrow transplant;[6–10] †inoperable bowel obstruction in patients with cancer;[11,12] †hypertrophic pulmonary osteo-arthropathy;[13] †ascites in cirrhosis and cancer;[14–16] †buccal fistula;[17] †death rattle (noisy respiratory secretions); †bronchorrhoea;[18] †reduction of tumour-related secretions.[16]

Pharmacology

Octreotide (and **lanreotide**) is a synthetic analogue of somatostatin with a longer duration of action.[19] Somatostatin is an inhibitory hormone found throughout the body. In the hypothalamus it inhibits the release of growth hormone, TSH, prolactin and ACTH. It inhibits the secretion of insulin, glucagon, gastrin and other peptides of the gastro-enteropancreatic system (i.e. peptide YY, neurotensin, VIP and substance P), reducing splanchnic blood flow, portal blood flow, GI motility, gastric, pancreatic and small bowel secretion, and increasing water and electrolyte absorption.[20]

In Type 1 diabetes mellitus, octreotide decreases insulin requirements. However, in Type 2 diabetes, octreotide suppresses both insulin and glucagon release, leaving blood glucose concentrations either unchanged or slightly elevated.[21,22] Thus, octreotide (with dextrose) has been suggested as treatment for refractory sulfonylurea-induced hypoglycaemia.[23]

Somatostatin acts as an inhibitory neurotransmitter in the CNS, has anti-inflammatory and analgesic effects and also inhibits cell proliferation.[24–26] Somatostatin analogues have a direct anticancer effect and improve prognosis in patients with neuroendocrine or solid tumours of the GI tract.[27–32] The combination of somatostatin analogues and targeted anticancer therapies (e.g. tyrosine kinase inhibitors) are now used in the treatment of some neuroendocrine tumours.

There are five somatostatin receptors ($SST_{1–5}$), each mediating a different biological action of somatostatin. Neuroendocrine tumours express various receptor profiles, but generally SST_2 or SST_5 predominate.[25] Octreotide and **lanreotide** bind with high affinity to SST_2 and SST_5 and with moderate affinity to SST_3.[25] New somatostatin analogues with different receptor affinity profiles are under investigation, e.g. **pasireotide**. Potentially, these could improve symptoms which are or have become refractory to octreotide (tolerance can occur after 12–18 months of use).[31]

Various radionuclides have been linked to somatostatin analogues for either diagnostic or therapeutic purposes. The latter is still in development and requires the tumour to demonstrate high uptake on a somatostatin receptor radionuclide scan. Best results are seen in fitter patients without significant liver involvement.[31]

The inhibitory, antisecretory and absorptive effects of octreotide are utilized in a wide range of clinical settings:

Hormone-secreting tumours: octreotide improves symptoms by inhibiting hormone secretion, e.g.:
• 5HT in carcinoid (improving flushing and diarrhoea)
• VIP in VIPomas (improving diarrhoea)
• glucagon in glucagonomas (improving rash and diarrhoea).

Inoperable bowel obstruction in patients with cancer: octreotide can provide rapid improvements in nausea and vomiting. The optimal dose has not been formally identified, but reports suggest < 50% of patients respond to the typical starting dose of 300microgram/24h,[33] and 75–90% respond to 600–800microgram/24h.[12,34] Although doses of up to 1,500microgram/24h have been used,[35] a dose of 600–800microgram/24h is generally sufficient to identify those likely to respond.[34,36] Benefit is less likely in obstruction of the gastric outlet or proximal small bowel.[33,37]

In comparisons with **hyoscine butylbromide** (60–80mg/24h; p.15), octreotide (300–800microgram/24h) provides more effective and rapid improvements in nausea and vomiting and reduction in NG tube output. However, in those patients responding to either drug, after about 4–6 days, overall symptom relief is similar, and NG tube removal possible with both.[34] (Although no head-to-head comparison has been published to date, it is likely that the same is true for **glycopyrronium**, p.12). **Lanreotide** has also been successfully used in patients with bowel obstruction due to peritoneal carcinomatosis.[38]

Ascites: octreotide 300microgram SC b.d. can suppress diuretic-induced activation of the renin-aldosterone-angiotensin system. Its use has improved renal function and Na^+ and water excretion in patients with cirrhosis and ascites receiving **furosemide** and **spironolactone** (p.68).[15,39]

Octreotide is also reported to reduce the rate of formation of malignant ascites.[14,16] In a pilot RCT of depot octreotide 30mg IM monthly for malignant ascites, the median time to next paracentesis was doubled (28 vs. 14 days), although this did not reach statistical significance. Nonetheless, patients receiving octreotide had significantly less abdominal bloating, abdominal discomfort and shortness of breath.[40]

Octreotide may interfere with ascitic fluid formation in various ways, including a reduction in splanchnic blood flow, or by inhibiting vascular endothelial growth factor which increases vascular permeability and also promotes angiogenesis and tumour growth. Octreotide could be considered in patients with rapidly accumulating ascites requiring frequent paracentesis despite diuretic therapy (if indicated; see **spironolactone**, p.68) and/or when an indwelling catheter is inappropriate or declined. Octreotide may also help resolve chylous ascites and/or pleural effusion from various causes.[41–49]

Other antisecretory effects: octreotide reduces salivary production and may be of use in salivary or buccal fistulas (see **hyoscine butylbromide** p.15, **hyoscine hydrobromide** p.17, and **glycopyrronium** p.12).[2,17] Experience of its use in death rattle is limited.[50] The use of octreotide led to rapid and complete control of bronchorrhoea (> 1L/24h) in a patient with diffuse adenocarcinoma of the lung.[18]

When given in conjunction with pancreatic surgery *for cancer* (but not for other conditions), octreotide reduces the risk of complications, e.g. fistula.[1] If enterocutaneous fistulas complicate abdominal surgery, somatostatin analogues reduce the time to closure and length of hospital stay.[3] However, in a review limited to pancreatic fistula, evidence of benefit was lacking.[51]

Octreotide is recommended first-line for severe chemotherapy- or radiotherapy-induced diarrhoea (i.e. an increase of ≥7 stools/day over baseline, hospital admission and IV fluids > 24h required), and second-line for less severe diarrhoea which does not respond to **loperamide** 16–24mg/24h (p.37).[9,10] For those who have experienced severe chemotherapy-induced diarrhoea, prophylactic depot octreotide is recommended for subsequent cycles.

Octreotide has also been used for the treatment of enterovesical fistula,[52] and to improve mucous discharge from rectal cancers.[16] However, in an RCT, octreotide failed to improve diarrhoea in patients with ileal pouch anastomosis (± pouchitis) following total colectomy for ulcerative colitis.[53]

Pain: octreotide is reported to have an analgesic effect in patients with cancer, e.g. in bone pain from metastatic carcinoid, in hypertrophic pulmonary osteo-arthopathy, pain arising from GI cancer, or when given IT.[13,54–56] However, a small RCT found octreotide to be no better than placebo.[57]

The development of somatostatin analogues which have greater affinity for the receptors considered predominantly responsible for an anti-inflammatory effect (SST1, SST4) may prove more effective.[24] Octreotide may also be of value in chronic pancreatitic pain caused by hypertension in scarred ducts.[58,59] Benefit could be secondary to its antisecretory action.[60] (Suppressing exocrine function by administering **pancreatin** supplements (p.60) can also reduce pain in patients with chronic pancreatitis).[61]

Miscellaneous: at doses far below those necessary for an antisecretory effect (e.g. 1microgram SC t.d.s.), octreotide protects the stomach from NSAID-related injury, probably via its ability to reduce NSAID-induced neutrophil adhesion to the microvasculature.[62] A systematic review casts doubt on the value of octreotide in the acute management of bleeding oesophageal varices.[63]

Uncontrolled data suggest somatostatin analogues may reduce transfusion requirements in patients with angiodysplasia of the GI tract.[64] Octreotide improves tolerance to being upright, in part by reducing splanchnic blood flow. Potentially this could benefit patients with postural hypotension caused by the loss of the ability to vasoconstrict the splanchnic blood vessels in response to standing.[65] Octreotide is used as an adjunct to IV dextrose in the treatment of hypoglycaemia caused by sulfonylurea overdose.[66]

Octreotide is generally given as a SC bolus or by CSCI[67] but can be given IV when a rapid effect is required. Octreotide has also been administered IT as an analgesic.[54] A long-acting depot formulation is also available but evaluation has been generally limited to hormone-secreting tumours.[68] Benefit from depot octreotide has been reported in an RCT for the prevention of chemotherapy-related diarrhoea[6] and in cancer patients with bowel obstruction.[69,70] **Lanreotide** is available in depot formulations only.

Onset of action 30min.
Time to peak plasma concentration 30min SC.
Plasma halflife 1.5h SC.
Duration of action 8h.

Cautions

In Type 1 diabetes mellitus, **insulin** requirements may be reduced by up to 50%; monitor blood glucose concentrations to guide dose reductions with both **insulin** and oral hypoglycaemic agents. Insulinoma: may exacerbate hypoglycaemia.

Cirrhosis, renal failure requiring dialysis (both lead to reduced elimination which may necessitate a dose reduction). May cause gallstones (although the manufacturer advises ultrasound examination of the gallbladder before treatment and every 6–12 months thereafter, this is generally not necessary in palliative care). Avoid abrupt withdrawal of short-acting octreotide after long-term treatment (may precipitate biliary colic caused by gallstones/biliary sludge).

May cause bradycardia, conduction defects or arrhythmias; use with caution in at-risk patients. Monitor thyroid function during long-term treatment (may cause hypothyroidism).

Drug interactions

Octreotide increases the bio-availability of **bromocriptine** by about 40% (consider when using the combination in acromegaly).[71]

Octreotide markedly reduces plasma **ciclosporin** concentrations and inadequate immuno-suppression may result. Increase the **ciclosporin** dose by 50% before starting octreotide, and monitor the plasma concentration daily to guide further adjustments.[71]

Undesirable effects

Dry mouth, flatulence (lowers oesophageal sphincter tone), nausea, abdominal pain, diarrhoea, steatorrhoea (GI undesirable effects may be reduced by administering octreotide between meals or at bedtime), impaired glucose tolerance, hypoglycaemia (shortly after starting treatment), persistent hyperglycaemia (during long-term treatment), gallstones (10–20% of patients on long-term treatment), pancreatitis (associated with gallstones).

Dose and use

Octreotide is painful if given as a SC bolus injection. Warming the ampoule or vial to body temperature before injection by holding it in the hand reduces the pain. With CSCI, to reduce the likelihood of inflammatory reactions at the skin injection site, dilute to the largest volume possible, preferably in 0.9% saline (see p.699).

The dose varies according to the indication (Table 1). To maximize the benefit (convenience and cost) of the multidose vials, the starting doses have been given in convenient fractions of 1mg (e.g. 250–500microgram rather than 300–600microgram). If necessary, the dose should be titrated upwards; higher doses are generally well tolerated.[72] However, after the desired response has been achieved, it may be possible to reduce to a lower maintenance dose.

Table I Dose recommendations for SC octreotide

Indication	Starting dose[a]	Maximum dose[b]
Hormone-secreting tumours		
Acromegaly	100–200microgram t.d.s.	600microgram/24h[20]
Carcinoid, VIPomas, glucagonomas	50microgram once daily or b.d.	1,500microgram/24h; rarely 6,000microgram/24h[73]
Intractable diarrhoea (including that caused by chemotherapy and radiotherapy)	250–500microgram/24h	1,500microgram/24h,[9,10,74] occasionally higher
Intestinal obstruction	250–500microgram/24h	750microgram/24h, occasionally higher
Tumour-antisecretory effect	50–100microgram b.d.	600microgram/24h[16]
Ascites	250–500microgram/24h	600microgram/24h[14]
Bronchorrhoea	250–500microgram/24h[18]	
Hypertrophic pulmonary osteo-arthopathy	100microgram b.d.[13]	

a. doses 'rounded' to maximize benefit from multidose vials
b. 'unrounded' doses derived from the literature.

CSCI compatibility with other drugs: There are 2-drug compatibility data for octreotide in 0.9% saline with **diamorphine, haloperidol, hyoscine butylbromide, hyoscine hydrobromide, midazolam, morphine sulfate, ondansetron**, and **oxycodone**.
  Incompatibility may occur with **dexamethasone** or **levomepromazine**. More details and 3-drug compatibility data can be found in the extended appendix section of the on-line PCF on www.palliativedrugs.com
  For compatibility charts for mixing drugs in WFI see Appendix 3, p.821.

Depot formulation

A depot formulation of octreotide 10–30mg, given every 4 weeks is available (Sandotatin LAR®). Higher (40–60mg) or more frequently administered (3 weekly) doses are sometimes required.[72] This has a relative bio-availability of about 60% compared to SC octreotide. Generally, the depot formulation is used only when symptoms have first been controlled with SC octreotide. Patients who have not previously received SC octreotide should have a test dose of 50–100microgram SC and, provided there are no unacceptable undesirable effects, then switch to the depot injection. The starting dose for those patients with acromegaly or gastroenteropancreatic tumours who have received a test dose or who are adequately controlled is 20mg every 4 weeks. The depot formulation requires deep IM injection into the gluteal muscle; to minimise irritation use alternate sides for subsequent injections.

  In acromegaly, stop the SC dose of octreotide when the first depot injection is given; for other neuro-endocrine tumours continue the SC dose for a further 2 weeks.

  In a survey, 40% of clinicians reported the use of depot formulations in the management of cancer-related bowel obstruction.[75] There is limited published experience of their use in this setting, although benefit in a small number of patients with ovarian cancer for up to 15 months has been reported.[69] A reduction in NG tube output and symptomatic benefit is evident within 24h.[70] The use of **lanreotide** long acting injection in bowel obstruction from peritoneal carcinomatosis has recently been explored in a double-blind, placebo-controlled RCT.[38]

Lanreotide

Patients can be started directly on either of the long acting formulations. However for palliative care, use of the Somatuline Autogel® may be preferable as it is given by deep SC injection into the superior, external quadrant of the buttock:
- start with 60mg every 4 weeks for the first 3 months
- if necessary, increase to 120mg every 4 weeks.

Supply

For full details of storage and reconstitution details, see manufacturer's SPC.

For prolonged storage, keep all *unopened* ampoules, vials and pre-filled syringes in a refrigerator. Once opened, a multidose vial can be kept for up to 2 weeks at room temperature for day-to-day use.

Octreotide (generic)

Injection (as acetate) 50microgram/mL, 1mL amp = £4; 100microgram/mL, 1mL amp = £7; 500microgram/mL, 1mL amp = £34 (note: based on BNF pricing this is more expensive than proprietary Sandostatin® ampoules).

Injection (as acetate) 200microgram/mL multidose vial, 1mg in 5mL = £70.

Sandostatin® (Novartis)

Injection (as acetate) 50microgram/mL, 1mL amp = £3; 100microgram/mL, 1mL amp = £6; 500microgram/mL, 1mL amp = £27 (note: based on BNF pricing this is cheaper than generic ampoules).

Injection (as acetate) 200microgram/mL multidose vial, 1mg in 5mL = £70.

Sandostatin LAR® (Novartis)

Depot injection (microsphere powder for aqueous suspension), octreotide (as acetate) 10mg vial = £427; 20mg vial = £706; 30mg vial = £903 (all supplied with diluent filled syringe) for deep IM injection every 28 days.

Lanreotide

Somatuline LA® (Ipsen)

Long acting injection (copolymer microparticles for aqueous suspension), lanreotide (as acetate) 30mg vial (with vehicle) = £323 for IM injection every 14 days.

Somatuline Autogel® (Ipsen)

Depot injection (prefilled syringe), lanreotide (as acetate) 60mg = £551; 90mg = £736; 120mg = £937 for deep SC injection into the superior, external quadrant of the buttock every 28 days.

1 Gurusamy KS *et al.* (2012) Somatostatin analogues for pancreatic surgery. *Cochrane Database of Systematic Reviews.* **6**: CD008370.
2 Spinell C *et al.* (1995) Postoperative salivary fistula: therapeutic action of octreotide. *Surgery.* **117**: 117–118.
3 Coughlin S *et al.* (2012) Somatostatin analogues for the treatment of enterocutaneous fistulas: a systematic review and meta-analysis. *World Journal of Surgery.* **36**: 1016–1029.
4 Dorta G (1999) Role of octreotide and somatostatin in the treatment of intestinal fistulae. *Digestion.* **60 (Suppl 2)**: 53–56.
5 Farthing MJ (1994) Octreotide in the treatment of refractory diarrhoea and intestinal fistulae. *Gut.* **35 (Suppl 3)**: s5–10.
6 Rosenoff SH *et al.* (2006) A multicenter, randomized trial of long-acting octreotide for the optimum prevention of chemotherapy-induced diarrhea: results of the STOP trial. *Journal of Supportive Oncology.* **4**: 289–294.
7 Crouch M *et al.* (1996) Octreotide acetate in refractory bone marrow transplant-associated diarrhea. *Annals of Pharmacotherapy.* **30**: 331–336.
8 Harris A (1992) Octreotide in the treatment of disorders of the gastrointestinal tract. *Drug Investigation.* **4**: 1–54.
9 Benson AB *et al.* (2004) Recommended Guidelines for the Treatment of Cancer Treatment-Induced Diarrhea *Journal of Clinical Oncology.* **22**: 2918–2926.
10 Maroun JA *et al.* (2007) Prevention and management of chemotherapy-induced diarrhea in patients with colorectal cancer: a consensus statement by the Canadian Working Group on Chemotherapy-Induced Diarrhea. *Current Oncology.* **14**: 13–20.
11 Mercadante S and Porzio G (2012) Octreotide for malignant bowel obstruction: twenty years after. *Critical Reviews inOncology/Hematology.* **83**: 388–392.
12 Ripamonti C and Mercadante S (2004) How to use octreotide for malignant bowel obstruction. *Journal of Supportive Oncology.* **2**: 357–364.
13 Nguyen S and Hojjati M (2011) Review of current therapies for secondary hypertrophic pulmonary osteoarthropathy. *Clinical Rheumatology.* **30**: 7–13.
14 Cairns W and Malone R (1999) Octreotide as an agent for the relief of malignant ascites in palliative care patients. *Palliative Medicine.* **13**: 429–430.
15 Kalambokis G *et al.* (2005) Renal effects of treatment with diuretics, octreotide or both, in non-azotemic cirrhotic patients with ascites. *Nephrology, Dialysis, Transplantation.* **20**: 1623–1629.
16 Harvey M and Dunlop R (1996) Octreotide and the secretory effects of advanced cancer. *Palliative Medicine.* **10**: 346–347.
17 Lam C and Wong S (1996) Use of somatostatin analog in the management of traumatic parotid fistula. *Surgery.* **119**: 481–482.
18 Hudson E *et al.* (2006) Successful treatment of bronchorrhea with octreotide in a patient with adenocarcinoma of the lung. *Journal of Pain and Symptom Management.* **32**: 200–202.
19 Lamberts SWJ *et al.* (1996) Octreotide. *New England Journal of Medicine.* **334**: 246–254.
20 Gyr K and Meier R (1993) Pharmacodynamic effects of sandostatin in the gastrointestinal tract. *Digestion.* **54**: 14–19.
21 Davies R *et al.* (1989) Somatostatin analogues in diabetes mellitus. *Diabetic Medicine.* **6**: 103–111.
22 Lunetta M *et al.* (1997) Effects of octreotide on glycaemic control, glucose disposal, hepatic glucose production and counterregulatory hormone secretion in type 1 and type 2 insulin treated diabetic patients. *Diabetes Research and Clinical Practice.* **38**: 81–89.

23 Dougherty PP and Klein-Schwartz W (2010) Octreotide's role in the management of sulfonylurea-induced hypoglycemia. *Journal of Medical Toxicology.* **6**: 199–206.

24 Heyles Z et al. (2006) Effects of the somatostatin receptor subtype 4 selective agonist j-2156 on sensory neuropeptide and inflammatory reactions in rodents. *British Journal of Pharmacology.* **149**: 405–415.

25 Pinter E et al. (2006) Inhibitory effect of somatostatin on inflammation and nociception. *Pharmacology and Therapeutics.* **112**: 440–456.

26 Patel YC (1999) Somatostatin and its receptor family. *Frontiers in Neuroendocrinology.* **20**: 157–198.

27 Rinke A et al. (2009) Placebo-controlled, double-blind, prospective, randomized study on the effect of octreotide LAR in the control of tumor growth in patients with metastatic neuroendocrine midgut tumors: a report from the PROMID Study Group. *Journal of Clinical Oncology.* **27**: 4656–4663.

28 Deming DA et al. (2005) A dramatic response to long-acting octreotide in metastatic hepatocellular carcinoma. *Clinical Advances in Hematology and Oncology.* **3**: 468–472; discussion 472–464.

29 Kouroumalis E et al. (1998) Treatment of hepatocellular carcinoma with octreotide: a randomised controlled study. *Gut.* **42**: 442–447.

30 Cascinu S et al. (1995) A randomised trial of octreotide vs best supportive care only in advanced gastrointestinal cancer patients refractory to chemotherapy. *British Journal of Cancer.* **71**: 97–101.

31 Walter T et al. (2012) New treatment strategies in advanced neuroendocrine tumours. *Digestive and Liver Disease.* **44**: 95–105.

32 Miljkovic MD et al. (2012) Novel medical therapies of recurrent and metastatic gastroenteropancreatic neuroendocrine tumors. *Digestive Diseases and Sciences.* **57**: 9–18.

33 Shima Y et al. (2008) Clinical efficacy and safety of octreotide (SMS201-995) in terminally ill Japanese cancer patients with malignant bowel obstruction. *Japanese Journal of Clinical Oncology.* **38**: 354–359.

34 Mystakidou K et al. (2002) Comparison of octreotide administration vs conservative treatment in the management of inoperable bowel obstruction in patients with far advanced cancer: a randomized, double-blind, controlled clinical trial. *Anticancer Research.* **22**: 1187–1192.

35 Weber C and Zulian GB (2009) Malignant irreversible intestinal obstruction: the powerful association of octreotide to corticosteroids, antiemetics, and analgesics. *American Journal of Hospice and Palliative Care.* **26**: 84–88.

36 Riley J and Fallon M (1994) Octreotide in terminal malignant obstruction of the gastrointestinal tract. *European Journal of Palliative Care.* **1**: 23–25.

37 Hisanaga T et al. (2010) Multicenter prospective study on efficacy and safety of octreotide for inoperable malignant bowel obstruction. *Japanese Journal of Clinical Oncology.* **40**: 739–745.

38 Mariani P et al. (2012) Symptomatic Treatment With Lanreotide Microparticles in Inoperable Bowel Obstruction Resulting From Peritoneal Carcinomatosis: A Randomized, Double-Blind, Placebo-Controlled Phase III Study. *Journal of Clinical Oncology.* **30**: 4337–4343.

39 Kalambokis G et al. (2006) The effects of treatment with octreotide, diuretics, or both on portal hemodynamics in nonazotemic cirrhotic patients with ascites. *Journal of Clinical Gastroenterology.* **40**: 342–346.

40 Jatoi A et al. (2012) A pilot study of long-acting octreotide for symptomatic malignant ascites. *Oncology.* **82**: 315–320.

41 Yildirim AE et al. (2011) Idiopathic chylous ascites treated with total parenteral nutrition and octreotide. A case report and review of the literature. *European Journal of Gastroenterology and Hepatology.* **23**: 961–963.

42 Widjaja A et al. (1999) Octreotide for therapy of chylous ascites in yellow nail syndrome. *Gastroenterology.* **116**: 1017–1018.

43 Ferrandiere M et al. (2000) Chylous ascites following radical nephrectomy: efficacy of octreotide as treatment of ruptured thoracic duct. *Intensive Care and Medicine.* **26**: 484–485.

44 Sharkey AJ and Rao JN (2012) The successful use of octreotide in the treatment of traumatic chylothorax. *Texas Heart Institute Journal.* **39**: 428–430.

45 Zhou DX et al. (2009) The effectiveness of the treatment of octreotide on chylous ascites after liver cirrhosis. *Digestive Diseases and Sciences.* **54**: 1783–1788.

46 Pfammatter R et al. (2001) Treatment of hepatic hydrothorax and reduction of chest tube output with octreotide. *European Journal of Gastroenterology and Hepatology.* **13**: 977–980.

47 Dumortier J et al. (2000) Successful treatment of hepatic hydrothorax with octreotide. *European Journal of Gastroenterology and Hepatology.* **12**: 817–820.

48 Lee PH et al. (2005) Octreotide therapy for chylous ascites in a chronic dialysis patient. *Nephrology (Carlton).* **10**: 344–347.

49 Mincher L et al. (2005) The successful treatment of chylous effusions in malignant disease with octreotide. *Clinical Oncology.* **17**: 118–121.

50 Clark K et al. (2008) A pilot phase II randomized, cross-over, double-blinded, controlled efficacy study of octreotide versus hyoscine hydrobromide for control of noisy breathing at the end-of-life. *Journal of Pain and Palliative Care Pharmacotherapy.* **22**: 131–138.

51 Gans SL et al. (2012) Systematic review and meta-analysis of somatostatin analogues for the treatment of pancreatic fistula. *British Journal of Surgery.* **99**: 754–760.

52 Shinjo T et al. (2009) Treatment of malignant enterovesical fistula with octreotide. *Journal of Palliative Medicine.* **12**: 965–967.

53 Van Assche G et al. (2012) Octreotide for the treatment of diarrhoea in patients with ileal pouch anal anastomosis: a placebo-controlled crossover study. *Colorectal Disease.* **14**: 181–186.

54 Penn RD et al. (1992) Octreotide: A potent new nonopiate analgesic for intrathecal infusion. *Pain.* **49**: 13–19.

55 Befon S et al. (2000) Continuous subcutaneous octreotide in gastrointestinal cancer patients: pain control and beta-endorphin levels. *Anticancer Research.* **20**: 4039–4046.

56 Katai M et al. (2005) Octreotide as a rapid and effective painkiller for metastatic carcinoid tumor. *Endocrine Journal.* **52**: 277–280.

57 De-Conno F et al. (1994) Subcutaneous octreotide in the treatment of pain in advanced cancer patients. *Journal of Pain and Symptom Management.* **9**: 34–38.

58 Donnelly PK et al. (1991) Somatostatin for chronic pancreatic pain. *Journal of Pain and Symptom Management.* **6**: 349–350.

59 Okazaki K et al. (1988) Pressure of papillary zone and pancreatic main duct in patients with chronic pancreatitis in the early state. *Scandinavian Journal of Gastroenterology.* **23**: 501–506.

60 Lembcke B et al. (1987) Effect of the somatostatin analogue sandostatin on gastrointestinal, pancreatic and biliary function and hormone release in man. *Digestion.* **36**: 108–124.

61 Draganov P and Toskes PP (2004) Chronic pancreatitis: controversies in etiology, diagnosis and treatment. *Revista Espanola de Enfermedades Digestivas.* **96**: 649–659.

62 Scheiman J et al. (1997) Reduction of NSAID induced gastric injury and leucocyte endothelial adhesion by octreotide. *Gut.* **40**: 720–725.

63 Gotzsche PC and Hrobjartsson A (2008) Somatostatin analogues for acute bleeding oesophageal varices. *Cochrane Database of Systematic Reviews.* **3**: CD000193.

64 Brown C et al. (2010) Somatostatin analogues in the treatment of recurrent bleeding from gastrointestinal vascular malformations: an overview and systematic review of prospective observational studies. *Dig Dis Sci.* **55**: 2129–2134.

65 Jarvis SS et al. (2012) A somatostatin analog improves tilt table tolerance by decreasing splanchnic vascular conductance. *Journal of Applied Physiology.* **112**: 1504–1511.

66 Glatstein M et al. (2012) Octreotide for the treatment of sulfonylurea poisoning. *Clinical Toxicology.* **50**: 795–804.

67 Mercadante S (1995) Tolerability of continuous subcutaneous octreotide used in combination with other drugs. *Journal of Palliative Care.* **11 (4)**: 14–16.

68 Scherubl H et al. (1994) Treatment of the carcinoid syndrome with a depot formulation of the somatostatin analogue lanreotide. *European Journal of Cancer.* **30A**: 1590–1591.

69 Matulonis UA et al. (2005) Long-acting octreotide for the treatment and symptomatic relief of bowel obstruction in advanced ovarian cancer. *Journal of Pain and Symptom Management.* **30**: 563–569.

70 Massacesi C and Galeazzi G (2006) Sustained release octreotide may have a role in the treatment of malignant bowel obstruction. *Journal of Palliative Medicine.* **20**: 715–716.

71 Baxter K (ed) (2008) Stockley's Drug Interactions. (8e). Pharmaceutical Press, London.

72 Ludlam WH and Anthony L (2011) Safety review: dose optimization of somatostatin analogs in patients with acromegaly and neuroendocrine tumors. *Advances in Therapy.* **28**: 825–841.

73 Harris A and Redfern J (1995) Octreotide treatment of carcinoid syndrome: analysis of published dose-titration data. *Alimentary Pharmacology and Therapeutics.* **9**: 387–394.

74 Cello J et al. (1991) Effect of octreotide on refractory AIDS-associated diarrhea. A prospective, multicenter clinical trial. *Annals of Internal Medicine.* **115**: 705–710.

75 Palliativedrugs.com (2010) Octreotide - What is your experience? Available from: www.palliativedrugs.com/download/100401_octreotide.pdf

Updated (minor change) June 2014

PROGESTOGENS BNF 6.4.1.2 & 8.3.2

Class: Sex hormones.

Indications: Authorized indications vary between products; consult SPC for details. Hormone therapy in endometrial cancer (use in breast, prostate and renal cancer has diminished);[1] anovulatory uterine bleeding; secondary amenorrhoea; mild–moderate endometriosis; †anorexia and cachexia in cancer and AIDS; †post-castration hot flushes in both women and men.

Contra-indications: Medroxyprogesterone acetate (**MPA**): oestrogen-progestogen-dependent cancer, hepatic impairment, history of (or high risk of developing) thrombo-embolism, active thrombophlebitis, undiagnosed abnormal vaginal bleeding, pregnancy (known or suspected).

Pharmacology

In addition to natural **progesterone**, there are several classes of synthetic progestogens, e.g. derivatives of retroprogesterone, progesterone, and 17α-hydroxyprogesterone (**cyproterone, MPA, megestrol acetate**).[2] Whereas all derivatives have a progestogenic effect on the uterus, there are differences in other biological effects (Table 1).

Table 1 Comparison of the biological effects of natural progesterone and selected synthetic progestogens[2]

Progestogen	Effect[a]		
	Androgenic	Anti-androgenic	Anti-mineralocorticoid
Progesterone	−	+	+
Cyproterone acetate	−	++	−
Megestrol acetate	+	+	−
MPA	+	−	−

++ = effect present; + = weak effect; − = no effect.

a. all the above possess similar progestogenic, anti-gonadotrophic, anti-oestrogenic and glucocorticoid effects.

In palliative care, progestogens are used mainly in selected patients with cachexia-anorexia, although their efficacy in cachexia is debatable (see next section). Progestogens may improve appetite by increasing levels of orexigenic neurotransmitters in the hypothalamus (e.g. neuropeptide Y), counteracting the anorexic effects of cytokines on the hypothalamus, or by interfering with the production of cytokines via their glucocorticoid anti-inflammatory effect.[3,4] In vitro, cytokine release from peripheral blood mononucleocytes are inhibited by both **MPA** and **megestrol acetate** in concentrations that would be achieved by daily doses of 1,500–2,000mg and 320–960mg respectively.[3] The release of serotonin was also inhibited and was considered one possible mechanism by which progestogens have an anti-emetic effect.[3]

Bio-availability of **MPA** and **megestrol acetate** is low (Table 2). Both **MPA** and **megestrol acetate** are highly protein-bound, mainly to albumin. **MPA** is metabolized extensively in the liver, and excreted mainly as glucuronides, whereas **megestrol acetate** is excreted mainly unchanged in the urine.

Table 2 Selected pharmacokinetic data[5,6]

	Medroxyprogesterone acetate	Megestrol acetate
Bio-availability	1–10%	No absolute data; reduced by 25% in fasting state
Time to peak plasma concentration	2–7h	3–5h
Plasma halflife	38–46h	24–42h

Cachexia and anorexia

Cachexia is common in cancer and other chronic diseases, impairing quality of life and increasing morbidity and mortality.[7] Cachexia is characterized by the loss of skeletal muscle ± body fat that cannot be fully reversed by conventional nutritional support. Loss of skeletal muscle is associated with impaired physical function and quality of life, whereas loss of fat (the body's main energy store) is associated with reduced survival. Recommended diagnostic criteria for cancer cachexia are:
- involuntary weight loss > 5% in the past 6 months, or
- weight loss > 2% in patients with either a BMI of < 20kg/m^2 or skeletal muscle sarcopenia (absolute muscularity < 5th centile of gender-specific norm).[8]

In cancer, a negative protein and energy balance is driven by the combination of reduced food intake (anorexia) and abnormal host metabolism resulting from factors produced by the cancer, e.g. proteolysis-inducing factor, or by the host in response to the cancer, e.g. cytokines.[9] One outcome of this is a chronic inflammatory state, as evidenced by a raised serum CRP, the level of which relates to the degree and rate of weight loss.[10] Cytokines such as interleukin-1 and tumour necrosis factor-α act on the hypothalamus and skeletal muscle leading to anorexia, inefficient energy expenditure, wasting of skeletal muscle and loss of body fat. Management needs to address both the reduced nutritional intake and the abnormal host metabolism; increasing nutritional intake alone is generally ineffective.[9,11–13]

Recent recommendations emphasize the importance of early identification and intervention, and recognize that once cancer cachexia is advanced (patient has severe muscle wasting, ongoing catabolism, WHO performance status 3–4, metastatic disease refractory to therapy and a prognosis of < 3 months) a response to treatment is unlikely, and that the focus in these circumstances should be on symptom relief and psychosocial support.[8]

Megestrol acetate is used to stimulate appetite and weight gain. A recent systematic review included 35 RCTs, totalling about 4,000 patients, mostly with cancer, AIDS (n = 475) or other conditions (n = 270).[14] It concluded that the quality of the evidence was very low. Nonetheless, when compared with placebo, **megestrol acetate** increased appetite in about 1/4 and weight (≈2kg) in about 1/12, but not overall quality of life. There was little difference in efficacy when compared with other drugs, e.g. **prednisolone**, except in patients with cancer where **megestrol acetate** resulted in greater weight gain. For appetite stimulation, 160mg/day is probably the optimum dose; for weight gain higher doses (480mg) appear more effective.[14] However, the RCTs used body weight as a primary outcome measure; none accurately evaluated changes in body composition (see below). Data from individual RCTs indicates that impotence occurred in 10–25% of men.[4,15–22] Further, oedema, thrombo-embolism and deaths were more frequent in the patients treated with **megestrol acetate**.[14] Similar findings were reported in a study in frail elderly patients[23] and, in consequence, enthusiasm for its use in this setting has declined.

In studies which have evaluated body composition, both **megestrol acetate** and **MPA** appear to increase fat mass, but not fat-free mass, the part which includes skeletal muscle.[4,15,16,24] Thus it is likely that the gain in weight with progestogens (and corticosteroids), rather than representing the ideal increase in skeletal muscle *and* fat, is a less helpful retention of fluid or increase in fat only. This could make mobilizing more difficult in an already debilitated patient. In addition, the catabolic effect of progestogens on skeletal muscle could further weaken the patient. Catabolism may result from the glucocorticoid effect of progestogens but they also suppress the amount and function of testosterone, which is anabolic.

Progestogens are much more expensive than **dexamethasone** or **prednisolone**. **Megestrol acetate** 800mg/day and **dexamethasone** 3mg/day are comparable with regard to appetite stimulation and non-fluid weight gain, although the latter was not accurately evaluated.[25] In this study, a high proportion of patients discontinued **dexamethasone** (36%) or **megestrol acetate** (25%) because of undesirable effects. **Dexamethasone** was more likely to cause cushingoid changes, myopathy, heartburn and peptic ulcers; **megestrol acetate** was associated with increased thrombo-embolism.[25] **Dexamethasone** is a fluorinated corticosteroid, a class which is more prone to cause muscle catabolism.[26] Thus, ideally, **dexamethasone** should be limited to short-term use only.

If long-term use of a corticosteroid is contemplated, a switch to the non-fluorinated **prednisolone** 10–20mg/day should be considered.[4] However, for patients expected to live months rather than weeks, progestogens may be more appropriate. Caution is still required as long-term progestogens can also cause cushingoid changes (25% of patients after 3 months in one study),[27] muscle catabolism and suppression of the hypothalamic-pituitary-adrenal axis. The latter may present with non-specific symptoms and a high level of clinical suspicion is required.[28] Additional corticosteroid replacement therapy would be a reasonable precaution in patients with serious infections or undergoing surgery.[4,29,30] Adrenal suppression is secondary to a central glucocorticoid effect on the hypothalamus and is dose-related; maximal suppression is seen with daily doses of **megestrol acetate** 200mg and **MPA** 1,000mg.[27]

In an attempt to improve outcomes, progestogens have been combined with other drugs, with the best evidence available for NSAIDs, e.g.:
- **megestrol acetate** 160mg t.d.s. + **ibuprofen** 400mg t.d.s.[31]
- **MPA** 500mg b.d. + **celecoxib** 200mg b.d.[32]
- **megestrol acetate** 160mg b.d. + **celecoxib** 300mg daily + l-carnitine + antioxidants.

Note: in this study **celecoxib** was administered as 200mg once daily alternating with 400mg once daily, but this is unnecessary if both 100mg and 200mg tablets are available.[33]

NSAIDs provide benefit by reducing the chronic inflammatory response, and some have used **indometacin** or **celecoxib** alone.[34,35] Compared with progestogen alone, the combinations lead to greater improvements in fatigue, quality of life and lean body mass.[33] However, similar benefit is obtained with the combination of **celecoxib** + l-carnitine + antioxidants with or without **megestrol acetate**, suggesting the latter adds relatively little.[36]

In conclusion, progestogens and systemic corticosteroids (see p.499) are useful *appetite stimulants* which can increase calorie intake and as such may be indicated in selected patients for anorexia. Progestogens may be better for long-term use than corticosteroids, but significant undesirable effects can occur. Starting doses should be low and titrated to the lowest effective dose. Both progestogens and corticosteroids are best *not* regarded as 'anticachexia' agents; any weight gain is likely to be because of an increase in fat and fluid retention, and the catabolism of skeletal muscle *increased*, particularly in inactive people.

Cautions

May suppress the hypothalamic-pituitary-adrenal axis.[37] Possibility of glucocorticoid effects. May cause or worsen diabetes mellitus.

MPA: discontinue if any of the following develop: jaundice, hepatic impairment, significant increase in blood pressure, thrombo-embolic event (e.g. stroke, myocardial infarction, DVT, pulmonary embolism), new onset migraine, severe visual disturbances. May exacerbate hypercalcaemia, migraine, epilepsy, asthma, cardiac and renal impairment.

Megestrol acetate: history of thrombophlebitis, severe hepatic impairment.

Undesirable effects

Thrombo-embolism (5%).

Frequency not stated: hyperglycaemia, depression, insomnia, fatigue, hypertension, oedema/fluid retention, nausea, vomiting, constipation, cushingoid changes, bone mineral density loss, reduced libido, impotence, altered menstruation, breast tenderness, urticaria, acne.

Rare (<0.1%): jaundice, alopecia, hirsutism.

Dose and use
Appetite stimulation

Given the relatively poor benefit:risk ratio (see above), the use of progestogens requires careful consideration, particularly in patients with conditions other than cancer or AIDS:

- start with **megestrol acetate** 80–160mg PO each morning
- if initial response poor, consider doubling the dose after 2 weeks[38,39]
- maximum dose generally 800mg PO/24h.

MPA 400mg PO each morning–b.d. is an alternative in countries where higher strength tablets are available (e.g. 100mg, 200mg and 400mg).

Hot flushes after surgical or chemical castration

- **MPA** 5–20mg b.d.–q.d.s. or
- **megestrol acetate** 80mg each morning; 40mg is used in countries where the 40mg tablet or oral suspension is readily available. The effect manifests after 2–4 weeks.[40]

Supply

Megestrol acetate
Megace® (Bristol-Myers Squibb)
Tablets (scored) 160mg, 28 days @ 160mg each morning = £20.
Tablets 40mg, 28 days @ 40mg each morning = £83 (unauthorized in the UK, can import via IDIS, 100 tablets = £296, see Appendix 1, p.817).
Oral suspension 40mg/mL, 28 days @ 160mg each morning = £127 (unauthorized in UK, can import via IDIS, 240mL bottle = £250, see Appendix 1, p.817).

Medroxyprogesterone acetate
Provera® (Pharmacia)
Tablets 2.5mg, 5mg, 10mg, 100mg, 200mg, 400mg, 28 days @ 5mg b.d. = £7; 28 days @ 400mg each morning = £59.

Climanor® (Resource Medical)
Tablets 5mg, 28 days @ 5mg b.d. = £7.

1 Decruze SB and Green JA (2007) Hormone therapy in advanced and recurrent endometrial cancer: a systematic review. *International Journal of Gynecology Cancer.* **17**: 964–978.
2 Schindler AE et al. (2003) Classification and pharmacology of progestins. *Maturitas.* **46 (Suppl 1)**: s7–s16.
3 Mantovani G et al. (1998) Cytokine involvement in cancer anorexia/cachexia: role of megestrol acetate and medroxyprogesterone acetate on cytokine downregulation and improvement of clinical symptoms. *Critical Reviews in Oncogenesis.* **9**: 99–106.
4 MacDonald N (2005) Anorexia-cachexia syndrome. *European Journal of Palliative Care.* **12 (Suppl)**: 8s–14s.
5 Par Pharmaceuticals *Data on file.*
6 Deschamps B et al. (2009) Food effect on the bioavailability of two distinct formulations of megestrol acetate oral suspension. *International Journal of Nanomedicine.* **4**: 185–192.
7 Laviano A et al. (2003) Cancer anorexia: clinical implications, pathogenesis, and therapeutic strategies. *Lancet Oncology.* **4**: 686–694.
8 Fearon K et al. (2010) Definition and classification of cancer cachexia: an international consensus framework. *Lancet Oncology.* **12**: 489–495.
9 Gordon JN et al. (2005) Cancer cachexia. *Quarterly Journal of Medicine.* **98**: 779–788.
10 Scott HR et al. (2002) The systemic inflammatory response, weight loss, performance status and survival in patients with inoperable non-small cell lung cancer. *British Journal of Cancer.* **87**: 264–267.
11 Davis MP et al. (2004) Appetite and cancer-associated anorexia: a review. *Journal of Clinical Oncology.* **22**: 1510–1517.
12 Ramos EJ et al. (2004) Cancer anorexia-cachexia syndrome: cytokines and neuropeptides. *Current Opinion in Clinical Nutrition and Metabolic Care.* **7**: 427–434.
13 Laviano A et al. (2005) Therapy insight: Cancer anorexia-cachexia syndrome–when all you can eat is yourself. *Nature Clinical Practice Oncology.* **2**: 158–165.

14 Ruiz Garcia V et al. (2013) Megestrol acetate for treatment of anorexia-cachexia syndrome. *Cochrane Database of Systemic Reviews.* **3**: CD004310.

15 Loprinzi CL et al. (1993) Phase III evaluation of four doses of megestrol acetate as therapy for patients with cancer anorexia and/or cachexia. *Journal of Clinical Oncology.* **11**: 762–767.

16 Simons JP et al. (1998) Effects of medroxyprogesterone acetate on food intake, body composition, and resting energy expenditure in patients with advanced, nonhormone-sensitive cancer: a randomized, placebo-controlled trial. *Cancer.* **82**: 553–560.

17 Jatoi A et al. (2002) Dronabinol versus megestrol acetate versus combination therapy for cancer-associated anorexia: a North Central Cancer Treatment Group study. *Journal of Clinical Oncology.* **20**: 567–573.

18 Jatoi A et al. (2003) On appetite and its loss. *Journal of Clinical Oncology.* **21 (Suppl 9)**: 79–81.

19 Jatoi A et al. (2004) An eicosapentaenoic acid supplement versus megestrol acetate versus both for patients with cancer-associated wasting: a North Central Cancer Treatment Group and National Cancer Institute of Canada collaborative effort. *Journal of Clinical Oncology.* **22**: 2469–2476.

20 Kropsky B et al. (2003) Incidence of deep-venous thrombosis in nursing home residents using megestrol acetate. *Journal of the American Medical Directors Association.* **4**: 255–256.

21 Garcia VR and Juan O (2005) Megestrol acetate-probably less effective than has been reported! *Journal of Pain and Symptom Management.* **30**: 4; author reply 5–6.

22 Payne C (2012) Interventions for fatigue and weight loss in adults with advanced progressive illness. *Cochrane Database of Systematic Reviews.* **1**: CD008427.

23 Bodenner D et al. (2007) A retrospective study of the association between megestrol acetate administration and mortality among nursing home residents with clinically significant weight loss. *American Journal Geriatric Pharmacotherapy.* **5**: 137–146.

24 Loprinzi C et al. (1993) Body-composition changes in patients who gain weight while receiving megestrol acetate. *Journal of Clinical Oncology.* **11**: 152–154.

25 Loprinzi CL et al. (1999) Randomized comparison of megestrol acetate versus dexamethasone versus fluoxymesterone for the treatment of cancer anorexia/cachexia. *Journal of Clinical Oncology.* **17**: 3299–3306.

26 Faludi G et al. (1966) Factors influencing the development of steroid-induced myopathies. *Annals of the New York Academy of Sciences.* **138**: 62–72.

27 Willemse PH et al. (1990) A randomized comparison of megestrol acetate (MA) and medroxyprogesterone acetate (MPA) in patients with advanced breast cancer. *European Journal of Cancer.* **26**: 337–343.

28 Dev R et al. (2007) Association between megestrol acetate treatment and symptomatic adrenal insufficiency with hypogonadism in male patients with cancer. *Cancer.* **110**: 1173–1177.

29 Naing KK et al. (1999) Megestrol acetate therapy and secondary adrenal suppression. *Cancer.* **86**: 1044–1049.

30 Lambert C et al. (2002) Effects of testosterone replacement and/or resistance exercise on the composition of megestrol acetate stimulated weight gain in elderly men: a randomized controlled trial. *Journal of Clinical Endocrinology and Metabolism.* **87**: 2100–2106.

31 McMillan DC et al. (1999) A prospective randomized study of megestrol acetate and ibuprofen in gastrointestinal cancer patients with weight loss. *British Journal of Cancer.* **79**: 495–500.

32 Cerchietti LC et al. (2004) Effects of celecoxib, medroxyprogesterone, and dietary intervention on systemic syndromes in patients with advanced lung adenocarcinoma: a pilot study. *Journal of Pain and Symptom Management.* **27**: 85–95.

33 Maccio A et al. (2012) A randomized phase III clinical trial of a combined treatment for cachexia in patients with gynecological cancers: evaluating the impact on metabolic and inflammatory profiles and quality of life. *Gynecologic Oncology.* **124**: 417–425.

34 Bosaeus I et al. (2002) Dietary intake, resting energy expenditure, weight loss and survival in cancer patients. *Journal of Nutrition.* **132 (Suppl 11)**: 3465s–3466s.

35 Lai V et al. (2008) Results of a pilot study of the effects of celecoxib on cancer cachexia in patients with cancer of the head, neck, and gastrointestinal tract. *Head & Neck.* **30**: 67–74.

36 Madeddu C et al. (2012) Randomized phase III clinical trial of a combined treatment with carnitine + celecoxib +/- megestrol acetate for patients with cancer-related anorexia/cachexia syndrome. *Clinical Nutrition.* **31**: 176–182.

37 Villarroel et al. (2008) Megestrol acetate-induced adrenal insufficiency. *Clinical Translational Oncology.* **10**: 235–237.

38 Donnelly S and Walsh TD (1995) Low-dose megestrol acetate for appetite stimulation in advanced cancer. *Journal of Pain and Symptom Management.* **10**: 182–183.

39 Vadell C et al. (1998) Anticachectic efficacy of megestrol acetate at different doses and versus placebo in patients with neoplastic cachexia. *American Journal of Clinical Oncology.* **21**: 347–351.

40 Loprinzi CL et al. (1996) Megestrol acetate for the prevention of hot flashes. *New England Journal of Medicine.* **331**: 347–352.

Updated (minor change) May 2014

DANAZOL   BNF 6.7.2

Class: Anabolic steroid, 17α-alkyl androgen.

Indications: Endometriosis, severe pain in benign fibrocystic breast disease, †hereditary angioedema,[1,2] †pruritus associated with obstructive jaundice, †idiopathic immune thrombocytopenia, †gynaecomastia.

Contra-indications: Thrombo-embolic disorders; severe cardiac, hepatic or renal impairment (*except when indicated for* cholestatic pruritus, see p.797; androgen-dependent tumour; undiagnosed genital bleeding; porphyria; pregnancy; breast-feeding.

Pharmacology

Danazol is a chemically modified testosterone. It suppresses the pituitary-ovarian axis by inhibiting the pituitary output of gonadotrophins. The beneficial effect of 17α-alkyl androgens in hepatic (cholestatic) pruritus was discovered serendipitously some 60 years ago when the co-incidental use of **methyltestosterone** in a patient with primary biliary cirrhosis resulted in relief from the associated pruritus.[3] Hepatic pruritus is central in origin and is associated with enhanced opioidergic tone, secondary to the increased production of endogenous opioids.[4-6] In intrahepatic cholestasis, an opioid antagonist such as **naloxone** or **naltrexone** (see p.450) is the treatment of choice.[7]

It is possible that, when opioids are needed for concurrent cancer pain, a 17α-alkyl androgen is one alternative.[8] The mechanism of action is uncertain, but 17α-alkyl androgens are directly toxic to hepatocytes.[9-11] Thus, it is possible that danazol causes focal cell damage which limits the ability of the cholestatic liver to produce enkephalins. Androgens themselves can cause cholestatic jaundice,[12,13] and have occasionally caused severe hepatic impairment.[14,15] By mouth, 17α-alkyl androgens (e.g. **methyltestosterone**) are more bio-available than other androgens (e.g. **testosterone**) because of the reduction in first-pass hepatic metabolism in androgens with a 17α-alkyl radical.[16] Danazol also has additional effects on the liver which are not shared by **testosterone**.[17] The antipruritic effect is maintained even if the cholestasis is exacerbated by the androgen itself.[16] Androgens and oestrogens sometimes relieve non-specific pruritus in the elderly.[18]

A recent meta-analysis suggests that anabolic steroids may increase body weight and lean body mass in HIV-infected individuals, though the change is small and may not be clinically significant.[19]
Bio-availability 11% (fasting), 44% (after lipid-rich meal);[20] doubling the dose increases the plasma concentration by only 35–40%.
Onset of action 5–10 days in hepatic pruritus.
Time to peak plasma concentration <2h.
Plasma halflife 4.5h (single dose); >24h (multiple doses).
Duration of action >24h.

Cautions

Hepatic or renal disease, fluid retention, cardiovascular disease, hypertension, epilepsy, diabetes mellitus, lipoprotein disorder, polycythaemia, migraine. Discontinue if female virilization occurs (may become irreversible if treatment continued), or if symptoms of raised intracranial pressure or thrombo-embolism arise. Monitor LFTs and FBC every 6 months during long-term treatment. May cause false results with thyroid function tests. If contraception is required, a non-hormonal method will be necessary.

Drug interactions

Danazol inhibits CYP3A4 and may enhance the activity of several drugs, including **carbamazepine**, **ciclosporin**, **warfarin**, and possibly **tacrolimus**. It can cause insulin resistance.

The concurrent use of danazol and a statin has been associated with acute renal impairment, pancreatitis and rhabdomyolysis.[21,22]

Undesirable effects

Related to inhibition of the pituitary-ovarian axis: amenorrhoea, hot flushes, sweating, reduction in breast size, reduced libido, vaginitis, emotional lability.
Related to androgenic activity: acne, oily skin or hair, mild hirsutism, deepening of the voice, androgenic alopecia, and rarely clitoral hypertrophy. Paradoxically, testicular atrophy may occur.
Other effects: include dizziness, seizures, benign intracranial hypertension (rare), thrombotic events, nausea, severe hepatotoxicity (occasional), muscle cramps, photosensitivity.

Dose and use
Pruritus
Moisturizing the skin with an emollient is always the first step. In patients with an extrahepatic obstruction (e.g. because of pancreatic cancer, lymphadenopathy), the treatment of choice is generally stenting of the bile duct.

When this is not feasible or when associated with intrahepatic cholestasis, one of several drugs can be used, and the choice depends on both individual circumstances and local fashion:
- **naltrexone** 12.5–250mg once daily[5-7]
- **rifampicin** 150–300mg once daily[23]
- **paroxetine** 5–20mg once daily[24]
- danazol 200mg once daily–t.d.s. with food.[25]

Benefit from danazol is generally seen after about 5–10 days.[26] Androgenic changes may be ameliorated by reducing the dose from once daily to 3 times weekly or even less.[16]

Alternative 17α-alkyl androgens in some countries (not UK) include:
- **norethandrolone** 10mg b.d.–t.d.s.
- **methyltestosterone** 25mg once daily SL.

Supply

Danazol (generic)
Capsules 100mg, 200mg, 28 days @ 200mg once daily = £33 (note: based on BNF pricing, this is more expensive than proprietary danazol capsules).

Danol® (Sanofi-Aventis)
Capsules 100mg, 200mg, 28 days @ 200mg once daily = £15 (note: based on BNF pricing, this is cheaper than generic danazol capsules).

Paroxetine (generic)
Tablets 20mg, 30mg, 28 days @ 20mg once daily = £2.50.

Seroxat® (GSK)
Tablets (scored) 10mg, 20mg, 30mg, 28 days @ 10mg once daily = £12.
Oral suspension (sugar-free) 10mg/5mL, 28 days @ 10mg once daily = £9.

Rifampicin (generic)
Capsules 150mg, 300mg, 28 days@ 150mg once daily = £6.

Rifadin® (Sanofi-Aventis)
Capsules 150mg, 300mg, 28 days@ 150mg once daily = £5.
Oral syrup 100mg/5mL, 28 days @ 150mg once daily = £6.

Also see naltrexone, p.456.

1 Hosea SW and Frank MM (1980) Danazole in the treatment of hereditary angioedema. *Drugs*. 19: 370–372.
2 MacFarlane JT and Davies D (1981) Management of hereditary angio-oedema with low-dose danazol. *Br Med J (Clin Res Ed)*. 282: 1275.
3 Ahrens E et al. (1950) Primary biliary cirrhosis. *Medicine*. 29: 299–364.
4 Jones E and Bergasa N (1990) The pruritus of cholestasis. From bile acids to opiate agonists. *Hepatology*. 11: 884–887
5 Jones E and Dekker L (2000) Florid opioid withdrawal-like reaction precipitated by naltrexone in a patient with chronic cholestasis. *Gastroenterology*. 118: 431–432.
6 Jones EA and Bergasa N (2004) The pruritus of cholestasis and the opioid neurotransmitter system. In: Z Zylicz et al. (eds) *Pruritus in advanced desease*. Oxford University Press, Oxford, pp. 56–68.
7 Jones E and Bergasa N (1999) The pruritus of cholestasis. *Hepatology*. 29: 1003–1006.
8 Twycross RG et al. (2003) Itch: scratching more than the surface. *Quarterly Journal of Medicine*. 96: 7–26.
9 Welder A et al. (1995) Toxic effects of anabolic-androgen steroids in primary rat hepatic cell cultures. *Journal of Pharmacological and Toxicological Methods*. 33: 187–195.
10 Ohsawa T and Iwashita S (1986) Hepatitis associated with danazol. *Drug Intelligence and Clinical Pharmacy*. 20: 889.
11 Fermand JP et al. (1990) Danazol-induced hepatocellular adenoma. *American Journal of Medicine*. 88: 529–530.
12 Boue F et al. (1986) Danazol and cholestatic hepatitis. *Annals of internal medicine*. 105: 139–140.
13 Silva MO et al. (1989) Danazol-induced cholestasis. *American Journal of Gastroenterology*. 84: 426–428.
14 Elsharkawy AM et al. (2012) Cholestasis secondary to anabolic steroid use in young men. *British Medical Journal*. 344: e468.
15 Piekarska A and Wojcik K (2009) Modern anabolics and anticatabolics: The scope of the hepatologist's knowledge. *Experimental and Clinical Hepatology*. 5: 7–11.
16 Lloyd-Thomas H and Sherlock S (1952) Testosterone therapy for the pruritus of obstructive jaundice. *British Medical Journal*. ii: 1289–1291.
17 Fernandez L et al. (1994) Stanozolol and danazol, unlike natural androgens, interact with the low affinity glucocorticoid-binding sites from male rat liver microsomes. *Endocrinology*. 134: 1401–1408.
18 Feldman S et al. (1942) Treatment of senile pruritus with androgens and estrogens. *Archives of Dermatology and Syphilology Chicago*. 46: 112–127.
19 Johns KKJ et al. (2005) Anabolic steroids for the treatment of weight loss in HIV-infected individuals. *Cochrane Database of Systematic Reviews*. 4: CD005483.

20 Sunesen VH *et al.* (2005) Effect of liquid volume and food intake on the absolute bioavailability of danazol, a poorly soluble drug. *European Journal of Pharmaceutical Sciences.* **24**: 297–303.

21 Hsieh CY and Chen CH (2008) Rhabdomyolysis and pancreatitis associated with coadministration of danazol 600 mg/d and lovastatin 40 mg/d. *Clinical Therapeutics.* **30**: 1330–1335.

22 Andreou ER and Ledger S (2003) Potential drug interaction between simvastatin and danazol causing rhabdomyolysis. *Canadian Journal of Clinical Pharmacology.* **10**: 172–174.

23 Ghent C and Carruthers S (1988) Treatment of pruritus in primary biliary cirrhosis with rifampin. Results of a double-blind crossover randomized trial. *Gastroenterology.* **94**: 488–493.

24 Zylicz Z *et al.* (2003) Paroxetine in the treatment of severe non-dermatological pruritus: a randomized, controlled trial. *Journal of Pain and Symptom Management.* **26**: 1105–1112.

25 Twycross RG and Zylicz Z (2004) Systemic therapy: making rational choices. In: Z Zylicz *et al.* (eds) *Pruritus in advanced disease.* Oxford University Press, London, pp. 161–178.

26 Sherlock S and Dooley J (1993) *Diseases of the Liver and Biliary System* (9e). Blackwell Scientific, Oxford.

Updated May 2012

*THALIDOMIDE   BNF 8.2.4

Class: Biologic response modifier.

Indications: Multiple myeloma (with concurrent **melphalan** and **prednisone** as first-line treatment in patients ⩾65 years or ineligible for high dose chemotherapy), †cutaneous manifestations of lepromatous leprosy (erythema nodosum leprosum), †graft versus host disease (GVHD), †recurrent aphthous stomatitis (idiopathic, HIV-related, connective tissue disease (Behcet's syndrome)), †paraneoplastic sweating, †paraneoplastic and uraemic pruritus, †cachexia in HIV and cancer, †intractable GI bleeding, †intractable **irinotecan**-induced diarrhoea, †discoid lupus erythematosus, †prevention of graft rejection.[1–3]

Contra-indications: Because it causes severe congenital abnormalities (absent or shortened limbs), thalidomide is contra-indicated in pregnant women and in women with childbearing potential unless strict contraception is implemented (see Dose and use).[4]

Pharmacology

Thalidomide is an immunomodulator with anticytokine, anti-integrin, and anti-angiogenic properties.[5,6] It was withdrawn from use as a non-barbiturate hypnotic with anti-emetic properties in the early 1960s after it emerged that it was teratogenic (via binding cereblon, an E3 ligase protein).[7,8] Subsequently, it has been found to have immunomodulatory properties with potential for the treatment of various conditions.[9] However, its use is closely monitored and it is prohibitively expensive (see Supply).

Thalidomide inhibits the synthesis of the pro-inflammatory cytokine tumour necrosis factor α (TNF-α) by monocytes,[10] and stimulates interleukin-2 and interferon-γ production (thereby stimulating human T lymphocytes).[11] It also inhibits chemotaxis of neutrophils and monocytes. Thalidomide antagonizes PGE_2, PGF_2, histamine, serotonin, and acetylcholine.[12] It also affects several other mechanisms associated with inflammation and immunomodulation.[13] These properties probably account for the prevention of **irinotecan**-induced diarrhoea,[14] and the amelioration of paraneoplastic sweating[15] paraneoplastic pruritus,[16] and cough in idiopathic pulmonary fibrosis.[17]

An anti-inflammatory effect is also likely to explain benefit in the cachexia-anorexia syndrome in patients with cancer or HIV,[18–20] although high-quality evidence is limited.[21] Two small RCTs of thalidomide 100–200mg in patients with cancer found no overall benefit on body composition.[22,23] About half the patients experienced undesirable effects with the 200mg dose, particularly rash and drowsiness,[23] suggesting that a lower starting dose is advisable, i.e. 50–100mg at bedtime.

The main antiproliferative and pro-apoptotic effects of thalidomide (and its analogues) in cancer cells are downstream consequences of binding cereblon.[8,24–26] It also inhibits angiogenesis by suppressing vascular endothelial growth factor (VEGF), a potent angiogenic factor secreted by cancer cells in response to hypoxia. This property also provides the rationale underlying the use of thalidomide in refractory GI bleeding and epistaxis associated with underlying angiodysplasia.[27–31]

Analogues of thalidomide with similar anti-angiogenic, immunomodulatory and anti-inflammatory properties have been developed, e.g. **lenalidomide, pomalidomide** (not UK).[32] **Lenalidomide** is authorized as a second-line treatment with concurrent **dexamethasone**, in multiple myeloma.[33] In the USA it is also authorized for certain myelodysplastic syndromes which cause transfusion-dependent anaemia.[34] However, the analogues are also likely to carry serious teratogenic risk, are restricted in their availability, and are very expensive. Further, there is a dearth of experience with the analogues in symptom management and palliative care, and no obvious advantage over thalidomide.

The metabolism of thalidomide is by non-enzymatic hydrolysis in the plasma. Hepatic metabolism is minor. Studies in patients with hepatic and renal impairment have not been performed.

Bio-availability 67–93% PO in animals, no data in humans.

Onset of action varies from 2 days for lepromatous leprosy and paraneoplastic sweating to 1–2 months for GVHD and 2–3 months for rheumatoid arthritis.

Time to peak plasma concentration 2–6h, delayed by food.

Plasma half-life 6h (200mg/24h)–18h (800mg/24h).[13]

Duration of action 24h.

Cautions

Treat as a 'cytotoxic' when handling. Thalidomide potentiates the sedative properties of barbiturates and alcohol, and increases the likelihood of extrapyramidal effects with **chlorpromazine** and **reserpine**.[12] Thalidomide should be used cautiously with other drugs which cause drowsiness, neuropathy or reduce the effectiveness of oral contraception (e.g. HIV protease inhibitors, **rifampicin, rifabutin, phenytoin, carbamazepine**).[12,35]

Undesirable effects

Neuropathy

Low grade peripheral neuropathy occurs in >80% of patients receiving thalidomide, and severe neuropathy in 3–5%, generally after treatment lasting >6 months.[36,37] The incidence is higher in elderly patients, women, and in patients with pre-existing neuropathy or who are treated with neurotoxic chemotherapy, e.g. **vincristine, cisplatin, paclitaxel**.[37] Generally, the peripheral neuropathy presents as distal paraesthesia or dysaesthesia with or without sensory loss. Physical examination may be normal or show mildly decreased sensation in the distal limbs. Strength is usually preserved, but reflexes, particularly ankle jerks, may be depressed or absent. These symptoms, which are progressive, typically begin in the distal lower limbs and extend proximally and into the upper limbs.[38]

Although some studies have found a relationship between the cumulative dose and the occurrence of neuropathy,[39] others have not.[40] Nerve conduction studies typically show results consistent with a sensory axonal neuropathy. If a patient develops neuropathy, dose reduction or cessation may be required to decrease the likelihood of chronic painful neuropathy (see Dose and use).[41,42]

Some 80% of patients experience a mild decrease in bowel motility; this may reflect autonomic dysfunction, and can exacerbate constipation.[43]

Cardiovascular

Thalidomide and **lenalidomide** increase the risk of VTE in patients with multiple myeloma, particularly when used in combination with high-dose corticosteroids and/or chemotherapy, and thromboprophylaxis is recommended.[44] Both thalidomide and **lenalidomide** increase the risk of arterial thrombosis, e.g. myocardial infarction, stroke.[45] The MHRA recommends thromboprophylaxis for patients at increased thrombotic risk for the first five months of treatment.[45] Generally this is with LMWH or warfarin. Although aspirin has been used, UK guidelines advocate this only in patients with no other risk factors for VTE.[46,47]

Thalidomide is associated with arrhythmia, hypotension, and oedema. Sinus bradycardia, generally mild, has been reported in ≤25% of patients.[48] Severe sinus bradycardia occurs in only 1–3% of patients.[48] Mild peripheral oedema has been reported in 15%. Orthostatic hypotension and dizziness also have been reported with thalidomide.[49] A dose-dependent decrease in supine systolic and diastolic pressures is seen up to 2h after dosing.[50] However, symptom control doses should not affect blood pressure.

Skin

A pruritic and maculopapular rash may occur 10–14 days after starting treatment, starting on the trunk and extending to the back and proximal limbs. This is generally mild and resolves with the use of an emollient and dose reduction.[51] Severe skin reactions, such as Stevens-Johnson syndrome and toxic epidermal necrolysis, may also occur.[52] Skin complications seem more likely when thalidomide is combined with corticosteroids.

Other

These include drowsiness, seizures,[49] altered temperature sensitivity, irregular menstrual cycles, and hypothyroidism. Thalidomide can increase HIV viral load.[53] Myelosuppression is rare.

Tumour flare (a temporary increase in size of a cancerous lesion) may occur. When thalidomide is used to treat chronic lymphocytic leukaemia, some patients have experienced increased lymphadenopathy, enlargement of the spleen, and an increased lymphocyte count.[54]

Abnormal LFTs are common with **lenalidomide**. Serious (including fatal) instances of drug-related hepatitis have been reported in < 1% resulting in the recommendation for routine monitoring of LFTs (weekly for first 8 weeks and monthly thereafter).[55] Patients with multiple myeloma treated with thalidomide or **lenalidomide** have a small increased risk of a second primary malignancy.[56,57]

Dose and use

Thalidomide is prohibitively expensive and cost alone will severely limit its use. In palliative care, thalidomide should *never* be considered as a first-line treatment. Its use should be considered only when more conventional treatments have failed and a full review of the potential benefits and harms has been undertaken with specialist colleagues.

There are several potential uses for thalidomide in palliative care (Table 1).[58] Female patients prescribed thalidomide must be counselled about the need for contraception, and male patients must use a condom. Written consent should be obtained.[59] Contraception should be used for ≥4 weeks before starting, during, and for 4 weeks after stopping treatment. Regular pregnancy testing is advised throughout treatment. Because thalidomide is present in the semen of men treated with the drug, even after vasectomy a latex condom must be used during sexual intercourse with women of childbearing potential.[60]

Table 1 Potential uses of thalidomide in palliative care[a]

Indication	Dose
Aphthous ulcers in HIV+ disease	100–200mg at bedtime for 10 days[61]
Paraneoplastic sweating	100–200mg at bedtime[62,63]
Paraneoplastic and uraemic pruritus	100–200mg at bedtime[16,64,65]
Cachexia-anorexia in HIV+ disease and cancer	50–200mg at bedtime[18–20]
GI bleeding (associated with angiodysplasia/ radiation proctitis/cancer)	100–300mg at bedtime[30]
Intractable irinotecan-induced diarrhoea	400mg at bedtime[14,66]

a. Thalidomide is *not* the first-line treatment for any of these indications.

For dose modifications if peripheral neuropathy occurs (i.e. paraesthesia, weakness and/or loss of reflexes), see Table 2.[4]

Supply

In the UK, thalidomide is available through a strictly monitored Thalidomide Celgene pregnancy prevention programme (www.celgene.co.uk/hcp_thalidomide.aspx). Both prescribers and pharmacies must be registered with the programme to prescribe, order and supply thalidomide.

Lenalidomide is similarly monitored through the Revlimid pregnancy prevention programme (www.celgene.co.uk/hcp_revlimid.aspx).

Thalidomide Celgene® (Celgene)
Capsules 50mg, 28 days @ 50mg at bedtime = £299.

Lenalidomide
Revlimid® (Celgene)
Capsules 5mg, 10mg, 15mg, 25mg, 28 days @ 5mg at bedtime = £4,760.

Table 2 Dose changes in thalidomide-related neuropathy[a]

Grade	Impact of neuropathy	Dose modification[b]
1	No loss of function	Consider reducing dose if symptoms worsen
2	Interfering with function but not with activities of daily living	Reduce dose or interrupt treatment. If no improvement or further deterioration, stop treatment. If improves to grade 1 or better, restart treatment (if the benefit/risk ratio remains favourable)
3	Interfering with activities of daily living	Stop treatment
4	Disabling	Stop treatment

a. based on first-line use in multiple myeloma
b. monitor the patient regularly during treatment, e.g. monthly in women of child-bearing potential, otherwise every 3 months.

1 Calabrese L and Fleischer A (2000) Thalidomide: current and potential clinical applications. *American Journal of Medicine*. **108**: 487–495.
2 Chen M et al. (2010) Innovative uses of thalidomide. *Dermatologic Clinics*. **28**: 577–586.
3 Hello M et al. (2010) Use of thalidomide for severe recurrent aphthous stomatitis: a multicenter cohort analysis. *Medicine (Baltimore)*. **89**: 176–182.
4 Celgene (2013) Thalidomide Celgene 50mg Hard Capsules. SPC. www.medicines.org.uk
5 Jacobson J (2000) Thalidomide: a remarkable comeback. *Expert Opinion in Pharmacotherapy*. **1**: 849–863.
6 De Sanctis JB et al. (2010) Pharmacological properties of thalidomide and its analogues. *Recent Patents on Inflammation and Allergy Drug Discovery*. **4**: 144–148.
7 Marriott J et al. (1999) Thalidomide as an emerging immunotherapeutic agent. *Trends in Immunology Today*. **20**: 538–540.
8 Lopez-Girona A et al. (2012) Cereblon is a direct protein target for immunomodulatory and antiproliferative activities of lenalidomide and pomalidomide. *Leukemia*. **26**: 2326–2335.
9 Peuckmann V et al. (2000) Potential novel uses of thalidomide: focus on palliative care. *Drugs*. **60**: 273–292.
10 Sampaio E et al. (1991) Thalidomide selectively inhibits tumour necrosis factor alpha production by stimulated human monocytes. *Journal of Experimental Medicine*. **173**: 699–703.
11 Corral LG and Kaplan G (1999) Immunomodulation by thalidomide and thalidomide analogues. *Annals of the Rheumatic Diseases*. **58 (Suppl 1)**: 1107–113.
12 Radomsky C and Levine N (2001) Thalidomide. *Dermatologic Clinics*. **19**: 87–103.
13 Bousvaros A and Mueller B (2001) Thalidomide in gastrointestinal disorders. *Drugs*. **61**: 777–787.
14 Govindarajan R et al. (2000) Effect of thalidomide on gastrointestinal toxic effects of irinotecan. *Lancet*. **356**: 566–567.
15 Deaner P (2000) The use of thalidomide in the management of severe sweating in patients with advanced malignancy: trial report. *Palliative Medicine*. **14**: 429–431.
16 Smith J et al. (2002) Use of thalidomide in the treatment of intractable itch. Poster abstract 21. In: *Palliative Care Congress*; Sheffield, UK.
17 Horton MR et al. (2012) Thalidomide for the treatment of cough in idiopathic pulmonary fibrosis: a randomized trial. *Annals of internal medicine*. **157**: 398–406.
18 Gordon JN et al. (2005) Thalidomide in the treatment of cancer cachexia: a randomised placebo controlled trial. *Gut*. **54**: 540–545.
19 Davis M et al. (2012) A Phase II dose titration study of thalidomide for cancer-associated anorexia. *Journal of Pain and Symptom Management*. **43**: 78–86.
20 Reyes-Teran G et al. (1996) Effects of thalidomide on HIV-associated wasting syndrome: a randomized, double-blind, placebo-controlled clinical trial. *AIDS*. **10**: 1501–1507.
21 Reid J et al. (2012) Thalidomide for managing cancer cachexia. *Cochrane Database of Systematic Reviews*. **4**: CD008664.
22 Yennurajalingam S et al. (2012) The role of thalidomide and placebo for the treatment of cancer-related anorexia-cachexia symptoms: results of a double-blind placebo-controlled randomized study. *Journal of Palliative Medicine*. **15**: 1059–1064.
23 Wilkes EA et al. (2011) Poor tolerability of thalidomide in end-stage oesophageal cancer. *European Journal of Cancer Care (Engl)*. **20**: 593–600.
24 Eisen T (2000) Thalidomide in solid tumors: the London experience. *Oncology (Williston Park)*. **14 (Suppl 13)**: 17–20.
25 Eleutherakis-Papaiakovou V et al. (2004) Thalidomide in cancer medicine. *Annals of Oncology*. **15**: 1151–1160.
26 Latif T et al. (2012) Thalidomide and its analogues in the treatment of Multiple Myeloma. *Experimental Hematology and Oncology*. **1**: 27.
27 Bauditz J et al. (2004) Thalidomide for treatment of severe intestinal bleeding. *Gut*. **53**: 609–612.
28 Craanen ME et al. (2006) Thalidomide in refractory haemorrhagic radiation induced proctitis. *Gut*. **55**: 1371–1372.
29 Karajeh MA et al. (2006) Refractory bleeding from portal hypertensive gastropathy: a further novel role for thalidomide therapy? *European Journal of Gastroenterology and Hepatology*. **18**: 545–548.
30 Lambert K and Ward J (2009) The use of thalidomide in the management of bleeding from a gastric cancer. *Palliative Medicine*. **23**: 473–475.
31 Franchini M et al. (2012) Novel treatments for epistaxis in hereditary hemorrhagic telangiectasia: a systematic review of the clinical experience with thalidomide. *Journal of Thrombosis and Thrombolysis*.

32 Li S et al. (2010) Recent advances of IMiDs in cancer therapy. *Current Opinion in Oncology*. **22**: 579–585.

33 Richardson P et al. (2010) Lenalidomide in multiple myeloma: an evidence-based review of its role in therapy. *Core Evidence*. **4**: 215–245.

34 Castelli R et al. (2013) Immunomodulatory drugs: new options for the treatment of myelodysplastic syndromes. *Clinical Lymphoma Myeloma and Leukemia*. **13**: 1–7.

35 Thomas D and Kantarjian H (2000) Current role of thalidomide in cancer treatment. *Current Opinion in Oncology*. **12**: 564–573.

36 Dimopoulos MA and Eleutherakis-Papaiakovou V (2004) Adverse effects of thalidomide administration in patients with neoplastic diseases. *American Journal of Medicine*. **117**: 508–515.

37 Mileshkin L et al. (2006) Development of neuropathy in patients with myeloma treated with thalidomide: patterns of occurrence and the role of electrophysiologic monitoring. *Journal of Clinical Oncology*. **24**: 4507–4514.

38 Wulff CH et al. (1985) Development of polyneuropathy during thalidomide therapy. *British Journal of Dermatology*. **112**: 475–480.

39 Fullerton P and O'Sullivan D (1968) Thalidomide neuropathy: a clinical, electrophysiological, and histological follow up study. *Journal of Neurology, Neurosurgery and Psychiatry*. **31**: 543–551.

40 Chapon F et al. (1985) [Neuropathies caused by thalidomide]. *Rev Neurol (Paris)*. **141**: 719–728.

41 Gardner-Medwin J et al. (1994) Clinical experience with thalidomide in the management of severe oral and genital ulceration in conditions such as Behcet's disease. *Annals of Rheumatic Diseases*. **53**: 443–450.

42 Ochonisky S et al. (1994) Thalidomide neuropathy incidence and clinico-electrophysiologic findings in 42 patients. *Archives of Dermatology*. **130**: 66–69.

43 Grover JK et al. (2002) The adverse effects of thalidomide in relapsed and refractory patients of multiple myeloma. *Annals of Oncology*. **13**: 1636–1640.

44 Carrier M et al. (2011) Rates of venous thromboembolism in multiple myeloma patients undergoing immunomodulatory therapy with thalidomide or lenalidomide: a systematic review and meta-analysis. *Journal of Thrombosis and Haemostasis*. **9**: 653–663.

45 MHRA (2011) Thalidomide: risk of arterial and venous thromboembolism. *Drug Safety Update*. **4**. www.mhra.gov.uk/Safetyinformation.

46 Palumbo A et al. (2011) Aspirin, warfarin, or enoxaparin thromboprophylaxis in patients with multiple myeloma treated with thalidomide: a phase III, open-label, randomized trial. *Journal of Clinical Oncology*. **29**: 986–993.

47 Bird JM et al. (2011) Guidelines for the diagnosis and management of multiple myeloma 2011. *British Journal of Haematology*. **154**: 32–75.

48 Kaur A et al. (2003) Thalidomide-induced sinus bradycardia. *Annals of Pharmacotherapy*. **37**: 1040–1043.

49 Clark T et al. (2001) Thalidomid (Thalidomide) capsules: A review of the first 18 months of spontaneous postmarketing adverse event surveillance, including off-label prescribing. *Drug Safety*. **24**: 87–117.

50 Noormohamed F et al. (1999) Pharmacokinetics and hemodynamic effects of single oral doses of thalidomide in asymptomatic human immunodeficiency virus-infected subjects. *AIDS Research and Human Viruses*. **15**: 1047–1052.

51 Ng SS et al. (2002) Thalidomide, an antiangiogenic agent with clinical activity in cancer. *Biomedical and Pharmacology Journal*. **56**: 194–199.

52 Rajkumar SV et al. (2000) Life-threatening toxic epidermal necrolysis with thalidomide therapy for myeloma. *New England Journal of Medicine*. **343**: 972–973.

53 Marriott J et al. (1997) A double-blind placebo-controlled phase II trial of thalidomide in asymptomatic HIV-positive patients: clinical tolerance and effect on activation markers and cytokines. *AIDS Research and Human Retrovirus*. **13**: 1625–1631.

54 Chanan-Khan A et al. (2005) Results of a phase I clinical trial of thalidomide in combination with fludarabine as initial therapy for patients with treatment-requiring chronic lymphocytic leukemia (CLL). *Blood*. **106**: 3348–3352.

55 MHRA (2013) Lenolidomide (Revlimid): risk of serious hepatic adverse drug reactions - routine monitoring of liver function now recommended. *Drug Safety Update*. **6**. www.mhra.gov.uk/Safetyinformation

56 MHRA (2013) Thalidomide: risk of second primary malignancies. *Drug Safety Update*. **6**. www.mhra.gov.uk/Safetyinformation.

57 MHRA (2011) Lenolidomide (Revlimid): risk of a second primary malignancy - update. *Drug Safety Update*. **5**. www.mhra.gov.uk/Safetyinformation

58 Davis M and Dickerson E (2001) Thalidomide: dual benefits in palliative medicine and oncology. *American Journal of Hospice and Palliative Care*. **18**: 347–351.

59 Powell R and Gardner-Medwin J (1994) Guideline for the clinical use and dispensing of thalidomide. *Postgraduate Medical Journal*. **70**: 901–904.

60 Teo SK et al. (2001) Thalidomide is distributed into human semen after oral dosing. *Drug Metabolism and Disposition*. **29**: 1355–1357.

61 Jacobson J et al. (1997) Thalidomide for the treatment of oral aphthous ulcers in patients with human immunodeficiency virus infection. *New England Journal of Medicine*. **336**: 1487–1493.

62 Deaner P (1998) Thalidomide for distressing night sweats in advanced malignant disease. *Palliative Medicine*. **12**: 208–209.

63 Calder K and Bruera E (2000) Thalidomide for night sweats in patients with advanced cancer. *Palliative Medicine*. **14**: 77–78.

64 Goncalves F (2010) Thalidomide for the control of severe paraneoplastic pruritus associated with Hodgkin's disease. *American Journal of Hospice and Palliative Care*. **27**: 486–487.

65 Silva S et al. (1994) Thalidomide for the treatment of uremic pruritus: a crossover randomized double-blind trial. *Nephron*. **67**: 270–273.

66 Govindarajan R (2000) Irinotecan and thalidomide in metastatic colorectal cancer. *Oncology (Williston Park)*. **14 (Suppl 13)**: 29–32.

Updated June 2013

8: URINARY TRACT DISORDERS

TAMSULOSIN   BNF 7.4.1

Class: Uroselective α_1-adrenergic receptor antagonist (α_1 antagonist).[1]

Indications: Symptoms associated with benign prostatic hypertrophy (BPH), †radiation-induced urethritis, †before trial without catheter inserted for acute urinary retention in men,[2] †medical management of urinary stones.[3]

Contra-indications: Symptomatic postural hypotension.

Pharmacology

Tamsulosin is a selective competitive antagonist at post-synaptic α_{1A}- and α_{1D}-adrenergic receptors, causing smooth muscle relaxation in the prostate gland, bladder neck, and possibly the detrusor (i.e. the bladder itself).[4,5] Tamsulosin is metabolized in the liver, primarily by CYP2D6 and CYP3A4; <10% is excreted unchanged in the urine.

In BPH, smooth muscle hyperplasia is estimated to be responsible for nearly half of the obstructive component. Tamsulosin is prescribed for men with moderate–severe voiding lower urinary tract symptoms (voiding LUTS, e.g. urinary hesitancy, poor urinary stream, incomplete bladder emptying, terminal dribble) and a moderately enlarged prostate gland gland (<30g). Tamsulosin reduces functional prostatic obstruction and increases maximum urinary flow rate. RCTs show that tamsulosin improves LUTS by 20–50%, compared to 20–30% for placebo.[6]

Other less specific α_1 antagonists are available, e.g. **prazosin** (taken b.d.). Symptomatic and urodynamic efficacy is similar when taken at the highest dose possible without unacceptable undesirable effects. Tamsulosin causes less postural hypotension than **prazosin** when given alone or with commonly used antihypertensive drugs, e.g. **atenolol, enalapril** and **nifedipine**.[7,8] However, even with tamsulosin there is a risk of severe hypotension necessitating hospital admission in the first 4 weeks after starting treatment.[9]

For men with troublesome moderate–severe LUTS, a greater degree of prostatic enlargement (>30g) or a PSA >1.4nanogram/mL (surrogate marker for a prostate gland >30g)[10] and at risk of progressive obstruction, a 5α-reductase inhibitor, e.g. **dutasteride** or **finasteride**, should be considered. Whereas tamsulosin generally improves symptoms within days with a full response by 6 weeks, 5α-reductase inhibitors improve symptoms only after 3–6 months.[10,11] Combined treatment with α_1 antagonist and a 5α-reductase inhibitor is more effective than either agent alone but has higher incidence of undesirable effects than monotherapy, and generally is neither necessary nor appropriate in patients with a prognosis of only 2–3 months.[12]

15% of men with voiding LUTS associated with BPH also have significant storage LUTS (e.g. frequency, urgency and incontinence). Because tamsulosin may relax bladder smooth muscle, it may reduce detrusor instability and storage LUTS. However, if storage LUTS persist following a trial of tamsulosin, consider adding an anti-muscarinic (see **Oxybutynin** p.551). This has not been demonstrated to increase the risk of acute urinary retention, particularly in men with a post-voiding residual volume of <250mL.[13,14]

An alternative approach to the management of urinary hesitancy when urinary obstruction has been excluded, is to use either a muscarinic drug, e.g. **bethanechol** 10–25mg t.d.s., or an anticholinesterase, e.g. **distigmine bromide** (not UK) 5mg each morning (30min before breakfast) to stimulate bladder contraction. Because of different mechanisms of action, they can be used concurrently with tamsulosin.

Tamsulosin 400–800microgram/24h reduces external beam radiotherapy-induced LUTS (voiding, storage and mixed types) in patients with prostate cancer. When started at least 5 days before prostate radiation brachytherapy, tamsulosin also reduces short-term LUTS.[15]

Bio-availability m/r ~100% PO fasting, reduced by 30% p.c.;[4] Flomaxtra® XL 55–59%, not affected by food.

Onset of action m/r 4–8h; maximum benefit 4–8 weeks.

Time to peak plasma concentration 1h; m/r 4h fasting, 6h p.c.;[4] Flomaxtra® XL 4–6h, not affected by food.

Plasma halflife 5–7h; m/r 9–13h (healthy volunteers), 14–15h (elderly);[4] Flomaxtra® XL 19h (single dose), 15h (steady-state).

Duration of action <24h.

Cautions
Severe hepatic or renal impairment.

Drug interactions
Concurrent use with epidural **morphine**, **sildenafil** or other α_1 antagonist increases the risk of postural hypotension.

Tamsulosin is metabolized mainly by CYP2D6, and CYP3A4. Caution should be taken with concurrent use of drugs which inhibit or induce these enzymes, e.g. **erythromycin**, particularly in those who are poor CYP2D6 metabolizers (see Chapter 25, p.767).

Undesirable effects
For more information, see National Clinical Guidelines Centre information.[10]

Very common (>10%): dizziness, orthostatic hypotension, ejaculatory impairment.[11]

Common (<10%, >1%): headache, asthenia, drowsiness or insomnia, amblyopia, chest pain, rhinitis, sinusitis, pharyngitis, cough, bitter taste, nausea, abdominal discomfort, diarrhoea, back pain, reduced libido, impotence or erectile dysfunction.

Uncommon (<1%, >0.1%): syncope, palpitations, vomiting, constipation, rash, pruritus, gynaecomastia.

Very rare (<0.01%, >0.001%): priapism.

Dose and use
Hesitancy of micturition
- m/r tamsulosin 400microgram PO once daily (because absorption is significantly affected by food, take at the same time each day with respect to meals)
- if necessary, increase to 800microgram m/r once daily after 2–4 weeks.[4]

Trial without catheter in men with acute retention
- m/r tamsulosin 400microgram PO once daily for 1–3 days before catheter removal.[2]

Supply
Tamsulosin (generic)
Capsules m/r 400microgram, 28 days @ 400microgram once daily = £6.

Flomaxtra® XL (Astellas)
Tablets m/r 400microgram, 28 days @ 400microgram once daily = £10.

1 Hieble JP et al. (1995) International Union of Pharmacology. X. Recommendation for nomenclature of alpha 1-adrenoceptors: consensus update. Pharmacol Rev. **47**: 267–270.
2 Zeif HJ and Subramonian K (2009) Alpha blockers prior to removal of a catheter for acute urinary retention in adult men. Cochrane Database of Systematic Reviews. CD006744.
3 Lu Z et al. (2012) Tamsulosin for ureteral stones: a systematic review and meta-analysis of a randomized controlled trial. Urologica Internationalis. **89**: 107–115.
4 Lyseng-Williamson KA et al. (2002) Tamsulosin: an update of its role in the management of lower urinary tract symptoms. Drugs. **62**: 135–167.
5 Yamada S et al. (2011) alpha1-Adrenoceptors and muscarinic receptors in voiding function - binding characteristics of therapeutic agents in relation to the pharmacokinetics. British Journal of Clinical Pharmacology. **72**: 205–217.
6 Wilt TJ et al. (2003) Tamsulosin for benign prostatic hyperplasia. Cochrane Database of Systematic Reviews. **1**: CD002081.
7 Lowe FC (1997) Coadministration of tamsulosin and three antihypertensive agents in patients with benign prostatic hyperplasia: pharmacodynamic effect. Clinical Therapeutics. **19**: 730–742.
8 Michel MC et al. (1998) Tamsulosin: real life clinical experience in 19,365 patients. European Urology. **34 (Suppl 2)**: 37–45.
9 Bird ST et al. (2013) Tamsulosin treatment for benign prostatic hyperplasia and risk of severe hypotension in men aged 40–85 years in the United States: risk window analyses using between and within patient methodology. British Medical Journal. **347**: f6320.
10 NICE (2010) Lower urinary tract symptoms. The managment of lower urinary tract symptoms in men. Clinical Guideline. CG97. www.nice.org.uk
11 NHS (2010) Clinical knowledge summaries. LUTS in men, age related (prostatism). http://cks.nice.org.uk
12 Roehrborn CG et al. (2010) The effects of combination therapy with dutasteride and tamsulosin on clinical outcomes in men with symptomatic benign prostatic hyperplasia: 4-year results from the CombAT study. European Urology. **57**: 123–131.
13 Sarma AV and Wei JT (2012) Clinical practice. Benign prostatic hyperplasia and lower urinary tract symptoms. New England Journal of Medicine. **367**: 248–257.
14 MacDiarmid SA et al. (2008) Efficacy and safety of extended-release oxybutynin in combination with tamsulosin for treatment of lower urinary tract symptoms in men: randomized, double-blind, placebo-controlled study. Mayo Clinic Proceedings. **83**: 1002–1010.
15 Crawford ED and Kavanagh BD (2006) The role of alpha-blockers in the management of lower urinary tract symptoms in prostate cancer patients treated with radiation therapy. American Journal of Clinical Oncology. **29**: 517–523.

Updated January 2014

OXYBUTYNIN   BNF 7.4.2

Class: Antimuscarinic (anticholinergic).

Indications: Symptoms of an overactive bladder: urgency (with or without urge incontinence), frequency (>8 times/day) and/or nocturia (waking more than once at night to void).[1]

Contra-indications: Bladder outflow obstruction, GI obstruction including paralytic ileus, predisposition to narrow-angle glaucoma, and myasthenia gravis.

Pharmacology

Bladder muscle (detrusor) contains all subtypes of muscarinic receptor. M_2 and M_3 predominate, with M_2 outnumbering M_3 3:1. M_3 receptors are particularly important in relation to detrusor contraction; the function of M_2 receptors is less clear.

Oxybutynin hydrochloride has an antimuscarinic effect on bladder innervation. It is relatively selective for M_1 and M_3 receptor subtypes (see p.5). It also has a direct papaverine-like antispasmodic effect on the detrusor.[2] It inhibits bladder contraction, relieves spasm induced by various stimuli, increases bladder capacity, and delays the desire to void in patients with a neurogenic bladder. Oxybutynin also has a topical anaesthetic effect on the bladder mucosa.[3] Oxybutynin has an active metabolite N-desethyloxybutynin. It is not clear what proportion of its total effects are due to the metabolite. The plasma halflife of oxybutynin increases in the elderly, generally allowing smaller doses to be given.

Urinary antimuscarinics reduce frequency by 15–20% (vs. 10% with placebo); leakage episodes 45–75% (vs. 20–45%); urgency 40% (vs. 35%), and have subjective improvement rates of 40–70% (vs. 20–50%).[4,5] The absolute probability of continence after 4 weeks of treatment is 15–30%.[6]

Newer antimuscarinics, e.g. **solifenacin, darifenacin**, have higher M_3 receptor selectivity than older ones, e.g. oxybutynin and **tolterodine**.[7] They cause fewer undesirable effects and may have greater efficacy. In fact, compared with immediate-release oxybutynin, all other urinary antimuscarinics, and m/r and TD formulations of oxybutynin, are better tolerated.[5] However, although there is some evidence suggesting that m/r formulations and higher doses of some newer drugs (e.g. **fesoterodine** and **solifenacin**) have greater efficacy than oxybutynin,[1] this is not reflected in recent NICE guidelines.[6]

Oxybutynin (a tertiary amine) enters the CNS relatively easily, whereas **trospium** (a quaternary ammonium compound) does not. The M_1 receptor plays a significant role in modulating cognitive function. Thus, if an antimuscarinic with significant affinity for the M_1 receptor (as does oxybutynin) crosses the blood-brain barrier, it may cause cognitive impairment and delirium.

Newer antimuscarincs which are more M_3 selective should have fewer undesirable CNS effects.[8] In one of very few RCTs to examine this aspect, findings suggested that m/r oxybutynin causes greater cognitive dysfunction in elderly patients compared with **darifenacin**.[9]

Because of the low cost of generic immediate-release oxybutynin, it is still first-line treatment for overactive bladder, but ideally should not be prescribed for the frail elderly. If immediate-release oxybutynin is not tolerated, consider m/r or TD oxybutynin. Alternatively (and in the frail elderly), use one of the newer more selective antimuscarinics, e.g. **fesoterodine** or **darifenacin** (a once daily product).[6,10-12]

It may take four weeks to see the full response to treatment, thus the antimuscarinic should be reviewed after that, and then every 6 months to determine whether it is still needed.[13] For other options, see Box A.

Bio-availability 2–11% PO (immediate-release); increased by 50% with m/r tablets (with a corresponding reduction in the amount of N-desethyloxybutynin).[14]

Onset of action 30–60min PO (immediate-release).

Time to peak plasma concentration 30–60min PO (immediate-release); 4–6h (m/r, after first dose);[14,15] 24–48h TD.

Plasma halflife 2–3h PO (immediate-release); 4–5h in the elderly (immediate-release); 12–14h (m/r).[14,15]

Duration of action 6–10h PO (immediate-release); >24h (m/r); >4 days TD.

Box A Alternative drugs for urinary frequency and/or bladder spasms

Other drugs with antimuscarinic properties, e.g. amitriptyline or imipramine 25–50mg at bedtime.

Musculotropic drugs, flavoxate 200–400mg t.d.s.; less effective but fewer undesirable effects.

Short-term topical intravaginal oestrogens may improve incontinence and frequency in postmenopausal women with vaginal atrophy.[11]

For persistent nocturia without daytime urgency or frequency:
• consider a loop diuretic, e.g. furosemide 40mg once daily around 1700–1800h
• in patients <65 years, vasopressin analogues are of value, e.g. desmopressin; hyponatraemia is a possible complication (see Desmopressin, p.514).
• NSAIDs, e.g. naproxen 250–500mg b.d.[10]

Cautions
See Antimuscarinics p.5.

Drug interactions
Oxybutynin is metabolized extensively by CYP3A4 hepatic enzyme. Concurrent use of drugs which are strong inhibitors of this enzyme (see Chapter 25, p.767) could potentially cause toxicity, and necessitate a reduction in the dose of oxybutynin.

Undesirable effects
Antimuscarinic effects are common, including dry mouth, cognitive impairment and delirium, particularly in the frail and elderly (see Antimuscarinics, Box B, p.6); nausea and abdominal discomfort. Skin reactions are common with TD oxybutynin.

Dose and use
Immediate-release
- start with 5mg PO b.d.,
- if necessary, increase progressively to 5mg q.d.s.[11]
- in the over 60s and the very frail, these doses should be halved.

Modified-release
- start with 5mg PO once daily
- if necessary, increase in 5mg/day steps at weekly intervals
- maximum recommended dose 20mg once daily.

Note: remains of m/r tablets may appear in the patient's faeces ('ghost tablets'), but these are inert residues, and do not affect the efficacy of the products.

TD patches
- apply 1 patch (3.9mg/24h) twice weekly to clean, dry skin on abdomen, hip or buttock; avoid application to same site within 1 week.

Supply
Oxybutynin (generic)
Tablets 2.5mg, 3mg, 5mg, 28 days @ 5mg b.d. = £6.

Ditropan® (Sanofi-Aventis)
Tablets 2.5mg, 5mg, 28 days @ 5mg b.d. = £9.
Oral solution 2.5mg/5mL, 28 days @ 5mg b.d. = £26.

Modified-release
Lyrinel® XL (Janssen-Cilag)
Tablets m/r 5mg, 10mg, 28 days @ 10mg once daily = £27.

Transdermal
Kentera® (Orion)
TD patches 36mg (releasing 3.9mg/24h), 28 days @ 1 patch twice weekly = £27.

1 Madhuvrata P et al. (2012) Which anticholinergic drug for overactive bladder symptoms in adults. Cochrane Database of Systematic Reviews. 1: CD005429.
2 Andersson KE (2011) Antimuscarinic mechanisms and the overactive detrusor: an update. European Urology. 59: 377–386.
3 Robinson T and Castleden C (1994) Drugs in focus: 11. Oxybutynin hydrochloride. Prescribers' Journal. 34: 27–30.
4 Novara G et al. (2008) A systematic review and meta-analysis of randomized controlled trials with antimuscarinic drugs for overactive bladder. European Urology. 54: 740–763.
5 Chapple CR et al. (2008) The effects of antimuscarinic treatments in overactive bladder: an update of a systematic review and meta-analysis. European Urology. 54: 543–562.
6 NICE (2013) Urinary incontinence: The management of urinary incontinence in women. Clinical Guideline. CG171. www.nice.org.uk
7 Abrams P et al. (2006) Muscarinic receptors: their distribution and function in body systems, and the implications for treating overactive bladder. British Journal of Pharmacology. 148: 565–578.
8 Callegari E et al. (2011) A comprehensive non-clinical evaluation of the CNS penetration potential of antimuscarinic agents for the treatment of overactive bladder. British Journal of Clinical Pharmacology. 72: 235–246.
9 Kay G et al. (2006) Differential effects of the antimuscarinic agents darifenacin and oxybutynin ER on memory in older subjects. European Urology. 50: 317–326.
10 NICE (2010) The management of lower urinary tract symptoms in men Clinical Guideline. CG97. www.nice.org.uk
11 NICE (2009) Incontinence - urinary, in women. Clinical Knowledsge Summaries. http://cks.nice.org.uk
12 NHS (2010) LUTS on men, age related (prostatism). Clinical Knowledge Summaries. http://cks.nice.org.uk
13 Marinkovic SP et al. (2012) The management of overactive bladder syndrome. British Medical Journal. 344: e2365.
14 Gupta M and Sathyan G (1999) Pharmacokinetics of an oral once-a-day controlled-release oxybutynin formulation compared with immediate-release oxybutynin. Journal of Clinical Pharmacology. 39: 289–296.
15 Janssen-Cilag (2009) Lyrinel XL prolonged release tablet. SPC. www.medicines.org.uk

Updated April 2014

METHENAMINE HIPPURATE   BNF 5.1.13

Class: Urinary antiseptic.

Indications: Prophylaxis against UTI.

Contra-indications: Methenamine hippurate should not be used in severe renal impairment (creatinine clearance <10mL/min; eGFR <10mL/min/1.73m²), infection of the *upper* urinary tract (pyelonephritis), metabolic acidosis, hepatic impairment, severe dehydration, or gout.

Pharmacology

Unlike most antibacterials, methenamine does *not* act by impairing bacterial protein synthesis. Methenamine hippurate dissociates into methenamine and hippuric acid in an acid environment (pH <5.5). Methenamine is then converted to formaldehyde which is responsible for the bactericidal effect.[1,2] Most bacteria are sensitive to formaldehyde at concentrations of ≥20microgram/mL, and acquired resistance does not appear to develop.

Urea-splitting bacteria, e.g. *Pseudomonas aeruginosa*, produce ammonia which increases the alkalinity of urine. This could inhibit the formation of formaldehyde, and thereby reduce the effect of methenamine. However, hippuric acid helps maintain an acidic environment.

Prophylaxis against UTIs

Oral antibacterials are more effective than methenamine hippurate for prophylaxis.[3] However, caution must be exercised with antibacterials because of the risk of acquired resistance.

Evidence supporting the use of methenamine hippurate in treating or preventing symptomatic UTIs is limited. It may be more effective in patients with a normal renal tract (e.g. patients without bladder stones or neuropathic bladder).[4] However, trials have been conducted in disparate patient populations, using variable doses and follow up, making results difficult to generalize. As such, efficacy, indications, dose, and length of treatment, are unclear.[4]

An RCT in people after spinal cord injury (some with indwelling urethral or suprapubic catheters, some using intermittent self-catheterization, and some reflex voiding) compared prophylactic methenamine hippurate with **cranberry juice** and placebo for 6 months or until first symptomatic UTI, and found that the incidence of symptomatic UTIs was the same in all three groups.[5]

Prophylaxis against Catheter-associated UTI (CAUTI) or blockage

Bacterial colonization of indwelling catheters is common, occurring in ≤30% of patients catheterized for >7 days and almost 100% in those catheterized for >28 days. An intrinsic limitation of using urinary antiseptics to prevent CAUTI is that some urine-colonizing bacteria produce secretions which eventually thicken enough to form a protective biofilm attached to the catheter surface. This can embed both the bacteria and phosphate crystals in a matrix which is impervious to urinary antiseptics or acidifying catheter patency solutions.

In catheterized patients, formaldehyde remains in the bladder only for a short time. Intermittent clamping may increase the effectiveness of methenamine hippurate, although this has not been tested in an RCT. (Note: catheter clamping should be avoided in patients with spinal cord compression above spinal cord level T7, because of the risk of autonomic dysreflexia).

Methenamine hippurate given to patients catheterized for ≤ 7 days following gynaecological surgery and for several days after catheter removal is effective in preventing CAUTI.[4,6] However, benefit from urinary antiseptics for CAUTI in patients with long-term urethral catheters or who undergo regular intermittent catheterisation has not been established in an RCT.[3,6]

Although not recently investigated, methenamine hippurate may reduce the frequency of catheter blockage with long-term indwelling catheters. In an RCT published in 1980, methenamine hippurate doubled the interval between catheter changes from 1 to 2 weeks.[7] However, catheter technology has progressed since then, and much longer intervals are now expected between catheter changes, e.g. 2–3 months.

Bio-availability readily absorbed.

Onset of action >2h.

Plasma halflife 4h.

Duration of action no data.

Cautions

Methenamine hippurate should *not* be administered concurrently with:
- sulfonamides because of the risk of crystalluria
- alkalinizing agents (e.g. **acetazolamide, potassium or sodium citrate, sodium bicarbonate**) because of the need for an acid urinary environment.

Undesirable effects

Occasionally causes dyspepsia, nausea and vomiting, rash, pruritus.

With chronic use, the formaldehyde produced from methenamine may irritate and inflame the bladder mucosa, and lead to painful and frequent voiding, haematuria and proteinuria.

Dose and use

The optimum dose for a urinary antiseptic in patients with an indwelling catheter has not been determined. The recommended dose at some centres is methenamine hippurate 1g PO b.d.–t.d.s.[2,6] The tablets may be crushed and taken with milk or fruit juice (see Swallowing difficulties, p.725).

Supply

Hiprex® (Meda)
Tablets 1g, 28 days @ 1g b.d. = £13.

---

1 Strom JJ and Jun H (1993) Effect of urine pH and ascorbic acid on the rate of conversion of methenamine to formaldehyde. *Biopharmaceutics and Drug Disposition.* **14**: 61–69.

2 Sweetman SC *Martindale: The Complete Drug Reference.* London: Pharmaceutical Press www.medicinescomplete.com (accessed January 2014).

3 Grabe. M *et al.* (2013) European Association of Urology. Guidelines on urological infections. Available from: http://www.uroweb.org/guidelines/

4 Lee BS *et al.* (2012) Methenamine hippurate for preventing urinary tract infections. *Cochrane Database of Systematic Reviews.* **10**: Cd003265.

5 Lee BB *et al.* (2007) Spinal-injured neuropathic bladder antisepsis (SINBA) trial. *Spinal Cord.* **45**: 542–550.

6 Hooton TM *et al.* (2010) Diagnosis, prevention, and treatment of catheter-associated urinary tract infection in adults: 2009 International Clinical Practice Guidelines from the Infectious Diseases Society of America. *Clinical Infectious Diseases.* **50**: 625–663.

7 Norberg A *et al.* (1980) Randomized double-blind study of prophylactic methenamine hippurate treatment of patients with indwelling catheters. *European Journal of Clinical Pharmacology.* **18**: 497–500.

Updated January 2014

CRANBERRY JUICE

Class: Herbal remedy.

Indications: †Prophylaxis against urinary tract infections (UTIs).

Pharmacology

Cranberry juice inhibits bacterial adherence to the urinary tract mucosa by disrupting the binding of bacterial macromolecules to receptors on mucosal epithelial cells.[1,2] This effect, which has been shown *in vitro* in *Escherichia coli*, is produced by pro-anthocyanidins (PAC) and fructose present in cranberries.[3–5] Urinary pH is not important,[5] and the addition of **ascorbic acid** (vitamin C) is not necessary.

Cranberry juice has also been shown to have *in vitro* activity against *Staphylococcus aureus, Klebsiella pneumoniae, Pseudomonas aeruginosa* and *Proteus mirabilis*.[6] Blueberry juice also contains PAC, and may possess anti-adhesive activity, but clinical trials are lacking.[3] Theoretically, these natural juices could be a useful alternative to antibacterials for preventing UTIs, and could thus reduce the development of resistant organisms.[3]

The potential benefit of cranberry juice is limited to the prevention of UTIs; it does not cure established infection.[6,7] However, recent systematic reviews suggest that it is less effective than previously thought.[5,8] Although the largest and most recent analysis found a trend towards a reduction in UTI frequency in women with recurrent UTIs, this was not statistically significant. In other subgroups (e.g. older people, people undergoing radiation therapy for cervical or bladder cancer, people with neurological disorders and people using urinary catheters) cranberry products were no more effective than placebo or no treatment in preventing UTIs.[5] Many of the studies had poor adherence and/or high drop-out rates, suggesting that long-term consumption of cranberry juice is unacceptable to some patients, possibly because of issues with its palatability, calorie content, volume or price.

One reason for the lower efficacy noted in the updated Cochrane review may have been the use of cranberry products with insufficient PAC content.[5] A dose of 300mL/24h of cranberry juice (providing a PAC dose of 36mg/24h) is commonly used because this reduced bacteriuria and pyuria in early clinical studies.[5,9,10] However, processing cranberry juice into powder for use in capsules and tablets can adversely affect PAC content; thus careful standardization is required to ensure adequate potency of these products.[10] A study using standardized cranberry powders found that PAC doses of 18, 36 and 72mg/24h significantly reduced bacterial adhesion in a dose-dependent and a time-dependent manner. Although the effect of a single dose of 72mg is still apparent after 24h, it was suggested that 36mg b.d. could be a better regimen.[10]

Pharmacokinetic details not available.

Cautions

Diabetes mellitus: despite its bitter taste, cranberry juice has a high sugar content. Like many other fruits and berries, cranberry juice contains significant amounts of salicylic acid (7mg/L). Theoretically, large amounts of cranberry juice could trigger a reaction in people with **aspirin** allergy or **aspirin**-induced asthma.[6]

Drug interactions

Cranberry juice contains various anti-oxidants, including flavonoids, which are known to inhibit cytochrome P450 activity (see Chapter 25, p.767).[11] This was originally thought to explain several case reports, including one fatality,[12–15] in which the regular use of cranberry juice was linked to an increase in or fluctuation of INR values in patients taking **warfarin** (predominantly metabolized by CYP2C9).[16] These cases prompted the recommendation that the concurrent use of cranberry products and **warfarin** should be avoided, unless the benefit (prevention of UTI) outweighed the risks,[13,17] However, in other countries, e.g. Canada and the USA, the risk is not considered sufficiently high to issue a regulatory warning.[18,19]

Patients on stable **warfarin** doses who drank cranberry juice 250mL once daily for 1 week showed no significant increase in anticoagulant activity.[20] Further, in volunteers, drinking cranberry juice 200mL t.d.s. did not significantly affect the pharmacokinetic profiles of **warfarin**, **tizanidine** or **midazolam** (probes for CYP2C9, CYP1A2 and CYP3A4 respectively).[21]

On the other hand, the quantities of flavonoids in different commercial brands of cranberry juice may differ and it is unclear whether other mechanisms are also involved. Thus, an interaction with **warfarin** cannot be entirely ruled out, particularly if large volumes of cranberry juice are drunk regularly or when cranberry products other than juice are taken.[22–24] Accordingly, if a patient taking **warfarin** consumes large amounts of cranberry juice or takes other cranberry supplements, the INR should be monitored more closely.

Undesirable effects

In very large doses, e.g. 3–4L/24h of juice, cranberry can cause GI upset and diarrhoea. Consuming more than 1L/24h over a prolonged period may increase the risk of uric acid kidney stone formation (300mL of cranberry juice contains approximately 19mg of oxalate).[6]

Dose and use

Patients may prefer high-strength capsules or tablets (containing cranberry extract ≥200mg; PAC ≥10mg) because they avoid the high fluid volume, bitter taste and high sugar content of the juice.
Although uncertain, aim for PAC dose of 72mg/24h:
• fruit juice 300mL b.d.
• high-strength capsules or tablets; this is likely to mean ≥6 tablets/24h, e.g. 3 b.d. or 2 t.d.s.
Note: it may take ≥ 4 weeks for benefit to show.

Supply

All products are OTC.

High-strength capsules and tablets (cranberry extract ≥200mg/tablet; PAC ≥10mg/tablet)
Many products are available, e.g. HealthAid Cranberry Tablets® (HealthAid) contain 200mg of cranberry extract, equivalent to 5000mg of cranberry powder; standardized to provide a minimum of PAC 10mg/tablet.

1 Liu Y (2006) Role of cranberry juice on molecular-scale surface characteristics and adhesion behaviour of Escherichia coli. *Biotechnology and Bioengineering.* **93**: 297–305.
2 Liu Y et al. (2008) Cranberry changes the physiochemical surface properties of E.coli and adhesion with uroepithelial cells. *Colloids and Surfaces B: Biointerfaces.* **65**: 35–42.
3 Jepson R (2007) A systematic review of the evidence for cranberries and blueberries in UTI prevention. *Molecular Nutrition and Food Research.* **51**: 738–745.
4 Howell AB (2007) Bioactive compounds in cranberries and their role in prevention of urinary tract infections. *Molecular Nutrition and Food Research.* **51**: 732–737.
5 Jepson RG et al. (2012) Cranberries for preventing urinary tract infections. *Cochrane Database of Systematic Reviews.* **10**: CD001321.
6 Natural Medicines Comprehensive Database (2008) Cranberry. In: *Natural Medicines Comprehensive Database.* Available from: www.naturaldatabase.com
7 Tong H et al. (2006) Effect of ingesting cranberry juice on bacterial growth in urine. *American Journal of Health-System Pharmacy.* **63**: 1417–1419.
8 Wang CH et al. (2012) Cranberry-containing products for prevention of urinary tract infections in susceptible populations: a systematic review and meta-analysis of randomized controlled trials. *Archives of Internal Medicine.* **172**: 988–996.
9 Avorn J et al. (1994) Reduction of bacteriuria and pyuria after ingestion of cranberry juice. *Journal of the American Medical Association.* **271**: 751–754.
10 Howell AB et al. (2010) Dosage effect on uropathogenic Escherichia coli anti-adhesion activity in urine following consumption of cranberry powder standardized for proanthocyanidin content: a multicentric randomized double blind study. *BMC Infectious Diseases.* **10**: 94. Available from: www.biomedcentral.com
11 Hodek P et al. (2002) Flavonoids-potent and versatile biologically active compounds interacting with cytochromes P450. *Chemico-Biological Interactions.* **139**: 1–21.
12 Suvarna R et al. (2003) Possible interaction between warfarin and cranberry juice. *British Medical Journal.* **327**: 1454.
13 CSM (Committee on Safety of Medicines) (2004) Interaction between warfarin and cranberry juice: new advice. *Current Problems in Pharmacovigilance.* **30**: 10.
14 MHRA (2003) Possible interaction between warfarin and cranberry juice. *Current Problems in Pharmacovigilance.* **29**: 8.
15 Grant P (2004) Warfarin and cranberry juice: an interaction? *Journal of Heart Valve Disease.* **13**: 25–26.
16 Rettie AE et al. (1992) Hydroxylation of warfarin by human cDNA-expressed cytochrome P-450: a role for P-4502C9 in the etiology of (S)-warfarin-drug interactions. *Chemical Research in Toxicology.* **5**: 54–59.
17 MHRA (2009) Public assessment report. Warfarin: changes to product safety information December 2009. Available from: www.mhra.gov.uk/home/groups/pl-p/documents/websiteresources/con065506.pdf
18 Health Canada (2004) Suspected warfarin-cranberry juice interaction. *Canadian Adverse Reaction Newsletter.* **14**: 2.
19 Health Canada (2011) Cranberry. Available from: http://webprod.hc-sc.gc.ca/nhpid-bdipsn/monoReq.do?id = 71&lang = eng
20 Li Z et al. (2006) Cranberry does not affect prothrombin time in male subjects on warfarin. *Journal of the American Dietetic Society.* **106**: 2057–2061.
21 Lilja JJ et al. (2007) Effects of daily ingestion of cranberry juice on the pharmacokinetics of warfarin, tizanidine, and midazolam– probes of CYP2C9, CYP1A2, and CYP3A4. *Clinical Pharmacology and Therapeutics.* **81**: 833–839.
22 Aston JL et al. (2006) Interaction between warfarin and cranberry juice. *Pharmacotherapy.* **26**: 1314–1319.
23 Welch J and Forster K (2007) Probable elevation in international normalized ratio from cranberry juice. *Journal of Pharmacy Technology.* **23**: 104–107.
24 O'Mara N (2007) Does a cranberry juice-warfarin interaction really exist? Detail document. *Pharmacist's Letter/Prescriber's Letter.* **23**: 1–3.

Updated June 2014

CATHETER PATENCY SOLUTIONS   BNF 7.4.4

Indications: Catheter blockage.

General considerations

Catheters can block because of blood clots, bladder mucosal debris, small calculi and/or phosphate encrustations on the surface of an indwelling catheter. Encrustations are associated with colonization of the urine by urease-producing bacteria, e.g. *Proteus mirabilis*, *Pseudomonas aeruginosa* and *Klebsiella*. Urease breaks down urea to form ammonia, increasing the alkalinity of the urine and leading to the deposition of mainly phosphate crystals on the surface of the catheter.

Some bacteria produce secretions which eventually thicken enough to form a protective biofilm attached to the catheter surface. This can embed both bacteria and phosphate crystals in a matrix which is impervious to acidifying solutions or urinary antiseptics. Thus, repeated blockage with encrustation generally means that the catheter needs to be changed.[1,2]

The main purpose of a catheter patency solution is to reduce the frequency of catheter blockage. Although a Cochrane review found insufficient evidence to make firm recommendations,[3] the BNF states that **sodium chloride** 0.9% is generally adequate as a mechanical flush for removing mucosal debris or small blood clots, and that solutions containing **citric acid** 3% (e.g. **solution G**) may be helpful in dissolving retained blood clots.[4]

In a palliativedrugs.com survey, **sodium chloride** 0.9% was most commonly used for both flushing out cell debris or blood clots (75% of respondents) and treating or preventing encrustation (>50%). **Solution G** was next most popular for these indications (<10% and 20–25% respectively). Few respondents used other solutions.[5]

Irrigation does *not* cure catheter-associated urinary tract infection (CAUTI).[6,7] Although the BNF states that **chlorhexidine** 0.02% irrigation can be used in the management of common bladder infections, it is ineffective against most *Pseudomonas* species, and may irritate the bladder mucosa, and cause a burning sensation or haematuria.[4]

Use of irrigations or prophylactic antibacterials to prevent CAUTI is *not* recommended by NICE or current European nursing guidelines.[8,9] Consideration should be given to the long-term use of a PO urinary antiseptic to acidify the urine and to reduce the frequency of infection (see **Methenamine hippurate**, p.554).

Dose and use

To reduce the likelihood of encrustations causing a blockage, latex catheters should be changed:
- uncoated every 2 weeks
- teflon-coated every 4 weeks
- silicone-coated or hydrogel-coated, up to every 6 weeks, depending on manufacturer's instructions.[4,9]

If the catheter is to be left for longer periods, a silicone catheter should be used with a catheter patency solution.[4] These catheters are designed to remain in place for up to 3 months.[9]

Some patients are more prone to recurrent encrustation than others. If encrustations regularly cause blockage, keep a diary over ⩾ 3 re-catheterizations, calculate the average time for which a catheter remains patent, then schedule a catheter change before a blockage is likely.[2,9]

For flushing out blockages caused by mucosal debris or small blood clots:
- start with **sodium chloride** 0.9% p.r.n.
- if necessary, use routinely every few days or even every day[5]
- if this is inadequate for dissolving retained clots, change to **solution G**.

For prevention of phosphate encrustations or calculi:[1,5]
- start with **sodium chloride** 0.9% p.r.n. or **solution G** once or twice a week
- if necessary, increase frequency.

Commercially available sachets are preferable to using a bladder syringe, because they are less likely to force encrusted material (which contains bacteria) higher up the urinary tract.

Supply

This is not a complete list; see BNF for additional options.

Sodium chloride 0.9%
OptiFlo S® (Bard)
Sachet 50mL, 100mL = £3.50 for both sizes.

Uriflex S® (Coloplast)
Sachet 100mL = £3.50.

Uro-Tainer sodium chloride® (B. Braun Medical)
Sachet 50mL, 100mL = £3.50 for both sizes.

Solution G containing **citric acid** 3.23% with magnesium oxide, sodium bicarbonate and disodium edetate
OptiFlo G® (Bard)
Sachet 50mL, 100mL = £3.50 for both sizes.

Uriflex G® (Coloplast)
Sachet 100mL = £2.50.

Uro-Tainer Twin Suby G® (B. Braun Medical)
Dual-chamber sachet (each chamber contains 30mL) = £4.50.

1 Williams C and Tonkin S (2003) Blocked urinary catheters: solutions are not the only solution. *British Journal of Community Nursing.* **8**: 321–326.
2 Getliffe K (2002) Managing recurrent urinary catheter encrustation. *British Journal of Community Nursing.* **7**: 574, 576, 578–580.
3 Hagen S (2010) Washout policies in long-term indwelling urinary catheterisation in adults. *Cochrane Database of Systematic Reviews.* **3**: CD004012.
4 British National Formulary Section 7.4.4. Bladder instillations and urological surgery London: BMJ Group and Pharmaceutical Press www.bnf.org (accessed April 2014).
5 palliativedrugs.com (2010) Survey: urinary catheter patency solutions – do you use them? Available from: www.palliativedrugs.com/latest/december/urinary-catheter-patency-solutions-do-you-use-them.html
6 Getliffe K (1996) Bladder instillations and bladder washouts in the management of catheterized patients. *Journal of Advanced Nursing.* **23**: 548–554.
7 Pomfret I et al. (2004) Using bladder instillations to manage indwelling catheters. *British journal of Nursing.* **13**: 261–267.
8 NICE (2012) Infection control. Prevention of healthcare-associated infections in primary and community care. *Clinical guideline* CG139. www.nice.org.uk
9 Geng A (2012) Evidence-based guidelines for best practice in urological health care. Catheterisation. Indwelling catheters in adults, urethral and suprapubic. European Association of Urology Nurses, Arnhem, The Netherlands. Available from: www.uroweb.org/fileadmin/EAUN/guidelines/EAUN_Paris_Guideline_2012_LR_online_file.pdf

Updated April 2014

DISCOLOURED URINE

Patients need to be warned about drugs and other substances which can discolour urine (Box A). If the urine is red, it may be assumed to be blood, and cause alarm.

Box A Selected causes of discoloured urine[a]	
Black/dark brown Iron (ferrous salts) Methocarbamol	**Purple** Degradation of tryptophan by urinary 　bacteria (see text)
Brown/orange/yellow Aloe Carrots Cascara Chloroquine Chlorzoxazone (not UK) Dantrolene Fluorescein Heparin Nitrofurantoin Paprika Phenazopyridine (not UK) Quinine Retinol (vitamin A) Riboflavin (vitamin B2) Rifampicin Senna (pH dependent) Sulfasalazine Sulfonamides Tolcapone Warfarin	**Blue/green** Amitriptyline[1] Chlorophyll breath mints FD & C Dye No. 1 (used in foods and medicines) Hydroquinone Indometacin Magnesium salicylate Phenols Promethazine (injection) Propofol[2] *Pseudomonas aeruginosa* (pyocyanin; alkaline urine) Resorcinol Thymol Triamterene **Milky colour** Diffuse glomerular nephritis Lipids Neutrophils Phosphates Radiographic dyes Urates

continued

Box A continued

Brown/red/pink
Beetroot (alkaline urine)
Blackberries (acid urine)
Dantron
Daunorubicin
Doxorubicin
Entacapone
Ibuprofen
Levodopa-containing medicines, e.g. co-beneldopa (levodopa + benserazide)
   and co-careldopa (levodopa + carbidopa)
Metronidazole (acid urine)
Napthalene-based dyes in foods and medicines, e.g. Ponceau 4R
Nefopam
Phenolphthalein (alkaline urine)
Phenothiazines
Phenytoin
Rhubarb (pH dependent)
Senna (alkaline urine)

---

a. discolouration which occurs only when urine is left 'on standing' has not been included.

The colour-banding in Box A is approximate, i.e. a drug listed under 'brown/orange/yellow' will most likely cause discolouration at some point in that range. Sometimes the colour is pH dependent. Further information on causes of discoloured urine is available from: www.wrongdiagnosis.com/symptoms/urine_color_changes/causes.htm

Note: urine colour will vary according to the concentration or dilution of the urine. Colouring agents in processed food can also affect urine colour.

Purple urine bag syndrome is caused by the breakdown of dietary tryptophan metabolites by bacteria in urine, ultimately producing indigo (blue) and indirubin (red) in alkaline urine.[3–5] Chronic urinary tract infection, long-term catheterization, constipation and immobility are the main risk factors. Although harmless, purple urine bag syndrome causes the urine to develop a strong, unpleasant odour, which becomes more noticeable over time and in warm conditions. This distresses patients more than the discolouration. Changing the drainage bag more frequently, e.g. every 3 days rather than every 5–7 days, helps to avoid the build-up of the odour. Indwelling long-term catheters may also need changing more often than normal.[5]

---

1 Beeley L (1986) What drugs turn urine green? *British Medical Journal.* **293**: 750.
2 Leclercq P et al. (2009) Green urine. *Lancet.* **373**: 1462.
3 Al-Jubouri MA and Vardhan MS (2001) A case of purple urine bag syndrome associated with Providencia rettgeri. *Journal of Clinical Pathology.* **54**: 412.
4 Ribeiro JP et al. (2004) Case report: purple urine bag syndrome. *Critical Care (London, England).* **8**: R137.
5 Robinson J (2003) Purple urinary bag syndrome: a harmless but alarming problem. *British Journal of Community Nursing.* **8**: 263–266.

Updated March 2014

9: NUTRITION AND BLOOD

ANAEMIA

Anaemia is defined as a haemoglobin (Hb) concentration:
- $< 130g/L$ in men > 15 years old
- $< 120g/L$ in non-pregnant women > 15 years old.[1]

The normal range for Hb varies between populations. It is acceptable to use the lower limit of the normal range in the laboratory performing the test to define anaemia.

Anaemia is common in cancer and other forms of chronic disease. The main causes are:
- anaemia of chronic disease
- iron deficiency
- chemotherapy-induced anaemia
- vitamin B_{12} deficiency
- folate deficiency
- malignant infiltration of the marrow
- haemolytic anaemia
- renal failure.

The commonest form in cancer is anaemia of chronic disease (ACD). ACD is a paraneoplastic phenomenon caused by cytokine-mediated suppression of endogenous erythropoietin production and disturbance of iron homeostasis. Iron mobilization from stores in the reticulo-endothelial system is impaired and iron absorption from the duodenum reduced. This causes functional iron deficiency, but over time, impaired utilization of oral iron can lead to absolute iron deficiency, and iron-deficiency anaemia (IDA) with ACD.[2] There are no reliable peripheral blood tests for the diagnosis of ACD, so several parameters need to be measured (Table 1).

Table 1 Anaemia of chronic disease (ACD) vs. iron-deficiency anaemia (IDA)

	ACD	IDA
Red cell appearance	Normochromic, normocytic[a]	Hypochromic, microcytic
Plasma ferritin	High/high-normal	Low[b]
Transferrin saturation[c]	Low	Low/very low
Transferrin concentration[d]	Low/low-normal	High/high-normal
Reticulocyte count	Low	Low
Plasma iron	Low	Low

a. anaemia may become microcytic if long standing
b. ferritin reflects iron stores but rises during acute an phase response, e.g. to trauma, infection and some cancers; thus ferritin may be normal or elevated in patients with IDA and cancer or inflammatory illness
c. measurement derived from plasma total iron binding capacity (TIBC) and plasma iron. Reflects availability of iron to erythropoetic cells
d. effectively the same measurement as TIBC.

It is important to distinguish between the various types of anaemia because treatment differs. However, it is difficult to diagnose IDA in the presence of ACD because red cell indices are less reliable when there is co-existent illness. When patients have both ACD and IDA, the anaemia may be more severe and microcytic, and ferritin may be normal or raised. Alternative methods of diagnosing IDA in the presence of ACD, such as hepcidin assays and serum transferrin receptor assays, remain experimental.[3]

There are three potential treatment options:
• iron (oral or IV)
• intermittent blood transfusions[4]
• SC **erythropoietin**.

Where IDA alone is diagnosed, the underlying cause should be treated if possible and ferrous sulphate prescribed. If oral iron is not tolerated or a rapid response is required (e.g. in patients about to commence myelosuppressive chemotherapy), parenteral iron is indicated.

Where ACD alone is diagnosed, there is insufficient evidence to prescribe IV iron routinely as monotherapy. However, about 75% of patients respond to **erythropoietin**. In patients already transfusion-dependent, about half will become transfusion-independent.[5,6] However, because of increased tumour progression and reduced survival time in cancer patients treated with **erythropoietin**,[7,8] NICE now recommends that it (with IV **iron**) should be used only for:
• **platinum**-induced anaemia in women with ovarian cancer who are symptomatic with an Hb ≤8g/dL
• patients with profound cancer-treatment related anaemia which is likely to have an impact on survival but who cannot be given blood transfusions.[9]

Blood transfusion can cause a transfusion reaction and anaphylaxis, and may increase the risk of stroke, myocardial infarction, acute renal failure and cancer recurrence.[10] However, blood transfusion remains the most practical treatment for palliative care patients with symptomatic ACD, even if its effectiveness is difficult to determine.[11]

In patients with ACD and suspected IDA, a therapeutic trial of oral iron may be considered. Because absorption of oral iron is impaired by ACD, some centres give parenteral iron. However, there is insufficient evidence to support this approach and the impact of parenteral iron on cancer cell growth, inflammation and bacterial growth is unclear. Thus, blood transfusion remains the most practical treatment in patients with co-existent symptomatic ACD and IDA.[3,12,13]

1 WHO (2008) Worldwide Prevalence of Anaemia. 1993–2005.
2 Weiss G and Goodnough LT (2005) Anemia of chronic disease. New England Journal of Medicine. **352**: 1011–1023.
3 Cullis JO (2011) Diagnosis and management of anaemia of chronic disease: current status. British Journal of Haematology. **154**: 289–300.
4 MHRA (2008) Recombinant human erythropoietins: new recommendations for treatment in cancer. Drug safety update: **(2)** 1. www.mhra.gov.uk/safetyinformation
5 Seidenfeld J et al. (2001) Epoetin treatment of anemia associated with cancer therapy: a systematic review and meta-analysis of controlled clinical trials. Journal of the National Cancer Institute. **93**: 1204–1214.
6 Turner R et al. (2001) Epoetin alfa in cancer patients: evidence-based guidelines. Journal of Pain and Symptom Management. **22**: 954–965.
7 Steensma DP (2007) Erythropoiesis stimulating agents. British Medical Journal. **334**: 648–649.
8 Bohlius J (2009) Recombinant human erythropoiesis-stimulating agents and mortality in patients with cancer: a met-analysis of randomized trails. Lancet. **373**: 1532–1542.
9 NICE (2008) Epoetin alfa, epoetin beta and darbepoetin alfa for cancer treatment-induced anaemia. Technology appraisal guidance TA142. www.nice.org.uk
10 Aapro M et al. (2012) Prevalence and management of cancer-related anaemia, iron deficiency and the specific role of i.v. iron. Annals of Oncology. **23**: 1954–1962.
11 Preston NJ et al. (2012) Blood transfusions for anaemia in patients with advanced cancer. Cochrane Database of Systematic Reviews. **2**: CD009007.
12 Thomas DW et al. (2013) Guideline for the laboratory diagnosis of functional iron deficiency. British Journal of Haematology. **161**: 639–648.
13 National Comprehensive Cancer Network Practice Guidelines in Oncology (2014) Cancer and chemotherapy-induced anemia. http://www.nccn.org/professionals/physician_gls/PDF/anemia.pdf (accessed February 2014).

Updated April 2014

FERROUS SULFATE   BNF 9.1.1.1

Class: Elemental salt.

Indications: Prevention and treatment of iron deficiency anaemia.

Contra-indications: Anaemia not caused by iron deficiency; haemosiderosis, haemochromatosis.

Pharmacology

Ferrous salts are better absorbed than ferric salts. Because there are only marginal differences in terms of efficiency of iron absorption, the choice of ferrous salt is based mainly on the incidence of undesirable effects and cost. Some undesirable effects relate directly to the amount of elemental iron, and improved tolerance after switching to another salt may be because the elemental iron content is less (Table 1). M/r formulations are designed to reduce undesirable effects by releasing iron gradually as the tablet or capsule passes down the GI tract.[1] However, these products are likely to carry most of the iron past the first part of the duodenum into parts of the intestine where iron absorption is poor. Such products have little therapeutic advantage and should not be used.[2]

Table 1   Elemental ferrous iron content of different iron salts

Iron salt	Amount (mg)	Ferrous content (mg)
Ferrous fumarate	200	65
Ferrous sulfate, dried (anhydrous)	200	65
Ferrous sulfate	300	60
Ferrous gluconate	300	35

Dietary accessible (non-haem) iron absorption may be increased by a high intake of red meat, poultry, fish or **ascorbic acid** (e.g. from fruits) but reduced by a high intake of phytates (e.g. in whole-grain cereals), polyphenols (e.g. in tea and coffee), and **calcium** (e.g. in dairy products).[3]

Some oral formulations contain **ascorbic acid** or chelated iron. These modifications have been shown experimentally to produce a modest increase in the absorption of iron. However, the therapeutic advantage is minimal, and the cost may be increased.[2] Further, **ascorbic acid** may increase GI irritation. There is no clinical justification for the inclusion of other therapeutically active ingredients such as the B group of vitamins (except **folic acid** for pregnant women).

When treating iron deficiency, Hb should rise by about 10g/L/week. Epithelial tissue changes such as atrophic glossitis and koilonychia also improve but generally more slowly.

Drug interactions

Because of decreased absorption of iron, the other drug or both, ferrous sulfate should not be administered concurrently with antacids, bisphosphonates, **calcium** salts, **colestyramine**, **demeclocycline**, **levodopa**, **levothyroxine**, **penicillamine**, quinolone antibacterials, tetracyclines, and **zinc**.

Undesirable effects

Dyspepsia, nausea, epigastric pain, constipation and diarrhoea. Nausea and epigastric pain are dose-related but the relationship between dose and altered bowel habit is not so clear.[2] Elderly patients are more likely to develop constipation, occasionally leading to faecal impaction; m/r products are more likely to cause diarrhoea, particularly in patients with inflammatory bowel disease.

Note: liquid formulations may stain teeth. Urine and stools are discoloured (black), and this may result in a false positive faecal occult blood test.

Dose and use

The diagnosis of iron deficiency should be confirmed before iron supplements are prescribed (see Anaemia, p.561). The PO dose of **elemental iron** for iron-deficiency anaemia is 100–200mg/24h. This can be provided, for example, as dried (anhydrous) ferrous sulfate 200mg b.d.–t.d.s

(= elemental iron 130–195mg/24h). After the Hb has risen to normal, treatment should be continued for a further 3 months to replenish the iron stores.[4]

Doses >600mg/24h of dried (anhydrous) ferrous sulfate exceed the maximal absorption capacity and increase undesirable effects. If undesirable GI effects occur:

- reduce the dose
- take with food (but may reduce absorption by up to 50%)
- switch to an alternative iron salt with a lower elemental iron content
- switch to a liquid formulation (may be less damaging to GI mucosa)[5]
- dilute liquid formulations and swallow through a straw to prevent discolouration of the teeth.

Consider prophylaxis in patients at high risk of iron deficiency, e.g. those with a poor diet, malabsorption, and after total or sub-total gastrectomy; for example, prescribe dried (anhydrous) ferrous sulfate 200mg once daily (elemental iron 65mg).

Supply

Ferrous sulfate, dried (generic)
Tablets 200mg (65mg iron), 28 days @ 200mg t.d.s. (195mg elemental iron/24h) = £3.

Ferrous fumarate (generic)
Tablets 210mg (68mg iron), 28 days @ 210mg t.d.s. (204mg elemental iron/24h) = £2.50.
Oral suspension 140mg (45mg iron)/5mL, 28 days @ 280mg (10mL) b.d. (180mg elemental iron/24h) = £10.

Fersaday® (AmCo)
Tablets 322mg (100mg iron), 28 days @ 322mg b.d. (200mg elemental iron/24h) = £2.

Galfer® (Thornton & Ross)
Capsules 305mg (100mg iron), 28 days @ 305mg b.d. (200mg elemental iron/24h) = £1.50.
Oral syrup 140mg (45mg iron)/5mL, 28 days @ 280mg (10mL) b.d. (180mg elemental iron/24h) = £10.

Ferrous gluconate (generic)
Tablets 300mg (35mg iron), 28 days @ 600mg t.d.s. (210mg elemental iron/24h) = £12.

This is not a complete list; see BNF for more information.

---

1 Cancelo-Hidalgo MJ et al. (2013) Tolerability of different oral iron supplements: a systematic review. *Current Medical Research Opinion.* **29**: 291–303.
2 British National Formulary Section 9.1.1.1 Oral Iron. London: BMJ Group and Pharmaceutical Press. www.bnf.org (accessed April 2014).
3 Heath AL and Fairweather-Tait SJ (2002) Clinical implications of changes in the modern diet: iron intake, absorption and status. *Best Practice and Research Clinical Haematology.* **15**: 225–241.
4 Goddard AF et al. (2011) Guidelines for the management of iron deficiency anaemia. *Gut.* **60**: 1309–1316.
5 Ji H and Yardley JH (2004) Iron medication-associated gastric mucosal injury. *Archives of Pathology and Laboratory Medicine.* **128**: 821–822.

Updated May 2014

ASCORBIC ACID (VITAMIN C)　　　　　　BNF 9.6.3

Class: Vitamin.

Indications: Scurvy, †decubitus ulcers, †urinary infection.

Pharmacology

Ascorbic acid (vitamin C) is a powerful reducing agent. It is obtained from dietary sources of fresh fruit and vegetables, e.g. blackcurrants, kiwifruit, broccoli, red pepper and oranges. It cannot be synthesized by the body. It is involved in the hydroxylation of proline to hydroxyproline, which is necessary for the formation of collagen. The failure of this accounts for most of the clinical effects found in deficiency (scurvy), e.g. keratosis of hair follicles with 'corkscrew hair', perifollicular haemorrhages, swollen spongy infected and bleeding gums, loose teeth, spontaneous bruising and haemorrhage, anaemia and failure of wound healing. Repeated infections are also common. In healthy adults, a dietary intake of about 30–60mg/24h is necessary; in scurvy, a rapid clinical response is seen with ≥250mg/24h in divided doses.

Absorption occurs mainly from the proximal small intestine by a saturable process. In health, body stores of ascorbic acid are about 1.5g, although larger stores may occur with intakes higher than 200mg/24h. It is excreted as oxalic acid, unchanged ascorbic acid and small amounts of dehydro-ascorbic acid. Ascorbic acid is used to acidify urine in patients with alkaline urine and recurrent urinary infections.

A beneficial effect of megadose ascorbic acid therapy has been claimed for many conditions,[1] including the common cold, asthma, atherosclerosis, cancer, psychiatric disorders, increased susceptibility to infections related to abnormal leucocyte function, infertility and osteogenesis imperfecta. Ascorbic acid has also been tried in the treatment of wound healing, pain in Paget's disease and opioid withdrawal. There are few RCTs to substantiate these claims. A systematic review of vitamin C for the prevention and treatment of cancer found no evidence of benefit.[2] However, vitamin C deficiency is common in cancer patients, and low plasma concentrations are associated with shorter survival.[3]

Vitamin C alone or with β-carotene and vitamin E does not prevent the development of colorectal adenoma.[4] However, ascorbic acid does reduce the severity of a cold but not its incidence.[5] On the other hand, enthusiasm for high-dose ascorbic acid for HIV+ people waned after many died from disease progression.[6] Although it has been postulated that ascorbic acid might help prevent ischaemic heart disease, in contrast to other anti-oxidant vitamins, little benefit is seen in RCTs.[7,8] Of more concern are data which indicate that a total daily dose as small as 500mg has a pro-oxidant effect which could result in genetic mutation.[9]

Drug interactions

Aspirin reduces the absorption of ascorbic acid by up to a third. In patients with renal impairment, because of an increased risk of aluminium toxicity, avoid concurrent use of ascorbic acid and aluminium-containing products.

Undesirable effects

GI symptoms may occur at doses of >1g/24h.[10] Doses of >3g/24h may result in diarrhoea, acidosis, glycosuria, oxaluria, and renal stones. Tolerance may occur with prolonged use of large doses, resulting in symptoms of deficiency if intake is reduced.

In the past, some centres used undissolved effervescent ascorbic acid tablets (available OTC) for debriding the tongue. However, such use has fallen out of favour because the acidity may:
• exacerbate a sore or inflamed mouth
• contribute to the demineralization of teeth
• predispose to oral infections (see p.599).
Further, if not completely dissolved or swallowed when lying down, the tablets could cause localized oesophagitis.

Dose and use

Ascorbic acid is generally given PO; if this is not feasible or malabsorption is suspected, it can be given by SC or IM injection or IVI.

Vitamin C deficiency
• for florid scurvy, give 100mg PO t.d.s. (or 250mg once daily–b.d. parenterally) for 4 weeks
• otherwise, give 100mg PO once daily; continue indefinitely in undernourished patients, particularly the elderly.

Enhancement of healing
• 100mg PO b.d. for 4 weeks.

Acidification of urine
• 100–200mg PO b.d.; test urine with litmus paper until a constant acid result is obtained. Note: may alter the excretion of some drugs.

Supply

Ascorbic acid (generic)

Tablets 50mg, 100mg, 200mg, 500mg, 28 days @ 100mg t.d.s. = £4.
Injection 100mg/mL, 5mL amp = £4.50.

1 Ovesen L (1984) Vitamin therapy in the absence of obvious deficiency. What is the evidence? *Drugs.* **27**: 148–170.
2 Coulter ID et al. (2006) Antioxidants vitamin C and vitamin e for the prevention and treatment of cancer. *Journal of General Internal Medicine.* **21**: 735–744.
3 Mayland CR et al. (2005) Vitamin C deficiency in cancer patients. *Palliative Medicine.* **19**: 17–20.
4 Greenberg E et al. (1994) A clinical trial of antioxidant vitamins to prevent colorectal adenoma. Polyp Prevention Study Group. *New England Journal of Medicine.* **331**: 141–147.
5 Hemila H (1994) Does vitamin C alleviate the symptoms of the common cold? a review of current evidence. *Scandinavian Journal of Infectious Diseases.* **26**: 1–6.
6 Abrams D (1990) Alternative therapies in HIV infection. *AIDS.* **4**: 1179–1187.
7 Rimm E (1993) Vitamin E consumption and the risk of coronary heart disease in men. *New England Journal of Medicine.* **328**: 1450–1456.
8 Stampfer M (1993) Vitamin E consumption and the risk of coronary disease in women. *New England Journal of Medicine.* **328**: 1444–1449.
9 Podmore I et al. (1998) Vitamin C exhibits pro-oxidant properties. *Nature.* **392**: 559.
10 Beveridge C (2002) Basic Nutrition. In: C Repchinsky and C LeBlanc (eds) *Patient Self Care* (1e). Canadian Pharmacists Association, Ottawa, pp. 339–358.

Updated November 2014

PHYTOMENADIONE (VITAMIN K₁)   BNF 9.6.6

Class: Vitamin.

Indications: Vitamin K deficiency, reversal of anticoagulant effects of **warfarin** and other coumarins, †bleeding tendency in patients with hepatic impairment, †hypoprothrombinaemia induced by salicylates, sulfonamides, **quinidine**, **quinine** and antibacterials.

Pharmacology

Vitamin K is a fat-soluble vitamin. Phytomenadione (vitamin K₁) is the active form, and is present in green vegetables, dairy products and soya bean oil. In addition, vitamin K is synthesized by bacteria in the terminal ileum and colon.

Phytomenadione is necessary for the synthesis of coagulation factors II, VII, IX and X, and of proteins involved in bone calcification. Oral coumarins block the recycling of vitamin K metabolites in the liver, and thus block the synthesis of the coagulation factors. This block is circumvented by exogenous vitamin K.

Hepatic stores of vitamin K are depleted in <3 days of dietary restriction. In patients with advanced cancer, >20% are vitamin K deficient.[1] Patients who are malnourished, have fat malabsorption (e.g. in biliary obstruction or liver disease) or are having prolonged courses of antibacterials which sterilize the GI tract are at risk of deficiency and a rapid rise in prothrombin time (PT) and activated partial thromboplastin time (APTT).

Menadiol sodium phosphate is a water-soluble synthetic vitamin K analogue. It can be given PO to prevent vitamin K deficiency in patients with fat malabsorption or to correct dietary deficiency. (Note: phytomenadione and vitamin K analogues do *not* reverse heparin-induced anticoagulation, see p.89).

Hepatic failure

Phytomenadione is *not* indicated routinely in chronic hepatic failure because blood coagulation is 'rebalanced' by a reduction of both procoagulant and anticoagulant factors.[2] If a patient with hepatic failure develops surface bleeding (e.g. petechiae, purpura, multiple bruising, epistaxis, gum bleeding, bleeding from GI tract), PT should be checked, and if prolonged, phytomenadione is indicated. However, its use should be limited to conscious patients with a reasonable performance status for whom other supportive measures are deemed appropriate (e.g. blood transfusion). Phytomenadione should not be used in moribund patients in an attempt to prevent an imminent inevitable death.

Because vitamin K deficiency is rarely the primary cause of coagulopathy in hepatic failure, phytomenadione may only partially correct the PT. A persistently prolonged PT following administration of phytomenadione may indicate the existence of a clotting factor deficiency caused by impaired hepatic synthesis. Other underlying conditions may also contribute to the bleeding tendency, e.g. renal failure, sepsis.[2]

Plasma halflife 1.5–3h.

Cautions

Unless there is major bleeding, phytomenadione should generally not be given to patients with a prosthetic heart valve; fresh frozen plasma or **dried prothrombin complex** should be used instead.

Oral absorption of **menadiol sodium phosphate** is reduced by concurrent administration with **colestyramine** or **liquid paraffin (mineral oil)**.

Undesirable effects

Rarely, anaphylaxis after IV use.

Dose and use

Phytomenadione (Konakion® MM) is given by slow IV injection over at least 30sec, generally 3–5min, or by IVI diluted in 50mL of 5% glucose over 20–30min (protect from light). *Konakion® MM formulation must not be given IM.*

Reversal of warfarin anticoagulation
Use the British Society for Haematology guidelines.[3,4]

Major bleeding
- stop **warfarin** *and*
- give reconstituted **dried prothrombin complex** (factors II, VII, IX, X) 25–50 Units/kg IV *and*
- phytomenadione 5mg slow IV; check INR after 3h
- repeat the dose if necessary; re-check INR after 3h
- maximum dose = 40mg/24h.

Note: recombinant factor VIIa is *not* recommended for emergency reversal of anticoagulation. Fresh frozen plasma produces suboptimal anticoagulation reversal and should be used only if **dried prothrombin complex** is not available.

Minor bleeding INR > 5
- stop **warfarin** *and*
- give phytomenadione 1–3mg slow IV.

No bleeding but prolonged INR
- INR > 5, withhold 1–2 doses of **warfarin** and reduce maintenance dose
- INR ≥8, give phytomenadione 1–5 mg *by mouth* using the injection formulation, and recheck INR after 24h
- restart **warfarin** when INR < 5.

Vitamin K deficiency in malabsorption
Prevention:
- give **menadiol phosphate** 10mg PO once daily
- check PT after 3 days and, if still raised, increase the dose progressively up to 40mg once daily (rarely necessary) until maximal PT correction is achieved
- once maximal PT correction is achieved, give a maintenance dose of menadiol phosphate 10mg PO once daily and monitor PT regularly.[5]

If serious bleeding:
- phytomenadione injection (Konakion® MM) 10mg IV (see above)
- if IV access difficult, consider using the Konakion® MM *Paediatric formulation* 10mg which can be administered IM
- **dried prothrombin complex** IV may also be necessary.

Correction of a bleeding tendency in hepatic failure

- give **menadiol phosphate** 10mg PO once daily
- check prothrombin time after 3 days and, if still raised, increase the dose progressively up to 40mg once daily (rarely necessary) until maximal PT correction is achieved
- if **menadiol phosphate** unavailable, consider giving phytomenadione 2.5–10mg *by mouth* using the injection formulation.

If serious bleeding:
- give phytomenadione injection (Konakion® MM) 10mg IV (see above)
- then as for malabsorption above.

When maximal PT correction is achieved, stop menadiol phosphate and recheck PT if signs of surface bleeding return. In patients with hepatic impairment, the risk of venous thrombosis is often paradoxically increased. Thus, in this situation, **dried prothrombin complex** should be used only in emergency situations after specialist advice and with regular coagulation monitoring. Note: **desmopressin** may improve haemostasis in patients with hepatic platelet dysfunction (see p.514).

Supply

Phytomenadione
Konakion® MM (Roche)
Injection (colloidal) phytomenadione 10mg/mL in a mixed micelles vehicle, 1mL (10mg) amp = £0.50. *For IV or IVI use only, do not use IM. PO use is off-label.*

Konakion® MM Paediatric (Roche)
Injection (colloidal) phytomenadione 10mg/mL in a mixed micelles vehicle, 0.2mL (2mg) amp = £1. *Konakion® MM Paediatric may be administered PO, IM, IV.*

Menadiol phosphate (generic)
Tablets menadiol sodium phosphate equivalent to 10mg of menadiol phosphate, 7days @ 10mg once daily = £9.

Oral solution 5mg/5mL, 30mL = £162; unauthorized, available as a special order (see Appendix 1, p.817). *Note price based on specials tariff applied in community.*

1 Harrington DJ et al. (2008) A study of the prevalence of vitamin K deficiency in patients with cancer referred to a hospital palliative care team and its association with abnormal haemostasis. *Journal of Clinical Pathology.* **61**: 537–540.
2 Tripodi A and Mannucci PM (2011) The coagulopathy of chronic liver disease. *New England Journal of Medicine.* **365**: 147–156.
3 British National Formulary Section 2.8.2. Oral anticoagulants. London: BMJ Group and Pharmaceutical Press. www.bnf.org (accessed January 2014).
4 Makris M et al. (2012) Guideline on the management of bleeding in patients on antithrombotic agents. *British Journal of Haematology.* **160**: 35–46.
5 Jagannath VA et al. (2013) Vitamin K supplementation for cystic fibrosis. *Cochrane Database of Systematic Reviews.* **4**: CD008482.

Updated April 2014

POTASSIUM   BNF 9.2.1.1

Class: Elemental salt.

Indications: Hypokalaemia (<3.5mmol/L).

Pharmacology

In palliative care, hypokalaemia is most common in patients receiving non-potassium-sparing diuretics, particularly if also taking a corticosteroid. Hypokalaemia is also associated with chronic diarrhoea and persistent vomiting. Correction of hypokalaemia is important in patients taking **digoxin** or other anti-arrhythmic drugs because of the risk of an arrhythmia. Potassium supplements are seldom required with small doses of diuretics given to treat hypertension.

When larger doses of thiazide or loop diuretics are given to eliminate oedema, potassium-sparing diuretics (e.g. **amiloride**, **spironolactone**) rather than potassium supplements are preferable. Dietary supplements also help to maintain plasma potassium; 10mmol of potassium is contained in a large banana and in 250mL of orange juice.

When treating hypokalaemia, potassium chloride is generally the salt of choice because of associated hypochloraemia. However, occasionally, hypokalaemia is associated with a hyperchloraemic metabolic acidosis, and an alkalinizing salt will be preferable, e.g. potassium *bicarbonate* or potassium *citrate* (not UK). Co-existing hypomagnesaemia should always be corrected (see p.571).

Drugs are a common cause of hyperkalaemia in hospitalized patients (see Cautions), particularly in association with pre-existing or new renal impairment. When *mild–moderate* (i.e. 5.5–6.9mmol/L, with no ECG changes or symptoms), dose reduction or stopping the causal drug may be all that needs to be done. However, other causes may need to be considered, e.g. hypo-aldosteronism, tumour lysis syndrome, **digoxin** toxicity. Spurious results can also occur, e.g. as a result of haemolysis, marked leukocytosis or thrombocytosis. Repeating the sample and/or obtaining advice from the clinical chemistry laboratory may be necessary. For the treatment of *severe* hyperkalaemia, see below.

Cautions

Hyperkalaemia may result if used concurrently with drugs which increase the plasma potassium concentration, e.g. ACE inhibitors, potassium-sparing diuretics, potassium-containing laxatives (e.g. Movicol®) **ciclosporin**. Use smaller doses of potassium if there is renal impairment (common in the elderly).

Undesirable effects

Oesophageal or GI ulceration, nausea and vomiting. Liquid or effervescent formulations are distasteful.

Dose and use

The normal adult daily requirement and the typical dietary intake of potassium is 40–80mmol. Whenever possible, orange juice and bananas should be used as a palatable source of potassium (see Pharmacology above). To minimize nausea and vomiting, potassium supplements are best taken during or after a meal.

Slow-K® tablets must be swallowed whole to preserve the m/r mechanism. Because this is difficult for some patients, liquid or effervescent products are generally preferable.

Prevention of hypokalaemia

- potassium *chloride*, e.g. Sando-K® 1–2 tablets b.d. (24–48mmol/24h K$^+$) *or*
- prescribe a potassium-sparing diuretic, e.g. **amiloride** 5–10mg once daily (maximum 20mg once daily) or **spironolactone** 25–200mg/24h.

Treatment of hypokalaemia

- potassium *chloride*, e.g. Sando-K® 2 tablets t.d.s. (72mmol/24h K$^+$)
- if the patient is hyperchloraemic, prescribe potassium *bicarbonate* effervescent tablets BPC 1968 instead
- if hypokalaemia persists, investigate for possible magnesium deficiency (see p.571).

Emergency treatment of hyperkalaemia

Stop and think! Are you justified in correcting a potentially fatal complication in a moribund patient?

Urgent treatment is required when hyperkalaemia is severe ($\geq$7mmol/L) or with any level $\geq$5.5mmol/L accompanied by ECG changes (e.g. reduced or absent P waves, PR prolongation, QRS widening) and/or symptoms (e.g. muscle weakness, paraesthesia, palpitation). An approach is summarized in Box A.

However, this is only part of the management of hyperkalaemia and specialist advice should be obtained as necessary.

Supply

Potassium *chloride*
Sando-K® (HK Pharma)
Tablets effervescent potassium bicarbonate and chloride equivalent to potassium 470mg (12mmol K$^+$) and chloride 285mg (8mmol Cl$^-$), 28 days @ 2 t.d.s. (72mmol/24h K$^+$ and 48mmol/24h Cl$^-$) = £13.

Box A   Emergency treatment of severe hyperkalaemia[1-3]

Stop potentially contributory or antagonistic drugs
These include ACE inhibitors, potassium-sparing diuretics, NSAIDS and potassium-containing laxatives (e.g. Movicol®).

β-blockers and digoxin should also be stopped as they antagonize the effect of insulin and β$_2$ agonists (see below).

Reduce the risk of cardiac arrhythmia
This is always the first step.

Give calcium gluconate 10mL of 10% solution IV over 2min; any improvement in ECG abnormalities will be seen in <3min; *stop if bradycardia develops*

If necessary, repeat the same dose every 10min until improvement is obtained; some patients require up to 50mL

Duration of action is 30–60min, and further doses may be required.

Note. Calcium gluconate can precipitate digoxin toxicity; give in 100mL of 5% dextrose IV over 20min in patients using digoxin (seek specialist advice).

Shift potassium into cells
When hyperkalaemia is severe (≥7mmol/L), insulin is generally given.

β$_2$ agonists (e.g. salbutamol) can be as effective.

Both reduce the plasma potassium concentration by about 0.5–1mmol/L.

Some guidelines do not recommended β$_2$ agonists as a sole treatment because some patients, e.g. those who are dialysis dependent or using β-blockers or digoxin, are less likely to respond.

The combination of insulin with nebulized salbutamol is more effective than either alone, with the latter helping to reduce the hypoglycaemic effect of the insulin.

These interventions do not remove potassium from the body, but buy time for more definitive treatment to be carried out.

Insulin
- add 10 units soluble insulin (e.g. Actrapid®) to 50mL dextrose 50% and give IV over 5min
- onset of effect 15min, duration of action at least 1h and commonly 4–6h
- if it becomes necessary to repeat the dose of insulin, additional glucose is not required if plasma glucose is ≥15mmol/L.

β$_2$ agonist
- give salbutamol 10–20mg nebulized over 10–30min (10mg in patients with ischaemic heart disease)
- when a nebulizer is not available, use salbutamol 1,200microgram (12 puffs) inhaled over 2min via a spacer device
- onset of effect 5–30min, duration of action 2h or more.

Monitoring treatment
- recheck urea and electrolytes after 30min; if there is a good response, check again 1–2h after the last intervention
- when insulin used, check blood glucose after 30min and then q1h for 6h, as delayed hypoglycaemia can occur.

Other measures
If the combined approach above fails to work, emergency dialysis may be necessary to remove potassium from the body (if appropriate to the patient's overall circumstances).

Calcium polystyrene sulphonate resin (Calcium Resonium®) 15g PO q.d.s. is also used together with regular lactulose to increase potassium loss from the GI tract. However, it is *not* an emergency treatment because it has a slow onset of action (4–24h); it can also be poorly tolerated.

Modified-release
Slow-K® (Alliance)
Tablets m/r potassium chloride 600mg (8mmol K$^+$ and 8mmol Cl$^-$), 28 days @ 2 t.d.s. (48mmol/24h K$^+$ and Cl$^-$) = £3.50.

Potassium *bicarbonate*
Effervescent potassium tablets BPC 1968 (generic)
Tablets effervescent potassium bicarbonate 500mg, potassium acid tartrate 300mg (6.5mmol K$^+$), 28 days @ 2 q.d.s. (52mmol/24h K$^+$) = £161; dose depends on acid-base balance as well as plasma potassium concentration.

---

1 GAIN (Guidelines and Audit Implementation Network) (2008) Guidelines for the treatment of hyperkalaemia in adults. Available from: www.gain-ni.org/Library/Guidelines/hyperkalaemia_guidelines.pdf
2 Mahoney BA (2009) Emergency interventions for hyperkalaemia. *Cochrane Database of Systematic Reviews.* **3**: CD003235.
3 Mandelberg A et al. (1999) Salbutamol metered-dose inhaler with spacer for hyperkalemia: how fast? How safe? *Chest.* **115**: 617–622.

Updated June 2013

MAGNESIUM   BNF 9.5.1.3

Class: Metal element.

Indications: Hypomagnesaemia, constipation (see p.56), †arrhythmia, †eclampsia, †asthma, †myocardial infarction.

Pharmacology

Magnesium is the second most abundant intracellular ion after potassium. It is involved in numerous enzymatic reactions and is a co-factor for many biological processes, most of which use ATP. It is important for bone mineralization, muscular relaxation and neurotransmission. About half of the total body magnesium is in soft tissue, the other half in bone, with less than 1% present in blood.[1–3] Intracellular magnesium is mostly bound to ribosomes, phospholipids and nucleotides.[1]

The recommended total daily intake is about 6–12mmol/24h. However, magnesium intake is falling as the use of processed and fast-foods increases, and increasingly, people are failing to meet this requirement.[3,4] Thus, the incidence of chronic magnesium deficiency is probably increasing, with possible health implications, but is unrecognized because of the diagnostic limitations of serum magnesium (see below).[3,4]

Magnesium competes with calcium for absorption in the small intestine, probably by active transport. The normal serum magnesium is 0.7–1.1mmol/L. However, some have argued that for optimal health, the lower limit for serum magnesium should be considered to be 0.85mmol/L.[3] This is based on a progressive increase in the frequency of magnesium deficiency seen with serum levels between 0.85mmol/L and 0.75mmol/L (from <10% to 90%) which is associated with an increased risk of morbidity, e.g. impaired glucose tolerance, type 2 diabetes mellitus, and mortality, e.g. sudden cardiac death.[3,4] Most of the serum magnesium is in the ionized, active form, with about 30% bound to albumin and inactive. Hypoalbuminaemia may lead to artificially low serum magnesium levels.

Magnesium is excreted by the kidneys, 3–12mmol/24h. Magnesium and calcium share the same transport system in the renal tubules and there is a reciprocal relationship between the amounts excreted.

Magnesium deficiency can result from:
- *reduced intake*, e.g. an inadequate dietary intake (common)
- *reduced absorption*, e.g. small bowel resection, cholestasis, pancreatic insufficiency, diarrhoea, stoma, fistula, PPI (rare and generally with prolonged use, i.e. >1 year, see p.31)[5,6]

- *increased excretion*, e.g. alcoholism, diabetes mellitus, interstitial nephritis, diuretic phase of acute tubular necrosis, hyperthyroidism, hyperparathyroidism, hyperaldosteronism, drug-induced (aminoglycosides, **amphotericin**, anti-epidermal growth factor receptor monoclonal antibodies, **cisplatin**, **ciclosporin**, loop diuretics).

The risk of hypomagnesaemia with **cisplatin** is dose-dependent and increases with cumulative doses (40% cycle 1 → 100% cycle 6).[7] It can persist for 4–5 months, and sometimes years, after completing treatment.[8,9] Although generally mild and asymptomatic, it can be severe and symptomatic.

Hypomagnesaemia is an emerging toxicity of anti-epidermal growth factor receptor monoclonal antibodies, e.g. **cetuximab**, **panitumumab**.[10,11] The risk increases in the elderly, in those with a higher baseline serum magnesium, and with duration of treatment (e.g. 5% <3 months → 50% >6 months of **cetuximab**).[10] It is reversible, with magnesium levels returning to normal 4–6 weeks after discontinuation of treatment.[10]

When magnesium deficiency develops acutely, the symptoms may be obvious and severe, particularly muscle cramps, which aids diagnosis (Box A). In chronic deficiency, symptoms may be insidious in onset, less severe and non-specific.

In animal studies, magnesium deficiency results in an increased release of substance P and other mediators from nerve endings. These activate immune cells to release histamine and cytokines, producing a pro-inflammatory state and increased levels of oxygen-derived free radicals and nitric oxide. Manifestations include:[12–14]

- cutaneous vasodilatation → erythema and oedema
- leukocytosis
- inflammatory lesions in cardiac muscle
- atherogenesis
- increased levels of oxidative stress
- hyperalgesia.

In humans, the incidence of magnesium deficiency increases with aging (due to poor diet, reduced intestinal absorption, increased urinary loss etc.) and obesity. Magnesium deficiency, aging and obesity are all associated with low-grade inflammation and increased oxidative stress.This has led some to postulate that magnesium deficiency is a contributing factor to age- and obesity-related diseases such as diabetes mellitus, cardiac failure, some cancers (e.g. breast, colon), and hypertension.[13,15–18] In support of this, an inverse relationship between serum magnesium and CRP has been demonstrated in patients with cardiac failure, with magnesium supplementation attenuating the elevated CRP.[19] The underlying mechanisms remain to be clarified, but in part may relate to magnesium acting as a natural 'calcium antagonist'.[4] Thus, in magnesium deficiency, intracellular calcium levels increase, activating processes which contribute to inflammation.[17]

Serum magnesium is associated with muscle performance, e.g. in the elderly[20] and in patients with coronary artery disease.[21] In the latter, the use of magnesium supplements improved exercise capacity. However, evidence that the use of magnesium supplements or the correction of mild magnesium deficiency, e.g. in patients with diabetes, is of consistent benefit is lacking.[2]

Hypomagnesaemia (and hypokalaemia) are risk factors for drug-induced *torsade de pointes* arrhythmia. Thus, when using a drug known to prolong the QT interval, e.g. **methadone**, monitoring of serum electrolytes is generally recommended in patients with cardiac disease or other risk factors for prolonged QT, and in those at risk of electrolyte imbalance, e.g. because of vomiting, diarrhoea or diuretics (see p.759).[22]

Hypermagnesaemia is rare and is seen most often in patients with renal impairment who take OTC medicines containing magnesium. Serum concentrations >4mmol/L produce drowsiness, vasodilation, slowing of atrioventricular conduction and hypotension. Over 6mmol/L there is profound CNS depression and muscle weakness (Box A). Calcium gluconate IV is used to help reverse the effects of hypermagnesaemia.

When drugs such as **cisplatin** cause severe renal wasting of magnesium, hypomagnesaemia is generally present and aids diagnosis. If necessary, this can be confirmed by the high urinary excretion of magnesium (i.e. >1mmol/24h). In deficiency states which develop more insidiously the serum magnesium is an insensitive guide to total body stores and hypomagnesaemia is not always present.[23,24] In this situation, the finding of a low urinary excretion of magnesium (i.e. <0.5mmol/24h) may help the diagnosis. Currently, the best method for detecting magnesium deficiency is the magnesium loading test (Box B).[23,25,26]

If it is not possible to perform a magnesium loading test, hypokalaemia (± hypocalcaemia) not responding to potassium (± calcium) supplementation should raise the possibility of magnesium deficiency, and a trial of magnesium replacement therapy should be considered.[2] Magnesium deficiency results in hypokalaemia via increased potassium loss in the urine and hypocalcaemia by reducing the release of, and tissue sensitivity to PTH.[27]

Magnesium blocks calcium channels including the NMDA-receptor-channel and this probably accounts for its analgesic effect (Box C).[28–31] However, despite the overall positive outcome from numerous RCTs, the role of magnesium as an analgesic in palliative care is yet to be determined and ideally such use should be in the setting of a clinical trial.

Cancer cells preferentially accumulate magnesium, which is used to activate or inhibit various metabolic and genetic pathways in order to promote cell survival and proliferation.[56] Animal studies suggest that magnesium deficiency inhibits the growth of the primary cancer but exacerbates metastatic disease, possibly by enhancing inflammation.[56] The relevance of these findings for patients is unknown.

Box A   Symptoms and signs of magnesium deficiency and excess

Magnesium deficiency	**Magnesium excess**
Muscle	Muscle
weakness	weakness
tremor	hypotonia
twitching	loss of reflexes
cramps	Sensation of warmth (IV)
tetany (positive Chvostek's sign)	Flushing (IV)
Paraesthesia	Drowsiness
Apathy	Slurred speech
Depression	Double vision
Delirium	Delirium
Choreiform movements	Hypotension
Nystagmus	Cardiac arrhythmia
Seizures	Respiratory depression
Prolonged QT interval	Nausea and vomiting
Cardiac arrhythmia, including *torsade de pointes*	Thirst
Increased pain (?)	Hypermagnesaemia
Hypomagnesaemia (not always)	
Hypokalaemia	
Hypocalcaemia	
Hypophosphataemia	

Box B   The magnesium loading test[25]

Collect pre-infusion urine sample for urinary magnesium (Mg)/creatinine (Cr) ratio. Measure Mg and Cr in mmol/L; divide the Mg value by the Cr value to calculate the Mg/Cr ratio.

By IVI over 4h, give 0.1mmol/kg of elemental magnesium, using magnesium sulfate 50% (contains elemental magnesium 2mmol/mL; see Supply), diluted to 50mL with 5% glucose.

Simultaneously, start a 24h urine collection for magnesium and creatinine. Measure the total amounts of magnesium and creatinine excreted in mmol (*not* the concentrations in mmol/L).

Calculate % magnesium retention:

$$1 - \left[\frac{\text{24h urinary Mg (mmol)} - (\text{pre-infusion urinary Mg/Cr ratio (mmol/L)} \times \text{24h urinary Cr (mmol)})}{\text{dose of elemental magnesium infused (mmol)}} \right] \times 100$$

>50% retention implies definite deficiency.

Box C   Magnesium as an analgesic

A number of studies have explored the effects of magnesium, mainly as an adjuvant analgesic for postoperative pain, with mixed results.

A systematic review of 14 studies concluded that there is no convincing evidence of reduced postoperative pain intensity or decreased analgesic requirements when magnesium was used as an adjuvant.[32]

However, of numerous RCTs undertaken since this systematic review, all but two have reported reduced postoperative pain and decreased analgesic requirements.[23–46]

Further, eight RCTs of spinal magnesium have all reported lower pain scores and decreased analgesic requirements.[47–54]

In a RCT of PO magnesium in patients with neuropathic pain, although the frequency of pain paroxysms and the emotional component of behaviour improved, there was no overall difference in pain intensity or quality of life.[55]

Cautions

Generally, parenteral magnesium should not be given to patients with heart block or severe renal impairment. Risk of hypermagnesaemia in patients with renal impairment.

Undesirable effects

Flushing, sweating and sensation of warmth IV; diarrhoea PO. Also see features of magnesium excess in Box A.

Dose and use

Severe (serum magnesium <0.5mmol/L) and symptomatic hypomagnesaemia generally necessitates >1mmol/kg of magnesium; the route of choice is IV, given in divided doses over 3–5 days.[2,57]

Mild or asymptomatic hypomagnesaemia may be treated PO. If the cause of the magnesium deficiency persists, PO maintenance therapy will be needed.

In mild–moderate renal impairment reduce IV replacement doses by 50% and monitor plasma magnesium daily. In severe renal impairment, avoid IV replacement if possible.

Prevention of deficiency
- magnesium-rich foods, e.g. meat, seafood, green leafy vegetables, cereals and nuts
- potassium-sparing diuretics also preserve magnesium, e.g. **amiloride**.

IV correction of chronic deficiency

Because the degree of deficiency is difficult to determine from the plasma magnesium, replacement is empirical, guided by symptoms, plasma magnesium and renal function. Guidelines vary; the following are examples.

Serum magnesium <0.5mmol/L with symptoms (life-threatening), e.g. arrhythmia, seizure
- give 8mmol IV over 10–15min
- give as 4mL of magnesium sulfate injection 50% (elemental magnesium 2mmol/mL) diluted to 10mL with 0.9% saline or 5% dextrose
- follow with IVI replacement as below.

Serum magnesium <0.5mmol/L with symptoms (not life-threatening)
- on the first day give about 0.5mmol/kg IVI, then 0.25mmol/kg IVI daily for 2–5 days until the deficiency is corrected
- give as an appropriate dose of magnesium sulfate injection 50% (elemental magnesium 2mmol/mL) added to 250mL 0.9% saline or 5% dextrose (maximum concentration 0.2mmol/mL)

- infuse over a convenient time interval, e.g. 1.5h; ensure the infusion rate is restricted to ≤0.6mmol/min to avoid exceeding the maximum renal tubular resorption capacity for magnesium
- if undesirable effects occur, e.g. hypotension, increase the infusion time, e.g. up to 4h.

IV is the parenteral route of choice. If PO and IV routes are not feasible, options include (in order of preference):

- IM magnesium sulfate: in severe deficiency, give 0.25–0.5mmol/kg/24h as above in divided doses, e.g. multiple injections q4–6h of magnesium sulfate injection 50% (elemental magnesium 2mmol/mL); can be painful. Although dilution to 0.8mmol/mL is recommended by some, this further reduces the practicality of this approach
- CSCI magnesium sulfate: data are limited, but use of an isotonic solution is recommended, i.e. 25mmol of magnesium sulfate in 100mL WFI.[58,59]

Serum magnesium > 0.5mmol/L and < 0.75mmol/L without symptoms
Begin with a trial of PO replacement. The main limiting factor is diarrhoea, as magnesium salts are generally poorly absorbed PO and have a laxative effect. It is uncommon with doses < 40mmol/24h, and the risk is reduced by a gradual introduction and by taking magnesium with or after food. None of the PO products are authorized for magnesium deficiency and products include those used normally as antacids or laxatives, e.g.:

- magnesium oxide 400mg (elemental magnesium 10mmol) tablets:
  ▷ start with 400mg b.d. with food
  ▷ increase weekly by 400mg/day
  ▷ usual maximum 400mg q.d.s (40mmol/24h)
- magnesium hydroxide BP (Milk of Magnesia®) 5mL q.d.s with food (28mmol/24h).

Generally, 6–12months of treatment is required to fully correct a deficiency. If poorly tolerated or ineffective, use IV replacement as above.

PO maintenance
To prevent recurrence of the deficit, prescribe magnesium ~24mmol/24h in divided doses with food. PO is used unless poorly tolerated or ineffective, e.g. malabsorption.

Magnesium glycerophosphate is used in some centres. However, the formulations contain less elemental magnesium per tablet (4mmol) or per mL (1mmol) than other products, increasing the tablet/volume burden for patients. They are also more expensive, particularly in primary care (see supply).

Supply
This is not an exhaustive list.

Prices are approximate as they vary widely between manufacturer, quantities purchased and primary and secondary care.[60]

Magnesium *oxide*
Capsules 400mg, 28 days @ 400mg b.d. = £12. Unauthorized; available as a special order from Martindale, (see Appendix 1, p.817).

Magnesium *hydroxide*
Oral suspension (magnesium hydroxide mixture BP 415mg/5mL) elemental magnesium 7mmol/5mL, 28 days @ 5mL q.d.s = £4; *do not store in a cold place;* available OTC as Milk of Magnesia®.

Magnesium *glycerophosphate*
All products are unauthorized; available as a special order from various specials manufacturers (see Appendix 1, p.817).
Tablets elemental magnesium 4mmol; *some brands may be chewable,* 28 days @ 2 tablets t.d.s (24mmol/24h) = £40–£150.
Oral liquid elemental magnesium 1mmol/mL, 28 days @ 5mL q.d.s. (20mmol/24h) = £180–£425; *expiry of product can vary between manufacturers from 1–24 months.*

Magnesium *sulfate*
Oral powder elemental magnesium 4mmol/1g, 28 days @ 2g t.d.s (24mmol/24h) = £1; available OTC as Epsom Salts BP; dissolve in water.
Injection 20% (200mg/mL), elemental magnesium 0.8mmol/mL, 20mL amp = £14.
Injection 50% (500mg/mL), elemental magnesium 2mmol/mL, 2mL, 5mL and 10mL amp = £2.50, £3 and £1 respectively.
Injection (prefilled syringe) 50% (500mg/mL) elemental magnesium 2mmol/mL, 4mL, 10mL syringe = £8 and £5 respectively.

1   Romani A (2007) Regulation of magnesium homeostasis and transport in mammalian cells. *Archives of Biochemistry and Biophysics.* **458**: 90–102.
2   Martin KJ et al. (2009) Clinical consequences and management of hypomagnesemia. *Journal of the American Society of Nephrology.* **20**: 2291–2295.
3   Elin RJ (2010) Assessment of magnesium status for diagnosis and therapy. *Magnesium Research.* **23**: 1–5.
4   Rosanoff A et al. (2012) Suboptimal magnesium status in the United States: are the health consequences underestimated? *Nutrition Reviews.* **70**: 153–164.
5   MHRA (2012) Proton pump inhibitors in long term use: reports of hypomagnesaemia. *Drug Safety Update.* **5**. www.mhra.gov.uk/ Safetyinformation
6   Ito T and Jensen RT (2010) Association of long-term proton pump inhibitor therapy with bone fractures and effects on absorption of calcium, vitamin B12, iron, and magnesium. *Current Gastroenterology Reports.* **12**: 448–457.
7   Hodgkinson E et al. (2006) Magnesium depletion in patients receiving cisplatin-based chemotherapy. *Clinical Oncology.* **18**: 710–718.
8   Schilsky RL et al. (1982) Persistent hypomagnesemia following cisplatin chemotherapy for testicular cancer. *Cancer Treatment Reports.* **66**: 1767–1769.
9   Buckley JE et al. (1984) Hypomagnesemia after cisplatin combination chemotherapy. *Archives of Internal Medicine.* **144**: 2347–2348.
10 Costa A et al. (2011) Hypomagnesaemia and targeted anti-epidermal growth factor receptor (EGFR) agents. *Target Oncology.* **6**: 227–233.
11 Cao Y et al. (2010) Meta-analysis of incidence and risk of hypomagnesemia with cetuximab for advanced cancer. *Chemotherapy.* **56**: 459–465.
12 Mazur A et al. (2007) Magnesium and the inflammatory response: Potential physiopathological implications. *Archives of Biochemistry and Biophysics.* **458**: 48–56.
13 Tejero-Taldo MI et al. (2006) The nerve-heart connection in the pro-oxidant response to Mg-deficiency. *Heart Failure Reviews.* **11**: 35–44.
14 Maier JA (2012) Endothelial cells and magnesium: implications in atherosclerosis. *Clinical Science.* **122**: 397–407.
15 Barbagallo M et al. (2009) Magnesium homeostasis and aging. *Magnesium Research.* **22**: 235–246.
16 Nielsen FH (2010) Magnesium, inflammation, and obesity in chronic disease. *Nutrition Reviews.* **68**: 333–340.
17 King DE (2009) Inflammation and elevation of C-reactive protein: does magnesium play a key role? *Magnesium Research.* **22**: 57–59.
18 Song Y et al. (2005) Magnesium intake, C-reactive protein, and the prevalence of metabolic syndrome in middle-aged and older U.S. women. *Diabetes Care.* **28**: 1438–1444.
19 Almoznino-Sarafian D et al. (2007) Magnesium and C-reactive protein in heart failure: an anti-inflammatory effect of magnesium administration? *European Journal of Nutrition.* **46**: 230–237.
20 Dominguez LJ et al. (2006) Magnesium and muscle performance in older persons: the InCHIANTI study. *American Journal of Clinical Nutrition.* **84**: 419–426.
21 Pokan R et al. (2006) Oral magnesium therapy, exercise heart rate, exercise tolerance, and myocardial function in coronary artery disease patients. *British Journal of Sports Medicine.* **40**: 773–778.
22 Al-Khatib SM et al. (2003) What clinicians should know about the QT interval. *Journal of the American Medical Association.* **289**: 2120–2127.
23 Dyckner T and Wester P (1982) Magnesium deficiency - guidelines for diagnosis and substitution therapy. *Acta Medica Scandinavica.* **661**: 37–41.
24 Ismail Y and Ismail AA (2010) The underestimated problem of using serum magnesium measurements to exclude magnesium deficiency in adults; a health warning is needed for "normal" results. *Clinical Chemistry and Laboratory Medicine.* **48**: 323–327.
25 Ryzen E et al. (1985) Parenteral magnesium testing in the evaluation of magnesium deficiency. *Magnesium.* **4**: 137–147.
26 Crosby V et al. (2000) The importance of low magnesium in palliative care. *Palliative Medicine.* **14**: 544.
27 Anonymous (2013) Hypomagnesaemia. *Drugs and Therapeutics Bulletin.* **51**: 33–36.
28 Mauskop A et al. (1995) Intravenous magnesium sulphate relieves migraine attacks in patients with low serum ionised magnesium levels: a pilot study. *Clinical Science.* **89**: 633–636.
29 Tramer M et al. (1996) Role of magnesium sulphate in postoperative analgesia. *Anesthesiology.* **84**: 340–347.
30 Crosby V et al. (2000) The safety and efficacy of a single dose (500mg or 1g) of intravenous magnesium sulfate in neuropathic pain poorly responsive to strong opioid analgesics in patients with cancer. *Journal of Pain and Symptom Management.* **19**: 35–39.
31 Bondok RS and Abd El-Hady AM (2006) Intra-articular magnesium is effective for postoperative analgesia in arthroscopic knee surgery. *British Journal of Anaesthesia.* **97**: 389–392.
32 Lysakowski C et al. (2007) Magnesium as an adjuvant to postoperative analgesia: a systematic review of randomized trials. *Anesthesia and Analgesia.* **104**: 1532–1539.
33 Tauzin-Fin P et al. (2006) Intravenous magnesium sulphate decreases postoperative tramadol requirement after radical prostatectomy. *European Journal of Anaesthesiology.* **23**: 1055–1059.
34 Ozcan PE et al. (2007) Role of magnesium sulfate in postoperative pain management for patients undergoing thoracotomy. *Journal of Cardiothoracic and Vascular Anesthesia.* **21**: 827–831.

35 Mentes O et al. (2008) Effect of intraoperative magnesium sulphate infusion on pain relief after laparoscopic cholecystectomy. Acta Anaesthesiologica Scandinavica. 52: 1353–1359.

36 Ryu JH et al. (2008) Effects of magnesium sulphate on intraoperative anaesthetic requirements and postoperative analgesia in gynaecology patients receiving total intravenous anaesthesia. British Journal of Anaesthesia. 100: 397–403.

37 Dabbagh A et al. (2009) Intravenous magnesium sulfate for post-operative pain in patients undergoing lower limb orthopedic surgery. Acta Anaesthesiologica Scandinavica. 53: 1088–1091.

38 Kogler J (2009) The analgesic effect of magnesium sulfate in patients undergoing thoracotomy. Acta Clinica Croatica. 48: 19–26.

39 Turhanoglu S et al. (2009) Magnesium sulfate reduces postoperative morphine requirement after remifentanil-based anesthesia. Medical Science Monitor. 15: 15–19.

40 Hwang JY et al. (2010) I.V. infusion of magnesium sulphate during spinal anaesthesia improves postoperative analgesia. British Journal of Anaesthesia. 104: 89–93.

41 Saadawy IM et al. (2010) Lidocaine vs. magnesium: effect on analgesia after a laparoscopic cholecystectomy. Acta Anaesthesiologica Scandinavica. 54: 549–556.

42 Paech MJ et al. (2006) Does magnesium sulfate reduce the short- and long-term requirements for pain relief after caesarean delivery? A double-blind placebo-controlled trial. American Journal of Obstetrics and Gynecology. 194: 1596–1602; discussion 1602–1593.

43 Tramer MR and Glynn CJ (2007) An evaluation of a single dose of magnesium to supplement analgesia after ambulatory surgery: randomized controlled trial. Anesthesia and Analgesia. 104: 1349–1374.

44 Kiran S et al. (2011) Evaluation of a single-dose of intravenous magnesium sulphate for prevention of postoperative pain after inguinal surgery. Indian Journal of Anaesthesia. 55: 31–35.

45 Gupta SD et al. (2011) Effect of magnesium infusion on thoracic epidural analgesia. Saudi Journal of Anaesthesia. 5: 55–61.

46 Olgun B et al. (2012) The effects of magnesium sulphate on desflurane requirement, early recovery and postoperative analgesia in laparascopic cholecystectomy. Magnesium Research. 25: 72–78.

47 Bilir A et al. (2007) Epidural magnesium reduces postoperative analgesic requirement. British Journal of Anaesthesia. 98: 519–523.

48 Arcioni R et al. (2007) Combined intrathecal and epidural magnesium sulfate supplementation of spinal anesthesia to reduce post-operative analgesic requirements: a prospective, randomized, double-blind, controlled trial in patients undergoing major orthopedic surgery. Acta Anaesthesiologica Scandinavica. 51: 482–489.

49 Farouk S (2008) Pre-incisional epidural magnesium provides pre-emptive and preventive analgesia in patients undergoing abdominal hysterectomy. British Journal of Anaesthesia. 101: 694–699.

50 Ghatak T et al. (2010) Evaluation of the effect of magnesium sulphate vs. clonidine as adjunct to epidural bupivacaine. Indian Journal of Anaesthesia. 54: 308–313.

51 Yousef AA and Amr YM (2010) The effect of adding magnesium sulphate to epidural bupivacaine and fentanyl in elective caesarean section using combined spinal-epidural anaesthesia: a prospective double blind randomised study. International Journal of Obstetrics and Anesthesia. 19: 401–404.

52 Ouerghi S et al. (2011) The effect of adding intrathecal magnesium sulphate to morphine-fentanyl spinal analgesia after thoracic surgery. A prospective, double-blind, placebo-controlled research study. Annales Francaises d'Anesthethesie et de Reanimation. 30: 25 30.

53 Khalili G et al. (2011) Effects of adjunct intrathecal magnesium sulfate to bupivacaine for spinal anesthesia: a randomized, double-blind trial in patients undergoing lower extremity surgery. Journal of Anesthesia. 25: 892–897.

54 Khezri MB et al. (2012) Comparison of postoperative analgesic effect of intrathecal magnesium and fentanyl added to bupivacaine in patients undergoing lower limb orthopedic surgery. Acta Anaesthesiol Taiwan. 50: 19–24.

55 Pickering G et al. (2011) Oral magnesium treatment in patients with neuropathic pain: a randomized clinical trial. Magnesium Research. 24: 28–35.

56 Castiglioni S and Maier JA (2011) Magnesium and cancer: a dangerous liason. Magnesium Research. 24: S92–100.

57 Miller S (1995) Drug-induced hypomagnesaemia. Hospital Pharmacy. 30: 248–250.

58 UK Medicines Information (2010) How is acute hypomagnesaemia treated in adults? Medicines Q&A. 350.2: www.evidence.nhs.uk

59 UK Medicines Information (2011) Can magnesium sulphate be given subcutaneously? Medicines Q&A. 14.4: www.evidence.nhs.uk

60 Heuschkel S and Smith J (2012) Oral Magnesium preparations for the treatment and prevention of hypomagnesaemia. North Staffordshire Combined Healthcare NHS Trust Area Prescribing Committee. Version 1.

Updated June 2013

ZINC BNF 9.5.4 & 9.8.1

Class: Metal element.

Indications: Zinc deficiency (zinc sulfate), Wilson's disease (zinc acetate), †anorexia due to taste changes, †wound healing.

Pharmacology

Zinc is an essential trace element with multiple functions. It is present in > 300 enzymes, and has catalytic, structural and regulatory functions (Box A).[1–3] It occurs in all tissues, particularly muscle and bone, and to a lesser extent in skin and liver. Most is intracellular, and much is intranuclear. Plasma contains only 0.1% of the body's zinc, mostly bound to albumin.[4]

Box A   Physiological functions of zinc

Gene expression and cellular stability
Zinc-dependent RNA and DNA polymerases and reverse transcriptase
Cell proliferation and differentiation
Regulation of apoptosis (cell-specific; either increases or decreases)
Zinc-fingers transcription factors
Structural maintenance of biomembranes

Homeostasis and metabolism
Cellular signal and transmission
Hormone storage, synthesis and action, e.g. sex and thyroid hormones
Metabolism of proteins, carbohydrates and lipids
Tissue growth and repair
Neurosensory (cognition, behavioural response, taste, smell, appetite)

Anti-oxidant
Protects from free radical reactions
Component of super oxide dismutase (SOD)
Induces metal-binding protein production
Membrane stabilization

Anti-inflammatory
Inhibits expression of pro-inflammatory cytokines (IL-4, IL-6, and TNF-α)

Immune response
Thymulin activity
T-cell maturation and differentiation
Regulates cytokine production
Natural killer cell activity
T-lymphocyte activation
Direct effect on DNA for immune cell proliferation

Homeostasis is achieved primarily through regulation of the intestinal absorption. When dietary zinc is high, intestinal metal-binding proteins increase, and these slow absorption.[3] With a very high intake, secondary homeostatic mechanisms operate, e.g. increased renal excretion and redistribution of tissue zinc.[4]

There are no significant stores of zinc in the body and a constant dietary intake is essential. The UK reference nutrient intake (RNI) for daily dietary (elemental) zinc is 5.5–9.5mg in men and 4–7mg for women.[2,5] In contrast, the EU recommended daily allowance is 15mg.[2,6] Sources include meat, sea food, dairy products, wholegrain cereals, legumes and nuts. Bio-availability of dietary zinc is about 20–30%, and is lower from plant sources because of phytate-binding.[2]

Excessive intake is generally safe. However, acute and chronic poisoning has been reported.[3,7] Prolonged ingestion of high doses (50–300mg/24h elemental zinc) is associated with impaired immune function with leucopenia and neutropenia, sideroblastic anaemia and reduced ferritin levels. It can lead to secondary copper deficiency with increased LDL:HDL cholesterol ratio and HbA1c.[3,7] The safe upper levels for elemental zinc intake recommended in the UK are 25mg/day from supplements and 42mg/day in total (i.e. from supplements and diet combined).[6,7]

In the brain, the main effect of zinc is to reduce neuronal excitability.[8] However, as a consequence of various insults (e.g. trauma, ischaemia, hypoglycaemia) zinc may accumulate to toxic levels and cause neural damage and apoptosis. Zinc also appears to have a role in the pathogenesis of neurodegenerative disease. Thus, zinc-dependent proteins have been implicated in MND/AML, and zinc induces amyloid deposition in Alzheimer's disease.[8] It is concentrated in and around plaques, but no clinical benefit is seen with **clioquinol**, a metal protein-attenuating compound, which interacts with zinc and promotes solubilization of amyloid.[9]

Zinc concentrations can be measured in the cellular components of blood (RBC, mononuclear cells and platelets), plasma, urine, faeces, skin, hair and saliva. Cellular zinc is sensitive but measurement is complex.[10] Consequently, plasma concentration is widely used instead, with zinc deficiency defined as < 15micromol/L.[11] However, plasma zinc may not reflect total body zinc, and is influenced by various factors, e.g. plasma protein, drugs (see Cautions), infection, and inflammation.[2,7,10,12] Thus, when zinc deficiency is clinically suspected, even if the plasma zinc concentration is within the normal range, a therapeutic trial of replacement therapy should be considered.

Zinc deficiency can occur relatively rapidly as a result of inadequate dietary intake, poor intestinal absorption or increased loss due to conditions such as cancer, malabsorption, alcoholism, renal disease, sickle cell anaemia and AIDS. Metal-binding proteins, in addition to binding zinc and other heavy metals such as copper, have a protective role scavenging toxic metals and free radicals, and improving immunity. However, in stressful states, e.g. inflammation and with increasing age, levels increase and bind more intracellular zinc. Consequently, the persistent sequestration of zinc leads to reduced bio-availability and a relative deficiency state.[3,13] The effects of zinc deficiency are numerous and reflect its multifunctional role and importance in gene expression, protein synthesis and enzyme function (Box B).[2,3,13]

Box B Consequences of zinc deficiency

Immunological
Increased risk of infections due to impaired cellular immunity
Reduced neutrophils, monocytes, natural killer cells
Reduced T-helper₁ cytokines (IL-2 and IFN-γ)
Reduced thymulin activity
Increased inflammation secondary to increased pro-inflammatory cytokines, NO, COX-2 and NF-κB

Other cellular effects
Increased apoptosis
Increased oxidative stress with lipid peroxidation of mitochondrial membranes

Haematological
Defective platelet aggregation
Iron-deficiency anaemia

Neuropsychological
Impaired smell, taste and vision
Impaired cognition
Behavioural disturbance
Depression

Gastro-intestinal
Anorexia
Diarrhoea
Gastric acid and pepsin secretion causing mucosal damage

Hormonal
Thyroid hormone function
Hypogonadism and infertility

Dermatological
Dermatitis
Alopecia
Nail dystrophy
Delayed wound healing

There are conflicting reports regarding the relationship between zinc and cancer. Some studies show no effect, others a protective effect and some an increased risk. A possible explanation is that the proliferative and apoptotic actions of zinc are cell-specific. In prostate, ovarian, oesophageal, and hepatocellular cancers, for example, malignant cells are unable to accumulate zinc and this results in a loss of zinc-induced apoptosis. In these cancers, zinc deficiency would lead to an increased risk, and supplementation could have an anti-cancer effect.[14] In contrast, in breast and pancreatic cancers, malignant cells have a high zinc concentration which enhances cell proliferation.[15]

Zinc may have a contributory role in cachexia. Systemic inflammation affects zinc transporters in cell membranes, leading to zinc accumulation in the liver and also skeletal muscle where, it is suggested, it could enhance protein catabolism and inhibit protein synthesis.[16] Further, this redistribution is also proposed to cause a deficiency of zinc elsewhere, resulting in systemic features of zinc deficiency, e.g. anorexia, hypogonadism and impaired immunity, which are common features of cachexia.[16]

Zinc supplements are of benefit in the common cold. A Cochrane review concluded that, in otherwise healthy people, zinc lozenges and syrup reduce the severity and duration of symptoms if started within 24h of the onset of symptoms. Studies have used different doses (30–190mg/24h) for different lengths of time. However, lozenges have been widely studied with benefit from doses ⩾70mg/24h continued throughout the cold. Prophylactic supplementation cannot be recommended because of insufficient data.[17] Another systematic review concluded a dose-dependant effect and found zinc acetate to be more effective than other formulations.[18] Patients with impaired immunity have not been investigated.

In zinc-deficient patients, supplements promote wound healing.[2] However, a Cochrane review (based on poor quality studies) found no strong evidence of benefit on leg ulcer healing.[19] There is inconclusive or insufficient evidence regarding zinc's effectiveness as a treatment for male infertility.[2] It may be of benefit in slowing the progression of age-related macular degeneration.[20]

Supplementation improves zinc deficiency, disturbances of taste and smell, and dry mouth (xerostomia).[21,22] It can help idiopathic taste disorders [23] but not if drug-induced.[11] Supplements can also prevent or reduce radiotherapy-induced taste changes.[24] The beneficial effect on zinc-related anorexia is linked to an increase in leptin levels and by influencing the hypothalamic neuropeptides which regulate appetite.[25] The effect on leptin possibly involves increased cytokine production.[26] Zinc is also used to prevent the absorption of copper in Wilson's disease.

Cautions
Acute renal impairment (zinc may accumulate). If taken for prolonged periods, monitor zinc and copper plasma concentrations, FBC and plasma cholesterol to detect incipient zinc toxicity and copper deficiency.

Drug interactions
PO zinc decreases GI absorption of chelating agents (**penicillamine, trientine**), fluoroquinolone antibacterials, **iron**, and tetracyclines. Absorption of PO zinc is decreased by **calcium** and **iron** supplements, chelating agents (**penicillamine, trientine**), phosphorus-containing products, and tetracyclines. Separating administration times by 2–3h avoids these interactions.

Thiazides and loop diuretics increase the urinary excretion of zinc which, if used long-term, may lead to deficiency.

Undesirable effects
More common: gastric irritation, gastritis, dyspepsia, abdominal pain, nausea, vomiting, diarrhoea; these can be reduced by giving PO zinc with or after food.
Less common: headache, lethargy and irritability.

Dose and use
Zinc deficiency
- elemental zinc ⩽50mg PO t.d.s., e.g. zinc sulfate (Solvazinc®) 1 tablet (elemental zinc 45mg) dissolved in water once daily-t.d.s. p.c. *or*
- zinc sulfate 14.6mg/mL injection: give 2mL IVI once daily (elemental zinc 6.5mg).

Wilson's disease

Zinc *acetate* ± chelating agents (**penicillinamine, trientine**) under specialist supervision to decrease copper absorption from the GI tract in Wilson's disease.[2] See BNF section 9.8.1.

Supply

Zinc sulfate (generic)
Injection 14.6mg/mL (elemental zinc 3.25mg/mL), 10mL vial – £2.50.

Solvazinc® (Galen)
Tablets effervescent zinc sulfate monohydrate 125mg (elemental zinc 45mg), 28 days @ 1 tablet t.d.s. = £16.

Many zinc products are available OTC (citrate, gluconate, glycinate, oxide and sulphate salts) as dietary supplements and as symptomatic treatment for the common cold.

1 Frassinetti S et al. (2006) The role of zinc in life: a review. *Journal of Environmental Pathology, Toxicology and Oncology.* **25**: 597–610.
2 Mason P (2006) Physiological and medicinal zinc. *Pharmaceutical Journal.* **276**: 271–274.
3 Stefanidou M et al. (2006) Zinc: a multipurpose trace element. *Archives of Toxicology.* **80**: 1–9.
4 King JC et al. (2000) Zinc homeostasis in humans. *Journal of Nutrition.* **130**: 1360S–1366S.
5 COMA (1991) Committee on Medical Aspects of Food and Nutrition Policy. Dietary reference values for food energy and nutrients for the United Kingdom. Report of the panel on dietary reference values. HMSO, London.
6 Mason P (2003) Upper safety limits for vitamins - why have different authorities set different guidance? *Pharmaceutical Journal.* **271**: 55–57.
7 EVM (2003) Expert Group on Vitamins and Minerals. Risk assessment: zinc: In: Safe upper levels for vitamins and minerals. pp253–262. Food Standards Agency, London. Available from: www.food.gov.uk
8 Frederickson CJ et al. (2005) The neurobiology of zinc in health and disease. *Nature Reviews Neuroscience.* **6**: 449–462.
9 Sampson E et al. (2008) Metal protein attenuating compounds for the treatment of Alzheimers Disease. *Cochrane Database of Systematic Reviews.* **1**: CD005880.
10 Hambridge M (2003) Biomarkers of trace mineral intake and status. *Journal of Nutrition.* **133**: 948S–955S.
11 Heyneman CA (1996) Zinc deficiency and taste disorders. *Annals of Pharmacotherapy.* **30**: 186–187.
12 Alpers DH (1994) Zinc and deficiencies of taste and smell. *Journal of the American Medical Association.* **272**: 1233–1234.
13 Vasto S et al. (2007) Zinc and inflammatory/immune response in aging. *Annals of the New York Academy of Sciences.* **1100**: 111–122.
14 Prasad AS et al. (2009) Zinc in cancer prevention. *Nutrition and Cancer.* **61**: 879–887.
15 Franklin RB and Costello LC (2009) The important role of the apoptotic effects of zinc in the development of cancers. *Journal of Cellular Biochemistry.* **106**: 750–757.
16 Siren PM and Siren MJ (2010) Systemic zinc redistribution and dyshomeostasis in cancer cachexia. *Journal of Cachexia Sarcopenia Muscle.* **1**: 23–33.
17 Singh M and Das RR (2013) Zinc for the common cold. *Cochrane Database of Systematic Reviews.* **6**: CD001364.
18 Science M et al. (2012) Zinc for the treatment of the common cold: a systematic review and meta-analysis of randomized controlled trials. *Canadian Medical Association Journal.* **184**: E551–561.
19 Wilkinson E et al. (2012) Oral zinc for arterial and venous ulcers. *Cochrane Database of Systematic Reviews.* **8**: CD001273.
20 Evans JR (2006) Antioxidant vitamin and mineral supplements for slowing the progression of age-related macular degeneration. *Cochrane Database of Systematic Reviews.* **2**: CD000254.
21 Tanaka M (2002) Secretory function of the salivary gland in patients with taste disorders or xerostomia: correlation with zinc deficiency. *Acta Otolaryngolica Supplementum.* **134**–141.
22 Henkin RI et al. (1999) Efficacy of exogenous oral zinc in treatment of patients with carbonic anhydrase VI deficiency. *American Journal of Medical Sciences.* **318**: 392–405.
23 Heckmann SM et al. (2005) Zinc gluconate in the treatment of dysgeusia–a randomized clinical trial. *Journal of Dental Research.* **84**: 35–38.
24 Ripamonti C et al. (1998) A randomized, controlled clinical trial to evaluate the effects of zinc sulfate on cancer patients with taste alterations caused by head and neck irradiation. *Cancer.* **82**: 1938–1945.
25 Shay NF and Mangian HF (2000) Neurobiology of zinc-influenced eating behavior. *Journal of Nutrition.* **130**: 1493S–1499S.
26 Mantzoros CS et al. (1998) Zinc may regulate serum leptin concentrations in humans. *Journal of American College of Nutrition.* **17**: 270–275.

Updated (minor change) March 2014

10: MUSCULOSKELETAL AND JOINT DISEASES

DEPOT CORTICOSTEROID INJECTIONS   BNF 10.1.2.2

Indications: Inflammation of joints and soft tissues, †pain in superficial bones (e.g. rib, scapula, iliac crest), †intractable pain caused by spinal metastases, †malignant (peritoneal) ascites.

Contra-indications: Untreated local or systemic infection. Must not be given IV or IT.

Pharmacology

Corticosteroids have an anti-inflammatory effect; they reduce the concentration of algesic substances present in inflammation which sensitize nerve endings.[1] Further, in animal studies, when injected locally around an injured nerve, corticosteroids have been shown to have a direct inhibitory effect on the spontaneous activity associated with nerve injury.[2]

For many years depot injections of corticosteroids have been given epidurally in selected patients with non-malignant radicular (nerve root) compression pain associated with spinal pathology, e.g. lumbar disc herniation, sciatica.[3] However, a systematic review found only weak RCT evidence for their efficacy.[4] Even so, in patients with spinal metastases and intractable radicular pain, clinical experience indicates that ED depot corticosteroids are sometimes helpful.

Cautions

History of severe affective disorders (e.g. depression, bipolar disorder) or steroid-induced psychosis, epilepsy, glaucoma, myasthenia gravis, hypertension, CHF, predisposition to thrombophlebitis, peptic ulceration, diverticulitis, ulcerative colitis, severe hepatic impairment, renal impairment, hypothyroidism, osteoporosis.

Depot formulations may result in symptomatic hyperglycaemia for several days in patients with diabetes mellitus and suppression of the hypothalamic-pituitary-adrenal axis for up to 4 weeks. Injection under a rib may be complicated by a pneumothorax.

Corticosteroids may mask or alter the presentation of infection in immunocompromised patients; such patients should not receive live vaccines and, if exposed to chickenpox, should receive *Varicella zoster* immunoglobulin.

Undesirable effects

Undesirable effects associated with systemic corticosteroids can also occur with depot injections (see Systemic corticosteroids, p.504). These include antagonism of antihypertensive, antidiabetic and diuretic drugs, and increased risk of hypokalaemia if used concurrently with β2 agonists (e.g. **salbutamol**, **terbutaline**) or other potassium-wasting drugs.

Occasionally, a patient develops lipodystrophy (local fat necrosis) which results in an indentation of the overlying skin.

ED injection of **methylprednisolone acetate** (unauthorized route) has been associated with wound dehiscence and with loss of sphincter control.

Dose and use
Injection into and/or over a painful bone secondary[5]
- infiltrate the skin and SC tissues overlying the point of maximal bone tenderness with local anaesthetic
- with the tip of the needle pressing against the tender bone, inject depot **methylprednisolone** *acetate* 80mg in 2mL
- if there are 2 painful bones, inject 40mg at each spot; generally limit the total amount given at any one time to 80mg.

Also, for rib lesions, reposition the needle under the rib and inject 5mL of **bupivacaine** 0.5% to anaesthetize the intercostal nerve. Complete or good relief occurs in about 70% of patients. If of benefit, injections can be repeated if the pain returns but not within 2 weeks.

Epidural injection[3]
Depot **methylprednisolone** *acetate* 80mg in 2mL (unauthorized route). A single ED injection is given, followed if necessary by a further 1–2 injections at 3–4 week intervals. The effect of ED corticosteroids is unpredictable and may not peak until 1 week after an injection. Depot corticosteroids cannot be injected through an epidural bacterial filter. In some countries, depot **triamcinolone** or a *non-depot* formulation of **dexamethasone sodium phosphate** is used for ED injection.

Malignant (peritoneal) ascites
After a preliminary paracentesis, inject intra-abdominally:
- **triamcinoloneacetonide** 8mg/kg, up to a maximum of 520mg (13 vials) *or*
- **triamcinolonehexacetonide** (not UK) 10mg/kg, up to a maximum of 640mg *or*
- **methylprednisoloneacetate** 10mg/kg, up to a maximum of 640mg (8×2mL vials).

In an open study, the mean interval between paracentesis doubled to 18 days.[6]

Supply
Methylprednisolone *acetate*
Depo-Medrone® (Pharmacia)
Depot injection (aqueous suspension) 40mg/mL, 1mL vial = £3.50, 2mL vial = £6, 3mL vial = £9.

Triamcinolone *acetonide*
Kenalog® Intra-articular/Intramuscular (Squibb)
Depot injection (aqueous suspension) 40mg/mL, 1mL vial = £1.50.

1 Pybus P (1984) Osteoarthritis: a new neurological method of pain control. *Medical Hypothesis.* **14**: 413–422.
2 Devor M et al. (1985) Corticosteroids reduce neuroma hyperexcitability. In: HL Fields *et al.* (eds) *Advances in Pain Research and Therapy* Vol 9. Raven Press, New York, pp. 451–455.
3 McLain RF et al. (2004) Epidural steroids for back and leg pain: mechanism of action and efficacy. *Cleveland Clinic Journal of Medicine.* **71**: 961–970.
4 Armon C et al. (2007) Assessment: use of epidural steroid injections to treat radicular lumbosacral pain: report of the Therapeutics and Technology Assessment Subcommittee of the American Academy of Neurology. *Neurology.* **68**: 723–729.
5 Rowell NP (1988) Intralesional methylprednisolone for rib metastases: an alternative to radiotherapy? *Palliative Medicine.* **2**: 153–155.
6 Mackey J et al. (2000) A phase II trial of triamcinolone hexacetanide for symptomatic recurrent malignant ascites. *Journal of Pain and Symptom Management.* **19**: 193–199.

Updated April 2014

RUBEFACIENTS AND OTHER TOPICAL PRODUCTS   BNF 10.3.2

Indications: Soft tissue pains (rubefacients, topical NSAIDs), pain relief in osteo-arthritis of the hand or knee (**capsaicin** cream 0.025%, topical NSAIDs),[1] post-herpetic neuralgia (after lesions have healed) and diabetic neuralgia (**capsaicin** cream 0.075%), peripheral neuropathic pain in non-diabetic patients (**capsaicin** TD patch 8%), †notalgia paraesthetica, †severe skin reaction to an indwelling SC cannula and/or phlebitis (**kaolin** poultice).

Contra-indications: Inflamed or broken skin.
Capsaicin TD patch 8%: do not apply to the face or head.
Topical NSAIDs: if nasal polyps or history of asthma, angioedema, urticaria or acute rhinitis precipitated by aspirin or another NSAID.

Pharmacology

Rubefacients act by counter-stimulation of the skin, closing the pain 'gate' in the dorsal horn of the spinal cord.[2,3] Further benefit is obtained by the inclusion of **levomenthol (menthol)**. This cools the skin for several hours by acting on heat-sensitive transient receptor potential (TRP) channels expressed on sensory nerve endings.[4,5] **Levomenthol**-containing rubefacients have been used as 'home remedies' for tension headache, muscle spasm, and joint pain. (**Levomenthol** is also an ingredient in several topical antipruritic products, see p.618). Warm **kaolin** poultices also act by counter-stimulation, substituting the pleasure of warmth for the stinging/burning of the inflamed skin.

Capsaicin

Capsaicin is a naturally occurring alkaloid found in the fruits of various species of *Solanaceae* (the nightshade family) and in pepper plants of the genus *Capsicum* (chilli peppers).[6] It acts by depleting substance P (SP) at sensory nerve endings. In animals, **capsaicin** has also been shown to be neurotoxic, particularly for nociceptive C fibres.[7]

Application of **capsaicin** causes an initial release of SP from C fibres which manifests as a burning or stinging sensation (see Undesirable effects below) with subsequent depletion on continued use. Axonal transport of SP to synaptic terminals is reduced and synthesis inhibited.[8] **Capsaicin** may also elevate the thresholds for the release of SP and other neurotransmitters. Reduced availability of SP diminishes pain transmission. After stopping topical **capsaicin**, SP stores revert to pretreatment levels and neuronal sensitivity returns to normal.[9–11]

In an open study of topical **capsaicin** cream 0.025% in post-axillary dissection pain, 12/18 women reported benefit after 1 month, eight of whom had good or excellent responses; and, after 6 months, most still had good relief.[12] An RCT of **capsaicin** cream 0.075% for 6 weeks gave comparable results: 8/13 patients had ⩾50% improvement, five of whom had a good or excellent result.[13] Benefit was mainly in relation to stabbing pain.

In an RCT in 99 patients with persistent neuropathic pain after cancer surgery, **capsaicin** cream 0.075% produced a mean reduction in pain scores of >50%, compared with <20% for placebo. Improvement was seen most often in women with post-mastectomy pain.[14]

However, a systematic review was unable to reach a firm conclusion about benefit from 0.075% **capsaicin** cream in neuropathic pain generally.[15] NICE no longer recommends 0.075% **capsaicin** cream for post-herpetic neuralgia in primary care.[16]

A TD patch containing **capsaicin** 8% is available for non-diabetic painful neuropathy, e.g. post-herpetic or HIV. This was developed to deliver high-concentration **capsaicin** to the cutaneous nociceptors in a single application, thereby achieving rapid 'knock-out' of their function, as opposed to the periods of enhanced sensitivity and slow desensitization seen after repeated application of 0.025% and 0.075% creams. A systematic review found that TD **capsaicin** provided long-term pain relief after a single application. In post-herpetic neuralgia, NNTs were 8.8 and 7 for patients grading themselves as 'much or very much better' at 8 and 12 weeks respectively. NNT values for reductions in pain intensity of ⩾30% and ⩾50% at 8 and 12 weeks were between 10 and 12. In HIV-related neuropathy, the NNT for self-assessment as 'much or very much better' at 12 weeks was 5.8, and that for reduction in pain intensity of ⩾30% at 12 weeks was 11.[17] To date, no RCTs have been published comparing TD **capsaicin** patches with systemic adjuvant analgesics (see p.295). Cost alone is likely to restrict their use to specialist pain clinics.

Capsaicin cream is of benefit in histamine-related pruritus, aquagenic pruritus, and pruritus associated with uraemia, nodular prurigo, psoriasis and post-axillary dissection syndrome (see Topical antipruritics, p.618).[5,18] Benefit is also seen with pruritus caused by notalgia paraesthetica (nerve injury, often caused by entrapment, of the dorsal ramus of the T2–T6 thoracic nerves which causes pruritus and/or altered sensation in the areas of skin between or below the shoulder blade on either side of the back).[19,20]

Topical NSAIDs

Topical NSAIDs are of value for the relief of pain associated with soft tissue trauma, e.g. strains and sprains,[21-23] inflammation of superficial joints,[24] early osteo-arthritis of the hand or knee.[1]

Topically applied salicylates and some other NSAIDs can achieve local high SC concentrations and therapeutically effective concentrations within synovial fluid and peri-articular tissues similar to those seen after PO administration.[25-28]

A Cochrane review compared topical NSAIDs with placebo in *acute* musculoskeletal pain over 1–2 weeks and found that topical NSAIDs had an NNT of 4.5 when a 50% reduction in pain was used as the measure of clinical success. Topical **diclofenac**, **ibuprofen**, **ketoprofen** and **piroxicam** were effective, whereas **indometacin** and **benzydamine** were no better than placebo.[21] A second Cochrane review concluded that, in *chronic* musculoskeletal pain, rubefacients containing salicylates were less effective than topical NSAIDs; and, in *acute* musculoskeletal pain, they were little better than placebo.[29] However, different formulations of the same drug can result in major differences in effectiveness.[30]

Pharmacokinetic details for **capsaicin** products and topical NSAIDs are shown in Table 1.

Table 1 Pharmacokinetic details for capsaicin products and topical NSAIDs

	Capsaicin cream 0.025% and 0.075%	Capsaicin TD patch 8%	Topical NSAIDs
Onset of action	Counter-stimulation generally immediate. 1 week in osteo-arthritis but full effect may not be seen for ≤2months. 2–4 weeks in neuralgia	1–14 days in peripheral neuropathy	Product- and drug-dependent
Duration of action	No data; manufacturers advise applying q4–6h	≥12 weeks in peripheral and HIV-related neuropathy; manufacturers advise a 3-month gap between applications	Product and drug dependent; manufacturers advise applying b.d.–q.d.s.

Cautions

General

Avoid contact with eyes, mucous membranes, and inflamed or broken skin; discontinue if rash develops. Do not cover with occlusive dressings or tight bandages.

Capsaicin cream 0.025% and 0.075%

Avoid hot baths or showers immediately before application because this can enhance the burning sensation. Avoid inhaling the vapour from the cream. Wash hands immediately after application (unless treating the hands, in which case, wash them 30min after application).

*Capsaicin TD patch 8%

Unstable or poorly controlled blood pressure, heart disease (see Undesirable effects). The painful burning sensation may necessitate local cooling (e.g. with a cold compress) or systemic analgesia. Avoid inhaling the vapour from the patch. Special precautions are required for handling (see Dose and use).

Topical NSAIDs

History of peptic ulcer, renal disease or asthma. Wash hands immediately after application (unless treating the hands, in which case, wash them 30min after application). May cause photosensitivity, particularly **ketoprofen**. Avoid exposing the treated area to sunlight when using topical **ketoprofen** and for 2 weeks afterwards.

Provided very large amounts are not applied, because plasma concentrations are much lower, undesirable effects and drug interactions are much less likely with topical NSAIDs than with systemic NSAIDs. Conversely, skin reactions (e.g. rash) occur more commonly with topical NSAIDS.[1]

Undesirable effects

The commonest undesirable effect of **capsaicin** cream is tingling, stinging or burning at the site of application. This effect is thought to be related to the initial release of SP from C fibres. The stinging and burning generally decreases with continued applications, often clearing in a few days but sometimes persisting for >4 weeks. Some patients discontinue treatment because of this. Runny eyes and respiratory tract irritation, causing coughing and sneezing, may result from rubbing the eyes and/or inhaling **capsaicin** vapour when applying the cream. Breathlessness and exacerbation of asthma have occurred occasionally.

Almost all patients experience local erythema and a burning sensation with **capsaicin** TD patches, unless the area is pretreated with local anaesthetic (see Dose and use). Other common local effects (1–10% of patients) are itching, blistering, swelling and dryness. Uncommon symptoms (1–10 per 1,000 patients) include eye irritation, raised blood pressure, arrhythmia including atrioventricular block, palpitations, cough, throat irritation, loss of taste sensation, muscle spasm, reduced sensation in limbs, local wheals, prickling sensation and bruising.

Large quantities of topical NSAIDs have been associated with systemic effects (e.g. hypersensitivity, rash, asthma, renal impairment[31]) and potentiation of **warfarin**, occasionally leading to bleeding.[32] Local reactions include drying, reddening, burning sensations, and contact dermatitis. A Cochrane review found that, in short-term studies, topical NSAIDs and placebo produced a similar incidence of local reactions and systemic undesirable effects (about 6% and 3% respectively).[21]

Dose and use
Capsaicin cream 0.025–0.075%
- apply a pea-sized amount t.d.s.–q.d.s. (the manufacturers specify q.d.s. initially for the 0.025% cream), leaving at least 4h between applications.

The burning sensation associated with the application of **capsaicin** cream is intensified and/or prolonged when larger quantities are applied (particularly with the higher-strength) or if initially applied less frequently than t.d.s.–q.d.s. If the burning is severe, topical **lidocaine** or another local anaesthetic can be applied before **capsaicin** in the first few weeks of treatment.

Because heat and humidity influence dysaesthesia, patients should avoid excessive sweating and not take a hot bath immediately before application. Occlusion and tight bandaging should also be avoided.

Patients should apply the cream using gentle massage, avoiding contact with eyes, mucous membranes and broken/inflamed skin. *Patients must wash their hands after applying the cream to avoid subsequent unintentional contact with the eyes (unless treating the hands, in which case, wash them 30min after application).*

Capsaicin TD patch 8%
Health professionals should wear nitrile gloves when handling the patches and cleansing solution; latex gloves do *not* provide adequate protection. Also consider using protective masks and safety glasses to avoid accidental contact of aerosolized **capsaicin** particles with the eyes and mucous membranes, particularly when removing the patch:
- mark out the most painful areas with ink
- depending on the size of the painful areas, up to 4 patches may be applied simultaneously, or a patch may be cut to fit
- wash the skin in the treatment area with soap and water and dry thoroughly; any hair may be clipped but not shaved
- because most patients experience a burning sensation when the patches are applied, pre-treat the area with topical **lidocaine** or another local anaesthetic 1h before applying the patches; wash off the local anaesthetic cream/ointment and thoroughly dry the skin before applying the **capsaicin** patch
- leave patches in place for:
  ▷ 30min if applied to the feet
  ▷ 1h if applied elsewhere
  ▷ if necessary, disposable socks or an open-weave bandage can be used to keep the patch in place
- when removing patches, roll them inwards to enclose the remaining **capsaicin**
- use the cleansing gel supplied to remove any traces of **capsaicin** from the patient's skin, both after any accidental contact and after removing the patches; leave the gel on the skin for 1min, then wipe off
- wash the skin with soap and water after using the cleansing gel
- treatment can be repeated after 3 months if necessary.

Used patches, gloves, wipes, socks and bandages should be placed in a plastic bag and disposed of safely.

Topical NSAIDs
- generally apply b.d.–q.d.s.

Kaolin poultice
- warm the poultice before use
- generally apply b.d.

Supply

For **levomenthol** products, see Topical antipruritics, p.618.

Kaolin (generic)
Poultice 200g = £3.

Kaolin Poultice K/L Pack® (K/L)
Poultice 4×100g pouches = £7.

Capsaicin
Zacin® (Cephalon)
Cream 0.025%, 45g = £18.

Axsain® (Cephalon)
Cream 0.075%, 45g = £15.

Qutenza® (Astellas)
TD patch 8% (contains 179mg **capsaicin**), 1 patch (with cleansing gel) = £210.

Topical NSAIDs
Diclofenac
Voltarol Emulgel® (Novartis)
Gel containing **diclofenac diethylammonium** 1.16% (equivalent to **diclofenac sodium** 1%), 20g (hospital only) = £1.50; 100g = £6 (also available OTC).
Also see **diclofenac**, p.329.

Felbinac
Traxam® (Goldshield)
Foam 3.17%, 100g = £9.
Gel 3%, 100g = £8.

Ibuprofen (generic)
Gel 5%, 30g = £1.50, 50g = £2, 100g = £4.

Fenbid® Forte (Goldshield)
Forte gel 10%, 100g = £4 (smaller packs available OTC).

Ibugel Forte® (Dermal)
Forte gel 10%, 100g = £6.
Also see **ibuprofen**, p.335.

This is not a complete list; see BNF for more details.

1 NICE (2013) Osteoarthritis. *Clinical Knowledge Summaries.* http://cks.nice.org.uk
2 Melzack R and Wall P (1965) Pain mechanisms: a new theory. *Science.* **150**: 971–979.
3 Melzack R (1991) The gate control theory 25 years later: new perspectives on phantom limb pain. In: M Bond et al. (eds) *Proceedings of the VIth World Congress on Pain.* Elsevier Science, Amsterdam, pp. 9–21.
4 Peier AM et al. (2002) A TRP channel that senses cold stimuli and menthol. *Cell.* **108**: 705–715.
5 Patel T et al. (2007) Menthol: a refreshing look at this ancient compound. *Journal of the American Academy of Dermatology.* **57**: 873–878.
6 Towlerton GR and Rice AS (2003) Topical analgesics for chronic pain. In: AS Rice et al. (eds) *Clinical Pain Management: Chronic Pain.* Arnold, London, pp. 213–226.
7 Chung JM et al. (1993) Chronic effects of topical application of capsaicin to the sciatic nerve on responses of primate spinothalamic neurons. *Pain.* **53**: 311–321.
8 Gamse R et al. (1982) Capsaicin applied to peripheral nerve inhibits axoplasmic transport of substance P and somatostatin. *Brain Research.* **239**: 447–462.

9 Gamse R et al. (1981) Differential effects of capsaicin on the content of somatostatin, substance P, and neurotensin in the nervous system of the rat. *Naunyn Schmiedebergs Archives of Pharmacology.* **317**: 140–148.
10 Fitzgerald M (1983) Capsaicin and sensory neurones: a review. *Pain.* **15**: 109–130.
11 LaMotte RH et al. (1988) Hypothesis for novel classes of chemoreceptors mediating chemogenic pain and itch. In: R Dubner et al. (eds) *Proceedings of the Vth World Congress on Pain.* Elsevier, New York, pp. 529–535.
12 Watson C et al. (1989) The postmastectomy pain syndrome and the effect of topical capsaicin. *Pain.* **38**: 177–186.
13 Watson CPN and Evans RJ (1992) Post-mastectomy pain syndrome and topical capsaicin: a randomized trial. *Pain.* **51**: 375–379.
14 Ellison N et al. (1997) Phase III placebo-controlled trial of capsaicin cream in the management of surgical neuropathic pain in cancer patients. *Journal of Clinical Oncology.* **15**: 2974–2980.
15 Derry S and Moore RA (2012) Topical capsaicin (low concentration) for chronic neuropathic pain in adults. *Cochrane Database of Systematic Reviews.* **9**: CD010111.
16 NICE (2013) Post-herpetic neuralgia. *Clinical Knowledge Summaries.* http://cks.nice.org.uk
17 Derry S et al. (2013) Topical capsaicin (high concentration) for chronic neuropathic pain in adults. *Cochrane Database of Systematic Reviews.* **2**: CD007393.
18 Xander C et al. (2013) Pharmacological interventions for pruritus in adult palliative care patients. *Cochrane Database of Systematic Reviews.* **6**: CD008320.
19 Bernstein JE (1988) Capsaicin in dermatologic disease. *Seminars in Dermatology.* **7**: 304–309.
20 Breneman D et al. (1992) Topical capsaicin for treatment of hemodialysis-related pruritus. *Journal of the American Academy of Dermatology.* **26**: 91–94.
21 Massey T et al. (2010) Topical NSAIDS for acute pain in adults. *Cochrane Database of Systematic Reviews.* **6**: CD007402.
22 Mason L et al. (2004) Topical NSAIDs for chronic musculoskeletal pain: systematic review and meta-analysis. *BMC Musculoskeletal Disorders.* **5**: 28.
23 Moore R et al. (1998) Quantitative systematic review of topically applied non-steroidal anti-inflammatory drugs. *British Medical Journal.* **316**: 333–338.
24 Underwood M et al. (2008) Advice to use topical or oral ibuprofen for chronic knee pain in older people: randomised controlled trial and patient preference study. *British Medical Journal.* **336**: 138–142.
25 Mondino A et al. (1983) Kinetic studies of ibuprofen on humans. Comparative study for the determination of blood concentrations and metabolites following local and oral administration. *Medizinische Welt.* **34**: 1052–1054.
26 Chlud K and Wagener H (1987) Percutaneous nonsteroidal anti-inflammatory drug (NSAID) therapy with particular reference to pharmacokinetic factors. *EULAR Bulletin.* **2**: 40–43.
27 Peters H et al. (1987) Percutaneous kinetics of ibuprofen (German). *Aktuelle Rheumatologie.* **12**: 208–211.
28 Dominkus M et al. (1996) Comparison of tissue and plasma levels of ibuprofen after oral and topical administration. *Arzneimittelforschung.* **46**: 1138–1143.
29 Matthews P et al. (2010) Topical rubefacients for acute and chronic pain in adults. *Cochrane Database of Systematic Reviews.* **11**: CD007403.
30 Haroutounian S et al. (2010) Topical NSAID therapy for musculoskeletal pain. *Pain Medicine.* **11**: 535–549.
31 O'Callaghan C et al. (1994) Renal disease and use of topical NSAIDs. *British Medical Journal.* **308**: 110–111.
32 Makris UE et al. (2010) Adverse effects of topical nonsteroidal antiinflammatory drugs in older adults with osteoarthritis: a systematic literature review. *Journal of Rheumatology.* **37**: 1236–1243.

Updated May 2014

SKELETAL MUSCLE RELAXANTS BNF 10.2.2

Skeletal muscle relaxants are used to relieve painful chronic muscle spasm and spasticity associated with neural injury, e.g. paraplegia, post-stroke, multiple sclerosis, and sometimes motor neurone disease/amyotrophic lateral sclerosis (MND/AML),[1] and also troublesome cramp. †**Baclofen** is also used to relieve hiccup.

Spasticity
All skeletal muscle relaxants may reduce voluntary muscle power. This may be a disadvantage in people with hemiplegia or paraplegia if increased spastic muscle tone is what enables them to walk or function more independently. Thus, dose escalation to the maximum recommended dose should be spread out over 4–8 weeks to balance the benefits of reduced spasticity with possible loss of functional performance and independence.

In contrast, in patients unable to use their limbs because of severe spasticity or paralysis or motor weakness, the dose can be escalated more rapidly. For these patients, sedation is likely to be the dose-limiting factor.[2]

There is low level evidence that spasticity in multiple sclerosis can be improved by exercise programmes, magnetic stimulation and electromagnetic therapies.[3]

Cramp
Cramp has many potential causes (Box A), including drugs (Box B). In the case of diuretics, cramp is triggered by volume depletion $\pm$ electrolyte imbalance, i.e. loss of sodium and magnesium. Cramp associated with **cisplatin** possibly relates to the combined impact of hypomagnesaemia and peripheral neuropathy. In many cases, the mechanism is not known.

Box A   Causes of cramp[4]

Idiopathic
Exercise
Old age (nocturnal leg cramps)

Acute extracellular volume depletion
Diuertics
Excessive sweating ('heat cramps')
   generally with exertion
Haemodialysis
GI fluid loss (diarrhoea, vomiting)

Drugs (Box B)

Endocrine
Hypo-adrenalism
Hypothyroidism
Pregnancy

Lower motor neurone disorders
MND/ALS
Neuropathy
Post-poliomyelitis
Radiculopathy
Metabolic
Cirrhosis
Hypomagnesaemia
Renal impairment

Miscellaneous
Autoimmune disease (antibodies to
   voltage-gated potassium channels)
Hereditary disorders

Box B   Drug-induced cramps[4]

ACE inhibitors
   enalapril
   ramipril
Amitriptyline
Amphotericin B
β_2-Agonists
   salbutamol
   terbutaline
Bisphosphonates
   pamidronate
   zoledronic acid
Celecoxib

Chemotherapy
   cisplatin
   vincristine
Cimetidine
Clofibrate (not UK)
Diuretics
Lithium
Statins
Steroids
   beclometasone (by inhaler)
   medroxyprogesterone acetate
   prednisolone

As always, it is important to consider correcting the correctable. Cramp cannot be induced or sustained in a stretched muscle, and calf stretching movements (both active and passive) and exercise are useful non-drug measures particularly before going to bed,[4] despite the lack of a strong evidence base.[5,6]

Drug treatment of lower limb muscle cramp is similar to that of spasticity.[7] **Quinine** has traditionally been used to relieve nocturnal cramp, but this is now discouraged (Box C).

Box C   Quinine and cramp

Quinine is more effective than placebo in reducing the frequency and intensity of cramp at doses of 200–500mg/24h, most commonly 300mg.[8]

The most common minor undesirable effects were GI or headache (quinine 13% vs. placebo 9%).[8] With use up to 2 months, the incidence of major undesirable effects and withdrawal was not significantly greater for quinine than for placebo (1.5% vs. 1.4%).[8]

---

continued

Box C   *Continued*

Even so, various regulatory agencies consider that, because alternatives are available, the collective risks associated with using quinine for cramp are too high to permit continued routine use:
- rare but serious undesirable effects:
  ▷ thrombocytopenia → severe bleeding (several deaths have been reported)
  ▷ haemolytic-uraemic syndrome → permanent renal damage
- toxicity in overdose → permanent blindness or death
- serious drug interactions with, e.g. digoxin, warfarin.[9,10]

Consequently, the MHRA advises that quinine should not be used for nocturnal cramps unless the following criteria are all met:
- treatable causes have been ruled out
- non-drug measures have failed
- they regularly cause loss of sleep
- they are very painful or frequent.[9]

If quinine is considered necessary, suitable doses are:
- quinine *sulfate* 200mg at bedtime, increased if necessary to 300mg at bedtime
- quinine *bisulfate* (not UK) 300mg at bedtime (equivalent to *sulfate* 200mg).

During the early stages of treatment, patients should be monitored for signs of thrombocytopenia, e.g. unexplained petechiae, bruising or bleeding.

Treatment should be discontinued after 4 weeks if there is no benefit, and interrupted approximately every 3 months to re-evaluate benefit.[5,9]

Table 1   Skeletal muscle relaxants and spasticity

Drug	Starting dose	Maximum dose	Undesirable effects	Monitoring	Precautions
Diazepam	5mg at bedtime	60mg/24h	Weakness, sedation, cognitive impairment, depression	Accumulation; prolongation of plasma halflife with cimetidine	Abrupt cessation may → rebound anxiety and insomnia
Baclofen	5mg once daily–t.d.s.	20mg q.d.s.	Weakness, sedation, fatigue, dizziness, nausea, hepatotoxicity	Periodic LFTs	Abrupt cessation may → agitation, psychosis and seizures
Tizanidine	2–4mg at bedtime	12mg t.d.s.	Drowsiness, dry mouth, dizziness, hepatotoxicity	Periodic LFTs	Do not use with CYP1A2 inhibitors; caution with antihypertensives, clonidine or digoxin. Abrupt cessation may → rebound hypertension and tachycardia
Dantrolene	25mg once daily	100mg q.d.s.	Weakness, sedation, diarrhoea, hepatotoxicity	Periodic LFTs	

Choice of drug

Baclofen, diazepam, dantrolene and **tizanidine** are all currently approved for use in patients with spasticity. **Baclofen, diazepam** and **tizanidine** act principally on spinal and supraspinal sites within the CNS; **dantrolene** (and **quinine**) acts on muscle. There is no clear evidence that any one drug is superior to the others (Table 1).[11–13]

If there is no concurrent indication for a benzodiazepine, **baclofen** is generally a good choice as the first-line drug, particularly if long-term treatment is likely. The use of **diazepam** as a muscle relaxant is discussed in benzodiazepines (see p.152).

More invasive treatments for spasticity include IT **phenol**. This is neurotoxic and can cause urinary and faecal incontinence. The use of indwelling devices to deliver IT **baclofen** has generally superseded the use of **phenol**.[7,14]

Botulinum toxin (BTX) injections are largely reserved for treatment of contractures. The BTX-type A light chain acts as a zinc endopeptidase and interferes with acetylcholine release.[15] The toxin is injected into each spastic muscle separately and reduces spasticity in a dose-dependent manner.[16] Its use is rarely relevant in palliative care. It has been used in people with neurodegenerative disorders, e.g. MND/ALS to manage drooling and, less commonly, dysphagia secondary to upper oesophageal sphincter dysfunction.[17,18]

Anti-epileptics have been used to treat cramp unresponsive to more conventional approaches (Table 2).

Table 2 Anti-epileptics for treating cramp[a,4]

Drug	Dose
Gabapentin	300mg at bedtime;[19] up to 900mg t.d.s.[14,20]
Carbamazepine	100–200mg at bedtime[4]
Phenytoin	100–200mg once daily[4]

a. also see anti-epileptics, p.254.

1 Zafonte R et al. (2004) Acute care management of post-TBI spasticity. Journal of Head Trauma Rehabilitation. **19**: 89–100.
2 Noth J and Fink GR (2004) Spasticity. In: R Voltz et al. (eds) Palliative Care in Neurology (No. 69). Oxford University Press, Oxford, p. 154.
3 Amatya B et al. (2013) Non pharmacological interventions for spasticity in multiple sclerosis. Cochrane Database of Systematic Reviews. **2**: CD009974.
4 Miller TM and Layzer RB (2005) Muscle cramps. Muscle Nerve. **32**: 431–442.
5 NHS (2012) Clinical Knowledge Summary. Leg cramps. Available from: www.cks.nice.org.uk/leg-cramps
6 Blyton F et al. (2012) Non-drug therapies for lower limb muscle cramps. Cochrane Database of Systematic Reviews. **1**: CD008496.
7 Kita M and Goodkin D (2000) Drugs used to treat spasticity. Drugs. **59**: 487–495.
8 El Tawil S et al. (2010) Quinine for muscle cramps. Cochrane Database of Systematic Reviews. **12**: CD005044.
9 MHRA (2010) Quinine: not to be used routinely for nocturnal leg cramps Drug Safety Update. **3**. www.mhra.gov.uk/safetyinformation
10 FDA (2010) Qualaquin (quinine sulfate): New Risk Evaluation and Mitigation Strategy - Risk of serious hematological reactions. Available from: www.fda.gov/Safety/MedWatch/SafetyInformation
11 Shakespeare DT et al. (2003) Anti-spasticity agents for multiple sclerosis. Cochrane Database of Systematic Reviews. **4**: CD001332.
12 Chou R et al. (2004) Comparative efficacy and safety of skeletal muscle relaxants for spasticity and musculoskeletal conditions: a systematic review. Journal of Pain and Symptom Management. **28**: 140–175.
13 Baldinger R et al. (2012) Treatment for cramps in amyotrophic lateral sclerosis/motor neuron disease. Cochrane Database of Systematic Reviews. **4**: CD004157.
14 Royal College of Physicians (2004) Multiple Sclerosis: National clinical guidelines for diagnosis and management in primary and secondary care. Available from: www.rcplondon.ac.uk/bookshop
15 Brin M (1997) Dosing, administration and a treatment algorithm for use of botulinum toxin A for adult-onset of spasticity. Muscle and Nerve. **20 (Suppl 6)**: 208–220.
16 Royal College of Physicians of London (2009) Spasticity in adults: management using botulinum toxin. National guidelines. Available from: www.rcplondon.ac.uk/bookshop
17 Young CA et al. (2011) Treatment for sialorrhea (excessive saliva) in people with motor neuron disease/amyotrophic lateral sclerosis. Cochrane Database of Systematic Reviews. CD006981.
18 Regan et al. (2012) Botulinum toxin for upper oesophageal sphincter dysfunction in neurological swallowing disorders. Cochrane Database of Systematic Reviews. **7**: CD009968.
19 Serrao M et al. (2000) Gabapentin treatment for muscle cramps: an open-label trial. Clinical Neuropharmacology. **23**: 45–49.
20 Paisley S et al. (2002) Clinical effectiveness of oral treatments for spasticity in multiple sclerosis: a systematic review. Multiple Sclerosis. **8**: 319–329.

Updated April 2014

BACLOFEN

Class: Skeletal muscle relaxant.

Indications: Spasticity ± painful flexor muscle spasms of voluntary (skeletal) muscle resulting from spinal or CNS lesions, †hiccup.

Contra-indications: PO: Active peptic ulcer (baclofen stimulates gastric acid secretion). **IT:** treatment-resistant epilepsy.

Pharmacology

Baclofen is a chemical congener of the naturally occurring neurotransmitter, GABA.[1] It acts upon the GABA-receptor, inhibiting the release of the excitatory amino acids glutamate and aspartate, principally at the spinal level and also at supraspinal sites, thereby decreasing spasm in skeletal muscle.[2,3] It is preferable to **diazepam** for long-term use (e.g. in patients with chronic neurological disease such as multiple sclerosis) because it avoids the problem of **diazepam** dependence. Further, its use is not associated with tolerance; it retains its antispasmodic effects even after many years of continued use.[4] Baclofen relieves hiccup, possibly by a direct effect on the diaphragm.
Bio-availability >90% PO.
Onset of action 3–4 days.
Time to peak plasma concentration 0.5–3h.
Plasma halflife 3.5h; 4.5h in the elderly.
Duration of action 6–8h.[5]

Cautions

Withdrawal: abrupt withdrawal of PO baclofen may precipitate serious psychiatric reactions, e.g. agitation, confusion, hallucinations, paranoia, delusions, psychosis. Thus, discontinue by gradual dose reduction over 1–2 weeks, or longer if withdrawal symptoms occur.[6] Sudden withdrawal of IT baclofen or failure of the IT pump may lead to a potentially fatal withdrawal syndrome (see Chapter 21, Box A, p.716).

Use with caution in patients with severe psychiatric disorders, epilepsy, Parkinson's disease, respiratory impairment, stroke, history of peptic ulceration, renal or liver impairment (monitor LFTs), diabetes mellitus, hesitancy of micturition (may precipitate urinary retention), patients who use spasticity to maintain posture or to aid function. Drowsiness may affect skilled tasks and driving; effects of alcohol enhanced.

Undesirable effects

Very common (>10%): sedation, drowsiness, nausea.
Common (<10%, >1%): dizziness, fatigue, muscle hypotonia, pain or weakness, ataxia, tremor, insomnia, headache, visual disturbances, nystagmus, psychiatric disturbances, hypotension, respiratory depression, dry mouth, vomiting, constipation or diarrhoea, urinary frequency or incontinence, dysuria, hyperhidrosis, rash.
Uncommon, rare or very rare (<1%, >0.001%): paradoxical increase in spasticity, seizures (particularly in known epileptics), joint pain, hypothermia, paraesthesia, taste disturbance, abdominal pain, hepatic impairment, urinary retention, impotence.

Dose and use

The starting dose intervals and titration steps given here are more conservative than those in the SPC. Starting doses are the same for muscle spasm, spasticity and hiccup:
- start with 5mg b.d.–t.d.s. PO; the risk of GI irritation is less if taken after food (see Chapter 14, Box B, p.643)
- increase if necessary by 5mg b.d.–t.d.s. every 3 days but more slowly if troublesome undesirable effects, particularly in the elderly
- effective doses for hiccup are often relatively low, e.g. 5–10mg t.d.s., although it may be necessary to increase the dose to 20mg t.d.s.
- for spasticity, the effective dose is generally ⩽ 20mg t.d.s. (maximum 100mg/24h)
- effective doses for muscle spasm fall somewhere in the middle.

With spasticity, if no improvement with maximum tolerated dose after 6 weeks, *withdraw gradually over 1–2 weeks.*

An undesirable degree of hypotonia may occur, but can generally be relieved by reducing the daytime dose and increasing the evening dose.

An IT injection is available for specialist use in patients with severe chronic spasticity in whom PO treatment is ineffective or poorly tolerated (see Chapter 21, p.716).

Renal impairment

Note: the plasma creatinine concentration in patients with a low muscle mass is likely to overestimate renal function.

Because baclofen toxicity has been seen in patients with renal impairment, those with an eGFR of 30–60mL/min/1.73m^2 should start with low doses at long intervals and titrate to effect, and people with an eGFR of <30mL/min/1.73m^2 should be prescribed an alternative drug (e.g. **tizanidine, dantrolene**).[7] However, advice on suitable doses and dose intervals in renal impairment varies:
- the *Renal Drug Handbook (3e)* advises:
  - ▷ for patients with creatinine clearance (Cl$_{cr}$) 10–20mL/min, start with 5mg b.d. and then titrate to response
  - ▷ for patients with Cl$_{cr}$ <10mL/min, start with 5mg once daily then titrate to response[8]
- the manufacturer's SPC states that signs of overdose have been seen in renal patients taking >5mg once daily, and thus advises:
  - ▷ 5mg once daily for patients with renal impairment (degree not stated) or undergoing regular haemodialysis
  - ▷ baclofen should be used in patients with end-stage renal disease (CKD stage 5; GFR <15mL/min) only if potential benefit clearly outweighs risk, and with close monitoring for signs of overdose, e.g. drowsiness, lethargy.

Supply

Baclofen (generic)
Tablets 10mg, 28 days @ 10mg t.d.s. = £2.
Oral solution 5mg/5mL, 28 days @ 10mg t.d.s. = £14.
*IT injection 50microgram/mL, 1mL amp (for test dose) = £2; 500microgram/mL, 20mL amp (for use in implantable pump) = £49; 2mg/mL, 5mL amp (for use with implantable pump) = £49.

Lioresal® (Novartis)
Tablets (scored) 10mg, 28 days @ 10mg t.d.s. = £11.
Oral solution (sugar-free) 5mg/5mL, 28 days @ 10mg t.d.s. = £24; *raspberry flavoured.*
*IT injection 50microgram/mL, 1mL amp (for test dose) = £3; 500microgram/mL, 20mL amp (for use in implantable pump) = £59; 2mg/mL, 5mL amp (for use with implantable pump) = £59.

1 Zafonte R et al. (2004) Acute care management of post-TBI spasticity. *Journal of Head Trauma Rehabilitation.* **19**: 89–100.
2 Guelaud C et al. (1995) Baclofen therapy for chronic hiccup. *European Respiratory Journal.* **8**: 235–237.
3 Ramirez FC and Graham DY (1992) Treatment of intractable hiccup with baclofen: results of a double-blind randomized, controlled, crossover study. *American Journal of Gastroenterology.* **87**: 1789–1791.
4 Gaillard JM (1977) Comparison of two muscle relaxant drugs on human sleep: diazepam and parachlorophenylgaba. *Acta Psychiatrica Belgica.* **77**: 410–425.
5 Kochak GM et al. (1985) The pharmacokinetics of baclofen derived from intestinal infusion. *Clinical Pharmacology and Therapeutics.* **38**: 251–257.
6 CSM (Committee on Safety of Medicines and Medicines Control Agency) (1997) Reminder! Severe withdrawal reactions with baclofen can be prevented by gradual dose reduction. *Current Problems in Pharmacovigilance.* **23**: 6.
7 Su W et al. (2009) Reduced level of consciousness from baclofen in people with low kidney function. *British Medical Journal.* **339**: b4559.
8 Ashley C and Currie A (2009) *The Renal Drug Handbook* (3e). Radcliffe Publishing Ltd, Oxford.

Updated June 2014

DANTROLENE SODIUM   BNF 10.2.2

Class: Skeletal muscle relaxant.

Indications: Chronic severe spasticity of skeletal muscle.

Contra-indications: Hepatic impairment, particularly active liver disease, e.g. hepatitis or cirrhosis (may cause severe liver damage); acute muscle spasm or where spasm is useful in maintaining posture, balance or walking.

Pharmacology
Unlike **baclofen** and **diazepam**, dantrolene acts directly on skeletal muscle by binding to ryanodine receptors, thereby reducing the amount of intracellular calcium available for contraction.[1] It produces fewer central undesirable effects than **baclofen** and **diazepam** and, if necessary, can be used concurrently with these drugs in an attempt to produce a better balance between muscle relaxation and undesirable effects, e.g. unacceptable drowsiness.[2]
Bio-availability 35% PO.
Onset of action up to 1 week.
Time to peak plasma concentration up to 3h.
Plasma halflife 5–9h.
Duration of action no data.

Cautions
Compromised pulmonary function, particularly COPD; predisposition to or actual cardiovascular impairment. Drowsiness may affect the performance of skilled tasks, e.g. driving; effects of alcohol enhanced.

Because of the risk of hepatotoxicity with long-term use, discontinue if no benefit is observed after 6 weeks of treatment. Perform LFTs before starting treatment and then at regular intervals, e.g. monthly, throughout treatment; if possible, avoid concurrent use of other hepatotoxic drugs.

Undesirable effects
Drowsiness, dizziness, muscle weakness, general malaise, fatigue and diarrhoea (all generally transient). However, diarrhoea may be severe and may necessitate stopping dantrolene temporarily or permanently.
Common (>1%): Seizure, visual disturbances, speech disturbances, headache, pericarditis, pleural effusion, respiratory depression, nausea, vomiting, abdominal pain, anorexia, fever, skin rash, elevation of LFTs.

Severe hepatotoxicity develops rarely, most often after 1–12 months, and is more likely in people over 30 years old, women (particularly those taking oral contraceptives), and with doses >400mg/24h.[3] Fatalities have occurred only with doses >200mg/24h.[4,5]

Dose and use
The dose of dantrolene should be built up slowly:
- start with 25mg once daily
- initially increase by no more than 25mg/24h weekly
- above 100mg/24h, larger increments are permissible (see SPC)
- usual effective dose 75mg t.d.s.
- maximum recommended dose 100mg q.d.s.

Supply
Dantrium® (SpePharm)
Capsules 25mg, 100mg, 28 days @ 75mg t.d.s. = £43.
Oral suspension 25mg/5mL, 28 days @ 75mg t.d.s. = £258, (unauthorized; available as a special order, see Appendix 1, p.817); *price based on specials tariff in the community.*

1 Zafonte R et al. (2004) Acute care management of post-TBI spasticity. *Journal of Head Trauma Rehabilitation.* **19**: 89–100.
2 Krause T et al. (2004) Dantrolene–a review of its pharmacology, therapeutic use and new developments. *Anaesthesia.* **59**: 364–373.
3 Kim JY et al. (2011) Safety of low-dose oral dantrolene sodium on hepatic function. *Archives of Physical Medicine and Rehabilitation.* **92**: 1359–1363.
4 Utili R et al. (1977) Dantrolene-associated hepatic injury. Incidence and character. *Gastroenterology.* **72**: 610–616.
5 Wilkinson S et al. (1979) Hepatitis from dantrolene sodium. *Gut.* **20**: 33–36.

Updated April 2014

TIZANIDINE   BNF 10.2.2

Class: Skeletal muscle relaxant.

Indications: Spasticity in multiple sclerosis, spinal cord injury or disease.

Contra-indications: Severe hepatic impairment, patients for whom spasm is useful in maintaining posture, balance or walking, concurrent use with potent CYP1A2 inhibitors, e.g. **ciprofloxacin, fluvoxamine.**

Pharmacology

Tizanidine, like **clonidine**, is a central α_2 agonist within the CNS at supraspinal and spinal levels.[1] It inhibits spinal polysynaptic reflex activity. This reduces the sympathetic outflow which in turn reduces muscle tone. Tizanidine has no direct effect on skeletal muscle, neuromuscular junctions or monosynaptic spinal reflexes. Tizanidine reduces pathologically increased muscle tone, including resistance to passive movements, and alleviates painful spasms and clonus.[2] In spasticity, tizanidine is comparable in efficacy to **diazepam** and **baclofen**,[3] and has superior tolerability.[4]

Tizanidine is well absorbed but undergoes extensive first-pass metabolism in the liver to inactive metabolites which are mostly excreted by the kidneys. Wide interindividual variability in the effective plasma concentration means that the optimal dose must be titrated slowly over 2–4 weeks. Maximum effects occur within 2h of administration.[5]

Bio-availability 40% PO.
Onset of action 1–2h; peak response 8 weeks.
Time to peak plasma concentration 1.5h.
Plasma halflife 2.5h; up to $14h \pm 10h$ in renal failure.[6]
Duration of action 'relatively short' (manufacturer's SPC).

Cautions

Elderly; renal impairment; cardiovascular disorders; concurrent administration with drugs which prolong the QT interval. Administration with hypotensive drugs or **digoxin** may potentiate hypotension or bradycardia. Drowsiness may affect performance of skilled tasks, e.g. driving; effects of alcohol enhanced.

LFTs should be monitored monthly for the first 4 months in patients taking 12mg/24h or more; discontinue if liver enzymes remain persistently raised >3 times the upper limit of normal.

Avoid abrupt withdrawal, particularly after long-term use or high doses (risk of rebound hypertension and tachycardia); monitor blood pressure during withdrawal.

Drug interactions

Tizanidine plasma concentrations are increased by CYP1A2 inhibitors, potentially leading to severe hypotension. Avoid concurrent use with potent CYP1A2 inhibitors, e.g. **ciprofloxacin** (and possibly **enoxacin** (not UK)), **fluvoxamine**; use with caution with other CYP1A2 inhibitors, e.g. **cimetidine, norfloxacin, oestrogens, progestogens** (see Chapter 25, p.767).[7]

Undesirable effects

Drowsiness, weakness and dry mouth in more than two thirds of those taking it,[8] although drowsiness and weakness may be less than with **diazepam** and **baclofen.**[9]

Hypotension and dizziness, nausea and other GI disturbances. Less frequently insomnia, bradycardia, hallucinations and hepatotoxicity (rare in doses ≤ 12mg/24h).

Dose and use
Slow upward titration helps to reduce undesirable effects:
* start with 2mg once daily
* if necessary, increase by 2mg every 3–4 days
* doses above 2mg/24h should be divided, and given b.d.–q.d.s.
* effective dose generally ≤ 24mg/24h, in 3–4 divided doses
* maximum recommended dose = 36mg/24h.

In elderly patients and in those with severe renal impairment (creatinine clearance < 25mL/min) an even slower titration is recommended. Because of the prolonged plasma halflife in renal impairment, the manufacturer recommends slow titration with a *single* daily dose.

Avoid abrupt withdrawal; if possible, taper higher doses over several weeks (see Cautions).

Supply
Tizanidine (generic)
Tablets 2mg, 4mg, 28 days @ 8mg t.d.s. = £34.
Oral solution or suspension 2mg/5mL, 28 days @ 8mg t.d.s. = £470 or £437 respectively, (unauthorized; available as a special order, see Appendix I, p.817); *price based on specials tariff in community.*

1 Zafonte R et al. (2004) Acute care management of post-TBI spasticity. Journal of Head Trauma Rehabilitation. 19: 89–100.
2 Wallace J (1994) Summary of combined clinical analysis of controlled clinical trials with tizanidine. Neurology. 44 (11 Suppl 9): s60–s69.
3 Lataste X et al. (1994) Comparative profile of tizanidine in the management of spasticity. Neurology. 44 (11 Suppl 9): s53–s59.
4 Kamen L et al. (2008) A practical overview of tizanidine use for spasticity secondary to multiple sclerosis, stroke, and spinal cord injury. Current Medical Research and Opinion. 24: 425–439.
5 Wagstaff A and Bryson H (1997) Tizanidine. A review of its pharmacology, clinical efficacy and tolerability in the management of spasticity associated with cerebral and spinal disorders. Drugs. 53: 435–452.
6 Keyser E and Ohnhaus E (1986) Data on file. Pharmacokinetic study with Sirdalud (tizanidine, DS 103–282) in patients with renal insufficiency.
7 Baxter K and Preston CL. Stockley's Drug Interactions. London: Pharmaceutical Press www.medicinescomplete.com (accessed February 2014).
8 Nance P et al. (1997) Relationship of the antispasticity effect of tizanidine to plasma concentration in patients with multiple sclerosis. Archives of Neurology. 54: 731–736.
9 Smith H and Barton A (2000) Tizanidine in the management of spasticity and musculoskeletal complaints in the palliative care population. American Journal of Hospice and Palliative Care. 17: 50–58.

Updated April 2014

11: EAR, NOSE AND OROPHARYNX

MOUTHWASHES   BNF 12.3.4

Cleaning and freshening the mouth

Lemon glycerine mouth swabs should not be used because the lemon flavouring has a drying effect.[1]

For home use, one of the following rinses made in tepid water is generally satisfactory:
- 1/4 teaspoon of **sodium chloride** (table salt) in 1 cup (approximately 250mL)
- 1 teaspoon of **sodium bicarbonate** (baking soda) in 1 cup
- 1/2 teaspoon of **sodium chloride** and 2 tablespoons of **sodium bicarbonate** in 4 cups.[2]

Some centres use less **sodium bicarbonate**, e.g. 1/2 half a teaspoon each of **sodium chloride** and **sodium bicarbonate**. In hospital, **compound sodium chloride mouthwash BP** (containing both **sodium chloride** and **sodium bicarbonate**) is often used. **Sodium bicarbonate** is widely used as symptomatic treatment for mild oral mucositis.

Chlorhexidine mouthwashes are used to prevent/treat various oral infections (e.g. periodontal disease, oral candidosis),[3,4] and to sterilize dentures and other prostheses.[5] **Chlorhexidine** inhibits the formation of plaque on teeth, and thus is useful when toothbrushing is not possible. However, **chlorhexidine** does not remove established plaque; this requires professional dental cleaning.

Note: **chlorhexidine** is inactivated by ingredients in some toothpastes. Thus, if a patient is using both, the use of the mouthwash should be delayed for ⩾30min after using toothpaste. Further, because **chlorhexidine** binds to **nystatin** and leads to inactivation of both drugs, it is important to delay giving **nystatin** oral suspension for ⩾30min after using **chlorhexidine** mouthwash.[6]

Most brands of **chlorhexidine** mouthwash contain alcohol which may cause discomfort; diluting the mouthwash with an equal amount of water may reduce this;[5] however, an alcohol-free product is available. **Chlorhexidine** can stain the teeth and tongue, and this is exacerbated by drinking tea and coffee. The staining can be removed by professional dental cleaning.

Debridement

Generally, a coated ('furred') tongue is indicative of inadequate salivary gland function (most likely drug-induced) and/or mouth breathing. Initial treatment is thus frequent routine mouth care, e.g. sips or sprays of cold water, or sucking ice-cubes, and petroleum jelly to lips. When inadequate, consider the use of artificial saliva and/or saliva stimulant (see p.601 and p.602). Specific debridement is achieved by gentle brushing with a baby's soft toothbrush several times per day until the tongue is clean.

Hydrogen peroxide mouthwash is sometimes used as a non-specific cleansing agent; the 'frothing' action of the mouthwash encouraging disintegration of oral debris. However, it should be used sparingly because its use can delay healing.[7]

In the past, some centres used effervescent **ascorbic acid** tablets or pineapple for debriding. However, such use has fallen out of favour. Both agents are acidic, and thus may exacerbate a sore or inflamed mouth, contribute to the demineralization of teeth, and predispose to oral infections (see p.601).

Cautions

MHRA has issued an alert for products or medical devices containing **chlorhexidine** following reports of anaphylaxis, including one precipitated by the use of a **chlorhexidine** skin wipe.[8]

Dose and use

Rinse the mouth with the recommended volume, generally 10mL, for about 30–60sec and then spit out:

- **sodium chloride** or **sodium bicarbonate** mouthwashes can be used p.r.n.; dilute **compound sodium chloride BP** mouthwash with an equal volume of warm water
- **chlorhexidine** has a prolonged duration of action, and generally needs to be used only b.d., either undiluted or diluted with an equal volume of warm water
- use **hydrogen peroxide** mouthwash undiluted after meals and at bedtime.

Supply

Sodium chloride mouthwash, compound BP
Mouthwash containing **sodium chloride** 1.5%, **sodium bicarbonate** 1% in peppermint-flavoured chloroform water; can be prepared locally.

Chlorhexidine gluconate (generic)
Mouthwash 0.2%, 300mL = £3; *may contain alcohol.*

Corsodyl® (GSK Consumer Healthcare)
Mouthwash 0.2%, 300mL = £2, 600mL = £4; *original or mint flavour.*
Mouthwash 0.2%, 300mL = £2.50; *alcohol-free, mint flavour.*
Oral spray 0.2%, 60mL = £4; *mint flavour.*
Dental gel 1%, 50g = £1.50.

Hydrogen peroxide
Peroxyl® (Colgate Palmolive)
Mouthwash 1.5%, 300mL = £3.50.

1 Poland JM et al. (1987) Comparing Moi-Stir to lemon-glycerin swabs. *American Journal of Nursing.* **87**: 422–424.
2 National Cancer Institute (2010) Oral complications of chemotherapy and head/neck radiation (PDQ). Available from: www.cancer.gov/cancertopics/pdq/supportivecare/oralcomplications/
3 Chow A (2010) Oral bacterial infections. In: AN Davies and JB Epstein (eds) *Oral Complications of Cancer and its Management.* Oxford University Press, Oxford, pp. 185–193.
4 Finlay I and Davies A (2005) Fungal Infections. In: A Davies and I Finlay (eds) *Oral Care in Advanced Disease.* Oxford University Press, Oxford, pp. 55–71.
5 Sweeney P (2005) Oral hygiene. In: A Davies and I Finlay (eds) *Oral Care in Advanced Disease.* Oxford University Press, Oxford, pp. 21–35.
6 Barkvoll P and Attramadal A (1989) Effect of nystatin and chlorhexidine digluconate on Candida albicans. *Oral Surgery Oral Medicine and Oral Pathology.* **67**: 279–281.
7 Thomas GW et al. (2009) Mechanisms of delayed wound healing by commonly used antiseptics. *Journal of Trauma-Injury Infection and Critical Care.* **66**: 82–90; discussion 90–81.
8 MHRA (2012) All medical devices and medicinal products containing chlorhexidine. *Medical Device Alert.* MDA/2012/075 www.mhra.gov.uk/safetyinformation

Updated (minor change) March 2014

ARTIFICIAL SALIVA   BNF 12.3.5

Dry mouth (xerostomia) is managed by saliva stimulants or substitutes. Although 99% of saliva is water, the remaining 1% comprises a wide range of electrolytes and molecules which are important for saliva's many roles, e.g. lubricant, cleansing, antimicrobial, taste, digestion, buffering, and mineralization of teeth.[1] This may explain why sipping water gives only short-lived relief.

Artificial saliva is a poor substitute for natural saliva. Thus, *unless a main salivary duct is blocked*, a saliva stimulant is preferable. Chewing gum acts as a saliva stimulant and is as effective as, and preferred to, mucin-based artificial saliva.[2] The gum should be sugar-free and, in patients with dentures, low-tack, e.g. Orbit®.

If dry mouth remains a problem, **pilocarpine** or **bethanechol** should be considered (see p.602). Acidic products should *not* be used as saliva stimulants because they predispose to oral infection (e.g. dental caries, oral candidosis) and cause dimeneralization of the teeth (leading to dental erosion and dental pain). For patients who do not respond to, or cannot tolerate saliva stimulants, artificial saliva is an option.

The ideal artificial saliva should be easy to use, pleasant, effective and well tolerated.[3] Further, it should have a neutral pH and contain fluoride (to enhance remineralization of the teeth).[4]

Generally, RCTs indicate that mucin-based products are better tolerated and more effective than cellulose-based ones,[5-7] with some patients finding cellulose-based products no better than frequent sips of fluid.

The mucin comes from the stomach of pigs, and this may be an issue for some patients (e.g. Jews, Muslims, vegetarians). There is no good evidence that gels are more effective or last longer than sprays.

Undesirable effects

Unpleasant taste, irritation of the mouth, nausea and/or diarrhoea in ⩽ 30% of patients.[2,8]

Dose and use

PCF regards sugar-free chewing gum as the saliva stimulant of choice for most patients. For patients with dentures, it should be low-tack, e.g. Orbit®.

Artificial salivas with a neutral pH are preferred for long-term use. Artificial salivas or saliva stimulants with an acidic pH should be avoided.

The duration of effect of artificial salivas is relatively short, due to a combination of swallowing and evaporation. Thus, artificial salivas may need to be taken every 10–30min, and also before (and sometimes during) meals. Proprietary artificial salivas with a neutral pH include:
- AS Saliva Orthana® (mucin-based sprays and lozenges); ACBS classified (see supply)
- Biotène Oralbalance® gel
- BioXtra® gel; ACBS classified (see supply).

Supply

Biotène Oralbalance® gel can be prescribed for any condition given to causing dry mouth. However, AS Saliva Orthana® products, and BioXtra® gel are classified in the UK as borderline substances and have ACBS approval only for dry mouth associated with radiotherapy or sicca syndrome. The prescriber must endorse an NHS FP10 prescription for one of these products with 'ACBS', otherwise the Prescription Pricing Authority will investigate whether it has been issued for an approved indication.

Mucin-based (porcine)
AS Saliva Orthana® (AS Pharma)
Oral spray 50mL bottle = £5; 500mL refill = £35.
Lozenges 30 = £3.50.

Cellulose-based
Biotène Oralbalance® (GSK Consumer Health)
Saliva replacement gel 50g = £5.

BioXtra® (RIS Products)
Saliva replacement gel 40mL tube = £4, 50mL spray = £4.

1 Davies A (2005) Salivary gland dysfunction. In: A Davies and I Finlay (eds) *Oral Care in Advanced Disease*. Oxford University Press, Oxford, pp. 97–114.
2 Davies AN (2000) A comparison of artificial saliva and chewing gum in the management of xerostomia in patients with advanced cancer. *Palliative Medicine*. **14**: 197–203.
3 Epstein JB and Stevenson-Moore P (1992) A clinical comparative trial of saliva substitutes in radiation-induced salivary gland hypofunction. *Special Care Dentistry*. **12**: 21–23.
4 Davies A (2010) Salivary gland dysfunction. In: AN Davies and JB Epstein (eds) *Oral Complications of Cancer and its Management*. Oxford University Press, Oxford, pp. 203–223.
5 S'Gravenmade E et al. (1974) The effect of mucin-containing artificial saliva on severe exerostomia. *International Journal of Oral Surgery*. **3**: 435–439.
6 Vissink A et al. (1983) A clinical comparison between commercially available mucin- and CMC-containing saliva substitutes. *International Journal of Oral Surgery*. **12**: 232–238.
7 Visch L et al. (1986) A double-blind crossover trial of CMC- and mucin-containing saliva substitutes. *International Journal of Oral and Maxillofacial Surgery*. **15**: 395–400.
8 Davies A et al. (1998) A comparison of artificial saliva and pilocarpine in the management of xerostomia in patients with advanced cancer. *Palliative Medicine*. **12**: 105–111.

Updated June 2014

PILOCARPINE   BNF 11.6 & 12.3.5

Class: Parasympathomimetic.

Indications: Xerostomia (dry mouth) after radiotherapy for head and neck cancer, dry mouth (and dry eyes) in Sjögren's syndrome and †drug-induced dry mouth.

Contra-indications: Intestinal or urinary obstruction, or when increased intestinal or urinary tract motility could be harmful (e.g. after recent surgery); when miosis could be harmful (e.g. narrow-angle glaucoma, acute iritis); unstable asthma.

Pharmacology

Pilocarpine is a parasympathomimetic (predominantly muscarinic) drug with mild β-adrenergic activity which stimulates secretion from exocrine glands, including salivary glands.[1] A systematic review suggests that 40–50% of patients with radiotherapy-induced dry mouth respond to pilocarpine, with a time to response of up to 12 weeks.[2] However, undesirable effects are common, and were the main reason for withdrawal from studies (6–15% of patients taking 5mg t.d.s.).

About 90% of patients with drug-induced dry mouth respond to pilocarpine with benefit seen <24h.[3] In an RCT, half of the patients preferred pilocarpine because it was more effective, and half preferred the comparator **mucin**-based artificial saliva, mainly because it was a spray and not a tablet.[3] Undesirable effects were much more common in patients receiving pilocarpine (84% vs. 22%), which resulted in about a quarter of the patients withdrawing from the study. Alternatives to pilocarpine are used at some centres, e.g. **bethanechol**.[4–6]

Bio-availability 96% PO.
Onset of action 20min (drug-induced dry mouth); up to 3 months (after radiation).
Time to peak plasma concentration 1h.
Plasma halflife 1h.
Duration of action 3–5h (single dose).

Cautions

Pilocarpine may antagonize the effects of antimuscarinic drugs, e.g. inhaled **ipratropium bromide**. Concurrent use with β antagonists (β blockers) may cause cardiac conduction disturbances.

Cognitive or psychiatric disorder, epilepsy, parkinsonism. Miosis may affect vision and driving ability, particularly at night. Cardiovascular disease (changes in haemodynamics or heart rhythm), hyperthyroidism, COPD (increased bronchial smooth muscle tone, airway resistance and bronchial secretions). Peptic ulcer (increased acid secretion), gallstones or biliary tract disease (increased biliary smooth muscle contraction). Mild–moderate hepatic impairment (reduce dose); avoid in severe hepatic impairment (no human data on metabolism and excretion). Renal impairment (no reliable human data on metabolism and excretion), kidney stones (potential for renal colic). Increased sweating may exacerbate dehydration in patients unable to drink sufficient fluids.

Undesirable effects

Very common (>10%): headache, flu-like syndrome, nausea, urinary frequency, sweating.

Common (<10%, >1%): dizziness, asthenia, chills, blurred vision, eye pain, conjunctivitis, flushing, palpitations, hypertension (after initial hypotension), rhinitis, abdominal pain, dyspepsia, vomiting, diarrhoea or constipation, rash, pruritus.

Undesirable effects with **bethanechol** are similar to pilocarpine but generally less severe, either because the equivalent dose is less or the muscarinic receptor binding pattern of **bethanechol** is different.

Dose and use

The manufacturer recommends t.d.s. during or directly after meals. However, adding a dose at bedtime reduces the likelihood of the patient waking in the night with an excessively dry mouth.[7]

In drug-induced dry mouth 5mg q.d.s. is generally effective, but after radiotherapy 10mg q.d.s. may be needed:

- start with 5mg t.d.s. with meals and at bedtime, or 6mg if using eyedrop formulation; this is 3 drops of a 4% solution (much cheaper, see Supply)
- if necessary and if tolerated, increase the dose to 10mg q.d.s. after 2 days if the dry mouth is drug-induced, and after 4 weeks if radiation-induced
- if no improvement with 10mg q.d.s., stop after 4 days if the dry mouth is drug-induced, and after 12 weeks if radiation-induced.

In patients with mild–moderate hepatic impairment, possibly start on a lower dose, e.g. 5mg b.d., and increase to 5mg q.d.s. if well tolerated.

If **bethanechol** is used instead for drug-induced dry mouth:

- start with 25mg t.d.s. 30min before meals
- reduce to 10mg t.d.s. if patients experience excessive salivation.

Supply

Note: **Bethanechol** tablets are cheaper than pilocarpine tablets. However, it is cheaper still to give pilocarpine *eyedrops* PO. The use of the eyedrops in this way is off-label.

Pilocarpine (generic)
Eyedrops 4% (40mg/1mL), 10mL lasts 33 days @ 2 drops/4mg PO t.d.s. = £3.50.

Salagen® (Novartis)
Tablets 5mg, 28 days @ 5mg t.d.s. = £42.

Bethanechol
Myotonine® (Glenwood)
Tablets (scored) 10mg, 25mg, 28 days @ 25mg t.d.s. = £23.

1 Anonymous (1994) Oral pilocarpine for xerostomia. *Medical Letter on Drugs and Therapeutics.* **36**: 76.
2 Davies A and Shorthose K (2007) Parasympathomimetic drugs for the treatment of salivary gland dysfunction due to radiotherapy. *Cochrane Database of Systematic Reviews.* CD003782
3 Davies A et al. (1998) A comparison of artificial saliva and pilocarpine in the management of xerostomia in patients with advanced cancer. *Palliative Medicine.* **12**: 105–111.
4 Everett H (1975) The use of bethanechol chloride with tricyclic antidepressants. *American Journal of Psychiatry.* **132**: 1202–1204.
5 Epstein J et al. (1994) A clinical trial of bethanechol in patients with xerostomia after radiation therapy. A pilot study. *Oral Surgery, Oral Medicine and Oral Pathology.* **77**: 610–614.
6 Davies A (2005) Salivary gland dysfunction. In: A Davies and I Finlay (eds) *Oral Care in Advanced Disease.* Oxford University Press, Oxford, pp. 97–114.
7 Davies A (2014) *Personal communication.*

Updated June 2014

DRUGS FOR ORAL INFLAMMATION AND ULCERATION

BNF 12.3.1

'Oral stomatitis' is a term applied to diffuse inflammatory, erosive and ulcerative conditions affecting the mucous membranes of the mouth, whereas 'oral mucositis' tends to be restricted to stomatitis caused by local radiotherapy, chemotherapy or other anti-cancer modalities.

The causes of oral ulceration include trauma (physical, chemical), recurrent aphthous ulceration, infection, cancer, skin conditions, nutritional deficiencies, GI conditions, haematopoietic disorders and drug treatment (Box A). It is important to determine the cause so that, if appropriate, specific treatment is given as well as symptomatic treatment. For example, ill-fitting dentures which cause traumatic ulceration (and/or mucosal hyperplasia) should be relined, or ideally replaced.[1]

Box A   Drug-related oral ulceration

Alimentary	**Chemotherapy**	**Other**
Pancreatin	Bleomycin	Alendronic acid
	Doxorubicin	Allopurinol
Analgesics	5-Fluoro-uracil	Emepronium (not UK)
NSAIDs	Melphalan	Gold
	Mercaptopurine	Interferons
Antibiotics	Methotrexate	Interleukin-2
Aztreonam		Molgramostim
Clarithromycin	**Corticosteroids**	Penicillamine
Proguanil	Flunisolide (not UK)	Potassium chloride
Vancomycin		
Zalcitabine	**Psychotropics**	
	Carbamazepine	
Cardiac	Olanzapine	
Captopril	Phenytoin	
Isoprenaline (not UK)	Sertraline	
Losartan		
Nicorandil		
Phenindione		

Management strategy

The symptomatic management of oral inflammation and ulceration involves measures which:
* maintain oral hygiene
* relieve the pain
* protect ulcerated mucosa
* treat secondary infection
* reduce the inflammation.

Advice should be sought from an oral medicine specialist if unexplained ulceration persists for >3 weeks.

Maintain oral hygiene

Simple mouthwashes, e.g. water or 0.9% **saline**, can be soothing, help to maintain oral hygiene, and prevent secondary infection (see p.599). The temperature of the mouthwash appears to be important, with tepid ones being more soothing than cold or warm ones.

Pain relief

Topical analgesics
Topical analgesics include:
* local anaesthetics
* NSAIDs
* antihistamines
* opioids.

Local anaesthetics
The efficacy of topical local anaesthetics depends on the formulation, duration of application (at least 5min is required) and site of application. There are limited data to support their use in oral mucositis, and any effect is of short duration.[2] They are less effective in more keratinized areas of the mouth, e.g. the palate.[3]

Some systemic absorption of the local anaesthetic occurs, which is increased by mucosal inflammation. However, plasma concentrations are generally low, and toxicity has been reported only in exceptional circumstances (see p.71). With all topical local anaesthetics, care must be taken not to produce pharyngeal anaesthesia before meals because this could lead to aspiration and choking:
- **lidocaine** ointment 5% (has a water-miscible base), rubbed gently onto the affected areas a.c. and p.r.n.
- **lidocaine** spray 10% (Xylocaine®), applied thinly to the ulcer using a cotton bud a.c. and p.r.n. (unauthorized use).

Various OTC products are also available.

NSAIDs
Benzydamine, an NSAID, also has local anaesthetic and antimicrobial effects.[4,5] It is available as an oral rinse or spray, and can ease the discomfort associated with oral stomatitis. It is recommended for the prevention of oral mucositis secondary to radiotherapy:
- **benzydamine** 0.15% oral rinse (Difflam®), rinse or gargle 15mL for 20–30sec before spitting out, repeat q3h–q1.5h p.r.n. Dilute with an equal volume of water if the full-strength oral rinse causes stinging.[6,7]

Excessive use of **choline salicylate** dental gel or confinement under a denture can result in oral irritation and/or ulceration. Remove any dentures before use and wait ⩾30min before re-inserting:
- **choline salicylate** 8.7% oral gel (e.g. Bonjela®), apply 1–2cm by gentle massage q3h p.r.n.; maximum recommended dose 6 applications/day.

Other options include **diclofenac** dispersible tablets and **flurbiprofen** lozenges (can also result in oral ulceration).

Antihistamines
Diphenhydramine (not UK) is an antihistamine with a topical analgesic effect. It has been used for decades for oral mucositis, particularly in the USA,[8] as a locally prepared oral rinse. It is spread around the mouth and then swallowed or spat out after 2min, e.g.:
- **diphenhydramine** 25mg/5mL and **magnesium hydroxide** in equal parts, up to 30mL q2h
- **diphenhydramine** 12.5mg/5mL, **lidocaine** viscous 2% and an antacid in equal parts[8]
- **diphenhydramine** 12.5mg/5mL and **kaopectate** in equal parts (the latter helps mixture to adhere to the oral mucosa).

Some centres use **doxepin** (a TCA and a potent H_1- and H_2-receptor antagonist) instead. It is given as an oral rinse containing **doxepin** 25mg/5ml up to six times per day.[9] It must not be swallowed: a dose of this size several times per day would cause drowsiness and possibly other toxicity (also see p.618).

Opioids
Opioids have a topical analgesic effect on inflamed tissue and can be used as a mouthwash. Some recommend that the mouthwash is subsequently swallowed in order to combine a systemic analgesic effect with the topical one:
- locally prepared **morphine sulfate** 0.2% (2mg/mL) solution, take 10mg in 5mL q4h–q3h, hold in the mouth for 2min *and then spit out or swallow*; some patients need higher doses, occasionally 30mg q4h–q3h[10,11]
- locally prepared **morphine sulfate** 1–5mg/mL gel, initially 3mL q8h–q4h, hold in mouth for 10min *and then spit out or swallow* (see p.372).

Systemic analgesics
Systemic analgesics include non-opioids and opioids given as for other pains, balancing benefit against undesirable effects. For severe mucositis (patient unable to eat ± unable to drink) with inadequate pain relief from topical measures, a parenteral opioid should be administered either by patient-controlled analgesia, continuous infusion with p.r.n. boluses as required, or transdermal

administration (e.g. **fentanyl**).[6] Chemotherapy patients often have a permanent IV access which can be used.

Protect the ulcerated areas

Coating agents are of limited value because they can be difficult to apply and they do not relieve persistent oral inflammatory pain. However, by adhering to and coating the denuded surface, they may help to reduce contact pain, e.g. from eating or drinking. Available agents include:

- **carmellose (carboxymethylcellulose) sodium** (Orabase® paste, Orahesive® powder) apply the paste to, or sprinkle the powder onto, the sore area p.c.
- **polyvinylpyrrolidine** and **sodium hyaluronate** oral gel (Gelclair®) t.d.s. p.r.n., ideally 30–60min a.c.; mix contents of 1 sachet with 40mL water, rinse around mouth for at least 1min, gargle and then spit out
- **sucralfate** is *not* of benefit in radiation-induced oral mucositis,[12] but may help in other types of oral stomatitis; it can be given in a suspension 1g/5mL q.d.s.

Treat secondary infection

Antiseptic and antibacterial mouthwashes may help prevent or treat secondary infection, particularly with multiple ulcers not easily accessible to covering pastes:

- *prevention*: **chlorhexidine gluconate** mouthwash 0.2%, ideally alcohol-free (see p.599)
- *treatment*: **doxycycline** suspension 100mg in 10mL q.d.s. for 3 days (unauthorized use; prepared by mixing a dispersible tablet or the contents of a capsule with a small quantity of water) rinse around the mouth for 2–3min and then spit out.

Alternatively if available, **tetracycline** suspension 250mg in 10mL[13] or **minocycline** suspension 10mg in 5mL[14] can be prepared from capsules in the same way (not UK).

Reduce the inflammation

Topical corticosteroids are useful in the management of certain types of oral ulceration, e.g. recurrent aphthous ulceration (Box B). However, corticosteroids do *not* feature in the management of oral mucositis. Systemic corticosteroids are generally reserved for severe ulcerative conditions, e.g. pemphigus vulgaris.

Box B Treatment of aphthous ulcers

Corticosteroids

Corticosteroids are the mainstay of treatment. Use as soon as symptoms/ulcers appear; avoid in oral infections:

- hydrocortisone oromucosal tablets 2.5mg q.d.s. for up to 5 days; tablets are placed at the site of the ulcers and left to dissolve
- beclometasone metered-dose aerosol inhaler 50 or 100microgram sprayed into the mouth b.d., when a more potent corticosteroid is needed for difficult-to-reach sites such as the soft palate and oropharynx (unauthorized use)
- betamethasone soluble tablets 500microgram, dispersed in 20mL water and rinsed around the mouth q.d.s.; also suitable when a more potent corticosteroid is needed for difficult-to-reach sites (unauthorized use).

Supply

The following list is selective.

Topical analgesics
Lidocaine (generic)
Ointment 5% in a water-miscible base, 15g = £6.

Xylocaine® (AstraZeneca)
Spray 10%, 50mL = £6. Apply thinly to ulcer using cotton bud (unauthorized use).

Benzydamine (generic)
Oral rinse (mouthwash) 0.15%, 300mL = £6.
Oromucosal spray 0.15%, 30mL = £4.

Difflam® (3M)
Oral rinse (mouthwash) 0.15%, 300mL = £7; also available OTC.
Oromucosal spray 0.15%, 30mL = £4.

Choline salicylate dental gel BP
Bonjela® (Reckitt Benckiser)
Oral gel 8.7%, 15g = £2; also available OTC.

Diclofenac
Voltarol® (Novartis)
Tablets dispersible 50mg, 28 days @ 50mg t.d.s. = £25.

Flurbiprofen
Strefen® (Reckitt Benckiser)
Lozenges 8.75mg, 16 = £2.50.

Morphine
Mouthwash 0.2% (2mg/mL in water), locally prepared.
Oral gel 0.1–0.5% (1–5mg/mL), locally prepared.

Coating agents
Orabase® (ConvaTec)
Oral paste containing **carmellose sodium** 16.7%, **gelatin** 16.7% and **pectin** 16.7%, 30g = £2.

Orahesive® (ConvaTec)
Powder containing **carmellose sodium, gelatin** and **pectin**, equal parts, 25g = £2.50.

Gelclair® (Cambridge Laboratories)
Oral gel containing **polyvinylpyrrolidine** and **sodium hyaluronate**, 28 days @ 1 sachet t.d.s. = £132.

Sucralfate
Antepsin® (Chugai)
Oral suspension 1g/5mL, 250mL = £6; *aniseed or caramel flavour.*

Antiseptic and antibacterial mouthwashes
For **chlorhexidine gluconate** mouthwashes, see p.599.

Doxycycline (generic)
Capsules 100mg (as hyclate), 3 days @ 100mg q.d.s. = £2.

Vibramycin-D® (Pfizer)
Dispersible tablets 100mg, 3 days @ 100mg q.d.s. = £7.

Corticosteroids
Hydrocortisone (generic)
Oromucosal tablets 2.5mg (as sodium succinate), 5 days @ 1 q.d.s. = £4.50.

Beclometasone (generic)
Aerosol inhalation 50microgram/metered dose, 200-dose inhaler = £4; 100microgram/metered dose, 200-dose inhaler = £7.

Betamethasone (generic)
Tablets soluble 500microgram, 28 days @ 500microgram q.d.s. = £17.

Betamethasone
Betnesol® (UCB)
Tablets soluble 500microgram, 28 days @ 500microgram q.d.s. = £6.

1 Walls A (2005) Domiciliary dental care. In: A Davies and I Finlay (eds) *Oral Care in Advanced Disease.* Oxford University Press, Oxford, pp. 37–45.
2 Saunders DP *et al.* (2013) Systematic review of antimicrobials, mucosal coating agents, anesthetics, and analgesics for the management of oral mucositis in cancer patients. *Supportive Care in Cancer.* **21**: 3191–3207.
3 Meecham J (2005) Oral pain. In: A Davies and I Finlay (eds) *Oral Care in Advanced Disease.* Oxford University Press, Oxford, pp. 134–143.

4 Turnbull RS (1995) Benzydamine Hydrochloride (Tantum) in the management of oral inflammatory conditions. *Journal Canadian Dental Association.* **61**: 127–134.

5 Fanaki NH and el-Nakeeb MA (1992) Antimicrobial activity of benzydamine, a non-steroid anti-inflammatory agent. *Journal of Chemotherapy.* **4**: 347–352.

6 MASCC Oral mucositis guidelines: http://www.mascc.org/assets/Guidelines-Tools/mascc%20isoo%20mucositis%20guideline s%20summary%201feb2014.pdf

7 Kim J et al. (1985) A clinical study of benzydamine for the treatment of radiotherapy induced mucositis of the orpharynx. *International Journal of Tissue Reaction.* **7**: 215–218.

8 NIH Consensus Development Conference Statement (1989) Oral complications of cancer therapies, prevention and treatment. *NIH Consensus Statement.* **7**: 1–11.

9 Epstein JB et al. (2007) Management of pain in cancer patients with oral mucositis: follow-up of multiple doses of doxepin oral rinse. *Journal of Pain and Symptom Management.* **33**: 111–114.

10 Cerchietti LC et al. (2002) Effect of topical morphine for mucositis-associated pain following concomitant chemoradiotherapy for head and neck carcinoma. *Cancer.* **95**: 2230–2236.

11 Cerchietti L and Cerchietti L (2007) Morphine mouthwashes for painful mucositis. *Supportive Care in Cancer.* **15**: 115–116; author reply 117.

12 Keefe DM et al. (2007) Updated clinical practice guidelines for the prevention and treatment of mucositis. *Cancer.* **109**: 820–831.

13 Barrons RW (2001) Treatment strategies for recurrent oral aphthous ulcers. *American Journal of Health-System Pharmacy.* **58**: 41–50; quiz 51–43.

14 Gorsky M et al. (2007) Topical minocycline and tetracycline rinses in treatment of recurrent aphthous stomatitis: a randomized cross-over study. *Dermatology Online Journal.* **13**: 1.

Updated June 2014

CERUMENOLYTICS   BNF 12.1.3

Indications: Impacted earwax (cerumen).

Contra-indications: perforated ear drum, presence of myringotomy tubes (grommets), recent ear surgery.

Pharmacology

Cerumen impaction is defined as an accumulation of earwax which causes symptoms, prevents adequate examination of the ear, or both; it does not necessarily imply complete obstruction.[1,2] Symptoms associated with impacted earwax include deafness, tinnitus, fullness, itching, otalgia, discharge, and chronic cough. Asymptomatic earwax does *not* need to be removed.

Earwax is secreted to provide a protective film on the skin of the external ear canal. It is generally expelled naturally. The risk of impaction is increased in children, the elderly, people with learning disabilities, and when natural expulsion is obstructed, e.g. by anatomical abnormalities of the ear canal, hearing aids, or inappropriate use of 'cotton buds' to clean the ears.[1,3]

Cerumenolytics are classified as either water-based (e.g. water, 0.9% saline, 5% **sodium bicarbonate**), oil-based (e.g. **almond oil, olive oil**), or non-water/non-oil based (e.g. **urea-hydrogen peroxide**).[4] Water-based products are true cerumenolytics (i.e. break up keratin within earwax),[5] whereas oil-based products lubricate and soften the earwax. The mechanism of action of non-water/non-oil-based products is unclear.

Evidence is too limited to indicate if one type of cerumenolytic is more effective than any other.[1,6] Systematic reviews suggest that cerumenolytics can clear earwax in about one third of cases in 4 days, thereby obviating the need for syringing.[4,6] For these patients, self-treatment with clean tap water will be the most cost-effective treatment.

Syringing without pre-treatment with a cerumenolytic is effective in about three quarters of patients.[3,4,6] After pre-treatment, success approaches 100%.[1] Pre-treatment with water 15–30min before syringing is as effective as applying drops b.d. for several days.[4,7] It works in 'nearly all cases' and is more convenient for patients.[8]

Syringing can cause undesirable effects, including pain, minor damage to the external ear canal, and otitis externa; less commonly perforation of the tympanic membrane and vertigo (the latter generally if the water is too cold).[1]

In those few cases where syringing fails to remove the wax, commonsense dictates that drops should be continued for several more days before a further attempt.[3,8]

There is limited evidence to support any type of manual removal of earwax.[2] However, many practitioners consider manual techniques to be standard practice.

Management strategy

PCF regards water (tap or sterile) or 0.9% saline as the cerumenolytics of choice.

- use drops alone for at least 4 days (e.g. 3–4 drops b.d.)
- if this fails, proceed to syringing
- if this fails, use drops for 3–4 more days and syringe again
- if syringing fails on the second occasion, proceed to manual removal using curette, probe, forceps, suction or hook.

To minimize the risk of damaging the ear canal and tympanic membrane, manual removal after failed syringing is best undertaken by those with specialist training.[1,3]

Supply

Although OTC products are available, their relative effectiveness is unproven and they appear to be no better than water or 0.9% saline. Thus, none is recommended. Some proprietary products contain potentially irritant constituents.[2]

0.9% Saline (generic)
Injection (use as ear drops) 5mL = £0.50.
Nose drops (use as ear drops), 10mL = £1.50; available OTC.

1 Browning G (2008) Ear Wax. In: *BMJ Clinical Evidence*. Available from: www.clinicalevidence.bmj.com/ceweb/conditions/ent/0504/0504-get.pdf
2 Roland PS *et al.* (2008) Clinical practice guideline: cerumen impaction. *Otolaryngology — Head and Neck Surgery*. **139 (3 Suppl 2)**: S1–S21.
3 McCarter DF *et al.* (2007) Cerumen impaction. *American Family Physician*. **75**: 1523–1528.
4 Hand C and Harvey I (2004) The effectiveness of topical preparations for the treatment of earwax: a systematic review. *British Journal of General Practice*. **54**: 862–867.
5 Chalishazar U and Williams H (2007) Back to basics: finding an optimal cerumenolytic (earwax solvent). *British Journal of Nursing*. **16**: 806–808.
6 Burton MJ and Doree CJ (2009) Ear drops for the removal of ear wax. *Cochrane Database of Systematic Reviews*. **1**: CD004326.
7 Pavlidis C and Pickering JA (2005) Water as a fast acting wax softening agent before ear syringing. *Australian Family Physician*. **34**: 303–304.
8 Eekhof JA *et al.* (2001) A quasi-randomised controlled trial of water as a quick softening agent of persistent earwax in general practice. *British Journal of General Practice*. **51**: 635–637.

Updated June 2014

12: SKIN

EMOLLIENTS   BNF 13.2.1

Indications: Dry or rough skin.

Introduction

Emollients soften and increase the hydration of the outermost layer of the epidermis (stratum corneum). This increases the integrity and resilience of the skin and so helps to protect the skin from irritants, allergens, and microbes.[1] Emollients also hydrate skin by preventing loss of water. Older patients are particularly likely to develop dry skin (asteotic dermatitis). Other common causes include:
- varicose (stasis) dermatitis
- drying environments
- excessive washing
- diuretics
- drug reactions
- radiotherapy.

Types of emollients

Emollients vary in greasiness depending on the amount of oil and water they contain (Table 1). Creams and ointments are most commonly used. However, other formulations may be used for specific indications. The choice of emollient depends on many factors.

Ointments are greasy because of their structure, even when their water content is high. Anhydrous ointments provide an occlusive film of oil over the surface of the skin. The water trapped under the ointment passes back into the stratum corneum which then swells up, improving skin barrier function.

Some creams contain **propylene glycol** which gives a smoother texture, and facilitates application. The properties of oily lotions are comparable to creams but, because they are more liquid, they can be applied more easily to large areas and are easier to apply to hairy skin. Both creams and oily lotions have a cooling effect on the skin (heat lost by evaporation of the water content).

Humectants are substances which attract moisture to, and retain it in, the stratum corneum, e.g. **urea, glycerol, lactic acid, alpha-hydroxy acids** and **propylene glycol**.[2] Adequate hydration is generally obtained with creams containing **urea** 5–10%[3,4] and, for patients with only mild–moderate dryness, this may be more cosmetically acceptable than using an ointment. **Urea** at higher concentrations of 20–30% is antipruritic, breaks down keratin, decreases the thickness of the stratum corneum, and is used in scaling conditions such as ichthyosis.[3] However, humectants may be irritating, particularly on inflamed skin, when humectant-free creams or ointments may be preferable.

Proprietary emollients often contain additives and fragrances (perfumes) which are potentially allergenic (Table 2). Concern about **lanolin** is largely misplaced; many emollients contain refined ('hypo-allergic') **lanolin** which is rarely responsible for contact dermatitis.[5]

Table 1 Emollient formulations

	Ointments	Creams	Lotions	Sprays	Soap Substitutes	Bath additives
Description	Grease-based	Emulsions of water and oil; vary from more greasy products (water-in-oil, 'rich creams') to more aqueous ones (oil-in-water, 'light creams')	Solutions, suspensions or emulsions from which water evaporates leaving a thin coating of powder or oil	Oil in volatile silicone	May be in the form of creams, lotions or ointments	Oil; often contain an antimicrobial or antipruritic
Features	Increased absorption	Cosmetically acceptable Suitable for face and flexures May be used for large areas	Suitable for wet rashes and hairy areas Spread well Useful for soaks or wet dressings	Spray on, so application is quick No touching the skin No contamination from the hands	Unlike soaps, do not have detergent properties	Widely used despite the absence of scientific evidence of benefit
Potential limitations	Messy Difficult to apply to hairy areas May occlude hair follicles Perspiration can be trapped under the ointment, causing discomfort from excessive body heat and moisture Avoid applying to large areas	May contain fragrances or preservatives	Only emulsions containing oil have an emollient effect; other lotions are drying Often contain alcohol which will sting broken skin	Make skin and surfaces slippery		Make skin and surfaces slippery; particular care needed when bathing Additives can cause contact dermatitis if used excessively

Table 2 Potential skin allergens in emollients

Allergen	Comment
Fragrances (perfumes)[a,3,6]	
Preservatives (particularly parabens and cresols)[a,3,6]	In many creams and lotions, and in some ointments
Emulsifying agents and ointment bases (particularly sodium lauryl sulfate and cetostearyl alcohols) [a,3,6]	In many creams, lotions and ointments
Wool fat derivatives (includes lanolin)[a,3,6]	In many creams and ointments
Topical local anaesthetics	
Neomycin	
Ethyl alcohol	In some products and skin wipes
Rubber additives (plasticizers, preservatives)	Undersheets, elastic stockings, etc.
Paraphenylenediamine, chromates	In leather
Tea tree oil[7]	

a. Section 13.1.3 of the BNF lists potential sensitizers which mainly fall into these categories.

Cautions

Official advice states that emollients containing **arachis** (peanut) **oil** should not be used by patients with peanut or soya allergy.[8] However, unlike *crude* **arachis oil**, the *refined* oil used in pharmaceutical products is not allergenic, and thus is highly unlikely to cause allergic reactions in people with (whole) peanut allergy.[9,10]

Clothing and dressings in contact with paraffin-based emollients, e.g. **emulsifying ointment BP** or **liquid paraffin and white soft paraffin ointment NPF** (liquid paraffin in white soft paraffin 50/50), are easily ignited by a naked flame. The risk is increased when the products are applied to large areas of the body, and clothing or dressings become soaked with them. Patients should keep away from fire or flames, and not smoke when using these products, particularly if applying large quantities.[11]

In hairy patients prone to folliculitis, to reduce the risk of further episodes, creams and ointments should be applied using downward strokes in the direction of hair growth, particularly on the legs.[12]

Dose and use

Choice of emollient involves consideration of:
- patient preference
- area to be treated, e.g. ointments are generally acceptable for the legs and trunk but not the face, and ointment may be necessary for the thicker skin of the palms and soles
- ingredients; does it contain known or potential allergens?
- degree of dryness; very dry skin often requires an ointment initially
- packaging, e.g. patients with weak hands may find removing screw-top lids or squeezing tubes difficult
- patient's lifestyle
- season; ointments are less well tolerated in the summer
- cost-effectiveness; **aqueous cream BP** is the cheapest product but does not suit everyone.

Aqueous cream sometimes causes burning/stinging $\pm$ erythema when used as an emollient, rather than just as a soap substitute, particularly in children with atopic dermatitis (eczema).[13] This has been linked to sodium lauryl sulfate (SLS), an ingredient of the emulsifying wax BP used to prepare **aqueous cream**, but may be caused by other sensitizing ingredients. The reaction generally occurs within 20min of applying the cream, but is rarely severe. Should it occur, another proprietary emollient which does not contain SLS or emulsifying wax BP can be substituted, e.g. Diprobase® cream.[14]

Emollients should be applied as frequently as needed to keep the skin well hydrated. This is generally twice daily. Very dry skin may require more frequent applications. Enough emollient should be applied to make the skin glisten.[12] However, if the emollient is applied too thickly, it may make the patient uncomfortable, hot or itchy, and may stain clothing.

The emollient should be applied immediately after a bath or shower when the skin is most hydrated. The patient should shake off excess water or lightly dab dry with a soft towel, and then apply the emollient to the damp skin. Emollients are essential for maintaining skin condition and should continue to be used at least once daily even when the dryness has improved/resolved.

It is helpful to demonstrate the use of the recommended emollient (or one of comparable consistency) to the patient and the family or carers. This is particularly useful in patients with unsightly skin who may feel ostracized, and for whom physical contact (touch) generally provides real psychological benefit.

In practice, the best emollient is the one which a patient is happy to use. This implies that it is both cosmetically acceptable and effective, and preferably should not be expensive. For example, many patients like the silky feel of **colloidal oatmeal** (e.g. Aveeno®), particularly on their hands and face. Average quantities required for b.d. application for 1 week are shown in Table 3.

Table 3 Quantities required for b.d. application for 1 week

	Creams and ointments (g)	Lotions (mL)
Face	15–30	100
Groins and genitalia	15–25	100
Both hands	25–50	200
Scalp	50–100	200
Both arms or both legs	100–200	200
Trunk	400	500

A light cream (e.g. **aqueous cream BP**, Cetraben®, Diprobase®) or emollient lotion b.d. generally suffices with mild–moderate degrees of dryness (Table 4). For severe dryness an ointment will be needed (e.g. Hydromol®, Epaderm®).

Soap should not be used because of its drying effect on the skin. It contributes to the breakdown of the skin barrier by raising the pH; this enhances protease activity, inhibits lipid synthesis, and promotes bacterial colonization. Use instead a soap substitute (e.g. **aqueous cream BP, emulsifying ointment BP**, Cetraben® cream, Dermol® cream or lotion) or a proprietary soap-free cleanser (e.g. E45® Emollient Wash Cream or Oilatum® Shower Gel).

An emollient bath additive, such as Dermalo® or E45® Emollient Bath Oil, can also be used when bathing. It is advisable to use a bath mat to prevent slipping when using such products in the bath or shower.

When there is an active inflammatory skin condition causing redness and eroded or scaly skin, apply a topical corticosteroid b.d. to the affected area for 3–7 days or until the inflammation settles. In practice, topical corticosteroids are prescribed mostly for dermatoses of the face and hands. Current best practice is to apply the corticosteroid 30–60min before or after the emollient has been applied.

For the trunk, hands, feet or limbs, choose a moderately potent topical corticosteroid, e.g. **clobetasone butyrate** 0.05% or **betamethasone valerate** 0.025% ointment. Mild topical corticosteroids, e.g. **hydrocortisone** 1%, are generally used for the face.

If the inflamed skin is deeply cracked and secondary infection is suspected, a topical corticosteroid + a topical antifungal and/or antibacterial should be prescribed; various combination products are available. To minimize the risk of developing resistance, products containing antimicrobials must not be used p.r.n. but as a full course for 7 days.

If emollient-related contact dermatitis is suspected, patch testing with the standard set of potential allergens may identify an allergen. If allergy is confirmed, a product which does not contain the allergen (and, ideally, any other added preservatives or fragrances) should be prescribed. However, not all contact dermatitis is allergic; sometimes it is caused by direct chemical irritation.

Lymphoedema

Skin care is just one component of multimodal lymphoedema management.[15,16] The following advice must be applied within the broader management context.

The choice depends on the state of the skin but also on current fashion and local contracts:[17]
- if not obviously dry and flaky, a light cream, can be applied once daily–b.d. as a prophylactic measure, e.g. **aqueous cream BP** or an alternative (see Table 4)
- if the skin is dry ± cracked, apply **liquid and white soft paraffin ointment NPF (liquid paraffin in white soft paraffin** 50/50)
- if there is a build-up of scales wash the affected area with a light cream (see Table 4) using a circular motion in order to soften and lift off the scales; then apply **liquid and white soft paraffin ointment NPF**, and cover with a hydrocolloid dressing (e.g. Granuflex®) and bandage; repeat every 1–3 days until the skin condition is good
- if there are toe web fissures, take scrapings to look for fungus and, if present, treat appropriately, e.g. **clotrimazole** 1% or **terbinafine** 1% cream b.d. for 2 weeks.

Note:
- ointments are generally needed for only 1–2 weeks
- some people prefer coconut oil because it has a skin-cooling effect.

Table 4 Emollient and additive content of selected topical products[a]

	Wool fat derivatives e.g. lanolin	Soft paraffin (petrolatum) or liquid paraffin (mineral oil)	Sensitizing preservative	Fragrance
Ointments				
Emulsifying ointment BP	−	+	−	−
White soft paraffin BP	−	+	−	−
Liquid paraffin and white soft paraffin ointment NPF	−	+	−	−
Epaderm®	−	+	−	−
Hydromol®	−	+	−	−
Oils				
Coconut oil BP	−	−	−	−
Water-in-oil (rich) creams				
Hydrous ointment BP	+	+	−	−
Aquadrate®	−	+	−	−
Lipobase®	−	+	+	−
Unguentum M®	−	+	−	−
Oil-in-water (light) creams				
Aqueous cream BP	−	+	−	−
Aveeno®	−	+	+	−
Cetraben®	−	+	+	−
Dermol®	−	+	−	−
Diprobase®	−	+	+	−
E45®	+[b]	+	+	−
E45® Itch relief	−	+	+	−
Hydromol®	−	+	+	−
Ultrabase®	−	+	+	+
Zerobase®	−	+	+	−
Lotions				
Aveeno®	−	+	+	−
Dermol®	−	+	−	−
E45®	+[b]	+	+	−

a. products which do not contain wool fat derivatives or liquid/soft paraffin generally contain plant-based oils or fatty acid derivatives
b. hypo-allergenic lanolin.

Antipruritic emollients

If pruritus is caused by dry skin, rehydration of the skin will correct it. Thus, all emollients are antipruritic in this sense. However, some products have a specific antipruritic agent added, and can provide extra benefit in some patients (see p.618).

Supply

This is not a complete list; see BNF for additional options.

> **Pharmaco-economics**
> Before prescribing a relatively expensive proprietary product, check to see whether, content for content, there is a cheaper essentially equivalent product.

Emollients

Aqueous cream BP (generic)
Cream (oil-in-water) containing **emulsifying ointment BP** 30%, phenoxyethanol 1% in water, 100g = £1, 500g = £5.

Cetraben® (Genus)
Cream containing **white soft paraffin** 13.2%, **light liquid paraffin** 10.5%, 50g pump-dispenser pack = £1.50, 150g pump-dispenser pack = £4, 500g pump-dispenser pack = £6, 1kg pump-dispenser pack = £12.

Colloidal oatmeal
Aveeno® (J&J)
Cream 100mL = £4, 300mL pump-dispenser pack £7.
Lotion 500mL = £7.
Bath oil 250mL = £4.50.
All classified in the UK as borderline substances; prescriptions must be endorsed ACBS.

Dermol® (Dermal)
Cream containing **benzalkonium chloride** 0.1%, **chlorhexidine hydrochloride** 0.1%, **liquid paraffin** 10%, **isopropyl myristate** 10%, 100g = £3, 500g pump-dispenser pack = £7.
Lotion Dermol® 500, containing **benzalkonium chloride** 0.1%, **chlorhexidine hydrochloride** 0.1%, **liquid paraffin** 2.5%, **isopropyl myristate** 2.5%, 500mL pump-dispenser pack = £6.

Diprobase® (MSD)
Cream (oil-in-water) containing **liquid paraffin** 6%, **white soft paraffin** 15%, **cetostearyl alcohol** 7.2%, cetomacrogol 2.25%, 50g = £1.50, 500g pump-dispenser pack = £7.

E45® (Reckitt-Benckiser)
Cream (oil-in-water) containing **liquid paraffin** 12.6%, **white soft paraffin** 14.5%, **hypoallergenic lanolin** 1%, 50g = £1.50, 500g pump-dispenser pack = £6.
Lotion containing **light liquid paraffin** 4%, **white soft paraffin** 10%, **hypoallergenic lanolin** 1%, 200mL = £2.50, 500mL pump-dispenser pack = £4.50; *classified in the UK as a borderline substance; prescriptions must be endorsed ACBS.*

Epaderm® (Mölnlycke)
Cream containing **yellow soft paraffin** 15%, **liquid paraffin** 10%, **emulsifying wax** 5%, 50g pump-dispenser pack = £1.50, 500g pump-dispenser pack = £7.
Ointment containing **emulsifying wax** 30%, **yellow soft paraffin** 30%, **liquid paraffin** 40%, 125g = £4, 500g = £7, 1kg = £12.

Hydromol® (Alliance)
Cream containing **sodium pidolate** 2.5%, **liquid paraffin** 13.8%, 50g = £2, 100g = £4, 500g = £12.
Ointment containing **yellow soft paraffin** 30%, **emulsifying wax** 30%, **liquid paraffin** 40%, 125g = £3, 500g = £5, 1kg = £9.

Hydrous ointment BP (generic)
Cream (water-in-oil) containing dried **magnesium sulphate** 0.5%, **wool alcohols ointment** 50%, phenoxyethanol 1% in water, 500g = £5.

Liquid paraffin and white soft paraffin ointment NPF (generic)
Ointment containing **liquid paraffin** 50%, **white soft paraffin** 50%, 500g = £2.50.

Petroleum jelly (generic)
Ointment containing **white** or **yellow soft paraffin BP**, 100g = £0.50.

Unguentum M® (Almirall)
Cream (water-in-oil) containing **saturated neutral oil, liquid paraffin, white soft paraffin**, 100g = £3, 500g = £8.

With humectants
Aquadrate® (Alliance)
Cream (water-in-oil) containing **urea** 10%, 100g = £4.50.

E45 Itch Relief® (Crookes)
Cream (oil-in-water) containing **urea** 5%, **macrogol lauryl ether** 3%, 100g = £3.50, 500g pump-dispenser pack = £15.

Non-soap cleansers
Aqueous cream BP (generic)
See above, under emollients.

Emulsifying ointment BP (generic)
Ointment containing **emulsifying wax** 30%, **white soft paraffin** 50%, **liquid paraffin** 20%, 500g = £2.

E45® Emollient Wash Cream (Reckitt-Benckiser)
Wash cream containing **soap substitute, zinc oxide** 5% in emollient base, 250mL pump-dispenser pack = £3; *classified in the UK as a borderline substance; prescriptions must be endorsed ACBS.*

Oilatum®Shower Gel (Stiefel)
Shower gel containing **light liquid paraffin** 70%, 150g = £5.

Bath oils
Dermalo® (Dermal)
Bath oil containing **liquid paraffin** 65%, **acetylated wool alcohols** 5%, 500mL = £3.50.

E45 Emollient Bath Oil® (Crookes)
Bath oil containing **liquid paraffin** 91%, **cetyl dimeticone** 5%, 500mL = £5; *classified in the UK as a borderline substance; prescriptions must be endorsed ACBS.*

Mild topical corticosteroid
Hydrocortisone (generic)
Cream 1%, 30g = £2.50.

Mildison® (Astellas)
Cream 1%, 30g = £2.

Moderately potent topical corticosteroids
Betamethasone valerate
Betnovate-RD® (GSK)
Cream 0.025%, 100g = £3.50; *this is 1/4 of the strength of Betnovate® cream.*
Ointment 0.025%, 100g = £3.50; *this is 1/4 of the strength of Betnovate® ointment.*

Clobetasone butyrate
Eumovate® (GSK)
Cream 0.05%, 30g = £2, 100g = £6.
Ointment 0.05%, 30g = £2, 100g = £6.

Antifungal creams
Clotrimazole (generic)
Cream 1%, 20g = £1.50.

Terbinafine (generic)
Cream 1%, 15g = £2; 30g = £4.

For more antifungal products, see p.622 and the *BNF*.

1 Cork MJ and Danby S (2009) Skin barrier breakdown: a renaissance in emollient therapy. *British Journal of Nursing*. **18**: 872, 874, 876–877.
2 Kraft JN and Lynde CW (2005) Moisturizers: what they are and a practical approach to product selection. *Skin Therapy Letter*. **10**: 1–8.
3 Sibbald D (2002) Dermatitis. In: C Repchinsky (ed) *Patient Self-care (2e)*. Canadian Pharmacists Association, Ottawa, pp. 479–505.
4 Fluhr JW et al. (2008) Emollients, moisturizers, and keratolytic agents in psoriasis. *Clinics in Dermatology*. **26**: 380–386.
5 Hoppe U (ed) (1999) The Lanolin Book. Beierdorf AG, Hamburg.
6 Voegeli D (2008) Care or harm: exploring essential components in skin care regimens. *British Journal of Nursing*. **17**: 24–30.
7 Rubel DM et al. (1998) Tea tree oil allergy: what is the offending agent? Report of three cases of tea tree oil allergy and review of the literature. *Australasian Journal of Dermatology*. **39**: 244–247.
8 MHRA (2003) Medicines containing peanut (arachis) oil. *Current Problems in Pharmacovigilance*. **29**: 5.
9 Hourihane JO et al. (1997) Randomised, double blind, crossover challenge study of allergenicity of peanut oils in subjects allergic to peanuts. *British Medical Journal*. **314**: 1084–1088.
10 Keating MU et al. (1990) Immunoassay of peanut allergens in food-processing materials and finished foods. *Journal of Allergy and Clinical Immunology*. **86**: 41–44.
11 British National Formulary Section 13.2.1 Emollients. London: BMJ Group and Pharmaceutical Press www.bnf.org (accessed May 2014).
12 Lawton S (2009) Practical issues for emollient therapy in dry and itchy skin. *British Journal of Nursing*. **18**: 978–984.
13 Cork MJ et al. (2003) An audit of adverse drug reactions to aqueous cream in children with atopic eczema. *The Pharmaceutical Journal*. **271**: 747–748.
14 MHRA (2013) Aqueous cream: may cause skin irritation, particularly in children with eczema, possibly due to sodium lauryl sulphate content. *Drug Safety Update*: **6**. www.mhra.gov.uk/safetyinformation
15 Twycross R et al. (2009) *Symptom Management in Advanced Cancer* (4e). palliativedrugs.com, Nottingham, pp. 108–111.
16 Twycross R et al. (2000) *Lymphoedema*. Radcliffe Medical Press, Oxford.
17 Linnitt N (2000) Skin management in lymphoedema. In: RG Twycross et al. (eds) *Lymphoedema*. Radcliffe Medical Press, Oxford, pp. 118–129.

Updated June 2014

TOPICAL ANTIPRURITICS   BNF 13.2.1 & 13.3

Indications: Pruritus which fails to respond to an emollient and/or specific treatment.

Background

Pruritus may be caused by systemic disease (such as drug hypersensitivity, obstructive jaundice, endocrine disease, malignant disease), skin disease (e.g. eczema, urticaria, psoriasis, scabies) or drugs (e.g. opioids).

Dryness of the skin (xerosis) is the commonest cause of pruritus without an accompanying rash, and an emollient is the first-line treatment, p.611. Dryness is associated with normal ageing, inflammatory skin conditions (e.g. atopic dermatitis), systemic disease (e.g. hypothyroidism, renal failure), and cachexia and general debility in advanced cancer.

Whenever possible, the treatment of pruritus should be cause-specific.[1,2] For example, in skin disorders:

- scabies → treat patient and the whole family with topical **permethrin** (preferred) or **malathion**[3,4]
- atopic dermatitis → topical corticosteroid (+ emollient)[5]
- contact dermatitis → topical corticosteroid, identify causal substance and avoid further contact.

In systemic disorders or when caused by opioids, a range of options exist (see Chapter 28, p.793). A topical antipruritic should be considered only if a bland emollient and cause-specific treatment fail to relieve.

Although topical products are not convenient to apply regularly to the whole body, many patients with generalized pruritus have patches of more intense discomfort, and may benefit from more limited application.

Pharmacology

Traditional topical antipruritics include **phenol**, **levomenthol (menthol)** and **camphor** (see Chapter 28, p.797). **Phenol** 0.5–3% acts by anaesthetizing cutaneous nerve endings.

618   www.palliativedrugs.com

Levomenthol 0.5–2% and **camphor** 0.5–3% may relieve pruritus by cooling the skin by acting on heat- sensitive transient receptor potential (TRP) channels expressed on sensory nerve endings.[6,7] Cooling the skin is known to reduce the intensity of histamine-induced pruritus, and patients who suffer from chronic pruritic conditions such as atopic dermatitis, psoriasis and uraemic pruritus often find that cold showers reduce the pruritus. Authorized products containing these substances are available OTC. **Levomenthol** can be prescribed as **levomenthol cream BP**, or in countries where a commercial product is unavailable, **levomenthol** 1% can be added to an emollient, e.g. **aqueous cream BP**.[8]

Capsaicin is a naturally occurring alkaloid found in the fruits of various species of *Solanaceae* (the nightshade family) and in pepper plants of the genus *Capsicum* (chilli peppers).[9] It acts by depleting substance P at sensory nerve endings. **Capsaicin** products are useful in relieving neuropathic pain (see p.584). Benefit has also been reported in histamine-related pruritus, aquagenic pruritus, and pruritus associated with uraemia, nodular prurigo, psoriasis and post-axillary dissection syndrome.[6]

A Cochrane review of pruritus in adult palliative care patients also found benefit in uraemic pruritus, but the methodological quality of the studies was low, introducing a risk of bias and thus preventing meaningful interpretation of the results.[10] **Capsaicin** has also been used successfully in the treatment of intractable pruritus ani.[11]

In practice, **capsaicin** will be applied to relatively limited areas of the skin. It often initially causes localized burning and stinging. This irritation subsides with repeated use but patients may have difficulty continuing treatment. Patients should initially use **capsaicin** cream t.d.s.–q.d.s. (leaving at least 4h between applications; the manufacturers specify q.d.s. for the 0.025% cream) to overcome the irritation, after which the frequency of applications can be reduced. The topical anaesthetic **EMLA (eutectic mixture of local anaesthetics, lidocaine** 2.5% and **prilocaine** 2.5%), used in conjunction with **capsaicin**, may reduce the initial irritation.[12] Excessive use of **EMLA** may result in acute transient systemic local anaesthetic neurotoxicity.[13]

Polidocanol (macrogol lauryl ether) is an anionic detergent with local anaesthetic properties.[14] Benefit has been reported in patients with pruritus associated with atopic dermatitis, non-atopic dermatitis and psoriasis, with the regular application of a cream containing 5% **urea** and 3% **polidocanol** (E45® Itch Relief Cream).[15,16] Benefit has also been reported in patients with pruritus associated with chronic renal failure who regularly used a **polidocanol**-containing bath oil (Balneum Plus®).[17]

Crotamiton 10% lotion (Eurax®) has a mild antiscabetic effect which is probably the reason for its reputation as an antipruritic. However, in an RCT in patients with chronic pruritic dermatoses, **crotamiton** lotion was no more effective than its vehicle.[18]

Topical H_1 antihistamines, e.g. **diphenhydramine**, are of benefit only when the pruritus is cutaneous in origin and related to histamine release.[1] Topical **diphenhydramine** can cause contact dermatitis and photosensitivity; if used, limit to 3 days. Oral sedating H_1 antihistamines, e.g. **alimemazine, chlorphenamine, hydroxyzine** may be helpful if sedation is desirable in intractable pruritus, e.g. if itch is disturbing sleep (see Chapter 28, p.793).

A **coal tar**-based shampoo, e.g. Polytar®, has a long tradition of use with scalp pruritus. *Note: at the time of going to press, there was a long-term supply issue with Polytar® in the UK. It has not officially been discontinued, but is unlikely to be available again until 2016.*

Doxepin

Doxepin is a TCA which is a potent H_1- and H_2-receptor antagonist. Its affinity for H_2-receptors is 6 times that of **cimetidine**.[19] It is also antimuscarinic, and may antagonize the pruritic effects of substance P at skin receptors. **Amitriptyline** is similar in potency to **doxepin** as an H_1 antihistamine, but other TCAs are much less so.[20] Patients with chronic urticaria who do not respond to conventional H_1 antihistamines may well benefit from **doxepin** 10–75mg PO at bedtime.[21] Oral **doxepin** 10mg b.d. has also been found effective in patients with uraemic pruritus.[22]

Doxepin 5% cream is reported to be of benefit in some patients with atopic dermatitis[19,23,24] but long-term independent studies are lacking.[25] It is not generally suitable for children. It is possible that the benefit is systemic rather than topical. About 15% of patients complain initially of localized stinging or burning, and a similar proportion complain of drowsiness, secondary to systemic absorption.[23] The sedation may help the antipruritic effect.

Doxepin cream is less effective than systemic treatment[26] and, depending on the products prescribed, can be more expensive than **doxepin** capsules plus an emollient. Allergic contact dermatitis may occur.[23] Patients with contact allergy should not take the drug by mouth.[27]

Cautions

Because of:
- the risk of contact dermatitis, *discourage* the use of topical H_1 antihistamines and of local anaesthetics
- their drying effect, *discourage* the use of products containing **calamine** unless they contain oil (e.g. **calamine oily lotion BP**).

Calamine oily lotion BP contains *refined* **arachis** (peanut) **oil**, and official advice states that emollients containing **arachis** (peanut) **oil** should not be used by patients with peanut or soya allergy.[28,29] However, unlike *crude* **arachis oil**, the *refined* oil is not allergenic, and is highly unlikely to cause allergic reactions in people with (whole) peanut allergy.[30,31]

Polytar® products also contain traces of **arachis** (peanut) **oil** from the **coal tar** extraction process, and thus might cause allergic reactions in people with peanut or soya allergy.

Patients prescribed **doxepin**, either systemically or topically, should avoid the concurrent use of drugs which inhibit cytochrome P450, e.g. **cimetidine**, imidazole antifungals and macrolide antibacterials (see Chapter 25, p.767). As with other TCAs, MAOIs should be discontinued $\geqslant 2$ weeks before starting treatment with **doxepin**. Monitor carefully in patients with glaucoma, severe heart disease, cardiac arrhythmias, urinary hesitancy, severe liver disease or a history of mania. Because of the possibility of undesirable systemic effects, e.g. dizziness, antimuscarinic effects, headache, GI disturbances, avoid applying the cream to large areas of skin. The manufacturer recommends a maximum of 3g per application, covering no more than 10% of the body area.

Use

Because pruritus is commonly associated with dry skin, an emollient (moisturizer) should be tried first (see p.611). A light cream (oil-in-water), e.g. Cetraben®, Diprobase®, or an emollient lotion often suffices with mild–moderate degrees of dryness. **Aqueous cream BP** is an option but at many centres is used only as a soap substitute. Products containing **colloidal oatmeal** (Aveeno®) are popular because of their silky feel (see p.616). Storing creams and lotions in a refrigerator may increase benefit.

Levomenthol 0.5%–2% (or **camphor** 0.5–3%) in a bland emollient base can be applied topically t.d.s.–q.d.s. Proprietary products include **levomenthol** 0.5–5% in **aqueous cream** (Dermacool®).

Calamine lotion BP contains **phenol** 0.5%, and can be strengthened by adding a further 0.5%. Although the vehicle is drying, it can be formulated as an oily lotion. **Phenolated calamine lotion USP** contains **phenol** 1%. However, because it is unsightly, **calamine** is unlikely to be acceptable except on a short-term basis, e.g. in acute contact dermatitis.

Supply

Several products available OTC contain **levomenthol** and **camphor** (with contents as high as 11%). These are marketed for rheumatic aches and pains, sprains or minor sports injuries, e.g. Tiger Balm Red®. Others are mainly intended for use on insect bites and the unit size is small.

Levomenthol
Levomenthol cream BP
Cream 0.5%, 1%, 2% in **aqueous cream BP**, 50g (2% only) = £1.50, 100g (1% and 2% only) = £3.50, 500g (all strengths) = £15.

Dermacool® (Pern Consumer Products)
Cream 0.5%, 1%, 2%, 5% in **aqueous cream BP**, 100g tube, 500g pump pack, available OTC.

Deep Freeze® (Mentholatum)
Gel 2% (Cold Gel®), 100g, available OTC.
Spray 2% (Cold Spray®), 150mL spray can, available OTC.
Deep Freeze® is marketed for minor sports injuries.

With camphor
LitoZin® (Lanes Health)
Muscle rub cream containing **levomenthol** 4%, **camphor** 2%, **eucalyptus oil** 2%, **methyl salicylate** 9%, **turpentine oil** 7%, 28g, available OTC.

Radian B® (Thornton & Ross)
Muscle lotion containing **levomenthol** 1.4%, **camphor** 0.6%, **ammonium salicylate** 1%, **salicylic acid** (as methyl and ethyl esters) 0.54%, 250mL, available OTC.
Muscle rub cream containing **levomenthol** 2.54%, **camphor** 1.43%, **methyl salicylate** 0.42%, **capsicum oleoresin** 0.005%, 100g, available OTC.

Phenol
Chymol Emollient Balm® (Almus)
Ointment containing **phenol** 2.4%, **eucalyptus oil** 1.2%, **methylsalicylate** 0.8% and **terpineol** 4%, 40g, available OTC but supply currently uncertain.

Polidocanol (macrogol lauryl ether)
Balneum Plus® (Almirall)
Bath oil containing **soya oil** 83%, mixed **lauromacrogols** 15%, 500mL = £7.

E45 Itch Relief® (Crookes)
Cream (oil-in-water) containing **urea** 5%, **macrogol lauryl ether** 3%, 100g = £3.50; 500g pump-pack = £15.

Doxepin
Sinepin® (Marlborough)
Capsules 25mg, 50mg, 28 days @ 25mg, 50mg, 75mg at bedtime = £4, £6 and £9 respectively.

Xepin® (CHS)
Cream 5%, 30g = £12.

Oral sedating H_1 antihistamines include **alimemazine, chlorphenamine** and **hydroxyzine**; non-sedating ones include **cetirizine** and **loratadine**; see *BNF* for details and other options.

1 Zylicz Z et al. (eds) (2004) Pruritus in Advanced Disease. Oxford University Press, Oxford.
2 Twycross R et al. (2009) Symptom Management in Advanced Cancer (4e). palliativedrugs.com, Nottingham, pp. 321–329.
3 British National Forumulary Section 13.10.4. Parasiticidal preparations. London: BMJ Group and Pharmaceutical Press www.bnf.org (accessed March 2014).
4 Strong M and Johnstone P (2007) Interventions for treating scabies. Cochrane Database of Systematic Reviews. 3: CD000320.
5 Cork MJ (1999) Taking the itch out of eczema: how careful use of emollients can break the itch-scratch cycle of atopic eczema. Asthma Journal. 4: 16–20.
6 Patel T et al. (2007) Menthol: a refreshing look at this ancient compound. Journal of the American Academy of Dermatology. 57: 873–878.
7 Peier AM et al. (2002) A TRP channel that senses cold stimuli and menthol. Cell. 108: 705–715.
8 Anonymous (2005) Pharmacy information pointers. The preparation of menthol (1 per cent w/w) in aqueous cream BP. Pharmaceutical Journal. 274: 469.
9 Towlerton GR and Rice AS (2003) Topical analgesics for chronic pain. In: AS Rice et al. (eds) Clinical Pain Management: Chronic Pain. Arnold, London, pp. 213–226.
10 Xander C et al. (2013) Pharmacological interventions for pruritus in adult palliative care patients. Cochrane Database of Systematic Reviews. 6: CD008320.
11 Lysy J et al. (2003) Topical capsaicin–a novel and effective treatment for idiopathic intractable pruritus ani: a randomised, placebo controlled, crossover study. Gut. 52: 1323–1326.
12 Yosipovitch G and Hundley JL (2004) Practical guidelines for relief of itch. Dermatology Nursing. 16: 325–328; quiz 329.
13 Brosh-Nissimov T et al. (2004) Central nervous system toxicity following topical skin application of lidocaine. European Journal of Clinical Pharmacology. 60: 683–684.
14 Vieluf D et al. (1992) Dry and itching skin - therapy with a new preparation, containing urea and polidocanol. Zeitschrift fur Hautkrankheiten. 67: 816–821.
15 Hauss H et al. (1993) Comparative study of a formulation containing urea and polidocanol and a greasy cream containing linoleic acid in the treatment of dry, pruritic skin lesions [in German]. Dermatosen in Beruf und Umwelt Occupational and Environmental Dermatoses. 41: 184–188.
16 Freitag G and Hoppner T (1997) Results of a postmarketing drug monitoring survey with a polidocanol-urea preparation for dry, itching skin. Current Medical Research and Opinion. 13: 529–537.
17 Wasik F et al. (1996) Relief of uraemic pruritus after balneological therapy with a bath oil containing polidocanol (Balneum Hermal Plus). An open clinical study. Journal of Dermatological Treatment. 7: 231–233.
18 Smith E et al. (1984) Crotamiton lotion in pruritus. International Journal of Dermatology. 23: 684–685.
19 Drake L et al. (1994) Relief of pruritus in patients with atopic dermatitis after treatment with topical doxepin cream. The Doxepin Study Group. Journal of the American Academy of Dermatology. 31: 613–616.

20 Figge J et al. (1979) Tricyclic antidepressants: potent blockade of histamine H$_1$ receptors of guinea pig ileum. European Journal of Pharmacology. **58**: 479–483.

21 Figueiredo A et al. (1990) Mechanism of action of doxepin in the treatment of chronic urticaria. Fundamental and Clinical Pharmacology. **4**: 147–158.

22 Pour-Reza-Gholi F et al. (2007) Low-dose doxepin for treatment of pruritus in patients on hemodialysis. Iranian Journal of Kidney Diseases. **1**: 34–37.

23 DTB (2000) Doxepin cream for eczema? Drug and Therapeutics Bulletin. **38**: 31.

24 Breneman D et al. (1997) Doxepin cream relieves eczema-associated pruritus within 15 minutes and is not accompanied by a risk of rebound upon discontinuation. Journal of Dermatological Treatment. **8**: 161–168.

25 Hoare C et al. (2000) Systematic review of treatments for atopic eczema. Health Technology Assessment. **4**: 1–191.

26 Smith P and Corelli R (1997) Doxepin in the management of pruritus associated with allergic cutaneous reactions. Annals of Pharmacotherapy. **31**: 633–635.

27 Bonnel RA et al. (2003) Allergic contact dermatitis from topical doxepin: Food and Drug Administration's postmarketing surveillance experience. Journal of the American Academy of Dermatology. **48**: 294–296.

28 MHRA (2003) Medicines containing peanut (arachis) oil. Current Problems in Pharmacovigilance. **29**. 5.

29 Anonymous (2003) Peanut allergy research is published. Pharmaceutical Journal. **270**: 391.

30 Keating MU et al. (1990) Immunoassay of peanut allergens in food-processing materials and finished foods. Journal of Allergy and Clinical Immunology. **86**: 41–44.

31 Hourihane JO et al. (1997) Randomised, double blind, crossover challenge study of allergenicity of peanut oils in subjects allergic to peanuts. British Medical Journal. **314**: 1084–1088.

Updated June 2014

BARRIER PRODUCTS   BNF 13.2.2

Indications: Skin protection, napkin rash.

Introduction

Barrier products contain water-repellent substances which help to protect the skin, and prevent maceration and infection. They can be used around stomas and in the perineal and peri-anal areas in patients with urinary or faecal incontinence. Most barrier creams and ointments are silicone-, titanium- or **zinc oxide**-based.[1]

   Zinc and castor oil ointment BP and Siopel® contain refined **arachis** (peanut) **oil**. However, unlike crude **arachis oil**, the refined oil is not allergenic, and thus is highly unlikely to cause allergic reactions in people with (whole) peanut allergy.[2,3]

   A cream is less greasy than an ointment and is easier to apply and wash off, e.g. Drapolene® (**benzalkonium chloride** 0.01% and **cetrimide** 0.2% in **white soft paraffin, cetyl alcohol** and **wool fat**) and Sudocrem® (**zinc oxide** 15%, hypoallergenic **lanolin** 4%). Some products include **dimeticone**, e.g. Conotrane®, or other water-repellent silicone.

   If a dressing is needed because of skin damage, a barrier product such as Cavilon No-Sting Barrier Film® will coat the skin with a film for ≤ 72h, and will prevent the dressing from adhering to the skin.

Cautions

If the damaged skin is infected, because barrier products prevent topical antimicrobials from penetrating the skin, delay their use until the infection has been treated.

Use

Ensure that infection is treated promptly with topical antifungals (more common) and/or antibacterials (less common).

Intertrigo

Intertrigo is an inflammatory dermatosis of skin folds primarily caused by skin on skin friction. Exacerbating factors cause skin maceration and inflammation, e.g. obesity, lack of air, heat and moisture. Secondary fungal or bacterial infection is common. The wet component is the most easily modified, and drying the involved skin is essential. Initial treatment may comprise:

- cleanse with a soap substitute (e.g. **aqueous cream BP, emulsifying ointment BP**, Cetraben® cream, Dermol® cream or lotion) or a proprietary soap-free cleanser (e.g. Dermol® Shower Emollient or Wash Emulsion, E45® Emollient Wash Cream or Oilatum® Shower Gel; see p.611)
- dry well; blow-drying with a hand-held hair dryer is generally effective
- if infection is likely and because fungal infection is more common, a topical broad-spectrum antifungal should be prescribed, e.g. **clotrimazole**

- if inflammation is present, a mild topical corticosteroid for 3–7 days often accelerates improvement, e.g. **hydrocortisone** 1% cream or ointment (see p.616); combination products containing both an antifungal and **hydrocortisone** 1% are available
- an absorbent powder, e.g. ZeaSORB® (**aldioxa** and **chloroxylenol**) may be helpful
- when the wetness and infection has settled, then begin to use a barrier product.

Protection around a stoma

Many products designed to protect the skin around a stoma from liquid effluent are available; a stoma-care nurse can advise on product selection. Sprays or wipes which dry to form a protective film are commonly used. An alcohol-free formulation is preferable because it is less likely to sting or irritate the skin.

Stoma therapists frequently use Comfeel® barrier cream prophylactically if the stoma effluent is liquid or if the stoma bag is being changed more than once daily. It is gently rubbed in and any excess wiped off. If the skin becomes red and sore, Cavilon No-Sting Barrier Film® is used instead.

A topical corticosteroid can be used short-term to treat moderate-severe inflammation. Foam products are well tolerated, e.g. Bettamousse® (off-label use; marketing authorization is for use as a scalp application).

Incontinence

After cleansing with a soap substitute and gently drying, apply a barrier product to the affected area whenever the dressing or padding is changed.[1]

Supply

The following is only a selection of the available products.

Ointments
Zinc and castor oil ointment BP (generic)
Ointment containing **zinc oxide** 7.5% in a **castor oil, arachis** (peanut) **oil, white beeswax** and **cetostearyl alcohol** base, 500g = £6.

Creams
Conotrane® (Astellas)
Cream containing **dimeticone 350** 22% and **benzalkonium chloride** 0.1%, 100g = £1, 500g = £3.50.

Drapolene® (Omega Pharma)
Cream containing **benzalkonium chloride** 0.01% and **cetrimide** 0.2% in a **white soft paraffin, cetyl alcohol** and **wool fat** base, 100g = £2, 200g = £3, 350g = £4.

Sudocrem® (Forest)
Cream containing **zinc oxide** 15%, hypoallergenic **lanolin** 4%, 125g = £2, 250g = £3.50, 400g = £5.

Stoma products
Comfeel® barrier cream (Coloplast)
Cream 60g = £5.

Cavilon No-Sting Barrier Film® (3M)
Foam applicator 5 × 1mL = £5; 5 × 3mL = £8.
Pump spray 28mL = £7.

Absorbent dusting powder
ZeaSORB® (Stiefel)
Dusting powder containing **aldioxia** 0.22%, **chloroxylenol** 0.5%, 50g = £2.50.

Antifungal products
Clotrimazole (generic)
Cream 1%, 20g = £1.50.

Canesten® (Bayer Consumer Care)
Cream 1%, 20g = £2, 50g = £3.50.
Solution 1%, 20mL = £2.50.
Spray 1%, 40mL = £5; *contains isopropyl alcohol.*

Miconazole (generic)
Cream 2%, 20g = £2, 45g = £2.

Daktarin® (Janssen-Cilag)
Cream 2%, 30g = £2.
Powder spray (Daktarin Aktiv®) 0.16%, 100g = £3.

Topical corticosteroids
For **hydrocortisone** 1%, see p.616.

Bettamousse® (RPH)
Foam (scalp application) containing **betamethasone valerate** 0.12%, 100g = £10.

Combined antifungal and topical corticosteroid products
Canestan HC® (Bayer Consumer Care)
Cream containing **clotrimazole** 1% and **hydrocortisone** 1%, 30g = £2.50.

Daktacort® (Janssen-Cilag)
Cream containing **miconazole** 2% and **hydrocortisone** 1%, 30g = £2.50.

---

1 Nazarko L (2007) Managing a common dermatological problem: incontinence dermatitis. *British Journal of Community Nursing.* 12: 358–363.
2 Keating MU et al. (1990) Immunoassay of peanut allergens in food-processing materials and finished foods. *Journal of Allergy and Clinical Immunology.* 86: 41–44.
3 Hourihane JO et al. (1997) Randomised, double blind, crossover challenge study of allergenicity of peanut oils in subjects allergic to peanuts. *British Medical Journal.* 314: 1084–1088.

Updated April 2014

13: ANAESTHESIA

*KETAMINE

The use of ketamine is associated with neuropsychiatric, urinary tract and hepatobiliary toxicity. Although most reports involve long-term recreational abusers, it has also arisen after only 1–2 weeks of therapeutic use (Box A). Accordingly, the use of ketamine should be restricted to specialist pain and specialist palliative care services in patients who have failed to obtain relief from standard drug and non-drug treatments.

Class: General anaesthetic.

Indications: Induction and maintenance of anaesthesia; †neuropathic, inflammatory, ischaemic limb and procedure-related pain unresponsive to standard treatments.[1,2]

Contra-indications: Any situation in which an increase in blood pressure or intracranial pressure would constitute a hazard.

Pharmacology
Ketamine, a derivative of phencyclidine (PCP), is a dissociative anaesthetic which has analgesic properties in sub-anaesthetic doses.[2,3] Ketamine is the most potent NMDA-receptor-channel blocker available for clinical use, binding to the PCP site when the channels are in the open activated state (Figure 1).[3] It also binds to a second membrane-associated site which decreases the frequency of channel opening.[3]

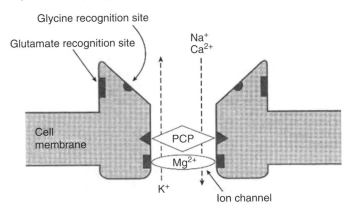

Figure 1 Diagram of the NMDA (excitatory) receptor-channel complex. The channel is blocked by Mg^{2+} when the membrane potential is at its resting level (voltage-dependent block) and by drugs which act at the phencyclidine (PCP) binding site in the glutamate-activated channel, e.g. dextromethorphan, ketamine, methadone (use-dependent block).[4]

The NMDA receptor-channel complex is closely involved in the development of central sensitization of dorsal horn neurons which transmit pain signals.[4] At normal resting membrane potentials, the channel is blocked by magnesium and is inactive.[3] When the resting membrane potential is changed as a result of prolonged excitation, the channel unblocks and calcium moves into the cell. This leads to neuronal hyperexcitability and results in hyperalgesia and allodynia, and a reduction in opioid-responsiveness. These effects are probably mediated by the intracellular formation of nitric oxide and cyclic guanosine monophosphate.[3]

The reduction in opioid-responsiveness arises from cross-talk between opioid receptors and the NMDA receptor-channel. Opioid receptor activation results in phosphorylation and opening of the NMDA receptor-channel leading to a cascade of events which ultimately down-regulates the opioid receptor and its effects, thereby contributing towards tolerance and hyperalgesia.[3]

In addition to blocking the NMDA receptor-channel, ketamine has other actions some of which may contribute to its analgesic effect. These include opioid-like and anti-inflammatory effects,[5] and interactions with:

- other calcium and sodium channels
- dopamine receptors
- cholinergic transmission
- noradrenergic and serotoninergic re-uptake (intact descending inhibitory pathways are necessary for analgesia).[2]

Ketamine is generally administered PO or SC/CSCI.[6,7] It can also be administered IM, IV, SL, intranasally, PR and spinally (preservative-free formulation).[8-15] However, for spinal routes, concerns have been raised about the potential for neurotoxicity.[16] Ketamine has been given by CIVI in adults and children in combination with opioids (**fentanyl, morphine**) ± **midazolam** to control intractable pain and agitation.[17-19]

Although in some countries both racemic ketamine and the S−enantiomer are available for clinical use, in the UK only the racemic mixture is marketed. However, it is possible to import the preservative-free S−entantiomer (see Supply). Because of its greater affinity and selectivity for the NMDA-receptor, the S−enantiomer as a parenteral analgesic is about 4 times more potent than the R−enantiomer, and twice as potent as the racemic mixture.[20-22] When equi-analgesic doses are compared, the S−enantiomer is also associated with lower levels of undesirable effects, e.g. anxiety, tiredness, cognitive impairment.[21,23]

About 90% of a parenteral dose of ketamine is excreted in the urine, mostly as conjugates of hydroxylated metabolites. Less than 5% is excreted unchanged via the faeces and urine. PO ketamine undergoes extensive first-pass hepatic metabolism mainly to norketamine (via CYP3A4), which is also a NMDA-receptor-channel blocker.[24] As an *anaesthetic*, norketamine is about one third as potent as parenteral ketamine. However, as an *analgesic* it is equipotent. The maximum blood concentration of norketamine is greater after PO administration than after an injection,[25] and in chronic use norketamine may be the main analgesic agent. Norketamine is further metabolized to dehydronorketamine.

Ketamine causes hepatic enzyme induction and enhances its own metabolism. The implications of this for the efficacy or tolerability of therapeutic ketamine is unknown. However, in abusers, it may contribute towards the relatively rapid tolerance to the desired 'high', with those taking it most days of the week reporting about a 7-fold increase in dose after the first 2 months of use.[26]

Ketamine causes tachycardia and intracranial hypertension. After anaesthetic use, most patients experience vivid dreams, misperceptions, hallucinations and alterations in body image and mood as emergent (psychotomimetic) phenomena, i.e. as the effects of a bolus dose wear off. These occur to a lesser extent with the sub-anaesthetic analgesic doses given PO or CSCI, and generally can be controlled by concurrent administration of a benzodiazepine (e.g. **diazepam, midazolam**) or **haloperidol**.[12,27,28] Sub-anaesthetic doses of ketamine are associated with impaired attention, memory and judgement, and it is used as a pharmacological model for acute schizophrenia.[3]

Although it is used as an analgesic in various clinical settings (including postoperatively[29,30]), the increasing concern about the potential for neuropsychiatric, urinary tract and hepatobiliary toxicity (Box A) will probably result in a decline in the use of ketamine for chronic non-cancer pain, and possibly cancer pain. In palliative care ketamine should generally be reserved for pain associated with hyperalgesia (and thus less responsive to standard analgesic drugs, including opioids and adjuvants, see p.295).

Chronic non–cancer pain

A review of sub-anaesthetic doses of ketamine for chronic non-cancer pain (mostly neuropathic but also ischaemic, fibromyalgia, post-whiplash, etc.) identified 29 RCTs and concluded that:
• ketamine provides relief
• undesirable effects can limit its use
• long-term use should be restricted to a controlled trial.[31]
A systematic review of analgesics for phantom limb pain reached similar conclusions.[32] There is RCT evidence of benefit in complex regional pain syndrome type 1, with relief persisting beyond the duration of the ketamine infusion.[33,34]

Cancer pain

A systematic review of ketamine as an adjunct to opioids in cancer pain found only two studies of sufficient quality[35,12] and concluded that there is insufficient robust evidence to assess potential benefits and harms.[36] Thus, in patients with cancer, evidence of ketamine's efficacy as an analgesic is mainly from case reports, retrospective surveys or uncontrolled studies in patients with refractory neuropathic, bone, and mucositis-related pain.[6,7,12,35,37–49]

Short-term 'burst' treatment with ketamine may sometimes have a relatively long-lasting effect (i.e. several days to weeks and occasionally for months).[45,47] For example, ketamine 100mg/24h by CIVI for 2 days in a cancer patient, repeated a month later, reduced opioid requirements by 70%.[50] Similarly, in non-cancer pain, patients taking regular strong opioids for ischaemic limb pain, a single 4h IV infusion of ketamine 600microgram/kg reduced opioid requirements during the next week.[51]

However, in a large case series, about a quarter of patients experienced severe undesirable effects from higher-dose 'burst' CSCI ketamine involving rapid dose escalation $100 \rightarrow 300 \rightarrow 500$mg/24h over 3–5 days.[45] Further, in a 5-day RCT in cancer patients using the same regimen, there was no difference in the proportion responding in the ketamine and placebo arms (about 50% in each, based on average pain score).[52] There were fewer treatment failures at the maximum dose (25 vs. 50%) but more undesirable effects and withdrawals due to toxicity (19 vs. 2%).[52] *These results suggest that rapid titration involving such doses of CSCI ketamine is generally inadvisable.*

Miscellaneous

PO/IV ketamine (generally in combination with **morphine** or **midazolam**) can provide analgesia in severe cancer treatment-related mucositis,[53] during painful procedures, e.g. change of dressings,[54–56] and orthopaedic emergencies.[57]

Topical ketamine has been applied to the skin in various non-cancer pains,[58,59] and used as an oral rinse in radiation-induced mucositits.[60]

Ketamine has a rapid antidepressant effect in patients with major depression, including a reduction in suicidal ideation. Following a single IV dose (500microgram/kg over 40min), up to 70% of patients respond, with improvements seen within hours and lasting a median of 18 days (range 4 days–12 weeks or more).[61,62] These effects are accompanied by a more rapid restoration of neuroplasticity than that seen with conventional antidepressants (see p.190). The exact mechanism is unclear but includes the release of brain-derived neurotrophic factor which helps to restore neuroplasticity, e.g. through the formation of new synapses.[61] Although case reports of benefit are emerging from the palliative care setting,[63–67] the use of ketamine to treat major depression is experimental, and should ideally be restricted to RCTs. Other drugs which act on the NMDA receptor-channel complex are undergoing clinical trials in depression.[68]

The use of CIVI ketamine has been explored in the treatment of refractory status epilepticus, but its possible use in clinical practice remains to be determined.[69]

Bio-availability 93% IM; 45% nasal; 30% SL; 30% PR; and 20% PO.[70,71]
Onset of action 5min IM; 15–30min SC; 30min PO.
Time to peak plasma concentration no data SC; 30min PO; 1h norketamine.[72]
Plasma halflife 1–3h IM; 3h PO; 12h norketamine.[73]
Duration of action 30min–2h IM; 4–6h PO, sometimes longer.[74]

Cautions

History of psychiatric disorder; epilepsy, glaucoma, hypertension, heart failure, ischaemic heart disease, CVAs, acute intermittent porphyria.[75] Raised intracranial pressure (e.g. as a result of head injury, intracranial tumour, hydrocephalus). Hyperthyroidism (increased risk of hypertension and tachycardia). Conditions causing excessive upper airway secretions; ketamine both increases salivation and sensitizes the gag reflex, leading on rare occasions to laryngospasm. Severe hepatic impairment (consider dose reduction).

Drug interactions

CYP3A4 inhibitors, e.g. **clarithromycin**, grapefruit juice, increase the plasma concentration of S–ketamine and reduce those of norketamine (not grapefruit juice); the clinical relevance of this is unclear.[76,77]

Plasma concentration of S–ketamine is decreased by potent CYP3A4 inducers, e.g. **rifampicin**, **St John's wort**. With PO S–ketamine, the area under the concentration-time curve is reduced by 60–85%.[78,79] Other potent inducers of CYP3A4 and CYP2B6 may have a similar effect.

Undesirable effects

Ketamine can be abused or diverted; careful monitoring is essential.

Dose-related psychotomimetic phenomena occur in about 40% of patients with CSCI ketamine, less with PO: euphoria, dysphasia, blunted affect, psychomotor retardation, vivid dreams, nightmares, impaired attention, memory and judgement, illusions, hallucinations, altered body image.

Delirium, drowsiness, dizziness, diplopia, blurred vision, nystagmus, altered hearing, hypertension, tachycardia, hypersalivation, nausea and vomiting. At higher anaesthetic doses, tonic-clonic movements are very common (> 10%) but these have not been reported after PO use or with analgesic parenteral doses.

Erythema and pain at injection site. Neuropsychiatric, urinary and hepatobiliary toxicity (Box A).

Box A   Ketamine and neuropsychiatric, urinary and hepatobiliary toxicity

Neuropsychiatric

There are no studies of neuropsychiatric effects in patients receiving therapeutic ketamine. Most participants in the studies below also abused multiple other drugs.

Long-term ketamine abusers have a dose-related increase in subclinical psychotic symptoms, e.g. delusions, dissociation and schizotypy. The relevance is uncertain; no definite link exists between ketamine abuse and psychosis.[80]

In frequent abusers of ketamine (⩾5 days/week), both short- and long-term memory are affected with dose-related impairments in visual recognition memory (tested by remembering patterns) and spatial working memory (tested by remembering which boxes contained hidden tokens).[80,81]

MRI changes were evident with *total estimated lifetime doses* of ⩽3g.[82,83] Functional MRI show dose-related alterations in the anterior cingulate cortex (decrease) and in the left precentral frontal gyrus (increase).[82]

These effects may be the consequence of long-term NMDA-receptor-channel blockade. Dopamine depletion in the prefrontal cortex, a key area involved in working memory, is also reported in those abusing ⩾200mg/week.[84] Ketamine is also directly neurotoxic, with dose-related MRI changes suggestive of disruption or damage to the white matter in the frontal and left temporoparietal regions.[83]

Memory impairments appear to improve with abstinence, but former abusers continue to score higher than controls on delusional symptoms.[80]

Urinary tract

In three patients with chronic pain, urinary symptoms developed after receiving ketamine PO 650–800mg/24h for 5–18 months.[85] In another patient, severe damage necessitated cystectomy after three years of ketamine PO 240mg/24h for chronic back pain.[86] However, urinary symptoms developed after only 9 *days* in a 16 year-old receiving ketamine PO 8mg/kg/24h.[87]

continued

Box A Continued

Urinary symptoms have been reported in abusers of 'street' ketamine, generally taken as powdered ketamine via nasal insufflation. The risk appears related to both dose and frequency of use.[88]

Symptoms include frequency, urgency, urge incontinence, dysuria, haematuria and lower abdominal pain.[88–90] The exact mechanism of the damage is unclear, but ketamine has a direct irritant effect on the upper and lower urinary tract.[91]

Investigations (e.g. cystoscopy and biopsy, CT urogram) may show interstitial cystitis, detrusor overactivity, decreased bladder capacity, vesico-ureteric reflux, hydronephrosis, papillary necrosis, and renal impairment. Irreversible damage leading to renal failure has occurred.

Animal studies have found an increased expression of P2X1 purinergic receptors (activated by ATP) but not muscarinic receptors on bladder smooth muscle, which may explain the reports of limited benefit from antimuscarinic antispasmodics.[92]

Consequently, when patients receiving therapeutic ketamine experience urinary symptoms without evidence of bacterial infection, practitioners should consider stopping the ketamine and seeking the advice of a urologist.

Symptoms generally settle several weeks after stopping ketamine. However, in some abusers, symptoms have persisted despite abstinence.[88,93]

Hepatobiliary
Abnormal LFTs have been associated with both ketamine abuse and therapeutic use, e.g. IV for maintenance anaesthesia (> 10h) or infusions for pain relief (≥4 days).[94–97] In the latter, although abnormal LFTs were sometimes apparent after 4–5 days, in others it occurred only with a second infusion some 2 weeks later.[97]

In abusers, abdominal pain has been reported and, in some, dilation or strictures of the common bile duct.[95,98,99]

The cause is unknown, but possibilities include a direct toxic effect of ketamine or a metabolite, or ketamine-related dysfunction of the sphincter of Oddi.[94,100]

With abstinence, the LFTs, abdominal pain and biliary duct dilation generally improve. Some recommend regular monitoring of LFTs during the long-term therapeutic use of ketamine.[97]

Dose and use

Because ketamine is associated with neuropsychiatric, urinary tract and hepatobiliary toxicity, prescription of ketamine as an analgesic should be restricted to specialists in pain or palliative care for patients who have failed to obtain adequate relief from standard non-drug and drug treatments, including the optimal use of opioids, non-opioids and adjuvant analgesics (see p.295). A toxicity monitoring form is available.[101]

In patients with a prognosis of more than a few weeks, once analgesia has been obtained, an attempt should be made to withdraw ketamine over 2–3 weeks. Benefit from a short course can last for weeks or even months, and can be repeated if necessary.[102] Thus, apart from patients with a prognosis of just days–weeks, long-term continuous ketamine should be used only as a last resort, i.e. in those patients with unsatisfactory analgesia from a short course approach.

Note: whole body hyperalgesia and allodynia may occur if ketamine is abruptly stopped after ≥3 weeks of use.[103]

All doses in this section relate to racemic ketamine.
Dose recommendations vary widely, but ketamine is often started low dose PO (see below). In some centres, an initial test dose is given to assess tolerability and efficacy. The prophylactic concurrent administration of a benzodiazepine or an antipsychotic is also routine in some but not all centres, where it is reserved for more select circumstances (see below). Long-term success, i.e. both pain relief and tolerable undesirable effects, varies from <20% to about 50%.[9,10,42,104]

Some practitioners routinely reduce the background opioid dose by 25–50% when starting parenteral ketamine. If the patient becomes drowsy, the dose of opioid should be reduced. If a patient experiences dysphoria or hallucinations, the dose of ketamine should be reduced and a benzodiazepine prescribed, e.g. **diazepam** 5mg PO stat & at bedtime, **lorazepam** 1mg PO stat & b.d., **midazolam** 5mg SC stat and 5–10mg CSCI, or **haloperidol**, e.g. 2–5mg PO stat & at bedtime, or 2–5mg SC stat and 2–5mg CSCI.[28] In patients at greatest risk of dysphoria (those with high anxiety levels), these measures may be more effective if given before starting ketamine.

When switching from CSCI to PO after just a few days, a conversion ratio of 1:1 should be used.[43,105] However, after weeks–months of use, some have found that a *smaller* total daily dose (25–50% of the parenteral dose) can maintain a similar level of analgesia, e.g. CSCI 400mg/24h → PO 150mg/24h.[41] In both instances, the patient should be monitored closely and the dose titrated accordingly. When switching from PO to CSCI or CIVI, it is advisable to commence on a small dose and titrate as required.

By mouth[6,7,106–108]

An oral solution can be obtained as a special order (see Supply) or prepared by a local pharmacy (Box B). When these options are not available, use direct from a vial or dilute for convenience (immediately before administration) to 50mg/5mL; add a flavouring of the patient's choice, e.g. fruit cordial, to mask the bitter taste.

- start with 10–25mg t.d.s.-q.d.s and p.r.n.
- if necessary, increase dose in steps of 10–25mg up to 100mg q.d.s.
- maximum reported dose 200mg q.d.s.[106,108]
- give a smaller dose more frequently if psychotomimetic phenomena or drowsiness occurs which does not respond to a reduction in opioid.

Box B   Preparation of ketamine oral solution: pharmacy guidelines

Use ketamine 100mg/mL 10mL vials because this is the cheapest concentration. Raspberry Syrup BP can be used for dilution but this is too sweet for some patients. Alternatively, use purified water as the diluent and ask patients to add their own flavouring, e.g. fruit cordial, just before use to disguise the bitter taste.

To prepare 100mL of 50mg/5mL oral solution:
- 10mL vial of ketamine 100mg/mL for injection
- 90mL purified water.

Store in a refrigerator with an expiry date of 1 week from manufacture.

Subcutaneous[7]

- typically 10–25mg p.r.n., some use 2.5–5mg
- if necessary, increase dose in steps of 25–33%.

CSCI[6,27,37,38,40,109]

Because ketamine is irritant, dilute to the largest volume possible, and consider the use of 0.9% saline as the diluent (see p.699). Consider the use of prophylactic **diazepam, lorazepam, midazolam** or **haloperidol** (see text above).

- start with 1–2.5mg/kg/24h
- if necessary, increase by 50–100mg/24h
- continue to titrate until adequate pain relief
- usual maximum 500mg/24h
- maximum reported dose 3.6g/24h.

CSCI compatibility with other drugs: There are 2-drug compatibility data for ketamine in WFI with **metoclopramide, midazolam** and **morphine sulfate**. For more details and 3-drug compatibility charts see Appendix 3, p.821.

There are 2-drug compatibility data for ketamine in 0.9% saline with **alfentanil, clonazepam, dexamethasone** (low-dose), **diamorphine, haloperidol, hydromorphone, levomepromazine, metoclopramide, midazolam, morphine sulfate** and **oxycodone**. For more details and 3-drug compatibility charts see the extended appendix section of the on-line PCF on www.palliativedrugs.com

Intravenous[7,110]
For cancer pain:
- typically 2.5–5mg p.r.n.

To cover procedures which may cause severe pain:
- 500microgram–1mg/kg (typically 25–50mg; some start with 5–10mg), given over 1–2min preceded by, e.g. IV **lorazepam** 1mg or IV **midazolam** 100microgram/kg (typically 5–10mg; some start with 1–2mg) to reduce emergent phenomena
- use a maximum concentration of ketamine 50mg/mL; 0.9% saline or 5% glucose are suitable diluents.

The right dose should provide analgesia within 1–5min lasting for 10–20min.

There is a risk of marked sedation when ketamine and a benzodiazepine are given concurrently. Use only if competent in airway management and the patient can be adequately monitored.
Procedures of longer duration may require ketamine CIVI; obtain advice from an anaesthetist.

CIVI[19,111,112]
Dilute to a concentration of 1mg/mL with 0.9% saline or 5% glucose.
- give a single 'burst' of 600microgram/kg up to a maximum of 60mg over 4h (reduce dose by 1/3–1/2 in elderly/frail patients); monitor blood pressure at baseline and then hourly:
  ▷ if necessary, repeat daily for up to 5 days
  ▷ if no analgesic response to an infusion, increase the dose of the next one by 30%
  ▷ further dose titrate according to response and/or undesirable effects
  ▷ repeat the above if the pain subsequently recurs.[102]

Or
- start with 50–150microgram/kg/h (typically 50–100mg/24h) and titrate as necessary (typical increments 25–50mg/24h)
- in one series of 46 patients with cancer:
  ▷ 20% responded to ≤100mg/24h
  ▷ typical dose 100–300mg/24h
  ▷ no psychotomimetic effects were seen with doses <300mg/24h.

Supply
All products are **CD** (currently Schedule 4 (part 1); under consultation to become Schedule 2 in 2014).

Ketamine (generic)
Oral solution or suspension (sugar-free) 50mg/5mL, 28 days @ 50mg q.d.s. = £215 or £135 respectively (unauthorized, available as a special order see Appendix 1, p.817, *price based on community specials tariff*).

Ketalar® (Pfizer)
Injection 10mg/mL, 20mL vial = £5; 50mg/mL, 10mL vial = £9; 100mg/mL, 10mL vial = £16. *Although use as an analgesic is unauthorized, ketamine injection can be prescribed both in hospitals and in the community. Community pharmacies can order ketamine injection through their usual Alliance Healthcare wholesale account. To initiate an account, contact head office (Tel: 020 8391 2323).*

Ketanest S®
Injection (preservative-free) S–ketamine hydrochloride (esketamine hydrochloride) *equivalent to S–ketamine base 5mg/mL, 10 x 5mL amp = £90; (unauthorized, available to import via IDIS, see Appendix 1, p.817); a doctor's letter with the reason why the preservative-free formulation is needed, GMC number and patients initials is required.*

1 Persson J et al. (1998) The analgesic effect of racemic ketamine in patients with chronic ischemic pain due to lower extremity arteriosclerosis obliterans. *Acta Anaesthesiologica Scandinavica*. **42**: 750–758.
2 Persson J (2013) Ketamine in pain management. *CNS Neuroscience and Therapeutics*. **19**: 396–402.
3 Mion G and Villevieille T (2013) Ketamine pharmacology: an update (pharmacodynamics and molecular aspects, recent findings). *CNS Neuroscience and Therapeutics*. **19**: 370–380.
4 Richens A (1991) The basis of the treatment of epilepsy: neuropharmacology. In: M Dam (ed) *A Practical Approach to Epilepsy*. Pergamon Press, Oxford, pp. 75–85.

5　De Kock M et al. (2013) Ketamine and peripheral inflammation. CNS Neuroscience and Therapeutics. **19**: 403-410.

6　Luczak J et al. (1995) The role of ketamine, an NMDA receptor antagonist, in the management of pain. Progress in Palliative Care. **3**: 127–134.

7　Kotlinska-Lemieszek A and Luczak J (2004) Subanesthetic ketamine: an essential adjuvant for intractable cancer pain. Journal Pain Symptom Management. **28**: 100–102.

8　Lin T et al. (1998) Long-term epidural ketamine, morphine and bupivacaine attenuate reflex sympathetic dystrophy neuralgia. Canadian Journal of Anaesthesia. **45**: 175–177.

9　Haines D and Gaines S (1999) N of 1 randomised controlled trials of oral ketamine in patients with chronic pain. Pain. **83**: 283–287.

10　Batchelor G (1999) Ketamine in neuropathic pain. The Pain Society Newsletter. **1**: 19.

11　Beltrutti D et al. (1999) The epidural and intrathecal administration of ketamine. Current Review of Pain. **3**: 458–472.

12　Mercadante S et al. (2000) Analgesic effect of intravenous ketamine in cancer patients on morphine therapy: a randomized , controlled, double-blind, crossover, double-dose study. Journal of Pain and Symptom Management. **20**: 246–252.

13　Carr DB et al. (2004) Safety and efficacy of intranasal ketamine for the treatment of breakthrough pain in patients with chronic pain: a randomized, double-blind, placebo-controlled, crossover study. Pain. **108**: 17–27.

14　Mercadante S et al. (2005) Alternative treatments of breakthrough pain in patients receiving spinal analgesics for cancer pain. Journal of Pain and Symptom Management. **30**: 485–491.

15　Yeaman F et al. (2013) Sub-dissociative dose intranasal ketamine for limb injury pain in children in the emergency department: a pilot study. Emergency Medicine Australasia. **25**: 161–167.

16　Vranken JH et al. (2005) Neuropathological findings after continuous intrathecal administration of S(+)-ketamine for the management of neuropathic cancer pain. Pain. **117**: 231–235.

17　Berger J et al. (2000) Ketamine-fentanyl-midazolam infusion for the control of symptoms in terminal life care. American Journal of Hospice and Palliative Care. **17**: 127–132.

18　Enck R (2000) A ketamine, fentanyl, and midazolam infusion for uncontrolled terminal pain and agitation. American Journal of Hospice and Palliative Care. **17**: 76–77.

19　Conway M et al. (2009) Use of continuous intravenous ketamine for end-stage cancer pain in children. Journal of Pediatric Oncology Nursing. **26**: 100–106.

20　Oye I et al. (1991) The chiral forms of ketamine as probes for NMDA receptor function in humans. In: T Kameyama (ed) NMDA receptor Related Agents: biochemistry, pharmacology and behavior. NPP, Ann Arbor, Michigan, pp. 381–389.

21　White PF et al. (1980) Pharmacology of ketamine isomers in surgical patients. Anesthesiology. **52**: 231–239.

22　Mathisen L et al. (1995) Effect of ketamine, an NMDA receptor inhibitor, in acute and chronic orofacial pain. Pain. **61**: 215–220.

23　Pfenninger EG et al. (2002) Cognitive impairment after small-dose ketamine isomers in comparison to equianalgesic racemic ketamine in human volunteers. Anesthesiology. **96**: 357–366.

24　Hijazi Y et al. (2002) Contribution of CYP3A4, CYP2B6, and CYP2C9 isoforms to N-demethylation of ketamine in human liver microsomes. Drug Metabolism & Disposition. **30**: 853–858.

25　Clements JA et al. (1982) Bio-availability, pharmacokinetics and analgesic activity of ketamine in humans. Journal of Pharmaceutical Sciences. **71**: 539–542.

26　Muetzelfeldt L et al. (2008) Journey through the K-hole: phenomenological aspects of ketamine use. Drug Alcohol Dependence. **95**: 219–229.

27　Hughes A et al. (1999) Ketamine. CME Bulletin Palliative Medicine. **1**: 53.

28　Giannini A et al. (2000) Acute ketamine intoxication treated by haloperidol: a preliminary study. American Journal of Therapeutics. **7**: 389–391.

29　Subramaniam K et al. (2004) Ketamine as adjuvant analgesic to opioids: a quantitative and qualitative systematic review. Anesthesia and Analgesia. **99**: 482–495.

30　Bell RF (2009) Perioperative ketamine for acute postoperative pain. Cochrane Database of Systematic Reviews 2006. **1** (Updated 2009).

31　Bell RF (2009) Ketamine for chronic non-cancer pain. Pain. **141**: 210–214.

32　Alviar MJM (2011) Pharmacological interventions for treating phantom limb pain. Cochrane Database of Systematic Reviews. CD006380.

33　Sigtermans MJ et al. (2009) Ketamine produces effective and long-term pain relief in patients with Complex Regional Pain Syndrome Type I. Pain. **145**: 304–311.

34　Schwartzman RJ et al. (2009) Outpatient intravenous ketamine for the treatment of complex regional pain syndrome: a double-blind placebo controlled study. Pain. **147**: 107–115.

35　Yang CY et al. (1996) Intrathecal ketamine reduces morphine requirements in patients with terminal cancer pain. Canadian Journal of Anaesthesia. **43**: 379–383.

36　Bell RF et al. (2012) Ketamine as an adjuvant to opioids for cancer pain. Cochrane Database Systematic Reviews. **11**: CD003351.

37　Oshima E et al. (1990) Continuous subcutaneous injection of ketamine for cancer pain. Canadian Journal of Anaesthetics. **37**: 385–392.

38　Cherry DA et al. (1995) Ketamine as an adjunct to morphine in the treatment of pain. Pain. **62**: 119–121.

39　Mercadante S (1996) Ketamine in cancer pain: an update. Palliative Medicine. **10**: 225–230.

40　Bell RF (1999) Low-dose subcutaneous ketamine infusion and morphine tolerance. Pain. **83**: 101–103.

41　Fitzgibbon EJ et al. (2002) Low dose ketamine as an analgesic adjuvant in difficult pain syndromes: a strategy for conversion from parenteral to oral ketamine. Journal of Pain and Symptom Management. **23**: 165–170.

42　Kannan TR et al. (2002) Oral ketamine as an adjuvant to oral morphine for neuropathic pain in cancer patients. Journal of Pain and Symptom Management. **23**: 60–65.

43　Benitez-Rosario M et al. (2003) A retrospective comparison of the dose ratio between subcutaneous and oral ketamine. Journal of Pain and Symptom Management. **25**: 400–402.

44　Fitzgibbon EJ and Viola R (2005) Parenteral ketamine as an analgesic adjuvant for severe pain: development and retrospective audit of a protocol for a palliative care unit. Journal of Palliative Medicine. **8**: 49–57.

45　Jackson K et al. (2010) The effectiveness and adverse effects profile of "burst" ketamine in refractory cancer pain. Journal of Palliative Care. **26**: 176–183.

46　Lauretti G et al. (1999) Oral ketamine and transdermal nitroglycerin as analgesic adjuvants to oral morphine therapy and amitriptyline for cancer pain management. Anesthesiology. **90**: 1528–1533.

47 Jackson K et al. (2001) 'Burst' ketamine for refractory cancer pain: an open-label audit of 39 patients. Journal of Pain and Symptom Management. 22: 834–842.
48 Lossignol DA et al. (2005) Successful use of ketamine for intractable cancer pain. Support Care Cancer. 13: 188–193.
49 James PJ et al. (2010) The addition of ketamine to a morphine nurse- or patient-controlled analgesia infusion (PCA/NCA) increases analgesic efficacy in children with mucositis pain. Paediatric Anaesthesia. 20: 805–811.
50 Mercadante S et al. (2003) Burst ketamine to reverse opioid tolerance in cancer pain. Journal of Pain and Symptom Management. 25: 302–305.
51 Mitchell AC and Fallon MT (2002) A single infusion of intravenous ketamine improves pain relief in patients with critical limb ischaemia: results of a double blind randomised controlled trial. Pain. 97: 275–281.
52 Hardy J et al. (2012) Randomized , double-blind, placebo-controlled study to assess the efficacy and toxicity of subcutaneous ketamine in the management of cancer pain. Journal of Clinical Oncology. 30: 11–17.
53 White MC et al. (2011) Pain management in 100 episodes of severe mucositis in children. Peadiatric Anesthesia. 21: 411–416.
54 Arroyo-Novoa CM et al. (2011) Efficacy of small doses of ketamine with morphine to decrease procedural pain responses during open wound care. Clinical Journal of Pain. 27: 561–566.
55 Kundra P et al. (2013) Oral ketamine and dexmedetomidine in adults' burns wound dressing–A randomized double blind cross over study. Burns. 39: 1150–1156.
56 Norambuena C et al. (2013) Oral ketamine and midazolam for pediatric burn patients: a prospective, randomized, double-blind study. Journal of Pediatric Surgery. 48: 629–634.
57 Cevik E et al. (2013) Comparison of ketamine-low-dose midozolam with midazolam-fentanyl for orthopedic emergencies: a double-blind randomized trial. American Journal of Emergency Medicine. 31: 108–113.
58 Finch PM et al. (2009) Reduction of allodynia in patients with complex regional pain syndrome: A double-blind placebo-controlled trial of topical ketamine. Pain. 146: 18–25.
59 Gammaitoni A et al. (2000) Topical ketamine gel: possible role in treating neuropathic pain. Pain Medicine. 1: 97–100.
60 Slatkin NE and Rhiner M (2003) Topical ketamine in the treatment of mucositis pain. Pain Medicine. 4: 298–303.
61 Salvadore G and Singh JB (2013) Ketamine as a fast acting antidepressant: current knowledge and open questions. CNS Neuroscience and Therapeutics. 19: 428–436.
62 Murrough JW et al. (2013) Antidepressant efficacy of ketamine in treatment-resistant major depression: a two-site randomized controlled trial. American Journal of Psychiatry. 170: 1134–1142.
63 Stefanczyk-Sapieha L et al. (2008) Intravenous ketamine "burst" for refractory depression in a patient with advanced cancer. Journal of Palliative Medicine. 11: 1268–1271.
64 Irwin SA and Iglewicz A (2010) Oral ketamine for the rapid treatment of depression and anxiety in patients receiving hospice care. Journal of Palliative Medicine. 13: 903–908.
65 Zanicotti CG et al. (2012) Mood and pain responses to repeat dose intramuscular ketamine in a depressed patient with advanced cancer. Journal of Palliative Medicine. 15: 400–403.
66 Grott Zanicotti C et al. (2013) Case report: long-term mood response to repeat dose intramuscular ketamine in a depressed patient with advanced cancer. Journal of Palliative Medicine. 16: 719–720.
67 Irwin SA et al. (2013) Daily oral ketamine for the treatment of depression and anxiety in patients receiving hospice care: a 28-day open-label proof-of-concept trial. Journal of Palliative Medicine. 16: 958–965.
68 Dolgin E (2013) Rapid antidepressant effects of ketamine ignite drug discovery. Nature Medicine. 19: 8.
69 Gaspard N et al. (2013) Intravenous ketamine for the treatment of refractory status epilepticus: a retrospective multicenter study. Epilepsia. 54: 1498–1503.
70 Chong CC et al. (2006) Bioavailability of ketamine after oral or sublingual administration. Pain Medicine. 7: 469–469.
71 Yanagihara Y et al. (2003) Plasma concentration profiles of ketamine and norketamine after administration of various ketamine preparations to healthy Japanese volunteers. Biopharmacentrics and Drug Disposition. 24: 37–43.
72 Grant IS et al. (1981) Pharmacokinetics and analgesic effects of IM and oral ketamine. British Journal of Anaesthesia. 53: 805–810.
73 Domino E et al. (1984) Ketamine kinetics in unmedicated and diazepam premedicated subjects. Clinical Pharmacology and Therapeutics. 36: 645–653.
74 Rabben T et al. (1999) Prolonged analgesic effect of ketamine, an N-methyl-D-aspartate receptor inhibitor, in patients with chronic pain. Journal of Pharmacology and Experimental Therapeutics. 289: 1060–1066.
75 Ward J and Standage C (2003) Angina pain precipitated by a continuous subcutaneous infusion of ketamine. Journal of Pain and Symptom Management. 25: 6–7.
76 Hagelburg N et al. (2010) Clarythromycin, a potent inhibitor of CYP3A, greatly increases exposure to oral S-ketamine. European Journal of Pain. 6: 625–629.
77 Peltoniemi MA et al. (2012) S-ketamine concentrations are greatly increased by grapefruit juice. European Journal of Clinical Pharmacology. 68: 979–986.
78 Peltoniemi MA et al. (2012) Rifampicin has a profound effect on the pharmacokinetics of oral S-Ketamine and less on intravenous S-ketamine. Basic and Clinical Pharmacology and Toxicology. 111: 325–332.
79 Peltoniemi MA et al. (2012) St John's wort greatly decreases the plasma concentrations of oral S-ketamine. Fundamental and Clinical Pharmacology. 26: 743–750.
80 Morgan CJ and Curran HV (2012) Ketamine use: a review. Addiction. 107: 27–38.
81 Morgan CJ et al. (2010) Consequences of chronic ketamine self-administration upon neurocognitive function and psychological wellbeing: a 1-year longitudinal study. Addiction. 105: 121–133.
82 Liao Y et al. (2012) Alterations in regional homogeneity of resting-state brain activity in ketamine addicts. Neuroscience Letters. 522: 36–40.
83 Liao Y et al. (2010) Frontal white matter abnormalities following chronic ketamine use: a diffusion tensor imaging study. Brain. 133: 2115–2122.
84 Narendran R et al. (2005) Altered prefrontal dopaminergic function in chronic recreational ketamine users. American Journal of Psychiatry. 162: 2352–2359.
85 Storr TM and Quibell R (2009) Can ketamine prescribed for pain cause damage to the urinary tract? Palliative Medicine. 23: 670–672.
86 Shahzad. K et al. (2012) Analgesic ketamine use leading to cystectomy: a case report. British Journal of Medical and Surgical Urology. 5: 188–191.

87 Gregoire MC *et al.* (2008) A pediatric case of ketamine-associated cystitis (Letter-to-the-Editor RE: Shahani R, Streutker C, Dickson B, et al: Ketamine-associated ulcerative cystitis: a new clinical entity. Urology 69: 810-812, 2007). *Urology*. **71**: 1232–1233.

88 Winstock AR *et al.* (2012) The prevalence and natural history of urinary symptoms among recreational ketamine users. *BJU International*. **110**: 1762–1766.

89 Chu PS *et al.* (2008) The destruction of the lower urinary tract by ketamine abuse: a new syndrome? *British Journal of Urology International*. **102**: 1616–1622.

90 Shahani R *et al.* (2007) Ketamine-associated ulcerative cystitis: a new clinical entity. *Urology*. **69**: 810–812.

91 Wood D *et al.* (2011) Recreational ketamine: from pleasure to pain. *British Journal of Urology International*. **107**: 1881–1884.

92 Meng E *et al.* (2011) Involvement of purinergic neurotransmission in ketamine induced bladder dysfunction. *Journal of Urology*. **186**: 1134–1141.

93 Cheung RY *et al.* (2011) Urinary symptoms and impaired quality of life in female ketamine users: persistence after cessation of use. *Hong Kong Medical Journal*. **17**: 267–273.

94 Ng SH *et al.* (2010) Emergency department presentation of ketamine abusers in Hong Kong: a review of 233 cases. *Hong Kong Medical Journal*. **16**: 6–11.

95 Wong SW *et al.* (2009) Dilated common bile ducts mimicking choledochal cysts in ketamine abusers. *Hong Kong Medical Journal*. **15**: 53–56.

96 Dundee JW *et al.* (1980) Changes in serum enzyme levels following ketamine infusions. *Anaesthesia*. **35**: 12–16.

97 Noppers IM *et al.* (2011) Drug-induced liver injury following a repeated course of ketamine treatment for chronic pain in CRPS type 1 patients: a report of 3 cases. *Pain*. **152**: 2173–2178.

98 Ng SH *et al.* (2009) Dilated common bile ducts in ketamine abusers. *Hong Kong Med J*. **15**: 157; author reply 157.

99 Seto WK *et al.* (2011) Ketamine-induced cholangiopathy: a case report. *American Journal of Gastroenterology*. **106**: 1004–1005.

100 Lee ST *et al.* (2009) Apoptotic insults to human HepG2 cells induced by S-(+)-ketamine occurs through activation of a Bax-mitochondria-caspase protease pathway. *British Journal of Anaesthesia*. **102**: 80–89.

101 Palliativedrugs.com (2013) Ketamine monitoring chart. *Document Library*. Pain (neuropathic): www.palliativedrugs.com.

102 Fallon M (2010) Personal communication.

103 Mitchell AC (1999) Generalized hyperalgesia and allodynia following abrupt cessation of subcutaneous ketamine infusion. *Palliative Medicine*. **13**: 427–428.

104 Enarson M *et al.* (1999) Clinical experience with oral ketamine. *Journal of Pain and Symptom Management*. **17**: 384–386.

105 Benitez-Rosario MA *et al.* (2011) A strategy for conversion from subcutaneous to oral ketamine in cancer pain patients: efficacy of a 1:1 ratio. *Journal of Pain and Symptom Management*. **10**: 1098–1105.

106 Clark JL and Kalan GE (1995) Effective treatment of severe cancer pain of the head using low-dose ketamine in an opioid-tolerant patient. *Journal of Pain and Symptom Management*. **10**: 310–314.

107 Broadley K *et al.* (1996) Ketamine injection used orally. *Palliative Medicine*. **10**: 247–250.

108 Vielvoye-Kerkmeer A (2000) Clinical experience with ketamine. *Journal of Pain and Symptom Management*. **19**: 3.

109 Lloyd-Williams M (2000) Ketamine for cancer pain. *Journal of Pain and Symptom Management*. **19**: 79–80.

110 Mason KP *et al.* (2002) Evolution of a protocol for ketamine-induced sedation as an alternative to general anesthesia for interventional radiologic procedures in pediatric patients. *Radiology*. **225**: 457–465.

111 Hocking G *et al.* (2007) Ketamine: does life begin at 40? *Pain Clinical Updates IASP*. XV. Issue 3.

112 Okamoto Y *et al.* (2012) Can gradual dose titration of ketamine for management of neuropathic pain prevent psychotomimetic effects in patients with advanced cancer? *American Journal of Hospice and Palliative Medicine*. **30**: 450–454.

Updated June 2014

*PROPOFOL BNF 15.1.1

Class: General anaesthetic.

Indications: Induction and maintenance of general anaesthesia, conscious sedation (diagnostic or therapeutic procedures, e.g. radiation therapy in children),[1] continuous sedation of intubated and mechanically ventilated patients $\geqslant$16 years on intensive care units, †refractory agitated delirium or intolerable distress in the imminently dying, †intractable nausea and vomiting.[2]

Contra-indications: Continuous sedation in children $\leqslant$16 years; when used for sedation in children in intensive care, the death rate increased 2–3 times.[3] Propofol 0.5% is contra-indicated for maintenance of general anaesthesia or continuous sedation in intensive care in adults and children, and maintenance of conscious sedation in children (diagnostic or therapeutic procedures).

Allergy to eggs, soya or peanuts (the available products contain purified egg phosphatide as an emulsifying agent and soya bean oil).[4]

Pharmacology

Propofol is an ultrafast-acting IV anaesthetic agent. It is rapidly metabolized, mainly in the liver, to inactive compounds which are excreted in the urine. The incidence of untoward haemodynamic changes is low. Propofol reduces cerebral blood flow, cerebral metabolism and, less consistently, intracranial pressure.[5] The reduction in intracranial pressure is greater if the baseline pressure is raised. On discontinuation patients rapidly regain consciousness (10–30min) without residual drowsiness.

In palliative care, propofol is occasionally used, when other approaches have failed, to relieve agitated delirium or intolerable distress in the imminently dying.[6] Careful titration generally permits 'conscious sedation', i.e. patients open their eyes on verbal command, possess intact autonomic reflexes, and tolerate mild noxious stimuli.[2] Such use has also been described in children at the end of life, and algorithms to assist physicians considering initiation of palliative sedation therapy in children have been suggested.[7,8]

Propofol also has an anti-emetic effect resulting in less postoperative vomiting compared with other anaesthetic agents.[9–11] Specific postoperative anti-emetic regimens have been designed.[12–14] Chemotherapy-related nausea and vomiting is also helped by adjunctive propofol.[15] In patients receiving non-platinum regimens who were refractory to a combination of **dexamethasone** and a $5HT_3$-receptor antagonist, propofol was of benefit in ≥80%.[16] In palliative care, propofol has also been used to relieve refractory nausea and vomiting in dying patients.[2] Most of the patients probably had bowel obstruction, and it was more effective in relieving nausea than vomiting.

Animal studies suggest that the mechanism of action of propofol as an anti-emetic is by inhibition of serotonin release by enhancing GABA activity, possibly by direct GABA-mediated action on $5HT_3$-receptors in the area postrema/chemoreceptor trigger zone.[17]

Propofol also has antipruritic, anxiolytic, bronchodilator, muscle relaxant and anti-epileptic properties. A possible role in refractory status epilepticus requires further clarification.[18,19] Transient excitatory phenomena are seen occasionally (e.g. myoclonus, opisthotonus, tonic-clonic activity), during induction or recovery when blood levels are low, and presumably at a time when inhibitory centres but not excitatory centres have been depressed.[5,20,21]

Onset of action 30sec.
Time to peak effect 5min.
Plasma halflife 2–4min initial distribution phase; 30–60min slow distribution and initial elimination phase; 3–12h terminal elimination phase. The terminal elimination halflife may increase with prolonged use.
Duration of action 3–10min after single IV bolus.[22,23]

Cautions

Risk of cardiorespiratory depression. Propofol clearance will reduce if cardiac output falls. Involuntary movements and seizures have been reported, particularly in epileptics, during induction or recovery.[20,24] With prolonged use in intensive care, the following have been reported: ECG changes, cardiac arrhythmia, heart failure, hepatomegaly, renal failure, rhabdomyolysis, metabolic acidosis, hyperkalaemia and hyperlipidaemia; when these occur in combination, it is termed a propofol infusion syndrome.

Although in intensive care use it is good practice to check plasma lipid levels in patients receiving propofol for ≥3 days, it is unnecessary in patients whose expected prognosis is only days.

Diprivan® contains disodium edetate (EDTA), a chelating agent which can reduce circulating concentrations and increase urinary losses of trace metals, e.g. zinc. Supplements should be considered for patients who are not imminently dying and who are likely to receive prolonged propofol treatment, particularly those at particular risk of deficiency, e.g. from fluid loss, catabolic states or infection.

Undesirable effects

Very common (>10%): local pain at the injection site.
Common (<10%, >1%): headache, hypotension, bradycardia, transient apnoea.
Uncommon (<1%, >0.1%): thrombosis, phlebitis.
Rare: epileptiform movements, propofol infusion syndrome, euphoria during recovery, misuse resulting in addiction and/or death. Concerns over a growing incidence among medical staff with access to propofol, e.g. anaesthetists, has prompted moves to designate propofol a controlled drug, particularly in the USA.[25–27]

Dose and use

Propofol is an emulsion of oil-in-water. This gives it a white appearance and makes it a potential growth medium. Diprivan® contains EDTA, a chelating agent which binds to divalent metal ions and reduces their availability for bacterial growth, replication and cell wall integrity. However, the concentration (0.005%) is sufficient only to *retard* microbial growth for up to 12h in the event of accidental contamination.[28] The generic products available in the UK contain no preservatives. Thus, with all propofol products, strict aseptic technique must be employed to prevent microbial contamination *and the container and IV line renewed every 6–12h, in accordance with the individual manufacturer's instructions.* The propofol products available in the UK must not be infused through a microbiological filter.

The use of propofol in palliative care should be restricted to units with access to the necessary expertise and equipment.

Undiluted propofol requires a computer-controlled volumetric infusion pump or IV syringe pump (see manufacturer's SPC for full details).

Undiluted propofol is given by CIVI as a 1% (10mg/mL) or 2% (20mg/mL) solution. Pain at the IV injection site is common but can be minimized by:
- using the antecubital vein (or a large vein in the fore-arm) instead of a hand vein[29,30]
- injecting **lidocaine** prior to the propofol infusion, alternatively for 1% propofol only, co-administration of the first dose with **lidocaine**: mix 20 parts propofol injection 1% with 1 part *preservative-free* **lidocaine** injection 0.5% (Diprivan® only) or 1% (Diprivan® and generic products) immediately before administration
- using 0.5% propofol (5mg/mL; Propofol-Lipuro®) for induction of anaesthesia or sedation for infusions of a maximum duration of 1h.

Note: *propofol 2% injection should not be mixed with* **lidocaine** *or any other drug.*

Diluted propofol injection 1% can be administered through a less sensitive infusion control device, e.g. an in-line burette or drop counter, after dilution with 5% glucose (Diprivan® and generic products) or 0.9% saline (generic products only; see SPCs for full details). Dilution is advised with less sensitive infusion control devices because the weaker concentration reduces the risk of severe overdose if the infusion runs fast. The concentration of propofol in the diluted solution must not be less than 2mg/mL because this can disrupt the emulsion. Diluted propofol should be used within 6h. *Propofol injection 2% should not be diluted.*

Compatibility: See the specific SPC for full details; formulations of propofol differ between manufacturers and compatibility data cannot be extrapolated from one product to another. Propofol injection 1% is compatible with certain concentrations of **alfentanil** (Diprivan® only) and **lidocaine**, and can be diluted with 5% glucose before use. *Propofol injection 2% should not be diluted or mixed with any other drugs.*

Both 1% and 2% propofol can be added through a Y-connector to a running infusion of 5% glucose, 0.9% saline or 4% glucose + 0.18% saline; the Y-connector should be placed as close to the injection site as possible.

Refractory agitated delirium or intolerable distress in the imminently dying

Consider propofol only if standard treatments have failed, i.e. a sedative antipsychotic + a benzodiazepine (Figure 1).[2,6,31–33] However, generally, **phenobarbital** should be used in preference to propofol because it is less complicated for clinical staff to titrate and monitor (see p.286).

Aim to titrate the dose until *conscious sedation* is achieved, i.e. patients open their eyes on verbal command but are not distressed by nursing interventions (e.g. mouth care, turning):
- remain with the patient throughout the initial titration process to ensure an effective and safe dose is found
- generally start with propofol 1mg/kg/h CIVI
- if necessary, increase by 0.5mg/kg/h every 5–10min until a satisfactory level of sedation is achieved; smaller dose steps can be used to fine-tune the treatment; most patients respond well to 1–2mg/kg/h
- to increase the level of sedation quickly, a bolus dose can be given by increasing the rate to 1mg/kg/*min* for 2–5min

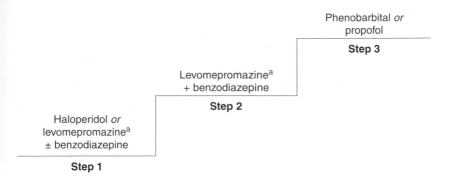

Figure 1 Drug treatment used at some centres for irreversible agitated delirium or intolerable distress in the imminently dying.

a. in countries where levomepromazine is not available, e.g. the USA, chlorpromazine is used instead.

- monitor the patient closely during the first hour of treatment with respect to symptom relief and/or level of sedation, and then after 2, 6, and 12h
- continue to monitor the effect of propofol and the level of sedation at least twice daily
- if the patient is too sedated (i.e. does not respond to a verbal command to open their eyes, shows no response to noxious stimuli) and/or there is evidence of drug-induced respiratory depression, the infusion should be turned off for 2–3min and restarted at a lower rate; occasionally this leads to a progressive reduction in dose because the patient has become unconscious as a result of their disease
- tolerance can develop, necessitating a dose increase, but generally not within 1 week
- long-term use of doses >4mg/kg/h is not recommended because of increasing risk of undesirable effects
- if the patient does not respond to propofol 4mg/kg/h alone, supplement with **midazolam** by CSCI
- it is important to replenish the infusion quickly when a container empties, because the effect of an infusion of propofol wears off after 10–30min
- *because propofol has no analgesic properties, analgesics should be continued.*

Intractable nausea and vomiting
The use of propofol as an anti-emetic should be considered only if all other treatments have failed (see p.241).[2] Dose titration is generally slower for intractable nausea and vomiting than for terminal agitation:

- remain with the patient for at least 10min following any dose change to ensure that excessive sedation does not occur
- generally start with propofol 0.5mg/kg/h CIVI
- if necessary, increase by 0.25–0.5mg/kg/h every 30–60min until a satisfactory response is obtained; smaller dose steps can be used to fine-tune the treatment
- most patients respond well to 0.5–1mg/kg/h; doses >1mg/kg/h may result in sedation
- monitor the patient closely during the first hour of treatment with respect to symptom relief and/or level of sedation and then after 2, 6, and 12h
- continue to monitor the effect of propofol and level of sedation at least twice daily
- if the patient is too sedated, the infusion should be turned off for 2–3min and then restarted at a lower rate
- if the patient responds well, reduce the infusion rate on a trial basis after 18–24h
- tolerance can develop, necessitating a dose increase, but generally not within 1 week
- it is important to replenish the infusion quickly when a container empties, because the effect of an infusion of propofol wears off after 10–30min
- when used solely for its anti-emetic effect in the last days of life, some centres reduce the dose of, or even discontinue, propofol when the patient becomes unconscious.

Supply

Propofol (generic; Propofol-Lipuro® and Propoven®)

Injection (emulsion) 5mg/mL (0.5%), 20mL amp = £3.50; *restricted to induction of general anaesthesia or induction of conscious sedationfor diagnostic and therapeutic procedures in adults and children, and short-term sedation in adults (1h maximum duration of infusion).*

Injection (emulsion) 10mg/mL (1%), 20mL amp = £4, 50mL infusion bottle = £10, 100mL infusion bottle = £19.

Injection (emulsion) 20mg/mL (2%), 50mL vial = £21.

Diprivan® (AstraZeneca)

Injection (emulsion) 10mg/mL (1%), 20mL amp = £1, 50mL pre-filled siringe 'Diprifusor TCI system' = £6.

Injection (emulsion) 20mg/mL (2%), 50mL pre-filled syringe 'Diprifusor TCI system' = £6.

'Diprifusor TCI system' is restricted to induction and maintenance of general anaesthesia in adults.

1　Harris EA (2010) Sedation and anesthesia options for pediatric patients in the radiation oncology suite. *International Journal of Pediatrics.* EPUB article ID 870921.

2　Lundstrom S et al. (2005) When nothing helps: propofol as sedative and antiemetic in palliative cancer care. *Journal of Pain and Symptom Management.* **30**: 570–577.

3　Anonymous (2001) Propofol (Diprivan) infusion: sedation in children aged 16 years or younger contraindicated. *Current Problems in Pharmacovigilance.* **27**: 10.

4　Hofer KN et al. (2003) Possible anaphylaxis after propofol in a child with food allergy. *Annals of Pharmacotherapy.* **37**: 398–401.

5　Mirenda J and Broyles G (1995) Propofol as used for sedation in the ICU. *Chest.* **108**: 539–548.

6　McWilliams K et al. (2010) Propofol for terminal sedation in palliative care: a systematic review. *Journal of Palliative Medicine.* **13**: 73–76.

7　Hooke MC et al. (2007) Propofol use in pediatric patients with severe cancer pain at the end of life. *Journal of Pediatric Oncology Nursing.* **24**: 29–34.

8　Anghelescu DL et al. (2012) Pediatric palliative sedation therapy with propofol: recommendations based on experience in children with terminal cancer. *Journal of Palliative Medicine.* **15**: 1082–1090.

9　Tramer M et al. (1997) Meta-analytic comparison of prophylactic antiemetic efficacy for postoperative nausea and vomiting: propofol anaesthesia vs omitting nitrous oxide vs total i.v. anaesthesia with propofol. *British Journal of Anaesthesia.* **78**: 256–259.

10　Sneyd JR et al. (1998) A meta-analysis of nausea and vomiting following maintenance of anaesthesia with propofol or inhalational agents. *European Journal of Anaesthesiology.* **15**: 433–445.

11　DeBalli P (2003) The use of propofol as an antiemetic. *International Anesthesiology Clinics.* **41**: 67–77.

12　Fujii Y et al. (2001) Small doses of propofol, droperidol, and metoclopramide for the prevention of postoperative nausea and vomiting after thyroidectomy. *Otolaryngology - Head and Neck Surgery.* **124**: 266–269.

13　Gan TJ et al. (1997) Determination of plasma concentrations of propofol associated with 50% reduction in postoperative nausea. *Anesthesiology.* **87**: 779–784.

14　Gan TJ et al. (1999) Patient-controlled antiemesis: a randomized, double-blind comparison of two doses of propofol versus placebo. *Anesthesiology.* **90**: 1564–1570.

15　Scher C et al. (1992) Use of propofol for the prevention of chemotherapy-induced nausea and emesis in oncology patients. *Canadian Journal of Anaesthesia.* **39**: 170–172.

16　Borgeat A et al. (1994) Adjuvant propofol enables better control of nausea and emesis secondary to chemotherapy for breast cancer. *Canadian Journal of Anaesthesia.* **41**: 1117–1119.

17　Cechetto DF et al. (2001) The effects of propofol in the area postrema of rats. *Anesthesia and Analgesia.* **92**: 934–942.

18　Rossetti AO (2007) Which anesthetic should be used in the treatment of refractory status epilepticus? *Epilepsia.* **48 (Suppl 8)**: 52–55.

19　Garcia Penas JJ et al. (2007) Status epilepticus: evidence and controversy. *Neurologist.* **13 (6 Suppl 1)**: S62–73.

20　Sneyd JR (1999) Propofol and epilepsy. *British Journal of Anaesthesia.* **82**: 168–169.

21　Meyer S et al. (2009) Propofol: pro- or anticonvulsant drug? *Anesthesia and Analgesia.* **108**: 1993–1994; author reply 1994.

22　Jungheinrich C et al. (2002) Pharmacokinetics of the generic formulation Propofol 1 Fresenius in comparison with the original formulation (Disoprivan 1). *Clinical Drug Investigation.* **22**: 417–427.

23　Fechner J et al. (2004) Comparative pharmacokinetics and pharmacodynamics of the new propofol prodrug GPI 15715 and propofol emulsion. *Anesthesiology.* **101**: 626–639.

24　AstraZeneca (2006) *Data on file.*

25　Wilson C et al. (2010) The abuse potential of propofol. *Clinical Toxicology.* **48**: 165–170.

26　Charatan F (2009) Concerns mount over misuse of anaesthetic propofol among US health professionals. *British Medical Journal.* **339**: b3673.

27　Monroe T et al. (2011) The misuse and abuse of propofol. *Substance Use and Misuse.* **46**: 1199–1205.

28　AstraZeneca (2010) *Personal communication.*

29　Wijeysundera DN and Kavanagh BP (2011) Prevention of pain from propofol injection. *British Medical Journal.* **342**: d1102.

30　Jalota L et al. (2011) Prevention of pain on injection of propofol: systematic review and meta-analysis. *British Medical Journal.* **342**: d1110.

31　Cheng C et al. (2002) When midazolam fails. *Journal of Pain and Symptom Management.* **23**: 256–265.

32　Moyle J (1995) The use of propofol in palliative medicine. *Journal of Pain and Symptom Management.* **10**: 643–646.

33　Mercadante S et al. (1995) Propofol in terminal care. *Journal of Pain and Symptom Management.* **10**: 639–642.

Updated (minor change) March 2014

14: GUIDANCE ABOUT PRESCRIBING IN PALLIATIVE CARE

In recent years, both national drug regulatory authorities and the general public have become increasingly concerned about the possibility of dangerous/life-threatening adverse drug reactions. Official documents and drug manufacturers' information often include a warning along the lines of:

'Use the lowest effective dose for the shortest possible time in order to reduce the risk of serious adverse events.'

This is, of course, one of the foundational principles of therapeutic drug use; it simply emphasises 'good practice'. Official documents and drug manufacturers' information also highlight when caution is necessary in relation to, for example, hepatic and renal impairment.

In palliative care, many patients are elderly and debilitated, and many have impaired organ function. Accordingly, in *PCF*, it is assumed that prescribers will adopt an appropriately cautious approach in relation to both dose and duration of treatment (also see *Getting the most out of PCF*, p.xv)

This chapter, in addition to offering general advice about 'safe prescribing', emphasizes the special needs of children and the elderly, and examines the impact of hepatic and renal impairment.

GENERAL PRINCIPLES

Drugs should be used only within the context of a systematic approach, which is encapsulated in the acronym **EEMMA**:
- *E*valuation of the impact of the illness on the patient and family, and of the causes of the patient's symptoms (often multifactorial)
- *E*xplanation to the patient before starting treatment about what is going on, and what is the most appropriate course of action
- *M*anagement: correct the correctable, non-drug treatment, drug treatment
- *M*onitoring: frequent review of the impact of treatment; optimizing the doses of symptom relief drugs to maximize benefit and minimize undesirable effects
- *A*ttention to detail: do not make unwarranted assumptions; listen actively to the patient, respond to non-verbal and verbal cues.

In palliative care, the axiom *diagnosis before treatment* still holds true. Even when cancer is responsible, a symptom may be caused by different mechanisms. For example, in lung cancer, vomiting may be caused by hypercalcaemia or by raised intracranial pressure (to name just two possible causes). Treatment often varies with the cause. Further, for many symptoms, the concurrent use of non-drug measures is equally important, and sometimes more important.

Attention to detail
Precision in taking a drug history
If a patient says, 'I take morphine every 4 hours', the doctor should ask, 'Tell me, when do you take your first dose?' 'And the second dose?', etc. It often turns out that the patient is taking morphine q.d.s. rather than q4h, and possibly p.r.n. rather than prophylactically.

A 90 year-old woman interpreted 'paracetamol four times a day' as meaning 0800h, 1200h, 1600h, and 2000h. She was pain-free during the day but regularly woke between 0200h and 0300h in excruciating pain - so much so that she dreaded going to bed at night. Retiming her medication, so that the doses were more equally spaced out around the clock (on waking, 1200h, 1800h, bedtime), resulted in a pain-free night.

"Think before you ink"

When prescribing any drug, particularly for patients already taking several other drugs, it is important for doctors to ask themselves:

'What is the treatment goal?'
'How can it be monitored?'
'What is the risk of undesirable effects?'
'What is the risk of drug interactions?'
'Can any of the patient's other drugs be stopped?'

Safe prescribing

Safe prescribing is a skill, and is crucial to success in symptom management. It extends to considering size, shape and taste of tablets and solutions, and avoiding doses which force patients to take more tablets, and/or open more containers, than would be the case if doses were 'rounded up' to a more convenient tablet size. For example, m/r **morphine** 100mg (one tablet, one container) is easier for the patient than 90mg (two tablets and two containers: 60mg + 30mg).

Safe prescribing requires good communication with patients, carers, and other professionals. Poor communication contributes to about half of preventable drug errors.[1] A lack of information and involvement may leave patients dissatisfied.[2]

Good communication includes clear documentation (e.g. allergies, co-morbidities, prescription writing).[3-5] The use of a patient's 'logbook' is to be encouraged; this would include important contact names and telephone numbers.

Safe prescribing practice is particularly important in palliative care where polypharmacy, debility, co-morbidities (e.g. renal impairment), involvement of multiple health professionals, and the use of higher risk medications are among the many factors which make such patients particularly vulnerable to problems with adherence (compliance), undesirable effects, medication errors, drug interactions and other potentially preventable burdens.

Keep it simple!

Many palliative care patients are taking 4–5 different drugs concurrently. Patients with diabetes and those with COPD, for example, may be taking 8–12 different ones. Drugs should be reviewed regularly to assess whether they are still necessary, e.g. long-term prophylactic medication such as statins, oral hypoglycaemics, antihypertensives (also see Chapter 16, p.670) to avoid problematic polypharmacy.[6]

A home medicines chart (see Figure 1 and Figure 2) is essential to prevent chaotic drug administration, e.g. one drug or other being taken in succession 'on the hour' throughout the day with hardly any respite.

Generally, the drug which needs to be taken most frequently should act as the 'anchor' drug and, as far as possible, other drugs linked to its administration times. However, antacids physically interact with many drugs, e.g. **azithromycin**, e/c products, quinolone antibacterials, **itraconazole** and tetracyclines, thereby reducing absorption. Accordingly, antacids should ideally be taken 2h before or after these drugs (see p.1, p.465 and p.510).

Although the SPC may indicate that an antibacterial should be given 'every 8 hours' or 'every 6 hours', generally for PO administration there is no need to be exact about this. Further, although patients with opioid-induced nausea are sometimes advised to take **metoclopramide** 30min before the opioid, in practice this is *rarely necessary.*

Some SPC and PIL indicate 'before food' (e.g. **lansoprazole**, p.34), or 'with/just after food' (e.g. NSAIDs, p.321) when this is not always necessary. Only when absolutely necessary should patients be asked to separate out drugs in relation to food. For example:

- when drug absorption is significantly affected by food. Box A lists drugs featured in *PCF* which, for maximal absorption, need to be taken either on an empty stomach or after food
- drugs which are known GI irritants. Box B lists those drugs featured in *PCF* for which food may reduce the risk or severity of undesirable GI effects.

In addition:

- drugs for diabetes and **pancreatin** should always be taken as recommended in relation to food/meal times
- in order to increase the contact time of the drug with the mucosa, food should not be taken immediately after drugs have been administered via the buccal mucosa (e.g. transmucosal **fentanyl**) or those used topically to treat oral ulceration or oropharyngeal candidosis.

Hospice Home Care

Name *Linda Barton*   **Age** *58*   **Date** *15 December 2014*

Tablets/Medicines	2am	On waking	10am	2pm	6pm	Bed time	Purpose
MORPHINE (Oramorph 2mg in 1mL)		10mL	10mL	10mL	10mL	20mL	pain relief
METOCLOPRAMIDE (10mg tablet)	1	1			1	1	anti-sickness
NAPROXEN (500mg tablet)			1			1	pain relief
SENNA (tablet)			2			2	for bowels
TEMAZEPAM (20mg tablet)						1	for sleep

If troublesome pain: take an extra 10mL of MORPHINE between regular doses.
If bowels remain constipated: increase SENNA to 3 tablets twice a day.

[Use this space for adding additional information,
e.g. further advice about 'rescue' medication]

- Keep this chart with you so you can show your doctor or nurse this list of what you are taking.
- Ask for a fresh supply of your medication 2–3 days before you need it.
- Sometimes your medication may be supplied in different strengths or presentations. If you have any concerns about this, check with your pharmacist.
- In an emergency, phone_____ and ask to speak to _____

Figure 1   Example of a patient's home medication chart (q4h).

Hospice Home Care

Name *Nicolas Crowthorne*   **Age** *65*   **Date** *15 December 2014*

Tablets/Medicines	Breakfast	Midday meal	Evening meal	Bedtime	Purpose
MAALOX PLUS (suspension)	10mL	10mL	10mL	10mL	for hiccups
MORPHINE (MST 100mg tablet)	1			1	pain relief
NAPROXEN (500mg tablet)	1			1	pain relief
SENNA (tablet)	2	2	2	2	for bowels
HALOPERIDOL (1.5mg tablet)				1	anti-sickness
DIAZEPAM (5mg tablet)				1	for sleeping and relaxation

If troublesome pain: take MORPHINE SOLUTION (2mg in 1mL) 10mL, up to every hour.
If troublesome hiccup: take extra 10mL of MAALOX PLUS, up to every 2 hours.

[Use this space for adding additional information,
e.g. further advice about 'rescue' medication]

- Keep this chart with you so you can show your doctor or nurse this list of what you are taking.
- Ask for a fresh supply of your medication 2–3 days before you need it.
- Sometimes your medication may be supplied in different strengths or presentations. If you have any concerns about this, check with your pharmacist.
- In an emergency, phone_____ and ask to speak to
_____.

Figure 2 Example of a patient's home medication chart (q.d.s.).

Box A Optimal absorption of drugs in relation to food[a,7,8]

Take on an *empty* stomach[b]
Antibacterials
  demeclocycline[c]
  doxycycline[c]
  flucloxacillin
  itraconazole *liquid*[d]
  phenoxymethylpenicillin
  tetracycline[c]
  rifampicin
  voriconazole
Bisphosphonates[c]
  ibandronic acid[c]
  sodium clodronate[c]
Propantheline

Take *with* or *just after* food
Cefuroxime
Itraconazole *capsules*[d]
Nitrofurantoin

---

a. these lists are limited to drugs featured in *PCF*
b. generally 30min before first food or drink of the day or 1h before and 2h after food at other times of the day
c. also avoid antacids, iron, zinc or milk for 2h before or after each dose to improve absorption
d. itraconazole liquid requires an empty stomach for full absorption, whereas food significantly improves the absorption of itraconazole capsules.

Box B Drugs for which food may reduce the risk of nausea/vomiting or GI irritation[a]

Baclofen
Corticosteroids
Etamsylate (not UK)
Metronidazole
Misoprostol
NSAIDs[b]

Iron
Potassium
Spironolactone
Tinidazole
Venlafaxine
Zinc

---

a. this list is limited to drugs which feature in the *PCF*
b. no substantial evidence.

Clear written instructions

Drug regimens should be written out in full for patients and/or families to work from. The recommendations published by the Royal Pharmaceutical Society[9] about the information to be recorded in writing when a patient transfers from one care provider to another also serve as a guide in relation to patients. Thus, the following should be written down on a purpose-designed chart:
• name of drug (generic and, if appropriate, also brand)
• formulation and strength
• reason for use ('for pain', 'for bowels', etc.)
• dose (x mL, y tablets)
• frequency and times to be taken.
For examples, see Figure 1 and Figure 2.

Advice should also include specific details about how to obtain further supplies. An alternative system will be necessary if both the patient and the immediate family cannot read.

Monitoring medication

It is often difficult to predict the optimum dose of a symptom relief drug, particularly opioids, laxatives and psychotropics. Further, undesirable effects put drug adherence in jeopardy. Thus, arrangements must be made for monitoring the effects of medication. The responsibility for monitoring must be clearly stated; shared decision-making is a definite risk factor for medication errors and problematic polypharmacy.[2,10]

Hypoalbuminaemia

Albumin binds acidic drugs, e.g. **phenytoin, warfarin, digoxin, naproxen** and **lorazepam**. When the albumin level is reduced by malnutrition, cirrhosis, nephrotic syndrome, end-stage renal disease, etc., the proportion of unbound (active) drug increases. This in turn increases the probability of toxicity with standard drug doses and normal total plasma drug concentrations, particularly with highly protein-bound drugs.

Most measured drug concentrations reflect the total drug concentration in the plasma (i.e. bound and unbound). Measuring free (unbound) levels of highly protein-bound drugs is not always possible but formulas to 'correct' for low plasma protein concentrations are available for some drugs. For example, to 'correct' the total phenytoin concentration in someone with hypoalbuminaemia the following formula can be used:[11]

$$\text{Corrected total phenytoin concentration} = \frac{\text{observed concentration}}{(0.02 \times \text{albumin}) + 0.1}$$

Acute phase proteins

α_1-acid glycoprotein (an acute phase protein) binds basic drugs, e.g. **lidocaine**, and when increased by infection, inflammatory disease, cancer, etc., the total plasma drug concentration will increase, but the proportion of unbound (active drug) may decrease or remain normal. Thus, a patient with an acute illness may have a high total **lidocaine** plasma concentration but a therapeutic or reduced unbound concentration. Reducing the dose to achieve a 'therapeutic' total concentration could result in loss of effect.

Compromise is sometimes necessary

It may be necessary to compromise on complete relief in order to avoid unacceptable undesirable effects. Antimuscarinic effects, e.g. dry mouth and visual disturbance, may limit dose escalation. Also, with inoperable bowel obstruction, it may be better to aim to reduce the incidence of vomiting to once or twice a day rather than to seek complete control.

Rescue ('as needed') medication

Patients need advice about what to do for intermittent symptoms, particularly break-through (episodic) pain. Generally, it is good practice to err on the side of generosity in relation to the recommended frequency of p.r.n. medication. However, it does depend on the class and formulation of the drug in question, and whether the patient is an inpatient or at home.

In all circumstances, it is important that the permitted frequency is stated clearly on the patient's medication chart (see Figure 1 and Figure 2), and also verbally explained to the patient and the family.

Patients taking regular m/r strong opioid medication at home

The *corresponding* immediate-release opioid analgesic formulation should also be prescribed q1h p.r.n. in an appropriate dose (see Chapter 5, p.293).

Patients taking regular immediate-release strong opioid medication at home

The *same* immediate-release opioid analgesic formulation should also be prescribed routinely q1h p.r.n.

With regular immediate-release strong opioids, if a patient needs an *occasional* rescue dose, say, 40min or less before the next regular dose is due, it may suffice to give the next regular dose early. However, opinion is divided. Some specialists say that a p.r.n. dose should be given, followed in due course by the regular dose.

Patients taking regular analgesic medication other than a strong opioid

Paracetamol and NSAIDs are often prescribed at the maximum recommended dose. In this case, an immediate-release opioid analgesic should be prescribed *q1h p.r.n.*, either a weak opioid or a low dose of a strong opioid.

Recommendations for anti-emetics, laxatives, and psychotropics have been given in their respective sections.

Inpatients

Recommendations can be more generous because there are trained personnel to monitor the effect of any additional medication, and thus prevent serious toxicity. For example, prescribing a range of permitted doses allows nurses to increase the amount given on their own initiative.

Example: Patient taking m/r **morphine** 100mg b.d.
Expected p.r.n. dose = 1/10–1/6 of total 24h dose, i.e. 20–30mg
Prescribe **morphine** immediate-release tablets/suspension 20–30mg q1h p.r.n.

In practice, nurses tend to start with the lower dose, but increase to the top of the range if necessary. If two consecutive top-of-the-range doses at the maximum permitted frequency are insufficient, medical advice should be obtained and alternative measures considered, e.g. rapid titration with IV **morphine** (see Box B, p.377 and Box C, p.378), with a subsequent upward adjustment of the regular PO dose.

INTERMITTENT SC DRUG ADMINISTRATION BY INFORMAL CARERS

Injections are regularly given by relatives and other informal carers to children or adults with, for example, diabetes mellitus or cystic fibrosis. In palliative care, there are occasions when it is helpful to train one or more relative, or other informal carer, to give intermittent SC injections (including **CD**s):
• regular medication which cannot be taken by a less invasive route
• emergency medication for symptoms which may develop particularly during a patient's last days. This may include insertion and priming of a cannula and/or preparation and administration of drugs via a previously inserted cannula.[12] Clear procedures are necessary to ensure the safety of the patient, support for the carer, and to comply with Nursing and Midwifery Council standards for medicines management (Box C).[13,14] Examples of procedures and documentation are available on www. palliativedrugs.com Document library, filed under Medication issues (Subcutaneous administration).

Box C   Procedures and safeguards for informal carers giving SC injections[12,15,16]
Careful evaluation of the situation by the healthcare team.
Informed consent obtained from the patient for administration by a named carer (signed if feasible).
Informal carers, particularly if qualified nurses or doctors, must not be pressured to give injections.
Both the patient and the carer should be able to opt out of the care arrangement at any time.
Carer's fears must be explored, including the possibility of the patient dying shortly after an injection.
Carers must: • be trained and assessed as competent, and documented in the patient's notes (together with the reason for using this approach) • be provided with written information for each drug, including the name, dose, indication, common undesirable effects, interval before a repeat dose is permitted, maximum number of injections/24h • keep a record of all injections given, including date, time, drug strength, formulation and dose, and name of person giving the injection • be provided with contact telephone numbers for both in- and out-of-hours.
Regular support and review of the situation must be carried out by a named health professional.
Close liaison with the primary health care team, and all out-of-hours services.

Some emergency medication can be given SL, rather than by injection. The same procedures and safeguards are needed when delegating the administration of any medicinal product to a relative or other informal carer.[14]

PRESCRIBING FOR CHILDREN

The background for this section is given in Box D. The general comments at the beginning of this chapter apply with equal force to children.

Box D Evaluation of symptoms in dying children

It is estimated that about 20 million children worldwide could benefit from palliative care.[17] In England, the prevalence rate for the under 20s is estimated to be 32 per 10,000 population aged 0–19.[18]

Although cancer is the second most common condition (after trauma) causing death in children, most children needing palliative care have diagnoses other than cancer. The largest group have neurological or neuromuscular disorders, e.g. hypoxic brain injury or inherited progressive metabolic, muscle or degenerative disease.

The need for palliative care may extend over many years, sometimes from the time of diagnosis, and is commonly needed in parallel with ongoing treatment of the underlying condition and of any intercurrent illness.

Evaluation is inherently more difficult than in most adults. Further, in children with life-limiting conditions, it is often difficult to identify the end-stage, particularly with disorders other than cancer.

Common problems include cerebral irritability, intractable seizures, skeletal muscle spasm, dystonia, pain, swallowing and feeding difficulties, gastro-oesophageal reflux, breathlessness and troublesome secretions.

Symptom evaluation is particularly difficult in children with cognitive impairment.[19,20] As far as possible, use self-reporting tools appropriate to the child's age and ability.[21–24]

A parent's report and staff observation are important.

Symptom scales and diaries aid continuity between different carers, and across different settings, e.g. home, school, hospital, hospice, and respite centre.

Ongoing care should be under the direction of a multiprofessional team,[25] including specialist paediatric palliative care,[26] ideally with advice from a paediatric pharmacist.

Individualized symptom management plans can facilitate communication and consistency of care across different settings.

As far as possible, drugs should be prescribed within the terms of their marketing authorization.[27] However, as in adult palliative care, there are many occasions when it is necessary to prescribe drugs 'off-label', i.e. beyond their authorized indications and/or routes of administration (see see p.xix). Indeed, because historically there has been little or no incentive to research the paediatric use of drugs, few are authorized for use in children or for indications for which they are regularly used.

Fortunately, there are several respected sources providing guidance about prescribing for children generally[28–31], for neonates[32] and more specifically in palliative care.[17,33,34] A Master Formulary is available from the Association for Paediatric Palliative Medicine.[35]

There is still a dearth of paediatric data for pharmacokinetics, pharmacodynamics, and drug safety.[36] In order to increase the body of knowledge, significant undesirable effects in children should be reported:

- in UK:
  - ▷ through the Yellow Card Scheme, www.yellowcard.gov.uk
  - ▷ through the PaedPalCare electronic care forum, www.togetherforshortlives.org.uk/professionals/care_provision/care_forum
- other countries have similar national and specialist reporting schemes, e.g.:
  - ▷ FDA Medwatch, www.fda.gov/safety/medwatch/default.htm(USA)
  - ▷ Medeffect, www.hc-sc.gc.ca/dhp-mps/medeff/index-eng.php (Canada)
  - ▷ Canadian Network of Palliative Care for Children, http://cnpcc.ca/
  - ▷ pediatric pain mailing list, http://pediatric-pain.ca/pediatric-pain-mailing-list (Canada)
- to www.palliativedrugs.com.

Extra care is required when prescribing for children:
- consider non-drug options, and prescribe only if there is a definite indication
- become familiar with a limited range of drugs and their effects in children
- simplify regimens as much as possible[6]
- try to avoid the need to administer drugs at school
- check dose calculations
- consider rounding down to the nearest dose that is practical to administer.

Children should be involved (at a level appropriate to their age and understanding) in decisions about taking drugs. Children are at increased risk of medication errors because of:
- lack of evidence-based data
- the diversity and rarity of their conditions
- the need to calculate and adjust the dose for the age and/or weight of the child
- the lack of suitable dose formulations
- variations in recommended doses and administration regimens
- inconsistent presentation of recommended dose information (e.g. microgram/kg per dose, microgram/kg/h, mg per dose, total 24h dose).

Particular care is required when prescribing in the neonatal period (prematurity and first 28 days of life) because of immature renal function and liver enzyme pathways, immature reticular activating systems, and differing volumes of distribution.

Deciding the dose

Paediatric dosing needs to be based on the physiological characteristics of the child, and the pharmacokinetics of the drug.[30,37] Dosing by age may be misleading, particularly in palliative care where, because of underlying disease, children are unlikely to be close to the mean weight for their age. Thus, generally, the dose is better determined by *body weight* than by age.

Using body surface area is more accurate because it tends to mirror physiological processes more closely, and this should be used particularly when calculating doses of cytotoxic drugs. Generally, doses in children should not exceed the maximum adult dose.

There is little evidence-based data for drug doses in children, and practice has often evolved from personal experience and case series. Flexible personalized schedules are acceptable for many drugs so as to make it as straightforward as possible for the child, and thus increase adherence to the regimen and minimize disruption to schooling and sleep. However, regular timing is important for some drugs, e.g. IV antibacterials.

Drug formulation and administration

Most children are able to take medicines orally, and many continue to do so throughout their illness. An oral liquid may be easier to administer than tablets or capsules, particularly for young children who are very unwell and/or have dysphagia. An oral syringe should be used for accurate measurement of oral liquids. However, some children may find tablets preferable to unpleasant tasting oral liquids, particularly if large volumes are needed.

Alternatively, it may be possible to mask the taste of unpleasant oral liquids/tablets by adding *small* quantities of food or fruit juice immediately before administration. However, medication should not be added to a feeding bottle or left mixed with food or fruit juice. For advice on suitable alternative formulations and ways of aiding administration, see Chapter 22, p.725 or discuss with a clinical pharmacist.

Many tablets (but *not* m/r ones) can be split, cut or crushed to aid dosing or administration. Although not recommended by the manufacturers, some matrix (but not reservoir) patches can be cut.[35]

The use of alternative routes of administration (buccal, intranasal, inhaled, PR, SC, IV) is relatively common in children. These routes avoid both degradation by gastric acid and first-pass metabolism by the liver. Some children already have a central venous line which can be accessed by carers. If available, this route is generally the most appropriate for continuous infusions. However, absorption can be affected by other factors, e.g. drug concentration and venous drainage of mucosal tissue, resulting in significant inter-patient variability in drug effect. With both buccal and intranasal administration, some swallowing of the drug is possible, leading to delayed absorption.[31]

IM administration is particularly distressing for children, and should generally be avoided. SC administration may be appropriate and acceptable for children, and is the route of choice for continuous infusions if there is no permanent central venous access.

Many seriously ill children are fed by nasogastric tube or gastrostomy, and these may provide an alternative route of drug administration (see Chapter 22, p.725). Vigilance is required because close to death GI absorption may be impaired. There is also the risk that drugs may continue to be administered via a feeding tube, even when no longer necessary or appropriate. Regular review is essential.

Pharmacokinetics and pharmacodynamics

Note: paediatric dosing based on weight alone may result in too small a dose in infants and children (because elimination does not change in direct proportion to weight), and too large a dose in neonates (who have immature drug elimination pathways).[38] Compared with adults, children under 12 years tend to absorb and metabolize drugs differently.

Neonates (< 1 month)

Relatively low renal and hepatic clearances, and higher volumes of distribution, result in a prolonged halflife for many drugs. This may necessitate lower doses at longer intervals (compared with infants and children, on a weight for weight basis). Neonates also have less fat and muscle, and increased bio-availability. Drugs primarily metabolized by the liver should be administered with extreme care until the age of 2 months.[37]

Immaturity also affects pharmacodynamics, e.g. there are postnatal changes in morphine receptors[39] and β_2-adrenoreceptors, but their clinical impact for prescribing purposes is poorly understood. Paradoxical reactions to benzodiazepines have also been observed in neonates, particularly in premature infants, probably due to a maturational effect of $GABA_A$ receptors.[40,41]

Infants and children (1 month-12 years)

Relatively high drug clearances, and normal volumes of distribution result in a shorter halflife for many drugs. This may necessitate relatively higher doses at shorter intervals (compared with adults). In infants, liver enzyme systems may still not be fully developed, and metabolic pathways may differ from those in older children. For example, **alfentanil, midazolam, morphine** all have longer halflives in infants (also in neonates).[37]

Monitoring drug concentrations

Monitoring plasma drug concentrations is generally of limited value, and additional venepunctures are distressing for children. Monitor the plasma concentration only when dose adjustment on a clinical basis is known to be inadequate, e.g. **gentamicin, phenobarbital, phenytoin, teicoplanin**.

Specific cautions when prescribing for children
Anti-epileptics

Many children with life-limiting or life-threatening conditions are on complicated anti-epileptic regimens. Interactions are common between anti-epileptics, and are mostly caused by liver enzyme induction or inhibition. They are variable and unpredictable and may increase toxicity without a corresponding increase in anti-epileptic effect. Anti-epileptics also have significant interactions with other drugs (see Anti-epileptics, p.254 and Chapter 25, p.767). Specialist paediatric neurology advice is recommended when titrating or reducing anti-epileptics in children.

Generally, anti-epileptic medication should *not* be stopped in the terminal phase, although absorption and administration may prove unpredictable. An alternative route of administration, and the addition or substitution of SC **midazolam** or **phenobarbital** may be necessary. Some anti-epileptics (**carbamazepine, clonazepam, diazepam, lorazepam, phenobarbital** and **valproate**) can be given PR, but may require dose adjustment.[42] For example, the dose of **carbamazepine** should be increased by 25% when converting from PO to PR.[43]

Rectal administration may also be possible for **lamotrigine**[44] and **vigabatrin**, but strong evidence is lacking.

Corticosteroids

In paediatric palliative care, the commonest reason for prescribing a corticosteroid is headache and vomiting caused by raised intracranial pressure associated with progressive intracranial tumours. Compared with adults, children seem to experience a more rapid onset of relatively severe undesirable effects (particularly cushingoid facies, proximal myopathy, weight gain, and changes in mood and behaviour).

Specialist paediatric palliative care teams now advocate short courses of corticosteroids (e.g. **dexamethasone** ≤500microgram/kg/day for 3–5 days for symptoms related to raised intracranial pressure):[35] this approach may often provide adequate symptom relief and causes less toxicity than continuous dosing. Following careful discussion of treatment goals, this can be repeated if necessary.[45]

Occasionally, continuous dosing may be required to achieve symptom control. In view of increased undesirable effects and increased difficulty in weaning a child off corticosteroids, continuous dosing should be at the lowest effective dose and for the shortest time possible.[46,47] A gastroprotective drug may need to be prescribed concurrently.

Codeine

Codeine is no longer recommended for the management of pain in children because of genetic variability in metabolism, affecting efficacy, undesirable effects and safety.[48,49] In particular, ultrafast metabolizers are vulnerable to potentially fatal respiratory depression. Recent World Health Organization guidance[50] now recommends for children a 2-step rather than 3-step analgesic ladder by removing the original second (weak opioid) step.

In Europe, codeine now has very limited indications for analgesic use in children: only for those > 12 years of age and only for short-term treatment of acute moderate pain if other medications are ineffective.[51,52] It should not be used in children known to be ultrafast metabolizers or those with conditions associated with breathing difficulties.

Strong opioids

Strong opioids can generally be used safely in children, just as in adults, although this may require careful explanation to parents and carers to allay fears. The transmucosal route (buccal, SL) is often used for p.r.n. doses of **morphine, diamorphine** or **fentanyl** to relieve break-through (episodic) pain. As in adults, doses of transmucosal fentanyl products should be titrated against the child's pain. The needed dose may not correlate closely with background opioid requirements, although these should be taken into account.

The use of some drugs is limited in children by the lack of an appropriate formulation. However, when a convenient strength is available, **fentanyl** and **buprenorphine** patches are being increasingly used as a convenient long-acting opioid formulation for children. In view of the risk of fatal respiratory depression, TD medications should be used only in children already taking opioids regularly. Particular care should be exercised if a child becomes pyrexial because this is likely to accelerate the rate of diffusion from the patch.

Other than with inappropriately used TD products, there is little evidence of opioids causing serious respiratory depression in children when the dose is individually titrated against a child's pain, except in neonates. In this group, there is a documented incidence of late respiratory depression (> 4h after administration of immediate-release **morphine**).[53] Compared with doses in children aged 2–12 years, the recommended doses per kg are lower in those under 2 years, and much lower in neonates (< 1 month).

Of the undesirable effects of opioids, pruritus and urinary retention are probably more common, and nausea probably less common than in adults (although this may be under-diagnosed).[54]

Phenothiazines

Although evidence is sparse, children may have an age-related increased risk of dystonic reactions with D_2 antagonists, e.g. phenothiazines and **metoclopramide** (see p.242, also see Chapter 26, p.781). Such drugs should be used with caution particularly in those <20 years old.[55,56]

PRESCRIBING FOR THE ELDERLY

Particular care is required when prescribing for the elderly.[57] The following should be kept in mind:[58,59]

- *avoid drugs whenever possible:* always consider non-drug options first; prescribe drugs only when clearly indicated
- *simplify regimens:* avoid complicated or frequent dose regimens; whenever possible give medication once daily or b.d.
- *limit the range of drugs:* become familiar with the use of a limited range of drugs and their effects in the elderly[6]
- use the recommended starting and maximum drug doses for elderly patients. If prescribing off-label, or no specific recommendations are made, consider starting at about 50% of the normal adult dose
- review treatment goals of each co-morbid disease and adjust treatments accordingly
- consider withdrawing drugs for co-morbid disease one at a time to assess impact on symptoms
- avoid treating undesirable drug effects with additional drugs if possible
- conduct regular medication reviews and discuss and agree all changes with the patient and/or carer.

Drug formulation and administration

Frail elderly patients may have difficulty swallowing tablets. They should be instructed to take tablets or capsules with fluid in an upright position to minimize the possibility of them remaining in the mouth or oesophagus, and causing ulceration (e.g. NSAIDs, **temazepam**). Alternative formulations (e.g. liquid) or routes of administration (e.g. SC) may be preferable (see Chapter 22, p.725).

Polypharmacy

Elderly patients are more likely to be receiving multiple drugs for existing comorbid conditions. The addition of more drugs for symptom relief may affect adherence, and increases the risk of drug interactions (see Chapter 25, p.767) and adverse reactions.

Presentation of adverse drug reactions in the elderly may be atypical and non-specific, and mistakenly be attributed to the onset of a new medical problem. Elderly patients taking five or more drugs are at significantly increased risk of falls and delirium. Thus, drugs should be reviewed regularly and any of doubtful benefit should be stopped. These include drugs for primary and secondary prevention which become irrelevant for a patient with a poor prognosis, e.g. statins,[6] and drugs which do not treat symptoms caused by an underlying disease.[60,61]

Pharmacokinetics

With increasing age, several changes occur which influence the pharmacokinetics of many drugs. The most important of these is the progressive decline in renal function. Drugs are excreted more slowly and a lower dose may suffice, particularly those with a narrow therapeutic ratio, e.g. **digoxin** (see Renal impairment, p.654). Acute illness, particularly accompanied by dehydration, can lead to a rapid further reduction in renal clearance.

Reduction in liver size and blood flow may reduce hepatic metabolism. Thus, drugs with significant first-pass metabolism, e.g. **morphine, amitriptyline, glyceryl trinitrate**, may have a higher bioavailability and faster onset, necessitating initiation at lower doses and dosing at less frequent intervals. Reduction in lean body mass and increase in body fat will alter distribution of lipophilic drugs e.g. benzodiazepines and **fentanyl**. When first given, these drugs will be stored in body fat, reducing their initial effect, but repeated administration may lead to prolonged release and significantly increased drug plasma levels.[60]

Pharmacodynamics

The aging body shows increased sensitivity to drugs, e.g. **warfarin** and centrally-acting drugs such as opioids, benzodiazepines and antipsychotics. This increases the risk of delirium, postural hypotension and falls (Box E).

Box E   Specific cautions when prescribing for the elderly[62]

Antimuscarinics
Falls, delirium, urinary retention, constipation (see p.6).

Antihypertensives, digoxin, psychotropics
Undesirable effects are more common. Use smaller doses and monitor closely.

Diuretics
Do not use long-term to treat simple gravitational or hypoproteinaemic oedema.

Hypoglycaemics
Chlorpropamide (not UK) and glibenclamide are best avoided because of their long halflives.

Night sedatives (hypnotics)
Cognitive impairment, delirium, falls, fractures. Use a short course of a drug with a short halflife. There is no evidence that zopiclone or zolpidem are better tolerated.

Nitrofurantoin
Pulmonary toxicity; lack of efficacy in patients with creatinine clearance < 60mL/min due to inadequate drug concentration in urine.

NSAIDs
Serious or fatal GI bleeding is more common. A special hazard in patients with heart disease (fluid retention) or renal impairment (may exacerbate). Use non-drug methods and paracetamol before prescribing an NSAID in low dose, e.g. naproxen 250mg b.d. or ibuprofen 200–400mg t.d.s.

Tricyclic antidepressants
Postural hypotension, sedation, delirium, falls and femoral fracture (see p.196)

Warfarin
A lower maintenance dose is generally required, and the outcome of bleeding is often more serious.

HEPATIC IMPAIRMENT

Because the liver is the main site for the metabolism of most drugs, hepatic impairment, particularly when moderate-severe, may lead to changes in pharmacokinetics and pharmacodynamics.[63] These changes can include:
- increased bio-availability
- accumulation of drugs or metabolites
- prolonged halflife
- disruption of the blood-brain barrier resulting in higher CNS concentrations of some drugs.[64,65]

Such changes result from how the liver disease impacts on drug:
- absorption, e.g. reduced bile salts in cholestasis → reduced absorption of lipid soluble drugs
- distribution, e.g.:
  ▷ ascites → increased volume of distribution of water-soluble drugs
  ▷ hypo-albuminaemia → increased level of active unbound drug in those which are highly protein-bound (also see correcting phenytoin levels in hypo-albuminaemia, p.644)
- metabolism, e.g.:
  ▷ decreased hepatic blood flow and drug extraction → increased bio-availability
  ▷ decreased function of cytochrome P450 and other enzymes (see below) → increased bio-availability

- excretion, e.g.:
  ▷ cholestasis → reduced elimination of drugs excreted in bile
  ▷ hepatic and renal impairment can occur concurrently (hepatorenal syndrome, see below) → necessitates further consideration and caution
- pharmacodynamics; there may be altered sensitivity to the effects of drugs, e.g.:
  ▷ antihypertensives → increased risk of hypotension
  ▷ diuretics → reduced response
  ▷ NSAIDs → increased risk of GI bleeding; fluid retention
  ▷ opioids, benzodiazepines, psychotropics → increased sedation; may precipitate encephalopathy (see below)
  ▷ oral anticoagulants → increased risk of bleeding
  ▷ oral hypoglycaemics → increased risk of hypoglycaemia.

Hepatic metabolism involves:[66]
- *phase I:* cytochrome P450 enzymes in the endoplasmic reticulum (see Chapter 25, p.767)
- *phase II:* various enzymes, e.g. glucuronyl transferases, in the endoplasmic reticulum and cytosol
- *phase III:* active drug transport across cell membranes, e.g. P-glycoprotein.

The effect of liver disease on drug metabolism depends on:
- *drug:* generally the liver converts active lipophilic drugs into inactive hydrophilic metabolites for excretion by the kidneys; sometimes pro-drugs are metabolized into active forms, e.g. **codeine → morphine**
- *disease severity:* because of the large hepatic reserve, impaired hepatic elimination only occurs in severe disease
- *enzymes:* generally phase II enzymes are affected less than phase I enzymes, which are also affected to different degrees, e.g. CYP1A2, 2C19 > 2A6, 3A4 > 2C9, 2E1
- *disease process:* e.g. acute hepatitis impairs phase I > phase III, whereas the opposite occurs in cholestasis; drugs excreted unchanged in the bile, e.g. **rifampicin, fusidic acid**, may accumulate in cholestasis.

Severe and rapidly deteriorating liver disease impairs renal function (hepatorenal syndrome). However, even moderate hepatic impairment reduces renal clearance and will necessitate a reduction in dose of renally excreted drugs.[67] Serum creatinine is an insensitive guide to glomerular filtration rate (GFR) in patients with cirrhosis (reduced muscle mass; reduced conversion of creatine → creatinine). Ideally, creatinine clearance should be used, but it can overestimate GFR in cirrhosis.[66]

Many drugs can precipitate hepatic encephalopathy by causing sedation (e.g. opioids, benzodiazepines and psychotropics), hypokalaemia (e.g. diuretics, corticosteroids), or constipation (e.g. opioids).

Thus, in liver disease, the metabolism of different drugs is not uniformly affected, and it is not possible to predict from routine LFTs how the metabolism of a particular drug will be impaired. Despite this, for many drugs, there are few data on the effects of hepatic impairment on their metabolism; often this is limited to changes in halflife which occur in cirrhosis.

The Child-Pugh score

The Child-Pugh total score gives a general indication of the degree of hepatic impairment in cirrhosis, and is mainly used as a prognostic aid (Table 1). It stratifies into three classes: total score 5–6 = A; 7–9 = B; ≥10 = C.

Table 1   Child-Pugh Criteria of Liver Disease (see text for classification)

Factor	Units	Score of 1	Score of 2	Score of 3
Serum bilirubin	micromol/L	<34	34–51	>51
	mg/dL	<2	2–3	>3
Serum albumin	g/L	>35	30–35	<30
	g/dL	>3.5	3–3.5	<3
INR		<1.7	1.7–2.3	>2.3
Ascites		None	Easily controlled	Poorly controlled
Hepatic encephalopathy		None	Minimal	Advanced

Clinical recommendations

Hepatotoxic drugs should be avoided or used with extra care. Drugs causing dose-related toxicity do so at lower doses in patients with hepatic impairment, and drugs producing idiosyncratic reactions do so more frequently. Information on the halflives in cirrhosis or hepatic impairment of selected drugs is available elsewhere.[68]

Analgesics: Non-opioids

A single-dose study of **paracetamol** in patients with liver disease found that, in mild liver disease, plasma halflife was similar to that in healthy controls (predictable considering that **paracetamol** is eliminated principally by glucuronidation) but that, in severe liver failure, its halflife was nearly doubled.[69]

Aspirin and **ibuprofen** have similar pharmacokinetics in patients with moderate–severe liver disease.[70,71] On the other hand, **naproxen** has a greatly increased halflife in patients with hepatic disorders,[72] and it is recommended that the dose is halved.[64]

Analgesics: Opioids

Except for **morphine** and **buprenorphine**, the major metabolic pathway for most opioids is oxidation. This is reduced in patients with hepatic cirrhosis, resulting in:

- decreased drug clearance, particularly for **alfentanil, dextropropoxyphene, pentazocine, pethidine** (meperidine), and **tramadol** and/or
- increased oral bio-availability caused by a reduced first-pass metabolism, for **dextropropoxyphene, dihydrocodeine, pentazocine** and **pethidine**.[73]

Codeine, dextropropoxyphene and **pethidine** are generally best not used in moderate–severe hepatic impairment.[74] Care also needs to be taken to avoid constipation with opioids, as increased bowel transit time can result in increased ammonia absorption, and precipitate encephalopathy.[75]

To a large extent, **tramadol** and **codeine** are pro-drugs activated by metabolism in the liver. They are both best avoided in moderate-severe liver impairment.

There have been several studies on the plasma clearance and elimination halflife of **morphine** in patients with various degrees of hepatic failure or cirrhosis. More recent studies have found a decreased plasma clearance and prolonged elimination halflife in patients with cirrhosis, compared with patients without liver disease, thus necessitating a reduction in dose and a decreased frequency of administration.[74,76,77]

In end-stage cirrhosis, **oxycodone** has severely impaired elimination which returns to within normal limits after liver transplantation.[78] **Oxycodone** is best avoided in severe cirrhosis. In contrast, **fentanyl** pharmacokinetics are not altered.[79] This may be because of the large volume of distribution of **fentanyl**, with only a small fraction in the central compartment for hepatic uptake. In this case, its terminal halflife would better reflect its slow release from tissue depots rather than its hepatic elimination.[79] Thus, **fentanyl** may be the opioid of choice in patients with moderate–severe liver failure or cirrhosis.

Anti-arrthymics

The halflife of **lidocaine** and **mexiletine** is tripled in cirrhosis. Thus, if used, reduce the dose to 25% of the usual dose.[80]

Antibacterials

Most of the commonly used antibacterials seem to be safe when used for patients with liver disease. Although there is generally no need to alter the dose of **ampicillin** in cirrhosis, patients with co-existing renal impairment may need a reduced dose.[81] **Ceftriaxone** and **metronidazole** show no significant change in pharmacokinetics in patients with severe liver disease.[80]

Rifampicin is used to palliate the symptoms of cholestatic pruritus; its elimination halflife has been shown to be almost doubled in patients with severe hepatic impairment compared with controls.[82]

Antidepressants

The halflife of **amitriptyline** is unchanged, so the dose is unchanged.[80] In contrast, the dose of **fluoxetine** should be halved, and **paroxetine** should be started at a reduced dose.

Anti-emetics

There are few data on the halflife life changes for **cyclizine, haloperidol, metoclopramide** or **prochlorperazine**. However, **metoclopramide** is reported to be safe in liver failure.[83]

Clearance of **ondansetron** is progressively reduced with increasing hepatic impairment. Patients with severe hepatic impairment should have their dose of this drug limited to 8mg/24h.[84]

Anti-epileptics

In the presence of liver disease **carbamazepine** should be avoided.[85] The halflife of **valproate** is significantly prolonged in cirrhosis and in acute hepatitis, but generally it is not necessary to adjust the dose.[86] Thus it may be used with caution. There are no data for **gabapentin** or **pregabalin**.

Antipsychotics

There are limited data on the antipsychotics. It is known that **chlorpromazine** has an unchanged halflife, but there may be increased sensitivity to its effects.

Benzodiazepines

Sedatives have been implicated as common precipitants of coma in patients with hepatocellular disease,[87] even in usual doses.[88]

Midazolam is extensively metabolized in the liver via oxidation.[89] Elimination is significantly reduced in cirrhosis. However, the hypnotic effects were reported to be similar in both cirrhosis and healthy controls. Even so, it is best to start with a reduced dose of **midazolam** in advanced cirrhosis, and titrate as necessary.[89]

The halflife of **diazepam** in cirrhosis more than doubles.[90] Given its long halflife in healthy subjects (⩽5 days, with an active metabolite with a halflife of ⩽8 days), it should be used with great caution, preferably only p.r.n.

In contrast, **oxazepam** was found to have unaltered disposition and elimination in acute viral hepatitis and mild–moderate cirrhosis.[87] This may be partly because conjugation of the drug occurs in organs other than the liver. However, in patients with severe decompensated cirrhosis and encephalopathy, clearance is decreased.[91] Thus, although **oxazepam** can be used in normal doses in mild–moderate liver disease, great caution must be exercised in severe liver impairment.

No changes in the halflife of **lorazepam** and **temazepam** were shown in patients with cirrhosis.[88,92] This is not surprising because they are also eliminated through glucuronidation as opposed to oxidation. Hence there should be little change in dose.

Diuretics

Spironolactone and **furosemide** are commonly used to control ascites and oedema, and both have no major change in their pharmacokinetics in liver disease.[93,94] However, over-vigorous treatment of ascites in such patients may lead to dehydration and oliguria, which may impair drug elimination and cause problems.[93]

RENAL IMPAIRMENT

Renal impairment has important effects on both the pharmacokinetic and pharmacodynamic properties of many drugs. The most important is the effect on excretion of a drug or its metabolites (if active) leading to:
- accumulation of drug or metabolite
- a prolonged halflife
- a longer time to reach steady-state.

This is relevant in relation to, for example, **digoxin**, **gabapentin** and **pregabalin**, **insulin**, **lithium**, **LMWH**, some opioids and their metabolites, e.g. morphine-6-glucuronide.

Other aspects of pharmacokinetics which may be affected include:
- hypo-albuminaemia can lead to an increase in the proportion of free drug in highly protein-bound drugs, resulting in a greater therapeutic effect and, if the serum drug concentration is used to monitor treatment, difficulty in interpreting the results, e.g. **phenytoin** (see p.644)
- reduced efficacy of some drugs acting on the kidneys, e.g. diuretics
- increased sensitivity to the therapeutic and undesirable effects of some drugs, even if elimination is unimpaired, possibly through increased permeability of the blood-brain barrier in the presence of uraemia, e.g. psycho-active drugs

• increased nephrotoxic effect of a drug, e.g. **allopurinol**, aminoglycosides, **ciclosporin, lithium,** NSAIDs; this may be particularly important for patients with mild–moderate renal impairment which is made worse by such drugs.

Some of these problems can be overcome by:
• avoiding drugs which are nephrotoxic
• using alternative drugs which are not renally excreted
• reducing the total daily maintenance dose of a renally excreted drug, either by reducing the size of the individual doses or by increasing the interval between doses
• taking special care with drugs with a narrow therapeutic index, where undesirable effects are likely with accumulation of the drug or its metabolites.

Advice about opioid choice in patients with renal impairment is given in the generic monograph on Strong opioids (p.367).

Principles of dose adjustment in renal impairment

The need for dose reduction in renal impairment depends on the extent to which the drug and any active metabolite are renally excreted and how serious any undesirable effects of the drug may be:
• for drugs with minimal undesirable effects, a simple scheme for dose reduction is sufficient, i.e. start low and monitor for efficacy and toxicity
• for drugs with a small safety margin, dose adjustments should be based on a measure of renal function, e.g. creatinine clearance, often estimated using the Cockcroft-Gault formula (see below)
• for drugs where both efficacy and/or toxicity are closely related to serum concentration, ongoing treatment must be adjusted according to clinical response and serum concentration, e.g. **gentamicin.**

Measuring renal function

The glomerular filtration rate (GFR) is the best overall measure of renal function, but the most accurate ways of measuring GFR are impractical for routine use. Serum creatinine concentration has traditionally been used as a proxy but is only a rough guide because a significant proportion of renal function may be lost before creatinine levels rise above the upper limit of normal, particularly in patients with a low body muscle mass or low protein intake. One approach is to use a formula-based *estimation* of GFR (eGFR), which takes into account some of the factors that complicate serum creatinine interpretation, e.g. Modification of Diet in Renal Disease (MDRD) study formula.[95]

Screening for, assessing and monitoring renal disease

The 4-variable (serum creatinine, age, sex, and ethnic origin) MDRD study formula is the nationally adopted standard in England.[57] It is more accurate than the Cockcroft-Gault formula with 90% of estimates <60mL/min/1.73m^2 within 30% of the true value. Changes in MDRD eGFR are more reliable than single estimates, with a decrease of $\geqslant15$% likely to represent a true change in renal function.[95] Five stages of renal disease are categorized according to MDRD eGFR (Table 2).[96]

The MDRD eGFR is expressed as a normalized value, i.e. what that individual's GFR would be if they had a body surface area of 1.73m^2. *Thus, the MDRD eGFR is not generally considered appropriate for considering drug clearance and dose adjustment because this should be based on an individual's absolute GFR.* For example, for individuals with a body surface area <1.73m^2, the MDRD eGFR could overestimate renal function and potentially lead to drug overdosing, with the converse being true for individuals with a body surface area >1.73m^2. The MDRD formula may also be misleading in situations where creatinine production, volume of distribution or excretion rate are altered, and in patients with a clearance of <50mL/min.[97] Further, it has not been validated for use in:
• children
• pregnancy
• acute renal impairment
• oedematous states
• malnourished patients
• muscle wasting disease states
• amputees.

Table 2 Diagnostic stages of renal disease

Stage	eGFR (mL/min/1.73m²)	Description[a]
1	>90	Normal renal function but renal disease based on urine findings, or presence of structural abnormalities or genetic trait
2	60–89	Mildly reduced renal function in the presence of renal disease (as above); in the absence of renal disease, an eGFR ≥60mL/min/1.73m² is considered normal
3	30–59	Moderately reduced renal function
4	15–29	Severely reduced renal function
5	<15	Very severe, established (end-stage) renal failure

a. evidence of damage or a reduced eGFR must be present for >3 months.

Thus, in palliative care patients who are elderly, malnourished, cachectic and/or oedematous, renal impairment may exist even when the serum creatinine or the MDRD eGFR are within normal limits, and it may be prudent to assume that there is at least mild renal impairment in such patients. Even when abnormal, the serum creatinine or the MDRD eGFR may both underestimate the actual degree of renal impairment.

Modifying drug dose based on renal function

In patients known to have chronic renal impairment or those at high risk of renal impairment, e.g. the elderly, and those with hypertension or diabetes, renal function should be checked before prescribing a drug which may need dose modification. A baseline serum creatinine and MDRD eGFR (bearing in mind the above limitations) can help to indicate the need for dose modification and serial measurements used to monitor the effect of the drug on renal function.

However, *when considering dose adjustment guidelines, creatinine clearance or an absolute MDRD eGFR should be calculated.* Because most dose adjustment guidelines are currently based on an estimated creatinine clearance using the Cockcroft-Gault formula, this should be used in preference. Alternatively, the MDRD eGFR can be converted to an absolute value:

Cockcroft-Gault formula

$$\text{Creatinine clearance} = \frac{F \times [140 - \text{age}] \times [\text{weight (kg)}]}{\text{serum creatinine (micromol/L)}}$$

F = 1.23 (male) or 1.04 (female)

Converting the MDRD eGFR to an absolute value:

Absolute eGFR (mL/min) = MDRD eGFR (mL/min/1.73m²) × (body surface area/1.73) (m²)

Body surface area (m²) = $\sqrt{((\text{height (cm)} \times \text{weight (kg)})/3600)}$

The Cockcroft-Gault formula, by taking weight rather than body surface area into account, tends to overestimate or underestimate creatinine clearance in obese and underweight patients respectively. As with the MDRD eGFR, it can be misleading in situations where creatinine production, volume of distribution or excretion rate are altered and similar precautions regarding the interpretation of results in palliative care patients will apply. It is not appropriate to use when renal function is changing rapidly.

Dose adjustment can then be made using the advice given in *PCF* or other resources such as the manufacturer's SPC, *The Renal Drug Handbook*,[98] *Drug Prescribing in Renal Failure*[99] and the *BNF.* It should be noted that the advice will vary.[100] For example, the *BNF* advice on dose adjustment is now generally expressed in terms of MDRD eGFR. Nonetheless, it points out that this:

• should not be used to adjust doses of nephrotoxic drugs or drugs with a narrow therapeutic index; use instead serum drug concentrations or creatinine clearance calculated using the Cockcroft-Gault formula
• should not be used to adjust drug doses in patients at both extremes of weight; use instead the absolute GFR or creatinine clearance calculated using the Cockcroft-Gault formula
• is not validated for use in children under 18 years.

PCF favours the dose adjustment guidance in *The Renal Drug Handbook* (generally based on creatinine clearance calculated using the Cockcroft-Gault formula) and reflects this unless stated otherwise. Nonetheless, given the limitations of the estimates of creatinine clearance, any guidance should be regarded only as useful approximations of a safe starting dose. Subsequent further adjustments are then based on response and undesirable effects, with monitoring of serum drug concentrations undertaken when appropriate.[101]

For *prescribing purposes*, renal impairment is generally arbitrarily divided into mild, moderate and severe, corresponding to creatinine clearances of 20–50mL/min, 10–20mL/min and <10mL/min respectively. However, the cut-off points vary slightly between sources.

When a drug dose modification has been necessary, or for drugs known to cause renal impairment, a clinical review and evaluation of renal function should be carried out within 2 weeks, or at any time if drug-induced nephrotoxicity is suspected, e.g. symptoms such as rash, arthralgia, oedema.[95]

Patients requiring dialysis

For guidance on drug use in dialysis, generally consult specialist renal pharmacists and/or the literature. For example, because dialysis can remove **gabapentin**, a low dose is given after each dialysis session.

TRANSDERMAL PATCHES AND MRI

Broadly speaking, TD patches contain the drug either in a reservoir or embedded within a matrix. This is protected by a backing on the outside, and a removable release-liner covering the adhesive surface to be applied to the skin. Some TD patches contain metal in their backing (Box F). This is potentially dangerous because, if such a patch is worn during MRI, the patient may develop a burn under the patch.[102,103]

Thus, TD patches with metal in the backing must be removed immediately before MRI, and replaced with a new patch immediately afterwards (Box F). Although some patches have metal in the release-liner, this is irrelevant because the release-liner is removed before application. *If in doubt, double-check.*

Box F is correct as of March 2014 for products distributed *in the UK.* For other countries, check the product literature, and/or contact the manufacturer directly.

Box F   TD patches (UK) and MRI, compiled from manufacturers' information (March 2014)

Need to remove before MRI	No need to remove before MRI
Some buprenorphine patches	Some buprenorphine patches
Hapoctasin®	BuTrans®, Transtec®
Clonidine	Capsaicin – Qutenza®
Catapres TTS®; not UK but may be	Estradiol ± progestogen HRT
imported, US product contains metal[104]	(hormone replacement therapy)
Hyoscine – Scopoderm TTS®	Elleste Solo MX®, Estraderm MX®,

continued

Box F   *Continued*

Some nicotine patches	Estraderm TTS®, Estradot®, Evorel®,
Boots NicAssist®, Lloyd's Pharmacy generic,	Evorel Conti®, Evorel Sequi®, FemSeven®,
NicAid®, Nicotinell TTS®, NiQuitin®	FemSeven Conti®, FemSeven Sequi®,
Rotigotine	Femtarix®, Progynova TS®
Neupro® for Parkinson's disease	Ethinylestradiol + norelgestromin for
or restless legs syndrome	contraception – Evra®
	Fentanyl
Contain metal salts; manufacturers	Durogesic DTrans® and all UK generics
advise removal before MRI	Glyceryl trinitrate
Diclofenac – Voltarol gel patch®	Deponit®, Minitran®, Nitro-Dur®,
Lidocaine – Versatis®	Transiderm-Nitro®
Some nicotine patches	Granisetron – Sancuso®
Boots NicAssist Translucent®,	Menthol – Deep Freeze®
Nicorette Invisi®	Some nicotine patches
Salicylic acid	NiQuitin Clear®, NiQuitin Pre-Quit Clear®
Scholl® callous removal pads, Scholl®	Oxybutynin – Kentera®
corn pads/plasters, Scholl® verruca	Rivastigmine – Exelon®
removal plasters	Testosterone – Intrinsa®

1   Rothschild JM et al. (2002) Analysis of medication-related malpractice claims: causes, preventability, and costs. *Archives of Internal Medicine.* **162**: 2414–2420.

2   Spinewine A et al. (2005) Appropriateness of use of medicines in elderly inpatients: qualitative study. *British Medical Journal.* **331**: 935.

3   Kanjanarat P et al. (2003) Nature of preventable adverse drug events in hospitals: a literature review. *American Journal of Health System Pharmacy.* **60**: 1750–1759.

4   Jones TA and Como JA (2003) Assessment of medication errors that involved drug allergies at a university hospital. *Pharmacotherapy.* **23**: 855–860.

5   Neale G et al. (2001) Exploring the causes of adverse events in NHS hospital practice. *Journal of the Royal Society of Medicine.* **94**: 322–330.

6   Duerden M et al. (2013) Polypharmacy and medicines optimisation: making it safe and sound. Kings Fund, London. www.kingsfund.org.uk

7   British National Formulary Appendix 3: Cautionary and advisory lables for dispensed medicines London: BMJ Group and Pharmaceutical Press www.bnf.org (accessed April 2013).

8   Sweetman SC. *Martindale: The Complete Drug Reference.* London: Pharmaceutical Press www.medicinescomplete.com

9   Royal Pharmaceutical Society (2012) Keeping patients safe when they transfer between care providers - getting the medicines right. Appendix 2: Good Practice Guidance for Healthcare Professionals. Final report. London.

10 Dean B et al. (2002) Causes of prescribing errors in hospital inpatients: a prospective study. *Lancet.* **359**: 1373–1378.

11 Ashley C and Currie A (2004) *The Renal Drug Handbook* (2e). Radcliffe Medical Press Ltd, Oxford.

12 NHS Lothian (2009) Patients and or carers administration of subcutaneous drugs by intermittent injections: adult palliative care. Protocol, procedure and teaching guideline version 2.

13 Nursing and Midwifery Council (2007) Standards for medicines management. Available from: www.nmc-uk.org

14 Lau DT et al. (2012) Hospice providers' key approaches to support informal caregivers in managing medications for patients in private residences. *Journal of Pain and Symptom Management.* **43**: 1060–1071.

15 Bradford and Airedale NHS Trust (2006) Subcutaneous drug administration by carers (adult palliative care). Available from: www.palliativedrugs.com document library

16 NHS National Prescribing Centre (2009) A guide to good practice in the management of controlled drugs in primary care (England) 3rd Edition.

17 International Children's Palliative Care Network (2008). Available from: www.icpcn.org.uk

18 Fraser LK et al. (2012) Rising national prevalence of life-limiting conditions in children in England. *Pediatrics.* **129**: e923–929.

19 Regnard C et al. (2007) Understanding distress in people with severe communication difficulties: developing and assessing the Disability Distress Assessment Tool (DisDAT). *Journal of Intellectual Disability Research.* **51**: 277–292.

20 Regnard C et al. (2003) Difficulties in identifying distress and its causes in people with severe communication problems. *International Journal of Palliative Nursing.* **9**: 173–176.

21 Herr K et al. (2006) Pain assessment in the nonverbal patient: position statement with clinical practice recommendations. *Pain Management Nursing.* **7**: 44–52.

22 Wong D and Baker C (1988) Pain in children: comparison of assessment scales. *Pediatric Nursing.* **14**: 9017.

23 von Baeyer CL and Spagrud LJ (2007) Systematic review of observational (behavioral) measures of pain for children and adolescents aged 3 to 18 years. *Pain.* **127**: 140–150.

24 von Baeyer CL (2009) Children's self-report of pain intensity: what we know, where we are headed. *Pain Res Manag.* **14**: 39–45.

25 EAPC Taskforce (2007) IMPaCCT: Standards for paediatric palliative care in Europe. *European Journal of Palliative Care.* **14**: 109–114.

26 Department of Health (2008) Better Care. Better Lives. Available from: https://www.gov.uk/government/organisations/department-of-health

27 AAP (American Academy of Pediatrics) (2006) Uses of drugs not described in the package insert (off-label uses). Available from: www.aap.org

28 Royal College of Paediatrics and Child Health (RCPCH) (2007) Medicines for Children (3e). RCPCH, London.

29 General Medical Council (GMC) (2007) 0-18. Guidance for all doctors. Available from: www.gmc-uk.org

30 British National Formulary for Children. London: BMJ Group and Pharmaceutical Press www.bnf.org (accessed April 2013).

31 Ballantine N and Bing Daglish E (2012) Chapter 17. Using Medications in Children. In: A Golman et al. (eds) Oxford Textbook of Palliative Care for Children 2e. Oxford University Press, Oxford.

32 Neonatal Formulary (2007) NNF5. Available from: www.neonatalformulary.com

33 Hain R and Jassal S (2010) Paediatric Palliative Medicine. Oxford Specialist Handbooks in Paediatrics. Oxford University Press, Oxford.

34 Jassal. S (2011) Basic symptom control in paediatric palliative care: the Rainbows Children's Hospice Guideleunes. 8e. Available from: http://www.togetherforshortlives.org.uk

35 Jassal S and Hain RD (2014) Association for Paediatric Medicine Master Formulary. Available from: www.appm.org.uk/10.html

36 Stephenson T (2005) How children's responses to drugs differ from adults. British Journal of Clinical Pharmacology. 59: 670–673.

37 Bartelink IH et al. (2006) Guidelines on paediatric dosing on the basis of developmental physiology and pharmacokinetic considerations. Clinical Pharmacokinetics. 45: 1077–1097.

38 Anderson BJ and Holford NH (2013) Understanding dosing: children are small adults, neonates are immature children. Archives of Disease in Childhood. 98: 737–744.

39 Nandi R et al. (2004) The functional expression of mu opioid receptors on sensory neurons is developmentally regulated; morphine analgesia is less selective in the neonate. Pain. 111: 38–50.

40 Waisman D et al. (1999) Myoclonic movements in very low birth weight premature infants associated with midazolam intravenous bolus administration. Pediatrics. 104: 579.

41 Ng E et al. (2002) Safety of benzodiazepines in newborns. Annals of Pharmacotherapy. 36: 1150–1155.

42 Smith S et al. (2001) Guidelines for rectal administration of anticonvulsant medication in children. Paediatric and Perinatal Drug Therapy. 4: 140–147.

43 Arvidsson J et al. (1995) Replacing carbamazepine slow-release tablets with carbamazepine suppositories: a pharmacokinetic and clinical study in children with epilepsy. Journal of Child Neurology. 10: 114–117.

44 Birnbaum AK et al. (2000) Rectal absorption of lamotrigine compressed tablets. Epilepsia. 41: 850–853.

45 Harrop E and Sen G (2010) The use of dexamethasone in children referred to a tertoary palliative care service who died from inoperable brain tumours over a 2 year period. What can we learn? Presented at - Cardiff International Conference for Paediatric Palliative Care.

46 Waterson G (2006) Corticosteroids in the palliative phase of brain tumours. Archives of Disease in Childhood. 86 (Suppl 1): A76.

47 Glaser AW et al. (1997) Corticosteroids in the management of central nervous system tumours. Kids Neuro-Oncology Workshop (KNOWS). Archives of Disease in Childhood. 76: 76–78.

48 Williams DG et al. (2001) Codeine phosphate in paediatric medicine. British Journal of Anaesthesia. 86: 413–421.

49 Tremlett M et al. (2010) Pro-con debate: is codeine a drug that still has a useful role in pediatric practice? Paediatric Anaesthesia. 20: 183–194.

50 World Health Organisation (2012) WHO guidelines on persisting pain in children with medical illnesses. Available from: www.who.int/medicines/areas/quality_safety/guide_perspainchild/en/

51 European Medicines Agency (2013) PRAC (Pharmacovigilance Risk Assessment Committee) recommends restricting the use of codeine when used for pain relief in children.

52 MHRA (2013) Codeine: restricted use as an analgesic in children and adolescents after European safety review. Drug Safety Update. 6. www.mhra.gov.uk/safetyinformation

53 Zernikow B et al. (2006) Paediatric cancer pain management using the WHO analgesic ladder-results of a prospective analysis from 2265 treatment days during a quality improvement study. European Journal of Pain. 10: 587–595.

54 Hain RDW (2006) Pharmacodynamics of morphine and M6G in children with cancer: analgesia and adverse effects. International Conference in Paediatric Palliative Care.

55 Grosset KA and Grosset DG (2004) Prescribed drugs and neurological complications. Journal of Neurology, Neurosurgery, and Psychiatry. 75 (Suppl 3): iii2–8.

56 van Harten PN et al. (1999) Acute dystonia induced by drug treatment. British Medical Journal. 319: 623–626.

57 DoH (2001) National Service Framework for Older People. HMSO, London.

58 Milton JC et al. (2008) Prescribing for older people. British Medical Journal. 336: 606–609.

59 Cruz-Jentoft AJ et al. (2012) Drug therapy optimization at the end of life. Drugs Aging. 29: 511–521.

60 Hubbard RE et al. (2013) Medication prescribing in frail older people. European Journal of Clinical Pharmacology. 69: 319–326.

61 Petrovic M et al. (2012) Adverse drug reactions in older people: detection and prevention. Drugs Aging. 29: 453–462.

62 Fink et al. (2012) American Geriatrics Society updated Beers Criteria for potentially inappropriate medication use in older adults. Journal of the American Geriatrics Society. 60: 616–631.

63 Bower M et al. (2010) Endocrine and metabolic complications of advanced cancer. In: Hanks G et al. (eds) Oxford Textbook of Palliative Medicine (4e). Oxford University Press, Oxford, pp. 1015–1033.

64 Williams RL et al. Naproxen disposition in patients with alcoholic cirrhosis. European Journal of Clinical Pharmacology. 27:291–6, 1984.

65 Garg RK (2005) Anesthetic considerations in patients with hepatic failure. International Anesthesiology Clinics. 43: 45–63.

66 Pirmohamed M (2006) Prescribing in liver disease. Medicine. 35: 31–33.

67 Morgan TR et al. (1995) Protein consumption and hepatic encephalopathy in alcoholic hepatitis. VA Cooperative Study Group #275. Journal of the American College of Nutrition. 14: 152–158.

68 Rhee C and Broadbent AM (2007) Palliation and liver failure: Palliative medications dosage guidelines. Journal of Palliative Medicine. 10: 677–685.

69 Forrest JA et al. (1979) Paracetamol metabolism in chronic liver disease. European Journal of Clinical Pharmacology. 15: 427–431.

70 Roberts MS et al. (1983) Pharmacokinetics of aspirin and salicylate in elderly subjects and in patients with alcoholic liver disease. European Journal of Clinical Pharmacology. 25: 253–261.

71 Juhl RP et al. (1983) Ibuprofen and sulindac kinetics in alcoholic liver disease. Clinical Pharmacology and Therapeutics. 34: 104–109.
72 Calvo MV et al. (1980) Naproxen disposition in hepatic and biliary disorders. International Journal of Clinical Pharmacology, Therapy and Toxicology. 18: 242–246.
73 Pond SM et al. (1980) Enhanced bioavailability of pethidine and pentazocine in patients with cirrhosis of the liver. Australian and New Zealand Journal of Medicine. 10: 515–519.
74 Tegeder I et al. (1999) Pharmacokinetics of opioids in liver disease. Clinical Pharmacokinetics. 37: 17–40.
75 Riordan SM and Williams R (1997) Treatment of hepatic encephalopathy. New England Journal of Medicine. 337: 473–479.
76 Crotty B et al. (1989) Hepatic extraction of morphine is impaired in cirrhosis. European Journal of Clinical Pharmacology. 36: 501–506.
77 Hasselstrom J et al. (1990) The metabolism and bioavailability of morphine in patients with severe liver cirrhosis. British Journal of Clinical Pharmacology. 29: 289–297.
78 Tallgren M et al. (1997) Pharmacokinetics and ventilatory effects of oxycodone before and after liver transplantation. Clinical Pharmacology and Therapeutics. 61: 655–661.
79 Haberer JP et al. (1982) Fentanyl pharmacokinetics in anaesthetized patients with cirrhosis. British Journal of Anaesthesia. 54: 1267–1270.
80 Bass NM and Williams RL (1988) Guide to drug dosage in hepatic disease. Clinical Pharmacokinetics. 15: 396–420.
81 Lewis GP and Jusko WJ (1975) Pharmacokinetics of ampicillin in cirrhosis. Clinical Pharmacology and Therapeutics. 18: 475–484.
82 Acocella G et al. (1972) Kinetics of rifampicin and isoniazid administered alone and in combination to normal subjects and patients with liver disease. Gut. 13: 47–53.
83 Uribe M et al. (1985) Successful administration of metoclopramide for the treatment of nausea in patients with advanced liver disease. A double-blind controlled trial. Gastroenterology. 88: 757–762.
84 Figg WD et al. (1996) Pharmacokinetics of ondansetron in patients with hepatic insufficiency. Journal of Clinical Pharmacology. 36: 206–215.
85 Micromedex (2005) Micromedex health series Vol 125. Available from: www.micromedex.com
86 Klotz U et al. (1978) Disposition of valproic acid in patients with liver disease. European Journal of Clinical Pharmacology. 13: 55–60.
87 Shull HJ et al. (1976) Normal disposition of oxazepam in acute viral hepatitis and cirrhosis. Annals of internal medicine. 84: 420–425.
88 Kraus JW et al. (1978) Effects of aging and liver disease on disposition of lorazepam. Clinical Pharmacology and Therapeutics. 24: 411–419.
89 Pentikainen PJ et al. (1989) Pharmacokinetics of midazolam following intravenous and oral administration in patients with chronic liver disease and in healthy subjects. Journal of Clinical Pharmacology. 29: 272–277.
90 Klotz U et al. (1975) The effects of age and liver disease on the disposition and elimination of diazepam in adult man. Journal of Clinical Investigation. 55: 347–359.
91 Sonne J et al. (1990) Glucuronidation of oxazepam is not spared in patients with hepatic encephalopathy. Hepatology. 11: 951–956.
92 Ghabrial H et al. (1986) The effects of age and chronic liver disease on the elimination of temazepam. European Journal of Clinical Pharmacology. 30: 93–97.
93 Abshagen U et al. (1977) Disposition kinetics of spironolactone in hepatic failure after single doses and prolonged treatment. European Journal of Clinical Pharmacology. 11: 169–176.
94 Verbeeck RK et al. (1982) Furosemide disposition in cirrhosis. Clinical Pharmacology and Therapeutics. 31: 719–725.
95 Anonymous (2006) The patient, the drug and the kidney. Drug and Therapeutics Bulletin. 44: 89–95.
96 Royal College of Physicians of London and Renal Association (2006) Chronic Kidney disease in adults: UK guidelines for identification, management and referral. Available from: www.renal.org
97 Holweger K et al. (2008) Novel algorithm for more accurate calculation of renal function in adults with cancer. Annals of Pharmacotherapy. 42: 1749–1757.
98 Ashley C and Currie A (2009) The Renal Drug Handbook (3e). Radcliffe Publishing Ltd, Oxford.
99 Brier M and Aronoff G (2007) Drug Prescribing in Renal Failure 5e. ACP Press, Philadelphia.
100 Vidal L et al. (2005) Systematic comparison of four sources of drug information regarding adjustment of dose for renal function. British Medical Journal. 331: 263.
101 Davison SN et al. (2010) Management of pain in renal failure. In: EJ Chambers et al. (eds) Supportive Care for the Renal Patient (2e). Oxford University Press, Oxford, pp. 139–188.
102 Institute for Safe Medication Practices (2004) Medication Safety Alert. Burns in MRI patients wearing transdermal patches. Available from: www.ismp.org/Newsletters/acutecare/articles/20040408.asp?ptr = y
103 MHRA (2007) Device Bulletin. Safety guidelines for magnetic resonance imaging equipment in clinical use. DB2007(03). MHRA and Department of Health, London, p. 46.
104 Hulisz DT (2008) Are topical patches safe during MRI or CT Scans? Medscape Pharmacists. Available from: www.medscape.com

Updated June 2014

15: OPIOID DOSE CONVERSION RATIOS

General approach

It is crucial to appreciate that conversion ratios are *never* more than an approximate guide. Thus, careful monitoring during conversion is necessary to avoid both underdosing and excessive dosing. Also see Opioid switching ('rotation'), p.365.

This chapter provides a summary of selected opioid dose conversion ratios. These can be used to calculate equivalent doses of opioids when switching from a weak opioid to **morphine**, or from one strong opioid to another. Caution is always necessary. Conversion ratios are *never* more than an approximate guide because of:
- wide interindividual variation in opioid pharmacokinetics; influencing factors include age, ethnicity, renal or hepatic impairment
- other variables including dose and duration of opioid treatment, direction of switch in opioid, nutritional status and concurrent medications
- their method of derivation, e.g. single dose rather than chronic dose studies using a range of clinical doses.

Careful monitoring is particularly necessary when:
- switching at high doses
- there has been a recent rapid escalation of the first opioid
- switching to **methadone**.

Explicit guidance on switching opioids is difficult because both the reasons for switching and the patient's circumstances differ. One guideline, based on expert consensus, recommends routinely reducing the calculated equivalent dose of the new opioid by 25–50% (see p.365). Various patient factors are then taken into account to modify the rule, e.g. no reduction in a young patient in severe pain switching at low dose, or an even bigger reduction in an older delirious patient in moderate pain switching at high dose.

Certainly, a dose reduction of at least 50% would seem prudent when switching at high doses (e.g. **morphine** or equivalent doses of $\geqslant$ 1g/24h), in elderly or frail patients, because of intolerable undesirable effects (e.g. delirium), or when there has been a recent rapid escalation of the first opioid (possibly due to opioid-induced hyperalgesia). In such circumstances, p.r.n. doses can be relied on to make up any deficit while re-titrating to a satisfactory dose of the new opioid.

A separate strategy is necessary for **methadone** (see p.433).

Determining the dose of the second opioid

Select the appropriate Table based on the routes of administration:

Route	Table	Page
PO to PO	1	663
PO to TD	2	664
PO to SC/IV	3	667
SC/IV to SC/IV	4	668

The Tables relate mainly to switching to or from **morphine**. If switching from an opioid other than **morphine** to another opioid, it will be necessary to convert the dose of the first opioid to **morphine** equivalents, and then use that quantity to determine the dose of the second opioid. With any switch:

- round the calculated dose up or down to the nearest convenient dose of the formulation concerned, e.g. tablet, TD patch, ampoule
- decide on an appropriate p.r.n. dose.

The conversion ratios in this chapter are based on referenced sources given in the various individual opioid monographs. Where these differ significantly from the manufacturers' recommended ratios, the latter are included for comparison.

Updated June 2014

Table 1 PCF recommended dose conversion ratios: PO to PO. Before use, see General approach (p.661)

Conversion	Ratio	Calculation	Example	Monograph
Codeine to morphine	10:1	Divide 24h codeine dose by 10	Codeine 240mg/24h PO → morphine 24mg/24h PO	Codeine, p.348
Dihydrocodeine to morphine	10:1	Divide 24h dihydrocodeine dose by 10	Dihydrocodeine 240mg/24h PO → morphine 24mg/24h PO	Dihydrocodeine, p.350
Hydrocodone to morphine	1.5:1	Divide 24h hydrocodone dose by 1.5 (decrease dose by 1/3)	Hydrocodone 60mg/24h PO → morphine 40mg/24h PO	Not UK
Tramadol to morphine	10:1	Divide 24h tramadol dose by 10	Tramadol 400mg/24h PO → morphine 40mg/24h PO	Tramadol, p.352
Morphine to hydromorphone	5:1	Divide 24h morphine dose by 5	Morphine 60mg/24h PO → hydromorphone 12mg/24h PO	Hydromorphone, p.430
	7.5:1[a]	*Divide 24h morphine dose by 7.5*	*Morphine 60mg/24h PO → hydromorphone 8mg/24h PO*	Hydromorphone, p.430
Morphine to methadone	Variable	See methadone, p.433		
Morphine to oxycodone	1.5:1	Divide 24h morphine dose by 1.5 (decrease dose by 1/3)	Morphine 60mg/24h PO → oxycodone 40mg/24h PO	Oxycodone, p.442
	2:1[a]	*Divide 24h morphine dose by 2*	*Morphine 60mg/24h PO → oxycodone 30mg/24h PO*	Oxycodone, p.442

a. italicized entries = manufacturers' recommendations.

Table 2 PCF recommended dose conversion ratios: PO to TD. Before use, see General approach (p.661)

Conversion	Ratio	Calculation	Example	Monograph
Morphine to buprenorphine	100:1	Multiply 24h morphine dose in mg by 10 to obtain 24h buprenorphine dose in microgram; divide answer by 24 to obtain microgram/h patch strength	Morphine 300mg/24h PO → buprenorphine 3,000microgram/24h → 125microgram/h; *round up to 70microgram/h × 2 or round down to* 70+35microgram/h patches	Buprenorphine, p.392
	75–115:1[a]	*Use the manufacturer's guidelines in SPC, summarized in Box A, p.665*		Buprenorphine, p.392
Morphine to fentanyl	100:1	Multiply 24h morphine dose in mg by 10 to obtain 24h fentanyl dose in microgram; divide answer by 24 to obtain microgram/h patch strength	Morphine 300mg/24h PO → fentanyl 3,000microgram/24h → 125microgram/h; give as 100+25microgram/h patches	Fentanyl, p.403
	100:1 or 150:1[a,b]	*Use the manufacturer's guidelines in SPC, summarized in Box B, p.666*	*For 150:1, the fentanyl dose will be smaller than that obtained with 100:1*	Fentanyl, p.403

a. italicized entries = manufacturers' recommendations
b. recommended ratio varies according to the duration of use of the previous strong opioid, see Box B, p.666.

For determining the appropriate p.r.n. morphine dose for patients receiving TD buprenorphine or TD fentanyl, see p.401 and p.411.

Box A Summary of manufacturers' recommendations for starting TD buprenorphine (for full details, see specific SPC)

BuTrans® 5, 10 and 20microgram/h TD buprenorphine patch
Patients aged 18 years and over
The lowest BuTrans® dose (BuTrans® 5microgram/h TD patch) should be used as the initial dose. Consideration should be given to the previous opioid history of the patient as well as to the current general condition and medical status of the patient.

Conversion from opioids
BuTrans® can be used as an alternative to treatment with other opioids. Such patients should be started on the lowest available dose (BuTrans® 5microgram/h TD patch) and continue taking short-acting supplemental analgesics during titration, as required.

Transtec® or Hapoctasin® 35, 52.5 and 70microgram/h TD buprenorphine patch
Patients over 18 years of age
The dose should be adapted to the condition of the individual patient (pain intensity, suffering, individual reaction). The lowest possible dose providing adequate pain relief should be given.

Conversion from opioids
Patients on a Step II (weak opioid) analgesic should begin with buprenorphine 35microgram/h TD. The administration of a non-opioid analgesic can be continued, depending on the patient's overall medical condition.

When switching from a Step III (strong opioid) analgesic to buprenorphine TD, the nature of the previous medication, administration and the mean daily dose should be taken into account in order to avoid the recurrence of pain. It is generally advisable to titrate the dose individually, starting with the lowest TD patch strength (35microgram/h). Clinical experience has shown that patients who were previously treated with higher doses of a strong opioid (approximately 120mg oral morphine per day) may start therapy with the next higher TD patch strength (i.e. 52.5microgram/h).

Sufficient supplementary immediate release analgesics should be made available during dose titration.

The necessary strength of buprenorphine TD must be adapted to the requirements of the individual patient and checked at regular intervals.

After application of the first buprenorphine TD patch the buprenorphine serum concentrations rise slowly and there is unlikely to be a rapid onset of effect. Consequently, a first evaluation of the analgesic effect should only be made after 24h.

The previous analgesic medication (with the exception of transdermal opioids) should be given in the same dose during the first 12h after switching to TD and appropriate rescue medication given on demand in the following 12h.

Box B Summary of manufacturer's recommendations for starting Durogesic DTrans® (for full details see SPC)[a]

Durogesic DTrans® 12/25/50/75/100microgram/h TD fentanyl patch
Adults:
Initial dose selection
The initial Durogesic DTrans® dose should be based on the patient's current opioid use and is recommended for use in patients who have demonstrated opioid tolerance. Other factors to be considered are the general condition and medical status of the patient.

In strong opioid-naïve patients, the initial dose of Durogesic DTrans® should not exceed 25microgram/h. However, due to limited clinical experience of its use in strong opioid-naïve patients, conversion to fentanyl TD is recommended only in those who are already opioid-tolerant.
In opioid-tolerant patients, the initial dose of Durogesic DTrans® should be based on the previous 24h opioid analgesic requirement. The recommended conversion ratio from oral morphine to Durogesic DTrans® varies according to the duration of use of the initial strong opioid as given below in Table 1 (several weeks) and Table 2 (highly opioid tolerant for a long period):

Table 1 Adults stabilized on strong opioid over *several weeks* (based on a conversion ratio of about 150:1)

Oral 24h morphine (mg/day)	Durogesic DTrans® (microgram/h)
<135	25
135–224	50
225–314	75
315–404	100
405–494	125
495–584	150
585–674	175
675–764	200
765–854	225
855–944	250
945–1034	275
1035–1124	300

Table 2 For highly opioid-tolerant adults on a stable and *well-tolerated* opioid regimen for a *long period* (based on a conversion ratio of about 100:1)

Oral 24h morphine (mg/day)	Durogesic DTrans® (microgram/h)
<44	12
45–89	25
90–149	50
150–209	75
210–269	100
270–329	125
330–389	150
390–449	175
450–509	200
510–569	225
570–629	250
630–689	275
690–749	300

Previous analgesic therapy should be phased out gradually from the time of the first patch application until analgesic efficacy with Durogesic DTrans® is attained. The initial evaluation of the analgesic effect of Durogesic DTrans® should not be made until the patch has been worn for 24h due to the gradual increase in serum fentanyl concentrations up to this time.

a. guidance varies between makes of TD fentanyl; see individual SPC.

Table 3 PCF recommended dose conversion ratios; PO to SC/IV. Before use, see General approach (p.661)

Conversion	Ratio	Calculation	Example	Monograph
Hydromorphone to hydromorphone	2:1	Divide 24h hydromorphone dose by 2	Hydromorphone 32mg/24h PO → hydromorphone 16mg/24h SC/IV	Hydromorphone, p.430
Methadone to methadone	2:1[a]	Divide 24h methadone dose by 2	Methadone 30mg/24h PO → methadone 15mg/24h SC/IV	Methadone, p.433
Morphine to alfentanil	30:1	Divide 24h morphine dose by 30	Morphine 60mg/24h PO → alfentanil 2mg/24h SC/IV	Alfentanil, p.385
Morphine to diamorphine	3:1	Divide 24h morphine dose by 3	Morphine 60mg/24h PO → diamorphine 20mg/24h SC/IV	Diamorphine, p.383
Morphine to hydromorphone	10–15:1	Divide 24h morphine dose by 10–15	Morphine 60mg/24h PO → hydromorphone 4mg/24h SC/IV	Hydromorphone, p.430
Morphine to methadone	Variable	See methadone, p.433		
Morphine to morphine	2:1	Divide 24h morphine dose by 2	Morphine 60mg/24h PO → morphine 30mg/24h SC/IV	Morphine, p.372
Morphine to oxycodone	2:1	Divide 24h morphine dose by 2	Morphine 60mg/24h PO → oxycodone 30mg/24h SC/IV	Oxycodone, p.442
Oxycodone to oxycodone	1.5:1[b]	Divide 24h oxycodone dose by 1.5 (decrease dose by 1/3)	Oxycodone 30mg/24h PO → oxycodone 20mg/24h SC/IV	Oxycodone, p.442
	2:1[c]	*Divide 24h oxycodone dose by 2*	*Oxycodone 30mg/24h PO → oxycodone 15mg/24h SC/IV*	Oxycodone, p.442

a. because mean oral bio-availability is 80% (range 40–100%), some centres use 1:1, e.g. methadone 30mg/24h PO → methadone 30mg/24h SC/IV, see p.433
b. because mean oral bio-availability is 75% (range 60–87%), some centres use a conversion ratio of 1.5:1 rather than 2:1
c. italicized entry = manufacturer's recommendation.

Table 4 PCF recommended dose conversion ratios; SC/IV to SC/IV. Before use, see General approach (p.661)

Conversion	Ratio	Calculation	Example	Monograph
Morphine to alfentanil	15:1	Divide 24h morphine dose by 15	Morphine 30mg/24h SC/IV → alfentanil 2mg/24h SC/IV	Alfentanil, p.385
Morphine to buprenorphine	30–40:1	Divide 24h morphine dose in mg by 30–40	Morphine 40mg/24h SC/IV → buprenorphine 1mg/24h SC/IV	Buprenorphine, p.392
Morphine to hydromorphone	5:1	Divide 24h morphine dose by 5	Morphine 30mg/24h SC/IV → hydromorphone 6mg/24h SC/IV	Hydromorphone, p.430
Morphine to methadone	Variable	See methadone, p.433		
Morphine to oxycodone	1:1	Use same dose as 24h morphine dose	Morphine 30mg/24h SC/IV → oxycodone 30mg/24h SC/IV	Oxycodone, p.442

16: DRUG TREATMENT IN THE IMMINENTLY DYING

In this chapter, in addition to the general discussion, advice is included about end-stage renal disease, heart failure and idiopathic Parkinson's disease (IPD). In essence, palliative care in all these situations is similar to palliative care in cancer, but with certain specific exceptions. These are detailed in the respective sections.

DIAGNOSING IMMINENT DEATH

In advanced cancer, if a patient is deteriorating without an obvious reversible cause:
- *month by month*, they probably have several months to live
- *week by week*, they probably have only weeks to live
- *day by day*, they probably have only days to live.

Estimating the prognosis in other end-stage diseases is generally less straightforward. However, in the absence of a reversible cause for deterioration, the following features collectively indicate that a patient probably has only days to live:
- physically wasted and profoundly weak → bedbound
- drowsy for much of the day → coma
- very limited attention span → disoriented (→ delirium)
- unable to take tablets or has great difficulty swallowing them
- little or no oral intake of food and fluid.[1,2]

Ideally, discussions about Advance Care Planning will already have taken place, and the carers will be aware of the patient's and family's wishes in relation to end-of-life care.[3] As death approaches, good communication becomes even more essential, both within the multiprofessional caring team and with the patient and family, particularly about uncertainties.

'GIVE DEATH A CHANCE'

In patients who are close to death it is often appropriate to 'give death a chance'. All patients must die eventually; ultimately nature will take its course. In this respect, the skill is to decide when the burdens of any life-sustaining treatment is likely to outweigh any benefits, and thus when to allow death to occur without further medical impediment. On the other hand, measures which provide comfort and symptom relief must be continued.

For example, an antibacterial is generally appropriate for the patient with advanced cancer who develops a chest infection when still relatively active and independent. However, in those who have become bedbound as a result of general progressive deterioration, and seem close to death, pneumonia should still be allowed to be 'the old person's friend'. In such circumstances it is generally appropriate *not* to prescribe an antibacterial (see p.461).

If it is difficult to make a decision, the '2-day rule' should be invoked, namely, if after 2–3 days of straightforward symptom management the patient is clearly holding his own, prescribe an antibacterial but, if the patient is clearly much worse, do not.

On the other hand, not all end-stage patients who develop a chest infection die from it. A few recover spontaneously, and some progress to a 'grumbling pneumonia' but no further. A continuing wet cough may cause distress and, possibly, loss of sleep. In circumstances when the patient is neither better nor worse after 3–4 days, an antibacterial may be indicated for symptom relief.

REVIEWING GOALS AND MEDICATION

When patients are clearly approaching death:
- *simplify medication:* particularly by stopping any remaining long-term prophylactic medication, e.g. statins, antihypertensives, oral hypoglycaemics, **warfarin**; and by stopping laxatives and antidepressants when the patient is moribund
- *anticipate and prescribe drugs p.r.n.* for common end-of-life problems, e.g. pain, breathlessness, vomiting, agitation, delirium, myoclonus, death rattle (see below)
- *prescribe drugs both PO and SC/IV*
- *review the need for IV hydration:* is it still appropriate? Can it be stopped?

In patients with insulin-dependent diabetes mellitus, the dose of **insulin** should be reduced as oral intake diminishes, and the regimen simplified. Once daily long-acting insulin is generally sufficient to avoid symptomatic hypo- or hyperglycaemia by keeping blood glucose levels between 6–15mmol/L (see p.522).

For advice about stopping **dexamethasone** in patients with intracranial malignancy, see p.507.

Finally, in the last days, some nursing procedures normally regarded as essential may be discontinued. For example, standard care of pressure areas may cause a moribund patient to become distressed. If so, such care should be reduced or stopped.

'AS NEEDED' MEDICATION

When a patient is likely to have difficulty with swallowing, non-PO as well as PO p.r.n. medication should be prescribed to cover common distressing situations. In some countries, SL, PR and TD products are preferred but, in the UK, SC injections are generally used. A typical pre-emptive regimen would include:
- **morphine** SC q1h p.r.n. (*dose depends on regular dose*) for pain, dyspnoea or cough
- **haloperidol** 1.5–5mg SC q1h p.r.n. for nausea and vomiting or agitated delirium
- **midazolam** 2.5–5mg SC q1h p.r.n. for anxiety or breathlessness; or, if seizures are likely, 10mg SC q1h p.r.n. (also see Anti-epileptics drugs, Box B, p.263)
- **hyoscine butylbromide** 20mg SC q1h p.r.n. for bowel colic or respiratory secretions in those too weak to expectorate.

Note: charting all these drugs 'q1h p.r.n.' facilitates rapid dose titration. However, if after several q1h doses there is no benefit or any benefit is short-lived, it is important to consider if an alternative or an additional drug is needed (also see Chapter 17, p.681).

Other drugs may be necessary in various circumstances, e.g. renal failure (see p.674), heart failure (see p.675), and Parkinson's disease (see p.676).

MAINTAINING COMFORT

Symptom relief in the last days of a patient's life is generally a continuation of what is already being done. However, previously well-managed symptoms can recur or new symptoms develop.[4–8] The same principles of management apply as before. However, because time is short, there is a greater need for urgency; tomorrow may be too late.

In patients close to death, incontinence is generally best managed by an indwelling urinary catheter.[9] This provides maximum comfort with minimum ongoing disturbance.

Pain

Most patients dying from cancer need a strong opioid. Expressed in oral **morphine** equivalents, data from several specialist palliative care centres indicate that:
- the median dose in the last 24h of life is 30–150mg
- individual dose requirements vary widely, e.g. 7.5–2,000mg/24h.[10–12]

Generally, pain will not be troublesome at the very end if relief has previously been good. However, even when the patient is close to death, careful evaluation is still necessary. Dying patients may call out to check whether someone is with them, that they are not alone. These cries may be misinterpreted as pain, and be a source of concern to family and carers.

Some patients show signs of discomfort when being turned in bed, even when apparently deeply unconscious, and may moan or cry out. Although, for example, this may be pain caused by joint stiffness, it could equally be an 'alarm response' to an unexpected disturbance. Disturbance distress is likely to be reduced by warning a patient (even when unconscious) of any intended interventions by describing the procedure to be undertaken, and by gentle slow handling.

Even so, new pains are relatively common in the last days.[6] Causes include:
- painful bedsore (consider the local application of a local anaesthetic gel ± topical **morphine**; see p.378)
- distended bladder (relieve by catheterization).

Occasionally, patients who have been taking an NSAID for metastatic bone pain suffer renewed pain after 12–24h if the NSAID is stopped when swallowing tablets is no longer possible. In this circumstance, an NSAID can be given as a liquid, suppository or injection (see p.322).

When a patient can no longer swallow medication PO, a strong opioid should be continued by an alternative route; abrupt discontinuation risks a renewed pain ± withdrawal symptoms, e.g. restlessness, diarrhoea.

Severe breathlessness

Patients often fear suffocating to death and a positive approach to the patient, their family and colleagues about the relief of terminal breathlessness is important:
- no patient should die with distressing breathlessness
- failure to relieve terminal breathlessness is a failure to utilize drug treatment correctly.

Because of the distress, inability to sleep and exhaustion, patients and their carers generally accept that drug-related drowsiness may need to be the price paid for greater comfort. However, unless there is overwhelming distress, deep sedation (reduced awareness/consciousness) is *not* the initial step. Some patients become mentally brighter when anxiety is reduced by light sedation (see p.379), and there is an associated improvement in their breathlessness. Even so, because increasing drowsiness also generally reflects a deteriorating clinical condition, it is important to stress the gravity of the situation and the aim of treatment to the relatives.

Drug treatment typically comprises:[13]
- parenteral administration of an opioid and a sedative-anxiolytic, e.g. **morphine** and **midazolam** by CSCI and p.r.n.
- **haloperidol** if the patient develops an agitated delirium (may be aggravated by a benzodiazepine; see p.672).

Death rattle (noisy respiratory secretions)

In most cases, an antimuscarinic is the drug of choice; see p.11.

Noisy tachypnoea in the moribund (without rattle)

Noisy tachypnoea in the moribund is distressing for the family and other patients, even though the patient is not aware. It represents a desperate last attempt by a patient's body to respond to irreversible terminal respiratory failure ± airway obstruction.

Consider alleviating the noise by reducing the depth and rate of respiration to 10–15/min with **diamorphine/morphine**, best initially titrated IV to identify an effective dose. This may be double, or even treble, the previously satisfactory analgesic dose. When there is associated heaving of the shoulders and chest, **midazolam** should be given as well, e.g. 5–10mg IV. The **diamorphine/morphine** ± **midazolam** can be repeated IV/SC hourly as needed.

Severe acute stridor as a terminal event

This may be caused by haemorrhage into a tumour pressing on the trachea. Administer **diazepam/midazolam** IV until the patient is asleep (5–20mg). If IV administration is not possible, alternatives include IM **midazolam** or PR **diazepam**.

Myoclonus

Multifocal myoclonus is a central pre-epileptiform phenomenon. It is exacerbated by hypoglycaemia and, in the moribund, may be caused or exacerbated by dopamine antagonists (antipsychotics, **metoclopramide**) and opioids (particularly at higher doses) or as a result of drug withdrawal (benzodiazepines, barbiturates, alcohol).

It is seen in cancer patients dying with encephalopathy associated with organ failure, e.g. renal failure, hepatic failure. It occurs with cerebral oedema and hypoxia, and also with hyponatraemia. Treat with a benzodiazepine (see p.152).

Grand mal seizure

See p.264.

Agitation and delirium

- mild delirium is not always easy to detect
- an antipsychotic is essential if a patient manifests features suggestive of delirium
- the use of a benzodiazepine alone may precipitate or exacerbate delirium[14]
- if in doubt, treat an agitated dying patient with both an antipsychotic and **midazolam**.

Delirium develops in most dying cancer patients as death approaches.[15,16] From a drug point of view, delirium is generally best treated with **haloperidol** ± **midazolam** given p.r.n. or by CSCI in an individually optimized dose. If delirium is not controlled on **haloperidol** ≤15mg/24h, a more sedating antipsychotic should be given instead, e.g. SC **levomepromazine** (see p.181).

Good practice dictates a step-by-step approach (Figure 1 and Box A); sedation is not 'all or none' but a continuum from p.r.n. sedation to continuous deep sedation.

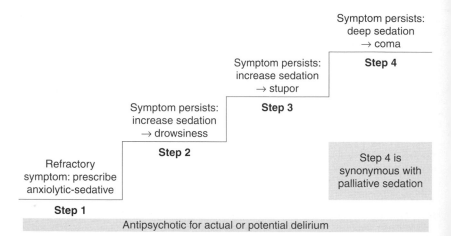

Figure 1 Progressive and proportionate treatment for an intolerable refractory symptom in an imminently dying patient.

Box A   Drugs for sedation in the imminently dying

For more information, see respective drug monographs.
First-line drugs
Midazolam
• start with 2.5–5mg SC stat and q1h p.r.n.
• if necessary, increase progressively to 10mg SC/IV stat
• maintain with CSCI/CIVI 10–60mg/24h.
Although some centres titrate up to 200mg/24h,[17] it is probably better to add in an antipsychotic before increasing above 30mg/24h (see p.158).

Haloperidol
• start with 2.5–10mg SC stat and q1h p.r.n. (1–5mg SC q1h in the elderly)
• maintain with CSCI 10–15mg/24h (see p.177).
If the patient fails to settle with 15mg/24h (in combination with midazolam), consider levomepromazine or, if latter not available, a third-line drug.

Second-line drugs
Levomepromazine
Generally given only if it is intended to reduce a patient's level of consciousness:
• start with 25mg SC stat and q1h p.r.n. (12.5mg in the elderly)
• if necessary, titrate dose according to response
• maintain with 50–300mg/24h CSCI.
Although high-dose levomepromazine (≥100mg/24h) is generally best given by CSCI, smaller doses can be conveniently given as an SC bolus at bedtime–b.d., and p.r.n. (see p.181).
Some centres use smaller doses first-line, e.g. 12.5mg SC stat and q1h p.r.n. (6.25mg in the elderly).

If levomepromazine is not available, use chlorpromazine; doses generally need to be higher, e.g. double those of levomepromazine.

Third-line drugs
Specialist use only; for patients who fail to respond to midazolam 60–120mg/24h together with either haloperidol 15mg/24h or levomepromazine 200mg/24h.
Phenobarbital
Because of the irritant nature of the injection and the volume after dilution, stat doses are generally given IM/IV, but can be followed by CSCI (see p.286).

Propofol
Propofol necessitates the use of an IVI and an appropriate variable-rate syringe driver (see p.634).[18]

Abrupt deep sedation is rarely necessary, e.g. sudden massive arterial haemorrhage. Particularly for existential distress, *respite* deep sedation for a few hours (up to 1–2 days in some centres) is an important step.[19]

In the imminently dying, it is uncommon to lighten the depth of the sedation once the patient is settled. However, at one centre, after the patient's distress has been relieved, medication is scaled down so that the patient is physically and mentally comfortable (albeit drowsy/sleeping for most/all of the time) but can be roused for short periods to permit meaningful communication:
'Our target in sedation is calming and comfort without lowering the level of consciousness deep enough to lose communication.'[17]

END-STAGE RENAL DISEASE

The two groups of patients for consideration in the last days of life are:
- those already on dialysis in whom a decision to stop dialysis has been made
- those who are chronic kidney disease (CKD) stage 5 (eGFR <15mL/min), and are being treated with maximum conservative management (i.e. all renal care except dialysis; this includes, for example, **erythropoietin**).

For the patient who stops dialysis the mean survival is 8–10 days, whereas the duration of survival in the conservatively managed group is very variable, ranging from weeks to more than a year. Indicators that death may be approaching are similar to other non-malignant conditions:
- declining physical function
- increasing dependence
- increasing number of symptoms.[20]

Patients with advanced kidney disease experience more symptoms than patients with advanced cancer, with a mean of 20 symptoms in the last month of life.[21] Common symptoms in the last days include:
- breathlessness (may relate to fluid overload and acidosis)
- myoclonic jerks and seizures (relate to both increased drug toxicity and uraemia)
- delirium (also relates to both increased drug toxicity and uraemia).

Other symptoms particularly associated with advanced kidney disease may continue to be a major problem, e.g. pruritus (see p.793) and restless legs. **Clonazepam** in low doses (i.e. a starting dose of 500microgram PO/SC at bedtime, increased to a maximum dose of 2mg/24h) is often helpful in relieving restless legs; myoclonus, and also neuropathic pain.

Occasionally, with severe fluid overload, if the patient still has a dialysis line in place, it may be appropriate to have a few hours of ultra-filtration to correct the overload.

Anticipatory prescribing
Note the following:
- some centres prescribe **fentanyl** (see p.403) or **alfentanil** (see p.385) instead of **morphine**; their lack of active metabolites is theoretically advantageous but it is uncertain if this outweighs the advantages of more cautious use of more familiar opioids
- indicate clearly that the prescribed strong opioid should be used for breathlessness as well as pain, possibly in association with low-dose **midazolam**, e.g. 2.5mg p.r.n q1h.
- halve the dose of **haloperidol**, **metoclopramide** and **midazolam** because of reduced clearance and the risk of accumulation, and an increased likelihood of dystonic reactions with **metoclopramide**
- do *not* use **hyoscine *hydrobromide*** for retained secretions/death rattle because of an increased risk of sedation and delirium; instead use **hyoscine *butylbromide*** (dose unchanged) or **glycopyrronium** (halve dose); see p.11.

Simplify long-term medication
Patients with advanced kidney disease typically take numerous drugs to manage the various aspects of their kidney disease and co-morbidities. These drugs can be divided into categories according to function (see below). When to stop drugs as the end of life approaches will depend on:
- how close to death they are
- the purpose of the drug
- likely effects from stopping it
- the burden of taking tablets.

Drugs for mineral and bone disease
Calcium and vitamin D preparations should be continued while the patient is swallowing or until they stop dialysis because of the risk of hypocalcaemia. This is particularly important for the patient who has had a parathyroidectomy. However, for those who have not and are taking **cinacalcet**, a calcimimetic, this may generally be stopped earlier. Phosphate binders can be reduced or stopped as intake reduces because their effect is on the food which is eaten.

Drugs for anaemia
For as long as it is desirable to maintain the haemoglobin for optimal symptom relief, **iron** (given as an infusion at dialysis) can be continued, as can **epoetin** until the final weeks.

Diuretics for fluid control

Patients may be taking high doses of diuretics, these should be continued if stopping them is likely to exacerbate symptoms.

Cardiovascular disease

End-stage kidney patients may be taking **aspirin** and antihypertensives. These are often continued until dialysis is stopped.

Drugs to maintain dialysis access

Warfarin should be continued until dialysis stops.

END-STAGE HEART FAILURE

In some *cancer patients*, congestive heart failure (CHF) is a significant cause of breathlessness. It is important to recognize this, and treat appropriately.

More detailed guidance about the care of patients with end-stage CHF is available from NICE[22] and elsewhere.[23–25] Resources include:

- *Supportive Care in Heart Failure*[26]
- *Heart Failure: from Advanced Disease to Bereavement*[27]
- *Heart Failure and Palliative Care: a team approach*[28]

This section provides guidance about which drugs can be stopped to ease a patient's 'tablet burden' without adversely affecting the level of comfort.[29] In end-stage CHF, it is important *not* to stop 'disease control' medication which also has an important contribution in symptom relief. Unlike cancer, where disease-specific treatment tends to become increasingly burdensome and futile (and possibly counterproductive), the continued disease-specific treatment of CHF generally continues to be essential for symptom management even when end-stage (Figure 2). If in doubt, obtain advice from the patient's cardiologist or specialist heart failure nurse.

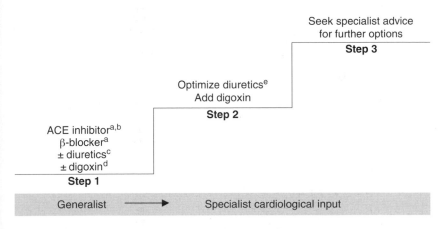

Figure 2 Synopsis of NICE guidance for drug treatment for CHF caused by left ventricular systolic dysfunction.[22]

a. in all patients who are stable, i.e. minimal or no signs of fluid overload or depletion, even if asymptomatic
b. if an ACE inhibitor is not tolerated, substitute an angiotensin-II antagonist, e.g. losartan
c. in patients with signs of fluid overload
d. in patients with atrial fibrillation
e. combine a loop diuretic with an aldosterone antagonist, i.e. spironolactone (see p.68) or eplerenone.

Drugs that improve survival and symptoms
Aldosterone antagonists, angiotensin-converting enzyme (ACE) inhibitors; angiotensin receptor blockers; β-blockers

These should generally be continued because there is good evidence that they slow progression of CHF, prolong survival, and improve symptom control.[30–36] Indications for considering a dose reduction or discontinuation on either a temporary or permanent basis are:
* symptomatic hypotension
* deteriorating renal function
* excessive tablet burden.

The patient's clinical condition, electrolytes and renal function should be monitored closely, and further dose adjustments made (up or down) as necessary (also see p.68).

Drugs that primarily improve symptoms in advanced disease
Loop diuretics

Furosemide (see p.63) and **bumetanide** are widely used.[37,38] Overall, they also increase survival. In very end-stage disease, the increasing dose required may exacerbate renal dysfunction. However, unless the patient becomes anuric or clinically hypovolaemic, a loop diuretic should be continued for symptom management. **Furosemide** by CSCI may reduce the need for hospital admission (see p.66).[39,40]

Anti-arrhythmic drugs

Anti-arrhythmic drugs can generally be considered for discontinuation at a relatively early stage. Most anti-arrhythmics lower blood pressure and can contribute to fatigue. However, if *symptomatic* tachycardias are present, or rate control is also helping angina symptoms, it may be best to continue. **Amiodarone** has a very long halflife (some 6 months) and thus can generally be stopped in end-stage CHF.

Anti-anginal agents

These can be discontinued if the patient has no angina. However, low-dose **isosorbide mononitrate**, with an 8h nitrate-free interval/24h, may help breathlessness.

Simplify long-term medication

Drugs for long-term prophylaxis and for co-morbid conditions need to be reviewed as in any other end-stage disease, bearing in mind the likely impact of discontinuation, e.g. **warfarin** (see p.86), thyroid replacement therapy. For drugs which may be detrimental as far as the heart failure is concerned but beneficial for a co-morbid condition, there will be need to review the potential balance between benefit and harm, e.g. NSAIDs. As always, an individual value judgement will be necessary.

Statins

Cholesterol-lowering drugs can generally be the first to be discontinued because they have no symptom-relieving properties.[41]

Antihypertensive drugs

These are generally inappropriate in end-stage disease.

Digoxin

In atrial fibrillation, **digoxin** may be important for rate control. Uncontrolled fast atrial fibrillation may be unpleasant for the patient and exacerbate symptoms. In patients in sinus rhythm, symptoms are less likely to worsen if digoxin is stopped.[42] If renal failure develops as the heart failure progresses, accumulation could lead to toxicity.

END-STAGE IDIOPATHIC PARKINSON'S DISEASE

Patients can die *with* concurrent idiopathic Parkinson's disease (IPD) or *from* IPD and, as such, patients can be at differing stages of disease as they approach death. One of the key challenges is trying to avoid centrally acting D_2 antagonists (e.g. antipsychotics, **metoclopramide**), because they exacerbate IPD, particularly rigidity and the consequential pain.

Although predicting prognosis in idiopathic IPD is often difficult, a progressive decline in physical status, continuing weight loss, recurrent infections, cognitive impairment, swallowing problems, and episodes of aspiration pneumonia strongly suggest that the patient has reached the end-stage. Given the unreliability of prognostication, frequent review is necessary. When deterioration is rapid, this may need to be daily (see p.670). Each patient requires careful individual evaluation; and, when possible, there should be ongoing liaison with an IPD specialist.

A rapid decline from diagnosis (within 3–5 years) with a poor response to **levodopa** could indicate a 'PD plus syndrome' (e.g. progressive supranuclear palsy, multisystem atrophy). Most of these patients die some 6–9 years after diagnosis. The approach to palliative care in these conditions is the same as for IPD.

In the last few days of life the patient with IPD is likely to be rigid, wasted, unable to swallow, and confused (delirium).[43] An attempt to continue dopaminergic drugs should be made in patients dying with concurrent IPD (see below). On the other hand, in patients dying from IPD, withdrawal of dopaminergic drugs is sometimes appropriate because of loss of efficacy and/or increased undesirable effects, e.g. agitation, delirium, hallucinations.[44]

Rigidity

Rigidity is not always a major issue for patients with end-stage IPD, and many tolerate a reduction in their often complex IPD drug regimens. On the other hand, important causes of rigidity towards the end of life are:
- not getting dopaminergic drugs on time
- an inability to swallow medication
- worsening IPD which is less dopamine-responsive.

Thus, if the patient can still swallow, ensure that medication is given on time, and consider prescribing p.r.n. doses of dispersible Madopar®, e.g. 62.5mg (= **benserazide** 12.5mg + **levodopa** 50mg).

If the patient is not able swallow, consider giving previous dopaminergic medication via an existing PEG or an NG tube. Alternatively, discuss the use of one of the following parenteral dopamine agonists with a PD specialist:
- TD **rotigotine**:
  ▷ start with a 2mg/24h patch; use a fresh site each day
  ▷ if necessary, after 1 week, increase to 4mg/24h
  ▷ maximum recommended dose = 8mg/24h
- SC **apomorphine**; also prescribe prophylactic **domperidone** to prevent almost inevitable nausea.[45]

Note: both **rotigotine** and **apomorphine** can cause delirium ± agitation; generally use only with guidance from a PD specialist.

Note: if dopaminergic medication is stopped, a CSCI of **midazolam** may help relieve rigidity. Optimal nursing care and gentle physiotherapy are also crucial.

Pain

Careful evaluation is needed to determine if pain is related to rigidity or to some other cause. Different pains often require different approaches to management:
- if related to rigidity, see above
- If not, consider:
  ▷ non-drug treatment (e.g. positioning, nursing care, physiotherapy, TENS, massage, heat) *and*
  ▷ drug treatment (see p.291).

Nausea and vomiting

Many drugs used for nausea and vomiting are D_2 antagonists, e.g. **metoclopramide, haloperidol, prochlorperazine** (see p.235), and ideally should be avoided in IPD because they will exacerbate rigidity and bradykinesia. Anecdotal reports suggest that **cyclizine** may also exacerbate IPD.

Anti-emetics least likely to exacerbate IPD are:
- **domperidone** (available as a suppository; not UK, see p.246)
- **ondansetron** (see p.251)
- **hyoscine *hydrobromide*** (see p.17), but may exacerbate delirium.

Despite being D$_2$ antagonists, it may be necessary to prescribe small doses of **levomepromazine** (e.g. 2.5–5mg at bedtime; see p.181) or **olanzapine** (e.g. 1.25–2.5mg at bedtime; see p.183) if all else fails.

Delirium and agitation

Remember: both **rotigotine** and **apomorphine** can cause delirium ± agitation.

There may well be need for a 'trade-off' between increased rigidity (and the consequential pain) and the relief of an agitated delirium. However, there are many potential causes for delirium and agitation in end-stage IPD and, as always, a systematic approach is necessary (see p.672):
- if feasible, treat any obvious underlying cause, e.g. constipation and/or urinary retention
- review dopaminergic drugs; discuss with the PD team the best order for stopping these
- this generally results in **levodopa** monotherapy, and perhaps reducing the dose of this as well
- if the patient can swallow, consider **quetiapine** (e.g. 25mg once daily–b.d.), an atypical antipsychotic available only as an oral product but the one least likely to cause extrapyramidal movement disorders
- if the patient cannot swallow, consider a benzodiazepine (see p.148), e.g.:
  ▷ **midazolam** 2.5mg SC p.r.n.
  ▷ **lorazepam** 0.5–1mg SC p.r.n.
  but be aware that this may sometimes exacerbate delirium
- if the situation remains unmanageable, prescribe an injectable antipsychotic, e.g. **levomepromazine** 6.25–12.5mg SC p.r.n (see p.181).

The use of **levomepromazine** will generally result in a reduction in the patient's level of consciousness, but will exacerbate PD less than **haloperidol**.

Some patients with PD also have dementia, commonly Alzheimer's or dementia with Lewy bodies (DLB).[46,47] Extra care needs to be taken in DLB. About 50% of such patients are oversensitive to antipsychotics and, if used, they will experience a marked exacerbation of the PD, reduced level of consciousness, increased delirium, and possibly neuroleptic (antipsychotic) malignant syndrome (see p.171).

AS DEATH APPROACHES

Even when there is nothing new to offer, it is important for the doctor to:
- continue to visit
- quietly indicate:
  'The important thing now is to keep you as comfortable as possible'
- continue to inform the family of the changing situation:
  'He is very weak now, but may still live for several days'
  'Although he seems better today, he's remains very weak... He could quickly deteriorate and die in just a few days'
- control agitation even if it results in sedation (see p.672)
- listen to the nurses.

1   Ellershaw JE et al. (1995) Dehydration and the dying patient. *Journal of Pain and Symptom Management*. **10**: 192–197.
2   Higgs R (1999) The diagnosis of dying. *Journal of the Royal College of Physicians of London*. **33**: 110–112.
3   Thomas K and Lobo B (eds) (2010) *Advance Care Planning in End of Life Care*. Oxford University Press, Oxford.
4   Fainsinger R et al. (1991) Symptom control during the last week of life on a palliative care unit. *Journal of Palliative Care*. **7**: 5–11.
5   Ventafridda V et al. (1990) Symptom prevalence and control during cancer patients' last days of life. *Journal of Palliative Care*. **6**: 7–11.
6   Lichter I and Hunt E (1990) The last 48 hours of life. *Journal of Palliative Care*. **6**: 7–15.
7   Wilkes E (1984) Dying now. *Lancet*. **1**: 950–952.
8   Exton-Smith AN (1961) Terminal illness in the aged. *Lancet* **2**: 305–308.
9   Fainsinger RL et al. (1992) The use of urinary catheters in terminally ill cancer patients. *Journal of Pain and Symptom Management*. **7**: 333–338.
10 Wilcock A and Chauhan A (2007) Benchmarking the use of opioids in the last days of life. *Journal of Pain and Symptom Management*. **34**: 1–3.

11 Good PD *et al.* (2005) Effects of opioids and sedatives on survival in an Australian inpatient palliative care population. *Internal Medicine Journal.* **35**: 512–517.

12 Thorns A and Sykes N (2000) Opioid use in last week of life and implications for end-of-life decision-making. *Lancet.* **356**: 398–399.

13 Navigante AH *et al.* (2006) Midazolam as adjunct therapy to morphine in the alleviation of severe dyspnea perception in patients with advanced cancer. *Journal of Pain and Symptom Management.* **31**: 38–47.

14 Breitbart W *et al.* (1996) A double-blind trial of haloperidol, chlorpromazine, and lorazepam in the treatment of delirium in hospitalized AIDS patients. *American Journal of Psychiatry.* **153**: 231–237.

15 Massie MJ *et al.* (1983) Delirium in terminally ill cancer patients. *Amercian Journal of Psychiatry.* **140**: 1048–1050.

16 Bruera E *et al.* (1987) Delirium and severe sedation in patients with terminal cancer. *Cancer Treatment Reports.* **71**: 787–788.

17 Muller-Busch HC *et al.* (2003) Sedation in palliative care - a critical analysis of 7 years experience. *BMC Palliative Care.* **2**: 2.

18 Lundstrom S *et al.* (2005) When nothing helps: propofol as sedative and antiemetic in palliative cancer care. *Journal of Pain and Symptom Management.* **30**: 570–577.

19 Cherny NI (1998) Commentary: sedation in response to refractory existential distress: walking the fine line. *Journal of Pain and Symptom Management.* **16**: 404–406.

20 Murtagh F and Sheerin N (2010) Conservative management of end-stage renal disease. In: Chambers EJ *et al.* (eds) *Supportive Care for the Renal Patient* (2e). Oxford University Press, Oxford.

21 Murtagh FE *et al.* (2010) Symptoms in the month before death for stage 5 chronic kidney disease patients managed without dialysis. *Journal of Pain and Symptom Management.* **40**: 342–352.

22 NICE (2010) Chronic heart failure: management of chronic heart failure in adults in primary and secondary care. *Clinical Guideline* CG108. www.nice.org.uk

23 Arnold JM *et al.* (2006) Canadian Cardiovascular Society consensus conference recommendations on heart failure 2006: diagnosis and management.[erratum appears in Canadian Journal of Cardiology. 2006 Mar 1;22(3):271]. *Canadian Journal of Cardiology.* **22**: 23–45.

24 Swedberg K *et al.* (2005) Guidelines for the diagnosis and treatment of chronic heart failure: full text (update 2005). European Heart Journal. Available from: 10.1093/eurheartj/ehi205

25 Hunt SA *et al.* (2005) Guideline Update for the Diagnosis and Management of Chronic Heart Failure in the Adult. ACC/AHA. Available from: http://circ.ahajournals.org/cgi/content/full/112/12/e154

26 Beattie J and Goodlin S (eds) (2008) Supportive Care in Heart Failure. In: *Supportive Care Series.* Oxford University Press, Oxford.

27 Johnson MJ *et al.* (2012) Heart failure: from advanced disease to bereavement. *End of Life Series.* OUP.

28 Johnson MJ and Lehman R (2006) *Heart Failure and Palliative Care: a team approach.* Radcliffe Publishing Ltd, Oxford.

29 Cleland JG *et al.* (2000) Polypharmacy (or polytherapy) in the treatment of heart failure. *Heart Failure Monitor.* **1**: 8–13.

30 Jong P *et al.* (2002) Angiotensin receptor blockers in heart failure: meta-analysis of randomized controlled trials. *Journal of the American College of Cardiology.* **39**: 463–470.

31 Shibata MC *et al.* (2001) Systematic review of the impact of beta blockers on mortality and hospital admissions in heart failure. *European Journal of Heart Failure.* **3**: 351–357.

32 The SOLVD Investigators (1991) Effect of enalapril on survival in patients with reduced left ventricular ejection fractions and congestive heart failure. The SOLVD Investigators. *New England Journal of Medicine.* **325**: 293–302.

33 Consensus Trial Study Group (1987) Effects of enalapril on mortality in severe congestive heart failure. Results of the Cooperative North Scandinavian Enalapril Survival Study (CONSENSUS). *New England Journal of Medicine.* **316**: 1429–1435.

34 The RALES Investigatgors (1996) Effectiveness of spironolactone added to an angiotensin-converting enzyme inhibitor and a loop diuretic for severe chronic congestive heart failure (the Randomized Aldactone Evaluation Study [RALES]). *American Journal of Cardiology.* **78**: 902–907.

35 Pitt B *et al.* (2003) Eplerenone, a selective aldosterone blocker, in patients with left ventricular dysfunction after myocardial infarction. *New England Journal of Medicine.* **348**: 1309–1321.

36 Pitt B *et al.* (1999) The effect of spironolactone on morbidity and mortality in patients with severe heart failure. Randomized Aldactone Evaluation Study Investigators. *New England Journal of Medicine.* **341**: 709–717.

37 McMurray JJ and Pfeffer MA (2005) Heart failure. *Lancet.* **365**: 1877–1889.

38 Faris R *et al.* (2006) Diuretics for heart failure. *Cochrane Database of Systematic Reviews.* CD003838.

39 Zacharias H *et al.* (2011) Is there a role for subcutaneous furosemide in the community and hospice management of end-stage heart failure? *Palliative Medicine.* **26**: 658–663.

40 Zatarain-Nicolas E *et al.* (2013) Subcutaneous infusion of furosemide administered by elastomeric pumps for decompensated heart failure treatment: initial experience. *Revista Espanola Cardiologia (Engl Ed).* **66**: 1002–1004.

41 McGowan MP and Treating to New Target Study G (2004) There is no evidence for an increase in acute coronary syndromes after short-term abrupt discontinuation of statins in stable cardiac patients. *Circulation.* **110**: 2333–2335.

42 Digitalis Invesitgation Group (1997) The effect of digoxin on mortality and morbidity in patients with heart failure. *New England Journal of Medicine.* **336**: 525–533.

43 Goy ER *et al.* (2008) Neurologic disease at the end of life: caregiver descriptions of Parkinson disease and amyotrophic lateral sclerosis. *Journal of Palliative Medicine.* **11**: 548–554.

44 National Council of Palliative Care (NCPC) Neurological Conditions Group (2011) Consensus statement for the management of symptoms in idiopathic Parkinsons's Disease (PD) and related conditions in the last few days of life.

45 Dewhurst F *et al.* (2009) The pragmatic use of apomorphine at the end of life. *Palliative Medicine.* **23**: 777–779.

46 McKeith IG *et al.* (2005) Diagnosis and management of dementia with Lewy bodies: third report of the DLB Consortium. *Neurology.* **65**: 1863–1872.

47 McKeith I (2002) Dementia with Lewy bodies. *British Journal of Psychiatry.* **180**: 144–147.

Updated June 2014

17: PRE-EMPTIVE PRESCRIBING IN THE COMMUNITY

Rapid access to drugs in the community is important to avoid crises at home and to reduce unwanted or unnecessary admissions in the last days of life.[1-3] Both enteral and parenteral formulations of drugs to relieve pain, nausea and vomiting, breathlessness, noisy respiratory secretions ('death rattle'), restlessness/agitation, delirium and seizures, need to be available.[4,5] The Department of Health (London) recommends that generally patients should be able to receive needed medication at the same time and in the same place as the out-of-hours consultation.[6] Ways of enabling this include:

- *Anticipatory prescribing*: encouraging prescribers to think ahead and prescribe extra medication to manage sudden changes in the patient's condition, or pro-actively prescribe injectable drugs commonly used at the end of life which are then available in the home on an 'if needed' basis[1,7]
- *Just in case* boxes: these are standard boxes containing drugs specifically prescribed for the patients, and left in the home.[8,9] Examples of the use of *Just in case* boxes are readily available.[6,10] The boxes generally contain a small selection of injectable drugs in a tamper-proof box, the choice based on local guidelines for care in the last days of life. Additional emergency supplies may be indicated for selected patients, e.g. for someone with MND/ALS (see below)[11] or a *Crisis haemorrhage* pack for those at risk of a major haemorrhage
- *Breathing Space* boxes: these are designed for patients with end-stage MND at risk of severe breathlessness, panic or choking. On request, the MND Association provides the box free of charge to the GP; it contains information for both the patient and the GP. The GP is asked to prescribe appropriate drugs, e.g. **midazolam**, **glycopyrronium** and **diamorphine**, and keep them in the box in the patient's home[11]
- *Palliative care emergency* kits: these contain various drugs and equipment which can be carried in an out-of-hours (OOH) service provider's car; this generally includes a wider range of drugs than in a *Just in case* box and also a syringe driver. To carry CDs they must able to demonstrate compliance with current Home Office regulations[12]
- *Extended pharmacy schemes*: nominated community palliative care pharmacies offer extended opening hours, and agree to carry an extended palliative care stock.

Examples of local practice are available in the Document library on www.palliativedrugs.com, filed under Medication issues (Out of hours issues).

Just in case boxes

The Gold Standards Framework (GSF) recommends the following for a *Just in case* box:

- SC formulations for pain, nausea and vomiting, agitation/restlessness and death rattle (2mL syringes and needles)
- ± rectal diazepam
- local prescribing algorithms
- signed permissions for medication administration
- patient information.[3,9]

Typical injectable drugs include:

- **diamorphine**, **morphine**, or **oxycodone** for pain
- **cyclizine**, **haloperidol** or **levomepromazine** for nausea and vomiting
- **midazolam** for agitation/restlessness
- **glycopyrronium**, **hyoscine** *hydrobromide* or **hyoscine** *butylbromide* for respiratory secretions.

Some boxes also include rectal **diazepam** or **lorazepam** tablets (for sublingual use).

A syringe driver may be left with the box.[6] WFI and a small sharps disposal container are also recommended.[10]

The cost of a *Just in case* box will depend on its contents, and how many amps of each drug are prescribed. Typically, a box will contain 2–5 amps of each injectable drug (Table 1).[8]

Table 1 Cost of Just in case drugs[13]

Drug	Strength and form	Cost/amp[a]
Diamorphine hydrochloride	5mg amp, powder for reconstitution	£2.50
	10mg amp, powder for reconstitution	£3
Morphine sulfate	10, 15, 20 and 30mg/mL; 1mL and 2mL amps	£1–4.50
Cyclizine	50mg/mL, 1mL amp	£1
Midazolam	2mg/mL, 5mL amp	£1
	5mg/mL, 2mL amp	£1
Hyoscine *hydrobromide*	400microgram/mL, 1mL amp	£3
	600microgram/mL, 1mL amp	£3
Glycopyrronium	200microgram/mL, 1mL amp	£1
	200microgram/mL, 3mL amp	£1.50
Diazepam rectal solution	5mg and 10mg rectal tube	£1.50

a. cost rounded up to nearest 50p.

If the patient is at risk of a crisis such as catastrophic haemorrhage, it is important to ensure that sufficient ampoules are provided to deal with this (should it occur), but not forgetting that non-drug measures are generally equally or more important.[14,15] If crisis medication is supplied (Table 2), it should be:
• readily available in the patient's home
• rapid in onset (2–5 min)
• already drawn up and kept in a fridge because there is rarely time to prepare an injection or calmly measure a SL dose
• if possible, given by the nearest carer, whether professional or informal (see Chapter 14, p.645). The 'nearest carer' will generally be a family member or other informal carer. Thus, it is necessary to train such carers to give medication SL or by injection, whichever is the case. (see Chapter 14, p.645).

In catastrophic haemorrhage, the SC route is inappropriate because of likely peripheral shutdown and unpredictable absorption. IV is ideal but, failing that, it should be given IM (deltoid may be quicker than gluteal).[16,17]

Table 2 Crisis drugs prepared in advance for a major haemorrhage in order of speed of onset

Drug	Route	Dose	Speed of onset
Midazolam	IV	10mg	2–3min (see p.157)
	IM	10mg	5–15min
Lorazepam	SL[a]	4mg (1mL)	5min (see p.162)
Midazolam	Buccal/SL[b]	10mg (2mL)	15min (see p.157)

a. use the contents of an ampoule for injection
b. if the 2mL volume of a 10mg dose of midazolam (both buccal liquid (Buccolam®) and injection products are 5mg/mL) exceeds what a patient can retain easily in their mouth, unauthorized 10mg/mL buccal products (e.g. Epistatus®) are available as a special order, see Appendix 1, p.817.

Boxes should generally be stored in a cool, dry, low-access area. **Lorazepam** injection needs refrigeration.

Procedures need to be in place to ensure the security of the box during the acquisition process, while stored in the patient's home, and during return to the pharmacy after use. In order to confirm that medication has not been unlawfully diverted, there must be an 'audit trail' documenting the ordering, dispensing and delivery of the drugs to the patient, and return of unused medication to the pharmacy.

A medication log included in the box can act as both an administration record and a stock balance sheet. The medication should be in a suitably robust container, fastened with a combination lock or a tamper-evident security tag. Unless specifically directed otherwise, it should be opened only by the community nurse who will be preparing the drugs for use by the patient/carer, or by a physician.

If the box is ordered before the last few days of life, there needs to be a robust procedure for reviewing the contents regularly, expiry dates, drug administration directions and medication doses as the patient's clinical condition changes. A prompt should be included in the box to ensure early medical review if any of the drugs are administered.[10] It is also essential that the patient and carer are told about:

- the contents of the emergency box
- the proper use of the medication, including training in the administration of SL/SC drugs when necessary (see Chapter 14, p.645)
- who to contact in the event of an emergency.

The administration of emergency medication in a patient's home at the end of life carries a high risk for error. In order to avoid confusion at the time of use, concise, well-written and illustrated *patient and carer information material* should be included in the box.

Palliative Care emergency kits for OOH services

The provision of and contents of Palliative Care emergency kits are dependent on the OOH service provider. The ideal is to 'keep it simple', i.e. to restrict the number of products to no more than 6–7. Some drugs will overlap OOH emergency medication needed in other clinical situations. Kits can be kept in the OOH provider's car, and also in OOH provider bases. Standardization across a geographical area is recommended, and helps staff to be familiar with what is available.

A starting point is the National OOH formulary palliative care core drug list:[19]

- **diamorphine** (injection)
- **cyclizine** (injection)
- **dexamethasone** (tablet)
- **hyoscine** *butylbromide* (injection)
- **ketorolac** or **diclofenac** (injection)
- **levomepromazine** (injection)
- **midazolam** (injection).

It is expected that these drugs will be part of a special locally available tamper-proof palliative care container. Local discussions will be necessary to determine optimum access. The quantities supplied should be enough to allow optimum symptom relief until formal review by palliative care team or GP.

Other drugs useful in palliative care appear in other sections of the National out-of-hours Formulary:

- **haloperidol** and **diazepam** (oral and injectable) are under 'Psychiatric emergencies'
- antacids, **domperidone** (oral), **glycerol** suppositories, anti-spasmodic agents, **loperamide**, **metoclopramide** (injectable), **phosphate** enema and **prochlorperazine** (buccal) are under 'Gastro-intestinal'
- **codeine** (oral), **diamorphine** (injectable), a locally negotiated NSAID (oral and injectable) and **paracetemol** (oral) are under 'Analgesics'
- **naloxone** is in its own section for opioid overdose.

Local guidelines for the use of these drugs for palliative care, contact numbers for specialist advice, equipment to allow administration (including syringe drivers), and guidance on any local arrangements for rapid access to higher strengths of **diamorphine** or other injectable strong opioids should be included with the kit or be easily accessible, remembering the wide range of care settings an OOH service provider may cover.

Extended pharmacy schemes

These generally involve networks of community pharmacies able to offer extended opening hours, and carrying a locally agreed palliative care stock list (Table 3). Some also agree to provide palliative care information, advice and an emergency contacts list for patients, carers and clinicians.[6]

Table 3 Lothian Community Pharmacy Palliative Care Networks Pan-Lothian Stock List October 2010[20]

Drug	Form	Strength	Quantity stocked
Alfentanil	Injection	1mg/2mL	1 × 10
Cyclizine	Injection	50mg/mL	2 × 5
Dexamethasone	Tablets	2mg	1 × 50
Dexamethasone (Organon)[a]	Injection	4mg/mL	1 × 10
Diamorphine hydrochloride	Injection	10mg	2 × 5
	Injection	30mg	2 × 5
	Injection	100mg	1 × 5
Diazepam	Rectal tubes	10mg/2.5mL	1 × 5
Fentanyl	TD patches	12microgram/h	1 × 5
	TD patches	25microgram/h	1 × 5
Glycopyrronium	Injection	200microgram/mL	1 × 10
Haloperidol	Injection	5mg/mL	2 × 5
Hyoscine *butylbromide* (Buscopan®)	Injection	20mg/mL	2 × 10
Hyoscine *hydrobromide*	Injection	400microgram/mL	1 × 10
Levomepromazine	Injection	25mg/mL	1 × 10
	Tablets[b]	6mg	1 × 28
Metoclopramide	Injection	10mg/2mL	2 × 12
Midazolam	Injection[c]	10mg/2mL	2 × 10
Morphine sulfate	Oral liquid	10mg/5mL	1 × 100mL
	Oral liquid	100mg/5mL	1 × 30mL
	Injection	10mg/mL	2 × 10
	Injection	30mg/mL	2 × 10
Morphine sulfate m/r (MST continus®)	Granules for oral suspension	30mg sachet	1 × 30
Oxycodone hydrochloride	Oral liquid	5mg/5mL	1 × 250mL
	Injection	20mg/2mL	1 × 5
Phenobarbital	Injection	200mg/mL	1 × 5
Sodium Chloride	Infusion[d]	0.9%	20 × 500mL
WFI (10mL amps)	Injection	–	2 × 10

a. dexamethasone 4mg/mL refers specifically to the Organon product. The comparable Hospira product contains dexamethasone 3.3mg/mL
b. levomepromazine 6mg tablets are unauthorized, available by special order from IDIS, see Appendix 1, p.817
c. the strength of midazolam stocked is 10mg/2mL; other strengths should not be used as they are too dilute for preparation of syringes for syringe drivers.

Achieving success

The success of any scheme will depend on generating and maintaining high levels of awareness across normal hours and OOH service providers. OOH service providers may employ large numbers of part-time staff working sporadic or infrequent shifts, covering the whole of emergency medicine, of which palliative care will be one small part. Straightforward up-to-date information about any local schemes for accessing drugs OOH needs to be integrated into induction and training sessions, any service handbooks, and be easily available at the point of need in service cars and at service bases.

1 Allanson H (2004) Delivering the out-of-hours review: securing proper access to medicines in the out-of-hours period. Department of Health. Available from: http://www.out-of-hours.info/documents.php
2 NICE (2004) Improving supportive and palliative care for adults with cancer. National Institute for Health and Clinical Excellence, London, UK. Available from: http://guidance.nice.org.uk/CSGSP
3 Gold Standards Framework (2010) Out of hours. Available from: www.goldstandardsframework.org.uk
4 Wowchuk SM et al. (2009) The palliative medication kit: an effective way of extending care in the home for patients nearing death. *Journal of Palliative Medicine.* 12: 797–803.
5 Dawkins L (2007) 'Just-in-case' medication boxes for palliative care patients. *End of Life Care.* 1: 65–69.

6 Allanson H (2008) Medicines in unplanned care toolkit. NHS Medicines Management Network Northwest and Department of Health.

7 Palmer E and Howarth J (2005) Palliative Care for the Primary Care Team (also available on gp-palliativecare.co.uk). In. Quay Books, London.

8 Amass C and Allen M (2005) How a "just in case" approach can improve out-of-hours palliative care. *The Pharmaceutical Journal.* **275**: 22–23.

9 Gold Standards Framework (2006) Check list of contents for "Just in Case Boxes". Available from: www.goldstandards framework.org.uk

10 Gold Standards Framework (2006) Examples of Good Practice Resource Guide - Just in case boxes. Available from: www.goldstandardsframework.org.uk

11 Motor Neurone Disease Association (2010) Breathing space kit. Available from: www.mndassociation.org

12 National Prescribing Centre (2009) A guide to good practice in the management of controlled drugs in primary care (England) 3rd edition. Available from: http://www.npci.org.uk/cd/public/docs/controlled_drugs_third_edition.pdf

13 British National Formulary London: BMJ Group and Pharmaceutical Press. www.bnf.org (accessed May 2014).

14 North Cumbria Palliative Care Service Crisis Management Group (2006) Guidance for healthcare staff for managing catastrophic haemorrhage. Available from: Document library www.palliativedrugs.com

15 Yorkshire Palliative Medicine Clinical Guidelines Group (2008) Guidelines on the management of bleeding for palliative care patients with cancer. Available from: Document library www.palliativedrugs.com

16 Lazebnik N et al. (1989) Intravenous, deltoid, or gluteus administration of meperidine during labor? *American Journal of Obstetrics and Gynecology.* **160**: 1184–1189.

17 British Association of Head and Neck Oncology Nurses (1999) Guidelines for carotid haemorrhage. Available from: http://www.bahnon.org.uk/Public/KnowledgeCentre/tabid/81/Default.aspx (subscription required).

18 Gold Standards Framework (2006) Check list for developing Just in Case boxes. Available from: www.goldstandards framework.org.uk

19 NHS Electronic drug tariff. Part XVIIC - National out-of-hours formulary. www.nhsbsa.nhs.uk/prescriptions (accessed May 2014).

20 Lothian Community Pharmacy Palliative Care Networks (2010) Pan-Lothian stock list October 2010. Available from: www.nhslothian.scot.nhs.uk

Updated (minor change) June 2014

18: MANAGEMENT OF POSTOPERATIVE PAIN IN OPIOID-DEPENDENT PATIENTS

Opioid-dependent patients include those using long-term opioids for:
- pain relief (mainly cancer but also non-cancer pain)
- long-term opioid maintenance for opioid dependence
- current substance misuse.

All such patients will require *additional opioids* to relieve *additional pain*. It is thus crucially important that pre-operative, peri-operative and postoperative doses take this into account, and that *extra amounts* of a strong opioid are prescribed. Generally, these will be larger than the typical doses used by non-opioid-dependent patients in these circumstances.[1] For example, if only typical postoperative doses are prescribed (e.g. **morphine** 2.5–10mg IV/SC q1h p.r.n.), patients who are tolerant to higher doses may experience little or no pain relief. However, opioid requirements vary widely and close monitoring is essential.

Because tolerance to undesirable effects, e.g. respiratory depression, develops more rapidly than to analgesia (often within days or 1–2 weeks at most), opioids can be safely titrated to the higher doses required in opioid-dependent patients.

Further, a sudden significant reduction in overall opioid dose may well precipitate an opioid withdrawal syndrome, possibly accompanied by *hyperalgesia*. This will magnify the postoperative pain and any other underlying pain. Thus, under-prescribing can lead to devastating overwhelming pain.

As far as possible, a multidisciplinary approach should be adopted, e.g. pre-operative consultation with the patient's substance misuse team, the anaesthetist and the acute pain team, to develop a pain management plan which should include intra-operative and postoperative monitoring, with dose adjustments made by an experienced anaesthetist. There are no uniform recommendations, but Box A outlines the general approach.[2–9] Addicts receiving maintenance therapy with **methadone** or high-dose SL **buprenorphine**, or **naltrexone** require additional considerations (see below).

Other classes of drugs used for analgesia, e.g. antidepressants, anti-epileptics, should also be continued with as little interruption as possible.[10]

Addicts receiving methadone maintenance therapy

Generally, **methadone** maintenance therapy is administered once daily, which is adequate to prevent opioid withdrawal symptoms for 24h, but not to relieve pain. In acute pain, generally the maintenance dose is continued at the same dose, but can be used to contribute towards analgesia *by halving the dose and administering it b.d.*[8] When the PO route cannot be used, SC or CSCI are alternative routes of administration (see p433).

Addicts receiving high-dose SL buprenorphine maintenance therapy

Buprenorphine acts as a partial agonist at the μ-opioid receptor, to which it binds with a higher affinity than other μ-opioid receptor agonists. Thus, when **buprenorphine** is present in sufficient amounts, it will antagonize the analgesic effects of other μ-opioid receptor agonists. This is likely only with the higher doses used SL for opioid maintenance, i.e. ≥16mg/day (see p.392). This has led some to advocate discontinuing high-dose SL **buprenorphine** 5–7 days before elective surgery to avoid compromising postoperative pain relief, and to manage withdrawal symptoms with **methadone** instead.[12] On the other hand, various μ-opioid receptor agonists have been successfully used for postoperative pain in patients on SL **buprenorphine** 2–32mg/day, although higher doses than usual may be required.[13–15]

Box A   Management of postoperative pain in opioid-dependent patients

1 Consider local anaesthetic or multimodal approaches to analgesia, e.g. regional blocks, paracetamol, NSAIDs, ketamine, clonidine, etc.

2 Identify the baseline opioid dose: in patients misusing opioids this may mean a 'best guess' estimate.

3 Generally, the baseline opioid dose should be continued as a regular prescription.

4 Reduce the baseline dose if:
   • the surgery will improve the pre-operative pain
   • the baseline opioid needs to be replaced by an alternative opioid; because of possible incomplete cross-tolerance, reduce the dose calculated from equipotency tables by at least 1/3, particularly when dealing with large doses, e.g. ≥ morphine 1g PO/24h or equivalent (see p.365).

5 Patients on m/r opioids PO can take them (and other analgesics) on the day of surgery, even if fasting, unless there is a specific contra-indication.[8]

6 If PO is not possible pre- or immediately postoperatively, an alternative route, e.g. CSCI or CIVI should be used to deliver the baseline dose. This can also be done via IV patient-controlled analgesia (PCA) (see point 12).

7 Before restarting m/r opioids PO, ensure that GI function has returned to normal. Gastric stasis can lead to delayed dissolution and drug absorption, followed by 'dose-dumping' when motility improves, with consequential overdose. Conversely, surgery which shortens GI transit time (e.g. small bowel resection) may render the use of m/r products inappropriate.

8 If the surgery is unlikely to lead to major changes in skin perfusion and the ongoing opioid requirements are unlikely to change, it is best to leave TD fentanyl patches in place, and give additional p.r.n. opioid.

9 If TD patches are removed, pain relief will persist for several hours because fentanyl is sequestrated widely throughout the body, particularly in adipose tissue (see p.403). Note: in postoperative patients, after a patch has been removed, the mean time for the plasma fentanyl concentration to drop below the minimum effective level is 16h, with a range of 2–23h.[11]

10 Continue long-term ED or IT pumps unchanged unless the surgery is expected to reduce the pain for which these are being used.

11 Prescribe an appropriate dose of a strong opioid for p.r.n. use; typically equivalent to 1/10–1/6 of the total daily dose.

12 With IV PCA, a larger bolus dose is generally necessary compared with the typical bolus dose of morphine 1mg. PCA can also be used to continuously deliver part or all of the baseline opioid dose.

Example
Patient on long-term morphine 300mg/day PO = 100mg/day IV = 4mg/h IV.
PCA background infusion = 2–3mg/h IV.
PCA bolus dose = 2mg IV with a 5min lockout period between doses.

With addicts, if there is considerable uncertainty about their opioid intake, it may be safer to underestimate both the background infusion dose and bolus dose required.

13 Close monitoring is required to:
   • identify inadequate dosing (unrelieved pain, withdrawal phenomena)
   • ensure rapid dose titration
   • prevent excessive dosing (sedation, respiratory depression)
   • ensure that bolus doses are not being misused.

For someone on high-dose SL **buprenorphine** who experiences acute pain unexpectedly, options include:
- regional anaesthesia
- optimizing the use of non-opioid analgesics (see Box A)
- prescribing a µ-opioid receptor agonist, e.g. IV **morphine, fentanyl**; higher doses than usual may be required
- progressively increasing the SL **buprenorphine** dose up to 24–32mg/day, and give in divided doses t.d.s.–q.d.s.[12,14]

Addicts receiving long-term naltrexone therapy

The opioid antagonist **naltrexone** is used to prevent relapse in opioid ex-addicts (by blocking the opioid 'high'), and in the treatment of alcohol dependence. It blocks all types of opioid receptor, and is long-acting. It thus prevents/blocks opioid analgesia. Analgesia for these patients is even more challenging (see Opioid antagonists, Box A, p.454).[16]

1 Rapp SE et al. (1995) Acute pain management in patients with prior opioid consumption: a case-controlled retrospective review. Pain. **61**: 195–201.
2 Macintyre PE (2001) Safety and efficacy of patient-controlled analgesia. British Journal of Anaesthesia. **87**: 36–46.
3 Roberts DM and Meyer-Witting M (2005) High-dose buprenorphine: perioperative precautions and management strategies. Anaesthesia and Intensive Care. **33**: 17–25.
4 Alford DP et al. (2006) Acute pain management for patients receiving maintenance methadone or buprenorphine therapy. Annals of Internal Medicine. **144**: 127–134.
5 British Pain Society (2006) Pain and substance misuse: improving the patient experience. A consensus document for consultation. British Pain Society, London. Available from: www.britishpainsociety.org
6 Macintyre PE and Ready LB (2006) Acute Pain Management - A Practical Guide (2e). Saunders Ltd., p. 272.
7 Mehta V and Langford RM (2006) Acute pain management for opioid dependent patients. Anaesthesia. **61**: 269–276.
8 Huxtable CA et al. (2011) Acute pain management in opioid-tolerant patients: a growing challenge. Anaesthesia and Intensive Care. **39**: 804–823.
9 British Pain Society (2010) Cancer pain management. British Pain Society, London. Available from: www.britishpainsociety.org
10 Farrell C and McConaghy P (2012) Perioperative management of patients taking treatment for chronic pain. British Medical Journal. **345**: e4148.
11 Grond S et al. (2000) Clinical pharmacokinetics of transdermal opioids: focus on transdermal fentanyl. Clinical Pharmacokinetics. **38**: 59–89.
12 Savage SR et al. (2008) Challenges in using opioids to treat pain in persons with substance use disorders. Addiction Science and Clinical Practice. **4**: 4–25.
13 Kornfield H and Manfredi L (2010) Effectiveness of full agonist opioids in patients stablized on buprenorphine undergoing major surgery: A case series. American Journal of Therapeutics. **17**: 523–528.
14 Heit HA and Gourlay DL (2008) Buprenorphine: new tricks with an old molecule for pain management. Clinical Journal of Pain. **24**: 93–97.
15 Macintyre PE et al. (2013) Pain relief and opioid requirements in the first 24 hours after surgery in patients taking buprenorphine and methadone opioid substitution therapy. Anaesthesia and Intensive Care. **41**: 222–230.
16 Vickers AP and Jolly A (2006) Naltrexone and problems in pain management. British Medical Journal. **332** (7534): 132–133.

Updated June 2014

19: ANALGESIC DRUGS AND FITNESS TO DRIVE

Several classes of centrally-acting analgesics have the potential to influence driving performance. Doctors have a duty of care to inform patients of this risk and advise them appropriately. As a minimum, patients should be reminded that it is their legal responsibility to ensure that they only drive if they feel 100% safe to do so. However, the impact of ceasing to drive can be considerable and impairment from stable doses of centrally-acting analgesics is not inevitable.

This chapter summarizes the evidence regarding the effect of opioids, anti-epileptics, antidepressants, benzodiazepines and cannabinoids on driving performance and the risk of a road traffic accident. Although the evidence is sometimes conflicting, the information provided here will assist health professionals when advising patients. Such advice will need to be tailored to individual circumstances, including the influence of the disease itself (e.g. risk of seizures), frailty, visual disturbances, the presence of pain, the possibility of pharmacokinetic interactions and the use of other sedative drugs (e.g. antimuscarinics).

Driving performance and drugs

Evaluating the impact of drugs on driving can be difficult. Driving performance is affected by multiple mechanisms from altered attention and reaction time to impaired judgment and risk taking. Studying actual or simulated driving, or surrogate laboratory markers of such skills, may not capture all influences on driving performance.[1,2] Although studying analgesic use among people involved in road traffic accidents avoids this problem, confounding factors include multiple drug use and impairment caused by pain and the illness itself.[3] Further, driving performance is impaired in some patients with chronic non-cancer pain not receiving centrally-acting medication.[4] Indeed, cognitive performance may improve with effective long-term opioid analgesia.[5,6] In a comparison of cancer patients (± **morphine** analgesia) with healthy volunteers, cognitive impairment was associated with cancer rather than **morphine**.[7]

Guidance for patients receiving a potentially sedating analgesic

In the UK, no distinction is made between illicit and prescribed drugs in terms of liability to prosecution for attempting to drive while intoxicated.[8] However, a Government consultation is currently underway for a new drug driving offence, to include a statutory defence for prescribed use of specified controlled drugs.

The evidence, summarized in Table 1, suggests that patients should be warned not to drive after starting and when titrating potentially sedating medication, or after taking a dose for break-through (episodic) pain. They should be warned that sedation will be increased by the concurrent use of alcohol (even within normal alcohol driving limits) or other sedating medication, whether obtained by prescription, over-the-counter, or for illicit use.

More specifically, patients receiving opioids, anti-epileptics and antidepressants can consider driving once a stable dose is achieved if they are not affected by drowsiness, nor impaired by the disease itself. If possible, use a less sedating drug, e.g. consider the use of an SSRI rather than a TCA when treating depression. For benzodiazepines, particularly if taken in the daytime and/or those with a long halflife, the risk is more persistent, and consideration should be given to using a less sedating alternative, e.g. an SSRI for anxiety, or not driving. The risk with stable doses of prescribed cannabinoids is unclear.

Providing the patient with written information also helps (Box A). Other examples of information leaflets are available at www.palliativedrugs.com; select Document library and search under Prescribing issues, Driving on medication.

Table I   Drugs and driving: a summary of the evidence

Class of drug	Impact on risk of a road traffic accident	Comments
Opioids	No increased risk with chronic use of a stable dose carefully titrated to avoid drowsiness and cognitive impairment[1,3,9–15]	Cognition and driving performance impaired for about 1 week after the start of treatment or after dose increments.[16,17] The risk is shared by weak opioids.[18] Additional transient impairment with doses for break-through (episodic) pain
Anti-epileptics	No increased risk with chronic use of a stable dose carefully titrated to avoid drowsiness and cognitive impairment[19]	Cognition impaired by multiple, high-dose anti-epileptics; marginally less with newer drugs (e.g. gabapentin) compared with older drugs (e.g. carbamazepine)[20,21]
Antidepressants	Sedative antidepressants double the risk in the elderly (>65 years) but not other age groups[19,22–25]	Sedative antidepressants impair performance for about 1 week after the start of treatment (mianserin ⩾2 weeks). SSRIs appear to cause less impairment[8,26]
Benzodiazepines	60–80% increase in risk[27]	Risk only partially decreases with time and is related to dose, halflife and concurrent alcohol. Risk from nocturnal use of shorter halflife hypnotic benzodiazepines is unclear[27,28]
Cannabinoids	Risk likely to be increased initially. The degree of tolerance to chronic use of stable doses of prescribed cannabinoids is uncertain	Most studies deal with illicit use, frequently confounded by alcohol consumption and risk-taking behaviours[29,30]

Box A   Example of a patient information leaflet: Strong painkillers and driving[11,13]

The medicines you are taking do not automatically disqualify you from driving in the United Kingdom. However, some painkillers can affect the speed of your reactions or general alertness. Both the label and the Patient Information Leaflet will warn you that drowsiness can occur. If receiving such medication, or other sedative drugs, it is important that you take the following precautions:

Do not drive
• unless you feel 100% safe to do so
• if you feel sleepy
• after taking other sedative drugs, whether or not recommended by your doctor, or after drinking alcohol
• after taking extra 'rescue' doses of a sedative painkiller, e.g. for at least 3 hours after an extra dose of morphine
• after starting or increasing the dose of a sedative painkiller; wait until any sleepiness wears off, generally about 5 days, but sometimes longer.

Restarting driving
You may try driving when you feel 100% safe to do so and you no longer feel sleepy. Begin by making a short trip:
• on roads that are quiet and familiar
• at a quiet time of day when the light is good
• with a companion who may take over driving if required.

continued

Box A Continued

If you and your companion are happy with your attentiveness, reactions and general ability, then you may start to drive. Do not exhaust yourself by driving long distances. If you are in any doubt, discuss with your doctor or other health professional.

Who to inform if you are planning to drive
- *your doctor*, who can warn you about medication which might affect the speed of your reactions or general alertness
- *your insurance company*, to be sure that you are covered (note: it may help if you send the company a copy of this leaflet).

Although you do not necessarily need to inform the DVLA that you are taking regular painkillers, in practice insurance companies generally advise this. However, in relation to cancer, the DVLA will need to be informed if you have a brain tumour, a secondary tumour in your brain or if you have had a fit or problems with eyesight. *If in doubt, discuss with your doctor or the DVLA medical advisory helpline* (0870 600 0301; and have your driving licence number ready).

Risk from specific analgesic drug classes
Opioids
Driving performance does not appear to be affected by stable doses of appropriately titrated strong opioids:[1,9–15]
- cognition returns to normal after about 1 week after the start of treatment or after dose increments[17]
- long-term opioid analgesia for cancer pain[15] and non-cancer pain[12,14] has little or no impact on surrogate laboratory measures of driving performance compared with:
  ▷ healthy volunteers[12]
  ▷ cancer patients not taking opioids[15]
  ▷ patients with various causes of cerebral impairment who had passed a standardized fitness-to-drive test[14]
- patients with non-cancer pain taking opioids at stable doses for ≥1 week do not differ from those not taking opioids or from healthy volunteers in tests of actual driving performance.[16]

The results of epidemiological studies are mixed.[27,32] However, an increased risk of road traffic accidents among drivers using opioid analgesics appears unlikely if confounding variables are taken into account:
- new vs. long-term use
- opioids vs. other psychotropics taken concurrently
- prescription vs. illicit use
- opioids vs. the pain itself.[3]

The optimal interval between dose initiation or increase and returning to driving is unclear and may vary between individuals and formulation used, e.g. steady-state plasma concentrations of TD **fentanyl** are generally achieved after 36–48h but, according to the manufacturers, this is sometimes achieved only after 6–12 days (see p.403).

Anti-epileptics
The use of multiple or high-dose anti-epileptics, particularly **phenobarbital** is associated with marked cognitive impairment. Newer drugs, e.g. **gabapentin**, may cause marginally less impairment than older drugs, e.g. **carbamazepine, valproate**.[20,21] However, in a case-control study, anti-epileptics were not associated with an increased risk of a road traffic accident.[19]

Antidepressants
Sedating antidepressants (e.g. **amitriptyline, doxepin, imipramine, mirtazapine, mianserin**) are associated with impaired driving performance in a standard on-the-road test. However, performance returned to baseline within 1 week except for **mianserin** when impairment remained at study end after 2 weeks.[26] In patients with neuropathic pain, impairment was present following the first dose of **amitriptyline** (25mg), but had returned to baseline when evaluated 2 weeks later.[4]

Although the DVLA generally advise that less sedating antidepressants are used where possible, e.g. SSRIs,[8] case-control studies suggest that they are not risk-free and caution is still required.[8,22–25,33,34]

Benzodiazepines

Benzodiazepines increase the risk of motor vehicle accidents by 60–80%. The risk is highest in those taking higher doses, drugs with a longer halflife, or concurrent alcohol.[26] The risk only partially decreases with time.[27]

Simulated driving tests show impaired reaction times, tracking and co-ordination with the acute use of benzodiazepines. In multiple-dose studies the degree of attenuation of impairment over time was variable.[32]

The risk from a bedtime dose of a hypnotic benzodiazepine with a short halflife is unclear; studies of airline pilots suggest that shorter-acting benzodiazepines do not cause a detectable sedating effect the following morning.[7] However, the results of case-control studies examining the risk of motor vehicle accidents are conflicting. **Zopiclone** is *not* a safer alternative.[26]

Cannabinoids

Most studies consider the risk from the illicit use of the whole cannabis plant. Interpretation is hampered by associated alcohol consumption, risk-taking behaviour (potentially a cause and/or effect of cannabis use), and methodological limitations. However, when taken together, these studies suggest that cannabis causes dose-dependent impairment of driving ability.[8,29,30] The risk of road traffic accidents is approximately doubled, and is further increased by concurrent alcohol consumption.[30] Some studies suggest a degree of insight into the impairment, and an ability to compensate partially for it (e.g. by driving more cautiously).

These studies are unlikely to reflect the risk associated with the use of stable doses of prescribed cannabinoids (see p.229). Stable doses may allow tolerance to impairment to develop, as with many psychotropics. For example, 6 patients with multiple sclerosis and painful spasticity showed no impairment of laboratory markers of driving ability after receiving **nabilone** 2mg/day for 4 weeks.[36] However, caution is necessary, particularly in physically debilitated patients, and they should be advised not to drive during initial dose titration. Once on a stable dose, and having evaluated the degree of psychomotor impairment caused by cannabinoids, restarting driving can be discussed.

1 Fishbain D et al. (2003) Are opioid-dependent/tolerant patients impaired in driving-related skills? A structured evidence-based review. *Journal of Pain and Symptom Management.* **25**: 559–577.
2 Verster JC and Roth T (2012) Predicting psychopharmacological drug effects on actual driving performance (SDLP) from psychometric tests measuring driving-related skills. *Psychopharmacology.* **220**: 293–301.
3 Fishbain D et al. (2002) Can patients taking opioids drive safely? A structured evidence-based review? *Journal of Pain and Palliative Care Pharmacotherapy.* **16**: 9–28.
4 Veldhuijzen DS et al. (2006) Effect of chronic nonmalignant pain on highway driving performance. *Pain.* **122**: 28–35.
5 Tassain V et al. (2003) Long term effects of oral sustained release morphine on neuropsychological performance in patients with chronic non-cancer pain. *Pain.* **104**: 389–400.
6 Jamison RN et al. (2003) Neuropsychological effects of long-term opioid use in chronic pain patients. *Journal of Pain and Symptom Management.* **26**: 913–921.
7 Clemons M et al. (1996) Alertness, cognition and morphine in patients with advanced cancer. *Cancer Treat Reviews.* **22**: 451–468.
8 Carter T (2006) *Fitness to Drive: A Guide for Health Professionals.* Royal Society of Medicine Press, London.
9 Kress HG and Kraft B (2005) Opioid medication and driving ability. *European Journal of Pain.* **9**: 141–144.
10 Brandman JF (2005) Cancer patients, opioids, and driving. *Journal of Supportive Oncology.* **3**: 317–320.
11 Pease N et al. (2004) Driving advice for palliative care patients taking strong opioid medication. *Palliative Medicine.* **18**: 663–665.
12 Sabatowski R et al. (2003) Driving ability under long-term treatment with transdermal fentanyl. *Journal of Pain and Symptom Management.* **25**: 38–47.
13 Chapman S (2001) The effects of opioids on driving ability in patients with chronic pain. *American Pain Society Bulletin.* **1**: 1.
14 Galski T et al. (2000) Effects of opioids on driving ability. *Journal of Pain and Symptom Management.* **19**: 200–208.
15 Vainio A et al. (1995) Driving ability in cancer patients receiving longterm morphine analgesia. *Lancet.* **346**: 667–670.
16 Byas-Smith MG et al. (2005) The effect of opioids on driving and psychomotor performance in patients with chronic pain. *Clinical Journal of Pain.* **21**: 345–352.
17 Bruera E et al. (1989) The cognitive effects of the administration of narcotic analgesics in patients with cancer pain. *Pain.* **39**: 13–16.
18 Bachs LC et al. (2009) The risk of motor vehicle accidents involving drivers with prescriptions for codeine or tramadol. *Clinical Pharmacology and Therapeutics.* **85**: 596–599.
19 Neutel I (1998) Benzodiazepine-related traffic accidents in young and elderly drivers. *Human Psychopharmacology.* **13(Suppl)**: s115–s123.
20 Aldenkamp AP et al. (2003) Newer antiepileptic drugs and cognitive issues. *Epilepsia.* **44 (Suppl 4)**: 21–29.

21 Brunbech L and Sabers A (2002) Effect of antiepileptic drugs on cognitive function in individuals with epilepsy: a comparative review of newer versus older agents. *Drugs.* **62**: 593–604.

22 McGwin G, Jr. *et al.* (2000) Relations among chronic medical conditions, medications, and automobile crashes in the elderly: a population-based case-control study. *American Journal of Epidemiology.* **152**: 424–431.

23 Barbone F *et al.* (1998) Association of road-traffic accidents with benzodiazepine use. *Lancet.* **352**: 1331–1336.

24 Leveille SG *et al.* (1994) Psychoactive medications and injurious motor vehicle collisions involving older drivers. *Epidemiology.* **5**: 591–598.

25 Ray WA *et al.* (1992) Psychoactive drugs and the risk of injurious motor vehicle crashes in elderly drivers. *American Journal of Epidemiology.* **136**: 873–883.

26 Ramaekers JG (2003) Antidepressants and driver impairment: empirical evidence from a standard on-the-road test. *Journal of Clinical Psychiatry.* **64**: 20–29.

27 Dassanayake T *et al.* (2011) Effects of benzodiazepines, antidepressants and opioids on driving: a systematic review and meta-analysis of epidemiological and experimental evidence. *Drug Safety.* **34**: 125–156.

28 Hemmelgarn B *et al.* (1997) Benzodiazepine use and the risk of motor vehicle crash in the elderly. *Journal of the American Medical Association.* **278**: 27–31.

29 UK Department for Transport (2000) Cannabis and driving: a review of the literature and commentary (No.12).

30 Asbridge M *et al.* (2012) Acute cannabis consumption and motor vehicle collision risk: systematic review of observational studies and meta-analysis. *British Medical Journal.* **344**: e536.

31 Twycross RG (1997) *Oral Morphine in Advanced Cancer* (3e). Beaconsfield Publishers, Beaconsfield.

32 Orriols L *et al.* (2009) The impact of medicinal drugs on traffic safety: a systematic review of epidemiological studies. *Pharmacoepidemiology Drug Safety.* **18**: 647–658.

33 Ravera S *et al.* (2011) Road traffic accidents and psychotropic medication use in The Netherlands: a case-control study. *British Journal of Clinical Pharmacology.* **72**: 505–513.

34 Rapoport MJ and Banina MC (2007) Impact of psychotropic medications on simulated driving: a critical review. *CNS Drugs.* **21**: 503–519.

35 Gunja N (2013) In the Zzz zone: the effects of Z-drugs on human performance and driving. *Journal of Medical Toxicology.* **9**: 163–171.

36 Kurzthaler I *et al.* (2005) The effect of nabilone on neuropsychological functions related to driving ability: an extended case series. *Human Psychopharmacology.* **20**: 291–293.

Updated June 2014

20: CONTINUOUS SUBCUTANEOUS DRUG INFUSIONS

CSCI in clinical practice

The administration of drugs by continuous subcutaneous infusion (CSCI) is common in palliative care in the UK, particularly in patients for whom swallowing medication has become increasingly difficult or impossible.[1,2]

Ambulatory battery-powered infusion devices are generally used to administer the CSCI.[2] These devices can also be used to administer medication by spinal infusion (see p.713).

CSCI is as effective as continuous IV infusion (CIVI),[3] and at least as good as intermittent bolus injections.[4] In settings where it is difficult to be certain that intermittent regular injections will be administered on time, CSCI is likely to provide better round-the-clock comfort.

Indications for CSCI

CSCI is not 'Step 4' on the analgesic ladder; it is a useful alternative route of administration in various circumstances,[5] including:

- persistent nausea and vomiting
- dysphagia
- bowel obstruction
- coma
- poor absorption of oral drugs (rare)
- patient preference.

Before setting up a CSCI, it is important to explain to the patient and family:

- the reason(s) for using this route
- how the infusion device works
- the advantages and possible disadvantages of CSCI (Box A).

Drugs used by CSCI

For most drugs, this route of administration is off-label (see p.xx).[6] However, there is extensive documented clinical experience of CSCI with many drugs used in palliative care. In addition, there are reports of other drugs given less frequently by this route, e.g. **diclofenac** (p.331), **furosemide** (p.66), **sodium valproate** (p.281).

For CSCI, the injectable formulation must be of a suitable concentration to deliver the required dose in a relatively small volume and also be relatively non-irritant. The risk of local irritation is increased when injectable formulations have a pH < 2 or > 11, or contain excipients which may themselves be irritant, e.g. some preservatives, solubilizing agents.

Although often administered by CSCI, several drugs with a long duration of action, e.g. **dexamethasone, levomepromazine** can be given as a bolus SC or IV injection once daily or b.d. (Table 1)[1]

Bolus SC injections should be given via a separate SC butterfly needle/cannula and *not* via a side-arm or port of a CSCI cannula or infusion line. This avoids potential problems with drug incompatibility or loss of symptom control caused by the flush replacing the CSCI contents of the infusion tubing.

Box A   Advantages and disadvantages of CSCI

Advantages
Saving nurses' time.
Round-the-clock comfort because plasma drug concentrations are maintained without peaks and troughs.
Less need for repeated injections.
Generally needs to be loaded once daily.
Control of multiple symptoms with a combination of drugs.
Independence and mobility maintained because the infusion device is lightweight and can be worn in a holster.
Patient preference.

Disadvantages
Initial cost of infusion devices.
Training of staff, together with need to maintain competency.
Lack of flexibility if more than one drug is being administered.
Lack of reliable compatibility data for some mixtures.
Possible inflammation and pain at the infusion site.
Although uncommon, problems with the infusion device can lead to break-through (episodic) pain (or other symptom) if the problem is not resolved quickly.

Table 1   Drugs which can be given once daily or b.d. instead of by CSCI

Drug	Plasma halflife (h)	Duration of action (h)
Clonazepam[a] (not UK)	20–60	≤12–24
Dexamethasone	3–4.5	36–54
Furosemide	0.5–2	6–8
Granisetron	10–11	≤24
Haloperidol	13–35	≤24
Levomepromazine[b]	15–30	≤24
Methadone[b]	8–75	≤12

a. for SC/IV bolus doses, dilute each 1mg/mL amp with 1mL WFI
b. relatively irritant SC

Prescribing CSCI

CSCI must be prescribed in the relevant section of the patient's drug chart. Some specialist units have separate CSCI drug charts (examples are available in the Document library of www.palliativedrugs.com); these must be linked or referred to in the patient's main drug chart. The prescription should specify:
• the dose of each drug to be administered over the infusion period (generally 24h)
• the diluent
• the final volume of the infusion.
Compatibility of the drug(s) and the diluent should be confirmed before the CSCI is set up; if it is not a routine combination, ideally, this should be documented in the patient's notes (see p.xxii).

If symptoms are controlled, start the CSCI 1–2h before the effect of the medication is due to wear off. If symptoms are uncontrolled, set up the CSCI immediately with stat doses of the same drugs.

Rescue medication

Appropriate doses of p.r.n. medication must also be prescribed. These are given via a separate SC needle/cannula (left *in situ* for this purpose) and flushed with compatible diluent (see below).

Drug doses
Converting from PO to CSCI

Drugs are generally *more* bio-available by injection than PO. This means that the dose of a drug given by CSCI will be *less* than the dose previously given PO, generally between 1/3 and 2/3 of the PO dose. The bio-availability data given at the end of the pharmacology section in the individual drug monographs serve as a guide to the appropriate reduction.

Thus, the dose of a drug with oral bio-availability of 75% should be reduced by a quarter when given SC, halved if 50% bio-available, and so on. Particular care should be taken with strong opioids (see p.667).

Converting from CSCI to PO

Some patients are able to revert from CSCI to PO medication, e.g. those being treated for nausea and vomiting. When this seems possible, convert the drugs sequentially rather than all at once. For example, convert the anti-emetic medication first and, if the nausea and vomiting do not recur, change the other medication 1–2 days later.

Remember: just as drug doses were reduced when starting CSCI, doses will generally need to be increased when reverting to PO. This is particularly the case with strong opioid analgesics, e.g. **morphine** 15mg/24h CSCI will need to be increased to **morphine** 30mg/24h PO.

The CSCI is generally discontinued when the first dose of the PO medication is administered. It is important to review p.r.n. medication, and to adjust it appropriately.

Converting from TD patches to CSCI (or vice versa)

As a general rule, TD **buprenorphine** or **fentanyl** patches should be continued when the need for supplemental opioid via CSCI is short-term, e.g. in the last days of life. It is simpler to supplement the patch with a CSCI of **morphine** or other opioid than to convert completely to a single alternative opioid. See the respective Quick Prescribing Guides for **buprenorphine** and **fentanyl** for more information, including the conversion of a CSCI opioid to a TD patch (p.401 and p.411).

Diluent

> *PCF recommends that generally WFI is used as the standard diluent of choice.* However, 0.9% saline should be considered if there is a potential or actual problem with inflammatory reactions at the skin injection site (see p.704).

The main purpose of diluents is to help reduce site irritation and enable drug delivery over a prescribed time. It is essential that the diluent is compatible with the drug(s) in the syringe. The SPC may indicate compatible diluents, particularly if a drug is authorized for CSCI. However, the information may not be comprehensive, and is unlikely to cover compatibility when drugs are mixed. Generally, either WFI or 0.9% saline can be used. They both have advantages and disadvantages (Table 2).

In the UK, WFI is widely used as the first-line diluent because it can be used to dilute all commonly used drugs in palliative care, including **cyclizine *lactate*** (see p.250) and higher concentrations of **diamorphine *hydrochloride*** (> 40mg/mL) or **haloperidol** (> 1mg/mL). There is also a wealth of supporting compatibility data and clinical experience for WFI (see Appendix 3, p.821).

For some drugs, e.g. **granisetron, hydromorphone, ketamine, ketorolac, octreotide** and **ondansetron**, more compatibility data exists with 0.9% saline and some prefer to use this as the diluent. Further, 0.9% saline would be a reasonable first-line diluent in those countries where **cyclizine *lactate*** or **diamorphine** are unavailable or not used.

Some centres in the USA use 5% glucose in water as the first-line diluent. However, this is acidic and unsuitable for very alkaline drugs, e.g. **dexamethasone, furosemide, ketorolac,** and **phenobarbital**.

To avoid confusion, consistency of practice within individual units is important.[8]

Table 2 Comparison of diluents

WFI	0.9% saline[7]
Advantanges	**Advantages**
Less chance of incompatibility	Isotonic. Preferable for diluting irritant drugs (potentially less infusion site reaction)
Generally more compatibility data available for commonly used drugs	
Disadvantages	**Disadvantages**
Large volumes are hypotonic, which may cause infusion site pain or skin reaction (generally not a problem in practice because infusion rates are so slow)	Incompatible with some drugs, e.g. cyclizine; higher concentrations of diamorphine >40mg/mL or haloperidol > 1mg/mL
	Generally less compatibility data available for commonly used drugs

Infusion volume

Factors influencing the final volume of the CSCI include the total volume of the drugs, the infusion device being used, the maximum rate of delivery, the intended infusion time and local guidelines. Greater dilution reduces:
- the risk of incompatibility
- the impact of priming a line (less drug in the 'dead space')
- injection site skin reactions from the drug.

For these reasons, 20mL syringes are now generally recommended as the minimum standard size to be used.

In deciding how much diluent to use, one approach, applicable to CME McKinley T34 syringe pumps, is to dilute the contents to a standard volume, e.g.:
- for a total drug volume <10mL, dilute to 15mL in a 20mL luerlock syringe
- for a total drug volume >10mL, dilute to 20mL in a 30mL luerlock syringe.

Additional dilution may be necessary when mixing drugs where compatibility depends on the final drug concentrations e.g. **cyclizine, dexamethasone, haloperidol, ketorolac** (see p.703, and footnotes of Charts 1–7, p.824–p.837).

In some situations, the total volume of drugs may exceed the maximum volume/24h that an infusion device can deliver, i.e. about 22mL or 34mL in a 30mL or 50mL syringe respectively for a CME McKinley T34 syringe pump. This is most likely with combinations which include higher doses of **fentanyl, metoclopramide, midazolam, morphine** or **oxycodone**. This problem can generally be circumvented by:
- using a more concentrated formulation (see below)
- changing the contents of the syringe driver more frequently, e.g. every 12h
- switching from **morphine** to **diamorphine** or **hydromorphone**
- using a different infusion device.[9]

When a cartridge/cassette/bag infusion system is used, a larger final volume is possible. Even so, some centres standardize to 50mL volume with a maximum rate of 2mL/h.

Caution is required when using a more concentrated formulation, e.g. **fentanyl** 5mg/mL, **oxycodone** 50mg/mL, **midazolam** 5mg/mL, because compatibility can differ from the normal strength formulation (Box B). Further, confusion between the normal and the more concentrated formulations has resulted in overdoses. Consequently, some organizations restrict their availability.[10]

Infusion duration

In the UK, CSCI syringes are generally timed to empty over 24h. The main reasons for this are:
- extrapolation of sterility guidelines from CIVI
- availability of stability and compatibility data
- standardization of practice (for safety reasons)
- tradition based on the limitations of older syringe drivers.

Generally, 24h is satisfactory in terms of both sterility, stability and practicality.[11,12]

For certain infusion devices, e.g. CADD pumps, elastomeric devices, stability and compatibility data may exist for a longer duration of infusion, e.g. 48–72h. Generally, these solutions are made up in aseptically controlled environments, e.g. pharmacy aseptic units to ensure sterility.

Infusion stability

Drug stability and compatibility are closely related. Stability describes how much of the drug remains in its original form in a given period of time. Compatibility describes whether the addition of a diluent or a drug causes a physical or chemical interaction. Various factors affect the stability of the drug in the CSCI and potentially could lead to incompatibility and impaired symptom control (Box B).

Box B   Factors affecting CSCI drug stability or compatibility[13–16]

Diluent (see p.699).

Final concentration of drug
The *concentration* of the drug in the solution (the *quantity* of the drug divided by the *total final volume*) should be checked against stability and compatibility data (see p.821).

Order of mixing
Particularly when compatibility is concentration dependent, e.g. dexamethasone should always be the last drug added to an already diluted and mixed syringe to reduce the risk of incompatibility.

Brand/formulation/strength of the drug
Injections contain various excipients, e.g. preservatives, diluents, stabilizing compounds, which can differ between brands, countries, and even between different strengths of the same drug, e.g. oxycodone (see p.838).

Duration of infusion
Note: the rate at which drugs degrade can be increased by:
Higher temperature: do not wear the infusion device under clothes
Exposure to light: e.g. levomepromazine turns pink/yellow; cover the infusion.

Adsorption onto delivery system material
E.g. ≤50% of a dose of clonazepam onto PVC tubing (see p.162).

Mixing drugs

The combination of two or more authorized (licensed) drugs results in a new unauthorized (unlicensed) product being formed. Doctors and other independent prescribers (nurse, pharmacist) can mix, and direct others to mix, drugs (including controlled drugs) for administration to a particular patient. Supplementary prescribers can mix and direct others to mix when part of a Clinical Management Plan (also see p.xx).[17]

In the UK, it is common practice to administer 2–3 different drugs in the same infusion device.[1,2,18] Some centres mix four or more drugs. However, the greater the number of drugs mixed, the greater the probability of compatibility problems. Accordingly, *PCF* recommends that generally no more than three drugs should be mixed in one syringe.

Drug compatibility

When mixing drugs it is essential to consider drug compatibility (Box C). Physical and/or chemical changes can occur which could lead to reduced efficacy.[19]

Box C Drug compatibility data

Physical compatibility

If mixing two or more drugs does not result in a physical change, e.g. discolouration, clouding or crystallization, they are said to be physically compatible.

Observational data

Data from many palliative care services about the visual appearance of various drug mixtures over the infusion period (generally 24h) have been collated for use in Appendix 3 (p.821). However, observational data are subjective and imprecise; generally, only major incompatibilities can be identified in this way.

Laboratory data

These are generally derived from microscopic examination of a drug mixture under polarized light at specified concentrations and several time points when kept under controlled conditions. Although more robust, these are not definitive; a solution may remain physically clear even when there is chemical incompatibility.[20]

Chemical compatibility

If mixing two or more drugs does not result in a chemical change leading to loss or degradation of one or more of the drugs, the mixture is said to be chemically compatible. Chemical compatibility data are generally obtained by analyzing the drug mixture by high-performance liquid chromatography (HPLC) at specified concentrations and several time points when kept under controlled conditions.

Occasionally, a drug combination has been shown to be chemically compatible but physically incompatible.

Ideally both physical and chemical compatibility data should be known. However, because of the infinite number of possible drug combinations, and a dearth of published chemical compatibility studies, generally, decisions are taken on the basis of physical compatibility, based on observational data and clinical experience.

Information sources

Information on CSCI compatibility can be obtained from several sources:
- *for infusions with WFI as a diluent:* Charts 1–7 (see Appendix 3, p.821) summarize the compatibility data for the more commonly used 2- and 3-drug combinations. They have been compiled from clinical observations in palliative care services in the UK, New Zealand and Australia, and from published compatibility data
- *for infusions with 0.9% saline as a diluent:* Charts 8–14 (see the extended appendix section of the on-line PCF on www.palliativedrugs.com) summarize the compatibility data for the more commonly used 2- and 3-drug combinations. They have been compiled from clinical observations in palliative care services in the UK, New Zealand and Australia, and from published compatibility data
- *Syringe Driver Survey Database* (SDSD) *on* www.palliativedrugs.com: this is a continually updated resource and contains observational compatibility data on mixing combinations of up to 4 drugs reported by health professionals. For this to be of maximum benefit, members are urged to donate information about both *successful* and *unsuccessful* combinations for which there are no previously published data
- *The Syringe Driver: Continuous Subcutaneous Infusions in Palliative Care*[18]
- www.pallcare.info
- *Handbook on Injectable Drugs.*[13]

Generally, these sources can only indicate if a drug combination is likely to be stable and compatible. Many factors affect drug compatibility and/or stability (see Box B) which helps explain conflicting reports. If there is doubt about the relevance of the compatibility data to the situation in which a given drug combination is to be used, advice should be obtained from a clinical pharmacist. Regular checks of the CSCI together with the patient's condition should always be undertaken (see p.705).

General principles for compatibility

When there is a lack of robust compatibility data for the prescribed drugs, the following general principles should be noted:

- generally, drugs with a similar pH are more likely to be compatible than those with widely differing ones (Table 3)
- most drugs are acidic in solution, however, **dexamethasone, diclofenac, furosemide, ketorolac, omeprazole** and **phenobarbital** are alkaline in solution and often cause compatibility problems (Table 3); as a result **diclofenac, furosemide, omeprazole** and **phenobarbital** should be administered separately and not be mixed with other drugs
- dilute to the maximum volume possible
- compatibility with **cyclizine** or **haloperidol** is often concentration dependent and they are more likely to cause problems at higher concentrations
- the risk of precipitation with **dexamethasone** is reduced if it is added last to an already dilute drug mixture. On the other hand, as already noted, **dexamethasone** has a long duration of action. Thus, except when it is being given to reduce the risk of skin reactions (see p.704), there is no real need to give it by CSCI (Table 1)
- occasionally, initial cloudiness or separation (precipitation) may occur which resolves on full mixing; however, ensure it fully resolves and monitor the infusion closely (note: delayed cloudiness can be caused by chemicals from the syringe or tubing leaching out)
- protect from direct sunlight (particularly levomepromazine) and heat
- the more drugs combined, the greater the risk of incompatibility; generally, PCF recommends a maximum of three drugs in one syringe
- checks in use should be undertaken more regularly (see p.705) monitoring both the infusion and expected clinical outcome. Where incompatibilities are found e.g. crystal formation, details should be submitted to the SDSD, to help build a database of evidence for drug combinations.

Table 3 Approximate pH values of parenteral drugs[13,21]

Drug[a]	pH	Drug[a]	pH
Alfentanil	4–6	Hyoscine *hydrobromide*	5–7
Buprenorphine	4–6	Ketamine	3.5–5.5
Clonazepam	3.6	Ketorolac	6.9–7.9
Clonidine	4–4.5	Levomepromazine	4.5
Cyclizine lactate	3.3–3.7	Lidocaine	5–7
Dexamethasone *sodium phosphate*	7–10.5	Methadone	3–6.5
Diamorphine[b]		Metoclopramide	4.5–6.5
Diclofenac	7.8–9	Midazolam	3
Fentanyl	4–7.5	Morphine *sulfate*	2.5–6.5
Furosemide	8–9.3	Octreotide	3.9–4.5
Glycopyrronium	2–3	Omeprazole	8.8–10.3
Granisetron	4.7–7.3	Ondansetron	3.3–4
Haloperidol	3–3.8	Oxycodone	4.5–5.5
Hydromorphone	4–5.5	Phenobarbital	9.2–10.2
Hyoscine *butylbromide*	3.7–5.5	Ranitidine	6.7–7.3

a. pH values may vary between each strength and different brands
b. powder for reconstitution; most stable when reconstituted so that the pH is 3.8–4.5.

Site of CSCI

See Box D. Traditionally an 18-gauge metal butterfly needle has been used, inserted at an angle of 30–45° into SC tissue. However, plastic/teflon cannula are increasingly used because they reduce the risk of site reactions and needle stick injury.[22–24]

Where possible use fine bore tubing with a small priming volume (preferably less than 0.3mL) and secure the tubing to the skin with a transparent semipermeable adhesive dressing (e.g. Tegaderm®), with a loop to reduce the likelihood of needle/cannula displacement.

Box D Siting a CSCI	
Areas to avoid Oedematous areas Skin folds Breast Broken, inflamed or infected skin Recently irradiated skin sites Cutaneous tumour sites Bony prominences Near a joint Anterior chest wall in cachectic patients Upper arm in bedbound patients who need turning Scarring	**Preferred sites** Anterior chest wall Anterolateral aspects of upper arms **Alternative sites** Anterior abdominal wall Anterior surface of the thighs

Infusion site problems

These occur in ≤25% of patients (Box E).[1,23] Apart from discomfort, local inflammation may impair drug absorption and thereby symptom control.

Box E   Causes of infusion site problems[18,25,26]
Anatomical site Local bruising (caused by needle/cannula) Irritant drug(s) Tonicity of the solution pH of the solution Incompatible drug–diluent mixture Allergy to nickel needle Glass particles from ampoules Sterile abscess Infection Infrequent resiting

With non-irritant drugs an infusion site may be satisfactory for ≥1 week (and occasionally 2–3 weeks).[23,27] Site reactions can be reduced by:

- use of a less irritant drug, e.g. **haloperidol** instead of **prochlorperazine** (Box F)
- considering the use of 0.9% saline as a diluent, when compatibility data exists (see p.699)
- diluting the solution as much as practical, this may include changing the syringe q12h instead of q24h to permit further dilution
- using a plastic cannula instead of a butterfly needle (always use in patients with a known metal allergy)
- changing the site prophylactically every 2–3 days; particularly if using irritant drugs
- applying **hydrocortisone** 1% cream to the skin around the needle entry site, and covering it with an occlusive dressing
- adding **dexamethasone** 1mg to the solution if compatibility data permits.[27]

Although the routine addition of **dexamethasone** has been recommended on the grounds that it extends the life of an infusion site by about 50%, the fact that some sites have lasted 2–3 weeks without **dexamethasone** means that routine use cannot be recommended.[27]

Box F Drugs which are irritant SC
Strongly irritant, do *not* give by CSCI Chlorpromazine Diazepam Prochlorperazine (sometimes given by SC bolus) **Relatively irritant by CSCI, precautions may be necessary**[a] Cyclizine Diclofenac Ketamine Ketorolac Levomepromazine Methadone Octreotide[b] Ondansetron Phenobarbital[c] Promethazine[c]

a. see text and respective monographs
b. painful if given as SC bolus; this is reduced if warmed to body temperature before injection
c. strongly irritant with risk of tissue necrosis if given by SC bolus injection.

Infusion devices

In the UK, ambulatory syringe drivers/pumps are the most commonly used devices for delivering drugs by CSCI. The use of cartridges/cassettes prepared by a pharmacist adds significantly to the cost. The CME McKinley T34 is the most frequently used syringe driver.[28,29] The older Graseby MS16A and MS26 syringe drivers lack the recommended safety features and by December 2015 they should no longer be used in the UK.[30,31]

Setting up the infusion device

Full instructions can be found in the manufacturer's instruction manuals. See also the Quick Clinical Guides on setting up a CME McKinley T34 syringe pump (p.706) and the Graseby MS16A and MS26A syringe driver (p.709); this is included for clinicians in countries where these are still used.

PCF recommends priming the infusion line before attaching it to the syringe pump. This uses approx. 0.3mL volume depending on the type of infusion line. This means that a small proportion of the dose drawn up for the patient will be lost in the 'dead space' when a new infusion is first set up. The final volume in the syringe should be noted and used to check the infusion rate (automatically calculated by some syringe drivers). Subsequent infusions given by the same line will not need priming, therefore the final volume and thus the infusion rate will be slightly different.

Checks in use

Specific record charts should be used for checking a CSCI; examples are available in the Document library of www.palliativedrugs.com. These record charts should be used in addition to the prescription chart. Checks should be documented within 1h of setting up the CSCI, and then q4h:
- is the device still working?
- is the correct rate still infusing?
- amount of time and volume of solution left, and whether the infusion is running to time (based on the preceding 4h)
- appearance of the solution in the tubing and syringe/cartridge/bag
- condition of the skin site
- battery status.

Do not remove the syringe/cartridge/bag from the infusion device to perform these checks. If checking indicates a problem, action should be taken and then documented, e.g. if the infusion needs to be resited (and hence reprimed), the time, the new site and the new infusion volume/syringe length should be recorded. Other comments might include details of incompatibility and mention of any mishaps, e.g. the delivery device found disconnected.

Quick Clinical Guide: Setting up a CME McKinley T34 syringe pump for CSCI

For full instructions, see the manufacturer's operation manual.

PCF recommends 'Lock on' mode for general use; this automatically provides an infusion duration of 24h.

PCF does *not* recommend the use of the automatic purge. Although designed to reduce the slack in the pump mechanism and achieve the correct flow rate more quickly (about 20min vs. 2h), it is more complex to set up and the clinical relevance of the time difference is unknown. Further, patients should have access to p.r.n. medication for the relief of any symptoms.

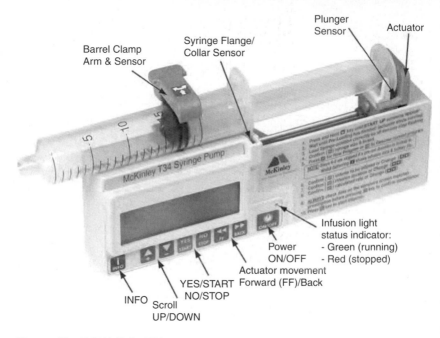

Figure The CME McKinley T34 syringe pump.

Additional equipment
- battery, PP3: 9V Alkaline/Lithium + spare battery (each lasts about 3–4 days)
- 20mL or 30mL luerlock syringe
- 100cm McKinley SC infusion line with integrated anti-free flow and anti-siphon valve (0.3mL priming volume)
- lock-box and key.

1 A CSCI may take 4–6h to provide effective symptom control. SC bolus doses of the appropriate rescue medication should be available to relieve any symptoms.

2 Fill a luerlock syringe with the drugs and dilute the contents to a standard volume, e.g. 15mL in a 20mL syringe with WFI, or when the volume of the undiluted drugs is > 10mL, to 20mL in a 30mL syringe. A larger final volume may also be required to ensure compatibility. For maximum fill volumes, see table below.

Syringe size	Maximum fill volume
20mL syringe	17mL
30mL syringe	22mL
50mL syringe[a]	34mL

a. the lock-box will not accommodate a 50mL syringe; however, the pump itself is still locked and thus can be used.

Note: dexamethasone should be the last drug added to an already dilute combination of drugs in order to reduce the risk of incompatibility.

3 The syringe should be made up immediately before use, using strict aseptic technique. Ensure adequate mixing has occurred; the solution should be clear and free from discoloration, crystals or precipitate.

4 Label the syringe, taking care not to completely obscure the solution. The label should be flat and unfolded to avoid obstructing the pump mechanism.

5 Attach the syringe to a McKinley infusion line and prime manually (this uses about 0.3mL) and note the remaining volume.

6 Insert the battery into the syringe driver.

7 Ensure the barrel clamp is down and the syringe is *not* connected.

8 Press and hold the **black** ON/OFF key until START UP screens appear.

9 Wait until pre-loading has finished (actuator stops moving).

10 Check the battery capacity by pressing the **blue** INFO key (use +/− keys to scroll to the battery status option) and the **green** YES key to view battery status.

At least 40% battery capacity is required for 24 hours. Change the battery if necessary, e.g. for community use. Switch off by holding down the **black** ON/OFF key until the screen goes blank, discard the battery, insert a new one and repeat steps 7–10.

11 The actuator will move automatically to the size of the last syringe used. If a different size syringe is required, use the FF/BACK keys to move the actuator to the correct position for syringe loading. Once the actuator has stopped moving, lift and rotate the barrel clamp arm, load the syringe (ensuring the plunger and syringe barrel are in the correct slots) and rotate and replace the barrel arm clamp.

12 The display screen will show if any of the 3 positioning points are not aligned correctly. If this is the case, remove the syringe and repeat step 11.

13 Ensure the pump has detected the correct syringe type and size, press the **green** YES key to confirm or use +/− keys to scroll and select the correct option.

14 A new programme *must* be set for each new syringe. If the pump gives the option of resuming a previous programme, it has been set up incorrectly. Do *not* take this option (press **red** NO key). Turn off the pump, remove the syringe and start again.

15 Check the correct infusion volume (as documented after priming) and duration (24 hours) is shown on the display. The rate is automatically calculated, but it is good practice to double check this by dividing the volume by the time. Press the **green** YES key if settings are correct.

16 Insert the cannula subcutaneously in the patient in a suitable position; secure and attach the syringe and infusion line to the cannula.

17 Press the **green** YES key to start the infusion.

The screen will continually show the time remaining for the infusion, the rate (mL/h) and the syringe selected.

18 Lock the keypad by pressing and holding the **blue** INFO key until the display shows Keypad LOCK ON.

19 Secure the pump in the lockbox provided. This cannot accommodate a 50mL syringe, but the pump itself can still be locked.

20 Protect the syringe from excessive sunlight and heat, e.g. electric blankets.

21 Regular checks on the progress, the visual appearance of the infusion and administration site should be performed and documented during the infusion. Do not remove the syringe from the pump to perform these checks. If checking indicates a problem, action should be taken and then documented. An infusion progress summary can be obtained whilst infusing by pressing the **blue** INFO key.

22 If there is a problem, an alert (short audible alarm and a screen message, infusion continues) or an alarm (continuous alarm, infusion stops and a red light appears above the **black** ON/OFF key) will activate. Refer to the trouble-shooting guide and manufacturer's operation manual for implications and actions.

23 Do not add drugs to a syringe or infusion line once the infusion has been commenced. Additional bolus drugs needed should be administered by a separate cannula.

Temporarily stopping and disconnecting the infusion

The infusion may sometimes need to be temporarily stopped (e.g. to change the battery) or disconnected (e.g. when the patient bathes/showers):
- unlock the keypad by pressing and holding the **blue** INFO key until the display shows LOCK OFF
- press the **red** STOP key to stop the infusion
- press and hold the **black** ON/OFF key to switch the pump off; leave the syringe attached to the pump
- *when temporarily disconnecting the infusion*: disconnect the infusion line at the cannula end; cap off both the infusion line and the cannula
- store syringe and infusion line safely; lock in a CD cupboard if it contains a CD.

After interruption:
- reconnect the infusion line to the cannula
- turn on the pump by pressing and holding the **black** ON/OFF key
- confirm the syringe size and brand
- press the **green** YES key to resume the infusion
- check and confirm the volume, duration and rate
- press the **green** YES key to start the infusion.

---

24 When the infusion is completed an alarm will sound and the infusion will stop. Unlock the keypad by pressing and holding the **blue** INFO key until the display shows keypad LOCK OFF. Press the **red** STOP key. Press and hold the **black** ON/OFF key to switch the pump off.

25 *If the next prescription is to be repeated exactly*, the same infusion line may be re-used as per local policy. Follow the guidance from step 1; at step 5 priming is not needed, remove the completed syringe from the pump, but leave it connected to the patient; at step 16, remove the old syringe from the infusion line and reconnect the infusion line to the new syringe; complete the remaining steps in the set up as before.

26 *If the next prescription is different (or changed mid-infusion)*, stop the infusion as in step 24, disconnect the infusion line from the patient *before* removing the syringe from the pump. Set up the next prescription from step 1 of the guidelines, using a new syringe and new infusion line.

Quick Clinical Guide: Setting up a Graseby MS16A or MS26 syringe driver for CSCI

For full instructions, see the manufacturer's operation manual.

The Graseby MS16A and MS26 syringe drivers do not have all of the safety features recommended by the UK NPSA and they have been withdrawn from use in the UK. This guide is provided solely for practitioners outside the UK, where these syringe drivers may still be used. PCF does *not* recommend the use of the MS26 boost facility because
- a single boost does not deliver an effective analgesic dose
- there is no lock-out period
- when multiple drugs are being infused, boosting is non-specific
- the infusion will run out before the scheduled changeover time.

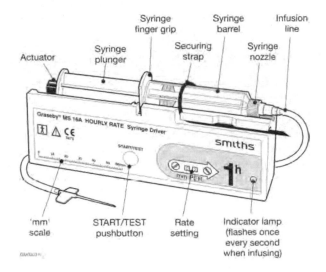

Figure   The Graseby MS16A hourly rate syringe driver.

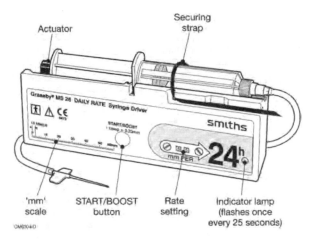

Figure   The Graseby MS26 daily rate syringe driver.

Additional equipment
- battery: 9V Alkaline + spare battery
- 20mL luerlock syringe
- SC infusion line with integrated anti-free flow and anti-siphon valve
- lock-box.

1 A CSCI may take 4–6h to provide effective symptom relief. SC bolus doses of the appropriate rescue medication should be available to relieve any symptoms.

2 Insert the battery and perform initial safety checks to ensure the correct syringe driver has been selected and is working correctly. Remove the battery until ready to commence the infusion.

3 Fill a luerlock syringe with the drugs and dilute the contents to the required volume using the millimetre length scale on the driver or ruler for reference. The MS16A and MS26 can deliver a maximum length of 60mm. However, many palliative care services standardize the length used at 48mm.

> The rate of delivery is based upon *a length of fluid in millimetres per unit time*; this allows any brand of syringe to be used. The rate is calculated differently between the MS16A (an *hourly* rate driver, i.e. delivers in **millimetres per hour**) and the MS26 (a *daily* rate driver, i.e. delivers in **millimetres per 24h**). Great care must be taken to ensure the rate of delivery is calculated accurately.

Note: dexamethasone should be the last drug added to an already dilute combination of drugs in order to reduce the risk of incompatibility.

4 The syringe should be made up immediately before use, using strict aseptic technique. Ensure adequate mixing has occurred; the solution should be clear and free from discoloration, crystals or precipitate.

5 Label the syringe, taking care not to completely obscure the solution. The label should be flat and unfolded to avoid obstructing the mechanism.

6 Calculate the delivery rate (see Box) and have it independently verified. Set the rate by adjusting the screws on the front of the driver using the tool provided. If using a standard delivery length of 48mm:
  Graseby **MS16A** *hourly* rate driver delivers in **millimetres per hour**.
  Set at **02** to run at 2mm/h over **24** hours.
  Set at **04** to run at 4mm/h over **12** hours.
  Graseby **MS26** *daily* rate driver delivers in **millimetres per 24 hours**
  Set at **48** to run at 2mm/h over **24** hours.
  Set at **96** to run at 4mm/h over **12** hours.

7 Connect the syringe to the infusion line and manually prime. Priming uses about 0.5mL and the contents of the delivery device will thus be delivered in less than the planned time, generally 24h. Re-measure and document this new length but do not adjust the set rate. Subsequent infusions which do not involve priming will last a full 24h.

8 Fit the syringe into the syringe driver with the flange of the syringe barrel in the vertical position. Slide the end plate up to the plunger of the syringe and secure the syringe with the rubber strap.

9 Attach the line to the butterfly cannula, or if using an existing line, attach the syringe to the line.

10 Re-insert the battery and an audible alarm sounds. Press and release the start button to silence the alarm and to activate the driver. Note: the syringe driver also makes this noise when:
  - the syringe is empty
  - the line set is blocked
  - the start/test button is held for 5sec (MS16A)
  - the start/boost button is held for 10sec (MS26).

Box Setting the rate of a Graseby syringe driver

MS16A *hourly* **rate driver**

$$Rate = \frac{measured\ 'length\ of\ volume'\ in\ mm}{delivery\ time\ in\ hours}$$

e.g. $\frac{48mm}{24h}$ = 2mm/h (48mm is about 8mL in a 10mL BD plastikpak syringe)

MS26 *daily* **rate driver**

$$Rate = \frac{measured\ 'length\ of\ volume'\ in\ mm}{delivery\ time\ in\ days}$$

e.g. $\frac{48mm}{1\ day}$ = 48mm/day

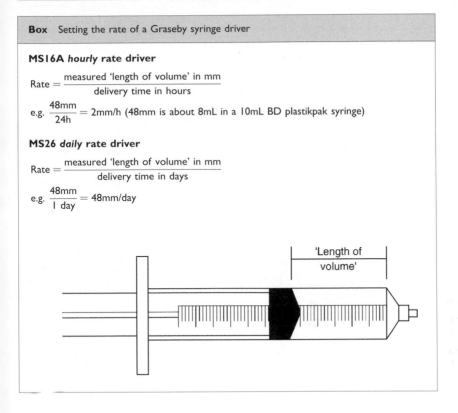

'Length of volume'

11 The light on the front of the driver should start flashing (every second for MS16A, every 25sec for MS26). If the light does not flash, consult the manufacturer's guidelines regarding battery replacement.

12 The clear plastic cover or lock-box should be carefully placed over the syringe driver. Ensure it is placed the correct way round to prevent accidental pressing of the start/boost button.

13 Protect the syringe from excessive sunlight and heat, e.g. electric blankets.

14 Regular checks on the progress, the visual appearance of the infusion and administration site should be performed and documented during the infusion. Do not remove the syringe from the driver to perform these checks. If checking indicates a problem, action should be taken and then documented.

15 Do not add drugs to a syringe or infusion line or increase the rate once the infusion has commenced. Additional bolus drugs needed should be administered by a separate cannula.

16 If the drug prescription is changed, discard the syringe in place and make up a new syringe. Use a new line and consider giving stat doses of appropriate medication if an immediate effect is needed by a separate cannula.

17 To stop a syringe driver, remove the battery. Always disconnect the line from the patient before removing the syringe from the driver.

1   Wilcock A et al. (2006) Drugs given by a syringe driver: a prospective multicentre survey of palliative care services in the UK. Palliative Medicine. **20**: 661–664.
2   O'Doherty CA et al. (2001) Drugs and syringe drivers: a survey of adult specialist palliative care practice in the United Kingdom and Eire. Palliative Medicine. **15**: 149–154.
3   Nelson KA et al. (1997) A prospective within-patient crossover study of continuous intravenous and subcutaneous morphine for chronic cancer pain. Journal of Pain and Symptom Management. **13**: 262–267.
4   Watanabe S et al. (2008) A randomized double-blind crossover comparison of continuous and intermittent subcutaneous administration of opioid for cancer pain. Journal of Palliative Medicine. **11**: 570–574.
5   Anderson SL and Shreve ST (2004) Continuous subcutaneous infusion of opiates at end-of-life. Annals of Pharmacotherapy. **38**: 1015–1023.
6   Fonzo-Christe C et al. (2005) Subcutaneous administration of drugs in the elderly: survey of practice and systematic literature review. Palliative Medicine. **19**: 208–219.
7   Schneider J et al. (1997) A study of the osmolality and pH of subcutaneous drug infusion solutions. Australian Journal of Hospital Pharmacy. **27**: 29–31.
8   Flowers C and McLeod F (2005) Diluent choice for subcutaneous infusion: a survey of the literature and Australian practice. International Journal of Palliative Nursing. **11**: 54–60.
9   Fudin J et al. (2000) Use of continuous ambulatory infusions of concentrated subcutaneous (s.q.) hydromorphone versus intravenous (i.v.) morphine: cost implications for palliative care. American Journal of Hospice and Palliative Care. **17**: 347–353.
10 Department of Health (2012) The never events list 2012-2013. https:www.gov.uk
11 British National Formulary Prescribing in palliative care and Appendix 6: Intravenous additives. London: BMJ Group and Pharmaceutical Press. www.bnf.org (accessed December 2013).
12 NPSA (National Patient Safety Agency) (2007) Promoting safer use of injectable medicines. Patient safety alert 20. www.nrls.npsa.nhs.uk
13 Trissel LA. Handbook on Injectable Drugs. Maryland USA: American Society of Health System Pharmacists www. medicinescomplete.com (accessed December 2013).
14 Kohut J, 3rd et al. (1996) Don't ignore details of drug-compatibility reports. American Journal of Health System Pharmacy. **53**: 2339.
15 Vermeire A and Remon JP (1999) Stability and compatibility of morphine. Int J Pharm. **187**: 17–51.
16 Schneider JJ et al. (2006) Effect of tubing on loss of clonazepam administered by continuous subcutaneous infusion. Journal of Pain and Symptom Management. **31**: 563–567.
17 National Prescribing Centre (2010) Mixing of medicines prior to administration in clinical practice - responding to legislative changes. Liverpool. Available from: www.npc.nhs.uk (archive website)
18 Dickman A and Schneider J (2011). The Syringe Driver: Continuous Subcutaneous Infusions in Palliative Care (3e). Oxford University Press, Oxford.
19 Foinard A et al. (2012) Impact of physical incompatibility on drug mass flow rates: example of furosemide-midazolam incompatibility. Annals of Intensive Care. **2**: 28.
20 Good PD et al. (2004) The compatibility and stability of midazolam and dexamethasone in infusion solutions. Journal of Pain and Symptom Management. **27**: 471–475.
21 Gray A et al. Injectable Drugs Guide. London: Pharmaceutical Press www.medicinescomplete.com (accessed November 2013).
22 Dawkins L et al. (2000) A randomized trial of winged Vialon cannulae and metal butterfly needles. International Journal of Palliative Nursing. **6**: 110–116.
23 Mitchell K et al. (2012) Incidence and causes for syringe driver site reactions in palliative care: A prospective hospice-based study. Palliative Medicine. **26**: 979–985.
24 Ross JR et al. (2002) A prospective, within-patient comparison between metal butterfly needles and Teflon cannulae in subcutaneous infusion of drugs to terminally ill hospice patients. Palliative Medicine. **16**: 13–16.
25 Oliver D (1991) The tonicity of solutions used in continuous subcutaneous infusions. The cause of skin reactions? Hospital Pharmacy Practice. **Sept**: 158–164.
26 Graham F (2006) Syringe drivers and subcutaneous sites: a review. European Journal of Palliative Care. **13**: 138–141.
27 Reymond L et al. (2003) The effect of dexamethasone on the longevity of syringe driver subcutaneous sites in palliative care patients. Medical Journal of Australia. **178**: 486–489.
28 Palliativedrugs.com (2014) Which syringe driver do you use? Available from: www.palliativedrugs.com
29 Freemantle A et al. (2011) Safer ambulatory syringe drivers: experiences of one acute hospital trust. International Journal of Palliative Nursing. **17**: 86–91.
30 NHS England (2013) Safer Use of Syringe Drivers. Quality Care Commission. www.cqc.org.uk/
31 NPSA (National Patient Safety Agency) (2010) Safer ambulatory syringe drivers. In: Rapid Reponse Report RRR019. www.nrls.npsa.nhs.uk

Updated April 2014

21: SPINAL ANALGESIA

Indications

Spinal analgesia is commonly used for obstetric or peri-operative pain relief but is relatively uncommon in palliative care.[1,2] Only 2–4% of cancer patients receiving specialist palliative care proceed to spinal analgesia because of inadequate pain relief with more standard systemic analgesia.[3–7] Typical indications for spinal analgesia include:
- systemic opioid intolerance (an unacceptable balance between efficacy and toxicity)
- refractory neuropathic pain (e.g. visceral neuropathic pain, lumbosacral plexopathy)
- pathological fracture in a patient close to death.

Spinal analgesia is effective in ≥50% of patients.[3,8–13] Good communication between the palliative care, pain, and primary care teams is essential.

Contra-indications

Uncorrected coagulopathy, systemic or local infection, raised intracranial pressure. Extra caution is necessary when there is:
- spinal deformity
- incipient spinal cord compression
- myelosuppressive chemotherapy.

Route, placement and delivery device considerations

Before insertion of a spinal catheter, baseline blood tests will help to evaluate fitness and exclude, for example, a coagulopathy. A neurological and cardiopulmonary examination provides a baseline for future reference if a problem arises.

Analgesics are delivered to the intrathecal (IT) or epidural (ED) space via an indwelling catheter placed by an anaesthetist. Commonly, the tube is tunnelled subcutaneously to emerge at a distant site, e.g. the supraclavicular fossa or flank, on the basis that this will reduce the risk of displacement and infection. This can be done using local anaesthesia ± sedation, but general anaesthesia is more comfortable for the patient.[7] However, simple placement without tunnelling (and without general anaesthesia) appears to be equally satisfactory.[14]

The preferred route and delivery device are influenced by local custom and the likely duration of use (Table 1). Although ED catheters are sometimes left in place for several months,[15] IT is the preferred route for long-term spinal analgesia expected to be necessary for more than a few weeks.[3] Devices vary in relation to fixed vs. variable delivery rates, patient-controlled boluses, and cost.

Table 1 Suggested route and delivery device

Likely duration of use	Route and device	Comments
≤3 weeks	External ED device (re-usable)	Fewer initial complications than IT (8% vs. 25%); less headache from CSF leakage[16]
3 weeks–3 months	External IT device (re-usable)	Fewer later complications than ED (5% vs. 55%); less catheter occlusion or migration[16]
≥3 months	Implantable IT device	More expensive initially, lower running costs; more cost-effective long-term[17]

Drugs delivered to the ED space diffuse through the meninges to reach the spinal cord and adjacent nerve roots. The level of the spinal cord at which the catheter is sited influences the area over which maximal analgesia is obtained. Migration or misplacement of ED catheters into the IT space (a rare event) will deliver an excessive dose resulting in significant toxicity and, unless recognized and treated urgently, may cause death secondary to respiratory arrest.

The IT route delivers drugs directly to the cerebrospinal fluid (CSF). Compared with the ED route, lower doses are required, thereby permitting the use of smaller devices and/or reducing the frequency of refilling (see below).[15] IT administration generally provides better pain relief than the ED route.[3,16,18,19] The area of analgesia is less dependent on the site of the catheter because drugs in the CSF automatically diffuse rostrally.

Although the same delivery devices can theoretically be used for SC, IV and spinal infusion, for maximum safety it is best to use a device specifically designed for spinal delivery.[4] Distinct pumps and connectors will reduce the potential for confusion in a patient receiving concurrent spinal and SC/IV infusions.[3,20] However, such recommendations must be weighed against the considerable advantage of staff using a delivery device with which they are familiar from frequent SC/IV use.

Clinical services caring for patients receiving spinal analgesia need clear procedures to be in place to minimize risk at all stages of treatment. An added problem is maintaining staff competence when such approaches are used infrequently. Clinical guidelines and 'refresher' training are both important.

Bolus vs. continuous infusion

Some centres give an initial bolus dose at the time of catheter placement before starting the infusion. If this includes a local anaesthetic (see below), this may cause transient loss of sensation, e.g. in the lower limbs, which patients may find unpleasant. Others just insert the catheter and start the continuous infusion. There is no evidence to suggest any major benefit from an initial bolus dose.[21]

Choice of drugs

Diamorphine/morphine, **bupivacaine** and **clonidine** are the most commonly used drugs (see below). Particularly in cancer-related neuropathic pain, opioids are generally combined from the outset with **bupivacaine** (or alternative local anaesthetic), and **clonidine** added subsequently if necessary. However, some units use **clonidine** from the outset.[22,23]

Health professionals should familiarize themselves with the guidance and supporting material relating to the legal implication of mixing medicines before administration[24,25] together with any local policy and practice.

Opioids

In the UK, **morphine** and **diamorphine** are widely used; the latter because of its solubility and lack of preservatives.[3,4,22,26–28] Because of concerns about precipitation with **diamorphine**, the British Pain Society recommends that **morphine** should always be used in Medtronic Synchromed® pumps.[4] However, there has been no formal comment about the simpler implanted Isomed pump or the Codman Archimedes. **Hydromorphone** is an alternative where **morphine** is poorly tolerated.[3–5,29,30]

Spinally administered opioids act locally and/or in the brain stem. The latter occurs through CSF diffusion and/or systemic redistribution. The advantages of spinal administration are greatest with hydrophilic opioids, e.g. **diamorphine**, **morphine** and **hydromorphone**. These are relatively slowly redistributed and so will remain longer in the CSF.[31] However, respiratory depression secondary to rostral spread within the CSF can be a late onset feature.

In contrast, the fentanils are highly lipid-soluble, and are rapidly redistributed systemically. Thus, spinal administration has fewer advantages over systemic use.[31] However, the lower risk of catheter tip granuloma may benefit some patients (see p.721).

There is considerable uncertainty about dose equivalents between routes.[3,21,32] Although there is a wide variation in response[33] the conversion factors for **diamorphine** and **morphine** in Table 2 will generally provide a safe initial spinal dose. In the example in Table 2, the appropriate p.r.n. dose of SC **morphine** will be (as usual) 1/10–1/6 of the SC equivalent of the IT dose, i.e. 30–50mg SC.[3,21,30]

Table 2 Suggested starting doses for spinal diamorphine and morphine

Total 24h SC opioid	Total 24h ED opioid dose	Total 24h IT opioid dose
Diamorphine x mg	x divided by 10	x divided by 100
Morphine y mg	y divided by 10	y divided by 100
Example:		
morphine 300mg	morphine 30mg	morphine 3mg

For patients who have not been on an established systemic opioid regimen, recommendations for an appropriate starting IT dose are shown in (Table 3).

Table 3 Suggested IT total daily drug doses (when not converting from an established systemic opioid regimen)

Drug	Starting doses	Typical range of final doses
Diamorphine	1–2mg	1–30mg
Morphine	1–2mg	1–30mg
Bupivacaine	5–12mg	5–30mg
Clonidine	5–15microgram	15–30microgram

Maximum opioid concentrations and daily doses have been proposed to minimize the risk of catheter tip granuloma formation (Table 4). These are less applicable if short-term use is anticipated, although granulomas have been reported after just 27 days.[34]

Table 4 Recommended maximum long-term IT drug concentrations and doses

Drug	Maximum concentration (mg/mL)	Maximum daily dose (mg)
Morphine	20	15
Hydromorphone	10	4
Bupivacaine	40	30
Clonidine	2	1

Local anaesthetic

Bupivacaine is the most widely used local anaesthetic for spinal analgesia.[3-5,30] It has inherent bactericidal properties which theoretically reduces the probability of infection.[30] Undesirable effects include dose-dependent motor and sensory impairment, affecting 4–13% and ≤7% of patients respectively, generally at doses > 15mg/day.[3,4,8-10,12]

Alternatives include **levobupivacaine** and **ropivacaine**. Both have similar efficacy and general tolerability to **bupivacaine**, and are less cardiotoxic.[35-38] On the other hand, they are not bactericidal, although in practice this appears *not* to result in more infections.

α-Adrenergic receptor agonist

When used, **clonidine** 15–30microgram/24h (IT) or 150–300microgram/24h (ED) is generally given concurrently with an opioid and a local anaesthetic. Benefit is seen particularly in neuropathic pain. Undesirable effects include dose-dependent hypotension and bradycardia (see p.76).[3,4,30] Abrupt cessation (e.g. because of pump failure) may cause severe rebound hypertension. Administer oral **clonidine** while seeking specialist advice.[5]

Other drugs

Baclofen is used for pain related to spasticity. An overdose can cause rostral progression of hypotonia, respiratory depression, coma and occasionally seizures.[39] Symptoms of underdosing are generally limited to a return of the patient's baseline spasticiy and rigidity. However, a life-threatening withdrawal syndrome can occur if IT **baclofen** is abruptly discontinued (Box A).

Box A   IT baclofen withdrawal syndrome

Cause
Sudden cessation of IT baclofen (e.g. delivery device failure; also see p.593). Reported with a wide range of doses (50–1,500microgram/24h).

Clinical features
Symptoms evolve over 1–3 days:
- prodromal pruritus or paraesthesia; ± priapism
- seizures (early and/or late onset)
- tachycardia, hypotension or labile blood pressure
- fever ($\rightarrow$ hyperthermia)
- dysphoria and malaise $\rightarrow$ decreased level of consciousness
- spasticity and rigidity greater than patient's baseline
- rhabdomyolysis $\rightarrow$ hepatic and renal failure, DIC
- coma ($\rightarrow$ death).

Management
Restart the IT baclofen infusion as soon as possible.
Cardiopulmonary support as indicated.
High-dose baclofen PO or by enteral feeding tube (up to 120mg/24h), see Chapter 22, Table 2, p.733.
If necessary, give a benzodiazepine by CSCI/CIVI (e.g. midazolam) titrated to achieve muscle relaxation, normothermia, stabilization of blood pressure and cessation of seizures.[a]

---

a. dantrolene is reported to improve spasticity but not other symptoms. Its use in this setting has been superseded by the benzodiazepines.

Spinal **ketamine** is associated with histological changes of uncertain significance within the cord.[5,41–44] Taken together with the risk of neuropsychiatric, urinary and hepatobiliary toxicity reported with PO and more traditional parenteral routes (see ketamine, p.625), the use of spinal **ketamine** in palliative care should be exceptional.

The spinal use of several other drugs has been reported, e.g. including **adenosine**, **gabapentin**, **midazolam**, **ketorolac**, **ziconotide** and **octreotide**.[5,45]

Drug compatibility

Unlike acute pain, with chronic intractable pain, a single drug given spinally is often inadequate. Combinations of **morphine** or **diamorphine** with **bupivacaine** ± **clonidine** are widely used, particularly with external devices.[8–10,18] Long-term compatibility data for drug combinations in both external devices (at room temperature) and implanted pump reservoirs (at body

---

temperature) are limited.[4] Several factors can affect drug stability and compatibility (see Chapter 20, Box B, p.701). It is important to check with a pharmacist that the compatibility data are relevant to spinal use, and to confirm what is the appropriate diluent.

When mixing drugs for long periods it is important to consider the material the delivery device is made of because this can affect drug stability, e.g. **diamorphine** should not be used in Synchromed pumps because of reports of precipitation.

Compatibility data at room temperature

There are compatibility data on the following combinations at room temperature:
- **diamorphine** with **bupivacaine** 4 weeks[46]
- **morphine sulfate** with **bupivacaine** or **clonidine** 2 months[47,48]
- **morphine sulfate** with **ropivacaine** 1 month[37]
- **hydromorphone** with **bupivacaine** 3 days[49]
- **fentanyl** with **ropivacaine**[37]
- **sufentanil** with **ropivacaine**[37]
- **clonidine** with **bupivacaine** 2 weeks[50]
- **clonidine** with **ropivacaine** 1 month.[37]

Compatibility data at body temperature

There are compatibility data on the following combinations at body temperature:
- **morphine sulfate** with **clonidine** ± **bupivacaine** ≤3 months in a SynchroMed® pump[51,52]
- **hydromorphone** 4 months in a SynchroMed® pump[53]
- **clonidine** with **hydromorphone** 1.5 months (only stability of **clonidine** evaluated).[54]

Ideally, delivery devices with mixtures to be administered over >24h should be prepared in a sterile environment, e.g. a licensed pharmacy unit. Drugs should be preservative-free.[4]

Undesirable effects and complications of spinal analgesia

These relate to:
- the drugs (Table 5)
- medical complications, e.g. bleeding, infection (Table 6)
- the delivery system (Table 6).[55]

Respiratory failure can result from central depression of respiratory drive (opioids) or impaired motor output to the respiratory muscles at the spinal level (**bupivacaine**). Rate of onset varies: systemic redistribution of the spinally administered opioid causes respiratory depression within minutes or hours, whereas diffusion through the CSF causes a delayed onset, occurring after 6–48h. Both **bupivacaine** and **clonidine** cause hypotension, the latter also causing bradycardia.

MRI can cause some types of implantable pumps to malfunction, e.g. Medtronic Synchromed®. This is related to the magnetic field strength of the scanner. Acccording to Medtronic Technical Services, no problems have been seen with Isomed® implanted pumps subjected to MR field strengths of up to 1.5 tesla.

Although the Medtronic Synchromed® may stop during an MRI scan, it generally restarts spontaneously afterwards. However, delays in restarting or alterations in pump programming have occurred. The MHRA has issued guidelines for dealing with this, and advises that when consultation with staff responsible for managing the pump has not been possible:
- an alternative imaging technique should be considered *or*
- the patient should be observed closely until it has been confirmed that the pump has restarted.[69,70]

Management of life-threatening complications

Clinicians caring for patients with spinal analgesia should be aware of potential life-threatening drug-related complications. Clinical areas should have access to resuscitation equipment including IV fluids, **naloxone** and **ephedrine** (Box B).

Table 5 Drug-related undesirable effects

Drug	Undesirable effect	Frequency (%)	Comment
Early onset and/or after titration			
Withdrawal of systemic opioids	Diarrhoea and intestinal colic		Partly avoidable if laxatives stopped and then re-titrated after change to spinal route
Opioids	Nausea and vomiting	33%[3,12,56,57]	
Opioids	Pruritus	10–15%	But rare when given with bupivacaine to patients already receiving systemic opioids
Bupivacaine	Motor or sensory disturbance; dose-dependent	4–13%	Persistent motor impairment, overall frequency in palliative care series[3,9,12]
Opioids, bupivacaine	Urinary retention	8–43%[3,8,57]	
Opioids, bupivacaine	Respiratory depression	0.1–2%[3,58]	
Bupivacaine, clonidine	Cardiovascular compromise	5–20%	Symptomatic hypotension; clonidine also causes bradycardia[3]
Late onset (also see p.360)			
Opioids[a]	Catheter tip granulomas	0.1%[34]	Seen in 3% of patients with long-term IT infusions; of these, > 80% were asymptomatic (also see p.721);[59] more common with ED infusions
Opioids	Decreased libido, ± disturbed menstruation	70–95%[60]	Endocrine effect seen with IT opioids if given > 1 year but may occur sooner. In patients with a long prognosis, measure testosterone and LH at baseline and annually in men, and estradiol, progesterone, LH and FSH in women[4]
Opioids	Hypocorticalism or growth hormone deficiency	15%[60]	
Opioids	Oedema	6–18%[4,11,61]	
Opioids	Immuno-modulation	Frequency uncertain[62]	Significance uncertain. May be more pronounced with systemic opioids

a. less commonly described with non-opioids.

Table 6 Non-drug complications of spinal analgesia

Undesirable effect	Frequency (%)	Comment
Traumatic catheter placement		
CSF leakage headache	25% of IT[19]	Less common in recent palliative series (0–7%), perhaps because of concurrent systemic analgesia[3,63] or more modern spinal needles[64]
ED haematoma	Rare	
Neurological tissue damage	≤0.004%[65,66]	
Infection		
Exit site infection	≤6%	In palliative care patients cared for at home or in palliative care units[3,9,63,67]
ED abscess	≤8%[3,7,12,67]	
Meningitis	≤3% [3,7,9,12]	
Delivery system		
Device-related complications	8–27%	E.g. catheter-related (fracture, kinking, displacement or withdrawal); pump failure (battery failure, mechanical failure, programming or refilling error). Rates, and propensity to human error, vary between pumps[3,55,56,61,68]

Box B Emergency management of life-threatening complications

Stop spinal infusion.
Administer oxygen.
Obtain IV access.
If patient arrests, follow local resuscitation procedures.

Respiratory depression (sedation often precedes bradypnoea)
Sit the patient up.
If respiratory rate ≤8 breaths/min, the patient is barely rousable, and/or cyanosed, administer 20microgram boluses of naloxone every 2min until respiratory status is satisfactory (see p.455).
Further boluses may be necessary because naloxone is shorter acting than morphine and other spinal opioids.

Hypotension[a] (systolic <80mmHg)
Lay patient flat (not head down).
Check heart rate: if <40 beats/min, treat bradycardia (below) or
If no evidence of fluid overload, give an IV fluid challenge, e.g. 500mL of a colloidal plasma expander over 30min.
Examine for alternative causes such as bleeding.
If no response to fluids, give ephedrine 6mg IV.

Bradycardia[a]
ECG monitoring, if available.
Administer atropine (0.6mg boluses IV, up to total 3mg).
If atropine ineffective, give ephedrine 6mg IV.

a. cardiovascular disturbance also occurs with IT baclofen withdrawal syndrome (see Box A).

Management of undesirable opioid effects

The transient undesirable effects seen when starting systemic opioids are also seen when starting spinal opioids *de novo* (see Strong opioids, Box B, p.361).[55] However, some undesirable effects are particularly associated with starting spinal opioid analgesia either *de novo* or after switching from a more traditional route.

Opioid discontinuation (diarrhoea, colic, sweating, restlessness)

Spinal delivery results in a massive reduction in the patient's total opioid dose. Laxatives should be discontinued and re-titrated. If peripheral withdrawal symptoms occur, the pre-spinal opioid should be given p.r.n. in a dose approximately 25% of the former pain-related p.r.n. dose.

Opioid-induced pruritus

This is generally a central reaction to opioids, and largely histamine-independent.[71–73] In surgical (opioid-naïve) patients who receive spinal opioids pre-operatively, the incidence is ≤80% but, in patients with chronic pain already taking opioids by another route, only 10–15%.[13,56,57] The incidence also depends on the opioid used; for example, with caesarean section, pruritus is much more common with epidural **morphine** than epidural **hydromorphone**.[74]

However, anecdotally in cancer patients receiving palliative care, the incidence of pruritus in such patients appears to be virtually zero,[75] possibly because of the concurrent use of **bupivacaine**.[76,77]

After spinal injection, pruritus typically spreads rostrally through the thorax from the level of the injection and is typically maximal in the face, but may be limited to the nose (more likely when **bupivacaine** is given concurrently).[78]

Although pruritus induced by either systemic or spinal **morphine** is relieved by **naloxone** or **naltrexone**, this risks reversal of analgesia.[79] In some countries, mixed κ agonists–μ antagonists are available (not UK) which, when given prophylactically, prevent **morphine**-induced pruritus (peri-operatively, after caesarian section) without decreasing analgesia:
- **butorphanol** IV or ED[80]
- **nalbuphine** IM[81]

Other options include pretreatment with either **tenoxicam** 20mg IV or **diclofenac** 100mg PR. These have been shown to reduce the incidence, intensity and duration of pruritus in surgical patients receiving spinal opioids.[82,83] However, compared with controls, those receiving a NSAID also had less pain and required significantly less opioid postoperatively. Thus, it is possible that the difference in opioid dose may explain the difference.

In lower limb orthopaedic surgery using IT **morphine** and **bupivacaine** anaesthesia, single pre-operative doses of either **gabapentin** 1200mg or **mirtazapine** 30mg were better than placebo at preventing pruritus, reducing the incidence from ~75% to ~50%, and reducing its severity and duration.[84,85]

Prophylactic 5HT$_3$ antagonists (mainly **ondansetron** 4–8mg IV) have also been shown to be of benefit.[86] Further, when given as treatment only to patients who developed pruritus (i.e. not prophylactically), **ondansetron** 8mg IV relieved pruritus in 70% in < 1h.[87] Accordingly, this is widely regarded as first-line treatment for spinal opioid-induced pruritus.

Note: prophylactically, **diphenhydramine** 25mg IV has been shown to be as effective as IV **ondansetron** but is not readily available in the UK.[88]

In summary, if spinal opioid-induced pruritus occurs in a palliative care patient, consider:
- **ondansetron** 8mg IV stat and p.r.n. (or 8mg b.d. PO for 2 days)
- switching to an alternative opioid
- if all else fails, ultra-low dose **naloxone**:
  ▷ titrate to effect using repeat bolus doses of 40microgram IV
  ▷ if pruritus recurs, give 1microgram/kg/h by IVI (also see Chapter 28, p.795).[77]

Urinary retention

Drug-related urinary retention may be transient; removal of the urinary catheter after 3–4 days is successful in three quarters of patients.[8] If persistent, may be because of the underlying disease.

Other complications
Suspected infection
Catheter-related infections can occur, often with coagulase + or – *Staphylococci*.

Exit site infection: transparent dressings allow the early identification of exit site erythema. Systemic and topical antibacterials should be started promptly; this reduces the incidence of deeper infection/meningitis.[3] However, prophylactic antibacterials should *not* be routinely used.

ED abscesses: present with fever, escalating pain (this is invariable; either the original pain and/ or back pain at the ED site), and new neurological impairment (80%).[12] Evaluation includes blood cultures, aspiration of fluid from the spinal catheter for microscopy and culture, neurological examination, identification of other potential sources of fever and MRI (see warning about MRI above). Seek early advice from a microbiologist and spinal or neurosurgeon. The risk increases with time. Distant non-healing wounds may be a risk factor.[7]

Meningitis: presents with fever and/or meningeal irritation (neck stiffness, stretch signs). Evaluation includes blood and line microscopy and cultures, WBC, neurological examination, and identification of other potential sources of fever. Also consider MRI, particularly if new neurological impairment is present (but see warning about MRI above). Spinal catheters need not be automatically removed and allow a means of obtaining CSF for culture.[3] Mild meningeal irritation can be a normal phenomenon post-procedure, and patients can be safely observed while awaiting CSF cultures if they are systemically well and the above reveal no evidence of infection.[89] A prolonged operation time when placing the catheter is a risk factor for serious catheter-related infection.[90]

New neurological impairment
It can be difficult to distinguish between new neurological signs and symptoms caused by complications of spinal analgesia and those caused by disease progresssion (Box C). Estimates of complication rates vary greatly, and often predominantly relate to peri-operative/obstetric spinal anaesthesia.[91] Disease-related neurological impairment is common: spinal cord compression occurs in ≤6% of patients receiving spinal analgesia.[3] ED metastases are present in ≤70% of patients with refractory cancer pain. They are associated with motor impairment, and higher **morphine** and **bupivacaine** dose requirements (although not higher pain scores). Those with spinal canal stenosis (50%) also have higher IT insertion complication rates.[92]

Box C Differential diagnosis of new neurological impairment in patients receiving spinal analgesia

Neurological damage caused by insertion of the catheter.
Bupivacaine-induced; dose-dependent, generally seen only when IT doses exceed 15mg/day,[4] but unmasking of incipient spinal cord compression can occur with lower doses.[4,93]
Disease progression, e.g. cauda equina or spinal cord compression.
Catheter complication, e.g. ED abscess or haematoma, catheter tip granuloma.

Evaluation
Neurological examination: to confirm the location of the problem: is it related to the catheter or could it be a separate second phenomenon?

Time of onset (after starting infusion):
- immediate: spinal medication, 'unmasking' of subclinical impairment, or neurological damage at insertion
- after days–weeks or longer: ED abscess, haematoma, or disease progression
- after several months–years: catheter tip granuloma.

Investigation: MRI = optimum (but see warning on p.717).

Catheter tip granulomas may present as catheter occlusion (manifesting as renewed and increasing pain) or local mass effects (spinal cord or cauda equina compression with associated pain). Generally occur 3 months–years after starting a spinal infusion; with the risk increasing with time.[59] Pain typically precedes neurological impairment, which develops gradually over days–weeks.[94]

Granulomas are more common with ED infusions than IT ones, and occur particularly with **morphine** or **hydromorphone** at higher concentrations.[5] The risk with **fentanyl** is probably lower. A granuloma caused by IT **baclofen** has been reported.[34] Granulomas often resolve spontaneously within a few months of discontinuing an infusion.

In the absence of neurological impairment, options include catheter tip relocation, opioid dose reduction and/or switching to **fentanyl** (but see p.715) or a non-opioid. Surgical excision may be necessary if symptoms persist or there is neurological impairment.[34]

Exacerbation of pain

A sudden increase in pain should be initially treated with p.r.n. opioid medication PO/SC while the cause is investigated. Possibilities include:
- worsening of the original pain
- development of a new pain because of:
  ▷ disease progression or co-morbidity
  ▷ spinal catheter-related abscess, haematoma or granuloma
- reduced effect of the infusion
  ▷ catheter dislodgement or disconnection
  ▷ delivery device malfunction.

Plain radiographs may show a kinked, dislodged or disconnected catheter. Catheter position and patency can be confirmed by injection of a radiological contrast agent after first aspirating the catheter dead-space to avoid delivery of the dead-space contents as a bolus. The contrast agent must be appropriate for CSF use: IT delivery of inappropriate radiological contrast agents can cause arachnoiditis *and death*.

Delivery device malfunction may involve:
- an empty syringe (problem with last refill, altered delivery rate or calendar error about next refill date)
- a problem with the pump itself (battery failure, mechanical failure)
- a problem with the catheter (kinking, fracture, displacement, occlusion).

If the spinal infusion includes **baclofen**, and sudden failure of drug delivery is suspected, be alert to the presence of a severe life-threatening withdrawal syndrome (see Box A). The sudden cessation of **clonidine** can cause severe rebound hypertension. Treat with oral **clonidine** while seeking specialist advice.[5]

Record keeping

It is recommended that monitoring charts are used with spinal infusions, comparable with those widely used for checking CSCI (see Chapter 20, p.705). The use of a spinal chart should be cross-referenced on the patient's main prescription chart, and should list the drugs being infused.

1 Kurita GP et al. (2011) Spinal opioids in adult patients with cancer pain: a systematic review: a European Palliative Care Research Collaborative (EPCRC) opioid guidelines project. *Palliative Medicine.* **25**: 560–577.
2 Hayek SM et al. (2011) Intrathecal therapy for cancer and non-cancer pain. *Pain Physician.* **14**: 219–248.
3 Baker L et al. (2004) Evolving spinal analgesia practice in palliative care. *Palliative Medicine.* **18**: 507–515.
4 British Pain Society (2007) Intrathecal drug delivery for the management of pain and spasticity in adults; recommendations for best clinical practice. The British Pain Society. Available from: www.britishpainsociety.org
5 Deer T et al. (2007) Polyanalgesic consensus conference 2007: Recommendations for the management of pain by intrathecal (intraspinal) drug delivery; report of an interdisciplinary expert panel. *Neuromodulation.* **10**: 300–328.
6 Tei Y et al. (2008) Treatment efficacy of neural blockade in specialized palliative care services in Japan: a multicenter audit survey. *Journal of Pain and Symptom Management.* **36**: 461–467.
7 Burton AW et al. (2004) Epidural and intrathecal analgesia is effective in treating refractory cancer pain. *Pain Medicine.* **5**: 239–247.
8 Sjoberg M et al. (1991) Long-term intrathecal morphine and bupivacaine in 'refractory' cancer pain. Results from the first series of 52 patients. *Acta Anaesthesiologica Scandinavica.* **35**: 30–43.
9 Mercadante S (1994) Intrathecal morphine and bupivacaine in advanced cancer pain patients implanted at home. *Journal of Pain and Symptom Management.* **9**: 201–207.
10 Sjoberg M et al. (1994) Long term intrathecal morphine and bupivacaine in patients with refractory cancer pain. Results from a morphine:bupivacaine dose regimen of 0.5:4.75 mg/ml. *Anesthesiology.* **80**: 284–297.
11 Hassenbusch S et al. (1995) Long-term intraspinal infusions of opioids in the treatment of neuropathic pain. *Journal of Pain and Symptom Management.* **10**: 527–543.
12 Smitt PS et al. (1998) Outcome and complications of epidural analgesia in patients with chronic cancer pain. *Cancer.* **83**: 2015–2022.
13 Smith TJ et al. (2002) Randomized clinical trial of an implantable drug delivery system compared with comprehensive medical management for refractory cancer pain: impact on pain, drug-related toxicity, and survival. *Journal of Clinical Oncology.* **20**: 4040–4049.

14 Linklater GT and Macaulay L (2005) Epidural analgesia in advanced cancer patients. *Anesthesia and Analgesia.* **100**: 600; author reply 600–601.

15 Chambers WA (2008) Nerve blocks in palliative care. *British Journal of Anaesthesia.* **101**: 95–100.

16 Crul BJP and Delhaas EM (1991) Technical complications during long term subarachnoid or epidural administration of morphine in terminally ill cancer patients: A review of 140 cases. *Regional Anesthesia.* **16**: 209–213.

17 Hassenbusch SJ et al. (1997) Clinical realities and economic considerations: economics of intrathecal therapy. *Journal of Pain and Symptom Management.* **14**: S36–48.

18 Nitescu P et al. (1990) Epidural versus intrathecal morphine-bupivacaine: assessment of consecutive treatments in advanced cancer pain. *Journal of Pain and Symptom Management.* **5**: 18–26.

19 Dahm P et al. (1998) Efficacy and technical complications of long-term continuous intraspinal infusions of opioid and/or bupivacaine in refractory nonmalignant pain: a comparison between the epidural and the intrathecal approach with externalized or implanted catheters and infusion pumps. *Clinical Journal of Pain.* **14**: 4–16.

20 NPSA (National Patient Safety Agency) (2011) Safer spinal (intrathecal), epidural and regional devices. *Patient Safety Alert Update:* PSA001. www.nrls.npsa.nhs.uk

21 Mercadante S (1999) Problems of long-term spinal opioid treatment in advanced cancer patients. *Pain.* **79**: 1–13.

22 Lee MA et al. (2001) A simple method of using epidural analgesia in palliative medicine. *Palliative Medicine.* **15**: 347–348.

23 Exner HJ et al. (2003) Epidural analgesia at end of life: facing empirical contraindications. *Anesthesia and Analgesia.* **97**: 1740–1742.

24 Department of Health (2010) Mixing of medicines prior to administration in clinical practice: medical and non-medical prescribing. HMSO, London. Available from: www.gov.uk

25 National Prescribing Centre (2010) Mixing of medicines prior to administration in clinical practice - responding to legislative changes. Liverpool. Available from: www.npc.nhs.uk (archive website)

26 Hassenbusch SJ et al. (2004) Polyanalgesic Consensus Conference 2003: an update on the management of pain by intraspinal drug delivery–report of an expert panel. *Journal of Pain and Symptom Management.* **27**: 540–563.

27 Chrubasik J et al. (1993) The ideal epidural opioid–fact or fantasy? *European Journal of Anaesthesiology.* **10**: 79–100.

28 Stein C (ed) (1999) Opioids in pain control. Basic and clinical aspects. Cambridge University Press, Cambridge.

29 Dougherty PM and Staats PS (1999) Intrathecal drug therapy for chronic pain: from basic science to clinical practice. *Anesthesiology.* **91**: 1891–1918.

30 Bennett G et al. (2000) Evidence-based review of the literature on intrathecal delivery of pain medication. *Journal of Pain and Symptom Management.* **20**: S12–36.

31 Bujedo BM (2014) Spinal opioid bioavailability in postoperative pain. *Pain Practice.* **14**: 350–364.

32 Sylvester R et al. (2004) The conversion challenge: from intrathecal to oral morphine. *American Journal of Hospice and Palliative Medicine.* **21**: 143–147.

33 Kedlaya D et al. (2002) Epidural and intrathecal analgesia for cancer pain. *Best Practice and Research Clinical Anaesthesiology.* **16**: 651–665.

34 Deer T et al. (2008) Management of intrathecal catheter-tip inflammatory masses: an updated 2007 consensus statement from an expert panel. *Neuromodulation.* **11**: 77–91.

35 Svedberg K et al. (2002) Compatibility of ropivacaine with morphine, sufentanil, fentanyl, or clonidine. *Journal of Clinical Pharmacy and Therapeutics.* **27**: 39–45.

36 Dahm P et al. (2000) Comparison of 0.5% intrathecal bupivacaine with 0.5% intrathecal ropivacaine in the treatment of refractory cancer and noncancer pain conditions: results from a prospective, crossover, double-blind, randomized study. *Regional Anesthesia and Pain Medicine.* **25**: 480–487.

37 Simpson D et al. (2005) Ropivacaine: a review of its use in regional anaesthesia and acute pain management. *Drugs.* **65**: 2675–2717.

38 Foster RH and Markham A (2000) Levobupivacaine: a review of its pharmacology and use as a local anaesthetic. *Drugs.* **59**: 551–579.

39 Coffey RJ et al. (2002) Abrupt withdrawal from intrathecal baclofen: recognition and management of a potentially life-threatening syndrome. *Archives of Physical Medicine and Rehabilitation.* **83**: 735–741.

40 Mohammed I and Hussain A (2004) Intrathecal baclofen withdrawal syndrome- a life-threatening complication of baclofen pump: a case report. *BMC Clinical Pharmacology.* **4**: 6.

41 Karpinski N et al. (1997) Subpial vacuolar myelopathy after intrathecal ketamine: report of a case. *Pain.* **73**: 103–105.

42 Benrath J et al. (2005) Long-term intrathecal S(+)-ketamine in a patient with cancer-related neuropathic pain. *British Journal of Anaesthesia.* **95**: 247–249.

43 Vranken JH et al. (2005) Neuropathological findings after continuous intrathecal administration of S(+)-ketamine for the management of neuropathic cancer pain. *Pain.* **117**: 231–235.

44 Vranken JH et al. (2006) Severe toxic damage to the rabbit spinal cord after intrathecal administration of preservative-free S(+)-ketamine. *Anesthesiology.* **105**: 813–818.

45 Deer T et al. (2008) Future directions for intrathecal pain management: a review and update from the interdisciplinary polyanalgesic consensus conference 2007. *Neuromodulation.* **11**: 92–97.

46 Mehta A and Kay E (1996) Admixtures' storage is extended. *Pharmacy in Practice.* **6**: 113–118.

47 Xu Quanyun A et al. (2002) Physical and chemical stability of low and high concentrations of morphine sulfate with clonidine hydrochloride packaged in plastic syringes. In: *International Journal of Pharmaceutical Compounding.* Jan–Feb: 66–69.

48 Trissel Lawrence A et al. (2002) Physical and chemical stability of low and high concentrations of morphine sulfate with bupivacaine hydrochloride packaged in plastic syringes. In: *International Journal of Pharmaceutical Compounding.* Jan–Feb: 70–73.

49 Christen C et al. (1996) Stability of bupivacaine hydrochloride and hydromorphone hydrochloride during simulated epidural coadministration. *American Journal of Health System Pharmacy.* **53**: 170–173.

50 Trissel LA (2010) *Handbook on Injectable Drugs* (16e). American Society of Health System Pharmacists, Maryland, USA.

51 Hildebrand KR et al. (2003) Stability and Compatibility of Morphine-Clonidine Admixtures in an Implantable Infusion System. *Journal of Pain and Symptom Management.* **25**: 464–471.

52 Classen AM et al. (2004) Stability of admixture containing morphine sulfate, bupivacaine hydrochloride, and clonidine hydrochloride in an implantable infusion system. *Journal of Pain and Symptom Management.* **28**: 603–611.

53 Hildebrand KR et al. (2001) Stability and compatibility of hydromorphone hydrochloride in animplantable infusion system. *Journal of Pain and Symptom Management.* **22**: 1042–1047.

54 Rudich Z et al. (2004) Stability of clonidine in clonidine-hydromorphone mixture from implanted intrathecal infusion pumps in chronic pain patients. *Journal of Pain and Symptom Management.* **28**: 599–602.

55 Naumann C (1999) Drug adverse events and system complications of intrathecal opioid delivery for pain: origins, detection, manifestations and management. *Neuromodulation.* **2**: 92–107.

56 Paice JA et al. (1996) Intraspinal morphine for chronic pain: a retrospective, multicenter study. *Journal of Pain and Symptom Management.* **11**: 71–80.

57 Winkelmuller W et al. (1999) Intrathecal opioid therapy for pain: Efficacy and outcomes. *Neuromodulation.* **2**: 67–76.

58 Rawal N et al. (1987) Present state of extradural and intrathecal opioid analgesia in Sweden. A nationwide follow-up survey. *British Journal of Anaesthesia.* **59**: 791–799.

59 Deer TR (2004) A prospective analysis of intrathecal granulomas in chronic pain patients: a review of the literature and report of a surveillance study. *Pain Physician.* **7**: 225–228.

60 Abs R et al. (2000) Endocrine consequences of long-term intrathecal administration of opioids. *Journal of Clinical Endocrinology and Metabolism.* **85**: 2215–2222.

61 Winkelmuller M and Winkelmuller W (1996) Long-term effects of continuous intrathecal opioid treatment in chronic pain of nonmalignant etiology. *Journal of Neurosurgery.* **85**: 458–467.

62 Budd K and Shipton E (2004) Acute pain and the immune system and opioimmunosuppression. *Acute Pain.* **6**: 123–135.

63 Mercadante S et al. (2007) Intrathecal treatment in cancer patients unresponsive to multiple trials of systemic opioids. *Clinical Journal of Pain.* **23**: 793–798.

64 Moen V et al. (2004) Severe neurological complications after central neuraxial blockades in Sweden 1990–1999. *Anesthesiology.* **101**: 950–959.

65 Aromaa U et al. (1997) Severe complications associated with epidural and spinal anaesthesias in Finland 1987–1993. A study based on patient insurance claims. *Acta Anaesthesiologica Scandinavica.* **41**: 445–452.

66 Cook TM et al. (2009) Major complications of central neuraxial block: report on the Third National Audit Project of the Royal College of Anaesthetists. *British Journal of Anaesthesia.* **102**: 179–190.

67 Holmfred A et al. (2006) Intrathecal catheters with subcutaneous port systems in patients with severe cancer-related pain managed out of hospital: the risk of infection. *Journal of Pain and Symptom Management.* **31**: 568–572.

68 Nitescu P et al. (1995) Complications of intrathecal opioids and bupivacaine in the treatment of "refractory" cancer pain. *Clinical Journal of Pain.* **11**: 45–62.

69 MHRA (2008) Implantable drug pumps manufactured by Medtronic - Synchro EL models 8626 and 8627 and SynchroMed II model 8637. *Medical Device Alert.* MDA/2008/2087. www.mhra.gov.uk/safetyinformation

70 MHRA (2009) Effects of MRI on implantable drug pumps. *Drug Safety Update.* **2**. www.mhra.gov.uk/safetyinformation

71 Reisine T and Pasternak G (1996) Opioid analgesics and antagonists. In: J Hardman et al. (eds) *Goodman and Gilman's The Pharmacological Basis of Therapeutics* (9e). McGraw-Hill, London, pp. 521–555.

72 Krajnik M (2004) Opioid-induced pruritus. In: Z Zylicz et al. (eds) *Pruritus in advanced disease.* Oxford University Press, London, pp. 84–96.

73 Tarcatu D et al. (2007) Are we still scratching the surface? A case of intractable pruritus following systemic opioid analgesia. *Journal of Opioid Management.* **3**: 167–170.

74 Chaplan SR et al. (1992) Morphine and hydromorphone epidural analgesia. *Anesthesiology.* **77**: 1090–1094.

75 Lynch L (2014) Personal communication.

76 Asokumar B et al. (1998) Intrathecal bupivacaine reduces pruritus and prolongs duration of fentanyl analgesia during labor: a prospective, randomized, controlled trial. *Anaesthesia and Analgesia.* **87**: 1309–1315.

77 Reich A and Szepietowski JC (2010) Opioid-induced pruritus: an update. *Clinical Experimental Dermatology.* **35**: 2–6.

78 Ballantyne J et al. (1988) Itching after epidural and spinal opiates. *Pain.* **33**: 149–160.

79 Kjellberg F and Tramer M (2001) Pharmacological control of opioid-induced pruritus: a quantitative systematic review of randomized trials. *European Journal of Anaesthesiology.* **18**: 346–357.

80 Du BX et al. (2013) Butorphanol prevents morphine-induced pruritus without increasing pain and other side effects: a systematic review of randomized controlled trials. *Canadian Journal of Anaesthesia.* **60**: 907–917.

81 Liao CC et al. (2011) Efficacy of intramuscular nalbuphine versus diphenhydramine for the prevention of epidural morphine-induced pruritus after cesarean delivery. *Chang Gung Medical Journal.* **34**: 172–178.

82 Colbert S et al. (1999) The effect of intravenous tenoxicam on pruritus in patients receiving epidural fentanyl. *Anaesthesia.* **54**: 76–80.

83 Colbert S et al. (1999) The effect of rectal diclofenac on pruritus in patients receiving intrathecal morphine. *Anaesthesia.* **54**: 948–952.

84 Sheen MJ et al. (2008) Preoperative gabapentin prevents intrathecal morphine-induced pruritus after orthopedic surgery. *Anesthesia and Analgesia.* **106**: 1868–1872.

85 Sheen MJ et al. (2008) Prophylactic mirtazapine reduces intrathecal morphine-induced pruritus. *British Journal of Anaesthesia.* **101**: 711–715.

86 Bonnet MP et al. (2008) Effect of prophylactic 5-HT3 receptor antagonists on pruritus induced by neuraxial opioids: a quantitative systematic review. *British Journal of Anaesthesia.* **101**: 311–319.

87 Borgeat A and Stimemann H-R (1999) Ondansetron is effective to treat spinal or epidural morphine-induced pruritus. *Anesthesiology.* **90**: 432–436.

88 Siddik-Sayyid SM et al. (2010) Ondansetron is as effective as diphenhydramine for treatment of morphine-induced pruritus after cesarean delivery. *Acta Anaesthesiologica Scandinavica.* **54**: 764–769.

89 Paice JA et al. (1997) Clinical realities and economic considerations: efficacy of intrathecal pain therapy. *Journal of Pain and Symptom Management.* **14 (Suppl 3)**: S14–26.

90 Byers K et al. (1995) Infections complicating tunneled intraspinal catheter systems used to treat chronic pain. *Clinical Infectious Diseases.* **21**: 403–408.

91 Bromage PR (1997) Neurological complications of subarachnoid and epidural anesthesia. *Acta Anaesthesiologica Scandinavica.* **41**: 439–444.

92 Appelgren L et al. (1997) Spinal epidural metastasis: implications for spinal analgesia to treat "refractory" cancer pain. *Journal of Pain and Symptom Management.* **13**: 25–42.

93 van Dongen RTM et al. (1997) Neurological impairment during long-term intrathecal infusion of bupivacaine in cancer patients: a sign of spinal cord compression. *Pain.* **69**: 205–209.

94 Miele VJ et al. (2006) A review of intrathecal morphine therapy related granulomas. *European Journal of Pain.* **10**: 251–261.

Updated June 2014

22: DRUG ADMINISTRATION TO PATIENTS WITH SWALLOWING DIFFICULTIES OR ENTERAL FEEDING TUBES

General principles

Simplifying drug therapy by reducing the number of medications and frequency of administration is particularly important for patients who are not able to swallow solids or for whom administering drugs by an enteral feeding tube (EFT) is being considered.

Modifying a product in a way not specified in the manufacturer's SPC renders its use off-label, e.g. emptying out the contents of a capsule. Thus, if available, appropriate alternative formulations of those drugs still considered necessary should be used, e.g. a soluble tablet or an oral liquid instead of a solid tablet (or an alternative authorized drug).

Administering drugs by EFT is generally off-label, and consideration should also be given to using an alternative authorized route, e.g. PR, SC, IV.[1,2] However, administration by EFT may be preferable from a practical or personal point of view.

Drug therapy, the formulations used, and swallowing ability should be kept under review, particularly before inpatient discharge. Training and detailed written instructions regarding the supply, preparation and administration of each drug should be given to the patient and/or carer and primary care team.[3]

Guidance on minimizing wrong route errors when giving drugs by PO or other enteral route has been published by the UK National Patient Safety Agency (NPSA).[4] Only enteral syringes should be used to draw up and administer oral liquids. Many local guidelines stipulate once only use. NPSA has also produced guidance on testing the position of nasogastric tubes.[5]

The administration of drugs by EFT is considered a level 3 skill for care workers in care homes. Staff must be adequately trained.[6,7] General guidance for the administration of drugs by EFT is given in the Quick Clinical Guide.

Choosing a suitable formulation

When planning to change to an alternative formulation or administer a drug by EFT, guidance should be obtained from a pharmacist. For those with impaired swallowing a Speech and Language Therapist (SALT) should also be consulted in order to understand the degree of swallowing impairment and perform a risk assessment.[8] Taking into account the balance of risks and uncertainties for drug administration to these patients, the choice of formulation in descending order of preference generally comprises:

- authorized soluble tablet or oral liquid
- effervescent tablet or dispersed tablet (authorized or off-label)
- oral liquid prepared by local pharmacy or special order
- dispersed capsule contents or crushed tablet
- injection (given PO or by EFT).

However, there are considerations and disadvantages for each of these options which can vary according to the drug prescribed, the patient's clinical need and the practical situation. These issues are summarized in Table 1. Thus, every drug needs to be assessed individually to determine which would be the most appropriate formulation, i.e. do not simply convert all solid dose medication to oral liquids. Table 2 contains a list of the formulations available for palliative care drugs with authorized and off-label alternatives for patients with swallowing difficulties and EFT.

Table 1 Summary of the issues to consider when choosing a suitable formulation

Formulation	Considerations / Disadvantages
Soluble tablet	Availability Sodium content, may be high Cost
Authorized oral liquid	Excipients causing undesirable effects Bio-availability and dosing frequency Viscosity and particle size Volume and palatability Cost
Effervescent tablet or dispersed tablet (authorized or off-label)	Sodium content, may be high Particle size Practicality Cost of authorized formulations
Locally prepared or special order oral liquid	As for authorized oral liquid *plus*: shelf-life/expiry storage conditions continuity of supply reduced quality assurance variable formulations between special order manufacturers higher cost than authorized oral liquid
Dispersed capsule contents (authorized or off-label) or crushed tablet	Occupational exposure Particle size Practicality Reduced dose ($\leqslant$20% lost with crushing) Risk of using an inappropriate formulation, e.g. m/r and causing destruction of m/r mechanism, more rapid absorption, and danger to patient
Injection given PO or by EFT	Osmolality/hypertonicity/unsuitable pH Excipients unsuitable for PO administration Risk of wrong route error Continuity of supply in the community Cost

Option 1: Authorized soluble tablet or oral liquid

If available, soluble tablets are generally the preferred option. Soluble tablets dissolve *completely* when placed in 10mL water to give a solution of the drug in contrast to effervescent, dispersible or orodispersible tablets which disperse in water or in the mouth to give particles (see option 2 below).

Liquid formulations are not always suitable as direct substitutes for solid dosage forms for several reasons:

- *excipients causing undesirable effects:* many oral liquid formulations contain excipients which in large volumes can cause osmotic diarrhoea, particularly with jejunal administration, e.g. sorbitol $\geqslant$15g/24h. The normal osmolality of GI secretions is 100–400mosm/kg, but many liquid formulations are >1,000mosm/kg.[9,10] Reduce osmolality by diluting with as much water as is practical. Some liquid formulations contain alcohol, e.g. Oramorph®, **loperamide, phenobarbital, ranitidine**

- *altered bio-availability and/or dosing frequency:* an oral liquid formulation may have a different bio-availability from the corresponding solid formulation, e.g. **citalopram, phenytoin, sodium fusidate**, necessitating a different dose. When converting from a m/r formulation to an immediate-release oral liquid, the dose and/or frequency may need to be changed
- *viscosity and particle size of suspensions:* patients may be unable to swallow a highly viscous formulation or particulate suspension. EFT are easily blocked by a highly viscous formulation, e.g. **amoxicillin-clavulanate**, mineral oil, syrups or by particles from a suspension, e.g. **ciprofloxacin, clarithromycin**. Viscosity may be reduced by diluting with 30–50mL water if practical [10]
- *large volumes:* from high doses or multiple drugs may be impractical, unpalatable and costly.

Option 2: Effervescent tablet or dispersed tablet (authorized or off-label)

Do not administer a formulation by EFT if it has failed to disperse into small, barely visible particles or has an oily residue. Sediment and oily films increase the risk of blocking EFTs (Box A).[10,11]

Effervescent tablets and authorized dispersible tablets disintegrate in water to particle/granule form. Many standard tablets will also disperse or dissolve when mixed with 10mL water even if not marketed as dispersible/soluble. Although off-label, this is often the most practical option for both patients with swallowing difficulties and those with EFT (Box A). However, for any tablets dispersed in water the following should be noted:

- fractional dosing from effervescent or dispersed tablets is not recommended due to inaccuracy
- the resulting particles/granules may be too large for administration by fine-bore EFT
- this option is unsuitable for patients unable to swallow biphasic preparations, i.e. solids and liquids together.

Box A Guidelines for preparation of dispersed formulations for EFT administration[1,3]

Information about the preparation of each medication should be documented on the prescription and in the patient's notes.

Prepare each drug separately.

Place the tablet(s) or capsule contents into the barrel of a 50mL enteral syringe;use a large container/drug pot for effervescent formulations.

Add 10mL of tap water (50mL for effervescent formulations), allow to disperse, then mix well:
- use sterile water for jejunal tubes or immunocompromised patients
- if using a drug pot or other container, once dispersed, draw up the contents using a 50mL enteral syringe; this reduces the risk of rupture of the EFT.

Inspect the contents of the enteral syringe to ensure that there are no large particles that might block the EFT.

Administer each drug separately via the EFT (see p.732).

If using a drug pot or other container, rinse with water, draw up with the same enteral syringe and administer the rinsings through the tube.

To ensure the patient receives the whole dose, use the same enteral syringe to draw up and administer the flush (see p.732).

Thoroughly clean any drug pots/containers/tablet crushers with hot soapy water according to local policy to avoid cross-contamination.

Do not:
- use hot water for drug dispersion as this may alter bio-availability
- leave dispersed medicines lying around unlabelled.

Orodispersible tablets are designed to disperse on the tongue and are generally swallowed with the saliva without water. Some orodispersible formulations may be more suitable than others for patients with swallowing difficulties and may depend on the extent of dysphagia. The formulations, dose equivalences and administration of orodispersible tablets vary depending on the drug concerned. Individual product details should be consulted before using by EFT.

Buccal, sublingual and most oromucosal formulations are designed to be absorbed by the oral mucosa and not the GI tract, thus bypassing first-pass hepatic metabolism. These may be suitable alternatives for patients with swallowing difficulties but are unsuitable for EFT administration. Check if the formulation is intended for buccal or enteral administration to prevent wrong route errors.

Option 3: Locally prepared or special order oral liquid
An oral liquid formulation prepared locally or by special order (see Appendix 1, p.817) may be an alternative if an authorized product is not available or not suitable.[12] The same issues as for authorized oral liquids need to be considered (see Table 1). However, it may be possible for an experienced pharmacist to alter a formulation with careful consideration for quality, storage and shelf-life and thus make it more suitable.[12] Continuity of supply after a patient has returned home, short shelf-life, storage conditions (e.g. refrigeration), differences in formulation between manufacturers and higher cost often make this option impractical.

Option 4: Dispersed capsule contents or crushed tablet
Opening capsules in order to disperse the contents is generally off-label and risks topical and inhaled exposure of the contents to the health professional. It is not recommended for certain drugs, e.g. antibiotics, cytotoxics, prostaglandin analogues or hormone antagonists. There are also risks to the patient if unsuitable formulations are used, e.g. m/r formulations may be harmful if accidentally chewed or crushed, or if the contents are irritant, e.g. **demeclocycline**.

A few capsules contain liquid contents, e.g. **nifedipine**. Because of the small volume of the contents (which varies between brands), it is not recommended that these are used as a source of a drug for swallowing difficulties or EFT administration.

It is sometimes feasible to add the contents of some capsules to water for administration by EFT, or to soft food, fruit juice or other liquids to aid those with swallowing difficulties. The manufacturer's SPC should be consulted to ensure that this will not cause problems with absorption or cause undesirable effects. Small quantities of soft food or liquids, e.g. a tablespoon (15mL), should be used to ensure that the entire dose is administered.

Crushing tablet/capsule contents to facilitate dispersion is *not* generally necessary as many tablets and capsule contents will disperse sufficiently in water without crushing (see option 2). Crushing can be dangerous for certain formulations (Box B) and care must be taken to ensure that this is safe for both the patient and health professionals. There is also significant risk of loss of dose or subsequent cross contamination. Thus, crushing should be considered a last resort and avoided unless specifically recommended by a pharmacist.[1]

Box B Formulations which must not be crushed or chewed

Do not crush
M/r formulations (including m/r capsule contents) because this will destroy the m/r mechanism and result in dangerous dose peaks and troughs.[10,11,13–15]

E/c (gastro-resistant) formulations (including e/c capsule contents) because this will destroy the e/c properties of the formulation, may alter bio-availability, and may block the tube.[10,11,14,15]

Cytotoxics, prostaglandin analogues, hormone antagonists or antibiotics because there are risks to the staff through inhalation and/or topical absorption.[10,11,15]

Buccal or sublingual formulations because their bio-availability may be dramatically reduced if absorbed by the GI tract.[10,11,15]

Option 5: Injection (given PO or by EFT)
Formulations for injection are often unsuitable for enteral administration. This may be for one or more of several reasons:

- high osmolality or hypertonicity; the high solute concentration can cause osmotic diarrhoea
- unsuitable pH of the formulation or acidic conditions of the stomach chemically degrading the drug, e.g. **omeprazole**
- formulation with a different salt of unknown bio-availability
- an additive which is irritant to the GI tract, e.g. polysorbate 80 (Tween®80) in **amiodarone**[1,16]
- risk of IV administration by mistake[4]
- cost.

Generally, all injections suitable for enteral administration should be diluted before administration, e.g. with 30–50mL water by EFT. Bio-availability between the solid dose form and the injection solution may be different and alter clinical response, e.g. more rapid absorption and higher peak levels may occur.

Specific considerations for EFT
Testing of tube position before drug administration
Fatalities from aspiration have occurred as a result of incorrect placement of nasogastric (NG) tubes.[7,17] Thus, even when placement devices are used, it is essential that correct NG tube position is confirmed *before anything is administered via the tube*. This includes water for activating lubricant to facilitate removal of the placement device. Use specific CE marked pH paper for testing gastric contents to confirm pH is within the 'safe' range of 1–5.5.[5] Radiographic confirmation in accordance with specific NPSA guidance is necessary only when there is doubt.

Correct NG tube position should be confirmed before each feed, before each drug administration and at least once daily. A break in feeding of 1h is required before testing. However, for patients on continuous feeding, multiple drug administration times, or on acid-suppressing drugs (e.g. antacids, H₂ antagonists and PPIs) this is impractical. Providing initial tube placement has been correctly confirmed and there is no reason to suspect displacement, tube position should be confirmed by observation of the external tube length and positioning in accordance with NPSA guidelines.[5]

Nasoduodenal and nasojejunal tubes are usually inserted under some form of guidance (e.g. endoscopic, radiological) to ensure correct tube placement. Initial confirmation of position should be undertaken as per local guidelines. Subsequent confirmation of tube position should be undertaken by observation of the external tube length (see above); testing with pH paper is not appropriate.

Semi-permanent and permanent devices, e.g. gastrostomy tubes, do not require repeated confirmation of position.

Site of drug delivery
The position of the tube may alter bio-availability, e.g. with jejunal tubes, absorption may be unpredictable because of the effects of pH or because the tube may extend beyond the main site of absorption of the drug, e.g. **cephalexin, metronidazole benzoate**.[1,9] Care should also be taken with drugs that have a narrow therapeutic range, e.g. **digoxin, warfarin, phenytoin** and other anti-epileptics.[9] Drugs which undergo extensive first-pass hepatic metabolism may have greater systemic effects because of increased absorption from direct delivery to the jejunum, e.g. opioids, TCAs.[2] Undesirable effects may also be increased because of rapid delivery into the jejunum. The acid barrier of the stomach is bypassed with jejunal tubes, some centres use aseptic technique to reduce the risk of infective diarrhoea.

Function of the tube
Drugs should not be administered if the tube is on free drainage or suction.[10]

Number of lumens
Ensure the correct lumen is used with multilumen tubes; some tubes have one lumen terminating in the stomach and another in the jejunum. *Do not use an aspiration gastric decompression port for drug administration.*

Lumen size
The outer diameter of an EFT is measured by the French gauge (1 French unit = 0.33mm).[2] However, the internal diameter of equivalent French gauge tubes varies between manufacturers. The tube material also affects the internal lumen size, e.g. silicone and latex tubes have thicker walls and therefore narrower internal lumens. Narrow lumen, e.g. 5–12 French, or long tubes,

e.g. NJ), are more likely to block, particularly with thick oral syrups and suspensions with large particles. Wide bore tubes require larger flush volumes.

Flushing the tube

This is essential to minimize drug interactions with the feeds. Water is the standard flush; use sterile water for jejunal tubes or immunocompromised patients because the acid barrier in the stomach is bypassed.[1] Tubes should be flushed before, in between drugs, and after drug administration ideally with 30mL water.[1,18] Use a 50mL enteral syringe to reduce the risk of tube rupture which can be caused by smaller syringes. Flush slowly with a push-pause technique to prevent leaving a coating of feed on the internal tube surface. Record the total flush and drug volume administered.

Feeding regimen

With continuous feeding and multiple drug administration periods, it may be necessary to adjust the feeding rate to compensate for the breaks in feed administration. If possible, the drug schedule should be rationalized, aiming for once daily drug administration to allow time for adequate nutrition.[2]

Bulk-forming laxatives

Do not administer by EFT because they may block the tube; use an enteral feed with a high-fibre content instead.[10]

Drug interactions and complications with EFT

Drugs can interact with food in many ways.[19,20] Enteral feeds can cause different problems associated with bio-availability, physical compatibility, and chemical interactions. Because they are in liquid form, the content, consistency and pH is very different to normal diet and variable between brands.

Drugs should *never* be added to enteral feeds because this increases the risk of incompatibility, microbial contamination, tube blockage, and underdosing or overdosing if the feed rate is altered.[21] However, complications can still arise from:

- *binding of drugs to the internal surface of the tube reducing absorption*, e.g. **carbamazepine**,[22] **clonazepam**, **diazepam**, **phenytoin**; minimize by diluting with 30–50mL water and flushing as per Quick Clinical Guide (see p.732).
- *physical interaction with the feed causing coagulation*, particularly if the drug formulation is acidic, i.e. pH < 4.[10] This applies to many syrups,[2] and risks tube blockage and reduced drug absorption. Abdominal distension caused by excessive gas production from effervescence has been reported when sodium bicarbonate solutions, used to deliver PPI formulations, have come into contact with the feed[23]
- *chemical interaction between the drug and feed causing a non-absorbable drug–feed complex*, e.g. bezoar (insoluble concretion) formation with **sucralfate**, in the tube or in the stomach.[24,25] Do not prescribe **sucralfate** by EFT
- *chemical interaction between the drug and the feed resulting in reduced drug available for absorption*, e.g. **carbamazepine**, **ciprofloxacin**, **digoxin**, **penicillins**, **phenytoin**, **theophylline**, **warfarin**.[26] A feed break of at least 1h before and after each drug is recommended to minimize the risk of reduced absorption
- *indirect drug or nutrient interactions*, e.g. the **vitamin K** or **eicosapentanoic acid** content of a feed affecting the action of **warfarin**[19] (also see p.814)
- *the effects of malnutrition on drug pharmacokinetics*.

Usual considerations for physical and chemical drug-drug interactions must also be taken into consideration, particularly if rationalizing drug administration to once or twice a day.

Flushing the tube effectively, diluting potentially problematic formulations, inserting a feed break as outlined in the Quick Clinical Guide (see p.732) and choosing an appropriate formulation will reduce the risk of dangerous interactions. Clinically, the most important interactions are those drugs with a narrow therapeutic range, e.g. **digoxin**, **theophylline**, **warfarin**, **phenytoin** and other anti-epileptics; these may warrant monitoring plasma concentrations. Clinical response should also be monitored closely. Appropriate precautionary measures may need to be taken if the feed is discontinued, particularly if dose adjustments were made because of an interaction.

Administration of e/c (gastro-resistant) and m/r formulations by EFT

Generally, these products should *not* be administered by EFT because of the risk of blocking the tube. However, some capsules/granules/compressed tablets contain e/c or m/r granules for which specific procedures have been developed to allow administration of the coated granules by EFT, e.g. **esomeprazole** gastro-resistant tablets and gastro-resistant granules for oral suspension (Nexium®), **lansoprazole** orodispersible tablets (Zoton FasTab®), certain m/r **morphine** formulations (MST Continus® suspension and Zomorph® capsules) **omeprazole** capsules (Losec®) and **theophylline** m/r capsules (Slo-Phyllin®). See the manufacturer's SPC and/or specialist information for details (Table 2).[1] In order to avoid dangerous dose peaks and troughs or tube blockage, it is essential that:

- the recommended procedure is strictly adhered to and is used only for that *specific* formulation and brand
- the correct tube size and type is used
- extreme care is taken to avoid crushing the coated granules, thereby destroying the coating
- clinical response is monitored closely.

Unblocking EFTs

Tube blockage may be caused by the feed, e.g. stagnant or contaminated feed, or by incorrect drug administration, e.g. particle blockage or interaction between the feed and drug. It can be minimized by effective flushing and choosing an appropriate formulation. It is more likely with narrow lumens; a 35% incidence of blockage in patients with 8 French tubes has been cited.[27] Many tubes can be unblocked using 15–30mL water in a 50mL syringe and a push-pull action, although this may take 20–30min. Excessive force must not be used to unblock a tube because of the danger of perforation. Care must be taken as unblocking a tube may result in bolus drug administration from residual drug in the tube.

Various other agents have anecdotally been used to unblock tubes, e.g. carbonated drinks or cranberry juice. However, these are acidic solutions and can make the situation worse by causing feed coagulation,[10] and are no longer recommended.[1] Pancreatic enzymes help only if the blockage is caused by the feed. Sodium bicarbonate needs to be added to activate the enzymes, which may not be practical. Re-insertion of guide-wires is not advisable unless under specialist supervision.[1]

For blockages which do not resolve with water, consult a specialist nutrition nurse if available.

Quick Clinical Guide: Administration of drugs by enteral feeding tube

Before drug administration

1 The administration of drugs by an enteral feeding tube (EFT) is considered a level 3 skill for care workers in care homes. Staff must be adequately trained.

2 Drug charts should state the specific route of administration, e.g. nasogastric (NG), nasojejunal (NJ), and specify the lumen to be used to prevent wrong route errors.

3 Check that there is documented confirmation that the EFT was correctly positioned following insertion. For NG tubes, use CE marked pH paper intended for testing human gastric contents (safe range pH1–5.5 after a 1h break in feeding) or, when there is doubt, by approved radiographic confirmation in accordance with NPSA guidelines.

4 If practical, reconfirm correct NG tube position before each drug administration. For patients on continuous feeding, multiple drug administration times or on acid-suppressants (antacids, H_2 antagonists, PPIs), if correct tube placement confirmed initially and there is no reason to suspect displacement, confirm tube position by observation of the external tube length (in accordance with NPSA guidelines); likewise for NJ tubes.

5 The patient should be in a sitting position to prevent regurgitation and pulmonary aspiration.

6 To prevent accidental parenteral administration, use enteral syringes, i.e. syringes which cannot be connected to IV catheters, ports or other parenteral devices. A 50mL enteral syringe reduces the risk of rupture of the EFT.

7 All EFT lumens should be clearly labelled.

> Do not use 3-way taps or syringe tip adaptors because these can inadvertently result in connection safeguards being bypassed.

Drug administration

> Do not add drugs to enteral feeds because this increases the risk of incompatibility, microbial contamination, tube blockage, and underdosing or overdosing if the feed rate is altered.

8 Stop the feed and ensure any other ports are closed and airtight.

9 Flush the EFT using a **push-pause** action with 15–30mL of water (*use sterile water throughout if jejunal tube or immunocompromised patient*). This helps to clear the tube and prevent physical interactions with the feed which could result in coagulation and blockage of the tube.

10 Check if a specific time interval is needed before and after administration to achieve maximal absorption and/or reduce the risk of chemical interactions.

11 Administer the most suitable formulation of each drug separately (see Choosing a suitable formulation, Box A, p.727 and Table 2, p.733).
   • a 50mL enteral syringe reduces the risk of rupture of the EFT; a 2mL or smaller enteral syringe can be used for very small quantities to accurately measure the dose.
   • flush between each drug with 15–30mL of water.

12 After drug administration, flush the EFT using a **push-pause** action with 15–30mL of water.

13 Resume feeding after any necessary feed break (see point 10).

After drug administration

14 Document the total volume of fluid given (including flushes) on a fluid balance chart.

15 Monitor the clinical response, particularly if:
   • changing from m/r to normal-release formulations
   • the drug has a narrow therapeutic range
   • the bio-availability of the drug differs between solid dose form and liquid.

Table 2 Information on alternative enteral formulations available for administering drugs to patients with swallowing difficulties or by EFT[1,28–31]

Drug	Authorized soluble tablet or oral liquid available	Tablet/capsule contents may disperse sufficiently for 8Fr NG tube[a,b]	Oral liquid can be prepared by local pharmacy or special order	Injection can be diluted and administered PO or by EFT	Comments
Acetylcysteine	No			Yes	
Amiloride	Yes	Yes			Sugar- and sorbitol-free oral solution
Aminophylline[a]	No	No	Yes	Yes	Consider discontinuing therapy due to dosing complexities. Give aminophylline injection orally as a diluted oral solution,[1] take care converting from m/r to immediate-release or convert oral aminophylline total daily dose to oral *unauthorized* theophylline liquid (aminophylline 250mg PO = theophylline 200mg PO) and split into t.d.s regimen (see theophylline below). Monitor blood levels
Amiodarone	No	No	Yes[f]	No	A 25mg/5mL suspension[f] or 200mg/5mL suspension can be prepared.[30] Injection contains irritant Tween 80
Amitriptyline	Yes	No	Yes[c,e]		Sugar- and sorbitol-free oral solution
Amlodipine	No	Yes	Yes[e,f]		A 1mg/mL suspension can be prepared (90 day shelf-life)[f] or with 1% methylcellulose in syrup (56 day shelf-life).[1] Disperse tablet for intrajejunal administration
Amoxicillin	Yes			Yes	Dilute oral suspensions with an equal volume of water to reduce viscosity for EFT use
Antacids	Yes				Not recommended by EFT as can coagulate with feed; not needed with jejunal tube
Ascorbic acid	No	Yes (effervescent)			Add effervescent tablets to 50mL water
Aspirin	No	Yes (dispersible)			Use dispersible tablet

continued

Table 2 Continued

Drug	Authorized soluble tablet or oral liquid available	Tablet/capsule contents may disperse sufficiently for 8Fr NG tube[a,b]	Oral liquid can be prepared by local pharmacy or special order	Injection can be diluted and administered PO or by EFT	Comments
Baclofen	Yes	Yes	Yes[d]		Authorized oral liquids are viscous and contain sorbitol (2.75g/5mL Lioresal®) dilute with an equal volume of water for EFT use. Dispersing tablets is preferable particularly for intrajejunal administration
Bethanechol	No		Yes		A 5mg/mL suspension with cherry syrup can be prepared (60 day shelf-life)[i]
Calcium & vitamin D	No	Yes (effervescent)			Use effervescent granules or effervescent tablet and add to 50mL water. The solution can crystallize and calcium can bind to phosphate in enteral feed. Flush EFT well to avoid
Carbamazepine[a]	Yes	Yes			Oral liquid contains sorbitol (1.25g/5mL Tegretol®). Dilute with an equal volume of water to reduce adherence to EFT. Monitor for increased undesirable effects particularly with intrajejunal administration
Carbocisteine	Yes				
Cefalexin	Yes				Dilute oral suspensions with equal volume of water to reduce viscosity for EFT use. Avoid opening capsules/crushing tablets due to risk of cephalosporin sensitization
Cefradine	Yes				Avoid opening capsules/crushing tablets due to risk of cephalosporin sensitization
Celecoxib	No	Yes			
Chlorphenamine	Yes				

continued

Table 2 Continued

Drug	Authorized soluble tablet or oral liquid available	Tablet/capsule contents may disperse sufficiently for 8Fr NG tube[a,b]	Oral liquid can be prepared by local pharmacy or special order	Injection can be diluted and administered PO or by EFT	Comments
Chlorpromazine	Yes	No	Yes[d]		Some oral liquids contain sorbitol. Handle with care to avoid contact sensitization; do not crush tablets
Cimetidine	Yes	Yes (effervescent)		Yes (Tagamet®)	Some oral liquids contain sorbitol (Dyspamet® 2.8g/5mL, Tagamet® negligible). Use effervescent tablet added to 30mL water, or diluted liquid for intrajejunal administration. Tagamet® and Dyspamet® disperse but no information on suitability for EFT
Cinnarizine	No	Yes			
Ciprofloxacin	Yes	Yes (Ranbaxy, Generics)	Yes[c]		Authorized oral suspension not recommended for EFT because too viscous and granular. Disperse tablet with 30–50mL sterile water not tap water (to avoid ion chelation). Stop feed for 1h before and 1–2h after dose. Do not administer with iron or zinc
Citalopram	Yes	Yes (Generics)			10mg of tablet equivalent to 8mg of oral liquid (4 drops). Oral liquid should be mixed with water for EFT, or water/orange/apple juice for PO use; contains alcohol (0.01 units/mL)
Clarithromycin[a]	Yes	Yes		No	Dilute oral liquid with an equal volume of water for EFT. Do not use EFT less than 9Fr gauge
Clindamycin	No	Yes (capsules)	Yes[e]		Avoid inhalation of the capsule contents
Clomipramine[a]	No	Yes			
Clonazepam	Yes	Yes (Rivotril®)	Yes[d,e,f]	Yes	Authorized oral solutions 500microgram/5mL and 2mg/5mL contain alcohol (0.01 units/5mL) and must not be diluted. No information on suitability via EFT. Dilute all other formulations with 30–50mL water to reduce risk of binding to the tube. Disperse tablets for intrajejunal administration. Injection contains alcohol and other excipients

continued

Table 2 Continued

Drug	Authorized soluble tablet or oral liquid available	Tablet/capsule contents may disperse sufficiently for 8Fr NG tube[a,b]	Oral liquid can be prepared by local pharmacy or special order	Injection can be diluted and administered PO or by EFT	Comments
Clonidine	No	Yes (100microgram Catapres®)	Yes[d,e]	Yes (Catapres®)	Unauthorized 50microgram/5mL oral solution and suspension can be obtained via special order. An100microgram/mL formulation with simple syrup can be prepared (1 month shelf-life)[l]
Co-amoxiclav	Yes	No			Oral liquid not recommended for EFT because too viscous
Co-codamol	No	Yes (effervescent/dispersible)			Add effervescent/dispersible tablet to 50mL water
Co-codaprin	No	Yes (dispersible)			Add dispersible tablet to 50mL water
Co-danthramer	Yes				Slightly viscous liquid; may require a larger flush volume
Co-danthrusate	Yes				No information on suitability via EFT
Codeine phosphate	Yes		Yes[d]		Dilute authorized oral liquid with an equal volume of water to reduce viscosity for EFT use. Tablets disperse but no information on suitability by EFT. Some dispersible or effervescent formulations contain 20mmol sodium per tablet
Co-phenotrope	No	Yes (Lomotil®)			
Co-trimoxazole	Yes				Oral liquid (Septrin®) contains sorbitol and needs diluting 3 times to reduce viscosity for EFT use
Cyclizine	No	Yes (Valoid®)	Yes[c,e]	Yes	Unauthorized 50mg/5mL oral solution and suspension can be obtained via special order
Cyproheptadine	No	Yes			
Cyproterone	No		Yes[d]		Tablets disperse but no information on suitability by EFT

continued

Table 2 Continued

Drug	Authorized soluble tablet or oral liquid available	Tablet/capsule contents may disperse sufficiently for 8Fr NG tube[a,b]	Oral liquid can be prepared by local pharmacy or special order	Injection can be diluted and administered PO or by EFT	Comments
Dantrolene	No		Yes[d,e]	No	Injection formulation may hydrolyse in the stomach. Capsule contents disperse but no information on suitability by EFT. Unauthorized 25mg/5mL or 100mg/5mL oral suspension can be obtained via special order
Demeclocycline	No	No			Capsule contents are irritant and only sparingly soluble. Absorption is reduced by calcium
Desmopressin	No	Yes (Desmotabs, DDAVP®)			DDAVP Melt® for SL use only, not for EFT administration
Dexamethasone	Yes	Yes (Organon)	Yes[d]	Yes	Authorized oral liquid contains sorbitol 500microgram/5mL
Dexamfetamine			Yes[e]		Unauthorized 5mg/5mL oral solution can be obtained via special order
Diamorphine	No		Yes		
Diazepam	Yes	Yes (APS)	Yes[d,e]	Yes	Dilute authorized oral liquid with an equal volume of water to reduce viscosity and risk of binding to the EFT. Disperse tablets for intrajejunal administration. Anecdotal evidence of using injection enterally; drug loss may occur due to binding to tube
Diclofenac[a]	No	Yes (dispersible)	Yes[e]		Use authorized dispersible tablet for EFT. Alternative unauthorized 10mg dispersible tablets or 50mg/5mL oral liquid (1 year shelf-life) available
Dicycloverine	Yes				Dilute oral liquid with an equal volume of water for EFT use
Digoxin	Yes				In theory 50microgram Lanoxin® oral liquid = 62.5microgram tablet, however in practice unlikely to be clinically important, monitor plasma concentrations if changing formulation or using a high-fibre feed. Oral liquid may cause diarrhoea. Lanoxin® tablets disperse but no information on suitability by EFT

continued

Table 2 Continued

Drug	Authorized soluble tablet or oral liquid available	Tablet/capsule contents may disperse sufficiently for 8Fr NG tube[a,b]	Oral liquid can be prepared by local pharmacy or special order	Injection can be diluted and administered PO or by EFT	Comments
Dihydrocodeine[a]	Yes				Dilute oral liquid with an equal volume of water for EFT use
Docusate sodium	Yes				Dilute oral liquid with an equal volume of water for EFT use
Domperidone	Yes	Yes (Co-Pharma, CP)	Yes[d]		Dilute oral liquid with an equal volume of water for EFT use. Contains sorbitol 2.3g/5mL. Consider dispersing tablets for intrajejunal administration
Doxepin	No	Yes (Sinepin®)			Use dispersible tablets, do not open capsules as contents are irritant
Doxycycline	No	Yes (dispersible)			
Erythromycin[a]	Yes	No			Dilute oral liquid with an equal volume of water for EFT use, some brands contain sorbitol. Tablets and capsule contents are e/c therefore not suitable for EFT
Esomeprazole	No	Yes (Nexium®)			Nexium® tablets and granules for suspension are authorized for administration via a gastric tube. The tablet contains a compressed core of e/c microgranules which can be dispersed and flushed via an 8Fr gauge NG tube. Do not crush. Strictly follow the procedure in the SPC to prevent tube blockage
Etamsylate (not UK)	No		Yes[d]		
Ferrous sulfate	No	No		No	Convert to an alternative iron salt oral liquid preparation. Ferrous sulfate 200mg = 3.3mL Niferex® or 7mL Galfer® or 12mL Sytron® (contains sorbitol 2g/5mL); dilute with an equal volume of water for EFT use

continued

Table 2 Continued

Drug	Authorized soluble tablet or oral liquid available	Tablet/capsule contents may disperse sufficiently for 8Fr NG tube[a,b]	Oral liquid can be prepared by local pharmacy or special order	Injection can be diluted and administered PO or by EFT	Comments
Flecainide	No	Yes (Generics)	Yes[c,e]	Yes	Use de-ionized/sterile water, *not tap water*. Note crushed tablets have a local anaesthetic effect. Do *not* dilute the injection or mix with alkaline solutions, e.g. chlorides, phosphates, sulfates. Unauthorized 25mg/5mL oral solution and suspension can be obtained via special order
Flucloxacillin	Yes	No		Yes (Berk, CP)	Dilute oral liquid with an equal volume of water for EFT use. Stop feed for 1h before and after dose. Avoid opening capsules due to risk of sensitization
Fluconazole	Yes	Yes (50mg capsule)	Yes[d]	No	Do not use the 150mg capsule contents
Fludrocortisone	No	Yes (Florinef®)			
Fluoxetine	Yes				Capsule contents can be dispersed but no information on suitability via EFT
Furosemide	Yes		Yes[d]		Authorized oral liquid is alkaline and may coagulate with other acidic preparations. Flush EFT well to avoid. Lasix® tablets disperse but no information on suitability via EFT. SL use may be an option (see p.64)
Gabapentin	Yes	Yes (Neurontin®)			The authorized oral solution contains propylene glycol and other excipients, which in high doses may exceed WHO daily intake limits
Glibenclamide	No	Yes (APS)	Yes[d]		Daonil® tablets disperse but no information on suitability via EFT
Gliclazide[a]	No	Yes (Alpharma, CP, Generics)	Yes[d,e]		When administering dispersed tablets by EFT, there may be residue left in the oral syringe, which is unlikely to be active drug due to high solubility. Flush EFT well to avoid blockage. Unauthorized 40mg/5mL and 80mg/5mL oral suspension can be obtained via special order

continued

Table 2 Continued

Drug	Authorized soluble tablet or oral liquid available	Tablet/capsule contents may disperse sufficiently for 8Fr NG tube[a,b]	Oral liquid can be prepared by local pharmacy or special order	Injection can be diluted and administered PO or by EFT	Comments
Glycopyrronium	No	No	Yes[e]	Yes	Tablets disperse coarsely and may leave sediment. Unauthorized oral formulations can be obtained via special order or can be made locally from glycopyrronium powder or injection (see p.13). Cost of bulk powder may be prohibitive
Granisetron	No	Yes (Kytril®)	Yes[f]	Yes	250microgram/5mL suspension can be prepared.[f] TD patch available
Haloperidol	Yes				Serenace® tablets disperse but no information on suitability by EFT
Hydrocortisone	No	Yes	Yes[e]	Yes (Efcortesol®)	Injection contains significant amounts of phosphate. Unauthorized 5mg/5mL or 10mg/5mL oral suspension can be obtained via special order
Hydromorphone[a]	No				Do not administer contents of m/r capsules by EFT due to high risk of blockage
Hyoscine butylbromide	No	No	Yes[e]	Yes	Injection may be stored for 24h in a refrigerator once opened. Unauthorized 10mg/5mL oral solution and suspension can be obtained via special order
Hyoscine hydrobromide	No		Yes[e]	Yes	Unauthorized 300microgram/5mL or 500microgram/5mL oral solution and suspension can be obtained via special order. TD patch available
Ibuprofen[a]	Yes	No			Oral liquid contains sorbitol 500microgram/5mL, dilute with an equal volume of water (more for intrajejunal administration) to reduce viscosity for EFT use
Imipramine	No		Yes[c]		Tofranil® disperse but particles may be too large for EFT use
Ispaghula husk					Do not administer due to high risk of blockage, consider using a high-fibre feed

continued

Table 2 Continued

Drug	Authorized soluble tablet or oral liquid available	Tablet/capsule contents may disperse sufficiently for 8Fr NG tube[a,b]	Oral liquid can be prepared by local pharmacy or special order	Injection can be diluted and administered PO or by EFT	Comments
Itraconazole	Yes				Stop the feed for 2h before and after dose. Oral liquid contains sorbitol and is acidic. Flush EFT well to avoid coagulation. Absorption via jejunum may be reduced
Ketamine	No		Yes[e]	Yes	A 50mg/5mL oral solution using the injection formulation can be prepared by pharmacy, 7 day shelf-life (see p.630). Unauthorized 50mg/5mL oral solution and suspension can be obtained via special order
Ketorolac	No	Yes (Toradol[®])			Dilute oral liquid with 2–3 times volume of water for EFT use
Lactulose	Yes				Dilute oral liquid with 2–3 times volume of water for EFT use
Lamotrigine	No	Yes	Yes[d,f]		Use authorized dispersible tablet. A 5mg/5mL suspension can be prepared[f]
Lansoprazole	No	Yes (FasTab[®]), and capsules	Yes		Add orodispersible tablet (FasTab[®]) to 10mL of water and administer by EFT using a push-pull technique to keep the granules suspended. Do not crush For tubes smaller than 8Fr, open capsules and mix e/c granules with 10mL of 8.4% sodium bicarbonate, (14 day shelf-life in a refrigerator if locally prepared by pharmacy)[l]
Levetiracetam	Yes	Yes (500mg Keppra[®])			Use the oral liquid for EFT
Levomepromazine	No	Yes (Nozinan[®])	Yes[d]	Yes	Tablet dispersion is coarse and may block tubes smaller than 8Fr
Lofepramine	Yes				Dilute oral liquid with an equal volume of water for EFT use; contains sorbitol 1.4g/5mL
Loperamide	Yes				Oral solution contains alcohol

continued

Table 2 Continued

Drug	Authorized soluble tablet or oral liquid available	Tablet/capsule contents may disperse sufficiently for 8Fr NG tube[a,b]	Oral liquid can be prepared by local pharmacy or special order	Injection can be diluted and administered PO or by EFT	Comments
Loratadine	Yes				Dilute oral liquid with an equal volume of water for jejunal administration to reduce osmolarity
Lorazepam	No	No	Yes[d,e]		Tablets do not disperse easily. Tablets (Genus brand) and injection can be used sublingually. Unauthorized 1mg/5mL oral solution and suspension can be obtained via special order
Macrogols	Yes				May not be suitable for EFT use due to the large volume required to dissolve the powder
Magnesium glycerophosphate	No		Yes[e]		Unauthorized 1mmol/mL oral solution can be obtained via special order (intermittent supply). Various unauthorized tablets available, some will disperse but no information on suitability by EFT
Mebeverine[a]	Yes				135mg tablet = 15mL oral liquid 50mg/5mL. Most effective when given 20min before food
Medroxy-progesterone acetate	No	Yes (Provera® 5mg, 100mg)	Yes[d]		
Megestrol acetate	No	Yes (Megace®)	Yes[d,e]		Unauthorized 40mg/mL oral suspension can be imported via IDIS
Melatonin[a]	No		Yes[e]		Unauthorized oral solutions and suspensions can be obtained via special order
Menadiol sodium phosphate	No		Yes[d,e]		Tablets disperse but no information on suitability by EFT. Unauthorized 5mg/5mL oral solution and suspension can be obtained via special order
Metformin[a]	Yes	Yes (Glucophage® sachets)	Yes[d]		Sachets disperse fully in 20mL of water for EFT, (manufacturer recommends 150mL for PO use)
Methadone	Yes				No information on suitability via EFT

Table 2 Continued

Drug	Authorized soluble tablet or oral liquid available	Tablet/capsule contents may disperse sufficiently for 8Fr NG tube[a,b]	Oral liquid can be prepared by local pharmacy or special order	Injection can be diluted and administered PO or by EFT	Comments
Methenamine	No				Tablets are authorized to be crushed and mixed with milk or fruit juice for swallowing difficulties. No information on suitability by EFT
Methylpred-nisolone	No	Yes (Medrone®)		Yes (Solu-Medrone®)	
Metoclopramide[a]	Yes			Yes	Some liquids may contain sorbitol. Maxolon® tablets disperse but no information on suitability by EFT
Metronidazole	Yes	No	Yes		Dilute authorized oral liquid with an equal volume of water for NG use and stop feed for 1h before the dose to allow gastric pH to recover to metabolize the benzoate salt. The benzoate salt is metabolized in the stomach, therefore *not* suitable for jejunal use. A 50mg/mL suspension with cherry syrup can be prepared (60 day shelf-life);[1] it does not require a break in feeding and is more suitable for intrajejunal administration
Midazolam	No		Yes[e]	Yes	Authorized 5mg/mL oromucosal solution for *buccal* use available as unit dose preparation. Unauthorized 10mg/mL oromucosal solution for *buccal* use can be obtained via special order. Injection can be used via PO, buccal, intranasal and PR routes; injection can be diluted with apple or blackcurrant juice, chocolate sauce or cola for PO administration
Mirtazapine	Yes	No			Use oral liquid; orodispersible tablets (Zispin SolTab®) are *not* recommended for EFT use because too granular
Misoprostol	No	No			Do not crush tablets because of occupational exposure risks to staff (see Box B)
Moclobemide	No	Yes (APS)			

continued

Table 2 Continued

Drug	Authorized soluble tablet or oral liquid available	Tablet/capsule contents may disperse sufficiently for 8Fr NG tube[a,b]	Oral liquid can be prepared by local pharmacy or special order	Injection can be diluted and administered PO or by EFT	Comments
Morphine[a]	Yes				Oral liquid can be used; 10mg/5mL contains alcohol (0.05 units/5mL). Dilute with an equal volume of water, for intrajejunal administration to reduce osmolarity
					The m/r granules in Zomorph® capsules are authorized for gastric administration via a 16Fr tube (internal diameter 2.5mm) with an open distal end or lateral pores (see SPC). Certain tubes have been found to cause problems.[8] The m/r granules should be mixed (do not crush) with 30mL water. Take great care to ensure that all the m/r granules are administered and are not crushed with the syringe plunger. Add extra water if necessary. There is some anecdotal data on using 8Fr tubes[1]
					The m/r granules in MST Continus® suspension sachets have been administered as above in tubes with 8Fr gauge or minimum internal diameter 1.05mm
					The m/r granules in MXL® capsules are not suitable for EFT administration
Nabilone	No				The capsule contents disperse but no information on suitability by EFT
Nabumetone	No	No			
Naltrexone	No		Yes[e]		Unauthorized 5mg/5mL oral suspension can be obtained via special order
Naproxen[a]	No	Yes	Yes[e]		Unauthorized 125mg/5mL or 200mg/5mL oral solution can be obtained via special order
Nefopam	No	Yes (Acupan®)			High risk of sediment when dispersing tablets, may not be suitable for EFT

continued

Table 2 Continued

Drug	Authorized soluble tablet or oral liquid available	Tablet/capsule contents may disperse sufficiently for 8Fr NG tube[a,b]	Oral liquid can be prepared by local pharmacy or special order	Injection can be diluted and administered PO or by EFT	Comments
Nifedipine[a]	No		Yes[e,f]		Consider an alternative product, e.g. amlodipine. Drawing up contents of liquid capsules not recommended, volumes vary between manufacturers, liquid is light sensitive, and risk of profound hypotension, particularly if converting from m/r preparation. Unauthorized 10mg/5mL oral suspension can be obtained via special order A 20mg/5mL suspension can be prepared using capsule contents[f,30]
Nitrazepam	Yes		Yes[e]		Dilute authorized oral liquid to reduce osmolality for intrajejunal use
Nitrofurantoin[a]	Yes	Yes	Yes[d]		Dilute authorized oral liquid with an equal volume of water for EFT use
Olanzapine	No	Yes (Zyprexa Velotab®)	Yes[e]		Unauthorized 2.5mg/5mL oral suspension can be obtained via special order
Omeprazole	No	Yes (Alpharma or Dexcel tablets); Losec MUPS®	Yes	Yes	A 2mg/mL formulation with 20mg capsule contents and 10mL 8.4% sodium bicarbonate can be prepared by pharmacy (45 day shelf-life in a refrigerator)[1] Orodispersible tablet (Losec MUPS®) can be added to 25mL of water and administered by EFT using a push-pull technique to keep the granules suspended. Do not crush. Suitable for 8Fr gauge Tablets (Alphyarma, Dexcel) disperse; larger doses may be required in gastric administration as this method destroys the e/c coating Contact Astra Zeneca for details of use of injection or infusion via EFT

continued

Table 2 Continued

Drug	Authorized soluble tablet or oral liquid available	Tablet/capsule contents may disperse sufficiently for 8Fr NG tube[a,b]	Oral liquid can be prepared by local pharmacy or special order	Injection can be diluted and administered PO or by EFT	Comments
Ondansetron	Yes			Yes	Oral liquid contains sorbitol 3g/5mL. Zofran® tablets disperse but no information on suitability by EFT or of the orodispersible tablet (Zofran Melt®). The injection is acidic, flush well to avoid coagulation with feed
Orphenadrine	Yes		Yes[c]		Authorized oral liquids contain sorbitol, 0.45g/5mL (Rosemont) and 1.75g/5ml (Biorphen®). Disipal® tablets disperse but no information on suitability by EFT
Oxybutynin[a]	Yes	Yes (Tillomed)	Yes[d,e]		Authorized oral liquid contains sorbitol 1.3g/5mL. Ditropan® may disperse but no information on suitability by EFT. Cystrin® may leave sediment and be unsuitable for EFT use. TD patch available
Oxycodone[a]	Yes				Significant anecdotal reports of use of liquid preparation by EFT
Paracetamol	Yes	Yes (dispersible/effervescent)			Add dispersible tablet to 50mL of water; consider sodium content
Paroxetine	Yes				Dilute oral liquid with an equal volume of water for EFT use, contains sorbitol
Phenobarbital	Yes		Yes[d,e,f]		Authorized elixir contains alcohol (0.38units/10mL dose). An unauthorized 50mg/5mL alcohol-free suspension can be obtained via special order or locally prepared. Dilute oral liquids with an equal volume of water for intrajejunal administration to reduce osmolarity. Tablets may disperse but no information on suitability by EFT
Phenoxymethyl-penicillin	Yes				Stop feed for 2h before and 1h after dose

continued

Table 2 Continued

Drug	Authorized soluble tablet or oral liquid available	Tablet/capsule contents may disperse sufficiently for 8Fr NG tube[a,b]	Oral liquid can be prepared by local pharmacy or special order	Injection can be diluted and administered PO or by EFT	Comments
Phenytoin	Yes	Yes (Flynn; capsules)	Yes[e]		Stop feed for 2h before and after dose and flush tube with 50mL water to minimize interaction with feed. Convert to once daily dose. Phenytoin *base* 30mg/5mL oral suspension (Epanutin®); 90mg (15mL) = 100mg phenytoin *sodium* tablet/capsule, shake liquid well, then dilute dose with 30–50mL water, administer and flush. An unauthorized concentrated oral liquid 90mg/5mL is available. Flynn hard capsule contents will disperse. Monitor plasma levels and adhere to a consistent protocol. Jejunal absorption is poor
Phytomenadione	No			Yes (Konakion MM®)	The injection is incompatible with certain types of siliconized syringes. Braun syringes are known to be compatible
Piroxicam	No				Add dispersible tablet (Feldene Melt®) to 50mL water, no information on suitability by EFT
Pilocarpine	No		Yes		
Potassium supplements[a]	Yes	Yes (effervescent)			Flush EFT well to prevent physical interaction with feed. Add effervescent tablets to 50mL water. Oral liquid contains sorbitol 2g/5mL and may cause diarrhoea, dilute with 50–100mL water, not recommended for intrajejunal administration
Prednisolone[a]	Yes	No	Yes[d]		
Pregabalin	Yes	Yes (Lyrica® capsules)			

continued

Table 2 Continued

Drug	Authorized soluble tablet or oral liquid available	Tablet/capsule contents may disperse sufficiently for 8Fr NG tube[a,b]	Oral liquid can be prepared by local pharmacy or special order	Injection can be diluted and administered PO or by EFT	Comments
Prochlorperazine	Yes	Yes (APS, Meridian)			Dilute oral liquid with an equal volume of water for EFT use. Use effervescent granules or disperse tablets for intrajejunal administration. Stemetil® tablets disperse but no information on use by EFT
Promethazine	Yes	Yes (Phenergan®)			Dilute oral liquid with an equal volume of water for EFT use
Propantheline	No		Yes[e]		
Ranitidine	Yes	Yes (effervescent)	Yes[d]	Yes	Add effervescent tablets to 30mL water, consider sodium content Authorized oral liquid contains alcohol (0.04units/5mL) and sorbitol
Rifampicin	Yes		Yes[f]		Stop feed for 2h before and 30min after dose. Dilute authorized oral liquid with equal volume of water: Do not open capsules; risk of contact sensitization. A 125mg/5mL suspension can be prepared (7 day shelf-life)[f]
Risperidone	Yes	Yes (Risperdal®)			No information on suitability of orodispersible tablets (Quicklet®) via EFT
Senna	Yes		Yes[d]		Granules not suitable for administration by EFT
Sertraline	No	Yes (Lustral®)	Yes[e]		Coarse tablet dispersion may block tube, consider alternative drug. Note crushed tablets have a local anaesthetic effect
Sodium clodronate	No	Yes (Bonefos®)			Stop feed for 1h before and after dose. Both capsule contents and tablets disperse in water
Sodium fusidate	Yes				Sodium fusidate tablets 500mg = 750mg oral suspension. Oral liquid contains sorbitol

continued

Table 2 Continued

Drug	Authorized soluble tablet or oral liquid available	Tablet/capsule contents may disperse sufficiently for 8Fr NG tube[a,b]	Oral liquid can be prepared by local pharmacy or special order	Injection can be diluted and administered PO or by EFT	Comments
Sodium valproate[a]	Yes	Yes (Epilim® Crushable)		No	Dilute oral liquid with an equal volume of water for EFT use. Some formulations contain sorbitol. Consider dispersing crushable tablets for intrajejunal administration or dilute oral liquid 3–4 times
Spironolactone	No	Yes (Most generics, Aldactone®)	Yes[d,e,f]		Unauthorized oral formulations can be obtained via special order; dilute with an equal volume of water for EFT use. Disperse tablet for intrajejunal administration. A 125mg/5mL suspension can be prepared. Other suspension formulae are also available[29]
Sucralfate	Yes	Yes			Do not use sucralfate via EFT. Oral liquid *not* recommended due to high viscosity, bezoar formation and binding with feed; likely to block tube. Need to stop feed for 1h before and after dose; impractical for q4h schedule
Tapentadol[a]	Yes				
Temazepam	Yes				Oral liquid contains sorbitol
Tetracycline	No		Yes[f]		A 125mg/5mL suspension can be prepared (7day shelf-life).[f] Significant interaction with enteral feed makes four times a day dosing difficult by EFT
Theophylline[a]	No		Yes[e]		Convert total daily dose of m/r preparations to oral *unauthorized* liquid and split into t.d.s. regimen. Stop feed for 1h before and 1h after dose. Dilute oral liquid with an equal volume of water. Monitor plasma levels closely The m/r granules of Slo-phyllin® capsules can be administered via EFT, although may block smaller tubes. Take care not to crush There is some information on giving aminophylline injection orally[i]

continued

Table 2 Continued

Drug	Authorized soluble tablet or oral liquid available	Tablet/capsule contents may disperse sufficiently for 8Fr NG tube[a,b]	Oral liquid can be prepared by local pharmacy or special order	Injection can be diluted and administered PO or by EFT	Comments
Tizanidine	No	Yes (Zanaflex®)	Yes[e]		Unauthorized 2mg/5mL oral solution and suspension can be obtained via special order
Tolbutamide	No	No	Yes[d]		
Topiramate	No	Yes (Topamax® tablets)	Yes[e]		Do not use Topamax® Sprinkle capsules by EFT as the beads stick to the tube causing blockage. Unauthorized 25mg/5mL or 50mg/5mL oral suspension can be obtained via special order
Tramadol[a]	No	Yes (Ranbaxy capsules, Zydol® soluble, Zamadol Melt®)	Yes[f]		Use authorized dispersible tablets. Oral drops 100mg/mL available; further dilute with water. Zydol® capsule contents may disperse but no information on suitability by EFT. A 25mg/5mL suspension can be prepared
Tranexamic acid	No	Yes (Cyklokapron®, Manx)	Yes[d,e]	Yes	Unauthorized 500mg/5mL oral solution and suspension can be obtained via special order
Trazodone	Yes	Yes (Molipaxin 50mg capsules)			Dilute oral liquid with an equal volume of water for EFT use
Trimethoprim	Yes		Yes[d]		Administer the dose during a break in feeding if practical. Dilute authorized oral liquid with an equal volume of water for EFT use, some formulations contain sorbitol
Vancomycin	No	No		Yes	The reconstituted injection is authorized for oral and NG tube use (24h shelf-life time in fridge for enteral use)
Venlafaxine[a]	No	Yes (Efexor®)	Yes[e]		Unauthorized 37.5mg/5mL or 75mg/5mL oral solution and suspension can be obtained via special order

continued

Table 2 Continued

Drug	Authorized soluble tablet or oral liquid available	Tablet/capsule contents may disperse sufficiently for 8Fr NG tube[a,b]	Oral liquid can be prepared by local pharmacy or special order	Injection can be diluted and administered PO or by EFT	Comments
Warfarin	Yes	Yes	Yes[d]		Stop feed for 1h before and 1–2h after dose. INR may be affected by the varying content of vitamin K in feeds
Zinc	No	Yes (effervescent)			Add effervescent tablet to 10mL water. Jejunal administration may reduce bio-availability

a. do not use m/r or e/c preparations unless specifically indicated. Take care if converting from m/r to immediate-release preparations because dose, frequency and clinical effect may be different

b. use the brand or manufacturer if specified; different brands may not disperse sufficiently for 8Fr NG tube administration; dispersion time may take up to 5min and require agitation

c. a simple suspension using Diluent C suspending agent can be prepared by some local pharmacies with a 7 day shelf-life

d. a simple suspension using Keltrol (Diluent A) suspending agent can be prepared by some local pharmacies with a 7 day shelf-life

e. unauthorized product, available from 'specials' manufacturers or imported (see Appendix 1, p.817)

f. a simple suspension using 1:1 mixture of Ora-Plus and Ora-Sweet as a vehicle can be prepared by some local pharmacies, 28 day shelf-life unless otherwise stated[30]

g. tubes which should *not* be used for administration of Zomorph® capsules include: Mallinkrodt enral 205-09-1, Bioser 1147221, Vygon 39110 and Vygon 2395.09. Tubes known to be successful in administering Zomorph® capsules include Pharma Plast LEVIN CH/FG 18, Vygon 391.16, Ventrol 15016IT 85753, Ventrol 82316 16A, Bioser 1147239 and Sherwood 90L100A.

1 White R and Bradnam V (2010). *Handbook of Drug Administration via Enteral Feeding Tubes*. London: Pharmaceutical Press www.medicinescomplete.com (accessed December 2013).

2 Williams NT (2008) Medication administration through enteral feeding tubes. *American Journal of Health-System Pharmacy*. **65**: 2347–2357.

3 BAPEN (British Association of Parenteral and Enteral Nutrition) (2004) Administering drugs via enteral feeding tubes. A practical guide. BAPEN. Available from: www.bapen.org.uk

4 National Patient Safety Agency (2007) Promoting safer measurement and administration of liquid medicines via oral and other enteral routes. *Patient safety alert*. NPSA/2007/PSA/19: www.nrls.npsa.nhs.uk

5 National Patient Safety Agency (2011) Reducing the harm caused by misplaced nasogastric feeding tubes in adults and infants. *Patient safety alert and supporting information*. NPSA/2011/PSA002: www.nrls.npsa.nhs.uk

6 UK Medicines Information (2013) What are the therapeutic options for patients unable to take solid oral dosage forms. *Medicines QA* **294.3**. www.evidence.nhs.uk

7 National Patient Safety Agency (2012) Harm from flushing of nasogastric tubes before confirmation of placement. *Rapid Reponse Reprt*. NPSA/2012/RRR001: www.nrls.npsa.nhs.uk

8 Jackson LD et al. (2008) Safe medication swallowing in dysphagia: a collaborative improvement project. *Healthcare Quarterly*. **11**: 110–116.

9 Adams D (1994) Administration of drugs through a jejunostomy tube. *British Journal of Intensive Care*. **4**: 10–17.

10 Thomson F et al. (2000) Enteral and parenteral nutrition. *Hospital Pharmacist*. **7**: 155–164.

11 Gilbar P (1999) A guide to drug administration in palliative care (review). *Journal of Pain and Symptom Management*. **17**: 197–207.

12 Royal Pharmaceutical Society of Great Britain (2010) Good Practice Guidance on the procurement and supply of pharmaceutical specials. Available from: www.rpharms.com

13 Schier JG et al. (2003) Fatality from administration of labetalol and crushed extended-release nifedipine. *Annals of Pharmacotherapy*. **37**: 1420–1423.

14 Cornish P (2005) "Avoid the crush": hazards of medication administration in patients with dysphagia or a feeding tube. *Canadian Medical Association Journal*. **172**: 871–872.

15 Wright DN et al. (2006) Consensus guideline on the medication management of adults with swallowing difficulties. *Guidelines* London Connect Medical.

16 Sanofi Aventis (2008) *Medical information. Data on file.*

17 NHS England (2013) Placement devices for nasogastric tube insertion DO NOT replace initial position checks. Patient Safety Alert. NHS/PSA/W/2013/001: www.england.nhs.uk/patientsafety

18 Phillips NM and Nay R (2008) A systematic review of nursing administration of medication via enteral tubes in adults. *Journal of Clinical Nursing*. **17**: 2257–2265.

19 Baxter K, Preston CL Stockley's Drug Interactions London: Pharmaceutical Press, www.medicinescomplete.com (accessed January 2014).

20 Schmidt LE and Dalhoff K (2002) Food-drug interactions. *Drugs*. **62**: 1481–1502.

21 Engle KK and Hannawa TE (1999) Techniques for administering oral medications to critical care patients receiving continuous enteral nutrition. *American Journal of Health System Pharmacy* **56**: 1441–1444.

22 Clark-Schmidt AL et al. (1990) Loss of carbamazepine suspension through nasogastric feeding tubes. *American Journal of Hospital Pharmacy*. **47**: 2034–2037.

23 Freeman KL and Trezevant MS (2009) Interaction between liquid protein solution and omeprazole suspension. *American Journal of Health System Pharmacy*. **66**: 1901–1902.

24 Garcia-Luna PP et al. (1997) Esophageal obstruction by solidification of the enteral feed: a complication to be prevented. *Intensive Care Medicine*. **23**: 790–792.

25 Chugai Pharma UK (2010) Summary of product characteristics for Antepsin suspension SPC. www.medicines.org.uk

26 Wohlt PD et al. (2009) Recommendations for the use of medications with continuous enteral nutrition. *American Journal of Health System Pharmacy*. **66**: 1458–1467.

27 Marcuard SP and Stegall KS (1990) Unclogging feeding tubes with pancreatic enzyme. *Journal of Parenteral Enteral Nutrition*. **14**: 198–200.

28 Nottingham City Hospital NHS Trust Pharmacy (1998) Administering drugs to patients by artifical enteral methods. Data on file.

29 Palliativedrugs.com (2003) July Newsletter. Available from: www.palliativedrugs.com

30 Smyth J (2010) *The NEWT guidelines for administration of medication to patients with enteral feeding tubes or swallowing difficulties* (2e). Pharmacy Department, North East Wales NHS Trust.

31 BNF for Children London: BMJ Group and Pharmaceutical Press. www.bnf.org (accessed January 2014).

Updated (minor change) September 2014

23: NEBULIZED DRUGS

Nebulizers are used in asthma and COPD for both acute exacerbations and long-term prophylaxis (see Bronchodilators, p.105).[1-3] Other uses include the pulmonary delivery of antimicrobial drugs for cystic fibrosis, bronchiectasis and AIDS-related pneumonia. Nebulizers are also used in palliative care (see below). The aim is to deliver a therapeutic dose of a drug as an aerosol in particles small enough to be inspired within 5–10min. A nebulizer is preferable to a hand-held metered dose inhaler (MDI) when:

- a large drug dose is needed
- co-ordinated breathing is difficult
- MDIs + a spacer are ineffective
- a drug is unavailable in an inhaler.

In these circumstances, by improving drug delivery, a nebulizer can result in better symptom relief.[4] However, nebulizers are noisy, more expensive and less convenient than an MDI; they are also ineffective in patients with shallow breathing, and in those unable to sit up to at least 45°, i.e. semi-upright or more. The higher doses administered can also increase the risk of undesirable effects and their use should be carefully monitored, to ensure ongoing efficacy and tolerability.

Commonly used nebulizers are:

Jet: the aerosol is generated by a flow of gas from, for example, an electrical compressor or an oxygen cylinder. At least 50% of the aerosol produced at the recommended driving gas flow should be particles small enough to inhale.

Ultrasonic: the aerosol is generated by ultrasonic vibrations of a piezo-electric crystal.

Aerosol output (the mass of particles in aerosol form produced/min) is not necessarily the same as drug output (the mass of drug produced/min as an aerosol). Ideally, the drug output of a nebulizer should be known for each of the different drugs given. Various factors affect the drug output and deposition:

- gas flow rate (generally air at 6–8L/min but oxygen if treating acute asthma)
- chamber design
- volume (commonly 2–2.5mL, up to 4mL)
- residual volume (commonly 0.5mL)
- physical properties of the drug in solution
- breathing pattern of the patient.

The choice of nebulizer can be crucial, particularly when trying to produce an aerosol small enough to deliver a drug to the alveoli. Services that provide nebulizers will generally offer information, education and support for patients and their families (Box A). Information should include:

- a description of the equipment and its use
- drugs used, doses and frequencies
- equipment maintenance/cleaning
- action to take if treatment becomes less effective
- action to take and emergency telephone number to use if equipment breaks down.

Patients should be instructed to take steady normal breaths (interspersed with occasional deep ones) and nebulization time should be less than 10min or 'to dryness'. Because there is always a residual volume, 'dryness' should be taken as 1min after spluttering starts. In general, whereas a mask can be used for bronchodilators, *a mouthpiece should be used for other drugs to limit environmental contamination and/or contact with the patient's eyes.* However, a mask may be preferable in patients who are acutely ill, fatigued or very young, regardless of the nature of the drug. Patients' nebulizer technique should be checked periodically.[5]

Nebulizers can also be used in patients with long-term tracheostomies or receiving non-invasive ventilation. Portable battery-operated nebulizers may be used in aircraft at the discretion of the cabin crew, but the airline must be notified in advance (also see Oxygen, p.129).

Box A Advice about using a nebulizer at home

To help your breathing, your doctor has prescribed a drug to be used with a nebulizer. The nebulizer converts the drug into a fine mist which you inhale.

The apparatus
Your nebulizer system consists of the following parts:

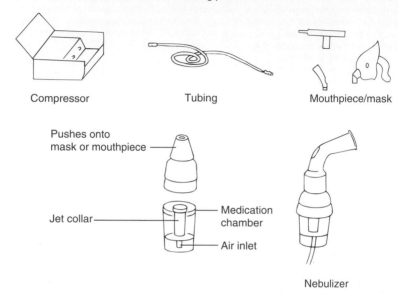

Compressor   Tubing   Mouthpiece/mask

Pushes onto mask or mouthpiece

Jet collar

Medication chamber

Air inlet

Nebulizer

The compressor is the portable pump which pumps air along the tubing into the nebulizer. The nebulizer is a small chamber for the liquid medicine, through which air is blown to make a mist.

The nebulizer has a screw-on top onto which the mask or mouthpiece is attached.

How to use your nebulizer
Place the medication in the nebulizer, replace the screw-on top and turn the compressor on. Inhale by mouthpiece or mask while breathing at a normal rate. Stop 1 minute after the nebulizer contents start spluttering or after a maximum of 10 minutes.

General advice
If you have a cough, the nebulizer may help you to expectorate, so have some tissues nearby.

You may wish to use the nebulizer before attempting an activity which makes you feel out of breath.

If the effects of the nebulizer wear off or you have any questions or concerns about it, please speak to your doctor or nurse.

Cleaning
Wash the mouthpiece/mask and nebulizer in warm water and detergent, then rinse and dry well. Ideally this should be done after every use, but *once a day as a minimum*. Attach the tube and run the nebulizer empty for a few moments after cleaning it to make sure the equipment is dry. Once a week, unplug and wipe the compressor and tubing with a damp cloth.

Table 1 Nebulized drugs and cancer-related cough or breathlessness[2,13]

Class of drug[a]	Indications	Scientific evidence	Comments
0.9% saline	Loosening of tenacious secretions	Limited[14]	Probably underused in this setting; may also help breathlessness
Mucolytic agents e.g. hypertonic saline	To thin viscous sputum	Enhances airway clearance in chronic lung diseases characterized by sputum retention	May result in copious liquid sputum which the patient may still not be able to cough up. May cause bronchospasm; begin with a low concentration, i.e. 3% and pretreat at risk patients with a bronchodilator[15]
Corticosteroids e.g. budesonide	Stridor, lymphangitis, radiation pneumonitis, cough after the insertion of a stent	None	Very limited clinical experience only; may not be more beneficial than use of inhaler or oral routes
Local anaesthetics e.g. lidocaine, bupivacaine	Cough, particularly if caused by lymphangitis carcinomatosa	Conflicting evidence for both breathlessness[16,17] and cough[6]	May cause bronchospasm; consider pretreating at risk patients with a bronchodilator.[6] Reduces gag reflex; risk of aspiration immediately after treatment
Opioids e.g. morphine, fentanyl	Breathlessness associated with diffuse lung disease	Despite supportive anecdotal evidence,[18] a systematic review indicates no advantage compared with 0.9% saline[19]	Not recommended; risk of bronchospasm
Bronchodilators e.g. salbutamol	Treatment of severe reversible airway obstruction	Extrapolated from patients with asthma and COPD	Try MDI + spacer first.[20,21] Use nebulizers only if trial of therapy shows real benefit
Furosemide	Breathlessness	Despite anecdotal reports of benefit (see p.63), the evidence does not support routine use[22]	Not recommended

a. a mask can be used for bronchodilators; a mouthpiece should be used for all other drugs to limit environmental contamination and/or contact with the patient's eyes. However, a mask may be unavoidable in those incapable of using a mouthpiece, e.g. when acutely ill, fatigued or very young.

Nebulizers in palliative care

Various drugs have been given by nebulizer to ease cough and breathlessness in advanced cancer (Table 1 and Table 2). However, apart from the use of bronchodilators for reversible airflow obstruction, there is often little evidence to support such use. Thus, some are not recommended by *PCF* for routine use; the remainder should be considered only when other avenues have failed, and reviewed after 2 days to check effectiveness (Table 1 and Table 2).

Table 2 Recommended uses of nebulized drugs in palliative care

Indication	Drug	Initial regimen	Dose titration	Comments
Tenacious secretions	Saline 0.9%	5mL p.r.n.	Up to q2h	
	Hypertonic saline 3%6 or 7%	4mL p.r.n. 4mL p.r.n.	Up to q.d.s. ⎱ Up to b.d. ⎰	Risk of bronchospasm
Reversible airway obstruction	Salbutamol	2.5mg q6h–q4h	Up to 5mg q4h	Risk of sensitivity to cardiac stimulant effects
Cough	*†Lidocaine 2% *†Bupivacaine 0.25%	5mL p.r.n. 5mL p.r.n.	Up to q.d.s. ⎱ Up to q.d.s. ⎰	Risk of bronchospasm Loss of gag reflex; nil by mouth for 1h after nebulization

When using **lidocaine** or **bupivacaine** for a dry cough (not recommended for breathlessness), in patients with asthma, consider pretreating with **salbutamol** because of the risk of initial bronchospasm.[6] After nebulized local anaesthetic, patients should be advised not to eat or drink for 1h because the reduced gag/cough reflex increases the risk of aspiration (also see Antitussives, p.142).

Because of lack of data, e.g. physico-chemical compatibility, and aerodynamic properties, manufacturers generally do not recommend mixing nebulizer solutions; thus most mixtures are off-label. However:[7–12]

- some ready-mixed combinations are commercially available, e.g. **salbutamol + ipratropium bromide** (generic and Combivent®)
- there are limited data indicating that 2-drug mixtures comprising one drug from any two of the classes below will be physically and/or chemically compatible (for all strengths):
  ▷ *β$_2$-adrenergic receptor agonists (β$_2$ agonists)*, **salbutamol** or **terbutaline** (Bricanyl®)
  ▷ *antimuscarinic*, **ipratropium bromide**
  ▷ *corticosteroids*, **budesonide** (Pulmicort®) or **fluticasone** (Flixotide®)
- solutions should be mixed immediately before use, using aseptic technique; if colour changes or cloudiness/precipitation occur, the mixture should be discarded
- if dilution is necessary, sterile 0.9% saline is generally best.

There is no information on 3-drug mixtures, and these cannot be recommended.

1 The Nebulizer Project Group of the British Thoracic Society Standards of Care Committee (1997) Current best practice for nebuliser treatment. *Thorax.* **52 (Suppl 2)**: s1–3.
2 European Respiratory Society (2001) Guidelines on the use of nebulizers. *European Respiratory Journal.* **18**: 228–242.
3 NICE (2010) Chronic obstructive pulmonary disease: management of chronic obstructive pulmonary disease in adults in primary and secondary care. *Clinical Guideline.* CG101. www.nice.org.uk
4 Tashkin DP et al. (2007) Comparing COPD treatment: nebulizer, metered dose inhaler, and concomitant therapy. *American Journal of Medicine.* **120**: 435–441.
5 Ari A and Restrepo RD (2012) Aerosol delivery device selection for spontaneously breathing patients: 2012. *Respiratory Care.* **57**: 613–626.
6 Slaton RM et al. (2013) Evidence for therapeutic uses of nebulized lidocaine in the treatment of intractable cough and asthma. *Annals of Pharmacotherapy.* **47**: 578–585.
7 UK Medicines Information (2013) Which commonly used nebuliser solutions are compatible? *Medicines Q&As.* 100.7: www.evidence.nhs.uk
8 Roberts G and Rossi S (1993) Compatibility of nebuliser solutions. *Australian Journal of Hospital Pharmacy.* **23**: 35–37.
9 McKenzie JE and Cruz-Rivera M (2004) Compatibility of budesonide inhalation suspension with four nebulizing solutions. *Annals of Pharmacotherapy.* **38**: 967–972.

10 Burchett DK *et al.* (2010) Mixing and compatibility guide for commonly used aerosolized medications. *American Journal of Health System Pharmacy.* **67**: 227–230.

11 Joseph JC (1997) Compatibility of nebulizer solution admixtures. *Annals of Pharmacotherapy.* **31**: 487–489.

12 Harriman A-M *et al.* (1996) Can we mix nebuliser solutions? Stability of drug admixtures in solutions for nebulisation. *Pharmacy in Practice.* Oct: 347–348.

13 Ahmedzai S and Davis C (1997) Nebulised drugs in palliative care. *Thorax.* **52 (Suppl 2)**: s75–s77.

14 Sutton PP *et al.* (1988) Use of nebulised saline and nebulised terbutaline as an adjunct to chest physiotherapy. *Thorax.* **43**: 57–60.

15 Pasteur MC *et al.* (2010) British Thoracic Society guideline for non-CF bronchiectasis. *Thorax.* **65 (Suppl 1)**: i1–58.

16 Winning A *et al.* (1988) Ventilation and breathlessness on maximal exercise in patients with interstitial lung disease after local anaesthetic aerosol inhalation. *Clinical Science.* **74**: 275–281.

17 Wilcock A *et al.* (1994) Safety and efficacy of nebulized lignocaine in patients with cancer and breathlessness. *Palliative Medicine.* **8**: 35–38.

18 Young IH *et al.* (1989) Effect of low dose nebulized morphine on exercise endurance in patients with chronic lung disease. *Thorax.* **44**: 387–390.

19 Jennings A *et al.* (2002) A systematic review of the use of opioids in the management of dyspnoea. *Thorax.* **57**: 939–944.

20 Congleton J and Muers MF (1995) The incidence of airflow obstruction in bronchial carcinoma, its relation to breathlessness, and response to bronchodilator therapy. *Respiratory Medicine.* **89**: 291–296.

21 Colacone A *et al.* (1993) A comparison of albuterol administered by metered dose inhaler (and holding chamber) or wet nebulizer in acute asthma. *Chest.* **104**: 835–841.

22 Newton PJ *et al.* (2008) Nebulized furosemide for the management of dyspnea: does the evidence support its use? *Journal of Pain and Symptom Management.* **36**: 424–441.

Updated March 2014

24: PROLONGATION OF THE QT INTERVAL IN PALLIATIVE CARE

The QT interval has attained greater clinical significance since it became apparent that various factors which prolong the QT interval, particularly drugs, predispose to a potentially fatal ventricular arrhythmia, *torsade de pointes*.

An accurate diagnosis of *torsade de pointes* is important because its management differs from other forms of ventricular tachycardia. Indeed, conventional drug treatments for ventricular tachycardia can exacerbate the underlying electrochemical derangement and perpetuate *torsade de pointes*.

Palliative care clinicians caring for patients with cardiac disease, or using **methadone**, need to be particularly aware of this phenomenon.

The QT interval lies on the electrocardiograph (ECG) between the beginning of the QRS complex (which marks the start of ventricular depolarization) and the end of the T wave (which marks the end of ventricular repolarization) (Figure 1).

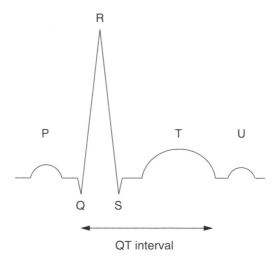

Figure 1 The QT interval.

The QT interval tends to be longer with slower heart rates. For comparative purposes, it is important to adjust ('correct') the observed QT interval to take account of this. The corrected value is designated QTc. Some ECG machines automatically calculate QTc, and this is a useful guide. However, automatic calculations can be inaccurate, particularly in the presence of atrial fibrillation, frequent ventricular ectopics, or a noisy trace. Thus, manual calculation of QTc is more accurate (Box A).[1] There are several ways of doing this, and local practice varies.[1,2]

Box A   Measuring the QT interval and calculating QTc[1]

ECG

A 12-lead ECG at 25mm/sec at 10mm/mV amplitude is generally adequate, taken after the patient has rested supine for about 5min.

Measure the QT interval together with the preceding RR interval in 3–5 heart beats from leads II and V5/V6.

Calculate the mean QT and RR interval from these 3–5 measurements.

Calculate QTc using one of the following formulas:
• Bazett's (exponential square root):

$$QTc = \frac{QT\,(sec)}{\sqrt{RR\,(sec)}}$$

• Fridericia's (exponential cube root):

$$QTc = \frac{QT\,(sec)}{\sqrt[3]{RR\,(sec)}}$$

Although Bazett's formula is the most widely used, Fridericia's may be more accurate at the extremes of heart rate.

Interpretation

QTc (msec)	Male	Female
Normal	<430	<450
Borderline	430–450	450–470
Abnormal	>450	>470

Note: These limits are to a certain extent arbitrary, and given a lack of international consensus, they vary between sources.

Obtain advice
Obtain cardiology advice if:
• the end of the T wave is difficult to determine, e.g. because of a U wave
• there is bundle branch block
• there is atrial fibrillation.

A prolonged QT interval is a pro-arrhythmic state associated with an increased risk of ventricular arrhythmia, particularly *torsade de pointes* (Figure 2); this is a form of polymorphic ventricular tachycardia of varying polarity which appears to wind around the baseline and hence its name. Short runs may cause palpitation or dizziness, longer ones syncope (generally without warning) or seizure-like activity; it can settle spontaneously within seconds or degenerate into fatal ventricular fibrillation.[3] Treatment includes cardioversion when haemodynamically compromised and **magnesium sulfate** IV (2g bolus followed by an infusion of 2-4mg/min).[3]

Additional premonitory ECG signs of *torsade de pointes* include T-U wave distortion (more exaggerated in a beat after a pause), T-wave alternans (marked alternate variation in size), new ventricular ectopics or couplets, and nonsustained polymorphic ventricular tachycardia initiated in the beat after a pause.[4]

The risk of *torsade de pointes* grows as the QT interval increases, particularly >500msec. A drug which leads to an increase in QTc interval of 20–60msec should also raise concern and, if by >60msec, serious concern about the risk of arrhythmia.[5]

Drugs prolong the QT interval mainly through potassium-channel blockade (particularly I_{Kr} 'rapid' subtype) by interfering with potassium currents in (enhanced) and out (reduced) of the cardiac myocytes, modifying their repolarization and prolonging the duration of the action

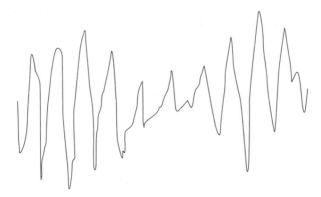

Figure 2 *Torsade de pointes.* Twisting complexes of ventricular tachycardia.

potential.[6] The resulting dispersion of intramural repolarization may promote triggered activity and re-entry, the electrophysiological substrate for *torsade de pointes*. Several drugs have been definitely linked with *torsade de pointes* (Box B). Concerns about safety have resulted in some drugs either having dose restrictions applied, e.g. **domperidone** (p.246), **citalopram/ escitalopram** (p.211), and **ondansetron** (p.251), or being withdrawn completely from the UK market, e.g. **astemizole, cisapride, sertindole, terfenadine, thioridazine.**

Box B Drugs available in the UK with a known risk of prolonged QT interval and *torsade de pointes*[a]

Anti-arrhythmic drugs	**Psychotropic drugs**
Amiodarone	Chlorpromazine
Disopyramide	Droperidol
Dronedarone	Haloperidol
Flecainide	Pimozide
Sotalol	Supiride
Antidepressant drugs	**Miscellaneous**
Citalopram	Anagrelide
Escitalopram	Arsenic trioxide
	Cocaine
Antimicrobial drugs	Domperidone
Levofloxacin	Methadone
Macrolides	Ondansetron
e.g. azithromycin, clarithromycin, erythromycin	Saquinavir
Moxifloxacin	Sevoflurane
Pentamidine	Toremifene
	Vandetanib
Antimalarial drugs	
Chloroquine	

a. for a full list, including those considered a possible or conditional risk, see www.azcert.org.

Apart from providing a list of drugs with a known risk of prolonged QT and *torsade de pointes*, the website www.azcert.org also identifies drugs considered 'possible risk' (insufficient evidence that authorized use causes arrhythmia) and 'conditional risk' (arrhythmia has occurred only under certain conditions, e.g. excessive dose, drug–drug interaction). The website also includes a list of drugs to be avoided by patients with congenital long QT syndrome.

The incidence of *torsade de pointes* is greatest with cardiac anti-arrhythmics, particularly those with class Ia or III activity. For some drugs, the risk becomes significant only with:[7,8]

- high doses
- IV administration
- a pharmacokinetic drug interaction (see Chapter 25, p.767)
- impaired metabolism:
  ▷ congenital, e.g. CYP2D6 poor metabolizers may be exposed to dangerously high plasma concentrations of risk-related drugs which are substrates for CYP2D6, even with normal doses e.g. **flecainide**
  ▷ acquired, e.g. hepatic or renal impairment.

The risk of drug-induced *torsade de pointes* is increased by the concurrent use of two or more drugs which prolong the QT interval, and is more likely to occur in the presence of other risk factors (Box C).[8] Some patients have a subclinical congenital long QT syndrome unmasked by a QT-prolonging drug.[3] Thus, the degree of prolongation of the QT interval is not only dose-related.

An additional contributory factor may be central sleep apnoea, which is associated with bradycardia and QT prolongation, and is reported to occur in 30% of patients on **methadone** maintenance.[9]

Box C   Main additional risk factors in drug-induced *torsade de pointes*

Female gender	Cardiac disease, e.g.:
Congenital long QT syndrome	• bradycardia <50 beats/min
Baseline prolonged QT interval	• left ventricular hypertrophy
Electrolyte imbalance:	• heart failure
• hypokalaemia	• recent conversion from atrial fibrillation
• hypomagnesaemia	• ventricular arrhychmia

Implications for practice

General recommendations to guide practice are given in Box D.[2]

Box D   A clinical approach to drug-induced QT prolongation

When using drugs known to prolong the QT interval, a prescriber needs to:

- understand the pharmacology of the drug, in particular factors which may lead to accumulation, e.g. drug–drug interaction, impaired elimination
- whenever possible, avoid the concurrent use of more than one drug which prolongs the QT interval
- use the lowest effective dose of the QT-prolonging drug
- evaluate and balance the potential benefit against the potential risk, taking into account the specific circumstances of the patient and the presence of other risk factors (see Box C), e.g.:
  ▷ in patients with a known (pre-existing) prolonged QT interval, avoid the use of all QT-prolonging drugs except under specialist guidance (see Box B)
  ▷ in patients with cardiac disease, drugs which prolong the QT interval should generally be avoided unless no suitable alternative exists
  ▷ in patients with cardiac disease, if a cardiac anti-arrhythmic known to prolong the QT interval is prescribed, consider undertaking an ECG before and after starting the drug, and regular monitoring of plasma potassium and magnesium concentrations to ensure these remain well within their normal ranges
  ▷ in patients without cardiac disease but with other risk factors, consider similar monitoring to above when using a QT-prolonging drug
  ▷ for advice about patients at the end of life and also methadone, see text

continued

Box D Continued

- explain to the patient (and family) the risk involved and the reasons for using the drug in question, to allow an informed decision to be made
- report instances of drug-related QT prolongation to the MHRA through the yellow card scheme at www.mhra.gov.uk/index.htm
- consider *torsade de pointes* as a possible cause of palpitations, syncope or seizure-like activity.

Palliative care patients in general may be at higher risk of a prolonged QT interval given the high prevalence of multiple drug use and metabolic disturbance. Polypharmacy is the norm in palliative care,[10] and using more than one drug concurrently increases the risk of drug interactions.[11–13] However, of 300 patients referred to a specialist palliative care unit who were not imminently dying, although 48 (16%) had a prolonged QT interval, only 2 (0.7%) had a severely prolonged uncorrected QT interval of >500msec (Figure 3).[5,14] Both patients had ischaemic heart disease and, if being considered for a QT-prolonging drug such as **methadone**, would have been identified by following the guidance to undertake an ECG in patients with one or more risk factors.

Nonetheless, a commonsense approach should prevail and the benefit of certain drugs used in the last days of life, e.g. **haloperidol**, is likely to far outweigh any risk, and an ECG is not required.[15]

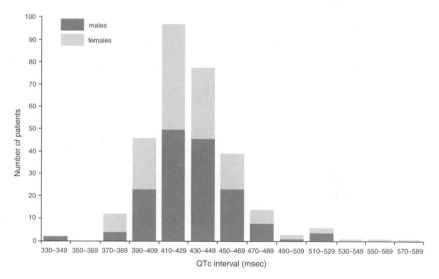

Figure 3 Distribution of the QT interval in 300 palliative care patients.[14]

Methadone

There have been longstanding concerns relating to the occurrence of serious adverse events with **methadone**, including deaths, from apparent unintentional overdose, particularly in the first 2 weeks of administration. As the use of **methadone** has increased, for both **methadone** maintenance and chronic pain, so has the number of deaths, disproportionately more than with other opioids, resulting in the US FDA issuing an alert to health professionals in 2006.[9] A major factor is considered to be a lack of knowledge among clinicians about the need to carefully monitor the use of **methadone**, particularly during the first 2–4 weeks (see Methadone, p.433). Although many of these deaths are likely to be a result of respiratory depression, *torsade de pointes* may be a contributing factor (Box E).

Box E   Methadone, prolonged QT and *torsade de pointes*

The association between methadone and prolonged QT was first reported in 1973.[16] The link with *torsade de pointes* was made in 2002 when it was described in 17 patients receiving a median dose of methadone of 330mg/day PO; all had QT > 500msec and most had other risk factors.[17]

Subsequently, methadone has been found to block ion channels associated with QT prolongation, and to increase the QT interval and the risk of *torsade de pointes* generally in a dose-dependent manner.[18]

However, although some found QTc unaltered by doses < 100mg/24h PO,[19] QTc > 500msec and *torsade de pointes* have been reported with daily doses as low as 30–40mg PO.[20] A review of 21 patients on methadone with confirmed prolonged QT and *torsade de pointes* found generally higher daily doses (median 130mg, range 40–700mg). However, multiple risk factors were common including female gender, heart disease, hypokalaemia, hypomagnesaemia, drug interaction, multiple QT-prolonging drugs, hepatic impairment, sinus bradycardia and cocaine misuse.[21] The frequent co-existence of other risk factors makes it difficult to quantify the risk from methadone alone and may explain the inconsistent dose-relationship seen between methadone and QT prolongation.

Although slight prolongation of the QT interval by methadone appears to be common, the clinical significance of this is unclear. A marked increase in QTc to > 500msec is seen in a small proportion of patients given methadone (generally about ≤ 5%, but 16% in one report).[18,20–24] The incidence of *torsade de pointes* and of *fatal torsade de pointes* is hard to quantify, but both are likely to be rare, e.g.:

- of the 400 adverse drug events for methadone reported to the MHRA between 1964 and 2009, 13 (3 fatal) were classified as cardiac; these included only one report each of *torsade de pointes* or ventricular fibrillation, both non-fatal; the deaths occurred after cardiopulmonary arrest or an unspecified fatal arrhythmia[25]
- the incidence of *non-fatal torsade de pointes* is estimated at 3 episodes/day per 1 million patients receiving methadone maintenance[26]
- the maximum mortality attributable to prolonged QT has been estimated to be 6 per 10,000 patient-years, based on the examination of deaths of patients receiving methadone maintenance therapy in Norway.[27]

IV methadone has been considered high-risk. In cancer patients receiving median IV doses of 430mg/day (range 2.4mg–2.4g):[28]

- two patients with prolonged QT died suddenly (although a definite link with *torsade de pointes* was not proven)
- QTc > 500msec occurred in a patient receiving as little as 10mg/day.

However, the formulation of methadone contained the QT-prolonging preservative chlorbutanol; this works synergistically with methadone to prolong the QT interval. Note: None of the methadone injections marketed in the UK contain chlorbutanol.

Guidelines to minimize the risk of cardiac toxicity with **methadone** are based largely on expert opinion, and recommendations vary.[15,18] Although some suggest routine ECG screening, this is debatable.[29,30] However, most advise an ECG in the presence of other risk factors for QT interval prolongation.[15,18] For example, since 2006, the SPC for **methadone** has recommended that it is used with caution in patients with any of the following risk factors for QT prolongation:

- a history of cardiac conduction abnormalities
- advanced heart disease or ischemic heart disease
- liver disease
- a family history of sudden death
- electrolyte abnormalities
- concurrent treatment with drugs which:
  - ▷ may cause electrolyte abnormalities
  - ▷ have a potential to prolong QT
  - ▷ inhibit CYP3A4 (see Chapter 25, p.767).

ECG monitoring is recommended in such patients before starting **methadone** and repeated when the dose is stabilized. Some guidelines suggest an annual ECG thereafter.[18] ECG monitoring is also recommended in patients without recognized risk factors for QT prolongation, before dose titration above 100mg/day PO and 1 week after such up-titration (an arbitrary dose, based on expert opinion; others suggest 120mg/day).[18] Monitoring of serum electrolytes, e.g. potassium, magnesium, is generally recommended in patients taking diuretics or at risk of hypokalaemia, e.g. because of vomiting or diarrhoea.

Other guidelines also recommend an ECG if other risk factors or cardiac symptoms (e.g. palpitation, dizziness, fainting spells, seizures) develop during treatment and highlight the importance of educating patients taking **methadone** to avoid where possible the use of other drugs which can prolong QT or inhibit **methadone** metabolism, and to urgently report cardiac symptoms.[31]

Guidance specific for palliative care is limited. In the USA, an expert group has developed a guideline for the use of *parenteral* **methadone** for chronic pain and in the palliative/hospice setting. Partly because of the increased risk presented by the preservative **chlorbutanol** (Box E), an ECG is recommended:

- before starting IV therapy and after 1 and 4 days of treatment
- when the dose is significantly increased
- if an additional risk factor for QT prolongation develops.[32]

Monitoring serum electrolytes in high risk patients and discussing the potential risks of prolonged QT and *torsade de pointes* with the patient and carers are also recommended. However, consideration of burden vs. benefit is paramount and, in those with life-limiting illness, the potential benefit of controlling otherwise refractory pain may far outweigh the risks, even when monitoring for arrhythmia is impractical.[32] A commonsense approach should prevail: ECG monitoring is generally irrelevant in the last days of life.[15]

On the other hand, for a patient with a reasonable prognosis, it may be appropriate to identify any risk factors for QT prolongation and consider ECG monitoring as recommended in the SPC. Nonetheless, research is required to establish the magnitude of the risk of *torsade de pointes* with **methadone** and the overall value of adopting such an approach in the palliative care setting.

If the baseline QT is prolonged, an alternative opioid should be considered. Further, if the QT interval increases to > 500msec when on **methadone**, generally it should be discontinued and an alternative used, e.g. SL **buprenorphine**. However, there has been a report of the successful use of parenteral **methadone** for analgesia in a patient with a prolonged QT interval.[33] Implantable cardioverter-defibrillators have also been used in addicts with *torsade de pointes* who needed to remain on **methadone**.[34]

Generally, **methadone** is available only as a racemic mixture. **S-methadone** is a more potent blocker of the potassium channels in the cardiac myocytes than **R-methadone**. CYP2B6 also displays stereoselectivity for the metabolism of **S-methadone**, and initial findings suggest that CYP2B6 poor metabolizers (found in about 6% of Caucasians and African-Americans) have higher levels of **S-methadone** and may thus be at greater risk of prolonged QTc.[35] The use of **R-methadone** may thus be safer in this respect but, at present, it is available only in Germany.[36,37]

1   Goldenberg I et al. (2006) QT interval: how to measure it and what is "normal". *Journal of Cardiovascular Electrophysiology.* 17: 333–336.

2   Al-Khatib SM et al. (2003) What clinicians should know about the QT interval. *Journal of the American Medical Association.* 289: 2120–2127.

3   Gupta A et al. (2007) Current concepts in the mechanisms and management of drug-induced QT prolongation and torsade de pointes. *American Heart Journal.* 153: 891–899.

4   Drew BJ et al. (2010) Prevention of torsade de pointes in hospital settings: a scientific statement from the American Heart Association and the American College of Cardiology Foundation. *Circulation.* 121: 1047–1060.

5   Committee for Proprietary Medicinal Products (1996) Points to consider: the assessment of the potential for QT interval prolongation by non-cardiovascular medicinal products. *European Agency for the Evaluation of Medicinal Products (EMEA).* CPMP/986/96.

6   Haverkamp W et al. (2000) The potential for QT prolongation and proarrhythmia by non-antiarrhythmic drugs: clinical and regulatory implications. Report on a policy conference of the European Society of Cardiology. *European Heart Journal.* 21: 1216–1231.

7   Idle JR (2000) The heart of psychotropic drug therapy. *Lancet.* 355: 1824–1825.

8   Zipes DP et al. (2006) ACC/AHA/ESC 2006 guidelines for management of patients with ventricular arrhythmias and the prevention of sudden cardiac death: a report of the American College of Cardiology/American Heart Association Task Force and the European Society of Cardiology Committee for Practice Guidelines (Writing Committee to Develop

guidelines for management of patients with ventricular arrhythmias and the prevention of sudden cardiac death) developed in collaboration with the European Heart Rhythm Association and the Heart Rhythm Society. *Europace*. **8**: 746–837.

9 Andrews CM et al. (2009) Methadone-induced mortality in the treatment of chronic pain: role of QT prolongation. *Cardiology Journal*. **16**: 210–217.

10 Twycross RG et al. (1994) Monitoring drug use in palliative care. *Palliative Medicine*. **8**: 137–143.

11 Bernard SA and Bruera E (2000) Drug interactions in palliative care. *Journal of Clinical Oncology*. **18**: 1780–1799.

12 Davies SJ et al. (2004) Potential for drug interactions involving cytochromes P450 2D6 and 3A4 on general adult psychiatric and functional elderly psychiatric wards. *British Journal of Clinical Pharmacology*. **57**: 464–472.

13 Wilcock A et al. (2005) Potential for drug interactions involving cytochrome P450 in patients attending palliative day care centres: a multicentre audit. *British Journal of Clinical Pharmacology*. **60**: 326–329.

14 Walker G et al. (2003) Prolongation of the QT interval in palliative care patients. *Journal of Pain and Symptom Management*. **26**: 855–859.

15 Wilcock A and Beattie JM (2009) Prolonged QT interval and methadone: implications for palliative care. *Current Opinion in Supportive and Palliative Care*. **3**: 252–257.

16 Stimmel B et al. (1973) Electrocardiographic changes in heroin, methadone and multiple drug abuse: a postulated mechanism of sudden death in narcotic addicts. *Proceedings of the National Conference on Methadone Treatment*. **1**: 706–710.

17 Krantz MJ et al. (2002) Torsade de pointes associated with very-high-dose methadone. *Annals of Internal Medicine*. **137**: 501–504.

18 Martin JA et al. (2011) QT interval screening in methadone maintenance treatment: report of a SAMHSA expert panel. *Journal of Addictive Diseases*. **30**: 283–306.

19 Stallvik M et al. (2013) Corrected QT interval during treatment with methadone and buprenorphine–relation to doses and serum concentrations. *Drug and Alcohol Dependence*. **129**: 88–93.

20 Stringer J et al. (2009) Methadone-associated QT interval prolongation and torsades de pointes. *American Journal of Health System Pharmacy*. **66**: 825–833.

21 Vieweg WV et al. (2013) Methadone, QTc interval prolongation and torsade de pointes: Case reports offer the best understanding of this problem. *Therapeutic Advances in Psychopharmacology*. **3**: 219–232.

22 Reddy S et al. (2010) The effect of oral methadone on the QTc interval in advanced cancer patients: a prospective pilot study. *Journal of Palliative Medicine*. **13**: 33–38.

23 Price LC et al. (2014) Methadone for Pain and the Risk of Adverse Cardiac Outcomes. *Journal of Pain and Symptom Management* (in press).

24 Huh B and Park CH (2010) Retrospective analysis of low-dose methadone and QTc prolongation in chronic pain patients. *Korean Journal Anesthesiology*. **58**: 338–343.

25 MHRA (2009) Personal communication.

26 Hanon S et al. (2010) Ventricular arrhythmias in patients treated with methadone for opioid dependence. *Journal of Interventional Cardiac Electrophysiology*. **28**: 19–22.

27 Anchersen K et al. (2009) Prevalence and clinical relevance of corrected QT interval prolongation during methadone and buprenorphine treatment: a mortality assessment study. *Addiction*. **104**: 993–999.

28 Kornick CA et al. (2003) QTc interval prolongation associated with intravenous methadone. *Pain*. **105**: 499–506.

29 Haigney MC (2011) First, do no harm: QT interval screening in methadone maintenance treatment. *Journal of Addictive Diseases*. **30**: 309–312.

30 Bart G (2011) CSAT's QT interval screening in methadone report: outrageous fortune or sea of troubles? *Journal of Addictive Diseases*. **30**: 313–317.

31 Office of Alcoholism and Substance Abuse Services (2009 March) Medical advisory panel position on QTc interval screening in methadone treatment. Available from: http://www.oasas.state.ny.us/Admed/cme/QTCinterval.cfm

32 Shaiova L et al. (2008) Consensus guideline on parenteral methadone use in pain and palliative care. *Palliative and Supportive Care*. **6**: 165–176.

33 Sekine R et al. (2007) The successful use of parenteral methadone in a patient with a prolonged QTc interval. *Journal of Pain and Symptom Management*. **34**: 566–569.

34 Patel AM et al. (2008) Role of implantable cardioverter-defibrillators in patients with methadone-induced long QT syndrome. *American Journal of Cardiology*. **101**: 209–211.

35 Eap CB et al. (2007) Stereoselective block of hERG channel by (S)-methadone and QT interval prolongation in CYP2B6 slow metabolizers. *Clin Pharmacol Ther*. **81**: 719–728.

36 Gaertner J et al. (2008) Methadone: a closer look at the controversy. *Journal of Pain and Symptom Management*. **36**: e4–7.

37 Ansermot N et al. (2010) Substitution of (R,S)-methadone by (R)-methadone: Impact on QTc interval. *Archives of Internal Medicine*. **170**: 529–536.

Updated (minor change) September 2014

25: VARIABILITY IN RESPONSE TO DRUGS

Variability in response to drugs

There is great inter-individual variability in the way people respond to a drug (Box A). For example, age-related decreases in liver mass, liver enzyme activity and hepatic blood flow result in a decrease in the overall metabolic capacity of the liver. This is of particular importance in relation to drugs which have a high 'hepatic extraction ratio', e.g. **amitriptyline, fentanyl, lidocaine, propranolol, verapamil**. The risk of toxicity from these drugs will be significantly higher in the elderly (also see Chapter 14, p.650). Similarly, an age-related decline in renal function can reduce the excretion of active drugs and metabolites, e.g. morphine-6-glucuronide and morphine-3-glucuronide, increasing the risk of toxicity (see Chapter 14, p.654).

Genetic variations, particularly those associated with cytochrome P450 (CYP450), are also important in either reducing or increasing the rate of drug metabolism (see below) Examples of how these manifest include:
- reduced or no response because of
  ▷ increased metabolism of an active drug to an inactive metabolite
  ▷ the failure to convert a pro-drug to its active form
- increased toxicity because of
  ▷ failure to metabolize an active drug to inactive metabolite(s)
  ▷ more rapid conversion to the active form or to a metabolite which is more active than the parent drug.

Other genetic variations, such as genes coding for receptors or drug transporters can also influence overall response, e.g. μ-opioid receptor or P-glycoprotein and opioids.

Drug–drug or drug–food interactions through induction or inhibition of CYP450 activity can cause similar manifestations to those resulting from genetic variation.

Variability in response to opioids

Many factors contribute to the inter-individual variation in response to opioids.[1–4]

μ-Opioid receptor

This is the key receptor mediating opioid analgesia.[5] Genetic variation in the μ-opioid receptor gene has been associated with variation in opioid response in acute post-operative pain,[6–8] chronic non-cancer pain,[9,10] and cancer pain.[11,12] However, meta-analysis of opioid pain studies showed no overall association with pain and only weak associations with **morphine** dose or undesirable effects.[13]

P-glycoprotein

The membrane-bound drug transporter P-glycoprotein influences drug absorption and drug excretion.[14,15] It limits the uptake of compounds from the GI tract, regulates the transfer of various drugs across the blood–brain barrier,[16] and influences drug excretion by the liver and kidneys. It is encoded by the ATP-binding cassette subfamily B member 1 (ABCB1) gene.

Box A Common factors affecting response to drugs

Adherence
Whether drug regimen adhered to or not

Genetic variation/polymorphism
Sequence variation including single nucleotide polymorphisms, gene deletions, gene duplications resulting in altered protein function, e.g. receptors, enzymes, drug transporters

Pharmacokinetics
Absorption
Distribution
Metabolism
Drug–drug interactions
Excretion

Pharmacodynamics
Receptor–drug interaction and effect
Drug–drug interactions
Decreased/increased receptor affinity due to concurrent disease state

Physiological factors
Gender
Age
Ethnicity
Hormonal changes
Circadian and seasonal factors

Environmental factors
Diet
Environmental toxins
Alcohol and recreational drugs
Smoking

Potential specific associations/concomitant disease
Diabetes mellitus
Gut microbiology
Hepatic cirrhosis
Malabsorption
Obesity

P-glycoprotein modulation of opioid CNS concentrations varies substantially between opioids, with **morphine, fentanyl**, and **methadone** being among those most affected.[17,18] In animals, removal ('knockout' mice) or inhibition (by **ciclosporin**) of P-glycoprotein activity enhances absorption and increases CNS concentrations of **fentanyl** and **morphine**, resulting in prolonged analgesia.[19] Thus, inhibitors of P-glycoprotein (e.g. **ciclosporin, clarithromycin, erythromycin, itraconazole, ketoconazole, quinidine, verapamil**) could increase CNS effects of opioids.

Variation in ABCB1 has been associated with increased pain relief with **morphine** in cancer pain[11] and decreased opioid requirements in mixed chronic pain.[10] Studies have shown conflicting results in relation to opioid-induced nausea and vomiting and other undesirable effects.[20–22]

Catechol-O-methyltransferase

Catechol-O-methyltransferase (COMT) is an enzyme which has a significant impact on the metabolism of several important neurotransmitters: dopamine, adrenaline (epinephrine) and noradrenaline (norepinephrine). The COMT gene is polymorphic, and < 25% of Caucasians have low activity variants.

One common variant in which the amino acid valine is substituted for methionine results in a 3–4 times decrease in COMT activity. It has been associated with increased pain sensitivity and higher μ-opioid system activation in experimental pain,[23,24] and increased **morphine** dose requirements in cancer patients.[25] Other variants of the COMT gene are associated with increased undesirable opioid effects, e.g. nausea and vomiting.[20,26,27]

Hepatic metabolism

Opioid metabolism takes place primarily in the liver. Opioids are metabolized via two main pathways, cytochrome P450 (CYP450) and UDP-glycosyltransferase (UGT; Table 1). Two phases of metabolism are generally described: phase 1 metabolism (modification reactions) and phase 2 metabolism (conjugation reactions).

The most important phase 1 reaction is oxidation, catalysed by the CYP450. The most important phase 2 reaction is glucuronidation, catalysed by the enzyme uridine diphosphate glucuronosyltransferase (UGT). Glucuronidation produces molecules which are highly hydrophilic and thus easily excreted by the kidneys.[28] Drug–drug interactions can occur from changes in CYP450 or UGT activity, although the latter are less well documented.

Table 1 Major opioid enzyme pathways

Drug	Pathway[a]			
	CYP2D6	CYP3A4/5	CYP2B6	UGT
Alfentanil		++		
Buprenorphine		++		+
Codeine	++			+
Dihydrocodeine	+			+
Fentanyl		++		
Hydrocodone	+			
Hydromorphone				++
Methadone		++	+	
Morphine				++
Oxycodone	+	+		
Oxymorphone		+		+
Sufentanil		++		
Tapentadol				++
Tramadol	++	++		

a. ++ for CYP pathways may result in clinically important drug–drug interactions (see Table 8).

Genetic polymorphism in cytochrome P450 (CYP450)

About 75% of all drugs are metabolized partly or completely by cytochrome P450 (Box B). Thus, variation in activity of the cytochrome P450 system can have a major impact on drug action.

Some 20–25% of drugs are affected by genetic variants of drug-metabolizing enzymes.[31] The bulk of the population will manifest a normal distribution in terms of the rate of drug metabolism, with activity ranging from well below-average to well above-average, but generally lumped together as extensive metabolizers (EM).[32] In addition, there are discrete genetic populations of individuals who fall beyond the ends of the spectrum. These are designated poor (PM) and ultra-rapid metabolizers (URM). More recently, intermediate metabolizers have been identified for some enzymes (Table 2).[29]

As a general rule, an URM may need a higher dose to obtain a therapeutic effect, and a PM a lower dose to prevent increased undesirable effects (Table 3).[31] Exceptions are 'pro-drugs' where metabolites are mainly responsible for the effect of the drug (see below). The effects of such genetic variations can be further modified by the co-administration of the relevant CYP450 inhibitor or inducer.

Of particular note is **codeine**, for which most of its analgesic effect results from partial conversion to **morphine** by O-demethylation catalysed by CYP2D6 (see p.348).[37,38] Compared with the general population (EM), a PM produces little or no **morphine** from **codeine**, and obtains little or no pain relief. On the other hand, undesirable effects are comparable in both categories.[39,40] At the other extreme, URM produce more **morphine**; this can lead to life-threatening opioid toxicity which, rarely, has been fatal in children.[41–44] Genetic variation involving CYP2D6 is also important in relation to **tramadol** (p.352) for which the (+) O-desmethyltramadol metabolite is responsible for the opioid analgesic effect. A PM produces little or none and thus obtains little or no benefit; conversely, an URM produces higher levels with a potential to cause opioid toxicity (see p.352).

Box B Cytochrome P450 (CYP450)[29,30]

CYP450 is a super-family of numerous enzymic proteins responsible for the oxidative metabolism of many drugs and some endogenous substances (e.g. fatty acids, eicosanoids, steroids, bile acids).

The root symbol used in naming the individual enzymes is CYP, followed by:
- a number designating the enzyme family (18 in humans)
- a capital letter designating the subfamily (44 in humans)
- a number designating the individual enzyme.

CYP450 enzymes exist in virtually all tissues, but their highest concentration is in the liver.

The enzymes concerned with drug metabolism are mostly CYP1–CYP3; these account for about 70% of the total CYP450 content of the liver.

The most important enzyme is CYP3A4, followed by CYP2D6 and CYP2C9

The presence of CYP3A4 in the wall of the GI tract is important; it probably acts in conjunction with P-glycoprotein, and together determine the extent of the intestinal metabolism of CYP3A4 substrates.

Table 2 Metabolizer status[33]

Category	Description	Possible impact
Poor (PM) *or* slow	Lacks functional enzyme (deletion of gene or non-functional variant)	Increased toxicity due to slower drug metabolism (e.g. haloperidol) *or* Therapeutic failure due to poor metabolism of a pro-drug to its active form (e.g. codeine)
Intermediate	Has two decreased-function enzymes or one decreased, one non-functional	Comparable to slow metabolizer but less marked
Extensive (EM) *or* rapid	Has at least one fully-functional enzyme	This is the norm
Ultra-rapid (URM)	Increased enzyme activity (duplication of gene or other mutation); relatively rare	Therapeutic failure due to faster drug metabolism *or* Increased toxicity due to faster conversion of parent drug to more active metabolite (e.g. tramadol) *or* pro-drug to active form (e.g. codeine)

Polymorphism in CYP3A4/5 may be of less clinical significance when considering opioid response.[45] Nonetheless, CYP3A4 activity varies up to 10 times and could be partly responsible for different dose requirements.[46] Opioids potentially affected are the fentanils, **methadone**, **oxycodone** and, to a lesser extent, **buprenorphine**.

Although genetic variation can result in serious consequences, pharmacogenetic testing is not routine, partly because it is not cost-effective, e.g. **warfarin** dosing.[47,48] However, in oncology, testing will determine if an individual is likely to respond to a specific drug, e.g. **cetuximab** (colorectal cancer), **trastuzumab** (breast cancer), and **dasatinib** (acute lymphoblastic leukaemia).

Table 3 Genetic polymorphism and PM/URM status[a,28,29,34–36]

Pathway	A selection of affected drugs	Population affected
CYP2D6 (debrisoquine hydroxylase)	β-Blockers (metoprolol)[b] Codeine[c] Tramadol[c] Oxycodone Debrisoquine Flecainide Tamoxifen[c] Antipsychotics (phenothiazines, haloperidol, risperidone) SSRIs (some, e.g. paroxetine) TCAs (imipramine, nortriptyline)[d]	Africans 0–34% Caucasians 5–10% Asians ≤ 1%
CYP2C9	NSAIDs Sulfonylureas (glipizide, tolbutamide) Phenytoin Warfarin	Caucasians 35% Asian/African < 1%
CYP2C19	Diazepam PPIs Clopidogrel[c] Antidepressants (imipramine, sertraline)	Asians 10–35% Africans 15% Caucasians 2–5%

a. there is roughly a similar number of URM as PM
b. 70% reduction recommended in PM; note also that co-administration with paroxetine (2D6 inhibitor) increases plasma concentrations four times
c. enzyme conversion produces active or more active metabolite
d. TCAs most likely to need a lower dose.

CYP450 drug–drug interactions

Pharmacokinetic drug–drug interactions mediated through increased or decreased activity of CYP450 enzymes are common, but the resultant clinical impact is difficult to predict.[29,49–50] Some drugs (inducers) increase the activity of specific CYP450 enzymes and others (inhibitors) decrease enzyme activity (see Table 8, p.775).

When CYP450 inhibitors or inducers are co-administered with drugs which are already affected by genetic polymorphisms they will either augment or mitigate the clinical effects of the genetic variation.

Induction

Onset and offset of enzyme induction is gradual, possibly 2–3 weeks, because:
- onset depends on drug-induced synthesis of new enzyme
- offset depends on elimination of the enzyme-inducing drug and the decay of the increased enzyme stores.

Induction of the rate of drug biotransformation generally leads to a decrease in the parent drug plasma concentration, and thus a *decreased effect*. However, if the substrate drug is an inactive pro-drug or metabolism produces a more active metabolite, induction will result in an *increased effect* and possible toxicity.

The impact of enzyme induction depends on the relative importance of the induced pathway to the substrate's metabolism, whether active metabolites are present, and on the concentration (dose) of the inducer. Sequential dose adjustments, either up or down, may be necessary to maintain the desired clinical effect of the affected drug;[29] converse dose adjustments may be required if the inducer is discontinued, e.g. **methadone** toxicity has occurred following discontinuation of **carbamazepine**, an inducer.[51]

Some anti-epileptics (e.g. **carbamazepine, phenobarbital, phenytoin**) and some other drugs (e.g. **dexamethasone, griseofulvin, rifampicin**) induce members of the CYP3A subfamily (Table 4). **Rifampicin** is the most potent clinically used inducer of cytochrome CYP3A. Some oestrogens are metabolized by CYP3A4/5, and induction by **rifampicin** (or another enzyme inducer) can cause oral contraceptive failure.

Table 4 Examples of drug interactions based on enzyme induction of CYP3A4/5

Substrate	Inducers	Outcome
Carbamazepine	Phenytoin	Metabolism ↑, effect ↓
Methadone	Carbamazepine, phenobarbital, phenytoin, rifampicin, St John's wort	Metabolism ↑, effect ↓ (possible recurrence of pain ± withdrawal symptoms)[52]
Midazolam	Carbamazepine, phenytoin	Metabolism ↑, effect ↓[53]
Phenytoin	Rifampicin	Metabolism ↑, halflife halved, effect ↓[54]
Protease inhibitors (for HIV)	St John's wort	Metabolism ↑, treatment failure[55–57]

Inhibition

Inhibition of drug biotransformation begins *within a few hours* of the administration of the inhibitor drug, leading to an increase in the plasma concentration and effect of the substrate drug, and increased toxicity, *except pro-drugs which will have a corresponding reduced effect*, e.g. **clopidogrel**. Table 5 gives examples of altered drug effects resulting from enzyme inhibition.

Table 5 Examples of drug interactions based on enzyme inhibition

Substrate	Inhibitors	Outcome
Codeine	Quinidine (not UK) (CYP2D6)	Biotransformation to morphine ↓, analgesic effect ↓[58]
Clopidogrel	PPIs (CYP2C19)	Biotransformation to active metabolite ↓, antithrombotic effect ↓[59–62]
Diazepam	Cimetidine (CYP3A4/5)	Metabolism ↓, effect ↑[63]
Lovastatin, (not UK) simvastatin	Clarithromycin, erythromycin (CYP3A4/5)	Metabolism ↓, risk of undesirable effects ↑ (e.g. raised CK plasma concentration, muscle pain, rhabdomyolysis)
Theophylline	Ciprofloxacin (CYP1A2)	Metabolism ↓ (18–113%), effect ↑[64]
TCAs	SSRIs (multiple CYP)	Metabolism ↓ (plasma concentrations ↑ 50–350%), effect ↑[65–67]
Warfarin	Fluvoxamine (CYP3A4/5)	Metabolism ↓ (plasma concentration ↑ 65%), effect ↑[68]

The mechanism of enzymatic inhibition is either reversible or irreversible. In reversible inhibition, the inhibitor drug (e.g. **cimetidine**, macrolide antibacterials) binds to the P450 enzyme and prevents the metabolism of the substrate drug.[69,70] The extent of inhibition of one drug by another depends on their relative affinities for the P450 enzyme, and the respective doses. In irreversible inhibition, the enzyme is destroyed or inactivated by the inhibitor drug or its metabolites (e.g. **chloramphenicol, spironolactone**).

CYP450 drug–drug interactions in palliative care

It can be challenging to determine the likelihood of drug–drug interactions in practice. Many patients receiving palliative care are elderly and have several chronic conditions, resulting in the use of numerous drugs, typically 7–8 (range 1–20).[71,72] This polypharmacy increases the likelihood of drug interactions involving CYP450, with possibly 15–20% of patients receiving a combination likely to produce a clinically relevant CYP-mediated interaction (Table 6).[71,72]

Table 6 Common drug combinations likely to produce clinically important CYP-mediated interactons in palliative care patients[71,72]

Drug combination	Likely outcome of the interaction[a]
Benzodiazepines[b]+ CYP3A4 inhibitor e.g. diazepam + itraconazole	Diazepam ↑
Benzodiazepines[b]+ CYP3A4 inducer e.g. diazepam + carbamazepine	Diazepam ↓
Corticosteroids + CYP3A4 inhibitor e.g. dexamathasone + clarithromycin	Dexamethasone ↑
Corticosteroids + CYP3A4 inducer e.g. dexamathasone + phenytoin	Dexamethasone ↓
Diazepam + omeprazole[c]	Diazepam ↑
Opioids[b] + CYP3A4 inhibitor e.g. oxycodone + fluconazole	Oxycodone ↑
Opioids[b] + CYP3A4 inducer e.g. fentanyl + carbamazepine	Fentanyl ↓

a. ↑ = drug effect increased; ↓ = effect decreased
b. which are full or part substrates of CYP3A4 (see Table 8, p.775)
c. inhibitor of CYP2C19 (see Table 8, p.775).

In one series, about 50% of the interactions involved corticosteriods, and 25% analgesics.[71] In a second series, the most frequently used inducers or inhibitors of CYP450 (and/or P-glycoprotein, or UGT) were **dexamethasone, esomeprazole, omeprazole, haloperidol, fluconazole, ciprofloxacin, carbamazepine, carvedilol** and **verapamil** (also see Table 8, p.775).[72] Interactions may be missed, e.g. recurrence of pain may be interpreted as disease progression rather than altered analgesic metabolism. The BNF (www.bnf.org) has a comprehensive list of drug interactions and their signifinance.

Serotonin toxicity can occur with an increase in serotoninergic transmission resulting from a drug–drug interaction, e.g. when the dose of an SSRI is being titrated upwards and another CYP2D6 or 3A4 inhibitor is added. Diagnosis depends on an accurate drug history and the presence of autonomic instability, neuromuscular signs (clonus, hyperreflexia) and cognitive-behavioural changes.

CYP450 drug–food interactions

An important interaction associated with CYP450 inhibition is a food–drug interaction involving grapefruit juice and CYP3A substrates administered PO, including some benzodiazepines (**diazepam, midazolam, triazolam**), some statins (**atorvastatin, lovastatin, simvastatin**), **buspirone, ciclosporin, felodipine, nifedipine, saquinavir** and **terfenadine**.[29,72–75]

Grapefruit juice contains several bioflavonoids (naringenin, naringin, kaempferol and quercetin) and furanocoumarins (bergamottin) which non-competitively inhibit oxidation reactions mediated by CYP3A enzymes in the wall of the GI tract.[74,76,77] The effect is unpredictable because the quantity of these components in grapefruit products varies considerably.[78,79]

The effect is maximal when grapefruit juice is ingested 30–60min before the drug. A single 250mL glass of grapefruit juice can inhibit CYP3A for 24–48h and regular intake continually suppresses GI CYP3A.[29,74] Thus, patients taking drugs metabolized by CYP3A are warned to avoid grapefruit juice, particularly if the drug has a narrow therapeutic index, e.g. **ciclosporin**. Pomelo, Seville orange and lime juices may also inhibit CYP3A;[80,81] apple juice has not been implicated.

Besides inhibiting CYP3A, naringin (and thus grapefruit juice) inhibits organic anion-transporting polypeptide 1A2 (OATP1A2), a carrier protein in the wall of the GI tract which is responsible for the uptake of several drugs. Orange juice (through its major flavonoid, hesperidin) has a similar effect[82] and possibly apple juice.[83] Drugs which may have their absorption reduced by this inhibition include some β-blockers (**atenolol, celiprolol, talinolol**), ciclosporin, **etoposide, fexofenadine, itraconazole**, and quinolone antibacterials (**ciprofloxacin, levofloxacin**).[82,83]

Case reports of serious adverse events related to grapefruit-drug interactions include:
• **amiodarone** → *torsade de pointes*
• **atorvastatin** and **simvastatin** → rhabdomyolysis.

Other drugs which may be affected by grapefruit include novel oral anticoagulants (**apixaban, rivaroxaban**), calcium channel blockers (**amlodipine, felodipine, verapamil**), CNS drugs (**quetiapine, buspirone**), cytotoxics (**nilotinib, lapatinib**), and immunosuppressants (**ciclosporin, tacrolimus, sirolimus**).[84] Interactions are generally drug-specific, not a class effect, and the BNF or SPC should be referred to for more information.

There is also concern that ingestion of cranberry juice may also modify drug action, mediated through flavonoids which specifically inhibit CYP2C9 (see p.555). **Warfarin** is an example of a drug which might be affected by this interaction and, indeed, early reports linked cranberry juice with adverse events associated with **warfarin**.[85-88] However, recent reports suggest that this interaction is unlikely to occur with the amounts of cranberry juice recommended for prophylaxis against UTIs.[89-92]

Nonetheless, an interaction with **warfarin** cannot be ruled out, particularly when large volumes of cranberry juice are drunk regularly, or when cranberry products other than juice are taken.[89,90,93] Thus, the INR should be monitored more closely in patients on **warfarin** if they consume large amounts of cranberry juice or take other cranberry supplements for prophylaxis against UTIs.[89]

Quantifying the effects of CYP450 inhibition and induction

Quantification of the effects of CYP450 inhibitors and inducers is still evolving. The more important enzymes for drug metabolism have generally accepted 'probe' substrates and potent inhibitors (Table 7), and these are used to determine reliable results for other drugs. Increasingly, data are becoming available which predict the clinical importance of drug–drug interactions. However, there is still much to be determined and, in palliative care where polypharmacy is the norm, a general awareness of potential interactions is important (Table 8).

Table 7 Examples of probe substrates and potent inhibitors

Enzyme	Substrate	Inhibitor
CYP3A4	Midazolam (PO)	Ketoconazole
CYP2D6	Dextromethorphan	Paroxetine
CYP2C9	Tolbutamide	None known
CYP1A2	Caffeine	Fluvoxamine
CYP2C8	Repaglinide	Gemfibrozil
CYP2C19	Omeprazole	Fluvoxamine

Table 8 CYP substrates, inhibitors and inducers (selected list)

Enzyme	Substrates	Inhibitors	Inducers
CYP1A2	Amitriptyline Caffeine Clomipramine Clozapine Ethinyloestradiol Imipramine Mirtazapine Olanzapine Paracetamol Propranolol Theophylline Tizanidine Trimipramine	Cimetidine Ciprofloxacin[a] Diltiazem Erythromycin (weak) Fluoxetine (weak)[b] Fluvoxamine[b] Mexiletine Norfloxacin (weak)[a] Paroxetine (weak)[b] Sertraline (weak)[b] Verapamil	Brassicas Charbroiled beef Smoking Omeprazole Phenobarbital Phenytoin
CYP2B6	Bupropion Ketamine Methadone Propofol		Phenobarbital Rifampicin
CYP2C8/9[c]	Amitriptyline Diclofenac Fluvastatin Glipizide Ibuprofen Imipramine Losartan Naproxen Phenytoin Piroxicam Tolbutamide Torsemide Warfarin Zafirlukast	Amiodarone Cimetidine Fluconazole[d] Fluvastatin (possibly) Metronidazole Miconazole Ritonavir Sulfamethoxazole Trimethoprim Zafirlukast	Barbiturates Carbamazepine Rifampicin St John's wort
CYP2C19[c]	Amitriptyline Citalopram Clomipramine Clopidogrel Diazepam Fluoxetine Imipramine Lansoprazole Moclobemide Nelfinavir Omeprazole Pantoprazole Pentamidine Phenytoin Proguanil Propranolol Sertraline	Cimetidine Esomeprazole Fluoxetine[b] Fluvoxamine[b] Ketoconazole[d] Lansoprazole Moclobemide Omeprazole Rabeprazole	Carbamazepine Phenytoin Rifampicin (possibly)

continued

Table 8 Continued

Enzyme	Substrates	Inhibitors	Inducers
CYP2D6[c]	Amitriptyline	Amiodarone	
	Carvedilol	Cimetidine	
	Clomipramine	Clomipramine	
	Clozapine	Flecainide	
	Codeine	Fluoxetine[b]	
	Desipramine	Fluvoxamine (weak)[b]	
	Dextromethorphan	Haloperidol	
	Dextropropoxyphene	Levomepromazine	
	Flecainide	Paroxetine[b]	
	Fluoxetine	Perphenazine	
	Haloperidol	Propafenone	
	Hydrocodone	Quinidine[e]	
	Imipramine	Sertraline (weak)[b]	
	Metoprolol	Tramadol[f]	
	Mexiletine		
	Mirtazapine		
	Nortriptyline		
	Ondansetron		
	Oxycodone		
	Paracetamol		
	Paroxetine		
	Perphenazine		
	Propafenone		
	Propranolol		
	Quinidine		
	Risperidone		
	Ritonavir		
	Sertraline		
	Timolol		
	Tramadol		
	Trazodone		
	Venlafaxine		
CYP2E1	Alcohol	Disulfiram	Alcohol
	Caffeine	Isoniazid	Isoniazid
	Isoniazid		Phenobarbital
	Paracetamol		
	Theophylline		
CYP3A4/5[g]	Alfentanil	Apixaban	Apixaban
	Alprazolam	Bromocriptine	Carbamazepine
	Amiodarone	Cimetidine	Dexamethasone
	Amitriptyline	Clarithromycin	Efavirenz
	Atorvastatin	Ciclosporin	Nevirapine
	Bromocriptine	Danazol	Phenobarbital
	Carbamazepine	Delavirdine	Phenytoin
	Cisapride	Dextropropoxyphene	Rifabutin
	Clarithromycin	Diltiazem	Rifampicin
	Clomipramine	Ergotamine	Rivaroxaban
	Clopidogrel	Erythromycin	St John's wort
	Clozapine	Ethinylestradiol	
	Codeine	Fluconazole[d]	
	Corticosteroids	Fluoxetine[b]	
	Ciclosporin	Fluvoxamine[b]	

Enzyme	Substrates	Inhibitors	Inducers
CYP3A4/5[g] (continued)	Diazepam	Grapefruit juice	
	Diltiazem	Indinavir	
	Erythromycin	Itraconazole[d]	
	Ethinyloestradiol	Ketoconazole[d]	
	Felodipine	Miconazole	
	Fentanyl	Midazolam	
	Imipramine	Nicardipine	
	Indinavir	Nifedipine	
	Lidocaine	Omeprazole	
	Loperamide	Paroxetine (weak)[b]	
	Losartan	Progesterone	
	Lovastatin	Quinidine	
	Methadone	Ritonavir	
	Midazolam	Rivaroxaban	
	Mirtazapine	Saquinavir	
	Nelfinavir	Sertraline (weak)[b]	
	Nifedipine	Testosterone	
	Omeprazole	Verapamil	
	Paracetamol	Zafirlukast	
	Phenytoin		
	Pimozide		
	Propafenone		
	Quinidine		
	Ritonavir		
	Saquinavir		
	Sertraline		
	Sildenafil		
	Simvastatin		
	Tamoxifen		
	Theophylline		
	Trazodone		
	Triazolam		
	Venlafaxine		
	Verapamil		
	Warfarin[h]		

a. relative inhibitory potency of fluoroquinolones: ciprofloxacin > norfloxacin > ofloxacin (almost none)
b. *in vitro* data suggest only moderate inhibition of SSRIs. CYP1A2 inhibition: fluvoxamine > all other SSRIs; CYP2D6 inhibition: paroxetine and fluoxetine > sertraline > fluvoxamine (almost none); CYP3A4 inhibition: fluvoxamine > fluoxetine > paroxetine and sertraline (almost none)
c. also genetic polymorphism, see Table 3, p.771
d. relative inhibitory potency of imidazoles: ketoconazole ≈ itraconazole > fluconazole (and possibly clotrimazole)
e. most potent CYP2D6 inhibitor
f. significant competitive inhibition of quinidine and propafenone metabolism has been documented with tramadol administration
g. expressed in GI mucosa resulting in substantial first-pass metabolism during absorption of some drugs
h. in patients taking warfarin, paracetamol ≥1300mg/24h for one week can increase the INR to >6 (but a total *weekly* dose of ≤2g has no effect); this is possibly a CYP450 interaction even though paracetamol is not listed above as a CYP inhibitor.

1 Droney J et al. (2011) Evolving knowledge of opioid genetics in cancer pain. Clinical Oncology. 23: 418–428.
2 Branford R et al. (2012) Opioid genetics: the key to personalized pain control? Clinical Genetics. 82: 301–310.
3 Ross JR et al. (2006) Clinical pharmacology and pharmacotherapy of opioid switching in cancer patients. Oncologist. 11: 765–773.
4 Somogyi AA et al. (2007) Pharmacogenetics of opioids. Clinical Pharmacology and Therapeutics. 81: 429–444.
5 Matthes H et al. (1996) Loss of morphine-induced analgesia, reward effect and withdrawal symptoms in mice lacking the mu-opioid-receptor gene. Nature. 383: 819–823.
6 Chou WY et al. (2006) Association of mu-opioid receptor gene polymorphism (A118G) with variations in morphine consumption for analgesia after total knee arthroplasty. Acta Anaesthesiologica Scandinavica. 50: 787–792.
7 Chou WY et al. (2006) Human opioid receptor A118G polymorphism affects intravenous patient-controlled analgesia morphine consumption after total abdominal hysterectomy. Anesthesiology. 105: 334–337.
8 Sia AT et al. (2008) A118G single nucleotide polymorphism of human mu-opioid receptor gene influences pain perception and patient-controlled intravenous morphine consumption after intrathecal morphine for postcesarean analgesia. Anesthesiology. 109: 520–526.
9 Janicki PK et al. (2006) A genetic association study of the functional A118G polymorphism of the human mu-opioid receptor gene in patients with acute and chronic pain. Anesthesia and Analgesia. 103: 1011–1017.
10 Lotsch J et al. (2009) Cross-sectional analysis of the influence of currently known pharmacogenetic modulators on opioid therapy in outpatient pain centers. Pharmacogenetics and Genomics. 19: 429–436.
11 Campa D et al. (2008) Association of ABCB1/MDR1 and OPRM1 gene polymorphisms with morphine pain relief. Clinical Pharmacology and Therapeutics. 83: 559–566.
12 Klepstad P et al. (2004) The 118 A > G polymorphism in the human mu-opioid receptor gene may increase morphine requirements in patients with pain caused by malignant disease. Acta Anaesthesiologica Scandinavica. 48: 1232–1239.
13 Walter C and Lotsch J (2009) Meta-analysis of the relevance of the OPRM1 118A>G genetic variant for pain treatment. Pain. 146: 270–275.
14 Schinkel AH (1997) The physiological function of drug-transporting P-glycoproteins. Seminars in Cancer Biology. 8: 161–170.
15 Marzolini C et al. (2004) Polymorphisms in human MDR1 (P-glycoprotein): recent advances and clinical relevance. Clinical Pharmacology and Therapeutics. 75: 13–33.
16 Davis MP et al. (eds) (2009) Pharmacogenetics and opioids. In: Opioids in Cancer Pain (2e). OUP, Oxford, pp. 287–299.
17 Dagenais C et al. (2004) Variable modulation of opioid brain uptake by P-glycoprotein in mice. Biochemical Pharmacology. 67: 269–276.
18 Barratt DT et al. (2012) ABCB1 haplotype and OPRM1 118A > G genotype interaction in methadone maintenance treatment pharmacogenetics. Pharmgenomics and Personalized Medicine. 5: 53–62.
19 Thompson SJ et al. (2000) Opiate-induced analgesia is increased and prolonged in mice lacking P-glycoprotein. Anesthesiology. 92: 1392–1399.
20 Ross JR et al. (2008) Genetic variation and response to morphine in cancer patients: catechol-O-methyltransferase and multidrug resistance-1 gene polymorphisms are associated with central side effects. Cancer. 112: 1390–1403.
21 Zwisler ST et al. (2010) The antinociceptive effect and adverse drug reactions of oxycodone in human experimental pain in relation to genetic variations in the OPRM1 and ABCB1 genes. Fundamental and Clinical Pharmacology. 24: 517–524.
22 Coulbault L et al. (2006) Environmental and genetic factors associated with morphine response in the postoperative period. Clinical Pharmacology and Therapeutics. 79: 316–324.
23 Kim H et al. (2006) Genetic polymorphisms in monoamine neurotransmitter systems show only weak association with acute post-surgical pain in humans. Molecular Pain. 2: 24.
24 Zubieta JK et al. (2003) COMT val158met genotype affects mu-opioid neurotransmitter responses to a pain stressor. Science. 299: 1240–1243.
25 Rakvag TT et al. (2005) The Val158Met polymorphism of the human catechol-O-methyltransferase (COMT) gene may influence morphine requirements in cancer pain patients. Pain. 116: 73–78.
26 Laugsand EA et al. (2011) Clinical and genetic factors associated with nausea and vomiting in cancer patients receiving opioids. European Journal of Cancer. 47: 1682–1691.
27 Kolesnikov Y et al. (2011) Combined catechol-O-methyltransferase and mu-opioid receptor gene polymorphisms affect morphine postoperative analgesia and central side effects. Anesthesia and Analgesia. 112: 448–453.
28 Smith HS (2009) Opioid metabolism. Mayo Clinic Proceedings. 84: 613–624.
29 Wilkinson GR (2005) Drug metabolism and variability among patients in drug response. N Engl J Med. 352: 2211–2221.
30 Sim SC (2005) Human Cytochrome P450 (CYP). Allele Nomenclature Committee. Available from: www.cypalleles.ki.se
31 Stamer UM et al. (2010) Personalized therapy in pain management: where do we stand? Pharmacogenomics. 11: 843–864.
32 Meyer U (1991) Genotype or phenotype: the definition of a pharmacogenetic polymorphism. Pharmacogenetics. 1: 66–67.
33 Sajantila A et al. (2010) Pharmacogenetics in medico-legal context. Forensic Science International. 203: 44–52.
34 Poulsen L et al. (1996) The hypoalgesic effect of tramadol in relation to CYP2D6. Clinical Pharmacology and Therapeutics. 60: 636–644.
35 Riddick D (1997) Drug biotransformation. In: H Kalant and W Roschlau (eds) Principles of Medical Pharmacology (6e). Oxford University Press, New York.
36 Williams DG et al. (2002) Pharmacogenetics of codeine metabolism in an urban population of children and its implications for analgesic reliability. British Journal of Anaesthesia. 89: 839–845.
37 Persson K et al. (1992) The postoperative pharmacokinetics of codeine. European Journal of Clinical Pharmacology. 42: 663–666.
38 Findlay JWA et al. (1978) Plasma codeine and morphine concentrations after therapeutic oral doses of codeine-containing analgesics. Clin Pharmacol Ther. 24: 60–68.
39 Eckhardt K et al. (1998) Same incidence of adverse drug events after codeine administration irrespective of the genetically determined differences in morphine formation. Pain. 76: 27–33.
40 Susce MT et al. (2006) Response to hydrocodone, codeine and oxycodone in a CYP2D6 poor metabolizer. Progress in Neuropsychopharmacology and Biological Psychiatry. 30: 1356–1358.
41 Gasche Y et al. (2004) Codeine intoxication associated with ultrarapid CYP2D6 metabolism. New England Journal of Medicine. 351: 2827–2831.
42 Koren G et al. (2006) Pharmacogenetics of morphine poisoning in a breastfed neonate of a codeine-prescribed mother. Lancet. 368: 704.
43 Kirchheiner J et al. (2007) Pharmacokinetics of codeine and its metabolite morphine in ultra-rapid metabolizers due to CYP2D6 duplication. Pharmacogenomics Journal. 7: 257–265.

44 Racoosin JA et al. (2013) New Evidence about an Old Drug - Risk with Codeine after Adenotonsillectomy. New England Journal of Medicine. 368: 2155–2157.

45 Pirmohamed M and Park BK (2003) Cytochrome P450 enzyme polymorphisms and adverse drug reactions. Toxicology. 192: 23–32.

46 Haddad A et al. (2007) The pharmacological importance of cytochrome CYP3A4 in the palliation of symptoms: review and recommendations for avoiding adverse drug interactions. Supportive Care in Cancer. 15: 251–257.

47 Kimmel SE et al. (2013) A pharmacogenetic versus a clinical algorithm for warfarin dosing. New England Journal of Medicine. 369: 2283–2293.

48 Pirmohamed M et al. (2013) A randomized trial of genotype-guided dosing of warfarin. New England Journal of Medicine. 369: 2294–2303.

49 Johnson MD et al. (1999) Clinically significant drug interactions. Postgraduate Medicine. 105: 193–222.

50 Samer CF et al. (2013) Applications of CYP450 testing in the clinical setting. Molecular Diagnosis and Therapy. 17: 165–184.

51 Benitez-Rosario MA et al. (2006) Methadone-induced respiratory impression after discontinuing carbamazepine administration. Journal of Pain and Symptom Management. 32: 99–100.

52 Kreek MJ et al. (1976) Rifampin-induced methadone withdrawal. New England Journal of Medicine. 294: 1104–1106.

53 Backman J et al. (1996) Concentrations and effects of oral midazolam are greatly reduced in patients treated with carbamazepine or phenytoin. Epilepsia. 37: 253–257.

54 Kay L et al. (1985) Influence of rifampicin and isoniazid on the kinetics of phenytoin. British Journal of Clinical Pharmacology. 20: 323–326.

55 Piscitelli SC et al. (2000) Indinavir concentrations and St John's wort. Lancet. 355: 547–548.

56 Henderson L et al. (2002) St John's wort (Hypericum perforatum): drug interactions and clinical outcomes. British Journal of Clinical Pharmacology. 54: 349–356.

57 Flexner C (2000) Dual protease inhibitor therapy in HIV-infected patients: pharmacologic rationale and clinical benefits. Annual Review of Pharmacology and Toxicology. 40: 649–674.

58 Sindrup S et al. (1992) The effect of quinidine on the analgesic effect of codeine. European Journal of Clinical Pharmacology. 42: 587–591.

59 MHRA (2009) Interactions between the use clopidogrel and proton pump inhibitors. Safety warnings and messages for medicines (6 July 2009). www.mhra.gov.uk/safetyinformation

60 Society for Cardiovascular Angiography and Interventions (2009) A national study of the effect of individual proton pump inhibitors on cardiovascular outcomes in patients treated with clopidogrel following coronary stenting: The Clopidogrel Medco Outcomes Study. Available from: www.scai.org

61 Juurlink DN et al. (2009) A population-based study of the drug interaction between proton pump inhibitors and clopidogrel. Canadian Medical Association Journal. 180: 713–718.

62 Ho M et al. (2009) Risk of adverse outcomes associated with concomitant use of clopidogrel and proton pump inhibitors following acute coronary syndrome. Journal of the American Medical Association. 301: 937–944.

63 Klotz U and Reimann I (1980) Delayed clearance of diazepam due to cimetidine. New England Journal of Medicine. 302: 1012–1014.

64 Nix D et al. (1987) Effect of multiple dose oral ciprofloxacin on the pharmacokinetics of theophylline and indocyanine green. Journal of Antimicrobial Chemotherapy. 19: 263–269.

65 Vandel S et al. (1992) Tricyclic antidepressant plasma levels after fluoxetine addition. Neuropsychobiology. 25: 202–207.

66 Finley P (1994) Selective serotonin reuptake inhibitors: pharmacologic profiles and potential therapeutic distinctions. Annals of Pharmacotherapy. 28: 1359–1369.

67 Pollock B (1994) Recent developments in drug metabolism of relevance to psychiatrists. Harvard Reviews of Psychiatry. 2: 204–213.

68 Tatro D (1995) Fluvoxamine drug interactions. Drug Newsletter. 14: 20ff.

69 Monaham B (1990) Torsades de Pointes occurring in association with terfenadine. Journal of the American Medical Association. 264: 2788–2790.

70 Honig P et al. (1993) Terfenadine-ketoconazole interaction. Pharmacokinetic and electrocardiographic consequences. Journal of the American Medical Association. 269: 1513–1518.

71 Wilcock A et al. (2005) Potential for drug interactions involving cytochrome P450 in patients attending palliative day care centres: a multicentre audit. British Journal of Clinical Pharmacology. 60: 326–329.

72 Kotlinska-Lemisezek A et al. (2014) Polypharmacy in patients wih advanced cancer and pain: a European cross-sectional study of 2282 patients. Journal of pain symptom management (in press).

73 Maskalyk J (2002) Grapefruit juice: potential drug interactions. Canadian Medical Association Journal. 167: 279–280.

74 Dahan A and Altman H (2004) Food-drug interaction: grapefruit juice augments drug bioavailability-mechanism, extent and relevance. European Journal of Clinical Nutrition. 58: 1–9.

75 MHRA (2004) Statins and cytochrome P450 interactions. Current problems in pharmacovigilance. 30: 1–2.

76 Rouseff RL (1988) Liquid chromatographic determination of naringin and neohesperidin as a detector of grapefruit juice in orange juice. Journal - Association of Official Analytical Chemists. 71: 798–802.

77 Gibaldi M (1992) Drug interactions. Part I. Annals of Pharmacotherapy. 26: 829–834.

78 Tailor S et al. (1996) Peripheral edema due to nifedipine-itraconazole interaction: a case report. Archives of Dermatology. 132: 350–352.

79 Fukuda K et al. (2000) Amounts and variation in grapefruit juice of the main components causing grapefruit-drug interaction. Journal of Chromatography B, Biomedical Sciences and Applications. 741: 195–203.

80 Savage I (2008) Forbidden fruit: interactions between medicines, foods and herbal products Pharmaceutical Journal 281: f17.

81 Baxter K (2008) Drug interactions and fruit juices. Pharmaceutical Journal. 281: 333.

82 Bailey DG et al. (2007) Naringin is a major and selective clinical inhibitor of organic anion-transporting polypeptide 1A2 (OATP1A2) in grapefruit juice. Clinical Pharmacology and Therapeutics. 81: 495–502.

83 Sampson M (2008) New reasons to avoid grapefruit and other juices when taking certain drugs. Report from the 236th National Meeting of the American Chemical Society. Philadelphia, August 19th 2008. Available from: www.eurekalert.org/pub_releases/2008-08/acs-nrt072308.php

84 Bailey DG et al. (2013) Grapefruit-medication interactions: forbidden fruit or avoidable consequences? Canadian Medical Association Journal. 185: 309–316.

85 Grant P (2004) Warfarin and cranberry juice: an interaction? Journal of Heart Valve Disease. 13: 25–26.

86 CSM (Committee on Safety of Medicines) (2004) Interaction between warfarin and cranberry juice: new advice. Current Problems in Pharmacovigilance. 30: 10.

87 MHRA (2003) Possible interaction between warfarin and cranberry juice. *Current Problems in Pharmacovigilance.* **29**: 8.
88 Suvarna R *et al.* (2003) Possible interaction between warfarin and cranberry juice. *British Medical Journal.* **327**: 1454.
89 O'Mara N (2007) Does a cranberry juice-warfarin interaction really exist? Detail document. *Pharmacist's Letter/Prescriber's Letter.* **23**: 1–3.
90 Aston JL *et al.* (2006) Interaction between warfarin and cranberry juice. *Pharmacotherapy.* **26**: 1314–1319.
91 Lilja JJ *et al.* (2007) Effects of daily ingestion of cranberry juice on the pharmacokinetics of warfarin, tizanidine, and midazolam–probes of CYP2C9, CYP1A2, and CYP3A4. *Clinical Pharmacology and Therapeutics.* **81**: 833–839.
92 Li Z *et al.* (2006) Cranberry does not affect prothrombin time in male subjects on warfarin. *Journal of the American Dietetic Society.* **106**: 2057–2061.
93 Welch J and Forster K (2007) Probable elevation in international normalized ratio from cranberry juice. *Journal of Pharmacy Technology.* **23**: 104–107.

Updated September 2014

26: DRUG-INDUCED MOVEMENT DISORDERS

Drug-induced movement disorders (extrapyramidal reactions) encompass:
- parkinsonism
- acute dystonia
- acute akathisia
- tardive dyskinesia.

The features of the various syndromes are listed in Box A.[1] Most extrapyramidal reactions are caused by drugs which block dopamine receptors in the CNS; these include all antipsychotics and **metoclopramide**.[2,3] The risk is associated with dose, pre-existing extrapyramidal signs, dementia and a genetic predisposition.[4,5] To minimize the risk, always use the lowest effective dose for the shortest duration possible.

Box A   Movement disorders associated with dopamine-receptor antagonists[1]

Parkinsonism
Coarse resting tremor of limbs, head, mouth and/or tongue
Muscular rigidity (cogwheel or lead pipe)
Bradykinesia, notably of face
Sialorrhoea (drooling)
Shuffling gait

Acute dystonias
one or more of
Abnormal positioning of head and neck (retrocollis, torticollis)
Spasms of jaw muscles (trismus, gaping, grimacing)
Tongue dysfunction (dysarthria, protrusion)
Dysphagia
Laryngopharyngeal spasm
Dysphonia
Eyes deviated up, down or sideways (oculogyric crisis)
Abnormal positioning of limbs or trunk

Acute akathisia
one or more of
Fidgety movements or swinging of legs
Rocking from foot to foot when standing
Pacing to relieve restlessness
Inability to sit or stand still for several minutes

Tardive dyskinesia
Exposure to antipsychotic medication for >3 months (>1 month if >60 years of age)
Involuntary movement of tongue, jaw, trunk or limbs:
- choreiform (rapid, jerky, non-repetitive)
- athetoid (slow, sinuous, continual)
- rhythmic (stereotypic)

Antipsychotic drugs differ in their propensity for causing extrapyramidal reactions (see p.168). A lower risk is associated with lower affinity for the D_2-receptor, D_2 partial agonism and/or $5HT_{2A}/5HT_{2C}$ antagonism.[6-8] Thus the risk is a spectrum (in descending order):
- **haloperidol** (the highest risk)
- phenothiazines (e.g. **levomepromazine**)
- **risperidone**
- **olanzapine**
- **quetiapine, clozapine** (the lowest risk).

However, their overall tolerability is comparable because lower rates of extrapyramidal reactions are offset by increased rates of sedation and/or undesirable metabolic effects (see p.168).[9]

Numerous other drugs have been implicated,[10-12] including most classes of antidepressants, **carbamazepine, diltiazem, 5-hydroxytryptophan, levodopa, lithium, methyldopa, ondansetron** and **valproate**.[13-15]

The link between extrapyramidal reactions and the serotoninergic system is partly caused by $5HT_{2A}$- and $5HT_{2C}$-receptors inhibiting dopaminergic neurones.[6] Thus, increased inhibition is seen in the propensity of SSRIs to induce such disorders, including akathisia,[16] whereas $5HT_{2A}$- and $5HT_{2C}$ antagonism reduces this propensity among some antipsychotics (see above).

Parkinsonism

Parkinsonism develops in 30–60% of patients treated long-term with antipsychotics.[4] It is most common in those over 60 years of age. It can develop at any stage but, except in patients with dementia, generally not before the second week.[4] There may be asymmetry in the early stages. The tremor of drug-induced parkinsonism typically:
- has a frequency of <8 cycles per second
- is worse at rest
- is suppressed during voluntary movements
- is associated with rigidity and bradykinesia (Box A).

This is different from drug-induced tremors of the hands, head, mouth or tongue which have a frequency of 8–12 cycles per second, and are best observed with hands held outstretched or mouth held open (Box B).

Treatment
- if possible, reduce or stop causal drug
- if caused by:
  ▷ **metoclopramide**, substitute **domperidone**
  ▷ an antipsychotic, switch to an alternative with a lower rate of extrapyramidal reactions (e.g. **quetiapine**)
- prescribe an antimuscarinic antiparkinsonian drug, e.g.:
  ▷ **orphenadrine** 50mg b.d. *or*
  ▷ **procyclidine** 2.5–5mg t.d.s. *or*
  ▷ **trihexyphenidyl** 2–5 mg once daily–t.d.s.

Box B Drug-induced (non-parkinsonian) tremor[17]

Anti-epileptics valproate	Lithium
	Methylxanthines
Antidepressants	caffeine
SSRIs	aminophylline
TCAs	theophylline
Antipsychotics	Psychostimulants
butyrophenones	dexamfetamine
phenothiazines	methylphenidate
β_2 Agonists	
salbutamol	
salmeterol	

Acute dystonia

Acute dystonias occur in up to 10% of patients treated with antipsychotics.[4,18] They are most common in young adults. They develop abruptly within days of starting treatment, and are accompanied by anxiety (Box A).

Treatment
- if possible, discontinue or reduce the dose of the causal drug
- if caused by **metoclopramide**, substitute **domperidone**
- if caused by an antipsychotic, switch to an alternative with a lower rate of extrapyramidal reactions (e.g. **quetiapine**).

For immediate relief, give an injection of:
- **diazepam** 5mg IV[19] or
- an antimuscarinic, e.g. **procyclidine** 5–10mg IV/IM or
- an antihistaminic antimuscarinic drug, e.g. **dimenhydrinate** or **diphenhydramine** 25–50mg IV/IM (both not UK).

With antimuscarinic drugs, benefit is typically seen in 10–20min. If necessary, repeat the injection after 30min. Continue treatment PO for 1 week with:
- **orphenadrine** 50mg b.d. or
- **dimenhydrinate** or **diphenhydramine** 25–50mg b.d.–q.d.s. (both not UK).

Acute akathisia

Akathisia is a form of motor restlessness in which the subject is compelled to pace up and down or to change the body position frequently (Box A).[20] It occurs in 20% or more of patients receiving typical antipsychotics.[4] The prevalence is no longer considered to be age-related, but younger patients may respond better to treatment than elderly ones.[4]

Akathisia can develop within days of starting treatment, and generally resolves within a week of stopping the causal drug. If the drug is continued, it may progress to parkinsonism. **Haloperidol** and **prochlorperazine** carry the highest risk.[21,22] It is uncommon for **metoclopramide** to cause akathisia.

Treatment
- if possible, discontinue or reduce the dose of the causal drug
- switch to an alternative antipsychotic with a lower rate of extrapyramidal reactions (e.g. **quetiapine**)
- if necessary, add **propranolol** 10mg t.d.s., increasing if necessary every few days to a maximum daily dose of 120mg (further benefit above this level is unlikely)[23]
- if the patient is very distressed, a benzodiazepine can be prescribed in addition for a few days, e.g. **diazepam** 5–10mg/24h,[19] **clonazepam** 0.5–1mg/24h, **lorazepam** 1–3mg/24h.

Although **propranolol**, a highly lipophilic non-selective β-adrenergic receptor antagonist (β-blocker), has a proven anti-akathisia effect, selective β_1-adrenergic receptor antagonists such as **atenolol** and **metoprolol** are either less or not effective.[23] This suggests that the effect is a central one, and/or that both β_1- and β_2-receptor antagonism is necessary to reduce akathisia.

Antimuscarinic antiparkinsonian drugs are sometimes helpful.[23] However, response in **haloperidol**-induced akathisia is less likely.[24] It has been suggested that benefit from antimuscarinic antiparkinsonian drugs occurs only if akathisia is associated with drug-induced parkinsonism.[25]

Diphenhydramine (not UK) may also be of benefit.[19] Other possible treatments include **amantidine**, **buspirone** and **clonidine**.[23,26]

Tardive dyskinesia

Tardive (late) dyskinesia is caused by the long-term administration of drugs that block dopamine receptors, particularly D_2-receptors.[27] It occurs in 20% of patients receiving a typical antipsychotic for >3 months, particularly in the elderly and in those on high doses, e.g. **chlorpromazine** 300mg/24h or more.[4,28] It is less common in patients receiving atypical antipsychotics (see p.168).[28] Tardive dyskinesia is also associated with the long-term use of **metoclopramide** (p.242).[29]

Tardive dyskinesia typically manifests as involuntary stereotyped chewing movements of the tongue and orofacial muscles (Box A). The involuntary movements are made worse by anxiety and reduced by drowsiness and during sleep.

Tardive dyskinesia is associated with akathisia in 25% of cases. In younger patients, tardive dyskinesia may present as abnormal positioning of the limbs and tonic contractions of the neck and trunk muscles causing torticollis, lordosis or scoliosis. In younger patients, tardive dyskinesia may occur if antipsychotic treatment is stopped abruptly.

Early diagnosis

'*Open your mouth and stick out your tongue.*'

The following indicate a developing tardive dyskinesia:

- worm-like movements of the tongue
- inability to protrude tongue for more than a few seconds.

Treatment

- if possible, discontinue or reduce the dose of the causal drug
- if caused by **metoclopramide**, substitute **domperidone**
- if caused by a typical antipsychotic, switch to an atypical antipsychotic
- withdraw antimuscarinics (it is exacerated by antimuscarinic antiparkinsonian drugs).[29]

Withdrawal of the causal drug leads to resolution in 30% in 3 months and a further 40% in 5 years. However, it is sometimes irreversible, particularly in the elderly. Seek specialist advice before initiating other drug treatments (e.g. **clonazepam**, ginko biloba).[30]

Paradoxically, increasing the dose of the causal drug may help temporarily, but should be considered only in desperation because it could subsequently exacerbate the dyskinesia.[29]

1 APA (American Psychiatric Association) (1994) Neuroleptic-induced movement disorders. In: *Diagnostic and Statistical Manual of Mental Disorders* (4e). American Psychiatric Association, New York, pp. 736–751.
2 Tonda M and Guthrie S (1994) Treatment of acute neuroleptic-induced movement disorders. *Pharmacotherapy.* 14: 543–560.
3 Jackson N et al. (2008) Neuropsychiatric complications of commonly used palliative care drugs. *Postgraduate Medical Journal.* 84: 121–126.
4 Caligiuri MR et al. (2000) Antipsychotic-Induced movement disorders in the elderly: epidemiology and treatment recommendations. *Drugs Aging.* 17: 363–384.
5 Tang S et al. (2009) MDPD: an integrated genetic information resource for Parkinson's disease. In: *Nucleic Acids Research.* Available from: http://nar.oxfordjournals.org/cgi/content/full/37/suppl_1/D858
6 Stahl SM (2013) Chapter 4: Psychosis and schizophrenia. In: *Essential Psychopharmacology: Neuroscientific Basis and Practical Applications* (4e). Cambridge University Press, USA, pp. 79–128.
7 Lieberman JA (2004) Dopamine partial agonists: a new class of antipsychotic. *CNS Drugs.* 18: 251–267.
8 Kapur S and Mamo D (2003) Half a century of antipsychotics and still a central role for dopamine D_2 receptors. *Progress in Neuro-psychopharmacology and Biology Psychiatry.* 27: 1081–1090.
9 Lieberman JA et al. (2005) Effectiveness of antipsychotic drugs in patients with chronic schizophrenia. *New England Journal of Medicine.* 353: 1209–1223.
10 Tarsy D and Simon DK (2006) Dystonia. *New England Journal of Medicine.* 355: 818–829.
11 Anonymous (1994) Drug-induced extrapyramidal reactions. *Current Problems in Pharmacovigilance.* 20: 15–16.
12 Zubenko G et al. (1987) Antidepressant-related akathisia. *Journal of Clinical Psychopharmacology.* 7: 254–257.
13 Anonymous (2009) Neuroleptic-induced extrapyramidal reactions. In: *Drugdex® Consults* Micromedex, Thompson Healthcare. Available from: http://www.micromedex.com/products/drugdex/
14 Matthews H and Tancil C (1996) Extrapyramidal reaction caused by ondansetron. *The Annals of Pharmacotherapy.* 30: 196.
15 Arya D (1994) Extrapyramidal symptoms with selective serotonin reuptake inhibitors. *British Journal of Psychiatry.* 165: 728–733.
16 Lane R (1998) SSRI-induced extrapyramidal side-effects and akathisia: implications for treatment. *Journal of Psychopharmacology.* 12: 192–214.
17 APA (American Psychiatric Association) (1994) Medication-induced postural tremor. In: *Diagnostic and Statistical Manual of Mental Disorders* (4e). American Psychiatric Association, New York, pp. 749–751.
18 Launer M (1996) Selected side-effects: 17. Dopamine-receptor antagonists and movement disorders. *Prescribers' Journal.* 36: 37–41.
19 Gagrat D et al. (1978) Intravenous diazepam in the treatment of neuroleptic-induced acute dystonia and akathisia. *American Journal of Psychiatry.* 135: 1232–1233.
20 White C and Jackson N (2005) Acute akathisia in palliative care. *European Journal of Palliative Care.* 12 (1): 5–7.
21 Kawanishi C et al. (2007) Unexpectedly high prevalence of akathisia in cancer patients. *Palliative and Supportive Care.* 5: 351–354.
22 Gattera J et al. (1994) A retrospective study of risk factors of akathisia in terminally ill patients. *Journal of Pain and Symptom Management.* 9: 454–461.
23 Miller CH and Fleischhacker WW (2000) Managing antipsychotic-induced acute and chronic akathisia. *Drug Safety.* 22: 73–81.
24 Van Putten T et al. (1984) Akathisia with haloperidol and thiothixene. *Archives of General Psychiatry.* 41: 1036–1039.
25 Braude W et al. (1993) Clinical characteristics of akathisia: a systematic investigation of acute psychiatric in-patient admission. *British Journal of Psychiatry.* 143: 139–150.
26 Poyurovsky M and Weizman A (1997) Serotonergic agents in the treatment of acute neuroleptic-induced akathisia: open-label study of buspirone and mianserin. *International Clinical Psychopharmacology.* 12: 263–268.
27 APA (American Psychiatric Association) (1992) *Tardive dyskinesia: a task force report of the American Psychiatric Association.* American Psychiatric Association, Washington, DC.

28 Jeste D (2000) Tardive dyskinesia in older patients. *Journal of Clinical Psychiatry.* **61 (Suppl 4)**: 27–32.
29 Margolese HC *et al.* (2005) Tardive dyskinesia in the era of typical and atypical antipsychotics. Part 2: Incidence and management strategies in patients with schizophrenia. *Canadian Journal of Psychiatry.* **50**: 703–714.
30 Bhidayasin R *et al.* (2013) Evidence-based guideline: treatment of tardive syndromes: report of the Guideline Development Subcommittee of the American Academy of Neurology. **81**: 463–469

Updated June 2014

27:   ANAPHYLAXIS

Anaphylaxis is an acute life-threatening systemic allergic hypersensitivity reaction. It develops rapidly in minutes or, at most, a few hours. It manifests as hypotension (fainting, collapse, loss of consciousness), and/or respiratory difficulty (laryngeal and bronchial constriction).[1]

Pathophysiology

Anaphylaxis is caused by the sudden release of numerous inflammatory mediators from mast cells and basophils into the systemic circulation. This results in:
- vasodilation, hypotension, capillary leakage (leading to cardiovascular collapse)
- mucosal and laryngeal oedema, bronchoconstriction (leading to respiratory difficulty).[1]

Most commonly, the allergic reaction results from the interaction of an allergen with specific IgE antibodies bound to mast cells and basophils, leading to the release of:
- preformed chemical mediators, e.g. chymase, histamine, tryptase
- newly synthesized mediators, e.g. cytokines, leukotrienes, platelet activating factor, prostaglandins.

Anaphylaxis may also be caused by other immunological mechanisms, e.g. IgG-antigen complexes. Some drugs, e.g. NSAIDs, can cause direct activation of mast cells. Other non-immunological triggers of anaphylaxis include exercise and cold.[2] Non-IgE reactions are sometimes called *anaphylactoid reactions*. However, in Europe, the term is no longer used. In terms of management, it is *not* necessary to identify the precise trigger; the difference is relevant only when investigations are being considered.[3–5]

Anaphylaxis is:
- specific to a given drug or chemically-related class of drugs
- more likely after parenteral drug administration
- more frequent in patients taking ß-blockers (see p.789), or who have **aspirin**-induced asthma or systemic lupus erythematosus
- more severe in patients with concomitant illness, particularly upper respiratory tract infections, chronic respiratory diseases.

Anaphylaxis is rare in palliative care. When it occurs, it is generally associated with antibacterials (see p.461) or an NSAID (see p.317). Although refined arachis (peanut) oil is unlikely to cause an allergic reaction, a possible case has been recorded in a woman with known peanut allergy who received an **arachis oil** enema.[6] **Chlorhexidine** has also been implicated, including after the use of a **chlorhexidine** skin wipe.[7]

Clinical features

Anaphylaxis is likely when the following criteria are met after exposure to a possible trigger:
- sudden onset and rapid progression of symptoms (minutes–few hours)
- life-threatening respiratory or circulatory problems
- skin and/or mucosal changes (Box A).[8]

Before progressing to life-threatening respiratory or circulatory problems, patients with a history of anaphylaxis may present with:
- sudden onset and rapidly progressing skin and/or mucosal changes plus GI symptoms (abdominal pain, colic, vomiting) *or*
- hypotension alone.[1,9]

The differential diagnosis of anaphylaxis is extensive but includes:
- life-threatening conditions, e.g. severe asthma, septic shock, seizure
- non life-threatening conditions, e.g. urticaria or angioedema, vasovagal episode, panic attack.[10]

Box A   Clinical features of anaphylaxis

Essential
Sudden onset of life-threatening circulatory *and/or* respiratory problems, e.g.

Circulatory problems
Tachycardia
Hypotension
Shock
Decreased consciousness
Cardiac arrest

Respiratory problems
Airway
   pharyngeal/laryngeal oedema
   hoarse voice
   stridor
Breathing
   breathlessness
   wheeze/bronchospasm (10%)
   cyanosis
   respiratory arrest

Probable
Skin/mucosal changes (80%):
   flushing or pallor
   erythema of skin
   itching
   urticaria
   angioedema[a], mostly face, hands, feet

Possible
Agitation
Confusion
Abdominal pain
Vomiting
Diarrhoea
Incontinence
Tingling of the extremities
Rhinitis
Conjunctivitis

---

a. angioedema is swelling in the dermis, subcutaneous and submucosal tissues.

Management

National guidelines vary; the advice here is based on guidance published by the UK Resuscitation Council[8,11] and NICE[7,11] Drugs and basic resuscitation equipment for treatment of anaphylaxis must be available in all clinical settings, either as part of a resuscitation kit or in an 'anaphylaxis box'. Urgent treatment with three drugs is required:

1. **Adrenaline** (epinephrine); *of paramount importance because it saves lives*

2. **Chlorphenamine** (or other H_1-antihistamine)

3. **Hydrocortisone** (Box B).

Adrenaline (epinephrine), a direct-acting sympathomimetic, is effective in attenuating anaphylaxis if given promptly and in sufficient dose.[8] Through its α_1-receptor agonist effects, it causes vasoconstriction, increases peripheral vascular resistance and reduces mucosal oedema. As a β_1 agonist, it increases the rate and force of myocardial contraction. As a β_2 agonist, it dilates bronchial airways, increases glycogenolysis and suppresses activity of mast cells, reducing the release of histamine and other inflammatory mediators.

   Adrenaline is given by IM injection (Box B). If there is doubt about the adequacy of the circulation, **adrenaline** can be given as a dilute IV solution, i.e. 1 in 10,000 (100microgram/mL), *using 50microgram (0.5mL) boluses, titrated to response.*

Note: if given too rapidly, IV **adrenaline** can cause ventricular arrhythmias, cardiac ischaemia, and hypertension. Thus, IV **adrenaline** should be given only by doctors experienced in its use and where full intensive care facilities are available.[8,12]

Box B   Management of anaphylaxis in adults

1 Discontinue administration of any potential causal agent, e.g. IVI of antibacterial or blood product.

2 **Adrenaline (epinephrine)** IM *every 5min* until blood pressure, pulse and breathing are satisfactory:
   • 1:1,000 (1mg/1mL), 500microgram (0.5mL) *or*
   • 300microgram (0.3mL) if an adrenaline (epinephrine) auto-injector is used.
   Administer into the anterolateral aspect of the middle third of the thigh.[6]
   If given promptly, patients rarely need >3 doses of 500microgram.[2]

3 Postion patient on back with legs elevated.

4 **Chlorphenamine** IM or IV to counter histamine-induced vasodilation and broncho-constriction:
   • 10mg over 1min
   • if necessary, repeat up to a maximum of 40mg/24h.[12]

5 **Hydrocortisone sodium succinate** IM or slowly IV over 1–10min:
   • 200mg for patients with bronchospasm, and for all severe or recurrent reactions to prevent further deterioration
   • *takes up to 6h to act.*

6 In severe cases of anaphylaxis, additional treatment (Box C) and transfer to hospital will be necessary.

7 If cardiorespiratory arrest occurs, start cardiopulmonary resuscitation if appropriate to the patient's circumstances (e.g. taking prognosis, stated wishes into consideration). Use doses of *diluted IV* **adrenaline** as recommended in Advanced Life Support guidelines; *IM* **adrenaline** is not recommended after a cardiac arrest.

Patients taking ß-blockers (ß-adrenergic receptor blocking drugs), TCAs or MAOIs

Patients taking ß-blockers, particularly non-cardioselective ones, are at increased risk of severe anaphylaxis because the ß-receptor-mediated effects of **adrenaline** are blunted. Further, unopposed stimulation of a-receptors, with reflex vagotonic effects, may lead to bradycardia, coronary artery constriction, *hypertension* and intracerebral haemorrhage. TCAs and MAOIs potentiate **adrenaline** and increase the risk of cardiac arrhythmias.

Previous UK anaphylaxis guidelines recommended halving the dose of **adrenaline** given to patients on ß-blockers, TCAs and MAOIs.[16] However, current guidelines note the large inter-individual variation in response to **adrenaline**, and this recommendation has been withdrawn. Patients on these drugs should be given a full initial dose of **adrenaline**, and further doses titrated according to the initial response.[8]

For patients taking ß-blockers and unresponsive to **adrenaline**, give **glucagon** 1–2mg SC, IM or IV every 5min, or as an IV infusion. **Glucagon** has ß-receptor independent inotropic, chronotropic and vaso-active effects.[8,11] These patients in particular may not respond to nebulized **salbutamol** and may require IV **salbutamol** or nebulized **ipratropium bromide** (see Box C).[8,12]

Follow-up

After the successful treatment of the acute event, other measures need to be considered (Box D).

Box C   Supplementary measures for anaphylaxis

Administer oxygen (>10L/min) if there is respiratory difficulty.

Insert an IV cannula or butterfly needle. If the patient is hypotensive give 0.9% saline 500mL–1L IV fluid over 10min.[13]   Repeat if blood pressure remains low.

If bronchospasm does not respond to three drug management (see Box B), give a nebulized ß$_2$ agonist, e.g. salbutamol 5mg, every 20min or as necessary.

If bronchospasm does not respond to nebulized salbutamol, consider a slow IV injection of salbutamol 250microgram diluted to 5mL with WFI, or a nebulized antimuscarinic bronchodilator, e.g. ipratropium bromide 500microgram, repeated as necessary.[4,12]

Occasionally, emergency tracheotomy and assisted respiration are necessary.

Some centres also give an H$_2$-receptor antagonist, e.g. ranitidine 50mg IV diluted to 20mL with 0.9% saline and given over 2min or 150mg PO stat.[14,15] However, H$_2$-receptors are involved only to a limited extent in anaphylaxis, and the use of an H$_2$-receptor antagonist in this situation is not essential.[8,9]

Monitor pulse, blood pressure, pulse oximetry and ECG tracings for ≥6h, ideally in a clinical area with full resuscitation facilities.

Box D   Follow-up

If the patient's prognosis is months rather than weeks, take a blood sample for mast cell tryptase as soon as possible after starting emergency treatment and a second sample not later than 4h after the onset of symptoms, and refer to an allergy clinic in due course.

If a patient has frequent idiopathic anaphylaxis, e.g. ≥2 in two months or ≥6 episodes in a year, continue both:
- **chlorphenamine** 4mg PO q6h (maximum 24mg/24h) for 2–3 months *and*
- **dexamethasone** 8mg once daily for 1 week and, then, if no further episodes of anaphylaxis or urticaria/angioedema occur, tail off over 2 weeks.[5,17]

Advise patients to avoid the suspected environmental, dietary or drug trigger.

Provide information about recognizing and managing an anaphylactic reaction.

Unless definitely caused by a drug or blood product, supply the patient with an **adrenaline** auto-injector, e.g. EpiPen.[18]

Adrenaline auto-injectors are device-specific in terms of injection technique, thus the patient should continue to use the same brand.

1   Simons FE *et al.* (2012) 2012 Update: World Allergy Organization Guidelines for the assessment and management of anaphylaxis. *Current Opinion in Allergy and Clinical Immunology.* **12**: 389–399.
2   Simons FE and Sheikh A (2013) Anaphylaxis: the acute episode and beyond. *British Medical Journal.* **346**: f602.
3   Simons FE (2010) Anaphylaxis. *Journal of Allergy and Clinical Immunology.* **125**: S161–181.
4   Khan BQ and Kemp SF (2011) Pathophysiology of anaphylaxis. *Current Opinion in Allergy and Clinical Immunology.* **11**: 319–325.
5   Greenberger PA (2007) Idiopathic anaphylaxis. *Immunology and Allergy Clinics of North America.* **27**: 273–293, vii–viii.
6   Pharmax (1998) *Data on file.*
7   MHRA (2012) All medical devices and medicinal products containing chlorhexidine. *Medical Devices Alert.* MDA/2012/075 www.mhra.gov.uk/Safetyinformation
8   Resuscitation Council (UK) (2008) Emergency treatment of anaphylactic reactions *Guidelines for healthcare providers.* www.resus.org.uk/pages/mediMain.htm
9   Simons FE *et al.* (2011) World Allergy Organization anaphylaxis guidelines: summary. *Journal of Allergy and Clinical Immunology.* **127**: 587–593 e581-522.
10 Rutkowski K *et al.* (2012) Anaphylaxis: current state of knowledge for the modern physician. *Postgraduate Medical Journal.* **88**: 458–464.
11 Soar J (2009) Emergency treatment of anaphylaxis in adults: concise guidance. *Clinical Medicine.* **9**: 181–185.
12 British National Formulary Section 3.4.3 Anaphylaxis. In. BMJ Group and Pharmaceutical Press www.bnf.org (accessed April 2013).
13 Annane D *et al.* (2013) Effects of fluid resuscitation with colloids vs crystalloids on mortality in critically ill patients presenting with hypovolemic shock: the CRISTAL randomized trial. *Journal of the American Medical Association.* **310**: 1809–1817.
14 Ellis AK and Day JH (2003) Diagnosis and management of anaphylaxis. *Canadian Medical Association Journal.* **169**: 307–311.
15 Mayumi *et al.* (1987) Intravenous cimetidine as an effective treatment for systemic anaphylaxis and acute allergic skin reaction. *Annals of Allergy.* **58**: 447–450.
16 McLean-Tooke AP *et al.* (2003) Adrenaline in the treatment of anaphylaxis: what is the evidence? *British Medical Journal.* **327**: 1332–1335.
17 Poon M and Reid C (2004) Best evidence topic reports. Oral corticosteroids in acute urticaria. *Emergency Medical Journal.* **21**: 76–77.
18 NICE (2011) Anaphylaxis. Assessment to confirm an anaphylactic episode and the decision to refer after emergency treatment for a suspected anaphylactic episode *Clinical Guideline.* CG134. www.nice.org.uk

Updated July 2014

28: DRUGS FOR PRURITUS

Pathophysiology

Although pruritus is limited to skin, conjunctivae or a mucous membrane (including the upper respiratory tract), the cause is not always peripheral (Box A).

Box A   A neuro-anatomical classification of pruritus

Peripheral causes
Cutaneous ('pruritoceptive'), e.g.
  skin diseases
  urticaria (most)
  stinging nettle rash
  insect bite reactions
  drug (± rash)
  cutaneous mastocytosis (rare)
Neuropathic, e.g.
  post-herpetic neuralgia

Central causes
Neuropathic, e.g.
  brain injury[1]
  brain abscess
  brain tumour[1]
  multiple sclerosis
Neurogenic, e.g.
  opioid
  cholestasis
  paraneoplastic
  Psychogenic

Mixed peripheral and central causes
Uraemia

Pruritogens

The afferent nerve fibres associated with peripheral causes of pruritus are a subset of C-fibres.[2,3] Their terminals are more superficial than the nociceptive C-fibres, close to the junction between epidermis and dermis and are stimulated by a wide range of pruritogens (Box B).

Box B   Chemical mediators of pruritus (pruritogens)

Amines, e.g.
  histamine
  serotonin
Opioids
Eicosanoids[a]
Cytokines
Proteases
Growth factors

Neuropeptides, e.g.
  substance P
  calcitonin-gene-related peptide (CGRP)
  bradykinin
  somatostatin
  vaso-active intestinal peptide (VIP)
  cholecystokinin

---

a. collective term for metabolites of arachidonic acid, including prostanoids and leukotrienes.

Studies suggest that there are two peripheral pathways for pruritus; one activated by histamine and the other by alternative pruritogens (e.g. cowhage spicules).[4] This helps to explain why some types of pruritus do not respond, or respond only weakly, to H_1 antihistamines.

Histamine
Histamine is an important chemical mediator of pruritus of cutaneous origin. Endogenous histamine released in the skin is mostly from mast cells and mediates pruritus via H_1-, H_4-[5,6] and possibly H_3-receptors.[7] Further, histamine probably also stimulates the formation of other pruritogens.[8]

H_4-receptors are also found in the spinal cord and brain.[9] Thus, histamine may be involved in some forms of central pruritus.

Proteases
Proteases are released from mast cells and keratinocytes and act on PAR2 receptors expressed on afferent neurones and keratinocytes.[10,11]

Serotonin/5HT
Serotonin/5HT is a weaker pruritogen than histamine.[12] Pruritus associated with spinal opioids is relieved by $5HT_3$-receptor antagonists.[13] Paradoxically, SSRIs (which have a serotonin/5HT *agonistic* effect) relieve pruritus associated with primary biliary cirrhosis,[14,15] cancer[16] and uraemia.[17]

Substance P
Substance P is released from mast cells and mediates pruritus via NK_1-receptors. The expression of these receptors is increased on keratinocytes in pruritic skin disease.[18] Aprepitant, an NK_1 antagonist, relieves pruritus in cancer patients receiving targeted anti-cancer drugs.[19]

Pruritus in systemic disease
Pruritus occurs in many systemic conditions (Box C), and may be caused by peripheral or central mechanisms, or both (Box D).

Box C   Systemic disease associated with pruritus[20]

Endocrine
Carcinoid syndrome
Diabetes mellitus (associated with genital candidosis)
Hyperparathyroidism (secondary to chronic renal failure)[a]
Hyperthyroidism
Hypothyroidism

Haematological
Leukaemia
Lymphoma
Mastocytosis
Multiple myeloma
Polycythaemia rubra vera

Hepatic
Cholestasis
Hepatitis
Primary biliary cirrhosis

Renal
Chronic renal failure

Other
AIDS
Cancer
Multiple sclerosis

a. correction of hypercalcaemia leads to the rapid relief; in other circumstances, hypercalcaemia is *not* associated with pruritus.

Box D   Causal factors in pruritus[a]

Cholestasis
Endogenous opioids ↑
Autotaxin[b] ↑
Serotonin release ↑

Old age
Dry skin
Mast cell degranulation[21] ↑
Skin sensitivity to histamine[21] ↑

Paraneoplastic
Histamine release from basophils
Serotonin release ↑
Immune response

Renal failure
Cytokines
Substance P release ↑
Skin divalent ions (Ca^{2+}, Mg^{2+}, PO_4^{2-}) ↑
Skin vitamin A ↑
Mast cell proliferation
µ- and κ-opioid receptor imbalance
Peripheral neuropathy

Targeted treatment with anti-EGFR drugs or tyrosine-kinase inhibitors
Secretion of stem-cell factors ↑ and accumulation of dermal mast cells in areas of skin rash
NK_1-receptors in mast cells and keratinocytes in inflamed areas[22] ↑

a. dry skin is often an important concurrent factor
b. causal role suggested by autotaxin concentration being considerably reduced by rifampicin.[23]

Drugs

All drugs have the potential to cause an allergic reaction which can cause pruritus, with or without a rash (Box E). The mechanism involves the release of histamine from mast cells. The pruritus responds to H_1 antihistamines (and stopping the offending drug).

Box E	Common allergic drug skin reactions	
Rashes		**Urticaria**
Cephalosporins		Cephalosporins
Penicillins		Penicillins
Phenytoin		Radio-opaque dyes
Sulfonamides		Sulfonamides

Opioid-induced pruritus

There are two types of opioid-induced pruritus. One is an allergic reaction related to cutaneous histamine release, and possibly occurs in only ~1% of patients receiving an opioid systemically. It responds to H_1 antihistamines and a switch in opioid.

Histamine is also released after an *intradermal* injection of an opioid (and responds to H_1 antihistamines). However, this is probably irrelevant in relation to pruritus associated with systemic opioids because *in vitro* studies indicate that the dose of **morphine** or **methadone** needed to release histamine from mast cells is some 10,000 times greater than the dose needed for μ agonist effects.[24]

The second type is a central reaction to opioids, and is less histamine-dependent.[25–27] In surgical (opioid-naïve) patients who receive spinal opioids pre-operatively, the incidence is ≤80% but, in patients with chronic pain already taking opioids by another route, only 10–15%.[28–30] The incidence also depends on the opioid used; for example, pruritus is four times more common with epidural **morphine** than epidural **hydromorphone**.[31]

However, anecdotally in cancer patients receiving palliative care, the incidence of pruritus in such patients appears to be virtually zero,[32] possibly because of the concurrent use of **bupivacaine**.[33,34]

Several hours after spinal injection, pruritus typically spreads rostrally through the thorax from the level of the injection and is typically maximal in the face, but may be limited to the nose (more likely when **bupivacaine** is given concurrently).[35]

Although pruritus induced by either systemic or spinal **morphine** is relieved by **naloxone** or **naltrexone**, this risks reversal of analgesia.[36] Other options are discussed in Chapter 21, p.720.

Management

Correct the correctable

Consider and treat:
- dry skin: very common in advanced cancer. Even when there is a probable endogenous cause, rehydration of the skin may obviate the need for specific measures (see Emollients, p.611)
- review the patient's medication: if a drug is the likely cause (Box E) it should be stopped, and an alternative prescribed if necessary (for opioids, see Table 1 below). With **penicillins** the pruritic rash may not appear until several days after the antibacterial has been stopped
- atopic dermatitis: topical corticosteroid and an emollient (see p.611)
- contact dermatitis: topical corticosteroid, identify causal substance, avoid further contact
- scabies: topical **permethrin** or **malathion** (see respective SPCs)
- cholestatic pruritus secondary to obstruction of the common bile duct: this resolves if the jaundice is relieved by inserting an intraductal stent via ERCP or other drainage procedure
- Hodgkin's lymphoma: radiotherapy and/or chemotherapy.

Non-drug treatment

Non-drug treatment includes the following measures:
- avoid soap; use moisturizing soap substitutes
- apply emollient b.d–t.d.s.

Table 1 Suggested treatment for specific causes of pruritus (UK)[a,b]

Condition	Step 1	Step 2	Step 3
Cholestasis[c]	Sertraline 50–100mg once daily A[15] or Rifampicin 150–600mg once daily A[49,50]	Danazol 200mg once daily–t.d.s.; if successful, titrate progressively downwards (e.g. to thrice weekly) after 2–3 weeks[51,52]	Naltrexone[d,e] 12.5–250mg once daily A[50,53]
Uraemia	If localized, capsaicin cream 0.025–0.075% once daily–q.d.s. A[38,39] or UVB phototherapy A[37]	Doxepin 10mg b.d. A[46] or Gabapentin 100–400mg after haemodialysis A[54–56]	Sertraline 50mg once daily B[17] or Naltrexone 50mg once daily A[e,f 57]
Systemic opioids (for spinal opioids, see Chapter 21, Box C, p.721)	Stat dose of H₁-antihistamine, e.g. chlorphenamine 4–12mg; if after 2–3h there is definite benefit, prescribe 4mg t.d.s. (for alternatives, see main text above) or a less sedative second generation H₁-antihistamine, e.g. cetirizine 10mg once daily/at bedtime[58]	Switch opioid, e.g. morphine →oxycodone[27,59]	Ondansetron 8mg PO b.d.
Hodgkin's lymphoma	Prednisolone 10–20mg t.d.s.	Cimetidine 800mg/24h[g] [60]	Carbamazepine 200mg b.d.[61]
Paraneoplastic, other causes, idiopathic	Sertraline 50–100mg once daily or Paroxetine 5–20mg once daily A	Mirtazapine 15–30mg at bedtime[62]	Thalidomide (see below When all else fails)

a. strength of recommendations: grade **A** is based on evidence from ≥1 RCTs, and grade **B** on well-designed non-randomized studies;[63] where no grade is given, the recommendation is based on case reports and/or expert opinion

b. given PO unless stated otherwise

c. in total bile duct obstruction, where bile duct stenting is impossible or unwanted

d. this is first-line treatment at some specialist liver centres

e. unsuitable for patients who need opioids for pain relief

f. RCTs give contradictory results: much benefit vs. no benefit (see *Commentary* below and Opioid antagonists, p.450)

g. in various haematological cancers, there are anecdotal reports of enhanced benefit when an H₁ antagonist and an H₂ antagonist are used in combination.

- discourage scratching: file finger nails, allow gentle rubbing
- avoid prolonged hot baths
- dry the skin by patting gently with a soft towel or use a hair dryer *on a cool setting*
- avoid overheating and sweating, particularly in bed at night
- increase air humidity in the bedroom to avoid skin drying
- in uraemia: UVB phototherapy.[37]

Drug treatment

Topical applications

Traditional topical antipruritics include **phenol** 0.5–3%, **levomenthol (menthol)** 0.5–2% and **camphor** 0.5–3% (see p.618). Although not practical to apply topical products over the whole body, some patients with generalized pruritus have areas of greater intensity and obtain benefit from the more selective application of a topical antipruritic.

In uraemic pruritus, **capsaicin** cream 0.025–0.075% once daily–q.d.s. may help.[38,39] Some patients find the burning sensation after application unacceptable (see p.584). Transdermal high-dose capsaicin has been reported to be of benefit in localized pruritus, e.g. brachioradial pruritus[40] and notalgia paresthetica.[41]

Although **doxepin** has also been used topically in various conditions, it has several disadvantages which limit such use (see p.618).

Systemic treatment

If the skin is inflamed as a result of scratching (but not infected), consider a corticosteroid, e.g. **dexamethasone** 2–4mg each morning or **prednisolone** 10–20mg each morning for 1 week.

Unless specific treatment is indicated, consider a trial of a sedative antihistamine either at bedtime (pruritus is generally worse at bedtime and through the night) or round the clock, depending on circumstances. Either an H_1-receptor antagonist or a phenothiazine with antihistaminic properties can be used:

- **chlorphenamine** 4mg t.d.s.–12mg q.d.s.; useful for rapid dose escalation to determine if an antihistamine is of benefit
- **promethazine** 25–50mg b.d.
- **hydroxyzine** 10–25mg b.d.–t.d.s.; 25–100mg at bedtime
- **alimemazine (trimeprazine)** 5–10mg b.d.–t.d.s.; 10–30mg at bedtime
- **levomepromazine** 6–25mg PO at bedtime.[42]

For some patients, a benzodiazepine is as effective as a sedative antihistamine.[43]

Doxepin, a TCA and potent H_1- and H_2-receptor antagonist, is a further alternative. Most TCAs have antihistaminic properties but **doxepin** is the most potent in this respect.[44] Some patients with chronic urticaria unresponsive to conventional H_1 antihistamines obtain relief from **doxepin** 10–75mg PO at bedtime.[45] In an RCT, **doxepin** 10mg b.d. PO was effective in patients with uraemic pruritus.[46]

Table 1 provides clinicians with a synopsis of possible treatments of choice. Some are supported by evidence from RCTs but, for others, the evidence is low level ('opinions and/or clinical experiences of respected authorities'). Further information is available elsewhere.[47,48]

Commentary

There appear to be similarities between neuropathic pain, pruritus and cough. The common theme being peripheral and central sensitization of the sensory nervous system. This may explain why a range of anti-epileptics and antidepressants have been reported as effective treatments for these very different symptoms. The persistence of pruritus in patients with myeloproliferative disorders despite disease control suggests central sensitization.

The inclusion of **carbamazepine** as an option for the treatment of pruritus with lymphoma or cancer is based on its successful use in just four patients (three with B-cell lymphoma and one with myeloma).[61] It had previously used with good effect in three patients with multiple sclerosis.[64]

Paroxetine, an SSRI, has been shown in an RCT to be of benefit in various situations (including solid cancers, haematological cancers, non-cancer disorders and idiopathic) but, because of its antimuscarinic effects and possible delirium in the elderly, **sertraline** is a better choice. (**Fluoxetine** and **citalopram** appear *not* to be effective). The antidepressant **mirtazapine**, an H_1-, $5HT_2$-, $5HT_3$-receptor antagonist, is reported anecdotally to be effective in pruritus associated with cancer and lymphoma.[62] Anecdotally, patients who fail to respond to an SSRI may respond to **mirtazapine**, and sometimes vice versa.

Although **ondansetron**, a $5HT_3$ antagonist, relieves pruritus induced by spinal opioids, it does *not* relieve cholestatic or uraemic pruritus.[65]

The classic hepatic enzyme inducer, **rifampicin**, in a dose of 300–600mg once daily has been shown to be of benefit in two RCTs lasting 1–2 weeks in patients with cholestatic pruritus.[49,50] Because of rare reports of severe hepatotoxicity with **rifampicin** and because of intolerance in cachectic patients, a lower starting dose is advisable, i.e. 150mg.

It has long been known that 17-α alkyl androgens relieve pruritus associated with cholestasis.[51,52] However, because they can be hepatotoxic, cholestasis (and thus the accompanying jaundice) may worsen. In patients with primary biliary cirrhosis this may be unwelcome. Over the decades several of this class of androgens have been withdrawn from the market for commercial reasons. **Danazol** is available in the UK but, in some countries, **methyltestosterone** (not UK) 25mg SL once daily will be a more convenient alternative.[51,52]

Significant benefit with **naltrexone** was seen in an RCT of uraemic patients with very severe pruritus[66] but not in patients with only moderate pruritus (also see Opioid antagonists, p.450).[67] Uraemic pruritus is multifactorial in origin (see Box D), and it is possible that μ- and κ-opioid receptor imbalance is significant only in very severe cases. This would fit with the results of a third RCT in which there was a subset of patients with uraemic pruritus who responded 'dramatically well' to **naltrexone**.[68] **Nalfurafine** (a κ agonist, not UK) 5microgram has been shown to be of benefit when given either IV after haemodialysis or PO once daily.[69,70]

Some patients with liver metastases and cholestasis produce endogenous opioids which may cause both pruritus and analgesia.[71] Anecdotally, although pain-free and not requiring opioids beforehand, some patients with cancer and cholestatic pruritus experience pain after treatment with **naltrexone**. Further, transient opioid withdrawal effects are common when PO **nalmefene**, an opioid antagonist, is used in cholestasis.[72]

Pruritus occurs in ≤ 50% of patients with polycythaemia vera. The treatment of choice is aspirin 300mg once daily–b.d. This is usually effective in < 30min, and the effect lasts 12–24h.[73]

Other options

In *en cuirass* breast cancer complicated by inflammation, local pruritus and pain, an NSAID may reduce both pruritus and pain.[74] An NSAID can also be helpful whenever there is inflammation present, either primary or secondary to scratching.

In cholestatic pruritus, the two RCTs which showed benefit with **colestyramine** (4g once or twice daily) were methodologically poor.[50] Many patients find **colestyramine** unpalatable, and it may cause nausea, vomiting and diarrhoea. It is not of value in complete large duct biliary obstruction.

Some recommendations are more or less specific to one particular disease. For example, **gabapentin** is a good choice in uraemic pruritus[54–56] whereas, in an RCT in cholestasis, **gabapentin** was less effective than placebo.[75] However, there are anecdotal reports of benefit in neuropathic pruritus and in pruritus of unknown origin.[76,77] Dose as for neuropathic pain (see p.272).

Aprepitant has been used successfully for the management of severe pruritus related to targeted biological cancer treatment with anti-EGFR antibodies and tyrosine-kinase inhibitors.[19] There are also case reports of benefit in other cancer patients.[78,79]

When all else fails

The treatments suggested for pruritus associated with 'other causes or idiopathic' (Table 1, bottom row) should be considered in all cases of intractable pruritus if the more specific options have failed to relieve.

Thalidomide 100–200mg at bedtime has been used successfully in paraneoplastic, Hodgkin's lymphoma and uraemic pruritus.[80–82] However, its cost is prohibitive, and it may cause severe neuropathy when used long-term (see p.543).

Midazolam may be of benefit in intractable central pruritus.[83,84] In one patient with cancer of the pancreas and cholestatic pruritus, CSCI midazolam was effective 'within a few hours' (2mg bolus followed by 1mg/h, increasing by 1mg/h every 15min p.r.n.), whereas **lorazepam** 1mg q6h or 2mg at bedtime (and several other psychotropic drugs) was ineffective.[84]

1 Dey DD et al. (2005) Central neuropathic itch from spinal-cord cavernous hemangioma: a human case, a possible animal model, and hypotheses about pathogenesis. Pain. 113: 233–237.
2 Schmelz M et al. (1997) Specific C-receptors for itch in human skin. Journal of Neuroscience. 17: 8003–8008.
3 Schmelz M et al. (2000) Which nerve fibers mediate the axon reflex flare in human skin? Neuroreport. 11: 645–648.
4 Namer B et al. (2008) Separate peripheral pathways for pruritus in man. Journal of Neurophysiology. 100: 2062–2069.
5 Dunford PJ et al. (2007) Histamine H4 receptor antagonists are superior to traditional antihistamines in the attenuation of experimental pruritus. Journal of Allergy and Clinical Immunology. 119: 176–183.
6 Cowden JM et al. (2010) The histamine H4 receptor mediates inflammation and pruritus in Th2-dependent dermal inflammation. Journal of Investigative Dermatology. 130: 1023–1033.
7 Sugimoto Y et al. (2004) Pruritus-associated response mediated by cutaneous histamine H3 receptors. Clinical and Experimental Allergy. 34: 456–459.
8 Yao G et al. (1992) Histamine-caused itch induces Fos-like immunoreactivity in dorsal horn neurons: effect of morphine pretreatment. Brain Research. 599: 333–337.
9 Strakhova MI et al. (2009) Localization of histamine H4 receptors in the central nervous system of human and rat. Brain Research. 1250: 41–48.
10 Steinhoff M et al. (2003) Proteinase-activated receptor-2 mediates itch: a novel pathway for pruritus in human skin. Journal of Neuroscience. 23: 6176–6180.
11 Reddy VB et al. (2008) Cowhage-evoked itch is mediated by a novel cysteine protease: a ligand of protease-activated receptors. Journal of Neuroscience. 28: 4331–4335.
12 Lowitt M and Bernhard J (1992) Pruritus. Seminars in Neurology. 12: 374–384.
13 Weisshaar E et al. (1997) Can a serotonin type 3 (5-HT3) receptor antagonist reduce experimentally-induced itch? Inflamm Research. 46: 412–416.
14 Browning J et al. (2003) Long-term efficacy of sertraline as a treatment for cholestatic pruritus in patients with primary biliary cirrhosis. American Journal of Gastroenterology. 98: 2736–2741.
15 Mayo MJ et al. (2007) Sertraline as a first-line treatment for cholestatic pruritus. Hepatology. 45: 666–674.
16 Zylicz Z et al. (2003) Paroxetine in the treatment of severe non-dermatological pruritus: a randomized, controlled trial. Journal of Pain and Symptom Management. 26: 1105–1112.
17 Shakiba M et al. (2012) Effect of sertraline on uremic pruritus improvement in ESRD patients. International Journal of Nephrology. 2012: 363901.
18 Chang SE et al. (2007) Neuropeptides and their receptors in psoriatic skin in relation to pruritus. British Journal of Dermatology. 156: 1272–1277.
19 Santini D et al. (2012) Aprepitant for management of severe pruritus related to biological cancer treatments: a pilot study. Lancet Oncology. 13: 1020–1024.
20 Greaves M (1992) Itching-research has barely scratched the surface. New England Journal of Medicine. 326: 1016–1017.
21 Guillet G et al. (2000) Increased histamine release and skin hypersensitivity to histamine in senile pruritus: study of 60 patients. European Academy of Dermatology and Venerology. 14: 65–68.
22 Gerber PA et al. (2010) Preliminary evidence for a role of mast cells in epidermal growth factor receptor inhibitor-induced pruritus. Journal of the American Academy of Dermatology. 63: 163–165.
23 Kremer AE et al. (2012) Serum autotaxin is increased in pruritus of cholestasis, but not of other origin, and responds to therapeutic interventions. Hepatology. 56: 1391–1400.
24 Barke K and Hough L (1993) Opiates, mast cells and histamine release. Life Sciences. 53: 1391–1399.
25 Reisine T and Pasternak G (1996) Opioid analgesics and antagonists. In: J Hardman et al. (eds) Goodman and Gilman's The Pharmacological Basis of Therapeutics (9e). McGraw-Hill, London, pp. 521–555.
26 Krajnik M (2004) Opioid-induced pruritus. In: Z Zylicz et al. (eds) Pruritus in advanced disease. Oxford University Press, London, pp. 84–96.
27 Tarcatu D et al. (2007) Are we still scratching the surface? A case of intractable pruritus following systemic opioid analgesia. Journal of Opioid Management. 3: 167–170.
28 Paice JA et al. (1996) Intraspinal morphine for chronic pain: a retrospective, multicenter study. Journal of Pain and Symptom Management. 11: 71–80.
29 Winkelmuller W et al. (1999) Intrathecal opioid therapy for pain: Efficacy and outcomes. Neuromodulation. 2: 67–76.
30 Smith TJ et al. (2002) Randomized clinical trial of an implantable drug delivery system compared with comprehensive medical management for refractory cancer pain: impact on pain, drug-related toxicity, and survival. Journal of Clinical Oncology. 20: 4040–4049.
31 Chaplan SR et al. (1992) Morphine and hydromorphone epidural analgesia. Anesthesiology. 77: 1090–1094.
32 Lynch L (2014) Personal communication.
33 Asokumar B et al. (1998) Intrathecal bupivacaine reduces pruritus and prolongs duration of fentanyl analgesia during labor: a prospective, randomized, controlled trial. Anaesthesia and Analgesia. 87: 1309–1315.
34 Reich A and Szepietowski JC (2010) Opioid-induced pruritus: an update. Clinical Experimental Dermatology. 35: 2–6.
35 Ballantyne J et al. (1988) Itching after epidural and spinal opiates. Pain. 33: 149–160.
36 Kjellberg F and Tramer M (2001) Pharmacological control of opioid-induced pruritus: a quantitative systematic review of randomized trials. European Journal of Anaesthesiology. 18: 346–357.
37 Gilchrest B et al. (1997) Relief of uremic pruritus with ultraviolet phototherapy. New England Journal of Medicine. 297: 136–138.
38 Breneman D et al. (1992) Topical capsaicin for treatment of hemodialysis-related pruritus. Journal of the American Academy of Dermatology. 26: 91–94.
39 Makhlough A (2010) Topical capsaicin therapy for uremic pruritus in patients on hemodialysis. Iranian Journal of Kidney Disease. 4: 137–140.
40 Zeidler. C et al. (2013) A capsaicin 8% patch for the treatment of brachioradial pruritus. Acta Derm Venereol. 93: 599–640.
41 Metz M et al. (2011) Treatment of notalgia paraesthetica with an 8% capsaicin patch. British Journal of Dermatology. 165: 1359–1361.
42 Closs S (1997) Personal communication.
43 Muston H et al. (1979) Differential effect of hypnotics and anxiolytics on itch and scratch. Journal of Investigative Dermatology. 72: 283.
44 Figge J et al. (1979) Tricyclic antidepressants: potent blockade of histamine H$_1$ receptors of guinea pig ileum. European Journal of Pharmacology. 58: 479–483.

45 Figueiredo A et al. (1990) Mechanism of action of doxepin in the treatment of chronic urticaria. Fundamental and Clinical Pharmacology. **4**: 147–158.

46 Pour-Reza-Gholi F et al. (2007) Low-dose doxepin for treatment of pruritus in patients on hemodialysis. Iranian Journal of Kidney Diseases. **1**: 34–37.

47 Misery. L et al. (eds) (2010) Pruritus. Springer, London.

48 Xander C et al. (2013) Pharmacological interventions for pruritus in adult palliative care patients. Cochrane Database of Systematic Reviews. **6**: CD008320.

49 Ghent C and Carruthers S (1988) Treatment of pruritus in primary biliary cirrhosis with rifampin. Results of a double-blind crossover randomized trial. Gastroenterology. **94**: 488–493.

50 Tandon P et al. (2007) The efficacy and safety of bile acid binding agents, opioid antagonists, or rifampin in the treatment of cholestasis-associated pruritus. American Journal of Gastroenterology. **102**: 1528–1536.

51 Ahrens E et al. (1950) Primary biliary cirrhosis. Medicine. **29**: 299–364.

52 Lloyd-Thomas H and Sherlock S (1952) Testosterone therapy for the pruritus of obstructive jaundice. British Medical Journal. **ii**: 1289–1291.

53 Wolfhagen F et al. (1997) Oral naltrexone treatment for cholestatic pruritus: A double-blind, placebo-controlled study. Gastroenterology. **113**: 1264–1269.

54 Razeghi E et al. (2009) Gabapentin and uremic itching in hemodialysis patients. Renal Failure. **31**: 85–90.

55 Gunal AI et al. (2004) Gabapentin therapy for pruritus in haemodialysis patients: a randomized, placebo-controlled, double-blind trial. Nephrology, Dialysis, Transplantation. **19**: 3137–3139.

56 Naini AE et al. (2007) Gabapentin: a promising drug for the treatment of uremic pruritus. Saudi J of Kidney Diseases and Translanation. **18**: 378–381.

57 Quan Phan N (2010) Antipruritic treatment with systemic u-opioid receptor antagonists; a review. Journal of the American Academy of Dermatology. **63**: 680–688.

58 Gaudy- Marqueste C (ed) (2010) Antihistimines. In: Pruritus. Springer, London, pp. 277–287.

59 Hassenbusch SJ et al. (2004) Polyanalgesic Consensus Conference 2003: an update on the management of pain by intraspinal drug delivery– report of an expert panel. Journal of Pain and Symptom Management. **27**: 540–563.

60 Aymard J et al. (1980) Cimetidine for pruritus in Hodgkin's disease. British Medical Journal. **280**: 151–152.

61 Korfitis C and Trafalis DT (2008) Carbamazepine can be effective in alleviating tormenting pruritus in patients with hematologic malignancy. Journal of Pain and Symptom Management. **35**: 571–572.

62 Davis M et al. (2003) Mirtazapine for pruritus. Journal of Pain and Symptom Management. **25**: 288–291.

63 BMJ Publishing Group (2009) Resources for authors. Checklists and forms: clinical management guidelines. Available from: http://resources.bmj.com/bmj/authors/checklists-forms/clinical-management-guidelines

64 Osterman PO (1976) Paroxysmal itching in multiple sclerosis. British Journal of Dermatology. **95**: 555–558.

65 To TH et al. (2012) The role of ondansetron in the management of cholestatic or uremic pruritus–a systematic review. Journal of Pain and Symptom Management. **44**: 725–730.

66 Peer G et al. (1996) Randomised crossover trial of naltrexone in uraemic pruritus. Lancet. **348**: 1552–1554.

67 Pauli-Magnus C et al. (2000) Naltrexone does not relieve uremic pruritus. Journal of the American Society of Nephrology. **11**: 514–519.

68 Legroux-Crespel E et al. (2004) A comparative study on the effects of naltrexone and loratadine on uremic pruritus. Dermatology. **208**: 326–330.

69 Wikstrom B et al. (2005) Kappa-opioid system in uremic pruritus: multicenter, randomized, double-blind, placebo-controlled clinical studies. Journal of the American Society of Nephrology. **16**: 3742–3747.

70 Kumagai H et al. (2012) Efficacy and safety of a novel k-agonist for managing intractable pruritus in dialysis patients. American Journal of Nephrology. **36**: 175–183.

71 Bergasa NV et al. (1994) Cholestasis in the male rat is associated with naloxone-reversible antinociception. Journal of Hepatology. **20**: 85–90.

72 Thornton J and Losowksy M (1988) Opioid peptides and primary biliary cirrhosis. British Medical Journal. **297**: 1501–1504.

73 Jackson N et al. (1987) Skin mast cells in polycuthaemia vera: relationship to the pathogenesis and treatment of pruritus. British Journal of Dermatology. **116**: 21–29.

74 Twycross RG (1981) Pruritus and pain on en cuirass breast cancer. Lancet. **2**: 696.

75 Bergasa NV et al. (2006) Gabapentin in patients with the pruritus of cholestasis: a double-blind, randomized, placebo-controlled trial. Hepatology. **44**: 1317–1323.

76 Kanitakis J (2006) Brachioradial pruritus: report of a new case responding to gabapentin. European Journal of Dermatology. **16**: 311–312.

77 Yesudian PD and Wilson NJ (2005) Efficacy of gabapentin in the management of pruritus of unknown origin. Archives of Dermatology. **141**: 1507–1509.

78 Vincenzi B et al. (2010) Aprepitant against pruritus in patients with solid tumours. Supportive Care in Cancer. **18**: 1229–1230.

79 Torres T et al. (2012) Aprepitant: Evidence of its effectiveness in patients with refractory pruritus continues. Journal of the American Academy of Dermatology. **66**: e14–15.

80 Silva S et al. (1994) Thalidomide for the treatment of uremic pruritus: a crossover randomized double-blind trial. Nephron. **67**: 270–273.

81 Smith J et al. (2002) Use of thalidomide in the treatment of intractable itch. Poster abstract 21. In: Palliative Care Congress; Sheffield, UK.

82 Goncalves F (2010) Thalidomide for the control of severe paraneoplastic pruritus associated with Hodgkin's disease. American Journal of Hospice and Palliative Care. **27**: 486–487.

83 Thomsen JS et al. (2002) Suppression of spontaneous scratching in hairless rats by sedatives but not by antipruritics. Skin Pharmacology and Applied Skin Physiology. **15**: 218–224.

84 Prieto LN (2004) The use of midazolam to treat itching in a terminally ill patient with biliary obstruction. Journal of Pain and Symptom Management. **28**: 531–532.

Updated June 2014

29: ORAL NUTRITIONAL SUPPLEMENTS

This section provides an overview of cachexia and the use of oral nutritional supplements in adults with cancer. It does not address nutritional supplements in children, patients with renal or hepatic failure, tube feeding or parenteral nutrition.

Introduction

Weight loss is a common adverse feature of cancer, associated with increased morbidity, poorer treatment tolerability and outcomes, and reduced survival. It generally occurs in the context of cancer cachexia, a multifactorial syndrome characterized by an ongoing loss of *skeletal muscle* mass ($\pm$ fat), leading to progressive functional impairment.[1] There is negative protein and energy balance driven by a variable combination of reduced food intake and abnormal metabolism, with no standard treatment available for the latter. Nutritional support alone can prevent or slow the rate of weight loss in patients with an inadequate intake, but this appears to be via an effect on fat rather than skeletal muscle mass.[2]

Screening

Whatever the cause of malnutrition, early detection and intervention is preferable and requires a multiprofessional pro-active approach. NICE guidance suggests that all patients should be screened for malnutrition when:
- admitted to hospital, and weekly thereafter
- admitted to care homes, and repeated if there is clinical concern
- first seen in outpatients, and repeated if there is clinical concern
- registering with a general practice.

As a minimum, screening should evaluate:
- the body mass index (BMI):

$$BMI = \frac{weight(kg)}{height^2(m)}$$

- percentage unintentional weight loss
- time over which nutrient intake has been unintentionally reduced and/or the likelihood of future impaired intake.[3]

Screening tools include the Malnutrition Universal Screening Tool (MUST) and the Nutritional Risk Screening Tool 2002.[4,5] Although not validated specifically for use in patients with cancer, they are easy to complete.[5,6] The Patient Generated Subjective Global Assessment is a specific tool for patients with cancer but requires more training and takes longer to complete.[7,8]

NICE guidance suggests nutritional support should be considered for patients with:
- BMI $< 18.5 kg/m^2$
- unintentional weight loss of $> 10\%$ in the last 3–6 months
- BMI $< 20 kg/m^2$ and unintentional weight loss of $> 5\%$
- inadequate oral intake for > 5 days
- malabsorption, increased nutrient losses, increased catabolism.[3]

Using these criteria, 30% and 60% of patients with thoracic or upper GI cancers respectively are malnourished even at the time of diagnosis.[9,10] Further, it could be argued that the remainder are at risk of malnutrition because of increased catabolism.

Recent cancer-specific recommendations have suggested lower thresholds for the diagnosis of cachexia, i.e. *any* of the following:
- weight loss $> 5\%$ over past 6 months
- BMI $< 20 kg/m^2$ and weight loss $> 2\%$
- sarcopenia and weight loss $> 2\%$.[1]

Ideally, patients identified by the screening process should then have their nutritional status assessed by an appropriately trained health professional (typically a dietitian) in order to produce an individualized nutrition care plan, which includes monitoring.[6,11] The assessment would take into account the patient's physical condition and prognosis, state of hydration, dietary intake, estimation of nutritional requirements, identification of underlying symptoms contributing to malnutrition (e.g. poor oral health or dentition, nausea, early satiety), and other psychosocial and dietary considerations.

Assessment and management

Guidelines on assessment and use of enteral nutrition in (Box A) are based on The European Society for Clinical Nutrition and Metabolism (ESPEN) guidelines on enteral nutrition (non-surgical oncology).[2]

Box A Guidelines on enteral nutrition by mouth or by tube

Nutritional assessment should be performed and nutritional support started when:
- malnutrition exists
- a patient is losing weight due to insufficient nutritional intake
- it is anticipated that the patient will be unable to eat for >7 days
- it is anticipated that food intake will be inadequate for >10 days
  ▷ <60% of estimated energy requirements or
  ▷ estimated as <50% of usual pre-illness intake (based on 24h recall of intake).

Daily energy requirements
When resting energy expenditure cannot be measured, daily total energy expenditure (TEE) can be estimated:
- ambulant patient: 30–35kcal/kg/day
- bedbound patient: 20–25kcal/kg/day.
These estimates are less accurate in patients who are severely underweight (underestimates TEE) or obese (overestimates TEE).

Daily protein
Generally 1–2g/kg/day.

Daily fluid requirement
Generally 30–40mL/kg/day, but consider losses caused by pyrexia, malabsorption, fistulas, high output stomas.

Goals of therapy
- prevent and treat malnutrition
- enhance effectiveness and reduce undesirable effects of anticancer treatment
- improve quality of life.

Route
The enteral route (PO or tube feeding when PO not feasible) is preferred to the parenteral route.[12]
Tube feeding can be delivered via transnasal or percutaneous (e.g. gastrostomy, jejunostomy) routes.
Tube feeding is preferable in patients with head and neck or oesophageal cancers causing dysphagia, or when severe radiation therapy-induced oral or oesophageal mucositis is anticipated (when the percutaneous route may need to be used).
The parenteral route is preferred when there is an increased risk of bleeding or infections from tube placement, e.g. in neutropenic or thrombocytopenic patients, or when the GI tract is not functioning.

continued

> **Box A** Continued
>
> **Formula**
> Standard nutrient composition formulas (1–1.5kcal/mL) should generally be used.
> For patients with early satiety or increased nutritional requirements, high-energy high-protein formulas may be preferable.
> Peri-operatively, ESPEN recommend formulas that provide immune-modulating substrates, e.g. arginine, ω-3 fatty acids, nucleotides. However, the evidence is contradictory.[13,14]
>
> **Drug treatment**
> In the presence of chronic systemic inflammation (evidenced by a raised CRP), drug treatments are recommended in addition to nutritional support. The anti-inflammatory effects of corticosteroids and progestogens can enhance appetite, improve metabolic derangements and quality of life.[15] They should be used for short periods only, weighing their benefits against their undesirable effects, particularly the risk of thrombosis with progestogens (see p.536).
> There are contradictory findings with the ω-3 fatty acid, eicosapentanoic acid (EPA), but benefit appears most likely when given in sufficient quantities (1.5–2g EPA/day) in combination with a high-protein and high-energy nutritional supplement.[16–19]
>
> **Peri-operative**
> All patients undergoing major abdominal surgery benefit from 5–7 days of nutritional support containing immune-modulating substrates, independent of their nutritional status. Patients at severe nutritional risk benefit from 1–2 weeks of nutritional support before major surgery.
>
> **Radiation therapy, chemotherapy, or stem cell transplant**
> Enteral nutrition support should be prescribed when general indications are met (see above). Patients undergoing head and neck or GI radiation should receive nutritional support to increase dietary intake and prevent therapy-associated weight loss.
>
> **End of life**
> Generally, hunger and the urge to eat are much diminished or absent in the last weeks/days of life.[20,21] Because cachexia is considered 'refractory' in patients with a limited prognosis, i.e. <3 months, the focus of care is on providing symptom relief, addressing patient and family eating-related distress, and the use of appetite stimulants when appropriate.[1] Small amounts of food can be offered as desired by the patient to alleviate hunger, and for pleasure and social purposes.[22]

Provision of oral nutrition support

Correct the correctable
If oral intake is to be improved, attention must be paid to:
- the ability to obtain and prepare food
- oral problems, e.g. xerostomia, mucositis, oral candidosis
- uncontrolled nausea and vomiting
- dysphagia.

Particularly in relation to neurogenic dysphagia, simple measures such as adding thickeners to liquids and to semi-solid foods may be enough. Generally, patients with swallowing difficulties which put them at risk of aspiration should be assessed by a speech and language therapist (SALT).

General advice
This includes:
- meal patterns, e.g. eat small amounts frequently
- substitute water-based drinks, e.g. tea, coffee with milk-based drinks, e.g. hot chocolate, malted drinks, milky coffee
- dietary fortification, e.g. use full-fat milk and cream, extra butter, margarine, oil and sugar (fats are the most concentrated source of energy)
- consider relaxing pre-imposed dietary restrictions, e.g. diabetic diet
- making use of microwave meals and convenience foods; quick and easy to prepare, often small portions, high in fat and salt. The latter may help patients with a reduced sense of taste.

Generally, weight gain is more likely with dietary advice and nutritional supplements than with dietary advice alone in patients with illness-related malnutrition.[23]

Appetite stimulants
See Progestogens (p.536) and Systemic corticosteroids (p.499).

Oral nutritional supplements
Oral nutritional supplements should be considered when a patient is unable to improve their nutritional intake by diet alone. Generally, they should supplement existing intake rather than replace it, e.g. 1–2 cartons/day of a 1.5kcal/mL milk-based nutritional supplement. However, some products are nutritionally complete and, if ingested in sufficient quantities, can be used as a sole source of nutrition (e.g. see Table 2, p.806).

Oral nutritional supplements are available in liquid, semi-solid or powder formulations. General prescribing guidelines are contained in Box B and product details in Table 1–Table 13, including thickeners and thickened drinks for use in patients with dysphagia. Generally, the supplements are ordered within the tables according to their energy density and protein content.

Product	Table	Page
Milkshake-style nutritional supplements	1	806
High-energy milkshake-style nutritional supplements	2	806
Savoury nutritional supplements	3	806
Milkshake-style nutritional supplements with fibre	4	807
Yoghurt-style nutritional supplements	5	807
Fruit juice-style nutritional supplements	6	807
High protein milkshake-style nutritional supplements	7	808
Semi-solid nutritional supplements	8	808
Powdered milkshake- and soup-style nutritional supplements	9	809
OTC nutritional supplements	10	810
Special application nutritional products	11	810
Modular carbohydrate, protein and fat supplements	12	812
Thickeners and thickened drinks	13	814

Energy content is given per unit and per mL and the protein content per unit. For other supplements, the nutritional content is given per 100mL or 100g as appropriate. Flavours frequently alter; check availability with the manufacturer. Unless otherwise stated, all products listed are Advisory Committee on Borderline Substances (ACBS) approved for patients with disease related malnutrition.

Box B   Guidelines for prescribing oral nutritional supplements

1 Ensure correctable underlying problems are addressed and general nutritional advice has been given.

2 Guided by the patient's preferences, provide a variety of formulations and flavours either separately or in commercially available starter packs, e.g.:
   - Fortisip® Range (Nutricia) contains Fortisip®, Fortijuce® and Fortisip Yoghurt Style® in various flavours
   - Ensure Plus Commence® (Abbott) contains Ensure Plus® in various flavours.

continued

Box B Continued

3 Provide information on how to use the supplements together with any special instructions, e.g.:
  • keep supplements chilled to improve palatability
  • use the straw provided with supplement to minimize unpleasant odour
  • use supplement as a between-meal snack, not as a meal replacement
  • maintenance of good oral hygiene
  • once opened, supplements can be stored in a refrigerator for up to 24h.

4 Review patient after one week:
  • prescribe the required number of cartons/units per day of the formulation and flavour(s) which are acceptable to the patient
  • if none are acceptable, try an alternative, e.g. juice-based or milkshake powder.

5 Review patient after 4 weeks of supplement use. If weight loss continues, seek advice from a dietitian. Monitoring should continue on a monthly basis until supplements are no longer required.

6 Patients with renal or hepatic failure, malabsorption, dysphagia, or at risk of refeeding syndrome should be referred to a dietitian.

The oral nutritional supplements listed are gluten-free and most are suitable for vegetarians. Those containing fish oils (EPA) and micronutrients or colourings derived from animal sources may not be acceptable to strict vegetarians. If uncertain with patients who have specific dietary restrictions, consult a dietitian or the manufacturers for advice.

Ingesting sufficient quantities orally may be difficult for patients with anorexia or taste changes and various strategies, including recipes suggested by the manufacturers, can be tried to aid compliance (Box C).

Box C Aiding compliance with milk- and juice-based supplements

Milk-based
Serve chilled ± ice
Add extra full-fat milk
Make a smoothie by adding fresh fruit
  and ice cream
Make into a jelly
Use instead of milk on cereals and
  in puddings (unflavoured)
Use to make custard/rice pudding
  (vanilla flavour)
Further recipes are available from:
www.abbottnutrition.co.uk
www.fresenius-kabi.co.uk
www.nestlehealthscience.co.uk
www.nutricia.co.uk
www.vitaflo.co.uk

Juice-based
Serve chilled ± ice
Add extra fruit juice
Make a spritzer by adding soda
  water/lemonade/carbonated water
Make into a jelly
Pour over fresh or tinned fruit
Freeze to make an ice lolly or ice cubes

Table 1 Milkshake-style nutritional supplements (suitable as a sole source of nutrition)[a,b]
Included for completeness: generally supplements with higher energy and protein content should be used.

Product	Unit size	Energy content	Protein content	Flavours/comments
Ensure® (Abbott)	250mL Can	250kcal (1kcal/mL)	10g	Chocolate, coffee, vanilla
Fresubin® Original Drink (Fresenius)	200mL Bottle	200kcal (1kcal/mL)	8g	Blackcurrant, chocolate, mocha, nut, peach, vanilla

a. avoid acidic citrus/tangy flavours in patients with a sore mouth
b. best served chilled.

Table 2 High-energy milkshake-style nutritional supplements (suitable as a sole source of nutrition)[a,b]

Product	Unit size	Energy content	Protein content	Flavours/comments
Fortisip® Compact (Nutricia)	125mL Bottle	300kcal (2.4kcal/mL)	12g	Apricot, banana, chocolate, forest fruit, mocha, strawberry, vanilla
Ensure Plus® Milkshake Style (Abbott)	220mL Bottle	330kcal (1.5kcal/mL)	14g	Banana, chocolate, coffee, fruits of the forest, orange, peach, raspberry, strawberry, vanilla, unflavoured
Fortisip® Bottle (Nutricia)	200mL Bottle	300kcal (1.5kcal/mL)	12g	Banana, chocolate, orange, strawberry, toffee, tropical, vanilla, unflavoured
Fresubin® Energy Drink (Fresenius)	200mL Bottle	300kcal (1.5kcal/mL)	11g	Banana, blackcurrant, cappuccino, chocolate, lemon, strawberry, tropical fruit, vanilla, unflavoured
Resource® Energy (Nestle)	200mL Bottle	300kcal (1.5kcal/mL)	11g	Apricot, banana, chocolate, coffee, strawberry-raspberry, vanilla

a. avoid acidic citrus/tangy flavours in patients with a sore mouth
b. best served chilled.

Table 3 Savoury-style nutritional supplements[a]

Product	Unit size	Energy content	Protein content	Flavours/comments
Fortisip® Savoury Multi Fibre (Nutricia)	200mL Cup	300kcal (1.5kcal/mL)	15g	Contains 4.6g (60:40 soluble:insoluble) fibre. Suitable as a sole source of nutrition; chicken
Ensure Plus® Savoury (Abbott)	220mL Bottle	330kcal (1.5kcal/mL)	14g	Suitable as a sole source of nutrition; chicken, mushroom

a. best served warmed, do not boil.

Table 4 Milkshake-style nutritional supplements with fibre (suitable as a sole source of nutrition)[a,b]

Product	Unit size	Energy content	Protein content	Flavours/comments
Fortisip® Compact Fibre	125mL Bottle	300kcal (2.4kcal/mL)	12g	Contains 4.5g fibre; mocha, strawberry, vanilla
Resource® 2.0 Fibre (Nestle)	200mL Bottle	400kcal (2.0kcal/mL)	18g	Contains 5g soluble fibre (50:50 FOS:GOS), do not exceed 4 bottles/day; apricot, coffee, strawberry, summer fruit, vanilla, unflavoured
Ensure Plus® Fibre (Abbott)	200mL Bottle	310kcal (1.6kcal/mL)	13g	Contains 5g fibre and fructo-oligosaccharides; banana, chocolate, raspberry, strawberry, vanilla
Fortisip® Multi Fibre (Nutricia)	200mL Bottle	300kcal (1.5kcal/mL)	12g	Contains 4.6g (60:40 soluble:insoluble) fibre; vanilla
Fresubin® Energy Fibre Drink (Fresenius)	200mL Bottle	300kcal (1.5kcal/mL)	11g	Contains 4g mixed fibre blend; banana, caramel, cherry, chocolate, strawberry, vanilla

a. useful for patients with constipation
b. shake well before use.

Table 5 Yoghurt-style nutritional supplements (suitable as a sole source of nutrition)[a,b]

Product	Unit size	Energy content	Protein content	Flavours/comments
Ensure Plus® Yoghurt Style (Abbott)	220mL Bottle	330kcal (1.5kcal/mL)	14g	Peach, strawberry
Fortisip® Yoghurt Style (Nutricia)	200mL Bottle	300kcal (1.5kcal/mL)	12g	Peach-orange, raspberry, vanilla-lemon

a. can be more palatable in patients with taste change (citrus/tangy flavours vs. sweet)
b. avoid acidic citrus/tangy flavours in patients with a sore mouth.

Table 6 Fruit juice-style nutritional supplements (not suitable as a sole source of nutrition)[a,b]

Product	Unit size	Energy content	Protein content	Flavours/comments
Ensure Plus® Juice (Abbott)	220mL Bottle	330kcal (1.5kcal/mL)	11g	Apple, fruit punch, lemon and lime, orange, peach, strawberry
Fortijuce® (Nutricia)	200mL Bottle	300kcal (1.5kcal/mL)	8g	Apple, blackcurrant, forest fruit, lemon, orange, strawberry, tropical
Fresubin® Juicy Drink (Fresenius)	200mL Bottle	300kcal (1.5kcal/mL)	8g	Apple, blackcurrant, cherry, orange, pineapple
Resource® Fruit (Nestle)	200mL Bottle	250kcal (1.3kcal/mL)	8g	Apple, orange, pear-cherry, raspberry-blackcurrant

a. may be preferable for patients with a dry mouth
b. avoid acidic citrus/tangy flavours in patients with a sore mouth.

Table 7 High protein milkshake-style nutritional supplements (not suitable as a sole source of nutrition)[a]

Product	Unit size	Energy content	Protein content	Flavours/comments
Fortisip® Compact Protein (Nutricia)	125mL Bottle	300kcal (2.4kcal/mL)	18g	Banana, mocha, strawberry, vanilla
Fresubin® 2kcal Fibre Drink (Fresenius)	200mL Bottle	400kcal (2kcal/mL)	20g	Contains 3g fibre; apricot-peach, cappuccino, chocolate, lemon, unflavoured, vanilla
Ensure® TwoCal (Abbott)	200mL Bottle	400kcal (2kcal/mL)	17g	Contains 2g FOS; banana, strawberry, vanilla, unflavoured
Fortisip® Extra (Nutricia)	200mL Bottle	320kcal (1.6kcal/mL)	20g	Chocolate, forest fruit, mocha, strawberry, vanilla
Fresubin® Protein Energy Drink (Fresenius)	200mL Bottle	300kcal (1.5kcal/mL)	20g	Cappuccino, chocolate, strawberry, tropical fruits, vanilla
Resource® Protein (Nestle)	200mL Bottle	250kcal (1.25kcal/mL)	19g	Apricot, chocolate, forest fruits, strawberry, vanilla
Fortimel® Regular (Nutricia)	200mL Bottle	200kcal (1kcal/mL)	20g	Chocolate, forest fruits, strawberry, vanilla

a. consider in patients with high protein loss or wounds when overall energy intake is adequate.

Table 8 Semi-solid nutritional supplements (suitable as a sole source of nutrition)

Product	Unit size	Energy content	Protein content	Flavours/comments
Fresubin® Creme (Fresenius)	125g Pot	230kcal (1.8kcal/g)	13g	Cappuccino, chocolate, praline, strawberry, vanilla
Forticreme® Complete (Nutricia)	125g Pot	200kcal (1.6kcal/g)	12g	Banana, chocolate, forest fruit, vanilla
Resource® Dessert Energy (Nestle)	125g Pot	200kcal (1.6kcal/g)	6g	Caramel, chocolate, vanilla
Resource® Dessert Fruit (Nestle)	125g Pot	205kcal (1.6kcal/g)	6g	Contains 1.6g fibre; apple, apple-peach, apple-strawberry
Fresubin® YOcreme (Fresenius)	125g Pot	187kcal (1.5kcal/g)	9g	Apricot-peach, biscuit, lemon, raspberry, unflavoured
Ensure® Plus Creme (Abbott)	125g Pot	171kcal (1.4kcal/g)	7g	Banana, chocolate, vanilla, unflavoured
Nutilis® Fruit Stage 3 (Nutricia)	150g Pot	206kcal (1.4kcal/g)	11g	Contains 3.9g fibre; apple, strawberry
ProSource® Jelly (Nutrinovo)	118mL Pot	90kcal (0.75kcal/mL)	20g	Fruit punch, orange

a. useful for patients with dysphagia.

Table 9 Powdered milkshake- and soup-style nutritional supplements (not suitable as a sole source of nutrition)[a,b,c]

Product	Unit size	Energy content	Protein content	Flavours/comments
Vitasavoury® 300 (Vitaflo)	50g Sachet	309kcal (6kcal/g)	6g	Reconstitute with hot water or whole milk; chicken, golden vegetable, leek and potato, mushroom
Vitasavoury® 200 (Vitaflo)	33g Cup	204kcal (6kcal/g)	4g	Reconstitute with hot water or whole milk; chicken, golden vegetable, leek and potato, mushroom
Calshake® (Fresenius)	87g Sachet	431kcal (5kcal/g)	4g	600kcal and 12g protein when reconstituted with full-fat milk (240mL); banana, chocolate, strawberry, unflavoured, vanilla, in boxes of 7
Scandishake Mix® (Nutricia)	85g Sachet	430kcal (5kcal/g)	4g	600kcal and 12g protein when reconstituted with full-fat milk (240mL); banana, caramel, chocolate, strawberry, vanilla, unflavoured, in boxes of 6
Enshake® (Abbott)	96.5g Sachet	434kcal (4.5kcal/g)	8g	600kcal and 16g protein when reconstituted with full-fat milk (240mL); banana, chocolate, strawberry, vanilla, in boxes of 6
Foodlink Complete (Foodlink)	450g Box	245kcal (4kcal/g)	12g	1 serving = 4 heaped dessert spoons. Reconstitute with full-fat milk or water (200mL); banana, chocolate, strawberry, vanilla with fibre, unflavoured
Fresubin® Powder Extra (Fresenius)	62g Sachet	260kcal (4kcal/g)	11g	397kcal and 18g protein when reconstituted with full-fat milk (200mL); with added vitamins and minerals; chocolate, strawberry, vanilla, unflavoured
Complan® Shake (Nutricia)	57g Sachet	250kcal (4kcal/g)	9g	385kcal and 16g protein when reconstituted with full-fat milk (200mL); With added vitamins and minerals; banana, chocolate, strawberry, vanilla, unflavoured

a. high palatability
b. some products are lower in vitamins and minerals compared with other supplements
c. milkshake style should be reconstituted using full-fat milk to optimize energy content.

Table 10 OTC nutritional supplements (not suitable as a sole source of nutrition)

Product	Unit size	Energy content[a]	Protein content	Comments
Complan (Nutricia)	57g Sachet	250kcal (4.4kcal/g)	9g	Reconstitute with 200mL hot or cold water/full-fat milk; banana, chicken, chocolate, strawberry, vanilla, unflavoured, in boxes of 4
Complan Smoothie (Nutricia)	250mL Carton	272kcal (1kcal/mL)	10g	Ready to drink; berry, tropical
BuildUp® Nutritious Soups (Nestle)	49g Sachet	200kcal (4.1kcal/g)	7g	Reconstitute with 150mL hot water/full-fat milk; contains 3.2g fibre; chicken, potato and leek, tomato, vegetable
BuildUp® Original (Nestle)	400g Tub	360kcal/100g (3.6kcal/g)	24g/100g	Use to fortify foods or as a drink; unflavoured
BuildUp® Nutritious Shakes (Nestle)	38g Sachet	130kcal (3.4kcal/g)	8g	Reconstitute with 200mL full-fat milk; contains 3g soluble fibre; banana, chocolate, strawberry, vanilla, in boxes of 4

a. unconstituted.

Table 11 Special application nutritional products[9,6]

Product	Unit size	Energy content	Protein content	Flavours/comments
Forti Care® (Nutricia)	125mL Bottle	200kcal (1.6kcal/mL)	11g	For use in patients with cachexia (pancreatic cancer and lung cancer undergoing chemotherapy). Contains eicosapentanoic acid (EPA), fibre and anti-oxidants. Recommended dose 3 bottles/day (providing 2.2g EPA); not nutritionally complete at this dose; cappuccino, orange-lemon, peach-ginger
Supportan® Drink (Fresenius)	200mL Bottle	300kcal (1.5kcal/mL)	20g	For use in patients with cachexia (pancreatic cancer and lung cancer undergoing chemotherapy). Contains eicosapentanoic acid (EPA) and docosahexanoic acid (DHA), anti-oxidants and fibre. Recommended dose 2 bottles/day (providing 2.85g EPA and DHA); cappuccino, tropical fruits
ProSure® (Abbott)	240mL Tetrapak	305kcal (1.3kcal/mL)	16g	For use in patients with cachexia (pancreatic cancer and lung cancer undergoing chemotherapy). Contains eicosapentanoic acid (EPA) and anti-oxidants. An intake of 1.5–2 cartons/day is required for benefit; not nutritionally complete at this dose; vanilla

continued

Table 11 Continued

Product	Unit size	Energy content	Protein content	Flavours/comments
Oral Impact® (Nestle)	74g Sachet	303kcal	17g	Contains immune-modulating substrates and soluble fibre (e.g. ω-3 fatty acids, arginine, nucleotides). Pre-operatively, 2–4 sachets a day (dissolved in 250mL of cool boiled water) recommended for 5–7 days; not nutritionally complete at this dose; citrus, coffee, tropical
Respifor® (Nutricia)	125mL Bottle	188kcal (1.5kcal/mL)	9g	For early intervention use in patients with COPD. Recommended dose 125mL t.d.s in combination with activity plan for 3 months; chocolate, strawberry, vanilla
Elemental E028 Extra Liquid® (SHS)	250mL Tetrapak	215kcal (0.9kcal/mL)	6g	A liquid elemental feed for patients with intractable malabsorption or radiation enteritis. Protein source is a mixture of essential and non-essential amino acids. Nutritionally complete; grapefruit, orange and pineapple, summer fruits
Elemental E028 Extra Powder® (SHS)	100g Sachet	427kcal/ 100g	13g/ 100g	An elemental feed for patients with intractable malabsorption or radiation enteritis. Protein source is a mixture of essential and non-essential amino acids. Nutritionally complete. Reconstitute with 100g powder in 500mL water; banana, orange, unflavoured
Survimed® OPD Drink (Fresenius)	200mL Bottle	200kcal (1kcal/mL)	9g	A peptide based sip feed for patients with malabsorption; nutritionally complete; vanilla
Peptamen® Vanilla Bottle (Nestle)	200mL Bottle	200kcal (1kcal/mL)	8g	For patients with impaired GI function. Contains protein source as peptides and fat is 70% medium-chain triglycerides to improve digestion and absorption. Nutritionally complete. Can be flavoured with 2 scoops of Nestle Nutrition Flavour Mix/100mL to improve palatability; banana, chocolate, coffee, lemon and lime, strawberry
Resource® OptiFibre® (Nestle)	250g Tub (5g per scoop) 10g Sachet	–	–	For use with patients who have constipation. Each scoop contains 4g and each sachet 6g of soluble fibre (partially hydrolyzed guar gum) which is mixed into hot or cold liquids and foods. Introduce gradually; begin with 1 scoop or 1/2 sachet and increase by 1 scoop or 1/2 sachet every 3 days. Recommended dose is 2 sachets/3 scoops/day, maximum 32g/day
Forceval® Capsules (Alliance)	15, 30 and 90 Cap pack	–	–	Multivitamin and mineral supplement given as 1 capsule daily. Capsule can be opened and contents mixed, for example, with a teaspoon of jam
Forceval® Soluble (Alliance)	30 Tablet pack	–	–	Effervescent multivitamin and mineral supplement given as 1 tablet daily

a. use with dietetic supervision
b. listed according to type.

Table 12 Modular carbohydrate, protein and fat supplements (not suitable as a sole source of nutrition)[a,b]

Product	Unit size	Energy Source	Energy content	Comments
Caloreen® (Nestle)	500g Tub	Carbohydrate	385kcal/100g	Glucose polymer powder to add to food and drinks; unflavoured
Polycal® Powder (Nutricia)	400g Tub	Carbohydrate	384kcal/100g	Glucose polymer powder to add to food and drinks; unflavoured
Maxijul® Super Soluble Powder (SHS)	132g Sachet, 200g, 2.5kg, 25kg Tub	Carbohydrate	380kcal/100g	Glucose polymer powder to add to food and drinks; recommended dilution 1:2; unflavoured
Vitajoule® (Vitaflo)	500g, 25kg Tub	Carbohydrate	380kcal/100g	Glucose syrup powder to add to food and drinks; unflavoured
Liquid Maxijul® (SHS)	200mL Carton	Carbohydrate	247kcal/100mL	Glucose polymer solution; can be used undiluted or diluted in drinks; orange, unflavoured
Polycal® Liquid (Nutricia)	200mL Bottle	Carbohydrate	247kcal/100mL	Glucose polymer solution; can be used undiluted or diluted in drinks; orange, unflavoured
Protifar® (Nutricia)	225g Tub	Protein	380kcal/100g 89g protein/100g	High-protein powder to add to food and drinks; unflavoured
Vitapro® (Vitaflo)	250g, 2kg Tub	Protein	390kcal/100g 75g protein/100g	High-biological value powdered protein to add to food and drinks; unflavoured
Fresubin® 5kcal SHOT (Fresenius)	120mL Bottle	Fat	500kcal/100mL	Long and medium-chain triglyceride fat emulsion. Recommended dose 30mL t.d.s–q.d.s; lemon, unflavoured
Liquigen® (Nutricia)	250mL Bottle	Fat	450kcal/100mL	Medium-chain triglyceride fat emulsion; unflavoured
Calogen® (Nutricia)	200mL, 500mL Bottle	Fat	450kcal/100mL	Long-chain triglyceride fat emulsion. Recommended dose 30mL t.d.s; banana, strawberry, unflavoured
Calogen® Extra (Nutricia)	200mL Bottle, 40mL Cup	Fat, carbohydrate	400kcal/100mL 5g protein/100mL	High energy fat emulsion with protein, carbohydrate, vitamins and minerals. Recommended dose 40mL t.d.s; strawberry, unflavoured
MCT Duocal® (SHS)	400g Tub	Fat, carbohydrate	497kcal/100g	Medium-chain triglyceride and carbohydrate powder to add to food and drinks; introduce gradually as tolerated; unflavoured
Super Soluble Duocal® (SHS)	400g Tub	Fat, carbohydrate	492kcal/100g	Fat and glucose polymer powder to add to food and drinks; unflavoured

continued

Table 12 Continued

Product	Unit size	Energy Source	Energy content	Comments
Duocal® Liquid (SHS)	250mL	Fat, carbohydrate	166kcal/100mL	Fat and carbohydrate emulsion; unflavoured
ProSource® Liquid (Nutrinovo)	100 × 30mL Sachet	Protein and carbohydrate	333kcal/100mL 33g protein/100mL (30mL sachet 100kcal, 10g protein)	Protein and energy liquid to drink as a 'shot' or to add to food and drinks; citrus-berry, orange, unflavoured
Pro-Cal® Powder (Vitaflo)	15g Sachet 510g, 1.5kg, 12.5kg Tub	Protein, fat, carbohydrate	667kcal/100g 14g protein/100g	Energy and protein powder to add to food and drinks; unflavoured
MCT Pro-Cal® (Vitaflo)	16g Sachet	Protein, MCT, carbohydrate	657kcal/100g 13g protein/100g	Energy, protein and MCT powder to add to food and drinks; unflavoured
Pro-Cal Shot® (Vitaflo)	250mL Bottle	Protein, fat, carbohydrate	334kcal/100mL 7g protein/100mL	Fat, protein and carbohydrate emulsion; banana, strawberry, unflavoured
Pro-Cal® Singles (Vitaflo)	30mL Pot	Protein, fat, carbohydrate	333kcal/100mL 7g protein/100mL (30mL pot 100kcal, 2g protein)	Fat, protein and carbohydrate emulsion; strawberry, unflavoured

a. use with dietetic supervision
b. listed according to type.

Table 13 Thickeners and thickened drinks[a,b]

Product	Unit size	Energy content	Comments
Fresubin® Thickened (Fresenius)	200mL Bottle	150kcal/100mL, 10g protein/100mL	Texture modified supplement drink in stage 1 and stage 2 consistency; strawberry, vanilla
Resource® Thickened Drinks (Nestle)	114mL Cup	89kcal/100mL	Ready to use, available in syrup and custard consistency; apple, orange
Nutilis® Complete (Nutricia)	125mL Bottle (Stage 1) 125mL Pot (Stage 2)	245kcal/100mL, 10g protein/100mL	Texture modified supplement drink; stage 1 and 2; strawberry, vanilla
Multi-thick® (Abbott)	250g Can	366kcal/100g	Modified maize starch. Can be used to thicken fluids and food
Nutilis® Clear (Nutricia)	175g Can	299kcal/100g	Maltodextrin, xanthangum and guar gum. Can be used to thicken foods and fluids. Fluids remain clear
Nutilis® Powder (Nutricia)	300g Can 12g Sachet	358kcal/100g	Modified maize starch. Can be used to thicken fluids and food
Resource® Thicken Up® (Nestle)	4.5g Sachet 227g Can	365kcal/100g	Modified maize starch. Can be used to thicken fluids and food
Resource® Thicken Up Clear® (Nestle)	1.2g Sachet 125g Can	306kcal/100g	Maltodextrin, xanthangum and potassium chloride. Can be used to thicken fluids and food. Fluids remain clear
Thick and Easy® Instant Food Thickener (Fresenius)	9g Sachet 225g, 4.5kg Tub	373kcal/100g	Modified maize starch. Can be used to thicken fluids and food
Vitaquick® (Vitaflo)	300g, 2kg Tub	391kcal/100g	Pre-gelatinized modified starch. Can be used to thicken fluids and food

a. for patients with dysphagia
b. listed according to type.

Cautions

Patients with renal or hepatic failure, malabsorption, dysphagia, or at risk of refeeding syndrome (see below) should be referred to a dietitian.

The high sugar content and acidity of some nutritional supplement drinks can encourage dental caries and patients should be advised on good oral hygiene, e.g. ingest the supplement relatively quickly and then clean teeth. However, sipping the supplement over a prolonged period may be unavoidable in patients with early satiety.

Generally, patients with diabetes can use nutritional supplements without problem. However, monitoring of blood sugars may be required when using supplements with a high carbohydrate content, e.g. carbohydrate modular supplements. Rarely, and generally in patients already taking large doses of additional vitamins, nutritional supplements have contributed to ingestion of harmful amounts of vitamins, e.g. vitamin B6 leading to sensory neuropathy. Drug-nutrient interactions may occur with:

- vitamin K, present in significant quantities in the nutritional supplement drinks, and **warfarin** → reduced anticoagulation
- eicosapentanoic acid, in Forticare®, Oral Impac®, Prosure®, and Supportan®, and **warfarin** → enhanced anticoagulation.[24,25]

Also see drug interactions and complications with enteral feeding tubes, p.730.

Refeeding syndrome

Refeeding syndrome is a potentially fatal condition caused by major shifts in fluids and electrolytes in malnourished patients who are started too rapidly on enteral or parenteral nutritional supplements.[26,27] Biochemically, refeeding syndrome is characterized primarily by hypophosphataemia.

During a period of starvation, the body adapts in various ways to cope with the lack of readily available carbohydrate, and switches to using fat and protein as the main source of energy. If malnutrition is prolonged, there are further hormonal and metabolic changes aimed at preventing protein and muscle breakdown. Several intracellular minerals become severely depleted (although plasma concentrations may remain normal).

During refeeding, glycaemia leads to increased insulin secretion and a series of sequential effects, including decreases in the plasma concentrations of phosphate, potassium, magnesium, and thiamine. If unrecognized and untreated, refeeding syndrome can result in life-threatening complications, including cardiac arrhythmia and multi-organ failure.[27] It is thus important that high risk patients should be managed by appropriately trained health professionals.

Although a regimen of rapid refeeding is unlikely in patients with advanced cancer and chronic oligophagia and/or cachexia, palliative care clinicians should be aware of the syndrome, and have a basic understanding of its management (Box D).

Box D   Risk factors for and management of refeeding syndrome[28]

Patients who have had very little or no nutritional intake for > 5 days are at risk of refeeding syndrome. It is associated with high morbidity and mortality and should be managed by appropriately trained health professionals.

High risk patients
Those with one or more of the following:
- BMI < 16kg/m^2
- unintentional weight loss of > 15% in the last 3–6 months
- little or no nutritional intake for > 10 days
- low plasma concentrations of PO4$^-$, K$^+$, Mg^{2+} before restarting feeding.

Or two or more of the following:
- BMI < 18.5kg/m^2
- unintentional weight loss > 10% within the last 3–6 months
- little or no nutritional intake for > 5 days
- a history of alcohol abuse or drugs, including insulin, chemotherapy, antacids and diuretics.

Management
For the first 2 days, patients who have had little or nothing to eat for ≥ 5 days should only be offered/given nutritional support estimated to meet ≤ 50% of their ideal requirements. After this, if biochemical parameters are satisfactory, it is safe to provide full nutrition.

If high risk:
- ensure adequate hydration
- before feeding, and for the next 10 days, administer:
  ▷ thiamine 200–300mg PO once daily
  ▷ strong compound vitamin B 1–2 tablets t.d.s. (or IV vitamin B once daily)
  ▷ multivitamin and mineral supplement PO once daily

continued

Box D Continued

- start nutritional support at ⩽10kcal/kg/day (5kcal/kg/day in extreme cases)
- increase intake progressively to achieve full nutritional requirements after 4–7 days
- if pre-feeding plasma concentrations are low, prescribe biochemical supplements:
  ▷ magnesium (e.g. 0.2mmol/kg/day IV, 0.4mmol/kg/day PO)
  ▷ phosphate (e.g. 0.3–0.6mmol/kg/day)
  ▷ potassium (e.g. 2–4mmol/kg/day).

Monitoring
Daily until stable, and then 2–3 times weekly: fluid balance, nutritional intake, biochemical parameters, and general physical and psychological condition.

---

1 Fearon K et al. (2011) Definition and classification of cancer cachexia: an international consensus. Lancet Oncology. 12: 489–495.
2 Arends J et al. (2006) ESPEN Guidelines on Enteral Nutrition: Non-surgical oncology. Clinical Nutrition. 25: 245–259.
3 National Collaborating Centre for Acute Care (2006) Nutrition Support in Adults: Oral nutrition support, enteral tube feeding and parenteral nutrition (No. 32). National Institute for Clinical Excellence, London.
4 Malnutrition Advisory Group (2003) The Malnutrition Universal Screening Tool. BAPEN, UK. Available from: www.bapen.org.uk/must_tool.html
5 Kyle UG et al. (2006) Comparison of tools for nutritional assessment and screening at hospital admission: a population study. Clinical Nutrition. 25: 409–417.
6 Davies M (2005) Nutritional screening and assessment in cancer-associated malnutrition. European Journal of Oncology Nursing. 9 (Suppl 2): S64–73.
7 Ottery FD (1996) Definition of standardized nutritional assessment and interventional pathways in oncology. Nutrition. 12: S15–19.
8 Bauer J et al. (2002) Use of the scored Patient-Generated Subjective Global Assessment (PG-SGA) as a nutrition assessment tool in patients with cancer. European Journal of Clinical Nutrition. 56: 779–785.
9 Chauhan A et al. (2007) NICE guidance for screening for malnutrition: implications for lung cancer services. Thorax. 62: 835.
10 Halliday V et al. (2010) Screening for malnutrition: implications for upper gastrointestinal cancer services. Journal of Surgical Oncology. 102: 543–544.
11 Thoresen L and de Soysa AK (2006) The nutritional aspects of palliative care. European Journal of Palliative Care. 13: 194–197.
12 Bozzetti F et al. (2009) ESPEN Guidelines on Parenteral Nutrition: non-surgical oncology. Clinical Nutrition. 28: 445–454.
13 Lobo DN et al. (2006) Early postoperative jejunostomy feeding with an immune modulating diet in patients undergoing resectional surgery for upper gastrointestinal cancer: a prospective, randomized, controlled, double-blind study. Clinical Nutrition. 25: 716–726.
14 Heyland DK et al. (2001) Should immunonutrition become routine in critically ill patients? A systematic review of the evidence. Journal of the American Medical Association. 286: 944–953.
15 Yavuzsen T et al. (2005) Systematic review of the treatment of cancer-associated anorexia and weight loss. Journal of Clinical Oncology. 23: 8500-8511.
16 Fearon KC et al. (2003) Effect of a protein and energy dense N-3 fatty acid enriched oral supplement on loss of weight and lean tissue in cancer cachexia: a randomised double blind trial. Gut. 52: 1479–1486.
17 Wilcock A (2005) Cachexia and omega-3 polyunsaturated fatty acids: the beginning of the end or the end of the beginning? Palliative Medicine. 19: 500–502.
18 Mazzotta P and Jeney CM (2009) Anorexia-cachexia syndrome: a systematic review of the role of dietary polyunsaturated Fatty acids in the management of symptoms, survival, and quality of life. Journal of Pain and Symptom Management. 37: 1069-1077.
19 van der Meij BS et al. (2010) Oral nutritional supplements containing (n-3) polyunsaturated fatty acids affect the nutritional status of patients with stage III non-small cell lung cancer during multimodality treatment. Journal of Nutritrion. 140: 1774-1780.
20 McCann RM et al. (1994) A comfort care for terminally ill patients: the appropriate use of nutrition and hydration. Journal of the American Medical Association. 272: 179–181.
21 Sarhill N et al. (2003) Evaluation of nutritional status in advanced metastatic cancer. Supportive Care in Cancer. 11: 652–659.
22 Antoun S et al. (2006) Artificial nutrition at the end of life: is it justified? European Journal of Palliative Care. 13: 194–197.
23 Baldwin C and Weekes C (2008) Dietary advice for illness-related malnutrition in adults. Cochrane Database of Systematic Reviews. 1: CD002008.
24 Baxter K and Preston CL Stockley's Drug Interactions. London: Pharmaceutical Press. www.medicinescomplete.com (accessed September 2012).
25 Holbrook AM et al. (2005) Systematic overview of warfarin and its drug and food interactions. Archives of Internal Medicine. 165: 1095–1106.
26 Mehanna HM et al. (2008) Refeeding syndrome: what it is, and how to prevent and treat it. British Medical Journal. 336: 1495-1498.
27 Boateng AA et al. (2010) Refeeding syndrome: treatment considerations based on collective analysis of literature case reports. Nutrition. 26: 156-167.
28 NICE (2006) Nutrition support in adults. Clinical guideline CG32. www.nice.org.uk

Updated (minor change) April 2014

Appendix 1: Obtaining unauthorized (unlicensed) products

The UK Medicines and Healthcare products Regulatory Agency (MHRA) is responsible for ensuring that medicinal products and medical devices are effective, safe and of appropriate quality. A medicinal product must have a marketing authorization (MA, formerly product licence; see p.xix), before it can be marketed. In the UK there is an exemption whereby an unauthorized product may be prescribed if there is a definite clinical need which cannot be satisfied by an existing authorized product.[1] Note: this is not the same as 'off-label use', which refers to the use of an authorized product beyond the specifications of its MA. Unauthorized products are generally those which:

- are authorized in another country but not in the UK and are imported into the UK by a specialist importing company, e.g. **hydromorphone** injection
- may be available from a UK manufacturer before an MA has been issued, e.g. if a patient wishes to continue an investigational product after a clinical trial
- have had an MA withdrawn but special provision has been made by the MHRA for a continued supply, e.g. **co-proxamol** (see dextropropoxyphene)
- require special-order manufacture into a suitable formulation, i.e. a 'special' (Box A).

When an unauthorized product is prescribed, clinicians need to know (or be made aware) that it does not have MA.[1] This can be forgotten particularly with readily available batch-made specials for local 'routine' specialist use, e.g. **ketamine** oral solution. Close collaboration between primary and secondary care health professionals is needed to ensure continuity of supply and product consistency for the patient.

Box A   Special-order manufactured formulations

A 'special' includes the following formulations:

- a locally prepared (extemporaneous) formulation made in a pharmacy under a pharmacist's direct supervision to fulfil a prescription for an individual patient, e.g. dilution of creams or ointments, some oral solutions
- a bespoke formulation made by a specials manufacturer holding a manufacturer's specials licence (MS) for an individual patient, without end product analytical testing, e.g. where a specific concentration is needed, as in some TPN and chemotherapy
- a formulation manufactured by a specials manufacturer holding an MS, produced in multiple quantities (batches) with end product analytical testing, e.g. some prefilled opioid syringes, ketamine oral solution.

An MS guarantees the sourcing of ingredients, product development, packaging and labelling, the manufacturing and ex-factory supply processes are to regulatory standards. It does not include formal evaluation of safety or efficacy.

To ensure the quality of the product, the Royal Pharmaceutical Society advises that a certificate of analysis (batch manufactured specials) or a certificate of conformity (bespoke products) should be requested by pharmacists with every product.

A certificate of analysis is evidence that critical parameters have been confirmed by retrospective physical, chemical or microbiological assay of a sample of the final product.

This differs from a certificate of conformity which is a signed statement by the manufacturer that they believe the product complies with the purchaser's specification.

Supply and record-keeping

The MHRA maintains a register of special-order manufacturers and specialist importing companies (http://tinyurl.com/cdslke). Licensed NHS hospital manufacturing units may also manufacture specials. A list of these units is included in the BNF. A database (*Pro-File*; www.pro-file.nhs.uk) provides information on products manufactured in the NHS but access is restricted to NHS pharmacy staff. The Association of Commercial Specials Manufacturers may also be able to provide information about commercial companies (www.acsm.uk.com).

Pharmacists should keep records of the source, quantity obtained, batch numbers and the quantity supplied of the unauthorized product, along with prescriber and patient details. They must also record and report any adverse reactions associated with their use.[1,2] Although pharmacists should record patient details (hence the commonly used term 'named patient supply'), there is no legal requirement to provide special-order manufacturers or specialist importing companies with this information[1]. When ordering, most companies require confirmation that the product is being supplied for a definite individual clinical need which cannot be satisfied by an existing authorized product.

In hospitals, some specials, e.g. **ketamine** oral solution, are used as standard supplies and kept as stock at ward level. Thus, they may be used without obtaining patient details; however, this is considered acceptable as long as the hospital formulary committee takes responsibility and appropriate governance is in place, e.g. a risk stratification and management plan.[2]

---

1 MHRA (2008) The supply of unlicensed relevant medicinal products for individual patients. In: *MHRA Products and Healthcare Regulatory Authority Guidance Note 14.* Available from: www.mhra.gov.uk (accessed 5 Sept 2012).

2 Anonymous (2010) Good practice guidance on the procurement and supply of pharmaceutical specials. *Pharmacy Professional.* **June**: 27–32.

Updated September 2012

Appendix 2: Taking controlled and prescription drugs to other countries

Some patients receiving palliative care travel to other countries and need to take medication with them. Two sets of laws need to be considered, those of the country from which they are leaving and those of the country or countries to which they are travelling. Detailed advice can be obtained from the regulatory authorities, embassies or consulates in the relevant countries.

UK Customs regulations

It is advisable to check for the latest Home Office guidance by contacting them directly or visiting the website:

The Home Office
Drugs Licensing and Compliance
4th Floor, Fry Building
2 Marsham Street
London SW1P 4DF
Tel: 020 7035 0484
Fax: 020 7035 6161
e-mail: DLCUCommsOfficer@homeoffice.gsi.gov.uk
https://www.gov.uk/controlled-drugs-licences-fees-and-returns

The UK customs regulations for travelling with prescribed drugs were simplified in 2008 and are the same for taking drugs out of or into the UK.

Leaving or entering the UK for <3 months and carrying <3 months supply
A covering letter from the prescribing doctor is:
- *required* for all controlled drugs in schedule 2, 3, 4 part I and part II
- *advised* for schedule 5 and all other prescribed medicines.
A list of controlled drug schedules is included in the BNF.[1]
The covering letter should state:
- the patient's name, address and date of birth
- the destination(s) and dates of outward and return travel
- the names, forms, strengths, doses and total amounts of the drugs being carried.

Leaving or entering the UK for ≥3 months or carrying >3 months supply
Patients should be advised to make contact with a doctor in the country in which they will be staying, and to obtain prescriptions for further supplies from that doctor. Otherwise they will need, *in addition* to a covering letter from their UK prescribing doctor, a personal import/export licence.

The import/export licence application form can be downloaded from the website above. Once completed, it must be posted or e-mailed to the Home Office Drugs Licensing and Compliance Unit along with a letter (in pdf format when e-mailed), on headed notepaper, from the doctor confirming the details given in the form are correct. At least 2 weeks should be allowed for processing. Applications from patients who are abroad, to import drugs into the UK, take longer.

For UK residents, the main limitation is likely to be the legislation of the country/countries to which they are travelling (see below).

All drugs should be kept in their original packaging and carried in the patient's hand luggage (together with the covering letter ± import/export licence) in case Customs want to examine them. Air passengers are generally allowed to carry up to 100mL of liquid in their hand luggage.

To carry more than 100mL may require prior approval from the airline and the departure airport; the medication should be presented at security for x-ray inspection and possible verification.

Travelling to or through other countries

It is important to fulfil the prescription and controlled drug import/export requirements for *all* the countries in which the patient will have to pass through Customs, otherwise entry may be refused.

The International Narcotics Control Board has produced a list of *suggested* maximum quantities of internationally controlled substances beyond which a traveller would require an import/export licence (Table 1). *However, patients should check the exact legal details and the quantities they are allowed to take into the country or countries before travelling with the relevant embassies or consulates, and the procedure for declaration at Customs.* For example, **codeine, dihydrocodeine** or **diamorphine** are not allowed in certain countries. A list of embassy contact details in the UK is available from the Home Office drugs website. It is also advisable to carry a duplicate copy of the prescription, preferably stamped by the pharmacy from which the drugs were obtained.

Table 1 Suggested maximum quantities of controlled substances for international travellers[a,b,2]

Drug	Quantity
Buprenorphine	300mg
Codeine	12g
Diazepam	300mg
Dihydrocodeine	12g
Fentanyl transdermal patches[b]	100mg
Fentanyl (other formulations)	20mg
Hydromorphone	300mg
Lorazepam	75mg
Methadone	2g
Methylphenidate	2g
Morphine	3g
Oxycodone	1g
Temazepam	600mg

a. this is not a complete list; see referenced source for more details
b. approximately, this adds up to 6 fentanyl 100microgram/h patches, and 8, 12, 24, 48 of the 75, 50, 25, 12microgram/h patches, respectively.

1 *British National Formulary* Guidance on Prescribing London: BMJ Group and Pharmaceutical Press www.bnf.org (accessed March 2013).
2 International Narcotics Control Board (2004) International guidelines for national regulations concerning travellers under treatment with internationally controlled drugs. www.incb.org

Updated June 2013

Appendix 3: Compatibility charts

PCF recommends that generally water for injection (WFI) is used as the standard diluent of choice because there is less likelihood of incompatibility. However, 0.9% saline should be considered when there is actual or potential for inflammation at the injection site (see Chapter 20, p.699).

Charts 1–7 and Table 1 summarize the compatibility data available for the more commonly used 2-drug and 3-drug combinations given by CSCI in WFI. Charts summarizing the compatibility data available for the more commonly used 2-drug and 3-drug combinations given by CSCI in 0.9% saline can be found in the extended appendix section of the on-line PCF on www.palliativedrugs.com

The charts have been compiled from clinical observations in palliative care services submitted to the www.palliativedrugs.com Syringe Driver Survey Database (SDSD) from the UK, New Zealand and Australia, and from published compatibility data (see reference list). The SDSD is a continually updated resource and contains more detailed observational compatibility data on mixing up to four drugs in either WFI or 0.9% saline.

A traffic light system has been devised for use in the clinical setting as a practical summary of the data available:

- *red* = do not use (available information indicates a compatibility problem)
- *amber* = proceed with caution (possible compatibility problem, depending on the order of mixing or drug concentrations)
- *green* = reported compatible (data may be observational, physical or chemical, i.e. may be practice- or evidence-based).

Multiple factors affect drug stability and compatibility, including drug concentration, brand/ formulation of the drug (e.g. compatibility for oxycodone 10mg/mL and 50mg/mL formulations differ), diluent, infusion time, exposure to light, ambient temperature, order of mixing and delivery system material (see Chapter 20, Box B, p.701). These factors probably explain why conflicting reports occur. *Regular monitoring of all CSCI drug combinations is essential*, even for those coded green. If there is doubt about the relevance of the compatibility data in any particular situation, e.g. at the extremes of dose and concentration, advice should be obtained from a clinical pharmacist.

Dexamethasone often causes compatibility problems. It should always be the last drug to be added to an already dilute combination of drugs, thus reducing the risk of precipitation. However, because **dexamethasone** has a long duration of action, it can generally be given as a bolus SC injection once daily.

Health professionals are urged to contact hq@palliativedrugs.com if their experience indicates that the code for a combination should be changed. Submissions to the SDSD of details of successful combinations for which there are no published data are also welcome.

Most of the information in these charts relates to the use of drugs outside the scope of their Marketing Authorization and health professionals using this information must satisfy themselves as to its appropriateness in any given clinical situation (also see p.xix). Further, health professionals should familiarize themselves with the guidance and supporting material relating to the legal implications of mixing medicines before administration (Department of Health, 2010 and National Prescribing Centre, 2010) together with any local policy and practice (also see p.xx).

Allwood M (1984) Diamorphine mixed with antiemetic drugs in plastic syringes. *British Journal of Pharmaceutical Practice.* **6**: 88–90.
Allwood M (1991) The stability of diamorphine alone and in combination with anti-emetics in plastic syringes. *Palliative Medicine.* **5**: 330–333.
Allwood M et al. (1994) Stability of injections containing diamorphine and midazolam in plastic syringes. *International Journal of Pharmacy Practice.* **3**: 57–59.
Al-Tannak NF et al. (2012) A stability indicating assay for a combination of morphine sulphate with levomepromazine hydrochloride used in palliative care. *Journal Clinical Pharmacy and Therapeutics.* **37**: 71–73.
Ambados F (1995) Compatibility of morphine and ketamine for subcutaneous infusion. *Australian Journal of Hospital Pharmacy.* **25**: 352.
Back I *Syringe driver database.* www.pallcare.info (accessed May 2013).
Barcia E et al. (2003) Compatibility of haloperidol and Hyoscine-N-butylbromide in mixtures for subcutaneous infusion to cancer patients in palliative care. *Supportive Care in Cancer.* **11**: 107–113.

Chin A et al. (1996) Stability of Granisetron hydrochloride with dexamethasone sodium phosphate for 14 days. American Journal of Health-System Pharmacy. 53: 1174–1176.

Department of Health (2010) Mixing of medicines prior to administration in clinical practice: medical and non-medical prescribing. Department of Health Gateway reference 14330. https://www.gov.uk

Dickman A and Schneider J. (2011) The Syringe Driver: Continuous Subcutaneous Infusions in Palliative Care (3e). Oxford University Press, Oxford.

Fawcett J et al. (1994) Compatibility of cyclizine lactate and haloperidol lactate. American Journal of Hospital Pharmacy. 51: 2292–2294.

Fielding H et al. (2000) The compatibility and stability of octreotide acetate in the presence of diamorphine hydrochloride in polypropylene syringes. Palliative Medicine. 14: 205–207.

Frimley Park Hospital NHS Trust (1998) Personal communication.

Gardiner P (2003) Compatibility of an injectable oxycodone formulation with typical diluents, syringes, tubings, infusion bags and drugs for potential co-administration. Hospital Pharmacist. 10: 354–361.

Good PD et al. (2004) The compatibility and stability of midazolam and dexamethasone in infusion solutions. Journal of Pain and Symptom Management. 27: 471–475.

Grassby P and Hutchings L (1997) Drug combinations in syringe drivers: the compatibility and stability of diamorphine with cyclizine and haloperidol. Palliative Medicine. 11: 217–224.

Grassby PF (1995) UK stability database (Apr 1995 and Jul 1997). Welsh Pharmaceutical Services, St. Mary's Pharmaceutical Unit, Corbett Road, Penarth, South Glamorgan.

Hagan R et al. (1996) Stability of ondansetron hydrochloride and dexamethasone sodium phosphate in infusion bags and syringes for 32 days. American Journal of Health-System Pharmacy. 53: 1431–1435.

Hines S and Pleasance S (2009) Compatibility of an injectable high strength oxycodone formulation with typical diluents, syringes, tubings, infusion bags and drugs for potential co-administration. European Journal of Hospital Pharmacy Practice 15: 32–38.

Hines S and Pleasance S (2011) Compatibility of injectable hydromorphone formulations with typical diluents, components of giving sets and drugs for potential co-administration. European Journal of Hospital Pharmacy Practice. 17: 47–53.

Huang E and Anderson RP (1994) Compatibility of hydromorphone hydrochloride with haloperidol lactate and ketorolac tromethamine. American Journal of Hospital Pharmacy. 51: 2963.

Hughes A et al. (1997) Ketorolac: continuous subcutaneous infusion for cancer pain. Journal of Pain and Symptom Management. 13: 315–317.

Ingallinera TS et al. (1979) Compatibility of glycopyrrolate injection with commonly used infusion solutions and additives. American Journal of Hospital Pharmacy. 36: 508–510.

Lau M-H et al. (1998) Compatibility of ketamine and morphine injections. Pain. 75: 389–390.

Lawson WA et al. (1991) Stability of hyoscine in mixtures with morphine for continuous subcutaneous administration. Australian Journal of Hospital Pharmacy. 21: 395–396.

LeBelle MJ et al. (1995) Compatibility of morphine and midazolam or haloperidol in parenteral admixtures. Canadian Journal of Hospital Pharmacy. 48: 155–160.

Mehta AC and Kay EA (1997) Storage time can be extended: A stability study of alfentanil and midazolam admixture stored in plastic syringes. Pharmacy in Practice. 7: 305–308.

Mendenhall A and Hoyt DB (1994) Incompatibility of ketorolac tromethamine with haloperidol lactate and thiethylperazine maleate. American Journal of Hospital Pharmacy. 51: 2964.

Middleton M and Reilly CS (1994) Do morphine and ketamine keep? The stability of morphine and ketamine separately and combined for use as an infusion. Hospital Pharmacy Practice. 4: 57–58.

Napp (2010) Personal communication.

Napp (2014) OxyNorm 10mg/mL solution for injection or infusion. SPC. www.medicines.org.uk

National Prescribing Centre (2010) Mixing of medicines prior to administration in clinical practice – responding to legislative changes. Available from www.npc.co.uk/policy/resources/mixing_of_medicines.pdf

Negro S et al. (2002) Physical compatibility and in vivo evaluation of drug mixtures for subcutaneous infusion to cancer patients in palliative care. Supportive Care in Cancer. 10: 65–70.

NHS Argyll and Clyde (2005) Syringe driver guidelines for Graseby MS26 (mm/24h). Available from: Document Library. www.palliativedrugs.com

NUH (Nottingham University Hospitals) NHS Trust (2002) Data on file. Hayward House, Nottingham.

Palliativedrugs.com (2006) Syringe Driver Survey Results. Newsletter Archive: June/July newsletter

Palliativedrugs.com Syringe Driver Survey Database www.palliativedrugs.com (accessed January 2014).

Pesko LJ et al. (1988) Physical compatibility and stability of metoclopramide injection. Parenterals. 5: 1–3, 6–8.

Peterson G et al. (1991) A preliminary study of the stability of midazolam in polypropylene syringes, Australian Journal of Hospital Pharmacy. 21: 115–118.

Pinguet F et al. (1995) Compatibility and stability of granisetron, dexamethasone, and methylprednisolone in injectable solutions. Journal of Pharmaceutical Sciences. 84: 267–268.

Regnard C et al. (1986) Antiemetics/diamorphine mixture compatibility in infusion pumps. British Journal of Pharmaceutical Practice. 8: 218–220.

Riley and Fallon (1994) Octreotide in terminal malignant obstruction of the gastrointestinal tract. European Journal of Palliative Care. 1: 23–25.

Sample E (2001) Personal communication. Burnaby Hospital, British Columbia, Canada.

Sanofi (2014) Nozinan injection. SPC. www.medicines.org.uk.

Schneider JJ (2001) Personal communication. Pharmacy Department, University of Newcastle, Callaghan, Australia.

Smith JC et al. (2000) The Stability of diamorphine and glycopyrrolate in PCA syringes. Pharmaceutical Journal. 265 (Suppl. R69).

Stewart JT et al. (1998) Stability of ondansetron hydrochloride and 12 medications in plastic syringes. American Journal of the Health-System Pharmacy. 55: 2630–2634.

Storey P et al. (1990) Subcutaneous infusions for control of cancer symptoms. Journal of Pain and Symptom Management. 5: 33–41.

Thomas B (2011) Personal communication. Pharmacist, LOROS (Leicestershire and Rutland Organisation for the Relief of Suffering) Hospice, UK.

Trissel LA Handbook on Injectable Drugs. Maryland, USA: American Society of Health-System Pharmacists www.medicinescomplete.com (accessed May 2013).

Trissel LA et al. (1994) Compatibility and stability of ondansetron hydrochloride with morphine sulphate and with hydromorphone hydrochloride in 0.9% sodium chloride injection at 4,22 and 32 degrees C. American Journal of Hospital Pharmacy. 51: 2138–2142.

Virdee H et al. (1997) the chemical stability of diamorphine and ketorolac in 0.9% sodium chloride stored in plastic syringes. *Pharmacy in Practice.* February: 82–83.

Walker SE et al. (1991) Compatibility of dexamethasone sodium phosphate with hydromorphone hydrochloride or diphenhydramine hydrochloride. *American Journal of Hospital Pharmacy.* **48**: 2161–2166.

Watson DG et al. (2005) Compatibility and stability of dexamethasone sodium phosphate and ketamine hydrochloride subcutaneous infusions in polypropylene syringes. *Journal of Pain and Symptom Management.* **31**: 80–86.

General key for charts

■ (black)	Do *not* use, *incompatible* at usual concentrations
□ (white outline)	Use with caution, compatibility may depend on order of mixing or drug concentrations
a,b,c, etc.	Some reports of *incompatibility*, but may be compatible at other concentrations (see footnotes)
■ (grey)	Reported compatible (data may be observational, physical or chemical, i.e. practice- or evidence-based)
?	No data. Please provide information on this combination to the Syringe Driver Survey Database (SDSD) www.palliativedrugs.com
■ (grey)	Not applicable or not generally recommended, e.g. seek specialist advice when combining multiple anti-emetics
#	Use non-PVC tubing; up to 50% of a dose of clonazepam is adsorbed by PVC tubing
##	Dexamethasone sodium phosphate can generally be given once daily by SC bolus injection. If given by CSCI, to minimize the risk of incompatibility, always add it last to a maximally diluted syringe
###	Compatibility data for oxycodone 10mg/mL formulation only; for 50mg/mL formulation, see Table 1, p. 838.

Alf	Alfentanil
Clzm	Clonazepam
Cyc	Cyclizine
Dex/Dexamethasone	Dexamethasone sodium phosphate
Dia	Diamorphine
Gly	Glycopyrronium
Gra	Granisetron
Hal	Haloperidol
HBBr	Hyoscine butylbromide
HHBr	Hyoscine hydrobromide
Hyd	Hydromorphone
Keta	Ketamine
Ketor	Ketorolac
Levo	Levomepromazine
Meto	Metoclopramide
Mid	Midazolam
MS	Morphine sulfate
MT	Morphine tartrate
Oct	Octreotide
Ond	Ondansetron
Oxy	Oxycodone 10mg/mL

Chart I Compatibility chart for two drugs in *WFI*.

Note: This chart summarizes the compatibility information available for drug combinations in **WFI** used for CSCI over 24h in palliative care units and the literature (see p.821). It includes compatibility data for oxycodone 10mg/mL formulation only; for 50mg/mL, see Table 1, p.838. It should be used in conjunction with the key and the footnotes. Further information about each combination may be found on the www.palliativedrugs.com Syringe Driver Survey Database (SDSD). Charts with drug combinations diluted in 0.9% saline can be found in the extended appendix section of the on-line PCF.

Chart 1 footnotes

All drug concentration values (mg/mL) specified below are the maximum *final* concentrations of each drug in the syringe after mixing and dilution reported compatible; at higher concentrations *incompatibility* has either been reported or may occur. For full reference details, see p.821.

a. alfentanil 0.24mg/mL + cyclizine 8.8mg/mL (Dickman *et al.* 2011, palliativedrugs.com 2014)

b. some observational reports of *incompatibility* from miscellaneous sources

c. cyclizine 8.33mg/mL + dexamethasone sodium phosphate 0.33mg/mL (Dickman *et al.* 2011, palliativedrugs.com 2014)

d. cyclizine up to 20mg/mL + diamorphine up to 20mg/mL, or cyclizine maximum 10mg/mL + diamorphine >20mg/mL, or cyclizine >20mg/mL + diamorphine maximum 15mg/mL (Grassby and Hutchings 1997)

e. cyclizine 8.82mg/mL + hydromorphone 5.8mg/mL (Hines and Pleasance 2011); one report of *incompatibility* at *lower* concentrations (Back 2013)

f. generally regarded as *incompatible*; one report of compatibility of low concentrations for a *12h* infusion of cyclizine 3.7mg/mL + hyoscine *butylbromide* 1.5mg/mL (palliativedrugs.com 2014)

g. cyclizine 8.82mg/mL + midazolam 0.88mg/mL (Back 2013, palliativedrugs.com 2014)

h. cyclizine 3mg/mL + oxycodone 9mg/mL; cyclizine concentrations between 3mg/mL and 8mg/mL may be used as long as the oxycodone concentration is reduced to below 3mg/mL by diluting with WFI (Napp 2010, Napp 2014)

i. dexamethasone sodium phosphate 0.15mg/mL + haloperidol 0.38mg/mL (Dickman *et al.* 2011, palliativedrugs.com 2014)

j. dexamethasone sodium phosphate 2mg/mL + hydromorphone 20mg/mL, or dexamethasone sodium phosphate >2mg/mL + hydromorphone 10mg/mL (Walker *et al.* 1991, Hines and Pleasance 2011)

k. dexamethasone sodium phosphate 0.11mg/mL + levomepromazine 2.78mg/mL (Dickman *et al.* 2011, palliativedrugs.com 2014)

l. diamorphine up to 50mg/mL + haloperidol 4mg/mL, or diamorphine 50–100mg/mL + haloperidol 3mg/mL (Grassby and Hutchings 1997)

m. diamorphine or morphine sulfate + midazolam generally regarded as compatible (palliativedrugs.com 2014, Dickman *et al.* 2011); one report of *incompatibility* for diamorphine (palliativedrugs.com 2014); microscopic precipitation may occur with morphine (LeBelle *et al.* 1995)

n. variable reports at higher concentrations, e.g. haloperidol 2.5mg/mL + hydromorphone 5mg/mL compatible (Huang and Anderson 1994), haloperidol 3mg/mL + hydromorphone 20mg/mL compatible (Hines and Pleasance 2011) but haloperidol 2mg/mL + hydromorphone 10mg/mL *incompatible* (Storey *et al.* 1990)

o. haloperidol <1mg/mL + morphine sulfate <10mg/mL (palliativedrugs.com 2014, Storey *et al.* 1990, Trissel 2006, LeBelle *et al.* 1995)

p. hydromorphone 0.5mg/mL + ketorolac 15mg/mL (Huang and Anderson 1994).

	Alf + Clzm#	Alf + Cyc	Alf + Dex##	Alf + Gly	Alf + Gra	Alf + Hal	Alf + HBBr	Alf + HHBr	Alf + Keta	Alf + Ketor	Alf + Levo	Alf + Meto	Alf + Mid	Alf + Oct
Cyclizine	a													
Dexamethasone##	?	?												
Glycopyrronium		?	?											
Granisetron	?	?	?	?										
Haloperidol		b	?		?									
Hyoscine Butylbromide	?	?	?		?									
Hyoscine Hydrobromide		?	?		?	?								
Ketamine	?	?	?	?	?	?	?	?						
Ketorolac	?	?	?	?	?	?	?	?	?					
Levomepromazine	?		?					?	?	?				
Metoclopramide	?		?			?			?	?				
Midazolam		c	?		?				?	?				
Octreotide	?	?	?	?	?	?	?	?	?	?			?	
Ondansetron	?	?	?	?		?	?	?	?	?			?	?

Note: This chart summarizes the compatibility information available for drug combinations in **WFI** used for CSCI over 24h in palliative care units and the literature (see p.821). It should be used in conjunction with the key and the footnotes. Further information about each combination may be found on the www.palliativedrugs.com Syringe Driver Survey Database (SDSD). Charts with drug combinations diluted in 0.9% saline can be found in the extended appendix section of the on-line PCF.

Chart 2 Compatibility chart for alfentanil: *three* drugs in ***WFI***.

Chart 2 footnotes

All drug concentration values (mg/mL) specified below are the maximum *final* concentrations of each drug in the syringe after mixing and dilution reported compatible; at higher concentrations *incompatibility* has either been reported or may occur. For full reference details, see p.821.

Note: Concentration dependent *incompatibility* reported with 2-drug combinations of **alfentanil + cyclizine** (see 2-drug chart, p.824).

a. alfentanil 0.53mg/mL + clonazepam 0.24mg/mL + cyclizine 8.82mg/mL (Dickman et al. 2011)

b. one report of *incompatibility* (Back 2013) but several other reports of compatibility (Dickman et al. 2011, palliativedrugs.com 2014)

c. alfentanil 3mg/mL + cyclizine 6mg/mL + midazolam 1.2mg/mL (Dickman et al. 2011).

Chart 3 Compatibility chart for diamorphine: *three* drugs in *WFI*.

Note: This chart summarizes the compatibility information available for drug combinations in **WFI** used for CSCI over 24h in palliative care units and the literature (see p.821). It should be used in conjunction with the key and the footnotes. Further information about each combination may be found on the www.palliativedrugs.com Syringe Driver Survey Database (SDSD). Charts with drug combinations diluted in 0.9% saline can be found in the extended appendix section of the on-line PCF.

Chart 3 footnotes

All drug concentration values (mg/mL) specified below are the maximum *final* concentrations of each drug in the syringe after mixing and dilution reported compatible; at higher concentrations *incompatibility* has either been reported or may occur. For full reference details, see p.821.

Note: Concentration dependent *incompatibility* reported with 2-drug combinations of **diamorphine + cyclizine** or **haloperidol** (see 2-drug chart, p.824).

a. diamorphine 5.88mg/mL + cyclizine 8.82mg/mL + dexamethasone sodium phosphate 0.71mg/mL (Dickman *et al.* 2011, palliativedrugs.com 2014)

b. diamorphine 56mg/mL + cyclizine 13mg/mL + haloperidol 2.1mg/mL (Grassby 1995, palliativedrugs.com 2014)

c. diamorphine 37mg/mL + cyclizine 8.82mg/mL + midazolam 2.35mg/mL (palliativedrugs.com 2014)

d. diamorphine 25mg/mL + dexamethasone sodium phosphate 0.35mg/mL + haloperidol 0.59mg/mL (Dickman *et al.* 2011)

e. diamorphine 3.53mg/mL + dexamethasone sodium phosphate 0.59mg/mL + metoclopramide 2.35mg/mL (Dickman *et al.* 2011)

f. diamorphine 35mg/mL + dexamethasone sodium phosphate 0.06mg/mL + ondansetron 1.41mg/mL (Dickman *et al.* 2011)

g. diamorphine 117.7mg/mL + haloperidol 0.59mg/mL + hyoscine *butylbromide* 3.53mg/mL (palliativedrugs.com 2014)

h. diamorphine 28mg/mL+ haloperidol 2mg/mL + midazolam 1mg/mL (palliativedrugs.com 2014).

Hyd + Clzm# Hyd + Cyc Hyd + Dex## Hyd + Gly Hyd + Gra Hyd + Hal Hyd + HBBr Hyd + HHBr Hyd + Keta Hyd + Ketor Hyd + Levo Hyd + Meto Hyd + Mid Hyd + Oct

Chart 4 Compatibility chart for hydromorphone: *three* drugs in *WFI*.

Note: This chart summarizes the compatibility information available for drug combinations in **WFI** used for CSCI over 24h in palliative care units and the literature (see p.821). It should be used in conjunction with the key and the footnotes. Further information about each combination may be found on the www.palliativedrugs.com Syringe Driver Survey Database (SDSD). Charts with drug combinations diluted in 0.9% saline can be found in the extended appendix section of the on-line PCF.

Chart 4 footnotes

All drug concentration values (mg/mL) specified below are the maximum *final* concentrations of each drug in the syringe after mixing and dilution reported compatible; at higher concentrations *incompatibility* has either been reported or may occur. For full reference details, see p.821.

Note: Concentration dependent *incompatibility* reported with 2-drug combinations of **hydromorphone + cyclizine, dexamethasone, haloperidol or ketorolac** (see 2-drug chart, p.824).

a. hydromorphone 1.67mg/mL + cyclizine 16.67mg/mL + octreotide 0.02mg/mL; *incompatibility* has been reported with cyclizine and octreotide see 2-drug chart, p.824 (Dickman 2011)

b. generally regarded as *incompatible*, despite observational reports of compatibility. as dexamethasone + midazolam 2-drug combination are *incompatible* although may be visually clear, see Chapter 20, Box C, p.702 (Good P 2004)

c. hydromorphone 3.75mg/mL + haloperidol 0.16mg/mL + ketamine 31.25mg/mL (palliativedrugs.com 2014)

d. hydromorphone 0.35mg/mL + haloperidol 0.06mg/mL + midazolam 0.23mg/mL (palliativedrugs.com 2014).

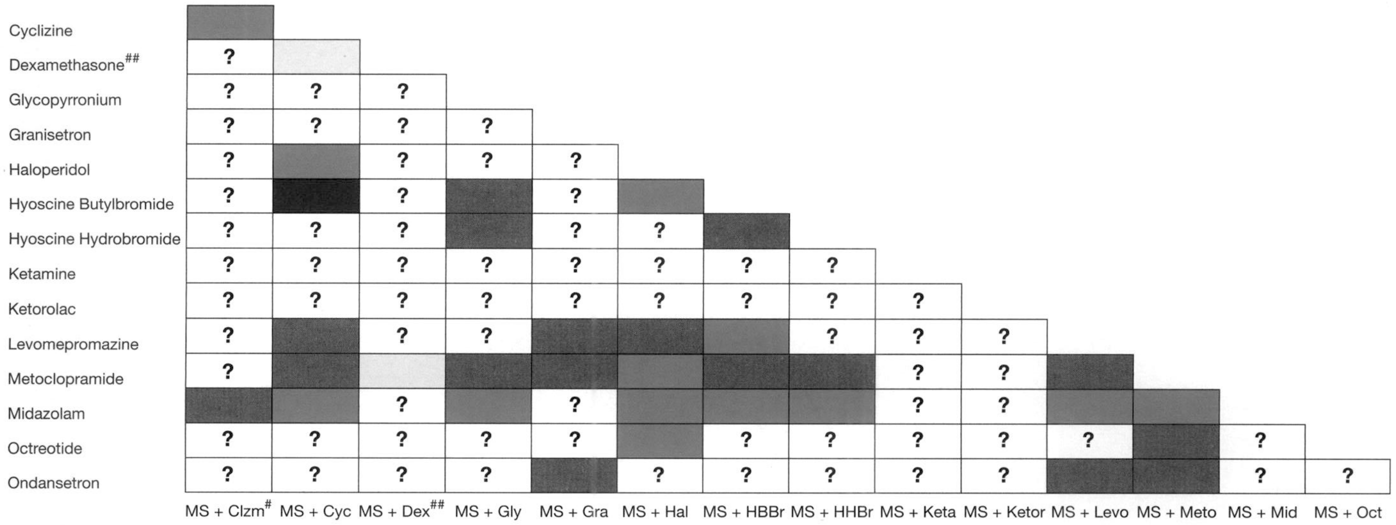

MS + Clzm# MS + Cyc MS + Dex## MS + Gly MS + Gra MS + Hal MS + HBBr MS + HHBr MS + Keta MS + Ketor MS + Levo MS + Meto MS + Mid MS + Oct

Row labels (top to bottom): Cyclizine, Dexamethasone##, Glycopyrronium, Granisetron, Haloperidol, Hyoscine Butylbromide, Hyoscine Hydrobromide, Ketamine, Ketorolac, Levomepromazine, Metoclopramide, Midazolam, Octreotide, Ondansetron

Note: This chart summarizes the compatibility information available for drug combinations in **WFI** used for CSCI over 24h in palliative care units and the literature (see p.821). It should be used in conjunction with the key and the footnotes. Further information about each combination may be found on the www.palliativedrugs.com Syringe Driver Survey Database (SDSD). Charts with drug combinations diluted in 0.9% saline can be found in the extended appendix

Chart 5 Compatibility chart for morphine sulfate: *three drugs in* **WFI.**

Chart 5 footnote

Note: Concentration dependent *incompatibility* reported with 2-drug combinations of **morphine sulfate** + **haloperidol** (see 2-drug chart, p.824).

	Oxy + Clzm[#]	Oxy + Cyc	Oxy + Dex[##]	Oxy + Gly	Oxy + Gra	Oxy + Hal	Oxy + HBBr	Oxy + HHBr	Oxy + Keta	Oxy + Ketor	Oxy + Levo	Oxy + Meto	Oxy + Mid	Oxy + Oct
Cyclizine	?													
Dexamethasone[##]	?	?												
Glycopyrronium	?	a	?											
Granisetron	?	?	?	?										
Haloperidol		b	?	?	?									
Hyoscine Butylbromide			?		?									
Hyoscine Hydrobromide		?	?		?									
Ketamine	?	?	?	?	?		?	?						
Ketorolac	?	?	?	?	?	?	?	?	?					
Levomepromazine			?	?					?	?				
Metoclopramide			?						?					
Midazolam		c	?		?					?				
Octreotide	?	?	?	?	?	?	?	?	?	?				
Ondansetron	?	?	?	?		?	?	?	?	?			?	

Note: Compatibility data for oxycodone 10mg/mL formulation only; for 50mg/mL formulation, see Table 1, p.838. This chart summarizes the compatibility information available for drug combinations in **WFI** used for CSCI over 24h in palliative care units and the literature (see p.821). It should be used in conjunction with the key and the footnotes. Further information about each combination may be found on the www.palliativedrugs.com Syringe Driver Survey Database (SDSD). Charts with drug combinations diluted in 0.9% saline can be found in the extended appendix section of the on-line PCF.

Chart 6 Compatibility chart for oxycodone 10mg/mL formulation: *three* drugs in ***WFI***.

Chart 6 footnotes

All drug concentration values (mg/mL) specified below are the maximum *final* concentrations of each drug in the syringe after mixing and dilution reported compatible; at higher concentrations *incompatibility* has either been reported or may occur. For full reference details, see p.821.

Note: Concentration dependent *incompatibility* reported with 2-drug combinations of **oxycodone + cyclizine** (see 2-drug chart, see p.824).

a. oxycodone 3.5mg/mL + cyclizine 7.5mg/mL + glycopyrronium 0.06mg/mL (Dickman *et al.* 2011, Napp 2010)

b. oxycodone 1.9mg/mL + cyclizine 7.14mg/mL + haloperidol 0.95mg/mL; higher concentrations have been reported compatible, but it is unclear whether the higher strength oxycodone formulation has been used (50mg/mL) which has a different compatibility profile (palliativedrugs.com 2014, Dickman *et al.* 2011, Napp 2010)

c. oxycodone 2.22mg/mL + cyclizine 8.33mg/mL + midazolam 0.28mg/mL; *incompatibility* with some 2-drug combinations of cyclizine + midazolam, see p.824 (Back 2013, palliativedrugs.com 2014, Napp 2010).

Clzm# + Meto   Cyc + Dex##   Cyc + Hal   Cyc + HBBr   Dex## + Mid   Gly + Keta   Gly + Levo   Hal + Mid   HBBr + Ketor   Levo + Mid

Haloperidol

Hyoscine Butylbromide

Hyoscine Hydrobromide

Ketamine

Ketorolac

Metoclopramide

Midazolam

Octreotide

Note: This chart summarizes the compatibility information available for drug combinations in **WFI** used for CSCI over 24h in palliative care units and the literature (see p.821). It should be used in conjunction with the key and the footnotes. Further information about each combination may be found on the www.palliativedrugs.com Syringe Driver Survey Database (SDSD). Charts with drug combinations diluted in 0.9% saline can be found in the extended appendix section of the on-line PCF.

Chart 7 Compatibility chart for non-opioids: *three drugs* in **WFI**.

Chart 7 footnotes

All drug concentration values (mg/mL) specified below are the maximum *final* concentrations of each drug in the syringe after mixing and dilution reported compatible; at higher concentrations *incompatibility* has either been reported or may occur. For full reference details, see p.821.

a. cyclizine 8.82mg/mL + dexamethasone sodium phosphate 0.71mg/mL + hyoscine *butylbromide* 2.35mg/mL (Dickman *et al.* 2011)

b. generally regarded as *incompatible* (NUH 2002); one report of compatibility (Back 2013)

c. generally regarded as *incompatible*; *incompatibility* reported with 2-drug combinations of cyclizine + hyoscine *butylbromide* and some 2-drug combinations of cyclizine + midazolam, see p.824 (NUH 2002, palliativedrugs.com 2014)

d. generally regarded as *incompatible*, despite observational reports of compatibility, as dexamethasone + midazolam 2-drug combination are *incompatible* although may be visually clear, see Chapter 20, Box C, p.702 (Good P 2004).

Compatibility information for oxycodone 50mg/mL formulation

When mixed with other drugs some differences in compatibility have been demonstrated for the 10mg/mL and 50mg/mL formulations of oxycodone solution for injection, e.g. with cyclizine (Gardiner 2003, Hines and Pleasance 2009). This may be due to the different ratios of excipients in each formulation. The manufacturer recommends that the compatibility information for each formulation is considered separately and not extrapolated from one formulation to another.

Chemical compatibility data between oxycodone 50mg/mL solution for injection and other drugs over 24h at room temperature are summarized in Table 1. Full details are available on the SDSD on www.palliativedrugs.com. Please submit details to the SDSD of successful combinations containing oxycodone 50mg/mL and, more important, details of combinations which were incompatible.

Table 1   Oxycodone 50mg/mL formulation compatibility with other drugs (Hines and Pleasance 2009)

	Oxycodone 250mg diluted[a]		Oxycodone 500mg undiluted	
	Dose (mg)	Concentration (mg/mL)	Dose (mg)	Concentration (mg/mL)
Cyclizine[b,c,d]	150	8.8	50	4.5
Dexamethasone sodium phosphate	20	1.2	40	2
Glycopyrronium	1.2	0.07	2.4	0.1
Haloperidol	7.5	0.4	15	1.2
Hyoscine butylbromide	30	1.8	60	4.6
Hyoscine hydrobromide	1.2	0.07	2.4	0.15
Ketamine	400	23.5	800	44.4
Levomepromazine	100	5.9	200	11.1
Metoclopramide	50	2.9	100	3.3
Midazolam	50	2.9	100	3.3

a. oxycodone 50mg/mL formulation, 5mL (250mg) mixed with the drug and diluted to 17mL with WFI or 0.9% saline; oxycodone final concentration 14mg/mL
b. use WFI only, incompatible with 0.9% saline
c. maximum concentrations found compatible for cyclizine and oxycodone 50mg/mL formulation; concentration dependent incompatibility found above this
d. for practical purposes, a cyclizine concentration of >4mg/mL to a maximum of 8mg/mL may be used if the oxycodone concentration is kept <14mg/mL by diluting with WFI (Napp, 2010).

Updated June 2014

Drug Index

Note: Main references are in **bold**.

Supplementary Topic Index

A textbook on pain and symptom management should be consulted for a full discussion of these topics.

Note:
1. **Words** in **bold type** indicate a chapter or an appendix.
2. **Numbers** in **bold type** indicate the main entry for that topic.